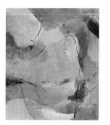

PSYCHIATRIC
NURSING

GET CONNECTED

To Content Updates, Drug Cards, and More!

Meet MERLIN *Merlin* Your online website

sign on at:

http://www.us.elsevierhealth.com/MERLIN/Keltner

what you will receive:

Whether you're a student or an instructor you'll find information just for you. Things like:
- Content Updates
- Drug Cards
- Author Information... and more

plus:

WebLinks

Hundreds of active websites keyed specifically to the content of this book. The Weblinks are continually updated, with new ones added as they develop.

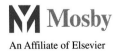 Mosby

An Affiliate of Elsevier

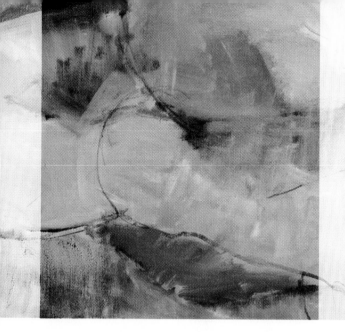

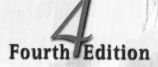

Fourth Edition

PSYCHIATRIC NURSING

Norman L. Keltner, EdD, RN, APRN
Professor
School of Nursing
University of Alabama at Birmingham
Birmingham, Alabama

Lee Hilyard Schwecke, RN, MSN, EdD
Associate Professor
School of Nursing
Indiana University
Indianapolis, Indiana

Carol E. Bostrom, MSN, APRN, BC
Clinical Assistant Professor
School of Nursing
Indiana University
Indianapolis, Indiana

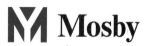 **Mosby**

An Affiliate of Elsevier

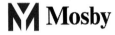

An Affiliate of Elsevier

11830 Westline Industrial Drive
St. Louis, Missouri 63146

PSYCHIATRIC NURSING

NOTICE

Psychiatric nursing is an ever-changing field. Standard safety precautions must be followed, but as new research and clinical experience broaden our knowledge, changes in treatment and drug therapy become necessary or appropriate. Readers are advised to check the most current product information provided by the manufacturer of each drug to be administered to verify the recommended dose, the method and duration of administration, and contraindications. It is the responsibility of the licensed prescriber, relying on experience and knowledge of the patient, to determine dosages and the best treatment for each individual patient. Neither the publisher nor the editor assumes any liability for any injury and/or damage to persons or property arising from this publication.

First Edition 1991. Second Edition 1995. Third Edition 1999.

ISBN-13: 978-0-323-01739-8
ISBN-10: 0-323-01739-8

Vice President and Publishing Director, Nursing: Sally Schrefer
Editor: Tom Wilhelm
Publishing Services Manager: Catherine Albright Jackson
Project Manager: Anne Gassett
Designer: Amy Buxton

GC/QWV

Printed in the United States of America

Last digit is the print number: 9 8 7 6 5 4 3

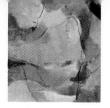

Contributors

David Barton Allen, RN, JD, MSHA, CHE
Assistant Hospital Director
University of Kentucky Medical Center
Lexington, Kentucky

Catherine S. Childers, MSN, RN, CNS
Clinical Nurse Specialist
Center for Psychiatric Medicine
University of Alabama Hospital
Birmingham, Alabama

Beverly K. Hogan, RN, MSN, CS
School of Nursing
University of Alabama at Birmingham
Birmingham, Alabama

Bette R. Keltner, RN, PhD, FAAN
Dean
School of Nursing and Health Studies
Georgetown University
Washington, D.C.

Regina Mims, BS, RN
Nurse Manager
Chilton Shelby Mental Health Center
Clanton, Alabama

Gordon Pugh, M Div, M Phil, MLAP, ICADC, BCC
Chaplain
Children's Hospital
Birmingham, Alabama
Program Director
Adventurelife! Counseling
Birmingham, Alabama

James Luther Raper, DSN, CFNP
Assistant Professor of Medicine and Nursing
University of Alabama at Birmingham
Birmingham, Alabama

Julia Balzer Riley, RN, MN, HNC
President, Constant Source Seminars
Ellenton, Florida
Co-Founder, Holistic Nursing Institute
Tucker, Georgia
Adjunct Faculty
Brenau University
Gainesville, Georgia
Continuing Education
Sarasota Technical Institute
Sarasota, Florida

Lawrence Scahill, MSN, PhD
Associate Professor
Yale Child Studies Center
Yale University School of Nursing
New Haven, Connecticut

Katherine E. Stewart, PhD, MPH
Assistant Professor of Preventive Medicine
University of Alabama at Birmingham
Birmingham, Alabama

Richard A. Sugerman, PhD
Professor of Anatomy
Chair, Department of Anatomy
Western University of Health Sciences
Pomona, California

Barbara Jones Warren, PhD, RN, CNS, CS
Associate Professor
College of Nursing
Ohio State University
Columbus, Ohio
President
American Psychiatric Nurses Association
Washington, D.C.

Judith A. Wilson, MS, RN, CS
Clinical Nurse Specialist
Center for Psychiatric Medicine
University of Alabama Hospital
Birmingham, Alabama

Sandra Jean Wood, MSN, RN, CS
Clinical Assistant Professor
School of Nursing
Indiana University
Indianapolis, Indiana

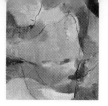

Reviewers

Charla Mae Andrews, RNC, MS
Spokane Community College
Spokane, Washington
Sacred Heart Medical Center
Spokane, Washington

Catherine L. Batscha, MSN, RN, CS
Lawrence Memorial Hospital/Regis College
 Collaborative ASN
Medford, Massachusetts

Judith Benvenutti, PhD, MPH, RN
Mississippi Gulf Coast Community College
Gulfport, Mississippi

Cheryl A. Boyd, PhD, CNS, CNP, RN, SANE
Shawnee State University
Portsmouth, Ohio

Barbara Kay Boyer, RN, BSN
Mental Health Institute
Independence, Iowa

Barbara Shelton Broome, RN, MSN, PhD, CNS
University of South Alabama
Mobile, Alabama

Rauda Gelazis, RN, PhD, CS, CTN
Ursuline College
Pepper Pike, Ohio

Milagros Y. Hall, RNC, BSN, CNA
Manhattan School, New York City Board of
 Education
New York, New York

Mildred Elizabeth Hathaway
York Technical College
Rock Hill, South Carolina
University of South Carolina
Lancaster, South Carolina

Connie S. Heflin, MSN, RN
Paducah Community College
Paducah, Kentucky

Dorothy J. Irvin, DNS, RN, CS
St. John's College
Springfield, Illinois

Susan L. Jones, PhD, RN, CS
Kent State University
Kent, Ohio

Melinda C. Keels, RN, MSN, ARNP
Itawamba Community College
Fulton, Mississippi

Deborah Klaas, PhD, RN
Sonoma State University
Rohnert Park, California

Mary Eileen Mueller, RN, MSN
Calhoun Community College
Decatur, Alabama

Leslie G. Oleck, MSN, RN, CS, LMFT
University of Indianapolis
Indianapolis, Indiana

Eris Field Perese, MS, RN
State University of New York at Buffalo
Buffalo, New York

Diann B. Sloan, PhD, MSEd, MSN
Northeast Mississippi Community College
Booneville, Mississippi

Linda S. Smith, MS, DSN, RN
Oregon Health and Science University
Klamath Falls, Oregon

Dorothy A. Varchol, RNC, MA, MSN
Cincinnati State Technical and Community College
Cincinnati, Ohio

Susan Mace Weeks, MS, RN, LMFT, LCOC
Texas Christian University
Fort Worth, Texas

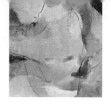

Preface

The first edition of *Psychiatric Nursing,* published in 1991, coincided with the dawning of the "decade of the brain." Quite frankly, when we wrote the prospectus for the book in late 1987, we never heard of the decade of the brain—but we anticipated it. From the beginning we emphasized the psychobiologic nature of mental disorders and the need for psychiatric nurses to grapple with these concepts without letting go of their traditional emphasis on the nurse-patient relationship. These ideas were first presented in an article featured in *Perspectives in Psychiatric Care* entitled "Psychotherapeutic Management: A Model for Nursing Practice." Alice R. Clarke was the editor of *Perspectives* at the time, and she enthusiastically embraced the idea of this "new" but old approach to psychiatric nursing. She "leapfrogged" this manuscript past others and published these ideas in the next edition. Alice understood the need for a change in thinking in psychiatric nursing practice. With this encouragement, a prospectus was developed for Mosby, and the Senior Nursing Editor, Linda Duncan, endorsed the model and issued a contract to publish a textbook based on this approach.

The psychotherapeutic management model simply states that psychiatric nurses have three tools:

- Themselves (e.g., therapeutic nurse-patient relationship)
- Medications
- Environment

This simple paradigm is informed by an in-depth understanding of psychopathology. Based on this model, it might be expected that the therapeutic language, psychotropic medications, and environmental considerations might change, depending on the patient's diagnosis. In other words, "One size does not fit all." For example, as the nurse develops an understanding of the psychopathology of schizophrenia, he or she recognizes that nursing interactions, medications, and environmental concerns for the patient are different from those of a patient suffering from a substance abuse disorder.

Although the psychotherapeutic management model is simple, implementation requires diligent study and practice. For example, to use the model the nurse must develop an understanding of the psychobiologic basis for mental disorders. However, for many students and for some faculty members, developing this understanding is a daunting task. Nonetheless, a solid grounding in psychobiologic concepts will elevate the nurse's level of practice. The same is true for psychopharmacology. This field is changing so rapidly that without an appreciation of basic concepts, the nurse is left bewildered and even unsafe.

We believe the straightforward approach to psychiatric care presented in *Psychiatric Nursing* is an effective method of care and is readily learned by students. New students can use the model almost immediately. The model directs students' attention toward important parameters of care. More experienced students and seasoned nurses can examine each intervention approach and the related psychopathologic factors to gain a deeper understanding and to refine their nursing care practice. The original article published in the 1980s captured the potential of this approach when it said, "Psychotherapeutic management is 'real world' nursing. Mastery of the components—psychopharmacology, therapeutic nurse-patient communication, and milieu management—grounded in psychopathological concepts is a challenging but achievable undertaking: one that will provide a model for productive psychiatric nursing and a distinct sense of professional achievement and role clarity for the psychiatric nurse" (Keltner, 1985).

Organization

The book is organized into eight units:

Unit I: Introduction to Psychiatric Nursing
Unit II: Continuum of Care
Unit III: Therapeutic Nurse-Patient Relationship
Unit IV: Psychopharmacology
Unit V: Milieu Management
Unit VI: Psychopathology
Unit VII: Special Therapies in Psychiatric Nursing
Unit VIII: Special Populations in Psychiatric Nursing

The crucial units are those that flesh out the three psychotherapeutic interventions (Units III, IV, and V) and the unit on psychopathology (Unit VI). Other units (e.g., electroconvulsive therapy in Unit VII) support the model or touch on issues not expressly addressed by the model.

New Content

In addition to the new full-color design, the fourth edition offers the following new content:

- Chapter 17, **Spirituality,** addresses how spirituality and beliefs regarding spirituality can affect patients and their treatment.
- Chapter 40, **Alternative and Complementary Therapies,** introduces what nurses need to know about the various alternative and complementary therapies associated with mental health and illness.
- Chapter 30, **Bipolar Disorders,** has been added to distinguish these disorders from depressive syndromes and to facilitate student comprehension of this important material.
- Discussions on **Antidepressant Drugs** and **Antimanic Drugs** have been split into two chapters (21 and 22) to make the material shorter and easier for students to digest.
- **Patient Education** is addressed more frequently and in greater detail throughout the text.
- **Diagnostic and Statistical Manual of Mental Disorders, text revision, (DSM-IV-TR)** diagnostic criteria are extensively used to prepare the student for interdisciplinary discussions and professional journal literature related to psychiatric care.
- New **Evolve web site** includes web links with content that is reviewed and updated quarterly. **Printable drug cards** are now provided on the web site and revised throughout the life of the fourth edition of *Psychiatric Nursing.*

Features

With students in mind, we have provided a number of tools to facilitate understanding and promote clinical competence. Many of the special features are distinctively designed.

- **Patient and Family Education** boxes in selected disorders chapters highlight the information the nurse needs to provide to the patient and family.
- **Critical thinking questions** are interspersed throughout the narrative to expand students' clinical reasoning skills.
- An *expanded* **study guide** in the back of the book includes multiple-choice study questions, case studies, and critical thinking questions. The built-in workbook reinforces students' comprehension of the content.
- **Key terms** unique to any particular chapter are grouped into a box format for easy reference, thus facilitating the understanding of chapter content.
- **Learning objectives** direct students to the important concepts in each chapter.
- **Family issues** boxes in selected chapters facilitate the students' awareness of the issues that families must confront when a member suffers from mental illness.

- **Clinical examples,** which are concise vignettes drawn from the authors' experiences, are interspersed throughout the text to provide realistic illustrations of specific content.
- **Case studies,** which are detailed depictions of psychiatric disorders, are used in selected chapters to help the student conceptualize the development of effective nursing care strategies.
- **Nursing care plans,** based on the six steps of the nursing process, are carefully developed from the case studies.
- **DSM-IV-TR** and related **North American Nursing Diagnosis Association** (NANDA) diagnoses are compared to help the students understand their interrelationship.
- **Key nursing interventions** are presented in the units on psychopharmacology (Unit IV) and psychopathology (Unit VI).
- **Drug side effects** and **nursing interventions** are provided in the section on psychopharmacology (Unit IV).
- All boxes and tables containing **pharmacologic content** are highlighted with a special symbol 🌡️ for emphasis and accessibility.
- **Key concepts** are placed at the end of each chapter to summarize important content.
- A **glossary** with current and usable definitions for key psychiatric terms is provided for quick reference.

Resources for the Instructor

A new **Instructor's Resource (CD-ROM),** available free to adopters of *Psychiatric Nursing,* includes the following:

- **Instructor's manual** with chapter summaries, chapter outlines, and open-book quizzes
- Completely revised computerized **test bank** with approximately 650 questions with correct answers, rationale for the correct answers, objectives, stages of the nursing process, and cognitive level
- Over 200 **PowerPoint slides** containing full-color figures from this textbook, as well as unique psychobiology slides from additional resources

Contact your local Mosby sales representative to obtain a copy of the Instructor's Resource.

As is true of all nursing text authors, our goal is to present accurate and meaningful information to the student without the distraction of sexist language. Where possible, we have made every attempt to avoid the use of sexist pronouns by using plural nouns and pronouns or "his or her" rather than risk stigmatizing by gender. To avoid awkwardness of style, we have sometimes referred to the nurse as "she" and the patient as "he."

Norman L. Keltner
Lee Hilyard Schwecke
Carol E. Bostrom

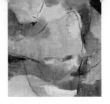

Acknowledgments

The fact that *Psychiatric Nursing* warrants a fourth edition humbles me. Past editions mention those who guided my thinking, encouraged me at the right time, or pushed me to develop my philosophy of and approach to psychiatric nursing care. I remember these individuals and their contributions to my life and others who mean so much. So, if my list grows long, it is because my debt runs high.

1963 Jeanne Lough, Stockton State Hospital: My first "psychiatric" teacher
1964 Vi Torres Lawrence, Delta College: Told me to shape up or ship out—old-fashioned motivation; Willie Smith, Mitch Patterson, and Dan Ramsey: fellow students at Delta College
1967 Army Nurse Corp: Where I learned the importance of an education
1970 Bette Keltner: Who married me against good advice
1971 John Bergey, Fresno State College: Encouraged me to pursue a Master's in psychiatry
1972 Jo Bacci, Stockton State Hospital: Gave me my first job as a teacher
1973 Sarah the Beara
1977 Amanda the Panda
1978 Jackie Johnson, Stanislaus State College, Department of Nursing
1981 Susan Leddy, University of Wyoming, College of Nursing
1982 Alex the Palex
1983 Opal Hipps, Baylor University, School of Nursing
1986 Nancy Cook, Cal State Bakersfield
1987 Alice Clarke, editor *Perspectives in Psychiatric Care:* Really liked my concept of "Psychotherapeutic Management," which led to this and other textbooks
1988 Linda Duncan and Jeff Burnham, Mosby
1989 Lee Schwecke and Carol Bostrom: Agreed to help me birth this book
1990 Rachel Booth, University of Alabama School of Nursing (UASON)
1994 Elizabeth Morrison, UASON: A real encourager
1998 Jeanne Allison and Jeff Downing, Mosby
2000 Psychiatric nursing faculty, UASON
2001 The Elsevier folks—Terri Wood, Cathy Ott, Jeanne Allison, and Dana Peick
2002 Bette Keltner: Still married to me against good advice

I also want to thank my students over the years. Many have given ideas on how to improve the book; others have indicated what we are doing right. I particularly want to thank those students who have taken the time to let me know that they actually have read the book. From the beginning I wanted a textbook that students would read. I keep hearing from students that they do.

NLK

This book would not have been possible without the hundreds of patients, victims, and survivors who were willing to share their pain, experiences, and successes. I also appreciate the students, faculty, and colleagues who questioned and challenged the content in the earlier editions and offered input for this edition. Norm Keltner, Carol Bostrom, and Sandy Wood deserve special mention for their insights and support. Over time, the staff of Community Hospital North Psychiatric Pavilion have helped me expand my knowledge and develop more effective intervention strategies. A sincere thank you to all who have touched my life and thereby influenced this book.

LHS

I dedicate the writing of this edition in memory of my parents, John and Henrietta Andruszko, and my uncle, Reverend William Gieranowski. They taught me to use my talents to help others in need, not only by their words but by the life they lived. Their faith has been a constant inspiration to me as I live my life. This textbook is also dedicated to the many individuals and families who have shared their joys and struggles with me. They believe that nurses are their primary advocates who understand and care for them. I hope this textbook will assist nurses in achieving some of the art and science of psychiatric nursing, regardless of where they practice.

A loving thank you to my husband, Paul, and my children, Melanie, Elizabeth, and Jonathan for always being there for me and with me.

CEB

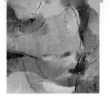

Detailed Contents

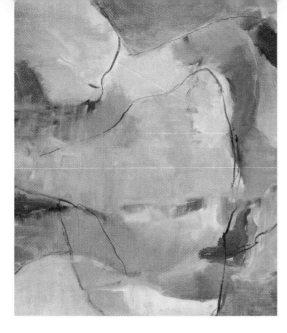

Introduction to Psychiatric Nursing

Norman L. Keltner

Learning Objectives

After reading this chapter, you should be able to:

- Describe the enormity of mental health concerns in both human and financial contexts.
- Explain the history of psychiatry as a foundation for current psychiatric nursing practice.
- Identify the significant changes that occurred during the period of the Enlightenment.
- Relate the contributions of early scientists to the current understanding of mental illness.
- Explain the impact of psychotropic drugs on psychiatric care.
- Analyze the immediate and long-term effects of the community mental health movement.
- Identify the specific strengths that enable psychiatric nurses to become effective in the new continuum of care.

"Some people's illnesses are so severe that they will always need asylum. A continuum of care is needed: from total freedom to total hospitalization, reflecting the diverse needs of mentally ill people"

Mona Wasow, professional social worker (MSW)
and mother of a mentally ill adult (1993)

Note to Students: *It is an interesting time to be studying psychiatric nursing. In June of 2001, we were all stunned by the news of a mother of five young children who was accused of killing her four boys: Luke, 2; Paul, 3; John, 5; Noah, 7; and her only daughter, Mary, 6 months. Andrea Yeats, 36 at the time, was said to suffer from postpartum depression (USA Today, 6/22/01). A few days later a woman in Italy was accused of stabbing to death her two sons, Giuseppe, 6, and Michele, 4 (Birmingham News, 7/01/01). Kuleva Jadranka, also 36, was said to have suffered "bouts of depression for years." A week later, former Representative Edward M. Mezvinsky of Pennsylvania pleaded innocent by reason of insanity to charges of fraud resulting from swindling $10 million from banks (Birmingham News, 7/06/01). It is speculated that Mr. Mezvinsky, 64, suffered from bipolar disorder. Whether you are sympathetic to these individuals or believe such considerations are a misuse of our freedoms, you have to admit that they provoke interest. All of these issues are complex and fall considerably outside the mainstream of psychiatric nursing care; nonetheless, they are related to what you will be studying in this text. Therefore although most of you will*

Key Terms

Asylum 1. A place of safety or sanctuary; a refuge; 2. An institution for the care of the mentally ill often associated with mistreatment and callousness.

Community mental health The application of the principles of psychiatric care to communities and groups of people. The goals of this effort are to maintain mental health, prevent mental illness when possible, and, when treatment is indicated, treat individuals in close proximity to their support systems.

Continuum of care Levels of care through which an individual can move, depending on the patient's needs at a given point in time.

Deinstitutionalization A shift in the location of treatment from large public hospitals to community settings.

Homelessness Individuals or whole families who may live exclusively on the streets or who may make use of community shelters, halfway houses, cheap hotels, or board-and-care homes.

Psychotropic drugs Medications used in the treatment of mental disorders.

not work full time in psychiatric nursing, you can learn a lot about mental illness, mental health, and yourself, and be better able to understand headlines in your morning papers by reading this book.

Epidemiologic evidence indicates that almost 6% of American adults over the age of 18 have a serious mental disorder in any 12-month period. When the full spectrum of mental and emotional disorders is incorporated, studies reveal that mental and addictive disorders affect approximately 25% of Americans each year. Table 1-1 provides a breakdown by diagnosis of the disorders prevalent at any time in American society, and Table 1-2 captures the costs of brain disorders in the United States, including both direct costs (e.g., medications) and indirect costs (e.g., lost wages). The pervasiveness of these maladies and the tremendous costs imply a great need for psychiatric professionals, including nurses, today and in the foreseeable future.

BENCHMARKS IN PSYCHIATRIC HISTORY

"And a certain woman...had suffered many things of many physicians, and had spent all that she had, and was nothing bettered, but rather grew worse" (Mark 5:25, 26, King James Version [1611]).

Table 1-1 12-Month Prevalence Rate of Mental Disorders in the United States

Diagnosis	Percentage of Population Over 17 Years of Age	Number of Persons
Anxiety disorders	12.6	20,034,000
Phobia disorders*	10.9	17,331,333
Mood disorders	9.5	15,143,000
Alcohol disorders	7.4	11,766,000
Major depression†	5.0	7,950,000
Drug disorders	3.1	4,929,000
Cognitive impairment	2.7	4,293,000
Obsessive-compulsive disorders	2.1	3,339,000
Antisocial disorders	1.5	2,385,000
Panic disorders*	1.3	2,067,000
Bipolar disorders†	1.2	1,908,000
Schizophrenia	1.1	1,749,000
Somatization	0.2	365,000

*Also calculated in anxiety statistics.
†Also calculated in mood disorders statistics.
From Regier DA et al: The de facto U.S. mental and addictive disorders service system: epidemiologic catchment area prospective, 1-year prevalence rates of disorders and services, *Arch Gen Psychiatry* 50:85, 1993; Surgeon General: *Mental health: a report from the Surgeon General*, Washington, DC, 1999, Department of Health and Human Services.

Table 1-2 Cost of Brain Disorders in the United States

Brain Disorder	Cost
Psychiatric disorders	$136,000,000,000
Alcohol abuse	90,000,000,000
Drug abuse	71,000,000,000
Dementia	113,000,000,000
Mental retardation	35,000,000,000
Total	445,000,000,000

National Foundation for Brain Disorders: *The cost of disorders of the brain*, Washington, DC, 1992, The Foundation.

The modern era of psychiatric care can be traced from events that occurred in England and France near the end of the eighteenth century, a time referred to as the Enlightenment. Before this time, the mentally ill were often regarded as no better than wild animals.

Rosenblatt (1984) writes of the ABCs of community response during this time: assistance, banishment, and confinement. Assistance, the least restrictive approach, provided food and money and often enabled the family to maintain its integrity as a unit. Banishment occurred in some communities, particu-

ITable 1-3I Benchmark Periods in Psychiatric History

Period	Key People or Developments	Significant Change in Thinking	Result(s)
Enlightenment			
~1790s	Pinel (1745-1826)—Unchained the mentally ill (1793) Tuke (1732-1822)—Established the York Retreat	The insane were no longer treated as less than human. Human dignity was upheld.	The asylum movement developed.
Scientific study			
~1870s	Freud (1856-1939)—Emphasized the importance of early life experiences in shaping mental health Kraepelin (1856-1926)—Developed classification of mental illness Bleuler (1857-1939)—Was optimistic about treatment	Humans could be studied, and that study held promise for treating and curing mental health problems.	The study of the mind and treatment approaches to psychiatric conditions flourished. The "Decade of the Brain" can be traced back to Kraepelin's thinking.
Psychotropic drugs			
~1950s	1949—Lithium 1950—Chlorpromazine 1952—Monoamine oxidase inhibitors (MAOIs) 1957—Haloperidol 1958—Tricyclic antidepressants (TCAs) 1960—Benzodiazepines	Some mental disorders are caused by chemical imbalances. If the chemical problem could be found through research, then a chemical cure could be found as well. In addition, people would no longer need to be confined.	A destigmatizing of mental illness occurred. Parents and others were not to blame. The term least restrictive environment evolved from this discovery.
Community mental health			
~1960s	Community Mental Health Centers Act (1963)	Individuals do not need to be hospitalized away from family and community. People have the right to be treated in their own community.	*Advantage:* Intervention in familiar surroundings has helped many people and is less expensive. *Disadvantage:* Homelessness is linked to deinstitutionalization, and many people "slip through the cracks" of the system.

larly when the deranged were strangers. Banishment led to wandering bands of "lunatics...living no one cared how, and dying no one cared where" (Rosenblatt, 1984). The infamous "Ship of Fools"—boatloads of the mentally disordered cast out to sea to find their "right minds"—occurred during this period.

Confinement was the most restrictive method of coping with the mentally ill, who were often chained. The old and the young, men and women, the insane, criminals, and paupers were indiscriminately mixed. The mentally ill were thought to be immune to normal biologic stressors such as cold, heat, and hunger. Patients were placed on display for the amusement of their caretakers and the paying public. For example, until 1770 a small fee was charged to visitors of St. Mary of Bethlem Hospital (Bedlam) in England. At Bedlam, treatments such as bleeding, bathing, vomiting and purging, and forced feedings were common "therapeutic" interventions (McMillan, 1997). At Bicétrè in France, the attendants served as "ringmasters," using whips to "encourage" their patients to perform (Rosenblatt, 1984). These warehouses for the tormented discouraged outside intrusion and attracted employees who were at the bottom levels of society, both socially and morally.

As the late 1700s approached, a day of enlightenment dawned: the establishment of the asylum. Four different periods stand out as benchmarks in the evolution of modern psychiatric care (Table 1-3):

Benchmark I: ~1790s
Benchmark II: ~late 1800s
Benchmark III: ~1950s
Benchmark IV: 1960s

During each of these four periods, the way of thinking about the mentally ill underwent significant changes, a result predominantly of certain individuals or specific events. After each period, events occurred that were important in their own right, but the inspirational sources of these events can be traced to the aforementioned benchmarks.

PERIOD OF ENLIGHTENMENT

"To consider madness incurable...is constantly refuted by the most authentic facts" (Philippe Pinel, December 11, 1794 [cited in Weiner, 1992]).

The modern era of psychiatric care began with two men, Philippe Pinel in France and William Tuke in England. In 1793 Pinel became the superintendent of the French institution, Bicétrè (for men), and later, the Salpêtrière (for women). Pinel was dismayed by the conditions he found and wrote of the patients, "They were abandoned to the incompetence of a callous director and to the cold brutality of servants who opposed a premeditated force of their own to impetuous acts of a blind and seemingly automatic violence" (Weiner, 1992). Soon after assuming leadership and motivated by scientific considerations, Pinel unchained the shackled, clothed the naked, fed the hungry, and abolished the whips and other instruments of cruel treatment. Simultaneously in England, William Tuke was planning a private facility that would ensure moral treatment for the mentally ill after he had witnessed the deplorable conditions in public facilities. In 1796, based on Quaker teachings, the York Retreat opened for patients, providing "a place in which the unhappy might obtain refuge—a quiet haven in which the shattered bark might find a means of reparation or safety" (Gollaher, 1995). Pinel and Tuke were responsible for this first benchmark of modern psychiatric care.

Asylum

The concept of the asylum developed from the humane efforts of Pinel and Tuke. The term *asylum* can mean protection, social support, or sanctuary from the stresses of life. A touring Chinese gymnast pleading for asylum is a good example of this definition. Currently, however, the term asylum most often provokes an image of mistreatment and neglect. It was the first definition that motivated Pinel, Tuke, and other similarly minded individuals.

Understanding that the mentally ill decompensated under stress, these individuals sought to provide an environment relatively free from stressors. Their language is inappropriate today—"madness," "lunacy," "insanity," "idiocy," "feeblemindedness"—but these were the accepted terms of their day. These early reformers were driven by a desire to improve the lot of abandoned, mentally ill persons and to provide asylum or sanctuary. An editorial in an 1803 issue of the *Alienest and Neurologist* made the following comment: "We owe the harmless lunatic a duty to save him from perpetual lunacy if we can. To leave him wholly to himself, even though he hurts no one, is not always kind. Such a course endangers incurable chronicity, and this is cruel to him" (Geller, 1992).

Dorothea Dix (1802-1887), the first major reformer in the United States, was instrumental in developing the concept of asylum and played a direct role in opening 32 state hospitals. Her efforts are invariably described as a crusade. Several years before launching her crusade, she visited Tuke's York Retreat. Undoubtedly, her impressions of Tuke's moral treatment influenced her concerns for the pain and suffering she had witnessed in her native land. Dix came to believe the greater citizenry, as represented by the government, had an obligation to their mentally ill brothers and sisters. She proposed to alleviate suffering with adequate shelter, nutritious food, and warm clothing. In Gollaher's (1995) exhaustive biography of Dix, he quotes from one of her Memorials, the documents she wrote to expose the terrible plight of the insane. From her Massachusetts Memorial, he notes:

> "*Concord:* A woman from the [Worcester] hospital in a cage in the almshouse. In the jail several, decently cared for in general but not properly placed in a prison. Violent, noisy, unmanageable most of the time.
> *Lincoln:* A woman in a cage.
> *Medford:* One idiotic subject chained, and one in a close [or narrow] stall for 17 years...
> *Granville:* One often closely confined...now losing the use of his limbs from want of exercise."

Although Dix is rightfully credited with being the first reformer with a nationwide perspective, other more regional sanctuaries had been established before her crusade. The first asylum in the United States was the Eastern Lunatic Asylum in Williamsburg, Virginia, founded in 1773. Other institutions followed, such as the Frankford Asylum near Philadelphia (1813), the Bloomingdale Asylum in New York (1818), and the Hartford Retreat in Connecticut (1824). The Philadelphia and New York asylums were established under Quaker influence and thus can be traced to Tuke.

The period of Enlightenment was short-lived. Within 100 years of the establishment of the first asylum, the reformers were being assailed as misusers and abusers of their charges. State hospitals were beset with problems. The first definition of asylum (sanctuary) had materialized in the form of hospitals' built-in rural settings. Patients were isolated geographically, socially, and, after release, from follow-up care. Patients were also isolated from public scrutiny, which enabled many large institutions to become closed systems. As might be guessed, the beneficence of the reformers was not shared by many "caretakers" who followed. Within a relatively brief period, the term asylum changed; it evolved from a place of refuge to a place of torment.

Today, a renewed interest in asylum as a place of rest and restoration exists. This concept can be considered in terms of the four Ps: parents, professionals, patients, and public, each of which has a stake in the discussion of asylum. Mona Wasow, MSW and the parent of a mentally ill adult, writes persuasively for the need of asylum: "Some people's illnesses are so severe that they will always need asylum. A continuum of care is needed: from total freedom to total hospitalization, reflecting the diverse needs of mentally ill people" (1993).

Critical Thinking Questions

1. Which of the two definitions of "asylum" do you believe is more prevalent in psychiatric nursing today?
2. What are some negative outcomes of deinstitutionalization that you have witnessed or with which you have been personally involved?

PERIOD OF SCIENTIFIC STUDY

The shift in focus from sanctuary to treatment is linked to the second benchmark in psychiatric care, personified by Sigmund Freud (1856-1939). Toward the last third of the nineteenth century, several scientists devoted themselves to understanding the mind and mental illness. The fruits of their labor held great promise, some of which is still unfulfilled. Nonetheless, the efforts forever changed the world's view: mental illness need not be suffered (however humanely patients were treated) but might be alleviated. In a sense, psychiatric care was popularized.

Early Scientists

Although Freud had the greatest impact on the world's view of mental illness, he neither thought nor worked in a vacuum. Other men and women had tremendous influence on this new enthusiastic and optimistic approach to mental illness. Emil Kraepelin (1856-1926) made tremendous contributions to the classification of mental disorders. Kraepelin was a true scientist whose descriptions of schizophrenia are classic and valuable reading. Eugene Bleuler (1857-1939) coined the term *schizophrenia* and added a note of optimism to its treatment. Still others, many of whom were colleagues or disciples of Freud, made significant contributions to the emerging field of psychiatry.

Freud's contributions still influence psychiatric care, although for a number of years, belittling his accomplishments was popular. Paraphrasing a statement made by Sir Isaac Newton (1642-1727): If we see far today, it is because we stand on the shoulders of giants.

Freud described human behavior in psychologic terms. He developed a theory of motivation, established the usefulness of talking (catharsis), explained the importance of dreams, and proposed to unlock the hidden parts of the mind. He introduced terms that are now daily fare, such as *psychoanalysis, id, ego, superego,* and *free association* and was able to do this because he felt free to study human beings. Charles Darwin's work caused him to view humans in a new context. From Freud's study evolved the work of others, many of whom studied with Freud. Alfred Adler, Carl Jung, Ernest Jones, Otto Rank, Helene Deutsch, Karen Horney, and Anna Freud (Freud's daughter) all made significant and, in most cases, lasting contributions to the field of dynamic psychiatry.

Freud's inspiration, however, reached far beyond those with whom he worked personally. Society in general is indebted to him, even though disagreement with his ideas has emerged. Freud challenged society to look at human beings objectively and fostered a milieu of thinking about the mind and mental disorders. (The selected theories of Freud, as well as other theorists' models of behavior, are presented in greater detail in Chapter 3.) Unit Three builds on these concepts and is devoted to the implementation of strategies for working with psychiatric patients.

PERIOD OF PSYCHOTROPIC DRUGS

From this milieu of theory and scientific thought came the third benchmark, which began approximately in 1950 with the discovery of psychotropic drugs. Chlorpromazine (Thorazine), an antipsychotic drug, and lithium, an antimanic agent, were introduced first, and imipramine (Tofranil), an antidepressant, was introduced a few years later. The impact of these drugs has been powerful. Patients who appeared beyond reach became less agitated and experienced a reduction in psychotic thinking. Depressed patients regained normal feelings. Hospital stays were shortened, and hospital environments improved. The widely held belief was that psychotropic drugs were truly miracle drugs. However, although psychotropic drugs have allowed many patients to be treated in less restrictive environments, many ethical, moral, and legal questions have arisen with this treatment modality. Unit Four is devoted to an understanding of the role of psychotropic drugs in the treatment of mental disorders.

PERIOD OF COMMUNITY MENTAL HEALTH

The notion that one benchmark period ended entirely before the next one began is inaccurate. Trends overlap as advocates of one view struggle to defend existing strategies while more dynamic forces emerge elsewhere. As the various treatment approaches were being developed in the milieu derived from Freud's theories, criticism grew, and the state hospital system continued its plunge into "psychiatric Siberia." The popular movie "The Snake Pit" (1948) portrayed a mindless, ineffective, and at times cruel system of care. In an even more devastating exposé, the book *The Shame of the States,* by Albert Deutsch (1948), vividly revealed with words and photographs the deplorable conditions in several large state hospitals in the United States.

Legislators were watching, reading, and listening; legislation was passed that would change the approach to psychiatric care. In 1946 President Tru-

man signed the National Mental Health Act, enabling the establishment of the National Institute of Mental Health (1949). In 1947 the Hill-Burton Act legislated funds to build general hospitals to include psychiatric units. This initiative began the effort to intervene early and shorten the length of hospitalization for psychiatric patients.

In 1961 the Joint Commission on Mental Illness and Health, appointed by President Kennedy, published a report entitled "Action for Mental Health." The report urged increased support for the state hospital system in recognition of the need for improved treatment of the mentally ill population. Opponents of the state hospital system overwhelmed supporters of this document. In fact, the more outspoken critics of the existing system pronounced the report as the cause of mental illness.

Rather than increasing monetary support for the state hospital system, a convergence of forces set the stage for this fourth benchmark period in psychiatric history:

1. The public's declining confidence in the state hospital system
2. The failure of various treatment approaches to eradicate mental illness
3. The legislative climate that had begun in the 1940s, emphasizing the civil rights of the mentally ill
4. The newfound faith in psychotropic drugs

These factors led to the enactment of the Community Mental Health Centers (CMHC) Act in 1963, which virtually destroyed the state hospital system. A deliberate shift was made from institutional to extrainstitutional care. The goal was deinstitutionalization of the state hospital system population. The aforementioned problem of geographic isolation was addressed with community treatment centers and community living arrangements (e.g., halfway houses). Keeping the mentally disordered individual closer to the family addressed the issue of isolation from family members. Isolation from follow-up care was remedied because various levels of care were available locally.

Eventually, community mental health programs were built to meet the needs of all people living within the boundaries of a designated (e.g., catchment) area. These programs had the following goals:

- Emergency care
- 24-hour inpatient care

- Partial hospitalization care
- Outpatient care
- Consultation and education for the population served by the center
- Screening services

Effect on Nursing

The community mental health movement broadened the scope of psychiatric nursing. No longer did the psychiatric nurse simply work in the hospital or inpatient setting. A whole range of opportunities became available to the psychiatric nurse, from working with the chronically mentally ill to working with the "worried well," (i.e., those with low self-esteem or those who are chronically unhappy) and from concentrating on individual treatment issues to focusing on broader social issues affecting mental health as well.

This professional evolution of care had both positive and negative effects on psychiatric nursing. On the positive side, the change broadened the understanding of and interest in mental health. With this interest and understanding came efforts to prevent problems and to develop strategies to maximize mental health. A negative effect, on the other hand, was the resultant confusion about mental illness. Specifically, the criteria for defining mental illness became less rigid and resulted in more and more "problems" being claimed as legitimate concerns of mental health professionals. For example, official diagnostic disorders now include mathematics disorder, hypoactive sexual desire disorder, sibling relational problem, and pathologic gambling disorder. Not all psychiatric nurses endorsed these "disorders" as legitimate psychiatric concerns; hence a certain professional confusion ensued. Were nurses psychiatric nurses, mental health nurses, or both? Undergraduate psychiatric nursing faculty members still debate this issue.

Deinstitutionalization

"The practice, over the past four decades, of releasing people with severe mental illnesses from institutions has been one of the largest social experiments in twentieth century America" (E. Fuller Torrey, 1997).

Deinstitutionalization refers to the depopulating of state mental hospitals. State hospitals reached their peak census in 1955 and then slowly began the process of trimming their census rolls. Important to understand is that the impetus for deinstitutionalization began as early as 1955. The roots of this process began with the growing concerns about asylum and were nurtured by some of the events previously discussed. A subtler factor was psychiatry's and psychiatric nursing's growing disillusionment with the chronically mentally ill and an embracing of the worried well.

These factors clearly laid the groundwork for deinstitutionalization; however, federal actions fully detonated the process. First, as discussed, was the CMHC Act of 1963. The second federal action was legislation that provided mentally disabled persons with an income while they were living in the community. This legislation was named Aid to the Disabled (ATD), now called Supplemental Security Income (SSI) and Social Security Disability Insurance (SSDI). The number of individuals with mental disorders receiving these benefits grew dramatically. Between 1986 and 1991 the number of workers with a mental disorder receiving SSDI increased by close to 50%, while the number of persons with mental disorders receiving SSI nearly doubled. Particularly controversial was the awarding of benefits to individuals with addictive disorders who often used these government funds to purchase more abused substances. Public concern and journalistic exposés led to termination of these benefits.

Shifting the Cost of Mental Illness

State governments soon found ATD, even when supplemented by the state, to be less costly than was public hospitalization because the federal government was paying for SSI, Medicare, and Medicaid. The federal share grew from 2% in 1963 to 62% by 1994 (Torrey, 1997). State financial incentives to treat effectively the severely mentally ill (SMI) declined as the involvement of the federal government increased.

Perhaps the final event in the deinstitutionalization movement was the change in commitment laws. Out of concern for the civil rights of mental patients, involuntary commitment to the state hospital became difficult (Rosenheck, 1997). The state had to demonstrate that the "accused" were a clear danger to themselves or to others. These sweeping changes were reactions to years of injustice wherein persons said to be mentally ill could be detained and involuntarily committed, with little recourse, for long

Box 1-1 | On Being Sane in Insane Places

Rosenhan wondered whether the "sane" could be distinguished from the "insane." He selected eight pseudopatients (people who pretended to be mentally ill) and instructed them to attempt to gain admission to public mental hospitals. The task was much easier than anyone had anticipated. Twelve hospitals in five states were used. The pseudopatient group consisted of a graduate student in psychology, three psychologists (including Rosenhan himself), a pediatrician, a psychiatrist, a painter, and a housewife; three were women and five were men. No one in the hospital knew of the deception.

The pseudopatients were trained to do the following:
1. Call the hospital and make an appointment.
2. On arriving at the hospital, tell the psychiatrist that they had been hearing voices.
3. On being asked to describe the voices, say that they were not sure but remembered the words "empty," "hollow," and "thud."
4. Other than giving this false information and false information about their names, occupations, and employers, be truthful and "normal." from that point forward.
5. Immediately on admission, cease simulating abnormal behavior and to behave "normally."
6. When asked how they were doing, respond "fine" and to inform the staff that they were no longer experiencing problems.

Despite behaving normally, none of the pseudopatients were discovered by the staff. However, approximately 25% of the other patients made comments about the pseudopatients' "sanity," and a few even guessed that the pseudopatients were doing some kind of undercover work. Rosenhan noted reluctance by the staff to see mental health in their patients. He stated, "Having once been labeled schizophrenic, there is nothing the pseudopatients can do to overcome the tag." Pseudopatient histories were written to support their diagnoses. In other words, psychiatrists saw problems that had never existed.

The pseudopatients were also asked to write down their observations. At first, they followed elaborate precautions to avoid detection; however, they were soon jotting down observations in front of the staff. The pseudopatients had discovered that no one was paying any attention to them.

Another part of the experiment was to determine the amount of time that was spent with patients. This amount was difficult to measure, thus a proxy behavior was substituted: time the nurses spent outside of the nurses' station. Nursing attendants had the highest percentage of time outside the station (11.3%). Rosenhan found that measuring registered nurse time outside of the nurses' station was impossible because it occurred so infrequently. Psychiatrists were even worse because they hid behind closed office doors; at least the patients were able to see the nurses. Rosenhan concluded, "Those with the most power have least to do with patients, and those with the least power are most involved with them."

Rosenhan decries the powerlessness and the depersonalization experienced by the pseudopatients. He remembered the way in which he was frequently awakened in the hospital at which he was admitted: "Come on you m-----f-----s, out of bed."

The pseudopatients were hospitalized on average for 19 days before they were deemed well enough for discharge. The range of stays was from 7 to 52 days.

From Rosenhan DL: On being sane in insane places, *Science* 179:250, 1973.

periods. (Rosenhan's classic study [1973] [Box 1-1] illustrates how difficult it was for a "sane" person to be discharged from a mental hospital.) The stage was set for rapid depopulation of state hospitals.

Depopulation of State Hospitals

The state hospital population reached its peak in 1955 with 558,922 patients (0.3% of the population). By 1997 the state hospital population had dropped to 70,000 patients (0.03% of the population) (Torrey, 1997), a decline of over 85%. Torrey asserts that 900,000 people would be in state hospitals today if the same proportions were in effect. Thus over 800,000 individuals who might have been hospitalized years ago are living outside such institutions. This decline has resulted in the closing of more than 50 state hospitals since 1970. Patients who remain hospitalized today require a high level of care, have few social relationships, are psychotic, and are typically acutely ill young men. Table 1-4 provides insights into where these people may be living.

Revolving-Door Effect

Although deinstitutionalization has slowed in the last few years, its effect on public mental hospitals is still profound. *Recidivism,* a term traditionally used to describe repeat criminal offenders, is now being used to describe the "revolving-door" effect of persons recycling through public mental hospitals. Although a significant reduction in beds has been achieved, admissions have increased considerably as a result of high rates of recidivism.

Table 1-4 Where Individuals with Severe Mental Illness Live

Location	Numbers (Approximate)
Nursing homes	1,000,000
Prison	150,000
State hospitals	70,000*
Homeless	200,000+†
Home with families, group or board-care homes, or on their own	50%

*See Depopulation of State Hospitals, p. 8.
†See Homelessness below.
National Institutes of Mental Health: *Mental health statistics,* Rockville, Md, 1993, Office of Consumer, Family, and Public Information, Center for Mental Health Services.
Torrey EF: The release of the mentally ill from institutions: a well-intentioned disaster, *Chron High Educ* 43(40):B4, 1997.

Community Effects

The effects of deinstitutionalization are also evident in community agencies. For example, emergency department use by acutely disturbed individuals has increased dramatically in the absence of the previous system. Emergency psychiatric services are sagging from the load they carry. General hospital psychiatric units are overwhelmed at times with a continuous flow of patients being admitted, discharged, or being observed for 23 hours (to avoid a full and costly admission). The mission of these hospitals has expanded because they have had to grapple with the new realities of health care. Many professionals believe that the typical patient is different as well. Compared with the patients of the 1960s and 1970s, today's patients are more aggressive. According to Ries (1997), approximately 4% to 8% of patients in psychiatric emergency departments are armed with weapons. Furthermore, approximately 1000 homicides are committed each year by SMI individuals who are not receiving adequate care (Torrey, 1997). Lastly, 10% to 15% of those in state prisons are SMI (Lamb, Weinberger, 1998).

HOMELESSNESS

Many psychiatric professionals believe that homelessness can be directly linked to deinstitutionalization. Twenty-five years ago, the most popular view held that homeless people (mostly Caucasian men) were skid-row bums, alcoholics, and hobos who chose to be homeless. The current view has altered that perception considerably. The current belief holds that the homeless are people (including entire families) who have been displaced by social policies over which they have no control. Perhaps 25% of the homeless are children, and another 25% are employed in low-paying jobs.

Estimates concerning the prevalence of mental illness among this population also vary. The consensus of opinion, however, is that 25% to 50% of adult homeless population has a psychosis, and that approximately the same number suffers from alcohol or drug abuse. Haugland, Siegel, and Hopper (1997) suggest that approximately 10% to 20% of homeless individuals have a dual diagnosis or suffer from both a mental illness and a substance abuse disorder.

People who are homeless and mentally ill present a challenge to the mental health system and to the political system in the United States; these individuals are usually single or divorced and have a weak social support system. The homeless SMI are found in parks, airport terminals, soup kitchens, jails, and general hospitals, often presenting a troubling specter. Furthermore, the economic windfall experienced by some Americans in recent years has not filtered down to the streets. Many homeless mentally ill persons have become bold in their efforts to survive, assaulting the sensitivities of passersby. From aggressive panhandling to embarrassing public elimination of bodily wastes, societal standards are being affronted. Although much of this alienating behavior is required for survival on the "mean" streets, it is behavior that offends mainstream America. The dilemma is real, and mental health professionals are searching for answers.

As mentioned, homeless people may live exclusively on the streets (the so-called street people), or they may live in community shelters, halfway houses, or board-and-care homes. A possible third group includes individuals who are able to stay for short periods in cheap hotels between nights in less accommodating surroundings. Still another significant group moves among homeless shelters, rehabilitation programs, jails, and prisons (Haugland et al, 1997).

Homelessness is an end-product of chronic mental illness and probably exacerbates it as well. Stated another way, many chronically ill persons end up on the streets because of their inability to succeed in a competitive society and, once they are on the streets, the stresses of homeless life compound their mental health problems; they are in a no-win situation. Hypothesizing that such a situation might exist,

Winkleby and White (1992) studied 1399 homeless adults in California and found that although 45.6% reported no impairment when they first became homeless, most of them eventually developed addictive and psychiatric disorders over time. As with many societal problems, some groups appear to fare worse than do others. Racial and ethnic minorities are overrepresented among the homeless.

Proponents of deinstitutionalization argue that these problems are not inherently a part of depopulating state hospitals but have resulted because the money has not followed the patient out of the hospital. Inpatient psychiatric treatment still accounts for a majority of mental health dollars in the United States; thus proponents argue that community mental health has never been given the financial base to realize its promise. Critics, on the other hand, point to the homeless and the disproportionate effect experienced by some minority groups as evidence of a need for change. Homelessness is more than a lack of shelter, the critics maintain; it is a lack of support systems that are available in the public mental hospital system.

EVOLUTION OF PSYCHIATRIC CARE CONCERNS

Psychiatry in general lost interest in the SMI as a result of the influx of psychoanalysts in the 1930s and 1940s (Miller, 1984). As Freud himself had discovered, his analytic approach was most helpful to persons with less severe problems and was not particularly helpful to psychotic patients. Thus as Freudian thinking influenced more psychiatrists and psychiatric nurses, a natural withdrawal from the SMI and a refocusing on individuals more amenable to treatment occurred. Public mental hospitals lost prestige as did the physicians and nurses working in them. Within the psychiatric nursing fraternity, staff nurses were not as highly valued as were those working in the therapist role. As participants in a self-fulfilling prophecy, the devalued inpatient psychiatric nurses in public hospitals, in many cases, became what they were perceived to be.

The mainstream of psychiatry and psychiatric nursing turned from chronically disturbed patients to individuals with lowered self-esteem, those who were striving to reach their potential, those who had not developed the ability to trust, and those who were existentially unhappy (Detre, 1987). Psychiatry

changed its focus from one extreme of the psychiatric care continuum (the SMI) to the other (the worried well) over a few decades. Social issues started to emerge as legitimate professional concerns. Psychiatry and psychiatric nursing became interested in issues such as poverty, racism, alternate lifestyles, and sexism at the professional level. Some clinicians perceive that this process of enlightenment and social relevance further distanced the mainstream of psychiatric care from persons most in need of that care.

Critical Thinking Question

It has been stated that the fields of psychiatry and psychiatric nursing lost interest in the SMI and became more interested in working with the worried well. Do you believe this is still true in psychiatric nursing? Support your answer.

HISTORY OF NURSING EDUCATION— THREE FIRSTS

First Psychiatric Nurse

The official history of psychiatric nursing began approximately 100 years ago. Linda Richards, the first American psychiatric nurse, was a graduate of the New England Hospital for Women. Richards spent much of her professional career developing nursing care in psychiatric hospitals and also directed a school of psychiatric nursing in 1880 at the McLean Psychiatric Asylum in Waverly, Massachusetts. Because of her efforts, more than 30 asylums had developed schools for psychiatric nurses by 1890.

First Psychiatric Nursing Textbook

In 1920, Harriet Bailey wrote the first psychiatric nursing textbook. The title of the book, *Nursing Mental Diseases,* reflects the appropriate terminology of the day. An important distinction about psychiatric nursing is that it was not brought into the greater nursing fold until the 1940s. Because psychiatric nurses were trained in state hospitals, they were allowed to work only in state hospitals. In 1937 the National League for Nursing (then called the National League for Nursing Education) recommended that psychiatric nursing be made a part of the curriculum of general nursing programs.

First Psychiatric Nursing Theorist

The views of an important figure in psychiatric nursing in the 1950s shaped and gave direction to psychiatric nursing practice and contributed to a professional climate. Hildegarde Peplau (1952, 1959) developed a model for psychiatric nursing practice. Her book, *Interpersonal Relations in Nursing* (1952), influences practice to this day. Her approach, heavily influenced by Harry Stack Sullivan, emphasizes the interpersonal dimension of practice. Peplau also wrote a history of psychiatric nursing that carefully traced the unfolding of the profession. Peplau may be the single most important historic figure in psychiatric nursing.

COMMUNITY-BASED CARE

The future of psychiatric care and psychiatric nursing will be linked to continuing efforts to prevent mental health problems and to treat existing disorders more effectively. Because of economic realities, much of that effort will be community based as part of a continuum of care. Nurses will need to continue to train for roles in the community while reestablishing a leadership role in inpatient services. An agenda for mental health has been established in the document *Healthy People 2010* (2000), developed by the U.S. Department of Health and Human Services.

Developing a Continuum of Care

In the early 1960s, mental health activists were successful in passing federal legislation that dramatically reshaped the way mental health services were delivered in the United States. Converging forces related to these changes have been previously discussed.

Specific problems associated with community mental health (CMH) were the liberalization of commitment laws, which allowed SMI patients to go untreated, and restrictive confidentiality rulings, which made discussing the difficult issues of treatment with family members a legal concern. As newspaper editorials, grassroots mental health organizations, and families have clamored about the obvious unmet needs of the SMI, the mental health and legal communities have rallied to respond. This insistence has culminated in thoughtful and deliberate dialogue among mental health professionals with the objective to make the mental health system work.

To make the system work, a seamless continuum of care must be developed that coordinates the activities of diverse treatment sources and facilitates movement between and among its entities. Until this seamless continuum is developed, many patients will slip through the cracks of the system as both bureaucratic dysfunction and corporate self-interest drain energies away from programs. Box 1-2 suggests the way in which the system is changing to develop this seamless continuum of care.

Role for Nursing in the Continuum of Care

CMH nursing has been in existence for many years. In 1982 the American Nurses' Association (ANA) defined the CMH nurse's role in the continuum of care as follows: "The nurse participates with other members of the community in assessing, planning, implementing, and evaluating mental health services and community services that include the promotion of the continuum of primary, secondary, and tertiary prevention of mental illness."

Nursing has an opportunity to assert itself at this point in psychiatric history because many values traditionally emphasized by psychiatric nursing fit with the concept of a continuum of care. For instance:

- Viewing the patient as a whole person
- Working with families
- Treating patients in their own homes
- Developing a relationship over time
- Educating patients about medications
- Assessing the environment for safety, hygiene, and supports

All of these traditional nursing activities position nurses to excel in the world of psychiatric care. Only time will tell whether the profession is up to the challenges ahead and is able to take advantage of its natural "fit" with today's health care realities.

|Box 1-2 | Systemic Changes

In the new health care reality, CMH must move rapidly away from some practices and toward new ways of conceptualizing the system.

- Away from symptom stabilization toward recovery and reintegration
- Away from a view that professionals have all the answers toward involving consumers and family members more
- Away from medication management toward holistic thinking (e.g., stabilizing housing, medical health, finances)

Critical Thinking Question

Many large numbers referring to both people and money have been discussed in this chapter. To help sensitize you to these numbers, consider the following: calculate the weeks, months, or years equivalent to 1 million, 1 billion, and 1 trillion seconds, and review the numbers referred to in the chapter with this concept in mind.

Key Concepts

1. Understanding the principles of psychiatric nursing is important because mental health problems affect approximately 25% of the population.
2. Modern psychiatry can be traced through four benchmark periods: Enlightenment, scientific study, psychotropic drugs, and CMH.
3. Historically, the mentally ill were banished and confined; but the period of Enlightenment ushered in an era in which the mentally ill were treated humanely.
4. The asylum movement (providing sanctuary from the hostile world) grew out of the humane emphasis of the period of Enlightenment and resulted in the development of state hospital systems.
5. During the period of scientific study, men such as Freud, Kraepelin, and Bleuler objectively studied human beings; this effort resulted in both psychodynamic and biologic understandings of mental disorders.
6. During the period of psychotropic drugs, antipsychotic drugs (chlorpromazine [Thorazine] in the early 1950s), antidepressant drugs (imipramine [Tofranil] in the late 1950s), and other drugs were developed and greatly contributed to the treatment of specific mental disorders.
7. The period of CMH began as a result of several converging factors including:
   - Hostility toward state hospitals
   - Psychotropic drugs
   - Civil rights
   - Financial incentives
8. Deinstitutionalization, which changed the locus of treatment from large public hospitals to the community, is a product of the CMH movement.
9. In 1955, over one-half million patients were in state hospitals; by 1997 approximately 70,000 were in these hospitals.
10. A high percentage of the nation's homeless has a diagnosable mental disorder. Critics of deinstitutionalization place some of the blame for homelessness on the CMH movement.
11. Psychiatric care and psychiatric nursing have evolved during the twentieth century. At one time, psychiatric nursing was closely associated with the care of the SMI but, similar to medicine, became professionally interested in the worried well. Today, some voices are challenging psychiatric nurses to return to caring for those most in need.
12. In 1920, Harriet Bailey wrote the first psychiatric nursing textbook, but Hildegarde Peplau's book, *Interpersonal Relations in Nursing*, has most influenced psychiatric nursing.
13. CMH nurses have a major role in the continuum of care because of their specific training in patient care, comprehensive services, patient education, and case management.

References

Birmingham News: *Ex-rep. Mezvinsky to plead insanity*, Page 3A, 7/6/01.

Birmingham News: *Woman examined after sons' deaths*, Page 11A, 7/1/01.

Detre T: The future of psychiatry, *Am J Psychiatry* 144:621, 1987.

Deutsch A: *The shame of the states*, New York, 1948, Harcourt Brace.

Geller JL: A historical perspective on the role of state hospitals viewed from the era of the "revolving door," *Am J Psychiatry* 149:1526, 1992.

Gollaher D: *Voice for the mad: the life of Dorothea Dix*, New York, 1995, The Free Press.

Haugland G et al: Mental illness among homeless individuals in a suburban county, *Psychiatric Services* 48(4):504, 1997.

Jones D: Kids' dad defends his wife, *USA Today*, 1A, 6/22/01.

Lamb HR, Weinberger LE: Persons with severe mental illness in jails and prisons: a review, *Psychiatric Services* 49:483, 1998.

McMillan I: Insight into Bedlam: one hospital's history, *J Psychosoc Nurs Ment Health Serv* 35(6):28, 1997.

Miller RD: Public mental hospital work: pros and cons for psychiatrists, *Hosp Community Psychiatry* 35:928, 1984.

National Foundation for Brain Disorders: *The cost of disorders of the brain*, Washington, DC, 1992, The Foundation.

National Institutes of Mental Health: *Mental health statistics*, Rockville, Md, 1993, Office of Consumer, Family, and Public Information, Center for Mental Health Services.

Peplau H: *Interpersonal relations in nursing*, New York, 1952, GP Putnam.

Peplau H: Principles of psychiatric nursing. In Arieti S, editor: *American handbook of psychiatry*, vol 2, New York, 1959, Basic Books.

Randolph F et al: Creating integrated service systems for homeless persons with mental illness: the ACCESS program, *Psychiatr Serv* 48(3):369, 1997.

Regier DA et al: The de facto U.S. mental and addictive disorders service system: epidemiologic catchment area prospective 1-year prevalence rates of disorders and services, *Arch Gen Psychiatry* 50:85, 1993.

Ries R: Advantages of separating the triage function from the emergency service, *Psychiatr Serv* 48(6):755, 1997.

Rosenblatt A: Concepts of the asylum in the care of the mentally ill, *Hosp Community Psychiatry* 35:244, 1984.

Rosenhan DL: On being sane in insane places, *Science* 179:250, 1973.

Rosenheck R: Disability payments and chemical dependence: conflicting values and uncertain effects, *Psychiatr Serv* 48(6):789, 1997.

Torrey EF: The release of the mentally ill from institutions: a well-intentioned disaster, *Chron High Educ* 43(40):B4, 1997.

U.S. Department of Health and Human Services: *Healthy people 2010,* Washington, DC, 2000, USDHHS.

Wasow M: The need for asylum revisited, *Hosp Community Psychiatry,* 44(3):207, 1993.

Weiner DB: Philippe Pinel's "Memoir on Madness" of December 11, 1794: A fundamental text of modern psychiatry, *Am J Psychiatry* 149(6):725, 1992.

Winkleby MA, White R: Homeless adults without apparent medical and psychiatric impairment: onset of morbidity over time, *Hosp Community Psychiatry* 43(10):1017, 1992.

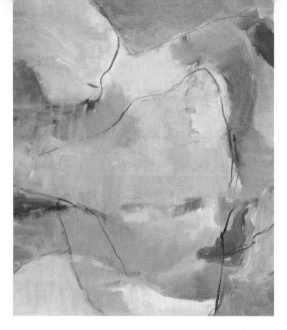

Chapter 2

Psychotherapeutic Management in the Continuum of Care

Norman L. Keltner

Learning Objectives

After reading this chapter, you should be able to:

- Describe the components of psychotherapeutic management.
- Explain the way in which the balancing of psychotherapeutic management components combine to form a powerful therapeutic model of care.
- Recognize the relationship between the continuum of care and the psychotherapeutic management model.

PSYCHOTHERAPEUTIC MANAGEMENT

Psychiatric nursing is in search of care delivery models that are not only effective for patient care, but can also capitalize on the uniqueness of the discipline. Psychotherapeutic management proposes a "real-world" approach to psychiatric nursing care that recognizes the interdependence of the mental health professions and exploits the strengths of psychiatric nursing. It answers the question, "What do psychiatric nurses do that is different from that of other mental health professionals, particularly social workers, psychologists, marriage and family counselors, and other therapists?" In 1979, Koldjeski wrote: "Psychiatric nurses must clearly demonstrate the exact nature of their practice and must differentiate their practice from the practice of other nonmedical mental health personnel." After Koldjeski's prescription, psychotherapeutic management was proposed as a model to clarify and distinguish the

role of the psychiatric nurse (Keltner, 1985). Psychiatric treatment can be divided into five basic categories: use of words (which encompass all forms of psychotherapy), drugs, environment, somatic therapies, and behavioral conditioning. Psychotherapeutic management emphasizes three of these categories: the psychotherapeutic nurse-patient relationship (words), psychopharmacology (drugs), and milieu management (environment), all of which must be supported by a sound understanding of psychopathology (Figure 2-1).

Stated another way, the student has three intervention tools:

1. Self
2. Psychotropic drugs
3. Environment

The particular intervention approach depends on the patient's psychopathology. For example, the nurse will learn to use different words when he or she speaks with a patient who is diagnosed with schizophrenia compared with a patient who is diagnosed with depression. More than likely, the patient with schizophrenia will require antipsychotic medications, whereas the depressed patient will receive antidepressant drugs, hence drug management is different. Finally, whereas the patient with schizophrenia may need an environment that reduces stressors, a key environmental concern for the depressed patient might be safety (e.g., suicide prevention). In other words, the psychotherapeutic management model recognizes that "one size does not fit all."

Key Terms

Behavior therapy A therapeutic approach that helps patients modify behavior by modifying or changing old patterns of behavior.

Continuum of care Levels of care through which an individual can move, depending on his or her needs at a given point in time.

Milieu Environment or setting.

Psychopathology The systematic study of mental disorders.

Psychotherapeutic management A model for nursing care that balances the three primary intervention modes that psychiatric nurses use: the therapeutic nurse-patient relationship (self), psychopharmacology (drugs), and milieu management (environment).

Psychotropic drugs Medication used in the treatment of mental disorders.

Therapeutic Refers to the communication of respect, a desire to help, and understanding to another person. Understanding includes knowledge of mental mechanisms, coping strategies, and stressors. Active listening is a crucial component of being therapeutic.

Therapy The means, usually with words, to cure or manage the course of a mental disorder. Nurses who practice psychotherapy are trained in a specific therapy model, for example, psychoanalysis or cognitive therapy.

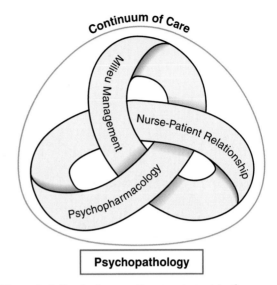

Figure 2-1 Psychotherapeutic management in the continuum of care.

Application of Psychotherapeutic Management Interventions

The application of psychopathology and the knowledgeable use of psychotherapeutic management skills extend beyond inpatient settings into a variety of care settings, such as outpatient programs, residential services, and home care. The needs of the individual and the setting in which care is delivered will influence the degree to which each of the components of psychotherapeutic management is used within the continuum of care (Figure 2-2).

For example, individuals with schizophrenia in an inpatient setting profit most when a therapeutic nurse-patient relationship, psychopharmacology, and a well-managed milieu are available. When one component is missing from the equation, treatment is compromised. Ordinarily, when psychotropic drugs and a well-managed milieu are subtracted from this equation, patients will decompensate into a pretreatment state. Similarly, when drugs and therapeutic communication are available (perhaps the

latter from only a few motivated staff members) but the overall environment is poorly managed, patients are left to fend for themselves and are drained of internal resources needed for healing. When inpatients receive only drug therapy but are denied therapeutic interaction opportunities in a well-managed milieu, a return to the inadequacies of custodial care takes place. In other words, all the components of the psychotherapeutic management equation must be present if patients are to realize fully the benefits of effective nursing intervention. However, one component may take precedence at a given point in time. For example, an individual with schizophrenia has missed his last appointment for his injection of haloperidol decanoate (Haldol decanoate). The nurse's priority might be to make a home visit to administer the injection. The psychopharmacology component is a priority at this time, but the nurse-patient relationship and milieu aspects are not ignored. Psychotherapeutic management endeavors to bring balance to practice and, with balance, role clarification, thus providing a valuable approach in both inpatient and outpatient settings.

CONTINUUM OF CARE

Unit Two deals with the continuum of care within which the psychotherapeutic management approach is implemented and includes providing services

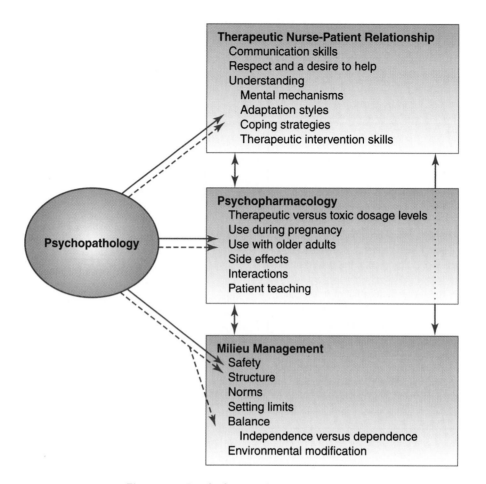

Figure 2-2 Psychotherapeutic management model.

based on the needs of the individual. The services span the continuum from health promotion through prevention, treatment, and rehabilitation. These services can be provided in a variety of settings. An important aspect of the continuum of care is that the individuals can be guided through treatment or services as their needs change. The individual's initial contact with the mental health system should involve the process of assessment and referral to the least restrictive, most effective, and most cost-conscious source of services. The multiple services may or may not involve the nurse as the primary caregiver; other disciplines or care providers may be responsible for a particular service. The psychotherapeutic management model has relevance in a variety of care settings and can be adapted by the nurse to any level of care.

The way in which the patient is guided to an appropriate level of care is based on a series of decisions (Figure 2-3). Traditionally, the nurse made these decisions as part of discharge planning before the patient's release from the hospital. Given current trends in mental health care, the decisions may be made by the nurse or other professionals during the "risk assessment phase."

Therapeutic Nurse-Patient Relationship

Differentiating therapy from being therapeutic is crucial for the student of psychiatric nursing. Therapy is the focus of graduate-level psychiatric nursing training, and the art of being therapeutic is the domain of undergraduate-level psychiatric nurses. Therefore when this course is completed, the student will not be a therapist but should be therapeutic.

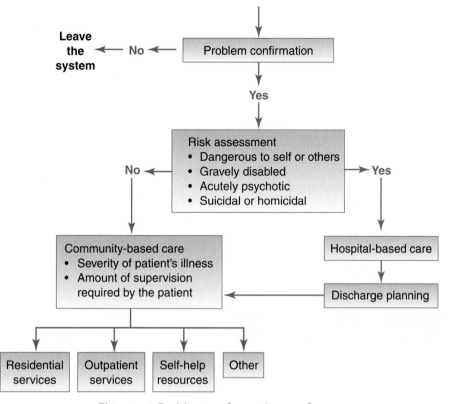

Figure 2-3 Decision tree for continuum of care.

Unit Three is devoted to this first dimension of psychotherapeutic management. The different emphases placed on words and the wide range of styles within the domain of words are discussed, specifically general communication skills (Chapter 9), the nature of the nurse-patient relationship (Chapter 10), nursing process (Chapter 11), anxiety, coping, and anxiety (Chapter 12), working with the aggressive patient (Chapter 13), working with groups of patients (Chapter 14), working with the families of patients (Chapter 15), working with patients from different cultures (Chapter 16), and dealing with the spiritual needs of patients (Chapter 17).

Psychopharmacology

Unit Four is devoted to the contribution of psychotropic drugs to psychiatric nursing, the responsibilities of the nurse, and essential information about these drugs. Psychopharmacology is an important dimension in psychotherapeutic management because psychotropic drugs have enabled millions of

people to live increasingly independent lives. Notably, drug intervention is neither always desirable nor appropriate. However, when drug therapy is indicated, patients typically respond more rapidly than they would without drugs.

The nurse who uses the nursing process model is able to assess patients' responses to medication, plan to respond to side effects should they occur, implement those plans, and evaluate for desired results. The nurse's pivotal role, particularly in an inpatient setting, allows intervention before serious drug-related problems occur. Additionally, the nurse dispenses medications and makes decisions regarding as needed (prn) medications. For these and other reasons, the nurse must have immediate access to information about psychotropic drugs.

Milieu Management

Milieu (or environment) management is a proactive approach to care that forges therapeutic benefits from patients' surroundings, whether in the home, hospital, or outpatient setting. The six environmental elements that nurses must consider in creating a therapeutic milieu include safety, structure, norms, limit setting, balance, and environmental modification. These elements may overlap; for example, safety is a component of all the other dimensions of milieu.

Nurses are the consistent force in the milieu. Kyes and Hofling (1974) state, "The interpersonal environment in which a patient lives may be therapeutic or nontherapeutic depending almost entirely on the interest and ability of the [nursing] staff." To this view, the authors add that the nurse is critical in guiding other staff members toward being therapeutic. Because human beings are incapable of not interacting with their environment, nurses must make these interactions therapeutic. Various aspects of milieu management are discussed in Unit Five.

> ### *Critical* Thinking Question
>
> Using the telephone book for your city, make a list of the mental health services available in your area. Which of these services would you use if your mother or father required psychiatric help?

PSYCHOPATHOLOGY

Unit Six on psychopathology provides the foundation on which the three components of psychotherapeutic management rest; it facilitates therapeutic communication in the nurse-patient relationship and lays the groundwork for an understanding of psychopharmacology and milieu management. Unit Six also includes information on the major mental disorders. Schizophrenia, depressive disorders, bipolar disorders, anxiety-related disorders, cognitive disorders, personality disorders, sexual disorders, substance-related disorders, dual diagnosis, and eating disorders are considered in separate chapters of Unit Six.

SPECIAL THERAPIES

Unit Seven on special therapies includes chapters on behavioral therapy, somatic therapies, and alternative and complementary therapies. Although these therapies are important dimensions of psychiatric care and are effective treatments, they do not have the universal clinical applications of the other categories of psychiatric treatment and are not emphasized in this text.

> ### *Critical* Thinking Question
>
> Based on your clinical setting, what is your evaluation of the components of the psychotherapeutic management model that you have observed?

SPECIAL POPULATIONS

Special populations in psychiatric nursing include victims of violence, child and adolescent psychiatric patients, older mentally ill adults, and patients who have human immunodeficiency viral (HIV) infections. Special populations are discussed in Unit VIII.

▌ Key Concepts

1. Psychotherapeutic management is a model of care that clarifies the nature of psychiatric nursing and differentiates psychiatric nursing practice from the practice of other disciplines.
2. In the continuum of care, the individual is guided to services based on specific needs at a given point in time.
3. The components of psychotherapeutic management include a therapeutic nurse-patient relationship, psychopharmacology, and milieu management, all of which are supported by a basic understanding of psychopathology.
4. The therapeutic nurse-patient relationship emphasizes the importance of the nurse to understand basic principles of therapeutic communication.
5. Being therapeutic is different from providing therapy in that therapeutic interactions should occur during every patient contact, whereas therapy indicates a more formal and structured interaction.
6. Psychopharmacologic understanding is important because nurses administer medication, make decisions about prn medication, and evaluate for therapeutic and adverse responses to medication.
7. Because human beings are incapable of not interacting with their environment, milieu management is an important nursing consideration. Nurses are uniquely responsible for developing patients' environment.
8. An understanding of psychopathology facilitates the nurse-patient relationship, lays the groundwork for understanding psychopharmacology, and provides a theoretical structure for milieu management.

References

Keltner NL: Psychotherapeutic management: a model for nursing practice, *Perspect Psychiatr Care* 23:125, 1985.

Koldjeski D: *Mental health and psychiatric nursing and primary health care: issues and prospects,* proceedings of the Fourth National Conference in graduate education in psychiatric and mental health nursing, Kansas City, MO, 1979, American Nurses' Association.

Kyes J, Hofling C: *Basic psychiatric concepts in nursing,* ed 3, Philadelphia, 1974, JB Lippincott.

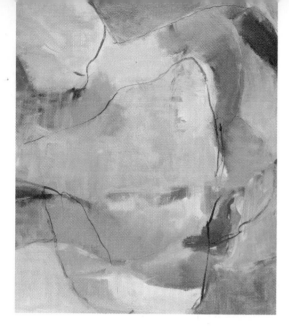

Chapter **3**

Models for Working with Psychiatric Patients

Lee H. Schwecke

Learning Objectives

After reading this chapter, you should be able to:
- Compare and contrast major therapeutic models that contribute to the understanding of psychiatric patients and their behaviors.
- Identify key concepts of the major therapeutic models.
- Describe the relevance of each therapeutic model to psychiatric nursing practice.

The following models of human behavior have been selected for discussion in this chapter because they provide basic concepts for working with psychiatric patients: psychoanalytic, developmental, interpersonal, cognitive-behavioral, reality therapy, and stress models. These models are summarized in Table 3-1 and throughout the chapter.

PSYCHOANALYTIC MODEL

The psychoanalytic model (Freud, 1936; Brill, 1938; Freud, Strachey, 1960) is a theory of the personality that originated with Sigmund Freud and emphasizes unconscious processes or psychodynamic factors as the basis for motivation and behavior. Freud believed that the personality is formed in early childhood and that knowledge of the way in which an individual's drives, instincts, psychic energy or libido, and psychosexual attitude are formed during the first 6 years of life is crucial to an understanding of the personality.

KEY CONCEPTS

Personality Processes

The personality consists of three processes—the id, the ego, and the superego—that function as a whole to bring about behavior. When these processes function in harmony, the individual experiences stability; when disharmony occurs, the individual is in conflict. The individual is all id at birth, wanting to experience only pleasure. This instinctual drive is known as the pleasure principle. Seeking pleasure involves primary process thinking, which enables the individual to strive for pleasure through the use of fantasies and images. The id is compulsive and without morals. The ego controls id impulses and mediates between the id and the reality.

The ego focuses on the reality principle and strives to meet the demands of the id while maintaining the well-being of the individual by distinguishing fantasy from environmental reality. Secondary process thinking comprises rational, logical thinking and intelligence. The ego is the part of the personality that experiences anxiety and uses defense mechanisms for protection. Heredity, environmental factors, and maturation influence the formation of the ego.

The superego is concerned with right and wrong, that is, the conscience; it provides the ego with an inner control to help cope with the id. The superego is formed from the internalization of what

Key Terms

Consciousness State of awareness of surroundings and experiences.

Ego Personality process that focuses on reality while striving to meet the needs of the id. The ego experiences anxiety and uses defense mechanisms for protection.

Euphoria Complete lack of tension, an exaggerated sense of well-being or happiness.

Free association In a therapeutic context, saying anything that comes to mind.

Id Personality process that wants to experience only pleasure, is impulsive, and is without morals.

Interpersonal security Relaxation of the tension of anxiety.

Irrational beliefs Beliefs that are not logical but influence feelings and behaviors.

Preconscious Memories that can be recalled to consciousness with some effort.

Primary appraisal Judgment that an individual makes about an event.

Reappraisal Appraisal judgments that are made after new or additional information has been received.

Satisfaction Relaxation of the tension of physiologic needs.

Secondary appraisal Evaluation that an individual makes about potential actions to be taken.

Superego Personality process that is concerned with right and wrong; the conscience. It provides the ego with an inner control to help cope with the id.

Terror State of extreme tension.

Transference Unconscious emotional reaction to a current situation that is actually based on previous experiences.

Unconscious Memories, conflicts, experiences, and material that cannot be recalled at will and are said to be repressed.

---

parents teach their children about right and wrong through rewards and punishments. Self-esteem is affected by the perception of a person's actions as good or right. Guilt and inferiority are experienced when the individual cannot live up to parental standards. Inner conflict results when the id, the ego, and the superego are striving for different goals.

Consciousness

Freud's concepts of the levels of consciousness are central in understanding problems of the personality and behavior. Consciousness, or material within an individual's awareness, is only one small part of the mind. The unconscious is a larger area and consists of memories, conflicts, experiences, and material that have been repressed and cannot be recalled at will. Preconscious material refers to memories that can be recalled to consciousness with some effort. Freud believed that uncovering unconscious material generates an understanding of behavior that enables individuals to make choices about behavior and thus improve mental health. Insight into the meaning of symptoms and behaviors facilitates change.

Defense Mechanisms

The ego usually copes with anxiety through rational means. When anxiety is too painful, the individual copes by using defense mechanisms to protect the ego and to diminish anxiety. When these mechanisms are used excessively, individuals are unable to face reality and do not solve their problems. Defense mechanisms are primarily unconscious behaviors; however, some are within voluntary control. Some common defense mechanisms are described in Table 3-2.

Painful feelings connected with childhood conflicts are often repressed. Later in life, as similar conflicts are once again experienced, repression fails and these feelings emerge, causing anxiety and discomfort. Freud defined three kinds of anxiety that form the basis of many mental illnesses. Reality anxiety stems from an external real threat. Neurotic anxiety deals with the fear that instincts will cause a person to do something to invite punishment, such as being promiscuous. Moral anxiety deals with guilt that is experienced when the individual acts contrary to the conscience, such as stealing money from a friend.

Goals of Psychoanalysis

The goals of Freudian psychoanalytic therapy are to bring the unconscious into consciousness enabling individuals to work through the past and understand their past and present behaviors. By overcoming repression and resistance to exploring feelings and thoughts, childhood experiences can be analyzed. Uncovering the causes of current behaviors leads to insight. Only then can individuals decrease their self-defeating behaviors and improve their mental health.

|Table 3-1| Therapeutic Models

Model	Assumptions	Goals and Approaches	Dialogue
Psychoanalytic (Freud)	Individuals are motivated by unconscious desires and conflicts. Personality is developed by early childhood. Illness results from childhood conflicts, and ego defenses are inadequate to cope with anxiety.	*Insight* into unconscious conflicts and processes Personality reconstruction	Patient: "All women hate me." Immediate response: "Tell me about one woman with whom you are having trouble."
	Change is a process of *insight*.	Using free association, dream analysis, and analyses of transference and resistance	*Insight*-oriented response: "Tell me about your relationship with your mother."
Developmental (Erikson)	Biologic, psychologic, social, and environmental factors influence personality development throughout the life cycle. *Growth* involves resolution of critical tasks at each of the eight developmental stages. Lack of resolution of tasks causes incomplete development and difficulties in relationships.	Mastering developmental tasks through achievement of insight; continued development through death Analyzing developmental issues, fears, and barriers to *growth* to achieve insight	Patient: "I can't do anything right. Help me." Immediate response: "I hear your doubt in yourself; but I did see you make a positive decision this morning."
	Change involves reexperiencing and resolving developmental crises. Change is a process of *growth*.	Facilitating mastery of developmental tasks with support and problem solving	*Growth*-oriented response: "I can help you look at ways to develop your self-confidence."
Interpersonal (Sullivan, Peplau)	Interpersonal relationships and anxiety facilitate development of the self-system. Development occurs in stages with changing types of relationships. Faulty patterns of relating interfere with security and maturity. Security operations protect against anxiety and interfere with learning.	Developing satisfactory relationships and maturity Relative freedom from the interference of anxiety Learning effective interpersonal skills	Patient: "I can't sit still. I'm too nervous." Immediate response: "Let's take a walk for a few minutes."
	Change is a process of *reeducation*.	Examining current interpersonal difficulties Using therapist-patient relationships as a vehicle for analyzing interpersonal processes and testing new skills Consensual validation, validation, reality testing, and reflecting positive appraisals	*Reeducation* response: "Let's talk about what kind of things make you nervous and what you can do about them."

Therapist's Role

The therapist uses free association (letting the patient say everything that comes to mind) such that repressed material can be identified and interpreted for patients. Dream analysis helps patients uncover the meaning of dreams, which also increases awareness about present behavior. Patients' inconsistencies and resistance to therapy are confronted. Transference (i.e., the unconscious emotional reaction based on previous experiences) that occurs in the current relationship is used to encourage working through feelings that would otherwise remain unconscious.

Relevance to Nursing Practice

In brief therapeutic encounters, the nurse must recognize and understand maladaptive defense mechanisms that patients use. The nurse carefully points

|Table 3-1 | Therapeutic Models—cont'd

Model	Assumptions	Goals and Approaches	Dialogue
Cognitive-behavioral (Beck, Ellis)	An individual has value simply because he or she exists. Individuals have potential for *rational* and irrational thinking.	Substituting *rational* beliefs for irrational ones Eliminating self-defeating behaviors	Patient: "My wife makes me so angry." Immediate response: "What did your wife do to make you angry?"
	Irrational beliefs produce irrational emotions and behaviors. Change involves changing beliefs to change feelings and behaviors.	Increased responsibility for feelings, behaviors, and change Challenging irrational beliefs Cognitive homework	*Cognitive-behavioral* response: "What is self-defeating about the statement you just made?"
	Change is a process of *rational* thinking.	Role playing and testing out new behaviors	
Reality therapy (Glasser)	An individual's most basic psychologic needs are to be loved (to be involved) and to feel worthwhile (to have respect from self and others). Needs must be met responsibly and within the context of reality. Responsibility is fulfilling one's needs without interfering with others who are fulfilling their needs. Illness results from irresponsible behavior.	Facing reality and developing standards for behaving responsibly Greater maturity, conscientiousness, and responsibility Being accountable for one's behaviors	Patient: "The stupid doctor revoked my pass for today." Immediate response: "What did you do that showed that you were not ready for a pass?"
	Change is a process of *relearning*.	Being open, warm, honest, and authentic; accepting of the patient as a person Becoming deeply involved with the patient Focusing on current behaviors and consequences Confronting irresponsible behaviors Assisting with *relearning* of responsible behaviors	*Relearning* response: "What behaviors do you think will be necessary before you will be given a pass?"
Stress (Selye, Lazarus)	Stress is any positive or negative occurrence or emotion requiring a response. Stress produces physiologic and psychologic responses. Inadequate handling of stress can lead to physical or mental illness or both.	Developing effective coping mechanisms	Patient: "I'm so tense, I can't sleep." Immediate response: "I have a relaxation exercise I can show you."
	Change is a process of *problem-solving*.	Reducing bodily tensions Increasing resources and social supports Managing stress Using biofeedback Using relaxation training	*Problem-solving* approach: "You've said you're worried about seeing your family tomorrow. Let's talk about what you might say to them."

out these mechanisms and works with patients to decrease these behaviors and increase adaptive ones. For an example, an individual who denies a problem with alcohol must recognize that an arrest for public intoxication, a pending divorce, and three job losses are, in fact, related to drinking and that abstinence from alcohol is the major adaptive coping mechanism needed. In long-term relationships, patients can be assisted with learning to think, feel, and behave according to their own individual values,

|Table 3–2| Defense Mechanisms

Defense Mechanism	Definition	Common Example	Patient Example
Repression	Unconscious and involuntary forgetting of painful ideas, events, and conflicts	A car accident victim is unable to remember details of the impact but was aware at the time.	Ms. Young, a victim of incest, no longer remembers the reason for which she has always hated the uncle who molested her.
Denial	Unconscious refusal to admit an unacceptable idea or behavior	A student initially refuses to admit that he is flunking a course despite an F on the first test.	Mr. Davis, who is alcohol dependent, believes that he can control his drinking if he so desires.
Suppression	Voluntary exclusion from awareness, anxiety-producing feelings, ideas, and situations	A college student states, "I cannot think about my wedding tonight. I have to study."	Michelle states to the nurse that she is not ready to talk about her recent divorce.
Rationalization	Attempts to make or prove that one's feelings or behaviors are justifiable	A student initially states, "I got a C on the test because the teacher asked stupid questions."	Mr. Jones, diagnosed with paranoid schizophrenia, states that he cannot go to work because his co-workers are mean, instead of admitting that his illness interferes with working.
Intellectualization	Using only logical explanations without feelings or an affective component	A wife explains to her husband about the dented car fender without showing any guilt at first.	Ms. Mann talks about her son's death from cancer as being merciful and shows no signs of her sadness and anger.
Identification	Conscious or unconscious attempt to model oneself after a respected person	When a little girl dresses up as her mother to play house, she tries to talk and act as her mother.	Sheila states to the nurse, "When I get out of the hospital, I want to be a nurse just like you."
Introjection	Unconsciously incorporating wishes, values, and attitudes of others as if they were your own	While her mother is gone, a young girl disciplines her brother exactly as her mother would.	Without realizing it, a patient talks and acts similar to his therapist, analyzing other patients.
Compensation	Covering up for a weakness by overemphasizing or making up a desirable trait	An academically weak high-school student becomes a star in the school play.	A patient with schizophrenia who is unable to talk to other patients becomes known for his expressive poetry.
Reaction formation	A conscious behavior that is the exact opposite of an unconscious feeling	An older brother who dislikes his younger brother still sends him gifts for every holiday.	Miss Marla, who unconsciously wishes her mother were dead, continuously tells staff that her mother is wonderful.

beliefs, and needs, not according to someone else's. As an example, a college student who is pursuing an engineering degree at the insistence of a domineering parent can be assisted in deciding his or her career goals, while developing the ego strength to withstand parental pressures. Patients may also need assistance with accepting their desires and drives as normal human phenomenon for which they need not feel guilt or shame and with choosing acceptable ways of expressing their desires and drives.

CLINICAL EXAMPLE

A middle-aged divorced woman projects blame for the divorce onto her husband. She now desires an intimate relationship but does not accept her sexuality and desires as normal. Nursing interventions focus on examining her role in fostering the divorce and accepting her sexual desires as a normal part of being human. The patient may also need guidance in selecting healthy, acceptable outlets for these desires.

|Table 3-2| Defense Mechanisms—cont'd

Defense Mechanism	Definition	Common Example	Patient Example
Sublimation	Channeling instinctual drives into acceptable activities	An adolescent with developing sexual interests takes a class on sexually transmitted diseases.	A former perpetrator of incest who fears relapse initiates a local chapter of Parents United.
Displacement	Discharging pent-up feelings to a less-threatening object	A husband comes home after a bad day at work and yells at his wife.	Ms. Faust attacks another patient after being told by her psychiatrist that she cannot have an 8-hour pass.
Projection	Blaming someone else for one's difficulties or placing one's unethical desires on someone else	An adolescent comes home late from a dance and states that her date would not bring her home on time.	Katrina states that she used marijuana while on pass because her boyfriend made her smoke it.
Conversion	The unconscious expression of intrapsychic conflict symbolically through physical symptoms	A student awakens with a migraine headache the morning of a final examination and feels too ill to take the test. She does not realize that 2 hours of cramming left her unprepared.	Mr. Jenson suddenly develops impotence after his wife discovers he is having an affair with his secretary.
Undoing	Doing something to counter-act or make up for a trans-gression or wrongdoing	After disciplining her son, a mother bakes his favorite cookies.	After accidentally eating another patient's cookies, Ms. Donnelly apologizes to the patients, cleans the refrigerator, and labels everyone's snack with their names.
Dissociation	The unconscious separation of painful feelings and emotions from an unacceptable idea, situation, or object	During a stressful class about domestic violence, a student finds herself daydreaming about the holidays.	A patient recalls that when she was sexually molested as a child, she felt as if she were outside of her body watching what was happening without feeling anything.
Regression	Return to an earlier and more comfortable developmental level	A 6-year-old child wets the bed at night since the birth of his baby sister.	Mr. Hivey has isolated himself in his room and has lain in a fetal position since his admission.

DEVELOPMENTAL MODEL

Erik Erikson (1963, 1968) built on Freud's psychoanalytic model by including psychosocial and environmental influences along with the Freudian psychosexual concepts. Erikson's developmental model spans the total life cycle from birth to death. He believed that each of his eight stages of development afforded opportunities for growth, even up to the acceptance of the person's own death.

KEY CONCEPTS

Each stage of development is an emotional crisis involving positive and negative experiences. Growth or mastery of critical tasks is the result of having more positive than negative experiences. Nonmastery of tasks inhibits movement to the next stage. Erikson believed that the drive of humans to live and grow is opposed by a drive to return to comfortable earlier states and behaviors; therefore he saw regression as a possibility.

Implied but not clearly described in Erikson's model is the concept of partial mastery of critical tasks in development. The degree of mastery of each stage is related to the degree of maturity that the adult attains. Deficits in development carried from one stage to the next progressively interfere with functioning until the individual is no longer capable of growing without emotionally returning to an earlier stage to resolve the crisis. For example, a person may develop enough trust in others to engage in superficial relationships but may not be able to develop intimacy with a spouse. Another person may have enough initiative to accept a job but lacks the industry to stay with it. An environmental or social tragedy can shake the early foundations of development, such as when divorce from a spouse threatens the individual's sense of trust in others and results in self-doubt.

Mastery of the critical tasks of each stage occurs more easily when it is chronologically appropriate. Overcoming delayed or incomplete development is difficult but possible.

Relevance to Nursing Practice

Most psychiatric patients demonstrate developmental delays or only partial mastery of the developmental stages preceding the stage expected for their chronologic age. The nurse conducts an assessment of the patient's level of functioning through the interpretation of verbal and nonverbal behaviors and identifies the degree of mastery of each stage up to the patient's chronologic age. The behavioral manifestations of problems are clues to issues to be addressed in working with the patient. For example, an adolescent is overwhelmed with shame about being sexually abused as a child. Mature intimate relationships will not be achievable until the shame and doubt are resolved through dealing more effectively with the memories and emotions related to the abuse. Although Erikson focused on the polarity of each developmental stage (e.g., trust-mistrust), as if the "positive" pole were the desirable task to be accomplished, it is now recognized that the extremes of either pole produce problems in functioning. For example, being overly trusting can result in being repeatedly taken advantage of by others. Adult manifestations of Erikson's stages are listed in Table 3-3. Nursing interventions with specific developmental issues are discussed in Chapter 10 on the nurse-patient relationship and in the chapters on specific disorders.

CLINICAL EXAMPLE

A patient is admitted involuntarily because he has stopped getting out of bed, eating, and taking his medicines. He is very suspicious of the nurse and the psychiatrist during the admission interviews. "My parents are just meddling in my business. I'm taking a vacation from work. If I just want to rest and lose weight, I have a right to do so." Initial nursing interventions focus on developing trust with the patient along with restarting his medicines.

INTERPERSONAL MODEL

Harry Stack Sullivan (1953) developed a comprehensive examination of interpersonal relationships called the interpersonal theory of psychiatry. Sullivan considered the healthy person as a social being with the ability to live effectively in relationships with others. Mental illness was viewed as any degree of lack of awareness of the processes in interpersonal relationships. Relationships were viewed as the source of anxiety, maladaptive behaviors, and negative personality formation.

KEY CONCEPTS

Sullivan conceived of the personality as an energy system in which the main goal is to reduce tension. Three types of tension were identified: the tension of needs (stemming from the physiochemical requirements of life), the tension of anxiety (stemming from interpersonal situations), and the tension of need for sleep. Theoretically, a person might vary from a state of complete lack of tension (euphoria) to a state of terror as a result of extreme tension, but Sullivan doubted that the pure extremes existed for very long after birth. The relaxation of the tension of needs is experienced as satisfaction, and the relaxation of the tension of anxiety is experienced as interpersonal security (Sullivan, 1953).

Self-System

Sullivan labeled the personality a "self-system" that develops relatively enduring patterns for avoiding or minimizing anxiety during interpersonal encounters and the meeting of biologic needs. Sullivan also believed that anxiety might be communicated empathically from one person to another. Anxiety activates behaviors that reduce it and help individuals differentiate among experiences (a process of

|Table 3-3 | Adult Manifestations of Erikson's Stages of Development

Life Stage	Adult Behaviors Reflecting Mastery	Adult Behaviors Reflecting Developmental Problems
I. Trust vs. mistrust (0-18 mo)	Realistic trust of self and others Confidence in others Optimism and hope Sharing openly with others Relating to others effectively	Suspiciousness or testing of others Fear of criticism and affection Dissatisfaction and hostility Projection of blame and feelings Withdrawal from others *or* Overly trusting of others Naive and gullible Sharing too quickly and easily
II. Autonomy vs. shame and doubt (18 mo-3 yr)	Self-control and willpower Realistic self-concept and self-esteem Pride and a sense of goodwill Simple cooperativeness Generosity tempered by withholding Delayed gratification when necessary	Self-doubt or self-consciousness Dependence on others for approval Feeling of being exposed or attacked Sense of being out of control of self and one's life Obsessive-compulsive behaviors *or* Excessive independence or defiance, grandiosity Denial of problems Unwillingness to ask for help Impulsiveness or inability to wait Reckless disregard for safety of self and others
III. Initiative vs guilt (3-5 yr)	An adequate conscience Initiative balanced with restraint Appropriate social behaviors Curiosity and exploration Healthy competitiveness Sense of direction Original and purposeful activities	Excessive guilt or embarrassment Passivity and apathy Avoidance of activities or pleasures Rumination and self-pity Assuming a role as victim or self-punishment Reluctance to show emotions Underachievement of potential *or* Lack of follow-through on plans Little sense of guilt for actions Excessive expression of emotion Labile emotions Excessive competitiveness or showing off
IV. Industry vs. inferiority (6-12 yr)	Sense of competence Completion of projects Pleasure in effort and effectiveness Ability to cooperate and compromise Identification with admired others Joy of involvement in the world and with others Balance of work and play	Feeling unworthy and inadequate Poor work history (quitting, being fired, lack of promotions, absenteeism, lack of productivity) Inadequate problem-solving skills Manipulation of others or violation of others' rights Lack of friends of the same sex *or* Overly high achieving or perfectionistic Reluctance to try new things for fear of failing Feeling unable to gain love or affection unless totally successful Being a workaholic
V. Identity vs. role diffusion (12-18 or 20 yr)	Confident sense of self Emotional stability Commitment to career planning and realistic long-term goals Sense of having a place in society Establishing relationship with the opposite sex Fidelity to friends Development of personal values Testing out adult roles	Lack of or giving up of goals, beliefs, values, productive roles Feelings of confusion, indecision, and alienation Vacillation between dependence and independence Superficial short-term relationships with opposite sex *or* Dramatic overconfidence Acting out behaviors (including alcohol and drug use) Flamboyant display of sex-role behaviors

Continued

|Table 3–3| Adult Manifestations of Erikson's Stages of Development—cont'd

Life Stage	Adult Behaviors Reflecting Mastery	Adult Behaviors Reflecting Developmental Problems
VI. Intimacy vs. isolation (18-25 or 30 yr)	Ability to give and receive love Commitments and mutuality with others Collaboration in work and affiliations Sacrificing for others Responsible sexual behaviors	Persistent aloneness or isolation Emotional distance in all relationships Prejudices against others Lack of established vocation; many career changes Seeking of intimacy through casual sexual encounters *or* Possessiveness and jealousy Dependency of parents or partner or both Abusiveness toward loved ones Inability to try new things socially or vocationally (staying in routine, mundane job, and activities)
VII. Generative lifestyle vs. stagnation or self-absorption (30-65 yr)	Productive, constructive, creative activity Personal and professional growth Parental and societal responsibilities	Self-centeredness or self-indulgence Exaggerated concern for appearance and possessions Lack of interest in the welfare of others Lack of civic and professional activities or responsibilities Loss of interest in marriage or extramarital affairs or both *or* Too many professional or community activities to the detriment of the family or self
VIII. Integrity vs. despair (65 yr to death)	Feelings of self-acceptance Sense of dignity, worth, and importance Adaptation to life according to limitations Valuing one's life Sharing of wisdom Exploration of philosophy of life and death	Sense of helplessness, hopelessness, worthlessness, uselessness, meaninglessness, or all Withdrawal and loneliness Regression Focusing on past mistakes, failures, and dissatisfactions Feeling too old to start over Suicidal ideas or apathy Inability to occupy self with satisfying activities (hobbies, volunteer work, social events) *or* Inability to reduce activities Overtaxing strength and abilities Feeling indispensable Denial of death as inevitable

Developed by L. Schwecke and S. Wood, Indiana University. Revised 2001.

learning). Severe anxiety (or panic) fails to convey information and produces confusion, even to the point of amnesia (Sullivan, 1953). Less severe anxiety informs the individual of the different situations and behaviors that cause and relieve tension. As the self-system is developing in infancy, it is initially organized into the "good me" when needs are satisfied, the "bad me" when needs are unmet and anxiety persists, and "not me" when anxiety is severe and information is not completely integrated into the personality on a conscious level.

As the infant moves to early childhood and develops language, the separate personifications of the self as good and bad begin to fuse into a sense of a whole individual with different behaviors in different situations. However, feedback from others (reflected appraisals) continues to shape the child's self-concept in positive and negative ways.

Because infants are unable to avoid "bad" caregivers or anxiety-producing situations, mechanisms called security operations develop to protect young children from anxiety. In somnolent detachment, sleep is used to avoid the anxiety. Apathy is an emotional detachment or numbing, even though the experiences are remembered. Selective inattention is a process of tuning out details associated with anxiety-producing situations. Dissociation prevents situations from integrating into conscious awareness. Converting anxiety to anger is another operation to reduce anxiety. The powerlessness experienced with anxiety is exchanged for a temporary feeling of power associated with anger directed outwardly.

Although these security operations protect against anxiety, they also interfere with the learning that normally occurs in interpersonal interactions (the socialization processes). For example, a child may use selective inattention to "tune out" a mother's suggestion about a more effective way to express anger. Focal awareness—the ability to grasp the details and meanings of situations and the behaviors of others—is necessary for adequate learning. Consensual validation is a process of verifying the accuracy of perceptions and meanings of events with others who are involved in those situations.

Personality Development

Sullivan's model includes a sequence of personality development focusing on tools or behaviors needed to accomplish developmental tasks. In infancy (birth to $1\frac{1}{2}$ years), for example, crying is a tool used to establish contact with others thus children can learn to count on others. In childhood ($1\frac{1}{2}$ to 6 years), language assists with learning to delay the gratification of needs. In the juvenile period (6 to 9 years), competition, compromise, and cooperation are tools for developing relationships with peers. In preadolescence (9 to 12 years), collaboration and the capacity for love assist in the development of a "chum" relationship with a person of the same sex. These same tools, along with sexual desire, facilitate learning to establish relationships with members of the opposite sex in early adolescence (12 to 14 years). The independence developed in early adolescence moves toward interdependence in later adolescence (14 to 21 years), and individuals learn to form lasting sexual relationships (Sullivan, 1953). Sullivan's development model did not describe changes beyond late adolescence.

Therapist's Role

For Sullivan, the focus of therapy is on patients' current interpersonal relationships and experiences. The goal of the therapy is to develop mature and satisfactory relationships that are relatively free from anxiety. The therapist-patient relationship is a vehicle for analyzing the patient's interpersonal processes and testing new skills in relating. The therapist takes an active role as a "participant observer" in experiencing patients' interpersonal problems. Although the focus of therapy is on patients' here-and-now problems, distortions that past experiences create, particularly "not me" experiences, are often revealed. The therapist helps correct these distortions with clear communications, consensual validation, and presentation of reality. In challenging a negative self-image, the therapist presents appraisals of patients as worthwhile, respectable individuals with rights, dignity, and valuable abilities. The focus of sessions is often on loneliness, fear of rejection, clarifying emotions and their causes, using anxiety for learning about the self and others, managing interpersonal frustrations, and developing self-respect.

Relevance to Nursing Practice

Hildegard Peplau (1952, 1963) played a significant role in applying Sullivan's concepts to nursing practice. Peplau saw a major goal of nursing as helping patients reduce their anxiety and convert it to constructive action. She elaborated on and applied to nursing Sullivan's concept of degrees of anxiety ("pure" euphoria, mild anxiety, moderate anxiety, severe anxiety, panic, terror states, and "pure" anxiety [Peplau, 1963]). Peplau described the effects of mild anxiety through panic levels on perception and learning (Chapter 12). She saw the nurse's role as helping patients decrease insecurity and improve functioning through interpersonal relationships that can be seen as microcosms of the way in which patients function in other relationships. For example, a patient says, "My wife always knows when I'm upset and wants to help me, but I just say nothing." The nurse might say, "What makes you anxious when you think about telling her the truth?" Specific applications of Sullivan's work as proposed by Peplau are presented in Chapter 10.

CLINICAL EXAMPLE

The nurse recognizes that a patient experiences increased anxiety whenever he is beginning a relationship with a woman. The patient complains about not knowing what to say or do when he is alone with her. "I'm so afraid of acting like an idiot that I get tongue-tied and sweaty. It's no wonder that I never see her again." Nursing interventions focus on specific sources of anxiety, overcoming insecurities, rehearsing social conversations with the nurse, and practicing social skills in a small group of patients.

COGNITIVE-BEHAVIORAL MODELS

Aaron Beck's cognitive therapy (1967) and Albert Ellis's rational-emotive therapy (RET) (1973) models focus on thinking and behaving rather than on expressing feelings. These models use a cognitive approach based on individual abilities to think, analyze, judge, decide, and do. Unlike Freud, who saw symptoms of disturbance as having been produced by childhood experiences, Ellis and Beck view individuals' present perceptions, thoughts, assumptions, beliefs, values, attitudes, and philosophies as needing modification or change (Beck, 1976; Ellis, 1973). Even distorted thinking learned from others in childhood can be unlearned. Individuals should value themselves simply because they exist and should not judge themselves by the way in which they perform or by the way in which they are rated by themselves and others.

KEY CONCEPTS

Beck and Ellis believe that individuals think both rationally and irrationally and that irrational beliefs or automatic thoughts are responsible for causing problems because self-defeating behaviors are maintained. Beck and Ellis also assert that individuals are capable of understanding their limitations and can change their values and beliefs while challenging their self-defeating behaviors. The repetition of irrational thoughts produces emotional disturbances that keep dysfunctional behaviors operant. Individuals who blame themselves and others and think and feel that something is "bad" maintain emotional disturbances. RET teaches individuals to stop blaming themselves and to accept themselves as they are with flaws and imperfections. Learning to change inappropriate emotions and self-defeating behaviors can be used to avoid anxiety. RET attacks problems from a cognitive, emotive, and behavioral standpoint by using the A-B-C theory of personality. A is the activating event, B is the belief about A, and C is the emotional reaction. A (event) does not cause C (emotions); rather, B (irrational beliefs about A) causes C. Intervention, then, is aimed at B (irrational beliefs) and is called D or disputing and changing irrational beliefs (Ellis, 1973). Similarly, Beck (1976) proposed examining the distorted perceptions, erroneous beliefs, self-deceptions, and blind spots that lead to "excessive, inappropriate emotional reactions" to events or stimuli. Reality testing and problem solving are aimed at correcting faulty cognitions and processes thus the individual develops "more realistic appraisals of himself and his world" (Beck, 1976).

According to Ellis (1973) and Beck (1976), most individuals subscribe to the following irrational beliefs and inappropriate rules for living:

- One should feel loved and approved by everyone.
- One must be totally competent to be considered worthwhile.
- Individuals have little ability to change or to control their feelings.
- Influences of the past should determine feelings in the present.
- Rejection or unfair treatment has catastrophic consequences.
- One is disliked when a disagreement exists with another.
- One should never make mistakes.
- Individuals who are obnoxious should be judged as rotten or bad.
- Being passive in life is easier than confronting difficulties and responsibilities.

Therapist's Role

The patient-therapist relationship is viewed as a collaborative effort to achieve goals for improved self-esteem, coping, relationships, and lifestyles (Beck, 1976). Because patients have many irrational "shoulds," "oughts," and "musts," the therapist actively and directly challenges these beliefs. The therapist demonstrates the degree to which their thinking is illogical. Humor is often used to confront the patient's irrational thinking. The therapist explains ways to replace irrational thinking with rational thinking to reduce dysfunctional feelings and behaviors. The process of therapy focuses on the present. Patients learn to take responsibility for their ideas and behaviors and eliminate disturbing behaviors. The therapist accepts patients as they are and does not allow patients to rate or condemn themselves. Homework assignments are given to focus on positive statements and behaviors and skill development. New, positive self-statements are encouraged to enable patients to begin to think, feel, and behave differently. Role-playing and modeling are also employed.

Relevance to Nursing Practice

Nurses help patients change irrational beliefs and reduce stress and anxiety through effective problem solving. Patients have many self-deprecating or negative feelings about themselves that the nurse can dispute by pointing out specific positive behaviors. As an example, a nurse, after listening to a patient discuss all his weaknesses, might say, "Let's work on a list of your positive qualities and strengths." Awareness of these qualities or aspects can facilitate patients' beliefs that they are worthwhile and have valuable characteristics. Self-blame and guilt can be reduced, and patients can feel better about themselves. One message is, "All of us make mistakes at times. Learning from these mistakes helps us grow and become more effective in relating to others." Patients who project blame can be shown that they alone are responsible for their behaviors. For example, alcoholics are skillful at blaming others for their problems when, in fact, they alone are responsible for continuing to drink and for the problems that result from drinking.

Other patients who continually function according to "shoulds," "musts," and "oughts" can be taught to act according to their personal wants and beliefs; they need not condemn themselves for being their own persons, and their anxiety and hostile feelings toward themselves and others can be eliminated when they can achieve feelings of comfort about themselves.

CLINICAL EXAMPLE

A depressed young man says to the nurse, "My friends have stopped coming around to see me. They say I'm always bragging about myself, but I feel like I have to prove myself to them and myself." Nursing interventions focus on the acceptance of himself as a worthwhile person with a few weaknesses but many positive qualities. Interventions also challenge his beliefs that he "must" be totally competent in front of others and never make mistakes.

REALITY THERAPY MODEL

William Glasser (1965) developed reality therapy because he believed patients and delinquents share the common characteristic of denying "the reality of the world around them" instead of fulfilling their needs responsibly within the context of reality and society. Glasser (1965) defined responsibility as "the ability to fulfill one's needs, and to do so in a way that does not deprive others of the ability to fulfill their needs." Glasser recognized that he could not change patients' histories or past relationship problems but that he could help them change current behaviors thus their futures could improve. He found that an improved sense of responsibility leads to improved mental health.

KEY CONCEPTS

According to Glasser (1965), all individuals continually strive to meet their needs. The two major psychologic needs are (1) to love and be loved (to have relatedness) and (2) to feel worthwhile (to have respect from the self and others). Implied in these needs are the needs for involvement and identity. Children develop a positive identity by being involved with others who teach right, wrong, and a sense of responsibility, while conveying that the children are worthwhile. Children then learn to be comfortable with and enjoy being around others.

Unfortunately, individuals do not always strive to meet their needs responsibly. An "incapacity or failure at the interpersonal level of functioning" may exist (Glasser, 1965). Glasser believed that illness results from behaving irresponsibly rather than the reverse and that anger, fear, depression, and anxiety are also the result of irresponsible behavior in relationships. Common forms of irresponsible behavior are violating one's morals, values, or standards; misinforming others about oneself or one's needs (being dishonest); shunning others because of fear of rejection; lying to oneself by rationalizing and excusing one's own behavior; not accepting the consequences of one's behavior; blaming others for problems; and, eventually, losing contact with reality (by denying it). Suicide and denial are major ways of avoiding reality and responsibility. Short-term pleasures such as those derived from alcohol and drugs also interfere with long-term satisfaction and happiness.

Therapist's Role

The goal of reality therapy is to help patients face reality and then to develop responsible behavior patterns, thus the patient's needs for love and worth can be met more effectively. Directing patients "toward greater maturity, conscientiousness, and responsibility" improves their potential for long-term happiness and pleasure (Glasser, 1965). Glasser emphasized the need for the therapist's authenticity, openness, honesty, responsibility, and deep involvement with patients. Initially, patients need warmth and uncritical acceptance as worthwhile persons who are cared about, even though their irresponsible behaviors, and the excuses for those behaviors, are not accepted. The unrealistic and irresponsible behaviors are actively confronted, even disciplined, while the patients as human beings and their positive behaviors are supported. Patients repeatedly evaluate whether their actions are getting the desired results and whether others are hurt in the process. Patients are asked to choose more effective behaviors and to design specific, realistic plans to try those behaviors. Plans that are unsuccessful are revised until accountability and responsibility are achieved.

Relevance to Nursing Practice

Psychiatric nurses are regularly involved in helping patients identify reality and factors that interfere with effectively meeting their needs. Reality testing is a common nursing intervention. An example is helping a patient understand that if he would like his wife to do something, he must be direct in saying it, instead of "hinting" about it as he has been doing. Nurses are routinely responsible for explaining the rules of a program or unit and for outlining expected and appropriate, as well as inappropriate, behaviors. The milieu of a program or unit is normally designed to foster improvements in independence and responsibility, which are rewarded with increases in privileges and freedom. Setting limits on unacceptable (irresponsible) behaviors benefits patients in the long term.

Even without labeling behaviors as irresponsible, nurses are accustomed to helping patients examine the consequences of specific behaviors, particularly in current relationships. For example, with a patient who typically cries instead of getting angry with her husband, the nurse might ask, "How does that solve your anger and your dislike of your husband's behavior?" Supportive confrontation encourages patients to make their own decisions about changes, choose their own solutions, and test new behaviors. This type of relearning process is described in Chapter 10 on the nurse-patient relationship.

CLINICAL EXAMPLE
During a group session with adolescents, they begin complaining about all types of parental and societal rules they dislike. A common theme among them is the (unrealistic) desire to be totally independent and free from all restrictions. The nurse asks them to point out the consequences of their recent rebellious behaviors. Begrudgingly, the teens identify continual arguments with parents, loss of friendships, disciplinary actions at school, arrests for alcohol or drug use, sexually transmitted diseases, suicide attempts, and psychiatric hospitalizations. The teens are then asked to identify specific and healthy future goals and the positive and responsible behaviors needed to achieve these goals.

STRESS MODELS

Stress models provide nurses with a framework for understanding the way in which stress affects individuals and their responses. The ability to adapt to stress leads to conflict resolution, whereas the inability to adapt effectively may result in physical or mental disorders or even death.

KEY CONCEPTS

Selye's Stress-Adaptation Model

Selye (1956) defined stress as wear and tear on the body. He developed a framework, the stress-adaptation theory, to explain the physiologic response to stress. Selye viewed stressors as any positive or negative occurrence, or any emotion requiring a response. Interaction with the environment and others inevitably produces stress. The type of response elicited depends on individual perception and definition of the stressor. However, Selye discovered, through objectively measuring structural and chemical changes in the body, that many individuals demonstrate the same symptoms regardless of the stressor. These changes became known as the general adaptation syndrome (GAS) and occur in three stages: alarm, resistance, and exhaustion. Selye did not elaborate on psychosocial changes, but his three stages can be correlated with the levels of anxiety (Chapter 12). The three stages of GAS are summarized in Table 3-4.

Alarm Reaction

Impinging any kind of stressor on individuals activates the preparation for "fight or flight." Individuals experience an increase in alertness so as to focus on the immediate task or threat and to mobilize resources and defenses to concentrate on the particular stressor. The levels of anxiety experienced are mild (+1) to moderate (+2). Learning and problem solving can occur. When the stressor continues and is not adaptively or effectively resolved, individuals experience the next stage.

Stage of Resistance

In this stage, individuals strive to adapt to stress. For adaptation to occur, the use of coping and defense mechanisms is increased. Problem solving and learning are difficult but can be accomplished with assistance. Psychosomatic symptoms such as headaches, ulcers, and colitis begin to develop. The levels of anxiety experienced are moderate (+2) to severe

|Table 3-4| Stress Adaptation Syndrome

Stage	Physical Changes	Psychosocial Changes
Stage I: Alarm reaction Mobilization of the body's defensive forces and activation of the potential for "fight-or-flight"	Release of norepinephrine and epinephrine causing vasoconstriction, increased blood pressure, and increased rate and force of cardiac contraction Increased hormone levels Enlargement of adrenal cortex Marked loss of body weight Shrinkage of the thymus, spleen, and lymph nodes Irritation of the gastric mucosa	Increased level of alertness Increased level of anxiety Task-oriented, defense-oriented, inefficient, or maladaptive behavior may occur
Stage II: Stage of resistance Optimal adaptation to stress within the person's capabilities	Hormone levels readjust Reduction in activity and size of adrenal cortex Lymph nodes return to normal size Weight returns to normal	Increased and intensified use of coping mechanisms Tendency to rely on defense-oriented behavior Psychosomatic symptoms develop
Stage III: Stage of exhaustion Loss of ability to resist stress because of depletion of body resources; fight, flight or immobilization occurs	Decreased immune response with suppression of T cells and atrophy of thymus Depletion of adrenal glands and hormone production Weight loss Enlargement of lymph nodes and dysfunction of lymphatic system If exposure to the stressor continues, cardiac failure, renal failure, or death may occur	Defense-oriented behaviors become exaggerated Disorganization of thinking Disorganization of personality Sensory stimuli may be misperceived with appearance of illusion Reality contact may be reduced with appearance of delusions or hallucinations If exposure to the stressor continues, stupor or violence may occur

From *Adult Health Nursing* by Kneisl/Ames, ©1986. Reprinted by permission of Pearson Education, Inc., Upper Saddle River, NJ.

(+3). When stressors become overwhelming, individuals experience the next stage.

Stage of Exhaustion

Exhaustion results from stress that lasts too long, is overwhelming, or may result from the individual's total inability to cope. Anxiety is experienced at the severe (+3) to panic (+4) levels. Defenses are exaggerated and dysfunctional, and the personality becomes disorganized, thinking becomes illogical, and decision making becomes ineffective. Delusions and hallucinations can occur with sensory misperception and a greatly reduced orientation to reality. Individuals may become violent, suicidal, or may be completely immobilized. In the case of immobilization, a severe level of anxiety may be present, but the individuals may not appear visibly anxious. Death may occur when exhaustion continues without intervention.

Lazarus's Interactional Theory

In contrast to Selye's emphasis on the physiologic effects of stress, Lazarus (1966) focuses on the psychologic aspects. According to Lazarus, psychologic

stress is "a relationship between the person and the environment that is appraised by the person as taxing or exceeding his or her resources and endangering his or her well-being" (Lazarus, Folkman, 1984). Lazarus believes that the basis of coping is not a result of anxiety, per se, but to the appraisal of threat. "Anxiety is the response to threat" (Lazarus, 1966). The significance of the threat or what it means to the individual is of primary importance. Different individuals perceive stressors differently. For one person, a particular event may be viewed as a challenge; for another, the same event may be viewed as a severe threat or problem. This personal evaluation of a stressor or event is based on cognitive appraisal.

Three types of cognitive appraisal have been identified. Primary appraisal refers to the judgment that individuals make about a particular event: What does it mean personally? What are its effects? Secondary appraisal is the individual's evaluation of the way to respond to an event. Possible strategies or solutions, as well as resources and supports, are examined. Reappraisal is further appraisal that is made after new or additional information has been received.

Numerous personal and environmental factors influence appraisal: commitments, beliefs, values, feelings, emotions, and views of what is important. A seemingly appropriate solution may not be useful because it conflicts with individual values and beliefs. For example, a passive wife may be unable to be assertive and confrontational with her husband because she was taught and believes that women should be quiet and submissive.

Stressful events often create demands with which individuals cannot effectively cope. Occasionally, personal resources or social supports are inadequate. Preferred methods of coping may be ineffective in resolving the problem and may actually result in more problems. Ineffective coping and the creation of additional problems result in additional stress and can lead to physical illness or mental illness or both.

Relevance to Nursing Practice

Stress theories provide a framework for the nurse to assess the effects of stress on patients and their coping processes. To assist patients with developing adaptive or effective coping methods, nurses must help patients identify and evaluate palliative, maladaptive, and dysfunctional behaviors that will enable the patients to become aware of the consequences of their behavior. Palliative mechanisms decrease the emotions without solving the problems. Maladaptive mechanisms do not manage the emotions sufficiently and do not solve the problems. Dysfunctional mechanisms create new or additional problems. (For additional explanation, see Chapter 12.)

Patients' appraisal of stressors or problems includes their perception of the stressors, the resources or supports they have to help them cope, and the way in which their beliefs and values influence that coping. For example, an individual who is independent, who has sufficient income and savings, a supportive family, and a belief that divorce is acceptable is likely to cope differently with a partner's affair than will an individual who is dependent, unemployed, without close family, and has a belief that divorce is not an option. In considering patients' perception of stressors, the nurse can facilitate cognitive restructuring or problem solving by helping patients choose adaptive and appropriate coping behaviors. Occasionally, the nurse will need to help initiate, encourage, and motivate patients to use adaptive behaviors. As an example, the nurse helps a patient who feels helpless and lonely share these feelings with a group of patients and ask for suggestions for fun (but less-threatening) activities with others. Together, the patient and the nurse can then evaluate the effectiveness of strategies used. When patients exhibit behaviors found in Selye's stage of exhaustion or are using primarily dysfunctional coping, the nurse is able to assess patients' inability to take constructive action; the nurse may be required to make decisions on behalf of patients. After patients gain some control over their situation, they can benefit from classes on stress management, problem solving, relaxation training, and biofeedback.

CLINICAL EXAMPLE
A male patient is admitted several weeks after his mother was diagnosed with terminal cancer. He is showing symptoms of misperceptions of reality, delusions, and hallucinations. The patient says, "I can't live without her. I'll lose the house. I can't work if she isn't there to get me up and going in the morning. No one else will help me." The nurse develops a care plan that focuses on (1) protecting the patient from harm and reducing the anxiety level, (2) offering emotion and stress management strategies, (3) engaging the patient in anticipatory grief work, (4) developing a new support system, and (5) designing specific plans for arising and getting ready each morning to be on time for work.

Critical Thinking Questions

1. How can an understanding of the therapeutic models assist you in working with psychiatric patients?
2. Which concepts and strategies derived from each of the therapeutic models have you observed being used with patients?

ECLECTIC APPROACH

Most psychiatric nurses adopt an eclectic approach with the therapeutic models presented in this chapter. Concepts from various models that best explain a patient's behaviors, problems, and needs are selected. For example, a recently divorced patient states, "I've screwed up my life. All I do is sit at home, cry, and sleep." The nurse might use the psychoanalytic model to identify that the patient is experiencing superego guilt and regression, the developmental model to understand the patient's dissatisfaction with self and withdrawal from others, or the cognitive-behavioral model to identify the "irrational belief" that one should never make mistakes. In the interpersonal model, the behavior of crying would be seen as a wish for contact with others and sleep as somnolent detachment. In the reality therapy model, the patient would be viewed as feeling unloved, having a loss of self-respect, and being depressed. Using the stress models, the focus is on redefining the meaning of the divorce and using adaptive coping strategies.

Critical Thinking Question

You are working with a patient who is recently divorced, afraid of making decisions, and suicidal. Which combination of concepts from the various theorists would you use in planning your nursing interventions?

Key Concepts

1. Concepts from various models provide frameworks for understanding patients' behaviors and problems.
2. Extensive use of defense mechanisms and maladaptive coping behaviors are assessed and understood by the nurse as inhibitors of healthy or adaptive responses. The nurse helps patients develop adaptive coping responses or behaviors.
3. Unresolved developmental issues interfere with patients' ability to solve problems and meet their own needs. Therefore these issues must be addressed in the nurse-patient relationship.
4. Peplau used Sullivan's concepts of anxiety as a critical part of her framework in the nurse-patient relationship.
5. According to the cognitive-behavioral model, replacing irrational beliefs with rational ones can reduce stress and anxiety.
6. Facing reality and self-responsibility are major goals of reality therapy.
7. Stress models explain many of the physiologic and psychologic responses to stress and are a basis for stress-reduction strategies.

References

Beck AT: *Depression: Chemical, experimental and theoretical aspects,* New York, 1967, Noeber Medical Division, Harper & Row.

Beck AT: *Cognitive therapies and the emotional disorders,* New York, 1976, International Universities Press.

Brill AA, editor: *The basic writings of Sigmund Freud,* New York, 1938, Random House.

Ellis A: *Humanistic psychotherapy: the rational-emotive approach,* New York, 1973, The Julian Press.

Erikson EH: *Childhood and society,* New York, 1963, WW Norton.

Erikson EH: *Identity: youth and crisis,* New York, 1968, WW Norton.

Freud S: *The problem of anxiety,* New York, 1936, WW Norton.

Freud S, Strachey J, editors: *The ego and the id,* New York, 1960, WW Norton.

Glasser W: *Reality therapy: a new approach to psychiatry,* New York, 1965, Harper & Row.

Kneisl CR, Ames SW: *Adult health nursing: a biopsychosocial approach,* Menlo Park, Calif, 1986, Addison-Wesley.

Lazarus RS: *Psychological stress and the coping process,* St Louis, 1966, McGraw-Hill.

Lazarus RS, Folkman S: *Stress, appraisal, and coping,* New York, 1984, Springer.

Peplau HE: A working definition of anxiety. In Burd SF, Marshall MA, editors: *Some clinical approaches to psychiatric nursing,* Toronto, 1963, Macmillan.

Peplau HE: *Interpersonal relations in nursing,* New York, 1952, GP Putnam.

Selye H: *The stress life,* St Louis, 1956, McGraw-Hill.

Sullivan HS: *Interpersonal theory of psychiatry,* New York, 1953, WW Norton

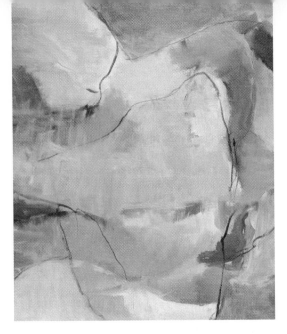

Chapter 4

Legal Issues

David B. Allen, Norman L. Keltner

Learning Objectives

After reading this chapter, you should be able to:

- Define the terms that apply to legal issues in psychiatric care.
- Define and discuss general legal principals and concepts.
- Describe the liability of the nurse in issues such as wrongful commitment, duty to warn, and master-servant rule.
- Identify landmark court rulings and their impact on psychiatric care.
- Define and discuss involuntary commitment issues and procedures.
- Define guardianship and conservatorship.
- Define and apply the concept of least restrictive alternative.
- Define and apply the concept of freedom from restraint and seclusion.
- Define and apply the concept of confidentiality.
- Define and apply the concept of the right to treatment and the right to refuse treatment.
- Articulate the competing interests of individual rights and the state's interest in maintaining the health and safety of its citizens.
- Identify and discuss corporate compliance issues in the health care setting.

The evolution of humane treatment of mentally ill persons roughly parallels that of advances made in the jurisprudence system. Historically, movement has been a slow, cautious process from viewing the mentally ill as demonic or weak-willed to viewing them as individuals with legitimate health care problems. Governmental systems and regulatory bodies thoughtfully attempt to achieve balance between the rights of the individuals against the rights of society at large. Although most people are aware of the difficulty in reaching this goal in criminal cases, they are less aware of the struggle for such a balance in psychiatric care.

This chapter focuses on the laws and regulations that affect psychiatric nursing practice and on the corresponding legal and public policy issues. Sources of these laws and regulations include the following:

1. The Constitution of the United States
2. Individual state and federal statutes
3. Precedent-setting legal cases
4. The Joint Commission on Accreditation of Health Care Organizations (JCAHO)
5. Centers for Medicare and Medicaid Services (CMS), formerly The Health Care Financing Administration (HCFA)

This chapter begins with a brief review of basic legal principals and sources of law that have influenced mental health delivery and serve as the basis for legally sound psychiatric nursing practice. The following topics will be reviewed:

1. Key legal terms
2. Common law, precedent-setting cases, statutory law, and administrative law
3. Tort law: negligence, assault and battery, and false imprisonment and related nursing liability
4. Contracts

Key Terms

Assault An act intended by the defendant to create a reasonable apprehension of harmful or offensive contact to another without consent.

Battery The harmful or offensive touching of another, the clothes of another, or anything else attached to another without consent.

Civil law The part of the legal system that is concerned with the legal rights and duties of private persons. Civil lawsuits can recapture monetary loss from professionals who have been guilty of false imprisonment, defamation of character, assault and battery, or negligence.

Common law—case law The term *common law* is applied to the body of principles that has evolved and continues to evolve and expand from judicial decisions that arise during the trial of actual court cases; law based on the outcome of cases.

Conservator One appointed by a court to manage the affairs of a person found to be incompetent and unable to manage his or her own affairs appropriately.

Corporate compliance A health care provider's responsibility to comply with governmental laws and regulations.

Criminal law The part of the legal system concerned with crime that is defined in state and federal statutes.

Gravely disabled Individuals who are unable to provide food, clothing, or shelter for themselves because of mental illness.

Informed consent Providing patients with information about specific treatments (including benefits, side effects, and possible risks) to enable them to make competent and voluntary decisions.

Involuntary commitment A commitment status in which a person who has the legal capacity to consent to mental health treatment refuses to do so and is involuntarily detained for treatment by the state. Three categories of involuntary commitment include evaluation and emergency care, certification for observation and treatment, and extended or indeterminate care.

Least restrictive alternative or least restrictive environment An environment that provides the necessary treatment requirements in the least restrictive setting possible. For example, a hospital setting is more restrictive than is a board-and-care setting. If the board-and-care setting provides the necessary treatment requirements for a person, then that environment would represent the least restrictive alternative.

Liable Found responsible and answerable by law and compelled to make restitution or satisfaction.

Malpractice Negligence by a professional. Malpractice is a civil action that can be brought against a nurse who has breached a standard of care that a reasonably prudent nurse would meet.

Master–servant rule As applied to the employer-employee relationship, this rule holds that the employer is responsible for the acts of employees as long as they are acting within the scope of their employment or authority.

Negligence The failure to do that which a reasonably prudent and careful person would do under the circumstances, or the doing of that which is reasonable and a prudent person would not do.

Power of attorney—limited or special A power of attorney is a written document in which one person—the principal—authorizes another person—the attorney in fact—to act on the principal's behalf. In a limited power of attorney, the attorney in fact is granted only those powers specifically defined in the document.

Probable cause Sufficient, credible facts that would induce a reasonably intelligent and prudent person to believe that a cause of action exists.

Restraint Any method of physically restricting a person's freedom of movement, physical activity, or normal access to his or her body.

Seclusion The involuntary confinement of a person alone in a room in which the person is physically prevented from leaving.

Standard of care The degree of skill, care, and diligence by members of the nursing professions, practicing in the same or a similar locality (Eskreis, 1998).

Statutory law Statutory law is written law emanating from a legislative body; the laws written by state authorities and federal legislative authorities that are passed in accordance with state and federal law.

Voluntary patients A status in which patients or a conservator or guardian requests treatment and signs an application for that treatment. These persons are also free to sign themselves out of the hospital.

Additionally, nursing's role in these and other legal issues will be presented throughout the chapter to help the student understand the applicable legal, regulatory, and compliance issues.

SOURCES OF LAW

The basic sources of law are common law, which is derived from judicial decisions; statutory law, which is created by the federal and state legislatures; and administrative law, developed by administrative agencies. When written laws are not completely clear or are contradictory to other laws, the judicial system is responsible for resolving these disputes. The resulting judicial decisions often influence legislative action to create an appropriate statute.

Common Law

The term common law is applied to the body of legal principles that has evolved and continues to evolve and expand from actual court cases. Many of these legal principles and rules have their origins in English common law.

The judicial system is necessary because having a law that covers every potential event that might occur is impossible. Moreover, the judicial system serves as a mechanism for reviewing legal disputes that arise in the written law and is an effective review mechanism for those issues in which the written law is silent or confusing and for situations in which issues involving both written law and common-law decisions occur.

Many of these rulings have influenced the current legal view of mental illness. Rules presented here, although they in no way form an exhaustive list of major court decisions, reflect decisions that have shaped the mental health treatment system and have served to improve patient care and protect the public.

1. The M'Naghten rule (1843) states that individuals who do not understand the nature and implications of murderous actions because of insanity cannot be held legally accountable for murder. This ruling was based on the case of Daniel M'Naghten, a Scotsman who felt persecuted by the ruling political party and attempted to kill the prime minister. Although he failed to kill the prime minister, he did shoot the Prime Minister's secretary. He was ruled not guilty by reason of insanity and was committed to an asylum. This case has provid-

Critical Thinking Questions

"Not guilty by reason of insanity" is a phrase that evokes passion in many people. Jeffrey Dahmer, the cannabilist murderer, did not say that he didn't do it. He said he was not guilty because he did not know what he was doing. His lawyers said he was not guilty by reason of insanity. What do you think about this concept? Do you believe this legal defense is often used? Is it reasonable to have such protection under the law?

ed a basis for legal decisions in American courts since 1851.

   Comment: When applied today, the M'Naghten criteria state generally that a person is not criminally responsible at the time of an act if, because of mental "disease or defect," the person did not know the nature and quality of the act, or if the person did know it, he or she did not know that the act was wrong. Because this standard focuses on the knowledge of "right or wrong," it is occasionally referred to as the "cognitive standard."

2. Rouse v. Cameron 373 F2d 451 (DC Cir 1966) was a case in which a man who pleaded not guilty by reason of insanity to the charge of illegally carrying a dangerous weapon was committed to a mental institution. After 4 years in the institution, the man argued that he was not receiving treatment (and therefore could not improve enough to be discharged). The court ruled that he had the right to treatment.

3. Whitree v. State of New York (1968) 290 NYS 2nd 486 was a case in which the plaintiff, Whitree, successfully sued the state of New York. Whitree was awarded $300,000 for damages incurred in his 14 years of hospitalization. The court ruled that he did not receive treatment and that, had he received adequate treatment, he could have been discharged 12 years earlier.

4. Wyatt v. Stickney 344 F Supp 373 (MD Ala 1972) was another case involving right to treatment. In this case, the entire mental health system of Alabama was sued for providing an inadequate treatment program. The court ruled that the Alabama mental health system must do the following at each institution:

- Stop using patients for hospital labor needs.
- Ensure a humane environment.
- Develop and maintain minimal staffing standards.
- Establish institutional human rights committees.
- Provide the least restrictive environment for each patient.

Comment: After nearly 30 years, this case was settled in 2000 under a consent decree that forces the state of Alabama to implement a wide range of mental health services at the local level.

5. Rogers v. Okin 478 F Supp (D Mass 1979) was a case in which patients at Boston State Hospital sought the right to refuse treatment. The ruling prohibited the hospital from forcing nonviolent patients to take medications against their will. The court based its decision on the constitutional right to privacy. Furthermore, this decision required patients or their guardians to give informed consent before drug treatment could begin. This case has significant implications for nurses who are tempted to "force" patients to take medications for "their own good."

6. Tarasoff v. The Regents of the University of California (1976) 17 Cal 3rd 425 further expanded the liability of mental health professionals. The court established a duty to warn of threats of harm to others. In this case, a patient confided to the therapist that he intended to kill an unnamed but readily identifiable girl when she returned from spending the summer in Brazil. The therapist notified campus police and requested their assistance in confining the man. The officers took the patient into custody but released him because he appeared rational. Shortly after her return from Brazil, the man, Prosenjit Poddar, killed Tatiana Tarasoff on October 27, 1969. Her parents successfully sued the University of California, claiming that the therapist had a duty to warn their daughter of Poddar's threats. More recent cases have expanded and amplified the Tarasoff decision (e.g., People v. Clark [1990], 50 Cal. 3d 583).

Comment: The duty to protect endangered third parties is now a national standard of practice, although some jurisdictions still hold that any disclosure of confidential information is a violation of patient rights.

7. Jackson v. Indiana 406 US 715 (1972) and Foucha v. Louisiana 60 USLW 4359 (1992). Justice White of the Supreme Court wrote, "Due process...requires that the nature of the commitment bear some reasonable relation to the purpose for which the individual is committed." Patients such as Jackson and Foucha were hospitalized presumably because they were both mentally ill and dangerous. This ruling recognized that persons who are no longer mentally ill no longer require hospitalization; and because other categories of criminal behavior do not require individuals to prove themselves as no longer dangerous, neither can such rigid criteria be used for the criminally insane (Appelbaum, 1993). More recent rulings indicate that sexual predator's (e.g., Megan's law) are exceptions.

Comment: The 14th Amendment of the Constitution of the United States forbids any state to "...deprive any person of life, liberty, or property without due process of law; nor [may it] deny...the equal protection of the laws."

Statutory Law

Statutory law is written law developed from a legislative body such as a state legislature. A statute can abolish any rule of common law by specifically stating the rule. Statutory law follows a chain of command with the Constitution of the United States being the highest in the hierarchy of enacted written law.

Article VI of the Constitution declares:

"This Constitution, and the Laws of the United States which shall be made in Pursuance thereof; and all Treaties made, or which shall be made, under the Authority of the United States, shall be the supreme Law of the Land; and the Judges in every State shall be bound thereby, any Thing in the Constitution or Laws of any State to the Contrary notwithstanding."

The meaning of this article is that the U.S. Constitution, federal law, and federal treaties take precedence over the constitutions and laws of states and local jurisdictions, such as state statutes.

Administrative Law

Administrative law is public law issued by administrative agencies authorized by statute to administer the enacted laws of federal and state governments. This branch of law controls the administrative operations of government. One example of these agencies is state boards of nursing. Obviously, monitoring and implementing these laws for federal and state legislative bodies would be difficult. For example, states boards of nursing have been created to issue guidelines for nursing practice, licensure, and compliance monitoring in the interest of public safety.

TORTS (CIVIL LAW)

Negligence

Negligence is a personal wrongdoing that is distinguished from a criminal law violation. Negligence is described as the failure to do or not to do what a reasonably careful person would do under the circumstances. Negligence is a form of conduct that is considered careless and is a departure from the standard of conduct generally imposed on reasonable persons.

The four elements that must be present for a plaintiff to recover damages caused by negligence are:

1. Duty to care
2. An obligation of reasonable care (i.e., standard of care)
3. Breach of duty
4. Injury proximately caused by breach of duty (i.e., proximate cause or causation)

All four of these elements should be present for plaintiffs to prevail in suits involving a negligent act. If proof exists of all four elements of negligence, then the plaintiffs are said to have presented a *prima facie* case of negligence, which will often enable them to win their cases.

Duty to care

Duty is defined as a legal obligation of care, performance, or observance imposed on a person who is in a position to safeguard the rights of others. This duty can arise from a special relationship, such as the relationship between a nurse and a patient. The duty to care can arise from a telephone conversation or it can arise out of a voluntary act of assuming the care of a patient. Duty can also be established by statute or contract between the physician and patient.

Reasonable care (standard of care)

A nurse, for example, who assumes the care of patients has the duty to exercise a standard of care, which is the degree of skill, care, and knowledge ordinarily possessed and exercised by other nurses in the care and treatment of patients. A nurse must be reasonable in the exercise of professional judgment as to the care rendered; however, reasonable judgment must not present a departure from the requirements of accepted nursing practice.

Breach of duty

Breach of duty is the failure to conform to or the departure from a required duty of care owed to a person. The obligation to perform according to a standard of care may encompass either doing or refraining from doing a particular act.

Proximate cause or causation

The fourth element necessary to establish negligence requires that a reasonable, close, and causal connection or relationship exists between the defendant's negligent conduct and the resulting damages suffered by the plaintiff. In other words, the defendant's negligence must be a substantial factor causing the injury. The mere departure from a proper and recognized procedure is insufficient to enable a patient to recover damages, unless the patient can show that the departure was unreasonable and the proximate cause of the patient's injuries. Foreseeability, as an element of negligence, is the reasonable anticipation that harm or injury is likely to result from an act or an omission to act. The test for foreseeability is whether anyone of ordinary prudence and intelligence should have anticipated the danger to another caused by his or her negligence.

Malpractice

A form of professional negligence is called malpractice. Malpractice claims can be brought against a variety of professions, including nurses. These claims against nurses are often the result of the nurse's failure to take measures to prevent harm to patients or a failure to maintain the standard of care of nurses in the community.

The psychiatric nurse is responsible for many significant decisions in the care of psychiatric patients. Lapses in attention to specific legal issues related to nursing practice can result in liability and suits against the nurse and the nurse's employer. Areas of concern that can lead to suits include inappropriate dissemination of confidential information, illegal confinement, failure to obtain consent for medication and other treatments, inadequate treatment, medication errors, and the breach of duty to warn of threatened suicide or harm to others.

Understanding the concept of the master-servant rule is vital to both clinical nurses and supervisors. Simply stated, an employer is responsible for the acts of the employee as long as the employee is acting within the scope and authority of employment. A nurse who exceeds clinical boundaries or fails to act as a reasonable and prudent nurse would in the same or similar circumstances incur liability to the employer. Understanding that unlicensed assistive personnel who exceed their clinical boundaries or authority and are under the direction or supervision of a nurse will cause liability to be incurred on the nurse is similarly critical.

Nursing implications

With the recent push to lower health care costs, the use of unlicensed assistive personnel (UAPs) has increased significantly. More nurses are finding themselves with job responsibilities that include delegating certain tasks to UAPs. When a nurse delegates, the authority to carry out the act on behalf of the nurse is conveyed to the assistant; however, the nurse remains accountable for the consequences of the act and for the adequate supervision of the assistant. When delegating, the nurse at a minimum should:

1. Know and follow the local hospital procedures to stay within his or her scope and authority.
2. Ensure that UAPs assigned have been fully trained and are qualified to carry out the tasks they are expected to perform.
3. Know the limitations and responsibilities of nursing practice of his or her state.

CLINICAL EXAMPLE
Clara Meyers, a 40-year-old woman with a history of recent depression with sleep deprivation and suicidal ideation, is admitted to your unit, is sedated, and placed on suicide precautions. The nurse assigns a new nursing assistant to check on the patient every 15 minutes for the entire shift. The nursing assistant, having checked the patient every 15 minutes for 2 hours and finding her asleep, decides that every 30 minutes is sufficient. The nurse who delegated this task was unaware that the new assistant had only general nursing assistant training and had never been oriented on a psychiatric unit. During the 30-minute period when the patient was left alone, she managed to get out of bed and go to the bathroom where she fell and fractured her pelvis. In the subsequent lawsuit, the nurse was identified as being liable for the UAP's poor decision that resulted in the fall.

DUTY TO WARN OTHERS

Another area of importance to psychiatric nurses is the "duty to warn of threatened suicide or harm." As noted, this duty is derived in part from the landmark case of Tarasoff v. The Regents of the University of California (1976) 17 Cal 3rd 425. Before the Tarasoff ruling, mental health professionals had no legal duty to warn of threatened suicide or harm to others. In 1976 the California Supreme Court issued the Tarasoff ruling, which states that failure to warn, coupled with subsequent injury to the threatened person, exposes the mental health professional to civil damages for malpractice. Although a number of clinicians have speculated that warning a potential victim may compromise the relationship with the patient, available evidence cannot support this assertion (Binder, McNeil, 1996). Based on this case and other rulings, the mental health professional must balance a duty to protect confidentiality with a responsibility to warn society of possible danger. Today, the Tarasoff ruling is supported by a litany of case law and is considered a national standard of care, holding that clinicians have a duty to warn third parties of possible danger (Limon v. Gonzaba, 940 S.W. 2d 326 [Tex. App.-San Antonio 1997]).

Nursing Implications

A nurse who is aware of a patient's intention to cause harm to self or others must communicate this information to other professionals and take steps to protect the potential recipient of harm. Not all comments or vague threats should be reported. The Tarasoff ruling specifies that a specific threat to a readily identifiable person or persons must be made. Whenever possible, a decision to communicate confidential patient communications should be discussed with the clinical team before taking action to ensure that patients' rights are balanced with those of third parties. Documentation in the patient's record is crucial for effective communication of this information. The nurse who fails to take prudent action can be held liable. One of the authors spoke with the patient represented in the following vignette. This is an example in which a spurned suitor became emotionally unstable and threatened his ex-girlfriend. This occurrence is not only fairly common, but it also often falls under the auspices of the mental health department to distinguish psychiatric aspects from criminal aspects.

CLINICAL EXAMPLE

Bud Hollman is a 36-year-old man with a history of mental illness that was successfully treated. He has maintained a steady job for the last 12 years. He has a history of abusing his wife over the last 7 years. His wife of 10 years has made a decision to divorce Mr. Hollman and end the abuse; she is currently in a safe house for abused women. Mr. Hollman is obsessed with his wife and with finding her. He goes to the homes of several friends and relatives searching for her. He is unsuccessful in finding her and becomes progressively more agitated. He is delusional, convinced that the only reason she left him is because she is possessed. When he fails to find her at her place of employment, he tells her fellow employees that she is demon possessed and that he intends to kill her. The police are called and Mr. Hollman is arrested. He is involuntarily committed for a 72-hour evaluation and is found to have a psychosis manifested by delusions. Mr. Hollman specifically tells the therapist of his wife's demonic possession and his plans to remove the demon. On review, the police and Mrs. Hollman are warned of his threats.

Intentional Torts: Assault, Battery, and False Imprisonment

Assault

The distinguishing feature between assault and battery is that assault is the apprehension of physical contact or the person's mental security, and battery is the actual physical contact. An assault is the deliberate threat coupled with the apparent present ability to do physical harm to another. No actual contact is necessary; it is the deliberate threat or attempt to injure another or the attempt by one to make bodily contact with another without his or her consent. To commit the tort of assault, two conditions must exist. First, the person who is attempting to touch another unlawfully must possess the apparent present ability to commit the battery, and second, the person who is threatened must be aware of or have actual knowledge of an immediate threat of a battery and must fear it.

Battery

A battery is an intentional touching of another's person, in a socially impermissible manner, without that person's consent. Battery is intentional conduct that violates the physical security of another. An act that would otherwise be considered as an assault may be permissible if proper consent has been given or if the act is in defense of oneself or of a third party. The receiver of the battery does not have to be aware that a battery has occurred. A clinical example of battery would be the force used in unlawful detention and/or inappropriate forceful restraint of a patient. Verbally threatening a patient that you are going to force them to take medication against the patient's will constitutes an assault.

False imprisonment

False imprisonment is the unlawful restraint of an individual's personal liberty or the unlawful restraint or confinement of an individual. The only necessity is that an individual who is physically confined to a given area experiences a reasonable fear that force, which may be implied by words, threats, or gestures, will be used to detain or to intimidate him or her without legal justification. Excessive force used to restrain a patient may produce liability for both false imprisonment and battery. In certain cases, preventing a patient from leaving a health-care facility may constitute false imprisonment. Persons who are wrongfully committed to a psychiatric facility may bring a civil suit for false imprisonment when probable cause is lacking and they are confined such that they cannot escape. The inappropriate use of restraint and seclusion or not allowing voluntary patients to leave when they are ready may also result in liability. A psychiatric facility should have a policy that defines the parameters of confinement, and the nurse must follow the policy guidelines.

CONTRACTS

Purpose of Contract

A contract is a special type of agreement, either written or oral, that involves legally binding obligations between two or more parties. A contract forces the parties involved to be specific in their understandings and expectations of each other. Contracts, particularly those in writing, serve to minimize misunderstandings and offer a means for the parties of a contract to resolve any disputes that may arise. To achieve this goal, formulating a contract that is clear, specific, and as simple as possible is important.

Elements of a Contract

A valid contract requires the following:

- Offer or communication of the offer. An offer is a promise by one party to do (or not to do) something if the other party will do (or not do) something. Not all statements or promises are offers.
- Consideration. Consideration is described in terms of legal detriment and legal benefit. Legal detriment is one's performance of an act not required by law or the forbearing from an act one has a right to do. The party who enjoys the result of another party's act or forbearance to act is said to have received a legal benefit.
- Acceptance. Acceptance requires a "meeting of the minds." The parties must understand and then agree on the terms of the contract.

In the clinical setting, patients commonly sign a series of contracts with the health care provider, physician, and with the institution or hospital. These contracts contain many terms and conditions focused primarily on patients' agreement to accept services from the health care provider in exchange for payment, usually received from a third-party insurance company. Deviations from legal norms in any of these three conditions invite invalidation of the contract and potential litigation.

COMMITMENT ISSUES

The decision to become a patient in a psychiatric facility is important. Patients must admit to themselves and to others that self-management is no longer a viable option for emotional stability. The paradox for individuals who require inpatient care is that the process of becoming a patient can itself cause anxiety and may be depressing. The psychiatric nurse should be aware of this aspect and the legal status of the patients in their charge.

Voluntary Patients

The vast majority of people with mental health problems are voluntary patients; that is, they seek help voluntarily. Although specific procedures vary from hospital to hospital and from state to state, basically, individuals or their therapists request admission, and patients sign the appropriate documents and contract, including a consent to treatment. When individuals are ready to leave the treatment setting, they sign themselves out. Most states have a grace period that allows professional staff the time and opportunity to assess patients before they leave voluntarily. Voluntary patients who want to sign themselves out can be placed on an involuntary commitment status by the court when the staff's assessment indicates a need for further treatment.

Involuntary commitment

Mental illness is not equivalent to incompetence (Trudeau, 1993). Competence involves the patient's ability to comprehend. Involuntary treatment means that an individual who has the legal capacity to consent to mental health treatment refuses to do so. In every state, individuals who are considered dangerous to self or others because of a mental disorder can be involuntarily treated for that mental disorder. The U.S. Supreme Court has repeatedly held, however, that the civil commitment process is subject to the restraints of the Fourteenth Amendment of the U.S. Constitution. The state must produce clear and convincing evidence to prove that a person is both mentally ill and dangerous. Failure to comply with these guidelines may render a commitment illegal (e.g., Vitek v. Jones, 1980). In approximately one half of the states, a third criterion—gravely disabled—is also cause (or required) for involuntary treatment. Involuntary treatment is divided into three common categories:

1. Evaluation and emergency care
2. Certification for observation and treatment
3. Extended or indeterminate care

Not surprisingly, involuntary treatment is the area of psychiatric care in which most legal issues develop. Although involuntary commitment usually implies inpatient care, it can also be applied to outpatient treatment (e.g., groups treated as a consequence for driving under the influence of alcohol).

Evaluation and emergency care

Individuals who meet any one of these three criteria (i.e., dangerous to self, dangerous to others, and gravely disabled) can be detained involuntarily for evaluation and emergency treatment in most states. An authorized person such as a police officer signs documents to place an individual under involuntary care. The length of the involuntary status varies from state to state; approximately 72 hours is the average.

Nursing implications

Because the law determines the length of this involuntary treatment period, staff must scrupulously adhere to legal time constraints. The nursing staff must be absolutely aware of the point at which the emergency treatment period is over and prepare the patient for discharge at that time. Patients may be asked to remain voluntarily in the facility; and if they refuse, they may then be asked to sign out against medical advice. The following clinical example provides a realistic vignette for involuntary detention.

CLINICAL EXAMPLE
Bill Wexler is a 52-year-old man who was informed that his job of 30 years is being eliminated. Although the job loss is part of a larger downsizing effort, Mr. Wexler is deeply and personally affected. Within a week, he begins to decompensate. He stops bathing and wears the same suit every day. He shows up for work 2 weeks after being terminated, not having bathed or shaved for a week and goes to his usual workspace. Another employee occupies the space, and Mr. Wexler demands that the worker move out of his space or he will throw him out. Efforts by other employees who know Mr. Wexler are unsuccessful in trying to calm him. He begins shouting that he is going to kill everyone in human resources and that he has a gun in the car and is going to get it. Security and the police are called and are successful in restraining Mr. Wexler after a brief struggle. Mr. Wexler is taken to the county emergency department and involuntarily committed for 72 hours.

On the other hand, Hegner (1996) describes the liability involved when involuntary commitment is unwarranted.

CLINICAL EXAMPLE
In McCobe v. City of Lynn, a federal court ruled that a psychiatrist was liable for the death of an older woman who was to be involuntarily committed. Ms. Zinger, a holocaust survivor, with eviction from her home imminent, was thought to be incapable of caring for herself. The police went to her home, and when Ms. Zinger refused to open her door, the police broke it down. In the struggle that ensued, Ms. Zinger suffered myocardial infarction and died.

Certification for observation and treatment

Each state has laws that provide for the certification for observation and involuntary treatment for mental illness. These laws, which differ from state to state, authorize a qualified expert to determine whether a person has a treatable mental disorder. A mental disorder can be defined as a condition that substantially impairs a person's thoughts, perception of reality, emotional process, judgment, or behavior. In most states, a qualified expert may be a physician, a psychiatrist, a master's-prepared nurse or social worker, or a psychologist. A treatable mental disorder indicates that the problem is amenable to and can improve with treatment. For example, a person who is hearing voices telling her to kill herself meets this criterion, whereas someone who is simply angry and threatening to kill someone may not.

During the certification process, a complaint or a probable cause statement is written, indicating that the person is a danger to self or others or is gravely disabled. The probable cause statement is required by the Fourth Amendment to the U.S. Constitution, which prohibits "search and seizure of a person without probable cause." In this context, probable cause means that known facts would lead an ordinary person to believe that the person detained is mentally disordered and is a danger to self or others or is gravely disabled. The probable cause hearing is not held to determine whether the person is mentally ill, but whether just cause exists to keep the person for treatment against his or her will.

If probable cause exists, individuals can then be detained for observation and treatment. These individuals must be informed of their rights on being certified for this level of involuntary care. The length of the observation and treatment periods varies from state to state.

Nursing implications

Patients must be released when no legal basis exists for continued confinement in the hospital. The hospital staff may suggest voluntary admission and, when it is refused, may require patients to sign out against medical advice. The staff cannot hold people simply because they believe the individual needs to be protected from themselves.

CLINICAL EXAMPLE

Mr. Banks, an 82-year-old well-nourished but dirty and malodorous man, was brought to the hospital by a social worker for psychiatric evaluation. Since his wife's death 3 years earlier, neighbors report that his house has been taken over by drug dealers and prostitutes. He is often seen outside at night, sleeping on the porch, despite cold weather. Furthermore, Mr. Banks has approached neighbors for food and has told them the drug dealers have taken his social security check. Mr. Banks insists he willingly allows others to live in his home and he enjoys the sex and drugs that come with the arrangement. He is alert, oriented, and no evidence of psychiatric disorder is found during evaluation. He declines offers to assist in finding safe housing, stating he wants to return to the lifestyle he missed during the years his wife kept him on the straight and narrow.

Extended or indeterminate commitment

Extended or indeterminate commitment is reserved for persons who need prolonged psychiatric care but refuse to seek such help voluntarily. These hospitalizations can last from 60 days to a great deal longer. These individuals are usually brought before a hearing officer, which is a major part of a system of checks and balances that decrease the possibility of someone being "railroaded" into a mental hospital.

Commitment of Incapacitated Persons

In most states, a procedure is required for establishing a conservator or guardian for gravely disabled persons (the conservatees). The legal system in the United States maintains that although a person may be undergoing severe mental and emotional upheaval (as in the clinical example of Mr. Wexler), that person is nonetheless recognized as competent before the law. The person who is identified as being gravely disabled, on the other hand, is viewed by the legal system as incompetent.

Gravely disabled is defined as the inability to provide food, clothing, and shelter for oneself because of a mental illness, which does not mean that all people living on the streets are gravely disabled nor that they should be hospitalized for "their own good." Judge David Bazelon addressed this concept in 1966: "Deprivations of liberty solely because of dangers to the ill persons themselves should not go beyond what is necessary for their protection" (Munetz, Geller, 1993). However, people with money in their pockets who cannot negotiate arrangements for food or shelter are gravely disabled.

Conservators and guardians

The appointment of a conservator or guardian is a serious legal matter, and full legal protection is provided for persons being evaluated for conservatee status. Proposed conservatees are entitled to representation by an attorney to challenge conservatorship. An appointed conservator or guardian may be given broad powers, including the right to order the conservatee to receive psychiatric treatment. Although technically patients might receive treatment against their will, a legal distinction exists between this kind of commitment and an involuntary commitment. That distinction is based on the premise that the conservator now speaks for the patient; hence the treatment is not involuntary. Conservators are legally obligated to act in the best interest of their conservatees.

Nursing implications

Because conservators speak for conservatees, the nurse must gain consent from conservators for decisions that are otherwise made by patients. A nurse who forgets to gain conservator approval may face legal consequences.

CLINICAL EXAMPLE

Ms. Park, a 73-year-old woman, is found by a social worker to be living in a filthy, roach-infested, older home. A neighbor who has not seen Ms. Park in several months calls the local department of human services. The neighbor explains that no one answers the door when she rings the doorbell. Ms. Park has lived there for years with her husband. Since he died 5 years ago, Ms. Park has lived alone. The stench of cats and cat feces is almost unbearable. Ms. Park is emaciated,

Continued

incoherent, and paranoid. The social worker decides to initiate involuntary commitment for Ms. Park to evaluate her mental and physical condition and her need for a conservatorship hearing.

PATIENT RIGHTS

In addition to the information that will be discussed in the following section, the Federal Register is a good source of information about patient rights and regulations that are published by the CMS. Aside from the legal and patient care issues, these rights must be assured for health care providers so as to participate in the Medicare and Medicaid programs. Box 4-1 outlines the current opinions that President George W. Bush has about patients' rights.

Right to Treatment with the Least Restrictive Alternative

The concept of the least restrictive alternative or least restrictive environment is central to the ideology of the deinstitutionalization movement (Munetz, Geller, 1993). People with mental health problems have the right to treatment of their problems in the least restrictive environment using the least restrictive means (i.e., without restraints and seclusion, unless necessary). This "right" has emerged from court decisions previously mentioned and has been articulated by President Carter's Commission on Mental Health in 1978 and is a key component of state statutes. Specifically, patients who are held against their will should not be detained without treatment, as occurred in the Whitree v. state of New York case described.

|Box 4-1| Principals for Patient Rights: President Bush's Opinion

THE WHITE HOUSE
Office of the Press Secretary
February 7, 2001
PRINCIPLES FOR A BIPARTISAN
PATIENTS' BILL OF RIGHTS

Patient Protections Should Apply to All Americans

A federal Patients' Bill of Rights should ensure that every person enrolled in a health plan enjoys strong patient protections. Because many states have passed patient protection laws that are appropriate for their states, deference should be given to these state laws and to the traditional authority of states to regulate health insurance.

A comprehensive federal Patients' Bill of Rights should provide patient protections such as:
- Access to emergency room and specialty care; direct access to obstetricians, gynecologists, and pediatricians
- Access to needed prescription drugs and approved clinical trials
- Access to health plan information; a prohibition of "gag clauses"
- Consumer choice and continuity of care protections
  Additional rights for patients should include the following:
- Patients should have a rapid medical review process for denials of care. The review process should ensure that doctors are allowed to make medical decisions and patients receive care in a timely manner.

- Patients should have the right to appeal a health plan's decision to deny care through both internal review and independent, binding external review.
- Slow and costly litigation should be a last resort.
- Patients should exhaust their appeals process first, allowing independent medical experts to make medical decisions and ensuring patients receive necessary medical care without the expense or delay of going to court.
- Federal remedies should be expanded to hold health plans accountable.
- After an independent review decision is rendered, patients should be allowed to hold their health plans liable in federal court if they have been wrongly denied needed medical care.
- Patient protection legislation should encourage, not discourage, employers to offer health care coverage.
- Employers, many of whom are struggling to offer health coverage to their employees, should be shielded from unnecessary and frivolous lawsuits and should not be subject to multiple lawsuits in state court. Increased litigation will only result in higher health care costs, potentially forcing employers to drop employee health coverage altogether. Only employers who retain responsibility for and make final medical decisions should be subject to suit.
  Americans want meaningful remedies, not a windfall for trial lawyers that result in expensive health care premiums and unaffordable health coverage. To protect patients' rights without encouraging excessive litigation, damages should be subject to reasonable caps.

Nursing implications

Typically, the nurse does not decide which treatment setting the patient will enter. However, the nurse has treatment responsibilities and can be held liable if the patient does not receive adequate treatment. The following clinical example illustrates the issue of the right to treatment using the least restrictive alternative.

CLINICAL EXAMPLE

Joe Kelly is a 56-year-old Vietnam veteran who suffers from posttraumatic stress syndrome characterized by periods of flashbacks and depression. After a flashback, Mr. Kelly is often confused and wanders about for days looking for friends he lost in the war. He poses no obvious danger to others or himself. His family is deceased, and he lives alone. When he is picked up by the police for loitering and evaluated by the social worker, Mr. Kelly insists on going home. His case, however, is heard before the court, which rules that he does not need commitment to a psychiatric unit but does need a temporary structured environment. The social worker finds a halfway house with the veteran's hospital, and Mr. Kelly agrees to temporary placement.

Right to Confidentiality of Records

Patient information is privileged material and should be treated confidentially. Both voluntary and involuntary patients are granted this legal consideration. Following this procedure is not always as easy as it might appear hence professional judgment is required. The guidelines in Box 4-2 provide a framework for mandatory confidentiality.

As straightforward as these guidelines are, they do not cover every situation or address exceptions. Jones (1993) points out that the rule of confidentiality is not absolute and uses the obvious example of a patient at risk for self-harm. Keeping this type of information confidential would constitute professional malpractice. Based on a U.S. Supreme Court ruling in Jaffe v. Redmond, the therapist-patient relationship is viewed as privileged, and the therapist need not divulge the content of therapy sessions even in a court of law (Appelbaum, 1993).

Nursing implications

The nurse should document in the nursing notes all confidential information that is released, including the date and circumstances under which disclosure was made, the names of the individuals or agencies receiving the disclosure and their relationships to the patient, and the specific information disclosed.

To release information about patients, a consent form must first be signed. Most states provide legal redress for patients should a nurse willfully disclose confidential information without the proper signature. The confidentiality of the patient's records should not be confused with the doctrine of privileged communication. Under this doctrine, a psychiatrist is not obliged to reveal the contents of sessions with the patient. This privilege is based on the understanding of the need for trust between physicians and patients. Most states do not include nurses under this provision.

The therapeutic modality of group therapy, which nurses often lead, is particularly vulnerable to violations of confidentiality. The group leader should always address this issue when starting a group or when a new member is introduced to the group. Nurses who lead group sessions must men-

---

Critical **Thinking Questions**

Some states have a category of commitment called "gravely disabled," whereas other states do not. Obviously, two firmly held views exist about this type of commitment. Does the state in which you live have this commitment category? Do you find the arguments more compelling for or against this commitment category?

|Box 4-2| Tips for Monitoring Confidentiality

1. Keep all patient records secure.
2. Carefully consider the content of all written entries.
3. Release information only with written consent.
4. Disguise clinical material when it is used for educational purposes.
5. Share information only with people who need to know, not with friends or in public areas.
6. Guard written material taken outside the clinical area.
7. Do not access written or electronic information out of curiosity.
8. Fax transmissions may be prohibited to unsecured areas in which a receipt error is a possibility.
9. Know to whom you are talking when relating patient information over the phone; "family" may be a reporter, boss, or insurance attorney.

tion the limitations to confidentiality that exist in the group format. Of course, after such a proclamation is made, forthrightness by group members concerning their thoughts, feelings, and behaviors may be potentially decreased. That staff not discuss patients in settings in which those without a clinical need to know can overhear those conversations is absolutely necessary.

CLINICAL EXAMPLE
Students frequently find themselves in the following situation. After developing a relationship with a patient, the student may hear, "I want to tell you something, but I don't want anyone else to know." What is the proper response? Is it a breach of the patient's right to confidentiality to tell others or to record what is said in the patient's chart? The student must let the patient know that anything said within the context of the nurse-patient relationship will be shared with other team members when appropriate.

Critical **Thinking Questions**

Confidentiality is stressed in nursing school but it may be violated. What should you do when one of your classmates is discussing a patient inappropriately? Is it a violation of confidentiality to discuss patients by name in a clinical conference?

Right to Freedom from Restraints and Seclusion

Throughout history, mechanical restraints and segregation have been used to manage the out-of-control behavior that accompanies some psychiatric disorders. Many people view physical restraint as synonymous with brutal custodial care (Appelbaum, 1999). Restraint is a broad term used to characterize any form of limiting a person's movement or access to his or her own body. The limits can be the result of physical holds, bedrails, laptrays, restraint devices, or medications. Seclusion is defined as the process of isolating a person in a room in which they are physically prevented from leaving. The real value of judiciously used restraint and seclusion to protect severely ill patients and those with whom they come in contact has been overshadowed in recent years by attention to injuries and deaths associated with their use. The U.S. Food and Drug Administration (FDA) estimates that at least

100 restraint-related deaths occur each year. In 1998 an investigative report in the Hartford Courant alleged that 142 deaths in psychiatric units, group homes, and residential facilities had been caused by the use of seclusion or restraint between 1988 and 1998. As a result of the dramatic case examples in the report, other media venues provided coverage drawing the attention from the lay public, advocacy groups, regulatory agencies, and members of Congress. In some instances, restraints and seclusion have been substituted for more appropriate management interventions. Patients' right to the least restrictive interventions to manage behavioral disturbances have been violated with resulting disability, injury, and death. The Omnibus Reconciliation Act of 1987 (OBRA) placed stringent limits on the use of physical and chemical restraints in nursing homes to ensure that their use was limited to medical necessity, not staff convenience. Many nursing homes have since implemented innovative strategies to preserve the safety of frail older adults, with a goal of becoming restraint free. JCAHO has developed standards to guide the use and efforts to reduce the use of restraints in both medical and psychiatric facilities. The CMS (formerly HCFA) has also published, within their Patients Rights document, strict rules for restraint and seclusion use in hospitals that receive Medicare and Medicaid funds (Federal Register, 1999).

Nursing implications

Restraint reduction is difficult to achieve given the prevalent belief that "a restrained patient is a safe one." Nurses who are aware of the potential negative physical, psychologic, and legal consequences associated with restraint and seclusion are more apt to look for alternate strategies. Most valuable are those interventions aimed at preventing a patient's escalation and loss of control. Attention to the nurse-patient relationship, therapeutic milieu, and principles of pharmacologic management can reduce the need for restrictive measures. Guidelines issued by CMS for restraint and seclusion use are substantially different for use in medically necessary and behavioral control situations. Although laws differ from state to state, general guidelines for use in psychiatry include multiple elements important for the nurse to document:

1. Staff members involved in decisions to restrain or seclude and those who apply or remove re-

straints must receive special training and demonstrate competency.

2. Alternatives to restraint and seclusion must be considered before their use.

3. Although nurses may be allowed to implement restraint or seclusion in emergent situations, a physician's order is required within 1 hour. Physician assistants and advanced practice nurses can also write restraint-seclusion orders (JCAHOnline. Accessed 5/24/02).

4. The least restrictive method or device possible must be chosen.

5. Nurses should carefully document events leading up to the intervention and justification for use.

6. Orders must contain the type restraint, rationale for use, and be time limited.

7. As needed (prn) orders are not permitted. Each episode must be based on eminent risk.

8. Restraint and seclusion are used for the shortest possible time. The nurse must tell the patients what behaviors are expected before release and reevaluate the patient at least every 2 hours for continued necessity.

9. Patients must be observed constantly during restraint and seclusion with documentation of safety and comfort interventions at least every 15 minutes. In a 1992 ruling, a U.S. district judge reaffirmed and strengthened some of the elements of the Wyatt v. Stickney case described earlier. Under this ruling, a patient in restraint and seclusion must be checked every 15 minutes and bathed every 24 hours.

10. Patients must be debriefed after restrictive interventions.

11. Patients have the right to request notification of a family member or other person in the event restraints or seclusion is implemented.

12. Death of any patient while in restraints, even when restraints did not contribute to death in the judgment of the health care provider, are required to be reported to the FDA.

Critical Thinking Question

Some psychiatric professionals believe the courts have gone too far in protecting the rights of patients and have actually set up barriers to effective mental health care. What do you think?

CLINICAL EXAMPLE

Kim Young is a 28-year-old Korean national married to an American serviceman who is currently assigned overseas. Ms. Young is extremely well versed in the American culture and language, as well as exceptionally bright and talented. Ms. Young has performed endless hours of volunteer work within her community and church. She is viewed as a person with boundless energy who never appears to stop. Her volunteer hours continue to increase, and she begins to preach in local bars and taverns. Her language becomes incoherent at times, and English and Korean are often mixed in the same sentence. When the owner of a local tavern calls the police after she refuses to leave, she begins to curse him and tries to hit him with a beer bottle. The police are able to restrain her, and she is involuntarily committed to a psychiatric unit. When approached by the staff, she spits, curses, and tries to strike them. Four-point physical restraint is ordered. Ms. Young requires seclusion and restraint thereafter for her aggressive behavior on several occasions. The nursing progress record (Box 4-3) and the restraint and seclusion nursing notes provide a record of her behavior and the nursing responses to that behavior.

| Box 4-3 | Nursing Progress Record

Time	Format
0210	Patient continues to pace hallway, dayroom, and room; at 0045, is asking for sleep medications. Patient states the best way to get well is walking.
0315	Patient refuses to go to room and tries to rest; pacing dayroom and at times kneeling as if in prayer.
0430	Patient is asleep on top of bed, naked; door is open.
0830	Patient refuses medication; appears very agitated.
0930	Patient is very agitated, tearing up another patient's magazine and throwing into trash. Patient is placed in seclusion.
1030	Agitation is escalated. When staff goes into room to check on the patient, she swings at staff and attempts to bite the nurse. Patient is placed in four-point restraint by four female and two male staff members. Patient states that she is being "raped" and that "Christ lives in me." Haldol 5 mg IM and Cogentin 2 mg IM is given.

Right to Give or Refuse Consent to Treatment

The final patient right to be explored is the right to give or refuse consent to treatment. Court rulings mentioned in this text provide legal precedents, and Rogers v. Okin provided the foundation for a patient's right to refuse treatment. Based on this and other constitutional arguments, New York State's highest court, the court of appeals, handed down a decision in 1986 that held in nonemergency situations, involuntary patients cannot be forced to take psychotropic medications. The decision, referred to as Rivers v. Katz, has led to diminished quality of care and has resulted in increased patient and staff injuries, according to a study by Ciccone and associates (1993).

The right of voluntary patients to refuse treatment has been recognized for a long time. When voluntary patients believe the treatment they are receiving is helpful, they can accept it; when they believe the treatment is not helpful, they can refuse it. Involuntary patients, on the other hand, have not always been understood to have the same right to refuse treatment. Through the years, many involuntary patients have been forced to take medications against their will. Legally, involuntarily admitted patients do not lose their right to give informed consent to the administration of psychotropic drugs. The key issue is whether patients have the capacity to give informed consent to the administration of these drugs. The court made the determination regarding drugs but does not respond to issues of need for alternative treatments. After the court decides that a person is not competent to understand the need for treatment, medications can then be imposed on that person. The way in which this decision is implemented varies from state to state.

In cases of a psychiatric emergency, medications can be given without consent to prevent harm to the patient or to others.

Nursing implications

Nurses administer medications to patients. Because it is not uncommon for patients to refuse medications and for nurses to coax those patients into taking medications, nurses must be sure that coaxing does not escalate to the point of forcing medications on a patient. Furthermore, although it might be tempting to hide medication in food or liquid when patients refuse them, these actions are considered "forcing." The deception is also counterproductive when trying to establish a therapeutic nurse-patient relationship. Factors that constitute a psychiatric emergency are also not always clear. Nurses may be liable should their interpretation of a psychiatric emergency differ from that of another professional or from that of a judge.

Suspension of Patient Rights

Occasionally, suspending rights for the protection of patients or of others and for therapeutic purposes is necessary. For instance, no units have unlimited telephone privileges, largely because this policy may be nontherapeutic.

Nursing implications

Suspension of a patient's rights requires the nurse to clearly document that allowing the patient to continue to exercise the specific right might result in harm to the patient or others. For example, suicidal patients' right to access personal belongings may be suspended because the belief exists that these patients might attempt to harm themselves with those objects. The nurse must document the concern and the suspension of this right in the nurse's notes.

ADVANCE DIRECTIVES FOR HEALTH CARE

A majority of states have recognized the rights of individuals to choose the type of medical treatment they receive in the event of a life-threatening medical condition, which is accomplished through use of living wills and health care directives. The U.S. Congress passed the Patient Self-Determination Act in 1991, which requires all health care facilities that serve Medicare or Medicaid patients to provide each of their adult patients written information regarding their right to make decisions about their medical care. These instructions must be consistent with the laws of each state. The patients are also made aware of the right to execute a living will or durable power of attorney. Both the living will and the health care directive list specific actions that the patient may choose to implement or not implement under the aforementioned life-threatening medical condition. Some examples are mechanical ventilator support or artificial nutrition. A durable power of attorney is a written document in which one person (the principal) authorizes another person (the attorney in fact) to act on the principal's behalf "in the event" the principal becomes unable to act on his or her own behalf secondary to a physical or mental disability. The disability causes this type of power of attorney to take effect.

Advance directives for mental health treatment are similar to medical care advance directives in many ways but have a number of additional challenges. The issue of ensuring competency at the time directives are executed is problematic, particularly for patients with fluctuating mental disorders. Nonetheless, in advance of a mental health crisis, individuals can issue directives about treatment in a number of areas, including but not limited to: (1) the use of specific medications including dose and route; (2) the use of specific treatment options, such as electroconvulsive therapy (ECT); (3) the use of behavior management including restraint, seclusion, and sedation; (4) a list of the individuals who are to be notified and allowed to visit; (5) a consent to contact health care providers and obtain treatment records; and (6) a willingness to participate in research studies (Srebnik, LaFond, 1999).

Nursing Implications

Nurses should be aware of the patient's right to establish advance directives for both physical and mental health care in the form of written statement of preference or by legal documentation of a durable power of attorney. Nurses should also be familiar with and follow employer procedures and laws that govern the way in which the patient is made aware of this right. The following actions are also important to ensure that patient's rights to self-determination are exercised:

1. Documentation in the medical record of either properly executed forms or a statement or signed waiver must be made indicating that the patient chooses not to exercise his or her right to provide advance directives.
2. That the attorney in fact chosen by the patient is consulted before making decisions regarding the patient in areas specified by the document.
3. Ensuring that all members of the health care team are made aware of advance directives and that they are considered in treatment planning.

CORPORATE COMPLIANCE

The term corporate compliance is used to describe a health care provider's responsibility to comply with governmental laws and regulations. Nearly

every health care provider receives some manner of federal or state funds under the Medicare and Medicaid programs and must therefore comply with the associated laws and regulations. Specifically, a growing number of antifraud and abuse requirements under the Medicare and Medicaid statutes have been enacted, as well as a number of federal and state laws. Much of the enforcement activity focuses on false billing and the associated statutes. The statute and summary of its contents are as follows:

1. Federal False Claims Act. Any false, fictitious, or fraudulent claim made in the course of seeking Medicare or Medicaid reimbursement.
2. Medicare and Medicaid fraud and abuse. An assortment of false billing activity, including double billing for the same service or equipment, billing for services that were not medically necessary, admitting a patient when medically unnecessary, and up-coding (i.e., billing for a service at a higher rate than that which was actually provided).
3. Antikickback statutes. Any type of remuneration or payment for a referral, including cash, excessive rent, paying the salary of an employee of the referring physician, and free goods or services.
4. Health Insurance Portability Act. This Act applies to all payers, not only Medicare and Medicaid, and makes engaging in health care fraud a crime (i.e., knowingly and willfully defrauding any health care plan or obtaining payment from health care plans by false or fraudulent pretenses).
5. Mail fraud and wire fraud statutes. Any misrepresentation that is part of a scheme calculated for the purpose of obtaining money or property and that uses the mails or wires (telephone lines) to carry out the scheme that violates these statutes.

In addition to these enforcement activities, most health care providers have published "Business Conduct Guidelines," which deal with honest and ethical conduct expectations. Because of the competitive nature of mental health care service provision, a temptation occasionally exists for persons so inclined to engage in inappropriate conduct to achieve desired business outcomes. To avoid misconduct, most health care providers require that employees undergo education and training in business conduct or "Corporate Compliance." Documenting services or products used by the patient is critical. Errors in entering patient charges or falsely documenting services a patient did in fact not receive can lead to civil and criminal sanctions.

In most practice settings, the nursing staff is responsible for completing a variety of forms that document the progress of patients and serve as legal records of the treatments patients received. Nursing notes, restraint and seclusion forms, medication records, and physician order sheets are only a few of the forms used. Careful attention to these records promotes communication among staff, enhances treatment, diminishes treatment errors (e.g., medication errors), and can protect the nurse in the case of legal action.

A critical point to remember is that the medical record will often be a key source of information used in any legal action against a health care provider. In addition to professional practice guidelines, most health care institutions will have written policies for documentation in the medical record. Being familiar with these guidelines and adhering to professional practice standards are important.

Key Concepts

1. The understanding of the rights of mentally ill persons has evolved over the centuries. Today, based on several precedent-setting legal decisions and laws, protection of the mentally ill person's rights has been established.
2. These landmark cases triggered several states to legislate the end of inappropriate, indefinite, and involuntary commitment to mental hospitals.
3. Three categories of commitment include:
   a. Voluntary patient: the person requests hospitalization and voluntarily agrees to be admitted.
   b. Involuntary commitment: a person with the legal capacity to consent refuses to do so and is treated against his or her will.
   c. Commitment of an incapacitated person: the treatment of a person who does not have the legal capacity to consent to treatment.
4. Patients under psychiatric care have many rights guaranteed by the Constitution of the United States and the constitutions of individual states.

5. Seclusion and restraint are special procedures for coping with assaultive and dangerous patients thus these patients can be isolated or mechanically restrained to prevent injury to the patient, other patients, or to staff.
6. Patients, even involuntarily admitted patients, must give informed consent before they are given psychotropic drugs and retain the right to refuse medication. Except for emergency situations, involuntarily admitted patients cannot be given medication against their will without judicial approval.
7. Psychiatric patients have the right to be treated in the least restrictive alternative or environment. In other words, if persons can receive appropriate care close to home in a community agency, then they cannot be forced to go to a public mental hospital far away from family and friends.

References

Appelbaum PS: Foucha v. Louisiana: when must the state release insanity acquittees? *Hosp Community Psychiatry* 44(1):9, 1993.

Appelbaum PS: Seclusion and restraint: Congress reacts to reports of abuse, *Psychiatr Serv* 50:881, 1999.

Appelbaum PS, Greer A: Confidentiality in group therapy, *Hosp Community Psychiatry* 44(4):311, 1993.

Binder RL, McNeil DE: Application of the Tarasoff ruling and its affect on the victim and the therapeutic relationship, *Psychiatr Serv* 47(11):1212, 1996.

Ciccone JR et al: Medication refusal and judicial activism: a reexamination of the effects of the Rivers decision, *Hosp Community Psychiatry* 44(6):555, 1993.

Eskreis TR: Seven common legal pitfalls in nursing, *AJN* 98:34, 1998.

42 CFR Part 482 Medicare and Medicaid Programs: Hospital conditions of participation: patients' rights; interim final rule, *Federal Register* 64(127):36069, 1999.

Hegner RE: Managed care carveouts for mental health and substance abuse, *J Am Psychiatr Nurs Assoc* 2:63, 1996.

JCAHOnline: www.jcaho.org/tip/j_online0502.html

Jones SL: More on confidentiality, *Arch Psychiatr Nurs* 7(3):123, 1993.

Munetz MR, Geller JL: The least restrictive alternative in the postinstitutional era, *Hosp Community Psychiatry* 44(10):967, 1993.

Srebnik D, LaFond J: Advance directives for mental health treatment, *Psychiatr Serv* 50(7):919, 1999.

Trudeau ME: Informed consent: the patient's right to decide, *J Psychosoc Nurs Ment Health Serv* 31(6):9, 1993.

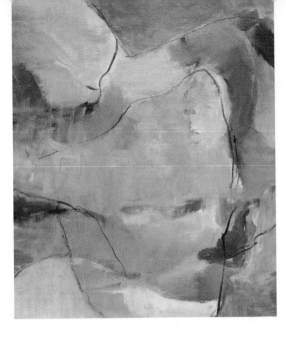

Chapter **5**

Psychobiologic Bases of Behavior

Richard A. Sugerman

Learning Objectives

After reading this chapter, you should be able to:

- Describe the importance of the psychiatric nurse's understanding of brain biology.
- Identify and describe gross neuroanatomic structures.
- Discuss the significance and role of five specific neurotransmitters in normal brain function.
- Identify the role of five specific neurotransmitters in schizophrenia, depression, anxiety, and dementia.

- Differentiate the functions of the sympathetic and parasympathetic nervous systems.
- Describe the function of the basal ganglia system and its significance for movement disorders.
- Discuss key psychobiologic assessment issues for the psychiatric nurse.

The central nervous system (CNS) is composed of the brain and the spinal cord. The brain can be further divided into the cerebrum, the brainstem, and the cerebellum. The brain weighs only approximately 3 to 4 pounds but contains 100 billion neurons, roughly the same number of stars that are in the Milky Way galaxy. The brain is incredibly complex, and a great deal about the brain remains that science does not know. What is known, however, is that many mental disorders that were formerly thought to be caused by psychosocial stressors or traumatic early life experiences or both are the result of altered or disordered brain biology. The National Foundation for Brain Research (1992) estimates that well over 650 brain disorders currently affect approximately 50 million Americans.

The U.S. Congress declared the 1990s the "decade of the brain." Before this time, psychiatric

nursing had been influenced primarily by the dominant ideas of the nineteenth century: the ideas of Freud, Bleuler, and Jung, asserting that mental disorders originate from psychodynamic causes. However, psychiatric nursing accepted the congressional mandate, and the 1990s witnessed significant changes in the education and practice of psychiatric nurses. Psychiatric nursing is now fully integrating biologic concepts and, consequently, is now being practiced holistically. The foundation of today's practice is understanding basic neuroanatomy and neurophysiology.

The objective of this chapter is to present a balanced view of biologic information, thus the student can coherently engage the rest of this book, can participate in interdisciplinary discussions, and can read the psychiatric literature with understanding. Understanding psychobiologic concepts enables the

Key Terms

Axons Long processes from the neuronal cell body that transmit impulses away from the cell.

Basal ganglia Large subcortical nuclei, including the caudate nucleus, putamen, and globus pallidus, which are responsible for modulating voluntary movement.

Cerebral cortex Narrow ribbon of gray matter that lies on the surface of the cerebrum. The gray matter lies "on top of" the white matter. The reverse is true in the spinal cord.

Coma Depressed consciousness during which even extreme stimulation of the RAS fails to cause a response.

Contralateral Opposite side of the body.

Corpus callosum Major connecting and communicating pathway between the hemispheres.

Dendrites Projections from the neuron that transmit impulses to the cell body.

Diencephalon Thalamus, hypothalamus, epithalamus, and metathalamus.

Extrapyramidal Outside the pyramidal system; the extrapyramidal-basal ganglia system modulates and supports voluntary movement.

Gray matter Composed of the cell bodies and dendrites of neurons.

Gyrus (gyri, *pl.*) Convolution of gray matter on the cerebrum.

Ipsilateral Same side of the body.

Lesion Injury to tissue.

Meninges Outer lining of the CNS composed of the dura mater, arachnoid, and pia mater.

Neuron Nerve cell.

Olfactory Pertaining to the sense of smell.

Pyramidal system Motor system for voluntary movement.

Sulcus (sulci, *pl.*) Groove separating gyri. Deep sulci are referred to as *fissures*.

White matter Composed of myelinated neuronal axons.

---

nurse to better assess patients' behaviors and plan appropriate nursing interventions. Specifically, the nurse should have an appreciation for the neuroanatomy of the brain, neurons and neurotransmitters, the autonomic nervous system, the ventricular system, and the clinical application of this information to major psychiatric disorders.

NEUROANATOMY OF THE BRAIN

The nervous system is divided into the CNS and the peripheral nervous system (PNS). The CNS (Figure 5-1) can be further divided into the brain and spinal cord. The brain is composed of the cerebrum, brainstem, and cerebellum.

Cerebrum

The cerebrum is divided into two cerebral hemispheres, which includes the diencephalon, and constitutes the bulk of the nervous system. The hemispheres are composed of a multitude of nervous system pathways, the cerebral cortex, certain limbic structures, and the basal ganglia. The hemispheres are interconnected by the corpus callosum. These structures are described in the following section.

Nervous system pathways

Some specialized neurons in the cerebral cortex transmit information via pathways throughout the CNS. A pathway is a bundle of these communicating neurons. In the CNS, a neuronal pathway (a

bundle of neurons) may be called a *tract*, a *fasciculus*, a *peduncle*, or a *lemniscus*. (In neuroanatomy, a single anatomic entity can have several names.) In the PNS, a neuronal pathway is called a *nerve*. Hence, cranial "nerve" III (CN III) is part of the PNS.

A number of large CNS pathways are readily apparent structures within white areas of the brain (white matter). For example, major pathways include the corpus callosum (Figures 5-2, 5-3), the internal capsule in each hemisphere (Figure 5-4, see also Figure 5-3), and the corona radiata (see Figures 5-3, 5-4). Although a great deal of public interest exists in differences between the right brain (visual-spatial, experiential tasks) and the left brain (language, mathematics, reasoning), many scientists now have a greater appreciation for the interrelatedness of the two hemispheres. The corpus callosum connects the two hemispheres and is the communication pathway between them. When the corpus callosum is severed, a split-brain syndrome develops. The internal capsule and the corona radiata are pathways through which motor and sensory information passes; for example, motor impulses from the motor cortex (precentral gyrus) to the foot pass through these pathways. In addition to these large pathways, many smaller tracts interconnect the four lobes of the cerebral cortex.

Cerebral cortex

The cerebral cortex is the outermost part of the brain and is composed of gray matter. The gray mat-

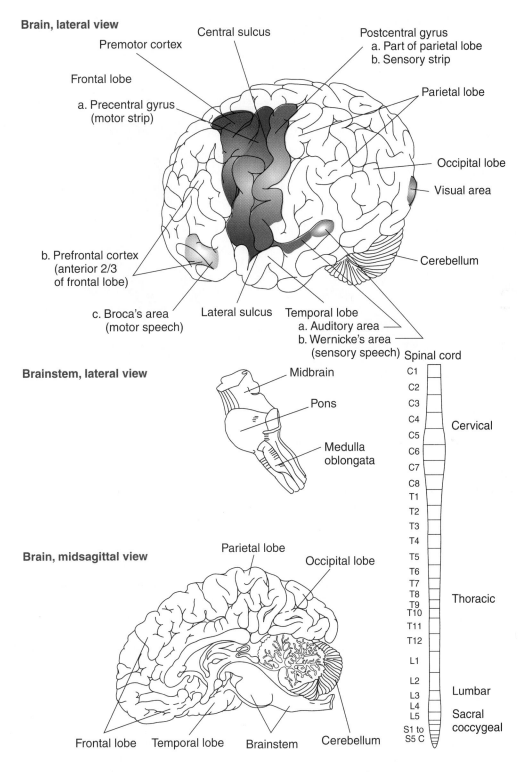

Figure 5-1 Expanded view of the central nervous system shows the major components (components are not to scale). (From Sugerman RA, Edmundson MJ, Robinson S: *Human anatomy,* Edina, Minn, 1979, Burgess.)

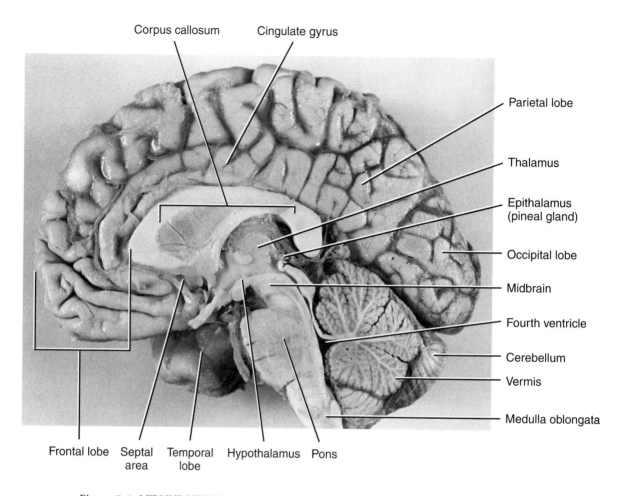

Corpus callosum   Cingulate gyrus

Parietal lobe

Thalamus

Epithalamus
(pineal gland)

Occipital lobe

Midbrain

Fourth ventricle

Cerebellum

Vermis

Medulla oblongata

Frontal lobe   Septal   Temporal   Hypothalamus   Pons
area   lobe

Figure 5-2 MIDLINE VIEW OF RIGHT HEMISPHERE. Anatomic sites are labeled.
(Photograph by Berto Tarin, Multimedia Department, Western University of Health Sciences.)

ter, actually taupe (gray-brown) in color, does the work of the brain. Gray matter consists of neuronal cell bodies, dendrites, and synapses and is not myelinated (myelinated axons make up the white matter). The cerebral cortex of the cerebrum is divided into four lobes: the frontal, temporal, parietal, and occipital lobes (see Figures 5-1, 5-2). Visual examination of the brain reveals the raised areas, or convolutions, and the grooves between these areas. Convoluted gray matter is referred to as a *gyrus* (plural, *gyri*), and the groove between two gyri is called a *sulcus* (plural, *sulci*). A deep sulcus is referred to as a *fissure*.

The net effect of this convoluted configuration is that more gray matter is provided to perform the work of the brain. This principle can be visualized by considering the coastline of Norway. If Norway did not have the fjords, its coastline would then be

rather small (i.e., approximately 1600 miles). However, because of the fjords, the actual coastline of Norway is extraordinary for a country of its size (i.e., approximately 12,500 miles). The gyri and sulci of the cerebral cortex are the "fjords" of the brain. The indentations provide for a much larger "coastline" of "working" gray matter than would be true if the brain's surface were smooth. The four lobes of the cerebral cortex are divided by three sulci.

Frontal lobes

The frontal lobes are divided into the *motor* (also called the *motor strip*), *premotor,* and *prefrontal areas.* The motor cortex lies immediately rostral to (in front of) the central sulcus (see Figure 5-1), which separates the frontal and parietal lobes. Because it lies in front of the central sulcus, the motor strip is also

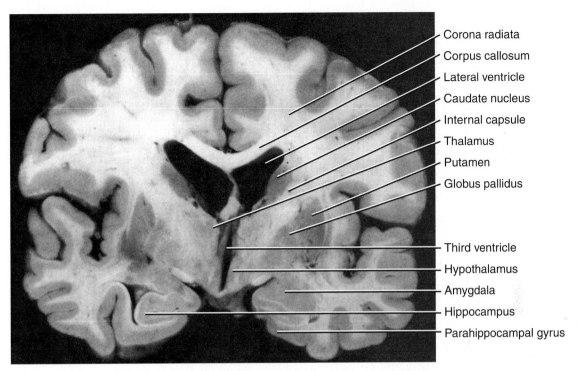

- Corona radiata
- Corpus callosum
- Lateral ventricle
- Caudate nucleus
- Internal capsule
- Thalamus
- Putamen
- Globus pallidus
- Third ventricle
- Hypothalamus
- Amygdala
- Hippocampus
- Parahippocampal gyrus

Figure 5-3 CORONAL SECTION OF THE CEREBRUM. Level of the hypothalamus is shown. (Courtesy Richard E. Powers, MD, University of Alabama, Birmingham, Brain Resource Program.)

called the *precentral gyrus.* The motor cortex controls voluntary motor activity, and the pathway (see Figure 5-4) from this area descends through the corona radiata and the internal capsule, crosses in the caudal brainstem, and synapses in the spinal cord. Approximately 80% of the corticospinal tract crosses over at the level of the lower brainstem (medulla oblongata), while the remaining 20% of the neurons descend down the spinal cord ipsilaterally (same side) before they cross over to the opposite side of the spinal cord. This remaining 20% of the corticospinal tract may be theoretically responsible for some limited motor recovery in patients with hemisected spinal cords; but the incidence of any actual recovery is rare at best. From the spinal cord, spinal nerves branch out into the periphery and connect to muscles. This system of voluntary movement is referred to as the *pyramidal system* or the *corticospinal tract* (pathway). The term *pyramidal* is used because many of the neurons in this tract pass through the pyramids of the lower (or caudal) brainstem (medulla oblongata). The extrapyramidal motor system lies outside the pyramids.

CLINICAL EXAMPLE

Think about wiggling the right big toe and then wiggle it. What is not known is the way in which a thought is translated into muscle movement. What is known is that this voluntary movement is a two-neuron system; that is, neurons from the motor cortex descend as described and synapse with spinal neurons. The spinal neurons project as a spinal nerve from the spinal cord and descend to the toe. The neurons from the motor cortex to the spinal cord are called *upper motor neurons* (see Figure 5-4). The neurons that project from the spinal cord down to the toe are *lower motor neurons.* Whether a disease is an upper motor neuron disease (e.g., stroke) or a lower motor neuron disease (e.g., polio) is clinically significant. An upper motor lesion normally results in a contralateral (body side opposite of the lesion) Babinski's sign. A lower motor neuron lesion normally results in flaccid paralysis.

The premotor area is associated with movement patterns for voluntary motor activity and with inhibiting lower motor neurons from overreacting to stimuli (Kandel, Schwartz, Jessell, 2000). This area

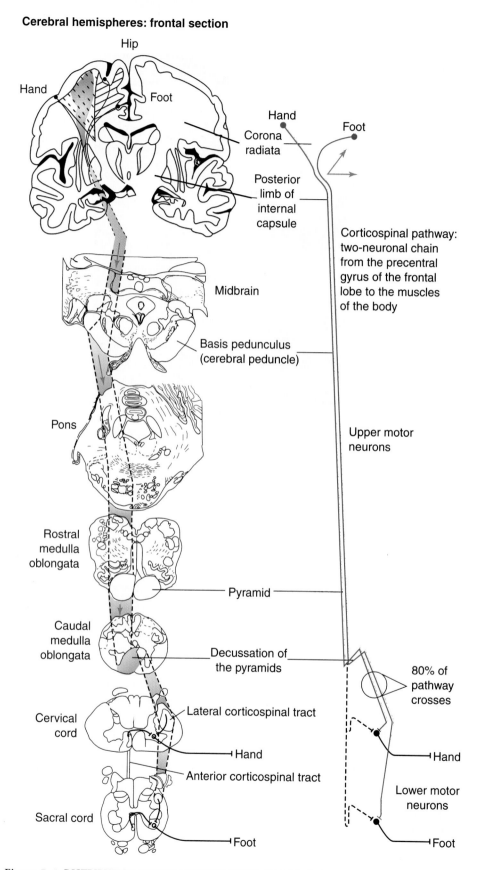

Cerebral hemispheres: frontal section

Hip

Hand

Foot

Hand

Foot

Corona radiata

Posterior limb of internal capsule

Corticospinal pathway: two-neuronal chain from the precentral gyrus of the frontal lobe to the muscles of the body

Midbrain

Basis pedunculus (cerebral peduncle)

Pons

Upper motor neurons

Rostral medulla oblongata

Pyramid

Caudal medulla oblongata

Decussation of the pyramids

80% of pathway crosses

Cervical cord

Lateral corticospinal tract

Hand

Hand

Anterior corticospinal tract

Lower motor neurons

Sacral cord

Foot

Foot

Figure 5-4 DISTRIBUTION OF THE CORTICOSPINAL TRACT. *Left,* Actual representation; *right,* schematic representation.

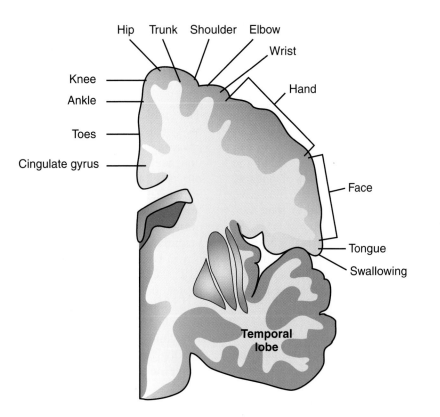

Figure 5-5 HOMUNCULUS OF THE PRECENTRAL GYRUS. This frontal section depicts the relative amount of cortex subserved in controlling the motor functions of various body areas.

is not under conscious control. Many movement disorders, including those associated with psychotropic drug use, arise from the premotor cortex and extrapyramidal system. Both the motor cortex and the premotor cortex are organized systematically (Kandel, Schwartz, Jessell, 2000). This arrangement is referred to as *somatotropic organization,* meaning simply that the area of the motor strip that controls a certain part of the body is relatively specific. This biologic reality has been visually depicted as a little person or, more commonly, a homunculus (Figure 5-5). Perhaps a word picture can best describe this specific pattern of voluntary motor localization. Think of a child hanging on the monkey bars with her head down and her feet hanging over the bar. Think of the top of the hemisphere as the bar, with the head hanging down laterally and one foot hanging down between the hemispheres.

The area of the motor strip where the head is located controls head movements, and the area where the foot hangs controls foot movements, and so on.

A health professional can give a physical examination to a person with a neurologic lesion (i.e., stroke, gunshot wound) and, using knowledge of the corticospinal tract and homunculus (see Figures 5-4, 5-5), can often predict the site of cortical lesions in the CNS. Knowing the location of the cranial nuclei allows the examiner to localize brainstem lesions. Two classic vascular lesions (Kiernan, 1998) in the brainstem illustrate the way in which a health care professional can diagnose a lesion site by understanding the location of brainstem structures. A patient who presents with ipsilateral paralysis of four of the six extraocular eye muscles and contralateral hemiparesis ("weakness" of all the body muscles on the opposite side) most likely had a vascular accident on one side of the midbrain toward the midline (see Figure 5-4, midbrain). A lesion affecting one half of the midbrain can affect the oculomotor nerve (lower motor neuron) and the corticospinal pathway (upper motor neuron), causing the observed signs. In a second example, a patient who presents with contralateral hemiparesis, ipsilateral loss of sensory position and discriminative touch, and ipsilateral paralysis of the tongue most likely had a vascular lesion on one side of the rostral medulla oblongata toward the midline (see Figure 5-4, rostral medulla oblongata). In both cases, the specific cranial nerves that have been damaged indicate the CNS level of these vascular accidents.

The prefrontal area of the cerebral cortex is responsible for thought, goal-oriented behavior, and inhibition. The frontal poles represent the seat of the personality; injuries in this area result in personality changes.

Temporal lobes

The temporal lobes lie inferior to the *lateral sulci* (the *lateral fissures of Sylvius*). Each temporal lobe is divided into an olfactory area, a primary auditory receptive area, secondary auditory association area, and a visual association area (Bear, Connors, Paradiso, 2001). Aphasias, both visual and auditory, are the result of damage to the temporal lobe. Individuals with visual aphasia cannot recognize words in print that they previously understood; the words are as unrecognizable as printed Russian would be to most people. People with auditory aphasia hear sounds but cannot associate the sounds with meaning.

Parietal lobes

The parietal lobes are posterior to the central sulcus. These primarily sensory-association areas contain a sensory strip (the postcentral gyrus) that roughly corresponds to the homunculus of the motor strip. The sensory areas interpret sensations. Caudal to this area are the association areas of the parietal lobes.

Occipital lobes

The occipital lobes are divided into visual receptive areas and visual association areas. In contrast to temporal lobe lesions, which can produce various types of visual aphasias, lesions in the occipital lobe's visual association cortex will result in loss of vision (blind-ness) from the contralateral visual field; that is, total damage of left side occipital visual association cortex results in loss of vision from the right visual field. The primary function of the occipital lobes is vision.

Limbic system

The limbic lobe forms the central core of the limbic system and is composed of the septal area, cingulate gyrus, and parahippocampal gyrus (see Figures 5-2, 5-3). The limbic lobe is built on the olfactory (smell) system. The *limbic system* is a broad term, referring to the limbic lobe and the structures that function with it: the frontal cortex, hypothalamus, amygdala, hippocampus, numerous tracts, brainstem nuclei, and the autonomic system. The way in which emotions and motivation are generated in the limbic system remains unclear. No specific anatomic areas exist that are correlated for love, hate, dislike, and so forth. Each emotion is likely diffusely linked to different limbic and nonlimbic areas. The limbic system controls the four Fs (feeding, fighting, fleeing, and fornicating), memory, the sense of pleasure, emotions, and motivation.

Limbic olfactory function

The first pathway discussed is the olfactory pathway, which is concerned with odor detection, feeding, and feeling pleasure. This chapter does not discuss odor detection beyond its relationship to limbic functions. Understanding the way in which significant smell relates to emotion is important. Large department stores have recognized for years that having a perfume display sells more than perfume alone.

Olfactory information is picked up by receptor neurons in the nasal cavity and transmitted to the olfactory bulbs, which are located directly under the surface of the frontal lobes. The olfactory bulbs project axons that synapse in the parahippocampal gyrus and a subdivision of the amygdala (see Figure 5-3).

Feeding functions

The septal area, which connects neuronally with the hypothalamus, is involved in several aspects of feeding (e.g., hypothalamic feeding and satiety centers). Experimentally, researchers can electrically stimulate or destroy these hypothalamic areas and affect whether an animal overeats or stops eating.

Fight or flight limbic function

The fight or flight pathway is composed of three major areas: amygdala, hypothalamus, and midbrain. Electric stimulation of these areas elicits rage behavior or flight. Bilateral destroying of the amygdala and selected areas in the hypothalamus can have a calming effect.

Memory limbic function

The limbic system is crucial to memory. The amygdala and the hippocampus, located deep in the temporal lobe, are key structures in the transfer of information from short-term to long-term memory (Bear, Connors, Paradiso, 2001). The *Papez circuit* consists of brain structures that are involved in the complex process by which memories are made and stored. Discussion of the Papez circuit is beyond the scope of this book; however, the reader should recognize that lesions along this circuit cause memory problems. For example, bilateral lesions of the hippocampus nuclei can be the result of anoxia from near drownings, and lesions of the mammillary bodies resulting in memory problems can occur in alcoholics because of a thiamine deficiency (i.e., Korsakoff's psychosis). These individuals frequently maintain long-term memory, but they cannot "make" new memories.

Amnestic states, amnestic dementias, punch-drunk syndrome, herpes encephalitis, and Alzheimer's disease involve dysfunction of the hippocampi and possibly other limbic structures (Boss, Stowe, 1986).

Pleasure

Electric stimulation of the reward pathway can cause animals and people to feel pleasure. Rats will press a bar repeatedly to receive electric stimulation to this pathway. The dopaminergic neurons projecting from the ventral tegmental area (VTA) (Figure 5-6) are of particular importance. These brainstem neurons project rostrally to the cortical and limbic areas, particularly the nucleus accumbens. Recently, investigators have hypothesized that cocaine and many other drugs produce effects by increasing the action of dopamine in the nucleus accumbens (Figure 5-7). The nucleus accumbens is said to be one of the brain's key pleasure centers. The nucleus accumbens is within the septal area (see Figure 5-2). Additionally, electric stimulation of the septal area has elicited sexual arousal in both animals and people. Likely, the nucleus accumbens, which is located in the septal area, is the nucleus responsible for sexual arousal (Heath, 1972).

Emotions and motivation functions

The emotions and motivation component includes the "feelings" about people, institutions, and life that affect behavior. For example, feelings help determine whether an act is right or wrong, good or bad, and whether a particular act will be performed. Most authors refer to these feelings as *visceral aspects of behavior.*

Basal ganglia

Strictly speaking, the basal ganglia (see Figure 5-3) are made up of three major nuclei: the caudate nucleus, the putamen, and the globus pallidus. These structures are also involved in motor functions. The putamen and globus pallidus together are referred to as the lentiform nucleus (lens shaped). The basal ganglia, or extrapyramidal system, including the substantia nigra (see Figure 5-6), resides between the midbrain and cerebral cortex and communicates back and forth about ongoing motor activity from the body. The basal ganglia system complements the pyramidal system. The pyramidal (or corticospinal) tract transmits commands for voluntary movement, and the basal ganglia system modulates these movements, maintains appropriate muscle tone, and adjusts posture. For example, when the hand is extended and the fingers are held still, slight oscillations of the fingers will occur. The basal ganglia system, which includes some motor pathways, works with the pyramidal system to keep these movements small.

The basal ganglia system balances excitatory and inhibitory neurons that have different neurotransmitters. Dopamine is the primary inhibitory neurotransmitter, and acetylcholine is the primary excitatory neurotransmitter. Gamma-aminobutyric acid (GABA) is another important inhibitory neurotransmitter in this system. Any significant decrease or increase in these neurotransmitters can result in basal ganglia (extrapyramidal) motor signs.

The basal ganglia system affects the contralateral side of the body. (A basal ganglia stroke affects the

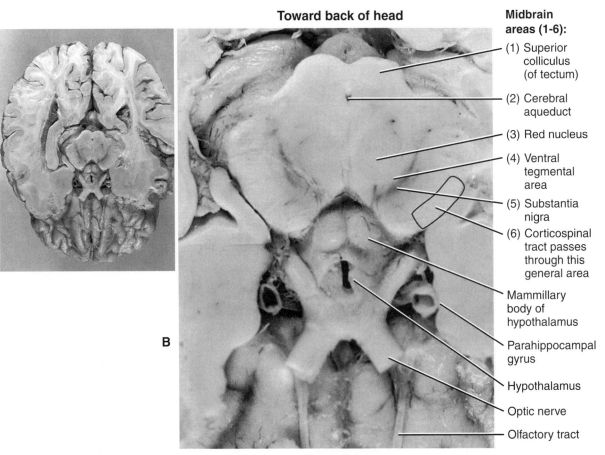

Toward back of head

Midbrain areas (1-6):

(1) Superior colliculus (of tectum)

(2) Cerebral aqueduct

(3) Red nucleus

(4) Ventral tegmental area

(5) Substantia nigra

(6) Corticospinal tract passes through this general area

Mammillary body of hypothalamus

Parahippocampal gyrus

Hypothalamus

Optic nerve

Olfactory tract

A

B

Toward face

Figure 5-6 A, Brain is sectioned transversely through the midbrain and parahippocampal gyri. B, Enlargement of the area through the midbrain is shown. (Photographs by Berto Tarin, Multimedia Department, Western University of Health Sciences.)

opposite side of the body.) Because this system maintains muscle tone and posture, movements are most noticeable during rest. For instance, Parkinson's disease, an extrapyramidal disorder, manifests with a resting tremor. These unwanted movements diminish with concentration and with intentional movement and are absent during sleep.

In summary, the pyramidal tract or corticospinal tract *controls* precise, voluntary movements; the basal ganglia, in conjunction with the cerebellum, *stabilize* motor movements. Lesions of the basal ganglia result in abnormal motor movements, such as those present in Parkinson's disease (resulting from decreased dopamine bioavailability from the substantia nigra) and Huntington's disease (chorea) (resulting from

alterations in GABA and the cholinergic system). All of the basal ganglia areas receive, integrate, and transmit motor information.

Critical **Thinking Questions**

1. What disease do you produce when you block the substantia nigra's dopamine from crossing the synapse at the next brain site (basal ganglia)?
2. What might happen to a person with an over-production of cerebral dopamine?
3. How might a pituitary gland tumor affect a person's hormone production, body development, and behavior? What signs or symptoms would you use to differentiate a left or right side cerebral hemisphere stroke?

Diencephalon

The diencephalon (see Figures 5-2, 5-3, 5-6) is made up of the thalamus, hypothalamus, epithalamus (including the pineal gland), and subthalamus. Although all of the nuclei of the diencephalon are important, only a brief review of the thalamus and the hypothalamus is provided in this text. The thalamus is the major sensory-basal ganglia relay nuclear area to and from the cerebral cortex. All sensory pathways, except the olfactory pathways, synapse in the thalamus (Kiernan, 1998). Sensory fibers ascend to and synapse in the thalamus and are then relayed to the cerebral cortex via the internal capsule and corona radiata (see Figure 5-3). The hypothalamus maintains homeostasis and is the controller of the autonomic nervous system. The hypothalamus (Kiernan, 1998) is a tiny, 4-gram structure positioned below the thalamus, which modulates visceral functions such as body temperature regulation, gastrointestinal activity, and cardiovascular functions. The hypothalamus also serves as a chemoreceptor by "sampling" cerebrospinal fluid and blood. The hypothalamus controls and influences functions such as food and water intake and endocrine secretion. The hypothalamus has two modes for affecting the pituitary gland. (The following numbers refer to Figure 5-8.) The first mode is (1) by the production of releasing and inhibiting hormones or factors that pass into the pituitary portal system (PPS), such as thyrotropin-releasing hormone or prolactin-releasing factor (PRF). These factors are transmitted to the anterior pituitary (2), where they cause the release or inhibition of anterior pituitary hormones into the blood of the PPS. The second mode is by the direct projection of hypothalamic neurons (3) into the posterior pituitary, where the neurons directly release their hormones (e.g., oxytocin) into the pituitary blood supply (4). Table 5-1 summarizes the hormonal cascade from the hypothalamus and some of the resulting clinical effects. As in the age-old question, "What came first, the chicken or the egg?" an increase or decrease in a specific hormone during mental illness fails to explain whether the changes are a cause of the illness or a result of the illness. Normally, all hormones are in careful balance. Additionally, lesions of the subthalamic nucleus can result in hemiballismus (Box 5-1).

Brainstem

The brainstem, cerebellum, and spinal cord reside beneath the cerebrum (see Figure 5-1). The brainstem is a collective term for the midbrain, pons, and

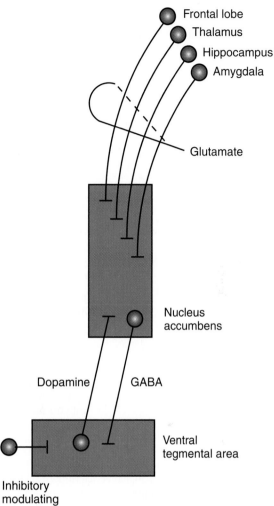

Figure 5-7 Mesolimbic pathway (system), which is identified as the primary pathway involved in substance abuse and in feeling pleasure. The ventral tegmental area (VTA) projects dopamine neurons to the nucleus accumbens. Opioids inhibit the modulating areas that affect the VTA and allow increased amounts of dopamine to be released in the nucleus accumbens, enhancing the reward aspects of the opioids. Glutamate neurons from the prefrontal cortex, thalamus, amygdala, and hippocampus project to the nucleus accumbens. A GABA pathway also exists from the nucleus accumbens to the VTA. The mesolimbic pathway includes many limbic structures. *GABA,* Gamma-aminobutyric acid.

medulla oblongata. The cerebellum is an expansive area attached to the posterior surface of the pons and resembles its Latin name, *little brain.* The most caudal portion of the CNS is the spinal cord (not

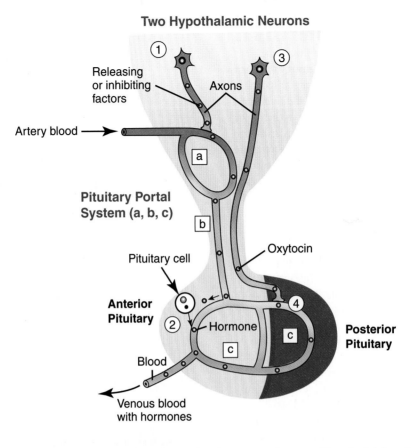

Figure 5-8 PITUITARY PORTAL SYSTEM (PPS). The PPS has a capillary bed *(a)* at the base of the hypothalamus, a capillary bed *(c)* in the pituitary gland, and a portal vein *(b)* in between. Hypothalamic neurons *(1, 3)* make hormones (i.e., neurotransmitters). Neuron *(1)* releases its hormone into capillary bed *(a)*, and the hormone descends through the portal vessel *(b)* into the pituitary gland capillary bed *(c)*. The hormone leaves the capillary bed and causes anterior pituitary gland cells to release specific hormones back into the capillary *(2)* for transport to glands or cells elsewhere in the body. A few hormones from the hypothalamus inhibit the production of pituitary gland cell hormones. Neuron *(3)* directly releases its hormone (e.g., oxytocin) into the posterior pituitary portion of the capillary bed *(c)*. The hormone again leaves in the blood *(4)* and travels to glands or cells elsewhere in the body.

discussed in this chapter). The reticular formation is an important pathway that spans the brainstem.

Midbrain

The midbrain (see Figure 5-6), which represents the continuation of the CNS below the cerebrum, is approximately 1.5 cm in length and is relatively narrow. The red nuclei and substantia nigra are large structures in the midbrain that can be easily distinguished on gross examination. The red nuclei in freshly cut brains are large, reddish, round balls; the

substantia nigra, as its name implies, is black. The black coloration is the result of melanin pigment found in neurons within the substantia nigra. From these dark cells, most of the brain dopamine is synthesized. In Parkinson's disease, these cells are depigmented, and less dopamine is produced. Dopamine deficiency causes the extrapyramidal motor disorders associated with Parkinson's disease. The VTA, which projects dopaminergic tracts to the limbic and corticol areas, is a midline structure medial and rostral to the red nucleus.

|Table 5-1| Classification of Neurotransmitters and Pathways

Neurotransmitter	Chemical Transmitter	Location Found	Major Pathways
Cholinergic systems	ACh	Myoneural junctions, autonomic ganglia, parasympathetic postganglionic neurons	Basal nucleus of Meynert to cerebral cortex, septal area (rostral to hypothalamus) to hippocampus
Monoamine systems	Catecholamines • Dopamine	Substantia nigra Ventral tegmental area	• Nigrostriatal • Mesolimbic • Mesocortical • Tuberoinfundibular
	• Norepinephrine	Locus ceruleus	Locus ceruleus (in pons) to thalamus, cerebral cortex, cerebellum, and spinal cord; lateral midbrain to hypothalamus and basal forebrain
	• Epinephrine	Red nucleus	Central tegmental tract
	Indolamine • Serotonin	Raphe nuclei	Central brainstem nuclei up to forebrain and down to spinal cord
Neuropeptides	Enkephalins Endorphins Substance P	Spinal cord, hypothalamus, midbrain Spinal cord, hypothalamus, midbrain Spinal cord, hypothalamus, and many other places	
	Somatostatin, VIP, CCK, ACTH, neurotensin, angiotensin II, and others		
Amino acids	GABA Glycine	Most common transmitter in brain Spinal cord, brainstem, and many other CNS areas	
	Glutamate Aspartate	Widely distributed in the CNS Hippocampus, dorsal root ganglion	

ACh, Acetylcholine; *ACTH*, adrenocorticotropic hormone; *CCK*, cholecystokinin; *CNS*, central nervous system; *GABA*, gamma-aminobutyric acid; *VIP*, vasoactive intestinal polypeptide. (From Keltner NL, Folks DG: *Psychotropic drugs*, ed 3, St Louis, 2001, Mosby.)
This table presents a simplified summary of many of the better-known neurotransmitters and, in general, where they are produced and released in the nervous system.

|Box 5-1| Differences Between Basal Ganglia and Cerebellar Movement Disorders

General Difference
- Cerebellar dysfunction: awkwardness of intentional movement
- Basal ganglia dysfunction: meaningless, unintentional movement that occurs unexpectedly

Cerebellar Disorders
1. Ataxia: awkwardness of posture and gait; lack of coordination; overshooting the goal when reaching for an object; inability to perform rapid, alternating movements, such as finger tapping; awkward use of speech muscles, resulting in irregularly spaced sounds
2. Decreased tendon reflexes on affected side
3. Asthenia: muscles tire easily
4. Intention tremor: noticed when intending to do something, such as reaching for a pencil
5. Nystagmus

Basal Ganglia Disorders
1. Parkinsonism: rigidity, bradykinesia, resting tremor, masklike face, shuffling gait
2. Chorea: sudden, jerky, and purposeless movements (e.g., Huntington's disease, Sydenham's chorea)
3. Athetosis: slow, writhing, snakelike movements, especially of fingers and wrists
4. Hemiballismus: a sudden, wild flailing of one arm

Adapted from Goldberg S: *Clinical neuroanatomy*, Miami, 1990, MedMaster.

Pons

The *pons,* which literally means bridge, forms a link between the midbrain and the medulla oblongata. The pons is a bulbous area approximately 2.5 cm in length that lies between the midbrain and the medulla oblongata and is anterior to the cerebellum. Some pathway fibers descending from the cerebrum pass through the midbrain and terminate in the pons. The pontine nuclei project motor and posture information to the cerebellum.

Medulla oblongata

The medulla oblongata is approximately 3 cm in length and narrows until it becomes continuous with the cervical spinal cord. Many cerebral cortex motor fibers that are in the midbrain and travel through the pons continue their descent on the anterior surface of the medulla oblongata; these fibers collectively form pyramidal shaped bulges known as the *pyramids.* The decussation of the pyramids—that is, the crossing over of the lateral corticospinal motor pathway contralaterally (to the opposite side)—takes place at the lower end of the medulla oblongata (see Figure 5-4). This crossing over is the reason that a right brain stroke results in left-side impairment. The medulla oblongata is responsible for many important functions, including respiration, regulation of blood pressure, partial regulation of heart rate, vomiting, and swallowing.

Reticular formation

A multineural pathway called the reticular formation resides within the brainstem. This pathway comprises a series of large nuclei, beginning within the midbrain, and extending through the pons and the medulla oblongata. The reticular formation may be thought of as a primitive brain buried deep within the brainstem. Input from most sensory pathways passes into the reticular formation, where it is integrated and then projected to areas such as the thalamus and hypothalamus. The reticular formation affects motor, sensory, and visceral functions.

The reticular activating system (RAS), which is part of the reticular formation, serves as a screening device that allows individuals to "tune out" some stimuli and attend to other stimuli. The ability to tune out is fortunate; otherwise, studying or even sleeping in some environments would be impossible. The RAS allows humans to fall asleep. The RAS is activated by sensory stimuli, pain, movement, feedback from the cortex, muscle tone, and sympathomimetic drugs (stimulants). Any of these factors help a person remain awake. Because of its many synapses, the RAS can be depressed easily. When a disruption occurs in the RAS and a person cannot sleep, psychosis can occur. When the RAS is "turned off," however, coma results. Some people have had their RASs deactivated, and no one knows how to reactivate it.

Cerebellum

The cerebellum (see Figures 5-1, 5-2) consists of two hemispheres separated by a central portion called the *vermis.* The cerebellar hemispheres and most of the vermis simultaneously receive sensory input from muscles and joints and receive motor signals from the cerebral cortex, indicating the way in which muscles are to be directed. Most of the cerebellum then communicates with the cerebral cortex through the thalamus to coordinate the final motor activity. Writing with a pen, reading a book, shooting a basketball, and climbing a mountain are possible because of a functioning cerebellum. Most of the cerebellum coordinates muscle synergy and activity but does *not* initiate movement. The second function of the cerebellum is the maintenance of equilibrium. Differences between movement disorders associated with cerebellar dysfunction and movement disorders associated with basal ganglia dysfunction are found in Box 5-1.

Cerebellar dysfunction can produce intention tremors that are on the same side of the body as is the lesion. Dissimilar to the basal ganglia resting tremors, which occur at rest, intention tremors occur when a person is asked to touch something, such as their own nose or a doctor's moving finger. These people have tremors when they attempt to concentrate on moving a limb.

NEURONS AND NEUROTRANSMITTERS

Neurons are the basic subunit of the nervous system. The brain contains *100 billion* neurons. The neuron is composed of a cell body with a large nucleus. The cell body and dendrites of the neuron make up the gray matter of the cortex and the brain nuclei. Neurons transmit information by sending action potentials, or waves of electric depolarization, down their processes to other neurons. Two processes project from the cell body: *dendrites* and *axons.* The dendrites receive impulses from other neurons and transmit these impulses to the cell body. Axons carry impulses away from the cell body to another neuron, muscle, or gland. Each neuron usually projects only one axon. Some axons are up to 3 feet in length but are microscopically thin. Some axons can synapse with thousands of dendrites, and the dendrites of one neuron can receive impulses from the axons of thousands of other neurons (Bear, Connors, Paradiso, 2001). The brain is extremely complex, and knowledge of this intricate wiring schematic continues to develop.

Neurons can be divided into three basic types: sensory neurons (or afferent neurons) that send messages to the CNS, motor neurons (or efferent neurons) that send messages from the CNS to the periphery, and association neurons (or interneurons) that lie between sensory and motor neurons. The vast majority of CNS neurons are association neurons. Most impulses (action potentials) travel from one neuron to another by sending a chemical called a *neurotransmitter* across a 20-nm space (the synapse), which separates these cells, to evoke the next action potential. Many drugs have their site of action in the nervous system in or around the synapse.

Neurotransmitters have been divided into four major groups or systems: cholinergic, monoamines, neuropeptides, and amino acids. Table 5-2 provides a summary of the four major groups of neurotransmitters. Specific examples for each group, the location of concentrations of these specific transmitters in the brain, and major pathways in the brain that use these neurotransmitters are found in this table. Neurotransmitters are thought to play major roles in some mental disorders (Table 5-3).

Table 5-2	Neurotransmitters and Related Mental Disorders*
Neurotransmitter	**Mental Disorder**
Increase (↑) in dopamine	Schizophrenia
Decrease (↓) in norepinephrine	Depression
Decrease (↓) in serotonin	Depression
Decrease (↓) in acetylcholine	Alzheimer's disease
Decrease (↓) in GABA	Anxiety

*This is a simplified explanation. A more refined explanation will be offered in appropriate chapters.

AUTONOMIC NERVOUS SYSTEM

The autonomic nervous system (Figure 5-9) is divided into the parasympathetic (craniosacral) and the sympathetic (thoracolumbar) nervous systems. The parasympathetic nervous system, which is a cholinergic system, conserves energy and is divided into cranial and sacral portions. The cranial part has neuronal components within the oculomotor (CN III), facial (CN VII), glossopharyngeal (CN IX), and vagus (CN X) cranial nerves; the sacral part is composed of neuronal elements located in the second through the fourth sacral spinal cord areas. Parasympathetic neurons are of particular interest to psychiatric nurses because of the many psychotropic drugs that have anticholinergic properties. Anticholinergic drugs block the function of these nerves; for example, CN III affects pupil and ciliary body constriction, CN VII affects tearing and salivation, CN IX affects salivation, and CN X affects the vagus nerve (e.g., the heart, gastrointestinal [GI] tract). Thus anticholinergic effects on these nerves cause dilated pupils, decreased lacrimation, dry mouth, tachycardia, and a slowed GI system, respectively.

The sympathetic nervous system expends energy and forms a continuous column running from the first thoracic to the third lumbar spinal cord areas. Although sympathetic neuron cell bodies are confined within portions of the thoracic and lumbar spinal cord, sympathetic neurons innervate effector organs throughout the body.

Both the sympathetic and the parasympathetic systems contain two neurons between the spinal cord and the effector organs. The first neuronal cell body is in the spinal cord, and its myelinated axon extends from the spinal cord to synapse with a peripheral neuron. The first neuron in the system is referred to as the *preganglionic neuron;* the second is the *postganglionic neuron.* Preganglionic neurons secrete acetylcholine as their neurotransmitter (see Figure 5-9). The postganglionic neurons send their unmyelinated axons to their effector organs: smooth muscle, cardiac muscle, or glands. Generally, the parasympathetic postganglionic neurons secrete acetylcholine, and the sympathetic postganglionic neurons secrete norepinephrine as their neurotransmitters.

The hypothalamus has both sympathetic and parasympathetic functions and is considered the high-

|Table 5–3| Hormonal Cascade from the Hypothalamus to Behavioral Effects

Hypothalamus-Made Hormones	Pituitary Gland	Target Gland or Hormone	Behavioral Affect
CRH	Stimulates production of two hormones: • ACTH • β-Endorphin	Adrenal gland, which produces cortisol and cortisol-related hormones ACTH drives cortisol production	1. Stress causes the release of cortisol 2. Depressed children have decreased diurnal cortisol secretory pattern 3. Depressed adolescents have increased cortisol around sleep onset 4. CRH increases in patient with PTSD 5. Patients with PTSD have a blunted ACTH response to CRH 6. β-Endorphin is involved in the endorphin pleasure pathway and thus feeling good
TRH	Stimulates production of TSH	Thyroid gland produces thyroxine and T_3	1. Adding T_3 to an antidepressant regimen may potentiate medication's response 2. In PTSD, T_3 is increased
GHIH (somatostatin)	Inhibits GH	GH stimulates body growth	Depressed children have blunted GH response to some drugs
ADH (vasopressin)	Released in pituitary portal system in pituitary	ADH affects renal tubules in kidneys for water retention	1. Involved in memory acquisition, storage, and retrieval 2. May be linked to polydipsic behavior in patients with schizophrenia
Oxytocin	Released in pituitary portal system in pituitary	Affects myoepithelial cells in mammillary glands for milk release	Involved in memory consolidation and retrieval
PRF	Stimulates production of prolactin	Mammillary glands, which produce milk	No significant effects
LHRH	Stimulates the production of two hormones: • LH • FSH	LH • Stimulates corpus luteum (female) to produce progesterone • Stimulates interstitial cells (male) to produce testosterone FSH • Stimulates follicle (female) to produce estrogen • Stimulates seminiferous tubules (male) to facilitate testosterone production	No significant effects

ACTH, Adrenocorticotropic hormone; *ADH*, antidiuretic hormone; *CRH*, corticotropin-releasing hormone; *FSH*, follicle-stimulating hormone; *GH*, growth hormone; *GHIH*, growth hormone-inhibiting hormone; *LH*, leutinizing hormone; *LHRH*, gonadotropin-releasing hormone; *PRF*, prolactin-releasing factor; *PTSD*, posttraumatic stress disorder; *TRH*, thyroid-releasing hormone; *TSH*, thyroid-stimulating hormone; T_3, triiodothyroxine.

This table lists (1) hypothalamic hormones and states whether they are releasing or inhibiting, (2) the specific hormones that they affect in the anterior pituitary gland (Griffin, Ojeda, 2000), (3) the way in which they affect that hormone production, (4) the target glands or body cells that are affected, and (5) the proposed affects of these hormones on behavior (Charney, Nestler, Bunney, 1999). Antidiuretic hormone and oxytocin are released directly into the blood thus they do not affect pituitary gland cells.

est autonomic center in the CNS. The hypothalamus can drive both systems selectively (see Figure 5-9).

VENTRICULAR SYSTEM

The brain "floats" in approximately 140 cc (approximately the volume of a small cup of coffee) of cerebrospinal fluid (CSF); however, the CNS produces approximately 800 cc of fluid per day. CSF circulates around the brain in the subarachnoid space and inside ventricles in the brain. Three connective tissue layers, known as *meninges,* cover the brain. The subarachnoid space is a narrow space between the middle meningeal layer (the arachnoid) and the innermost layer (the pia mater), which adheres to the brain. The thick outer layer, the dura mater, attaches to the inner surface of many bones of the skull. The ventricles form four spaces within the brain (see Figure 5-3). One large

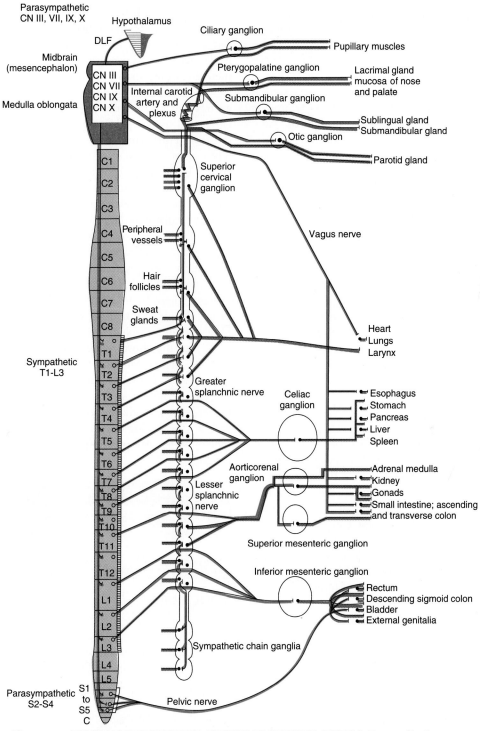

Figure 5-9 DIAGRAM OF THE ENTIRE AUTONOMIC NERVOUS SYSTEM. Preganglionic neurons are represented as green lines; the postganglionic neurons are represented as blue lines. The dorsal longitudinal fasciculus (DLF) (represented as a red line) interconnects the hypothalamus with parasympathetic and sympathetic autonomic neurons down to the sacral spinal cord level.

ventricle resides in each cerebral hemisphere, and small third and fourth ventricles are located, respectively, in the midbrain and between the pons and the cerebellum. The fourth ventricle communicates with the subarachnoid space. Eventually, the CSF in the subarachnoid space enters the vascular system through arachnoid villi that protrude into the superior sagittal sinus on the superior surface of the brain. If, for some reason, the arachnoid villi are compromised, such as from a head trauma or meningitis, the CSF then builds up quickly.

Enlargement of the ventricles occurs because of (1) blockage of the CSF outflow within or from the brain, (2) overproduction of CSF, (3) brain atrophy resulting from the death of large numbers of cortical neurons, and (4) neurodevelopmental problems. The first two problems are causes of hydrocephalus, while brain atrophy (neurodegeneration) is commonly found in chronic alcoholics and patients with Alzheimer's disease. Neurodevelopmental problems resulting in ventricular variance is thought to be associated with schizophrenia (Charney, Nestler, Bunney, 1999). In the case of neurodegeneration, creation of new space results in the ventricles enlarging to fill the void.

CLINICAL APPLICATION

As is stressed throughout this text, many mental disorders have biologic bases. A brief overview of these biologic influences is presented here, but the major discussion of these issues is found in the respective disorder chapter. This approach is in concert with the authors' view that the biologic context of mental disorders is intricately linked to symptoms and behaviors and is part of a holistic approach to understanding psychiatric patients. Placing most of the specific discussion of the psychobiologic parameters of mental disorders in a separate chapter titled "psychobiology" reinforces the mindset that this etiologic view is only one of many from which the student can select. The authors believe differently. Thus the student is urged to use this chapter to review brain anatomy and physiology and to apply this information to other chapters.

Schizophrenia

Several psychobiologic influences on schizophrenia have been proposed. First, researchers have noted that an increase in ventricular size is apparent in many people with schizophrenia (Charney, Nestler, Bunney, 1999). As mentioned, ventricles enlarge for one of four reasons. In schizophrenia, increased ventricle size is most likely related to neurodevelopmental reasons; that is, the brain around the ventricles has failed to develop, and the ventricles are enlarged to fill the empty space. This phenomenon is referred to as an increase in *ventricular brain ratios* (VBRs). Furthermore, in many individuals with schizophrenia, a decrease in the gray matter of the cortex and major subcortical nuclei is evident.

Other biologic differences found in people with schizophrenia include a decrease in cerebral blood flow, particularly in the prefrontal areas of the cortex. The term used to describe this condition is *hypofrontality* (Charney, Nestler, Bunney, 1999). Imaging technology that tracks blood flow and glucose metabolism has substantiated this physiologic change. These brain changes result in a decline in frontal cognitive functions, such as organizing, planning, learning, problem solving, and critical thinking.

By far, the most celebrated and widely known biologic theory for schizophrenia is the dopamine hypothesis. According to this theory, schizophrenia is caused by alterations of dopamine in the brain. Chapter 28 provides an elaboration of this theory and of the biologically related genetic theory of schizophrenia. Antipsychotics are discussed in Chapter 20.

> ### *Critical* Thinking Question
>
> In some patients with schizophrenia, a decrease in blood flow has been detected in the dorsolateral prefrontal area. If that were true, then what kind of symptoms might you expect to see?

Mood Disorders

Mood disorders are also thought to have a biologic basis. Decreased amounts of norepinephrine and serotonin, two important brain neurotransmitters, are thought to play a role in depression (see Table 5-3). Apparently, an overall deficiency exists in these neurotransmitters, and psychopharmacologic treatment is based on restoring these to optimal levels. More recent findings suggest that other neurotransmitters may also be factors in depression. For instance, some researchers find evidence for the involvement of acetylcholine, dopamine, and GABA.

Chapter 29 will present a discussion of these neurotransmitters, as well as the roles of receptor, thyroid, hypothalamic, and pituitary function in depression.

Anxiety Disorders

Anxiety disorders appear to have a biologic basis as well. Research indicates that drugs that activate GABA receptors, causing an inhibitory effect, can calm anxious patients. Other neurotransmitters, such as norepinephrine, dopamine, and serotonin, may also have roles in anxiety. Certainly, stimulation of the sympathetic system, which is accomplished by epinephrine, norepinephrine, and dopamine (see Table 5-2), causes an anxiety-like reaction. Anxiety disorders are discussed in Chapter 31.

Dementias

Dementias are directly related to brain pathology. Alzheimer's disease (AD), the leading cause of dementia in the United States, is caused by brain atrophy, which is demonstrated microscopically as neurofibrillary tangles and amyloid plaques. Patients with AD tend to have enlarged ventricles, narrowing of the cortical ribbon (gray matter), widening of the sulci, and decreases in the width of the gyri. Furthermore, a loss of cholinergic pathways is found in patients with AD, contributing to memory problems. Patients affected with AD forget facts, how to use words, and how to use common objects. AD and other dementias are discussed in Chapter 32.

Acquired Immunodeficiency Syndrome and Human Immunodeficiency Virus

Acquired immunodeficiency syndrome (AIDS) dementia is caused by a direct assault on the brain by the human immunodeficiency virus (HIV). HIV attacks the brain in two ways: it weakens and destroys T4 lymphocytes, which are part of the body's natural defense, exposing the brain to other pathogens; and it directly attacks the neuronal cell bodies and white matter of the brain. Because of the attack on white matter, AIDS can occasionally be mistaken for multiple sclerosis. AIDS dementia is discussed in Chapter 44.

Degenerative Diseases

Parkinson's disease is an example of a degenerative disease that affects both motor function and emo-tional stability. In parkinsonism, microscopic examination of the basal ganglia, specifically the caudate nucleus and the globus pallidus, reveals degenerative changes. The most significant change, however, is the deterioration of the substantia nigra, the chief synthesizing site of dopamine in the brain. The decreased availability of dopamine in the extrapyramidal system leads to tremor, bradykinesia, and rigidity. Parkinsonism is discussed in Chapter 19 and Chapter 32.

Demyelinating Diseases

Multiple sclerosis is an example of a demyelinating disease. In this disorder, both the myelin and eventually the axons break down (Brodal, 1998). This degeneration of myelin causes a variety of problems, including loss of sensation, muscle weakness, fatigue, double vision, and tingling in the extremities. People with multiple sclerosis also experience psychologic symptoms, undoubtedly related to demyelinization that occurs in the brain.

Anorexia Nervosa

Anorexia nervosa, a disorder characterized by the refusal to eat, appears to be associated with hypothalamic dysfunction. Anorexia nervosa is discussed in Chapter 37.

Trauma

Individuals who have experienced CNS trauma can experience brain insults that are similar to those found in dementia or parkinsonism. Victims of automobile accidents or gunshots, as well as boxers, can exhibit symptoms based on the nature of the injury. Individuals with an injury to the temporal lobe may experience memory loss or aphasia; those with a prefrontal lobe injury may experience personality changes or psychosis. Dementia pugilistica (punch-drunk syndrome), a dementia syndrome with the same molecular pathology as that of AD, can result from repeated blows to the head, for example, in the sport of boxing (Kiernan, 1998).

Chemical Dependency

The biologic pathways that might be responsible for the control that addictive substances have on people are just beginning to be understood. Current research suggests that the nucleus accumbens may be an important part of the addiction puzzle. Charney, Nestler, and Bunney (1999) discuss current studies on mechanisms involved in motivation and addiction.

Mitochondrial Deoxyribonucleic Acid Problems

Most people are familiar with a large number of genetic diseases that affect the psychologic health of individuals, such as Huntington's disease. Many other diseases have been credited with genetic predispositions similar to that of AD. These problems have their genesis in the deoxyribonucleic acid (DNA) of the chromosomes in each cell of our bodies. In 1988 scientists found that the DNA of mitochondria, the powerhouses of our body, can mutate and give rise to physical and psychologic problems (Wallace, 1997). These mutant mitochondria have been implicated in AD: mitochondrial encephalopathy, lactic acidosis, and strokelike episodes (MELAS); diabetes mellitus; among others. Dissimilar to chromosomes, mitochondria are passed to the ovum only by the mother. A variety of mutant mitochondria can result in a number of diseases. The mechanism is that the mutant mitochondria, which fail to properly produce the energy that cells need to function, increase in number over time and damage particular cells and body organs.

Critical Thinking Question

From what you have read in this chapter, can you defend Kraepelin's view of schizophrenia as a dementia? Explain.

Key Concepts

1. The brain is a complex organ composed of 100 billion neurons, and changes in its anatomy or physiology affect behavior. Holistic nursing care requires an understanding of the impact of brain dysfunction on behavior.
2. Many mental disorders that were formerly thought to have psychologic etiologic factors are now known to be influenced by brain dysfunction.
3. The nervous system is divided into the CNS and the PNS.
4. The CNS is divided into the brain and the spinal cord.
5. The nervous pathways in the brain are composed of myelinated axons (white matter) that connect and communicate among brain nuclei (gray matter).

6. The cerebral cortex is the outer layer of gray matter of the brain. Gray matter consists of neuronal cell bodies and is responsible for the work of the brain.
7. The two major neurotransmitters in the extrapyramidal system are dopamine (inhibitory) and acetylcholine (excitatory).
8. The pyramidal motor system controls precise movement; the basal ganglia motor system stabilizes motor movement.
9. The RAS involves degrees of consciousness. Sensory stimuli received in this system are forwarded to the thalamus. As stimulation of the RAS increases, the level of alertness increases.
10. Neurons are the basic subunit of the nervous system. The neuron consists of a cell body, *dendrites* that send information to the cell body, and a process called an *axon*, which transmits impulses away from the cell body.
11. Impulses travel from one neuron to another by sending a chemical called a *neurotransmitter* across a microscopic gap, known as a *synapse.*
12. The dopamine hypothesis postulates that schizophrenia results from increased levels of brain dopamine. Treatment is aimed at reducing those levels through the use of antipsychotic drugs. This broad view of causation is refined in Chapter 28.
13. The neurotransmitter theory of depression states that depression is related to decreased levels of norepinephrine or serotonin or both. This broad view of causation is refined in Chapter 29.
14. Anxiety disorders are likely related to alterations in GABA levels.
15. Dementias, specifically AD, are related to brain atrophy characterized by microscopic changes in the cortical neurons, neurofibrillary tangles, and amyloid plaques. A deficiency in the neurotransmitter acetylcholine occurs as well.

References

Bear MF, Connors BW, Paradiso MA: *Neuroscience: exploring the brain,* ed 2, Philadelphia, 2001, Lippincott-Williams & Wilkins.
Boss BJ, Stowe AC: Neuroanatomy, *J Neurosci Nurs* 18(4):214, 1986.
Brodal P: *The central nervous system,* ed 2, New York, 1998, Oxford University Press.
Charney DS, Nestler EJ, Bunney BS: *Neurobiology of mental illness,* New York, 1999, Oxford University Press.
Collins RC: *Neurology,* Philadelphia, 1997, WB Saunders.
Crow TJ: Schizophrenia as failure of hemisphere dominance for language, *TINS* 20:339, 1997.
Griffin JE, Ojeda SR: *Textbook of endocrine physiology,* ed 4, New York, 2000, Oxford University Press.

Heath RG: Pleasure and brain activity in man, *J Nerv Ment Dis* 154:3, 1972.

Kandel ER, Schwartz JH, Jessell TM: *Principles of neural science,* ed 4, New York, 2000, Elsevier.

Keltner NL, Folks DG: *Psychotropic drugs,* ed 3, St Louis, 2001, Mosby.

Kiernan JA: *Barr's: the human nervous system: an anatomical viewpoint,* ed 7, Philadelphia, 1998, Lippincott.

Kraepelin E: Clinical psychiatry: a textbook for students and physicians, New York, 1902, Macmillian (Translated by AR Deferdorf).

National Foundation for Brain Research: *The cost of disorders of the brain,* Washington, DC, 1992, The Foundation.

Sugerman RA, Edmundson MJ, Robinson S: *Human anatomy,* Edina, Minneapolis, 1979, Burgess.

Wallace DC: Mitochondrial DNA in aging and disease, *Sci Am* 277(2):40, 1997.

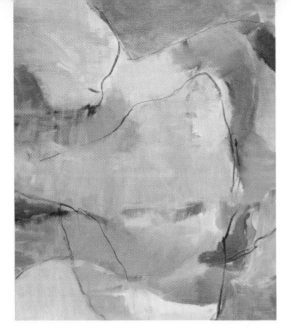

Chapter 6

Continuum of Care

Lee H. Schwecke, Carol E. Bostrom

Learning Objectives

After reading this chapter, you should be able to:
- Comprehend the concept of the continuum of care.
- Understand services necessary for prevention and treatment of mental disorders.
- Identify the impact of managed care on the continuum of care.
- Explain the importance of assessment in making decisions about referrals to various levels of care.

With the current trends in health care, mental health and psychiatric care are now evolving into a broader continuum of services. This unit provides an overview of the continuum of care, including chapters on hospital-based care and community-based care.

Nursing has a long history of involvement in health promotion, primary and secondary prevention, treatment, and rehabilitation. The challenge for psychiatric nursing involves the use of traditional knowledge and skills in nontraditional settings and programs. As reimbursement models, including managed care, influence the type and duration of services, nurses are learning to provide quality care in a holistic framework. For psychiatric nursing, short, crisis-oriented inpatient stays produce a demand for more intensive outpatient services. The continuum of care provides consumers a wide range of treatment modalities to assist the individual in achieving his or her optimal level of functioning.

Health promotion services are aimed at developing an improved level of well-being, such as with parent education classes. Primary prevention services, such as stress management and teen pregnancy classes, help individuals, who are identified as being at risk, to avoid health problems. Secondary prevention services offer early intervention when problems are identified, such as abuse in the family. Treatment services are aimed at diagnosis and treatment of actual health problems by providing hospital- and community-based care. Rehabilitation services attempt to prevent disability and relapse through programs such as educational groups, vocational and skills training, and halfway houses. (Collins, Diego, 2000).

Ideally, psychiatric mental health services should cover all areas within the spectrum. However, in reality, the focus is more heavily targeted at treatment and rehabilitation activities. Continued effort exists to integrate all levels of services into a seamless continuum of care thus an individual can move smoothly among them, while receiving quality of care. Quality indicators along the continuum of care are identified by Schreter (1997) and Trossman (1998) as:
1. Availability
2. Accessibility
3. Acceptability

4. Affordability
5. Accommodation (between client and services)
6. Appropriateness
7. Accountability

The role of nurses and other professionals is to assess the individual's current level of functioning to direct the person to the appropriate resources that will enhance quality of life and decrease fragmentation of care. Coordination of services for the individual necessitates multidisciplinary collaboration. Multidisciplinary care has been expanded to include not only professional staff, but also nonprofessionals, consumers, family, and a variety of nonpsychiatric resources, such as representatives from Medicare, Medicaid, nursing homes, group homes, medical clinics, and so forth.

MANAGED CARE

During the 1980s the high cost of health care became a major focus nationally. Models of care delivery, treatment approaches, and professional roles began to evolve to meet the demand of reducing costs. Today, managed care is one model of reimbursement that has assumed prominence.

Managed care is a system of entities that provides for reimbursement for services. Managed care also arranges the relationships between payers, providers, and consumers to monitor and influence both the behavior of mental health providers and the outcomes of care. Health maintenance organizations (HMOs), independent practice associations, and preferred provider organizations are examples of managed care. Preferred provider organizations restrict services to those offered by designated providers. In the public mental health system, care delivery is typically through HMOs and community mental health centers.

Managed care and private insurance have progressively dictated shorter lengths of hospital stay,

types of treatment, and even which medications may be prescribed. As a result, psychiatric treatment must be flexible, individualized, cost-effective, problem oriented, outcome based, and occur in the least restrictive setting. The goal is to help the individual achieve an optimal level of functioning in the least amount of time, while protecting the individual's right to freedom from harm (Marty, Chapin, 2000; Schreter, 2000).

IMPACT OF MANAGED CARE ON THE CONTINUUM OF CARE

The overall impact of managed care on the continuum of care has been a dramatic reduction in inpatient admissions and lengths of stay and course of treatment, although an inadequate range of community-based services remains (Smoyak, 2000b). More specific examples of the impact on the continuum of care are listed in Box 6-1. Hos-

| Box 6-1 | Impact of Managed Care on the Continuum of Care

Positive
- New innovative treatment modalities
- New levels of services within the community
- Decreased fraud
- More efficient use of treatment strategies
- Outcome-based treatment
- Improvement in coordinating services
- Incentives for health promotion and prevention services
- Increased involvement of consumers and their support systems in care decisions

Negative
- Inadequate reimbursement for some services, such as hospital-based care and long-term care
- Shifting of some consumers to nonmental health services, such as social services and the legal system
- Market-oriented and profit-driven care with ethical and legal issues
- Downsizing of psychiatric facilities and staff
- Difficulties in complying with guidelines and procedures of a variety of reimbursement plans
- Lack of genuine parity for mental health services

Adapted from Coffey J: Universal health coverage. Five good reasons why nurses should champion it, *Am J Nursing* 101(2):11, 2001; McKay ML: The growth of health care, *Am J Nurs* 101(1):24F, 2001; Smoyak SA: The history, economics, and financing of mental health care. Part 1: 17th to 19th centuries, *J Psychosoc Nurs* 38(9):26, 2000; Smoyak SA: The history, economics, and financing of mental health care. Part 3: the present, *J Psychosoc Nurs* 38(11):32, 2000; Trossman S: Quality managed care: a nursing perspective, *AJN* 98(6):56, 1998.

Key Terms

Continuum of care Levels of care through which an individual can move, depending on his or her needs at a given point in time.

Managed care A system of entities that arranges the relationships between payers, providers, and consumers; monitors and influences the behavior of the mental health providers and the outcomes of care; and reimburses for services.

pitals are now used primarily for acute and emergency situations, such as treating an individual who may be dangerous to self or others or both, helping with the person's inability to meet self-care needs, providing extensive or intensive evaluation, treating overdose or suicide attempt, treating combinations of medical and psychiatric problems, and managing acute detoxification or toxicity.

Some consumers and caregivers have doubts as to whether managed care is sufficiently meeting their needs. The tendency to restrict the types of services that will be reimbursed still exists, which leaves much of the financial burden of care to individuals and families who feel abandoned by health care systems and legislators (Smoyak, 2000b).

Critical Thinking Question

Identify resources in your local community that offer services for the prevention and treatment of mental health problems.

DECISION TREE FOR CONTINUUM OF CARE

To match the needs of individuals with appropriate services, comprehensive assessment is required. The decision to hospitalize an individual is only one aspect of deciding on the most appropriate referral for mental health problems (Figure 6-1). When inpatient psychiatric treatment is deemed as inappropri-

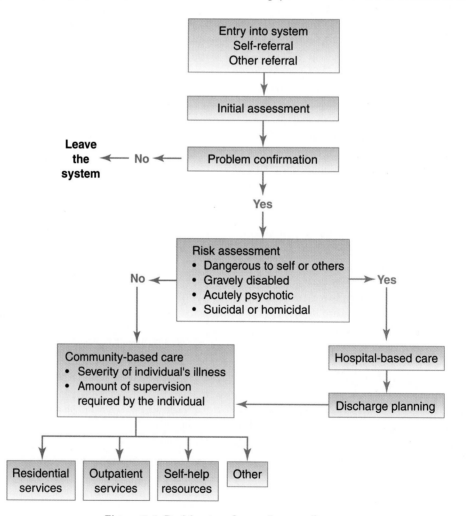

Figure 6-1 Decision tree for continuum of care.

ate, a determination must be made as to the level of care required. This type of decision making incorporates assessment of severity of symptoms, level of risk, level of functioning, intensity of supervision needed (e.g., safety), and type of treatment required to promote optimal level of functioning (Schreter, 2000). For example:

1. An individual with thoughts of suicide but without a plan might be managed effectively by attending a day-treatment program 5 days a week for 2 weeks.
2. An individual with a history of medication noncompliance who needs a place to live might be appropriately placed in a group home with 24-hour-a-day supervision.
3. An individual with alcoholism who has completed acute detoxification might need referral to outpatient counseling or a self-help group such as Alcoholics Anonymous.

For any individual, additional referrals along the continuum of care may be made if needs change.

ACCESSING THE CONTINUUM OF CARE

An individual may be referred to mental health services at the suggestion of a family physician; minister, priest, or rabbi; police; family; friends; or staff from the health clinic, emergency room, crisis service, or employee assistance program, to name a few. Self-referral is also a means by which individuals gain entry into the mental health system.

The individual and the care provider develop specific problem-oriented goals or outcomes based on objective data and subjective self-reports. Unfortunately, individuals may overestimate their progress toward the outcomes, or they may deny the need for follow-up care and fail to reach the outcomes. Because self-reports may be unreliable, more objective measures of outcomes are needed, such as compliance with medication and treatment, job attendance, and community living skills. The achievement of specific outcomes is critical for the issue of reimbursement by payers and for determining quality of care. However, only continually monitoring and valuing the quality indicators mentioned can maintain a seamless continuum of care.

Critical Thinking Question

Based on your interactions with patients, what factors would facilitate adequate quality care in terms of accessibility, availability, and acceptability?

Key Concepts

1. Emerging trends in health care are affecting the practice of psychiatric nursing.
2. The range of services is rapidly evolving to meet the needs of individuals with mental health problems.
3. Managed care has a major influence on the continuum of care.
4. The goal of managed care is to foster optimal functioning and health by providing the least expensive, least restrictive, and least intensive treatment.
5. Assessment of the individual's needs and level of functioning and the level of supervision the individual requires determines referral to hospital-based or community-based care.
6. Appropriate and specific outcome-based care is critical to optimizing the individual's level of functioning, as well as reimbursement.

References

Coffey J: Universal health coverage. Five good reasons why nurses should champion it, *Am J Nurs* 101(2):11, 2001.

Collins AM, Diego L: Mental health promotion and protection, *J Psychosoc Nurs* 38(1):27, 2000.

Marty DA, Chapin R: The legislative tenets of client's right to treatment in the least restrictive environment and freedom from harm: implications for community providers, *Community Ment Health J* 36(6):545, 2000.

McKay ML: The growth of health care, *Am J Nurs* 101(1):24F, 2001.

Schreter RK: Alternative treatment programs. The psychiatric continuum of care, *Psychiatr Clin North Am* 23(2):335, 2000.

Schreter RK: Essential skills for managed behavioral health care, *Psychiatr Serv* 48(5):653, 1997.

Smoyak SA: The history, economics, and financing of mental health care. Part 1: 17th to 19th centuries, *J Psychosoc Nurs* 38(9):26, 2000a.

Smoyak SA: The history, economics, and financing of mental health care. Part 3: the present, *J Psychosoc Nurs* 38(11):32, 2000b.

Trossman S: Quality managed care: a nursing perspective, *Am J Nurs* 98(6):56, 1998.

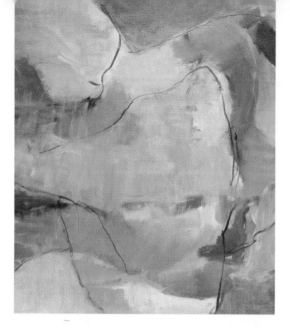

Chapter 7

Hospital-Based Care

Lee H. Schwecke, Carol E. Bostrom

Learning Objectives

After reading this chapter, you should be able to:

- Describe the impact of length of stay on hospital-based care.
- List the purposes of hospital-based care.
- Understand the types of care that may be available in hospitals.
- Comprehend the importance of discharge planning in hospital-based care.
- Identify the role of the nurse in implementing the psychotherapeutic management model in hospital-based care.

As a result of deinstitutionalization, primarily in the 1960s and 1970s (see Chapter 1), the inpatient care of patients with mental illness shifted away from large state or public hospitals to smaller, private facilities and psychiatric units within general hospitals located in the community. This planned reduction in state hospital beds has been reinforced because managed care and reimbursement issues have decreased the number of hospital beds for individuals with psychiatric disorders in all facilities. The length of stay (LOS) for each hospitalized individual has also decreased. The patients in hospitals now tend to be sicker and more diffi-cult to handle than they were in the past (Smoyak, 2000).

In the past, state institutions hospitalized patients for long periods, even up to a year or more. Now, LOS is more likely to be 1 to 2 months in state hospitals but much shorter in the more community-based, acute-care inpatient programs. For some of the seriously and persistently mentally ill and severely disabled individuals, state institutions or long-term hospitalization may be the least restrictive environment in which they can function.

Historically, patients admitted to acute care units often stayed 4 to 6 weeks. Today, LOS in the units is typically 3 to 5 days. Additionally, the LOS per year may be restricted, the dollar amount of coverage per year may be decreased, and co-payments may be increased (Smoyak, 2000). As reimbursement was decreased, hospital-based care, including medical, surgical, and other specialties, changed in the following areas: purpose and goals of hospitalization, a greater need for risk assessment before admission, implementation of more varied types of care, a change in staffing patterns, increased acuity of patients, and increased importance of discharge planning. Hospitals were the point of entry into the health care system, whereas the point of entry now can be anywhere along the continuum of care. As a result, a competent evaluation and triage is required for each individual who requests care (Schreter, 2000).

PURPOSES OF PSYCHIATRIC HOSPITAL-BASED CARE

The highest priority for admission to hospital-based care is safety for self and others, necessitating 24-hour supervision in a secure environment (Schreter, 2000), which includes individuals who are actively suicidal, self-mutilating, or threatening others with harm. Individuals who have attempted suicide are often transferred from the emergency room or medical intensive care unit to a psychiatric unit when medically stable.

Other individuals who require hospitalization include those who are at risk for accidental harm, that is, those who are gravely disabled (see Chapter 4). For example, individuals who are acutely psychotic or those who are confused and disoriented may not function well enough to meet their basic needs for food, clothing, shelter, medical care, or physical safety. In addition to safety and protection, hospitalization provides thorough medical and psychiatric evaluation to identify the underlying cause of their symptoms.

Another group that may be admitted includes individuals who are experiencing toxic reactions to medications or other substances and those who need medical intervention when withdrawal from substances might produce life-threatening conditions. Some individuals may be admitted for a medical evaluation or because the medical illness produces or complicates a psychiatric disorder.

The goals of hospital-based care are to assist individuals with attaining initial stabilization and a safe level of functioning and to assess for appropriate referrals for after-care. Attempts are made to interact with family or support systems or both to determine the individual's problems and needs, as well as to help the individual after discharge (Kirsch, 2000).

TYPES OF HOSPITAL-BASED CARE

Inpatient units vary from hospital to hospital and from community to community. For example, a small hospital may have only one closed (i.e., locked) inpatient unit that accepts all patients with all diagnoses. A larger hospital may offer more options for specialized care compared with the smaller hospital. Some common specialty care areas are described in Table 7-1.

An important type of inpatient service is the psychiatric intensive care unit (PICU). The PICU typ-

|Table 7-1| Types of Programming

Programming	Examples of Major Target Issues	Examples of Typical Groups
Age-Based		
Child	Family issues, developmental issues, peer relationships, academic issues, behavior management, life stresses, coping strategies	Feelings expression, self-esteem, story-telling, family education groups
Adolescent	Same as above plus intimate relationships, sexuality, substance abuse	Self-esteem, sexuality, conflict management, anger management, educational groups
Adult	Same as above plus acceptance of illness and medication compliance; social, occupational, and financial problem solving	Self-esteem, stress management, educational, activity groups
Older adult	Same as above plus aging processes, death and dying, retirement adjustment, disabilities and chronic illnesses, assistance in living issues	Spirituality, grief and loss, reminiscence, educational groups
Diagnosis-Based		
Acute or nonpsychotic or both	Insight into illness and life situations, problem solving, interpersonal relationships	Same as adult above plus problem-solving group
Chronic or psychotic or both	Symptom management, medication compliance, social skills, community living skills, vocational assessment	Same as adult above but on a more concrete level plus social skills, community-living skills, educational groups
Addictions	Dynamics of addiction, effects of addictions	Same as adult above plus self-help groups

ically has 8 to 10 beds with more safety precautions and more staff than other psychiatric units to handle at-risk behaviors, such as suicide, assault, self-mutilation, sexual acting out, arson, and escape. Seclusion and restraints may be used more often on this type of unit. The purpose of the PICU is initial symptom and behavior control so that individuals can then be transferred to more treatment-oriented units or programs. Group activities may or may not be provided. When group activities occur, the focus is typically reality or activity based.

DISCHARGE PLANNING

Hospital-based care uses multidisciplinary treatment conferences and discharge planning to ensure holistic care. Team members collaborate and coordinate inpatient care and determine after-care services within the continuum of care based on the individual's needs (Cesta, Falter, 1999). The team may include the psychiatrist, nurse, social worker, dietician, pharmacist, activity therapist, and chaplain. Consultations with other services, such as physical therapy, neurology, internal medicine, and after-care services, occur as needed. The individual has the opportunity to meet with any or all team members. The multidisciplinary team uses a decision tree in its discharge planning process (Cesta, Falter, 1999). (See Chapter 6) for discussion of the decision tree.) "The goal is to achieve the best match between the patient's clinical condition and the treatment options along the continuum" (Schreter, 2000).

Psychotherapeutic Management

Nurse-patient relationship

Nurses are the only members of the multidisciplinary team who provide 24-hour care during the hospital stay. Individuals admitted to psychiatric units today are more acutely ill than they were in the past and exhibit more severe psychopathology. With the aforementioned shorter LOS, within a day or two, the nurse must establish a therapeutic relationship, identify immediate needs, and provide holistic quality care. The nurse often begins to intervene while the individual is being admitted to the unit because of behaviors that are dangerous to self or others. Despite the individual's level of illness or the type of behaviors being exhibited, the patient must

quickly realize that the nurse is caring, empathetic, supportive, and helpful. The nurse may need to set limits on behaviors but, at the same time, convey respect and maintain the dignity of the individual.

After the individual acquires the sense of safety and is more able to control behavior, further assessment occurs. The nursing assessment must be direct, specific, and comprehensive. Gathering information from as many sources as possible is important. These sources include family, significant others, old charts and records, and professionals in outpatient services with whom the individual may have had contact.

Discharge planning has always been an important nursing role. With decreased LOS, life after hospitalization has become even more critical. Discharge planning begins at admission and is incorporated into the multidisciplinary treatment plan. For some individuals, discharge planning may be relatively simple, such as "return home with outpatient follow-up." For others, the discharge plan may be complex and involve a number of community services along the continuum of care, such as housing, medicine clinic, dental service, outpatient counseling, and a self-help group for the family. Although the nurse may not directly arrange for these services, the nurse coordinates this activity. Including the individual and the family or significant others in multidisciplinary conferences as much as possible is important, thus they can be involved in the development and implementation of goals, including those after discharge. For more information about the nurse-patient relationship, see Chapter 10.

Critical Thinking Question

You are admitting a 15-year-old boy to an inpatient unit because of alcohol and marijuana abuse, sexual promiscuity, and failing grades. These behaviors developed over the last 3 months after his father was diagnosed with terminal cancer. What types of programming would be most appropriate?

Psychopharmacology

The nurse is instrumental in obtaining the medication history: past and current medications and dosages, medication allergies, the individual's perspective on medication effectiveness, problems with side effects, and present and past compliance. An important role includes monitoring the effectiveness of medication, the presence of side effects, and educating the individual and family about the medication and side effects. The nurse must carefully assess the need for as-needed (prn) medication thus problem behaviors and symptoms can be alleviated as quickly as possible. The nurse emphasizes the importance of medication compliance in symptom management and control with the individual and family. (For specific information on medications, see Chapters 18 through 23.)

Milieu management

Traditionally, hospital-based care emphasized milieu therapy (see Chapter 24). Today, the milieu or inpatient environment remains therapeutic and supportive to encourage a return to adequate functioning in the community. The emphasis of milieu activities is on helping the individual cope with immediate needs and with stressors and problems in his or her home or living environment. "The inpatient stay should help the patient adapt to his or her external environment, not the inpatient milieu" (Johnson, 1997). Because of short-term stays, the need exists for structured milieus to include groups that are problem focused, goal oriented, and relevant to the needs of the individuals. Box 7-1 provides a sample daily schedule. The nurse assists the individual in applying information obtained in educational groups to his or her own situation. The nurse teaches the individual the best way to solve problems rather than focusing on resolving all problems before discharge. With these skills, hopefully the individual can continue to solve problems after discharge. Homework assignments, journal writing, and educational handouts provide even more structure in the milieu.

Critical Thinking Question

In a setting in which you have had experience, what roles of the nurse in a multidisciplinary team have you played?

Box 7-1 Sample of an Inpatient Daily Schedule*

7:00 AM	Wake-up and morning care
8:00 AM	Breakfast and free time
9:00 AM	Goal-setting group
10:00 AM	Stress-management group
11:00 AM	Exercise group
12:00 PM	Lunch and free time
1:00 PM	Medication education group
2:00 PM	Self-esteem group
3:00 PM	Addictions group
4:00 PM	Free time
5:00 PM	Dinner and goal review group
6:00 PM	Family education group
7:00 PM	Visiting or free time or both
9:00 PM	Free time
10:00 PM	Relaxation group
10:30 PM	Bedtime

*All group sessions last 40 minutes. Interactions with staff are expected between group sessions or during free time or both.

Key Concepts

1. The majority of hospital-based care is now provided on a short-term basis, focusing on crisis intervention and safety.
2. The over-arching goals of hospital-based care are provision of safety and discharge planning.
3. The type of hospital-based care available to individuals varies according to the size of both the hospital and the community.
4. Discharge planning begins at the time of admission and varies in complexity.
5. The psychotherapeutic management model is the most relevant approach to short-term hospitalization.

References

Cesta TG, Falter EJ: Case management: its value for staff nurses, *Am J Nurs* 99(5):48, 1999.

Johnson DR: Toward parsimony in the inpatient community meeting on a short-term unit, *Psychiatr Serv* 48(1):93, 1997.

Kirsch D: Developing outpatient mental health services for managed care, *Psychiatr Clin North Am* 23(2):403, 2000.

Schreter RK: Alternative treatment programs: the psychiatric continuum of care, *Psychiatr Clin North Am* 23(2):335, 2000.

Smoyak SA: The history, economics, and financing of mental health care. Part 3: the present, *J Psychosoc Nurs* 38(11):32, 2000.

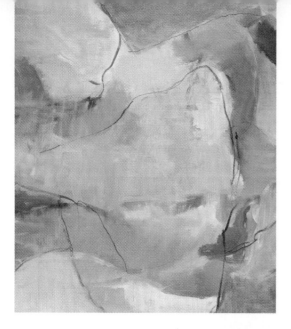

Chapter 8

Community-Based Care*

Carol E. Bostrom, Lee H. Schwecke

Learning Objectives

After reading this chapter, you should be able to:

- Identify the various levels of care within the continuum of care.
- Explain the value of psychotherapeutic management in the continuum of care.
- Define the concept of case management.
- Apply the nursing process to patients who are receiving case management services.

With the shift from hospital-based to community-based care, the range of community service has expanded. This chapter provides an overview of the types of services available within the continuum of care outside the hospital setting. Psychiatric services, in response to economic survival, are now delivered through partial programs, day treatment programs, intensive outpatient programs, and community-based centers (Tucker, Brust, 2000). Nurses have a potential role in any of the services because of their psychotherapeutic management skills, their knowledge of psychopathology, and their ability to adapt the use of the nursing process to any setting. Another valuable asset that nursing brings to the health care system is

its knowledge of reimbursement systems and budget restrictions. Using a holistic approach, nurses are able to deliver direct care to help reintegrate people with mental illness to community living, as well as advocate and link individuals to needed services using the case management approach (Gibson, 1999). Nurses can intervene in new community services in schools, nursing homes, workplaces, jails, and primary care offices, as well as in employee assistance programs (Schreter, 2000).

COMMUNITY-BASED SERVICES

Subacute Care

When inpatient hospitalization is unnecessary, individuals may be referred to outpatient services according to their needs, the amount of supervision that is appropriate, and which services will be reimbursed. The most restrictive service after inpatient hospitalization is subacute care. This level of care is appropriate when an individual requires 24-hour supervision but less intensive and less extensive services compared with inpatient hospitalization. Individuals are provided with beds, meals, medications, groups, and activities. Subacute care allows the individual autonomy and independence in choosing which activities and groups will be attended and which outside activities are appropriate, such as seeking employment and housing or applying for school or training or both.

---

*The section on case management is from a chapter previously written by Kris L. Wang.

Tiffany, a 23-year-old woman with borderline personality disorder and anorexia, describes herself as being in crisis because her boyfriend has left her. She has been unable to sleep or eat for the last 3 days and has superficial cuts on both wrists. After the cuts were cared for in the emergency room, she was taken to a subacute care unit. She received care for 4 days. On admission to the unit, she agreed to sign a "no-harm contract." She received wound care, an evaluation of her nutritional status, and assistance with sleep using relaxation tapes. She attended group sessions that focused on coping with anger and self-esteem issues. One evening she attended a "survivors of incest" group session in the community, which she had been previously attending. On discharge, Tiffany was referred back to her counselor at the neighborhood mental health clinic.

Partial Programs and Day Treatment

Individuals who need some supervision, structured activities, ongoing treatment, and nursing care may benefit from partial programs and day treatment. These programs vary in length from 4 to 8 hours per day and 1 to 5 days per week. Programming can occur during the day, evening, and night. Depending on the community, these programs may provide treatment for specific populations based on age (child, adolescent, adult, or older adult) or type of problem (addictions or chronic mental illness).

John, a 52-year-old man with severe depression resulting from the unexpected death of his wife, is discharged from the hospital but is unable to return to work. He attends a partial program for 2 weeks that meets from 10:00 AM to 3:00 PM, Monday through Friday. He attends groups that focus on exercise, spirituality, coping with losses, and self-esteem issues. Lunchtime provides an opportunity for socialization with program members.

Intensive Outpatient Programs

Intensive outpatient programs are designed to stabilize patients in the community by offering services at a greater level of intensity than do traditional outpatient programs (Schreter, 2000). The clubhouse model is based on a community-based rehabilitation model called Fountain House, which opened in New York City in 1948. This model focuses on supporting people with disabilities in their pursuit of recovery. The clubhouse model provides members with opportunities such as (1) daytime work-organized activities focused on its care and maintenance, (2) evening, weekend, and holiday leisure time activities, (3) support for employment, and (4) housing (Aquila et al, 1999).

Many new outpatient programs are based on the concept of recovery, which provides the consumer with control and responsibility for his or her life. Outpatient programs empower the consumer with the ability to maintain and improve in the major domains of life involving work, housing, relationships, and recreation. The recovery model emphasizes consumers' strengths and choices. Power and responsibility are shared in collaboration and involvement with friends, family, supports, and professionals (Jacobson, Curtis, 2000).

The assertive community treatment (ACT) is a comprehensive community-based service delivery model in which a team of professionals assumes direct responsibility for providing services needed by the consumer 24 hours a day, seven days a week. Services are provided in settings in which consumers' problems arise and support or skills are needed (Phillips et al, 2001). Multidisciplinary members, including nurses, operate as a team in sharing responsibility for providing comprehensive treatment and support to a specified number of consumers. Treatment and services include assistance with shopping, laundry, transportation, and housing. Supervising medication, monitoring health care, and responding to emergencies are a few of the many responsibilities that team members share. Team members also provide outreach to wherever the consumer lives, such as homeless shelters, the streets, and jails.

Traditional Outpatient Services

Traditionally, outpatient treatment has occurred in mental health clinics and private offices. The person providing counseling may be a psychiatrist, psychologist, social worker, clinical nurse specialist, nurse, or other professional. The number of visits per week or month varies according to the individual's needs. The typical pattern for an individual with a chronic mental illness may be a visit once a month with a counselor or case manager and periodic appointments with a psychiatrist for medication review. During these counseling visits, an assessment of needs for additional services is made to determine whether the individual needs more intense or a different type of service.

CLINICAL EXAMPLE

Larry, a 31-year-old man with the diagnosis of chronic undifferentiated schizophrenia, attends a community support program. He meets with his case manager every other week after he receives his haloperidol decanoate (Haldol Decanoate) injection from the nurse, who assesses for effectiveness of the medication and management of side effects. He also participates in a "social club," which offers lunch and social activities twice a week. The psychiatrist meets with him every 3 months for medication evaluation.

PSYCHIATRIC HOME CARE

Psychiatric home care services are available for the homebound because their illness or disability inhibits their leaving home to obtain services elsewhere. Home visits may occur in conjunction with other community-based services. Home care often serves individuals with severe and persistent mental illnesses and those with a combination of psychiatric and medical illnesses. Home care may be provided by traditional public and private home care agencies that have added psychiatric home services. Many psychiatric hospitals and community mental health centers have instituted home care programs.

CLINICAL EXAMPLE

Joe, an 80-year-old man with Alzheimer's disease, lives at home with his wife. The nurse assesses Joe's mental status and level of functioning. Assistance is given to Joe's wife in implementing safety measures in the home because of Joe's wandering behavior. The nurse assists with arranging respite care so that Joe's wife can go shopping and attend a weekly caregivers support group.

COMMUNITY OUTREACH PROGRAMS

Outreach services have been developed to reach individuals in areas in which a lack of traditional medical and social services exists. Programs such as mobile crisis teams are available that attempt to reach individuals, such as the homeless or transient groups (e.g., migrant workers and their families), who have had poor success with community-based services. Mobile programs that serve the needs of mentally ill individuals on the streets, under bridges, in parks, in missions, and at lunch programs exemplify outreach services. Some programs arrange for physician and nurse volunteers to operate a neighborhood clinic once or twice weekly to serve homeless individuals with medical or psychiatric needs or both.

RESIDENTIAL SERVICES

Residential services are available to individuals who need temporary or long-term housing. Most states have long-term care facilities for individuals needing prolonged 24-hour-a-day supervision. Length of stay may be 3 to 6 months or more. *Extended care facilities* (e.g., nursing homes) are available for people who require 24-hour-a-day supervision and medical nursing care. This level of care is often required for individuals with severe developmental disabilities, dementia, or acute and chronic medical illnesses.

Group homes may provide temporary or permanent housing for individuals with chronic mental disorders. Depending on the needs of the residents, staff may be present for 24 hours a day or less. Some group homes provide group therapy and structured activities, while others may provide only meals, a bed, and laundry facilities.

Traditionally, halfway houses were available for individuals with chemical dependency. Residents were expected to seek employment and participate in cooking and cleaning chores. Residents also attend self-help groups that meet on site, such as Alcoholics Anonymous. Some halfway houses may now be open to individuals with other problems.

Apartment living programs provide varying degrees of supervision and programming. Staff may be on site on a daily basis, offering group sessions and activities, or they may visit periodically to ensure medication compliance and attendance at various appointments.

CLINICAL EXAMPLE

Lois, a 63-year-old woman with the diagnosis of bipolar disorder mania, had been living with her son until her behaviors became unmanageable, which resulted from medication noncompliance. Because of her need for more supervision, she was placed in an apartment living program. A nurse visits her three times a week to monitor medication compliance. The nurse also assists her with keeping outpatient appointments.

Foster care and *boarding homes* are generally staffed by nonprofessionals but with professional supervision offered on an outpatient basis. Shelters provide room and board to the homeless. Some homes may provide services for specific populations, such as victims of violence or those with addictions.

Self-Help Groups

Self-help groups are another source of support on the continuum of care. Self-help group meetings are conducted by members, not professionals, and can occur on a weekly basis. Table 8-1 provides examples of types of self-help groups.

In providing holistic care, the nurse or other professional may assist the individual in linking with other community resources. The nurse may need to advocate and negotiate for services such as the following:

- Medical clinics
- Dental services
- Financial services
- Vocational services
- Transportation
- Housing
- Medicare and Medicaid
- Legal or justice system
- Church-related programs
- Employee assistance programs
- Consumer groups

|Table 8-1 | Self-Help Groups

Type of Group	Examples
Addiction-based	Alcoholics Anonymous Narcotics Anonymous Overeaters Anonymous
Survivor-based	Survivors of Suicide Incest Survivors Anonymous Adult Children of Alcoholics
Disorder-based	Eating disorders Bipolar disorder Families/caregivers support groups National Alliance for the Mentally Ill
Loss-based	Grief, divorce, bereavement support groups
Medically based (chronic or terminal illness)	Lupus, cancer, chronic fatigue, AIDS support groups
Prevention-based	Parenting, tough love support groups

> ### *Critical* Thinking Question
>
> Choose a patient with whom you are currently working. Given the services available on the continuum of care in the patient's community, which levels of care would be beneficial to the patient?

Psychotherapeutic Management

Psychiatric nursing advocates for the inclusion of nurses as members of the multidisciplinary team in any of the settings described in this chapter. Psychiatric nurses offer valuable contributions to community-based care because of their ability to adapt the nursing process and the psychotherapeutic management model of care to any setting.

Nurse-patient relationship

Developing a nurse-patient relationship in the community is challenging because of the decreased contact and time spent with the individual. Quickly establishing rapport and trust is critical to implementing the nursing process effectively and efficiently. Individuals are more likely to maintain contact with the nurse over time when they feel valued and respected, as well as feeling satisfied with their care. The nurse also uses the principles of developing the nurse-patient relationship in working with caregivers and family members. Developing collaborative relationships with other professionals is crucial for maintaining the continuum of care.

Psychopharmacology

In community-based settings, the individual and caregiver or family must have knowledge about medications and about the importance of taking these medications as prescribed. Noncompliance with medication is the major cause of relapse and rehospitalization. The nurse has a major role in teaching about medication effects, side effects, management of side effects, and the relationship between medication and symptom management. The nurse must be astute in recognizing early signs of both side effects and noncompliance to intervene quickly. To miss early signs of side effects can result in unnecessary patient discomfort (or worse). To miss noncompliance can lead to poor symptom management.

Milieu management

In community-based care, the principles of milieu management are adapted in assessing agencies, programs, and private homes. After assessing the individual's needs, the nurse is responsible for determining which services in the continuum of care would best meet the individual's needs in the least restrictive setting. Naturally, the nurse has less direct control and influence over environments in the community than they do in inpatient settings. Further economic factors affecting the health care system, individuals, and families may put constraints on environmental modifications that can be accomplished and the type of care that can be delivered. What this circumstance means is that the nurse adapts care based on limitations of the environment and availability of resources.

Critical Thinking Question

If you were to write a letter to your local congressperson, what would you say about the status of mental health care in your community?

CASE MANAGEMENT

Case management is "a collaborative process that assesses, plans, implements, coordinates, monitors, and evaluates options and services to meet an individual's health needs through communication and available resources to promote quality cost-effective outcomes" (Case Management Society of America, 1995). Nurses use this method to provide needed care and services to consumers, families, and groups along the continuum of care. Box 8-1 lists some important goals and purposes of case management. The nurse uses case management to increase continuity of care, ensure access to care, and provide direct cost-effective care. The nurse may assume multiple roles, such as teacher, counselor, advocate, and coordinator. The nurse must also possess key qualities to be effective, including warmth, sensitivity, creativity, empathy, and patience. These qualities facilitate independent living and enhance the quality of life. The nurse instills hope, encourages the individual's effort, and provides opportunities to pursue life goals (Adams, Partee, 1998). Intensive case management increases retention and compliance with treatment, reduces days of hospitalization, increases quality of

Box 8-1 Goals and Purposes of Case Management
Hope
Increased quality of life
Participation in treatment
Competency
Empowerment
Decreased readmissions to inpatient units
Increased social, vocational, and emotional functioning
Decreased burden on caregivers
Independence and growth
Community involvement
Adaptation to or recovery from mental illness
Satisfaction with environment
Continuous treatment
Cost-effective treatment

life, increases level of functioning, reduces use of community services, reduces costs of treatment, reduces symptoms, and increases consumer satisfaction (Bedell, Cohen, Sullivan, 2000).

NURSING PROCESS

The nursing process is the foundation of case management. Effective use of the nursing process in the areas of psychiatric rehabilitation, crisis intervention, home care, therapy, crisis intervention, consultation and liaison, resource linkage, and advocacy provides case management services for psychiatric patients (Figure 8-1). The nurse is skilled in synthesizing these components in an understandable and useful manner for patients.

Assessment

A comprehensive assessment of variables contributing to and interfering with recovery is crucial to the case management of psychiatric patients. The following areas are typically assessed:

- Medication compliance
- Social supports
- Family involvement
- Medical needs and limitations
- Skills
  - Cognitive
  - Vocational
  - Social
  - Problem solving
- Spiritual needs and concerns
- Coping abilities

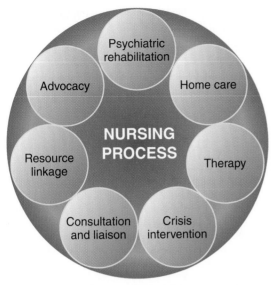

Figure 8-1 Case management components.

Outcome Identification and Planning

The nurse plans and prioritizes the appropriate care based on comprehensive assessment and nursing diagnoses. In the previous clinical example, the nurse prioritizes Mary's needs. The hand tremors must be addressed first, followed by Mary's ineffective use of leisure time and her financial needs. The nurse's plan includes (1) consultation with the psychiatrist regarding Mary's hand tremors, (2) working with Mary in structuring and using her leisure time in a healthful manner, such as using the library, and (3) linking Mary with the social worker for further exploration of financial resources and assistance.

Implementation

Many factors must be considered when prioritizing interventions, and the nurse must take a holistic approach when implementing these interventions. This consideration means recognizing and addressing the interconnectedness of factors in a patient's life (e.g., physical, mental, emotional, spiritual, environmental, financial). Another factor to consider is that by encouraging temporary dependency and compliance, the nurse enhances the prospect for greater independent functioning by the patient later in treatment.

In the previous clinical example, the nurse initiates the plan by building rapport and trust to establish the therapeutic relationship with Mary. The nurse arranges for a psychiatric evaluation before Mary leaves. An adjustment is made in Mary's haloperidol (Haldol), and she is given a prescription for benztropine (Cogentin), 1 mg bid prn. The nurse teaches Mary about the purpose and side effects of benztropine. During this discussion, Mary reports that she has insufficient funds to purchase both the benztropine and groceries. The nurse discusses the financial situation with Mary and discovers enough money for a 2-week supply of benztropine. The nurse then consults with the pharmacy to ensure that Mary can purchase a 2-week supply now and fill the remainder of the prescription at the beginning of the following month. The nurse then assesses Mary's transportation situation. Because the pharmacy is not on Mary's bus route, and because the cold weather prohibits walking, the nurse and Mary engage in problem solving. Mary agrees to call her sister before she leaves the clinic to obtain a ride to the pharmacy in the morning. The nurse also encourages Mary to ask Mary's sister to stop by the library and check out two books. Mary verbalizes agreement with this plan and believes it will be beneficial.

The nurse links Mary with the social worker by making an appointment for her in 2 weeks to discuss her financial situation. The nurse also evaluates Mary's areas of interest and develops a daily schedule with her based on these interests and routine daily living tasks (e.g., going to the library, reading, cooking, cleaning, bathing). This degree of nurse involvement increases Mary's dependence temporarily but has the potential for progressive independence in the future.

Evaluation

Evaluation is an ongoing process. Each intervention and overall patient status must be continually evaluated. Patients have changing needs, issues, and concerns. The nurse must be attuned to these changes during all interactions with patients. Responses to medication, including effectiveness and side effects, must be evaluated in an ongoing manner. For example, before Mary leaves the mental health clinic, the nurse evaluates the following:

- Mary's understanding of the medication changes, the desired responses, and the potential side effects
- Mary's plan for purchasing the benztropine
- The purpose, date, and time of the appointment with the social worker
- The purpose and understanding of using the library and the written schedule of daily activities

Key Concepts

1. Community-based services have evolved to meet the needs of individuals and families in the continuum of care.
2. The continuum of care includes inpatient hospitalization, outpatient services, residential care, self-help activities, and other resources.
3. The nursing process and the psychotherapeutic management approach can be adapted in any setting along the continuum of care.

4. The recovery model of care gives the consumer power and responsibility for his or her life.
5. The foundation of case management is the nursing process.
6. Case management is a method the nurse uses to provide care and services in various treatment settings along the continuum of care.

References

Adams SM, Partee DJ: Hope: the critical factor in recovery, *J Psychosoc Nurs Ment Health Serv* 36(4):29, 1998.

Aquila R et al: The rehabilitation alliance in practice: the clubhouse connection, *Psychiatr Rehabil J* 23(1):19, 1999.

Bedell JR, Cohen NL, Sullivan A: Case management: the current best practices and the next generation of innovation, *Community Ment Health J* 36(2):179, 2000.

Case Management Society of America: *Standards of practice,* Little Rock, Ark, 1995, CMSA.

Gibson DM: Reduced rehospitalizations and reintegration of persons with mental illness into community living: a holistic approach, *J Psychosoc Nurs Ment Health Serv* 37(11):20, 1999.

Jacobson N, Curtis L: Recovery as policy in mental health services: strategies emerging from the states, *Psychiatr Rehabil J* 23(4):333, 2000.

Phillips SD et al: Moving assertive community treatment into standard practice, *Psychiatr Serv* 52(6):771, 2001.

Schreter RK: Alternative treatment programs. The psychiatric continuum of care, *Psychiatr Clin North Am* 23(2):335, 2000.

Tucker S, Brust S: Establishing an empirically based psychiatric nursing practice in a rapidly changing health care environment, *J A Psychiatr Nurs Assoc* 6(4):112, 2000.

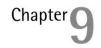

Chapter 9

Communication

Julia Balzer Riley, Bette R. Keltner,
Lee H. Schwecke

Learning Objectives

After reading this chapter, you should be able to:
- Understand major influences on communication.
- Distinguish between social and therapeutic communication.
- Identify goals of therapeutic communication.
- Discuss critical therapeutic communication issues.
- Describe a variety of techniques that facilitate patient-centered communication.
- State common causes of interference with therapeutic communication.

People grow in and through relationships. Relationships with patients help nursing students build positive interactive skills; however, each novel situation may still produce anxiety. Increased experience and a willingness to set aside personal concerns so as to be fully present with each unique person builds confidence and demonstrates the vital importance of communication (Suikkala, Leino-Kilpi, 2001). Most communication is a two-way process between two or more individuals. In nursing, this process is focused on patients' needs and problems. Professional or therapeutic communication is one of the means by which the nursing process is implemented to achieve quality patient care. In psychiatric nursing, therapeutic communica-

tion is one of the most important tools that nurses use to assist patients. It is the means for building trust, developing therapeutic relationships, providing support and comfort, encouraging growth and change, and implementing patient education.

As health care professionals, nurses rely on verbal, written, and electronic (computer) communication for sharing information, analyzing data, collaborating with other disciplines, and delivering services. Consequently, nursing requires a solid foundation in effective communication concepts and skills. For nurses who work with psychiatric patients (patients with alterations in thinking and behavior), the challenge of communicating is even greater. In psychiatric nursing, the goal is not only to understand patients and ensure that they understand the nurse, but also to teach patients more effective communication skills for interaction with mainstream society.

CATEGORIES OF COMMUNICATION

Communication is an interaction between two or more people that involves the exchange of information between a sender and a receiver. The product of communication is the message, which is to be interpreted by the receiver. Words (verbal or written) and behaviors (nonverbal) are the primary channels for communication. Sophisticated technology and electronic communication add additional challenges to clear communication (Balzer Riley, 2000).

Written Communication

Because written material is a primary means of acquiring and sharing information, mastery of language skills is imperative. All professions require some form of written reports, instructions, or sharing of findings and ideas. The skill of mastering vocabulary, grammar, and organization of ideas is critical.

Electronic Communication

Electronic communication requires special attention. The ability to send a quick e-mail can lead to less careful attention to the tone of the message and provides an easy way to deal with sensitive issues that are best handled face-to-face (Simpson, 1999). Internet access to consumer health information presents new challenges for the nurse's role as patient educator. Nurses serve as patient advocates to offer help in accessing and interpreting health information and its accuracy (Houston, Ehrenberger, 2001).

Speech and Behavior

In addition to sound, oral communication includes the mannerisms that modify the message. The timbre and tone of the voice have meaning. The rate and emphasis of speech affect the message. Body language can enhance or change the meaning of words. Verbal and nonverbal communication must match. Behaviors can negate a verbal message; for example, a patient is unlikely to (nor should) believe a nurse who says, "Yes, I will help you" with a frown and an angry tone of voice.

Dynamics of Therapeutic Communication

Therapeutic communication requires attention to multiple, interacting factors. At the core of therapeutic communication are the words and nonverbal behaviors that relate to patients' health needs and are exchanged between patients and the nurse. Figure 9-1 illustrates key variables in communication for the patient and the nurse. Viewing the patient and the nurse as a whole that operates within an environmental context is important. Communication is influenced (1) by the individual's personal experiences, gender, culture, values, and beliefs; (2) by the purpose of the interaction; and (3) by the physical and emotional context of the interaction. The nurse must communicate on patients' levels (according to their vocabulary, educational backgrounds, and the effects of their illnesses) without using a patronizing or condescending manner.

Interpretation of communication

Interpretation of a message is filtered through an individual's knowledge, experience, and biases. Some aspects of communication are more commonly understood than are others. Words are generally understood more precisely than are behaviors. Anyone who has studied a foreign language, however, appreciates that nuances are often lost in translation because of the limitations of words. All people should be considered as cultural beings who bring "differing values, beliefs, customs, and varying perspectives about illness causation, preferred methods of treatment, fears about illness, and expected outcomes" (Mendyka, 2000) to the health care setting. Both the nurse and the patient bring their own experiences to the relationship, which are different lenses through which each views an event. Having a broad knowledge of the effects of cultures is important if the nurse is to interpret accurately and respond appropriately to patient communications. (See Chapter 16 for cultural competence in psychiatric nursing.)

Patient communications often convey indirect messages or underlying themes about content, mood, or interaction issues. For example, a patient may spend 30 minutes describing his divorce of 3 years ago, two other broken relationships since then, having been laid off from his job, having to sell his house, and feeling as though he is a failure. The

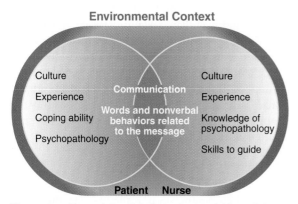

Environmental Context

Culture

Experience

Communication

Coping ability

Words and nonverbal behaviors related to the message

Psychopathology

Culture

Experience

Knowledge of psychopathology

Skills to guide

Patient   Nurse

Figure 9-1 Essential and influencing variables of the therapeutic communication environment.

underlying content theme might be interpreted as a series of major losses. As he describes all of these losses, he might convey anger or guilt or both. These mood themes would be congruent with the content theme. Feelings do not always match the content theme. If the patient were laughing as he described his losses, then his happiness would be considered as an incongruent mood theme.

Assessing for interaction themes involves examining the ways in which the patients relate to family, friends, other patients, and the staff. A patient might call the crisis center each time her roommate is out of town to complain about nervousness and loneliness. When her roommate returns, the patient is once again comfortable. The interaction theme may be assessed as one of dependency. The patient who plays one staff member against another and seeks attention by complaining about all of the other patients might be showing an interaction theme of manipulation. Themes are frequently the source of nursing diagnoses on which care plans are based.

Environmental considerations

The environment can facilitate or impede therapeutic communication. Factors such as noise level, privacy, type of furniture, space, and temperature can affect the quality of communication.

Proxemics refers to the way in which people perceive and use environmental, social, and personal space during interactions. Typically, boundaries of personal space for public and social communication

are more distant compared with those for intimate or therapeutic communication. However, illness and emotional factors such as suspiciousness, anxiety, perceptual distortions, aggressiveness, the genders of the two parties, and personal comfort will also influence the amount of space needed between the patient and the nurse. Patients are generally more comfortable when the nurse is at their eye level rather than standing over them. Face-to-face contact may not be as effective as is sitting at a slight angle to patients, which enables them to look away more easily (Dee, 1991). Some patients may require the presence of a table or an empty chair between themselves and the nurse to feel sufficiently safe to talk.

Physical considerations

Patients with certain physical problems may experience communication difficulties. For example, sensory limitations, developmental disabilities, speech impediments, pain, and physical deformities can interfere with clear communication. Patients with certain sensory limitations such as hearing loss may have compromised communication necessitating compensatory measures such as slow, face-to-face speech for lip reading. Developmental disabilities may seriously limit the ability of patients to comprehend and remember. Simple sentences with a single main idea may have to be repeated several times. Speech impediments or other problems may interfere with understanding patients' messages. Asking for repetition, clarification, and validation are important but can increase a patient's frustration when the practice becomes excessive. Having patients write their answers is an alternative when they are able to read and write. Physical pain often interferes with patients' abilities to think clearly and concentrate and may affect the sense of priority regarding problems to be addressed. Physical deformities and injuries, particularly facial ones, may inhibit the ability to talk and may interfere with the nurse's ability to concentrate on other problems.

Kinesics considerations

Kinesics is the study of body movements. Body language is the popular term that emphasizes the meaning of facial expressions, eye movements, gestures, and mannerisms. Interpretation of these may differ with various cultures (Mendyka, 2000). A variety of body language is used to indicate an individual's feelings. Avoiding prolonged eye contact is often used to disengage or ignore communication. Crossing the arms over the chest occurs many times when a person feels defensive (however, this also occurs when a person is cold). The nurse must be sensitive to these cues and interpret them in a global context of therapeutic communication. If the message appears inconsistent or confusing, exploring the meaning of body language may then be useful. For example, the nurse might say, "Many times, when people back away from someone, it is because they are afraid. Is there something that makes you fearful?"

Body language may communicate feelings or merely reflect a habit. Nurses must become aware of their own "body habits" and consider positive and negative meanings associated with these behaviors (Dee, 1991). Behaviors that communicate caring, confidence, and calmness should be cultivated. Sensitivity to and understanding of kinesics are important in interpreting messages from a patient but should be viewed as cues rather than as diagnostic tools. Again, validating the meaning of the patient's behavior with the patient is crucial (Dee, 1991).

> ### *Critical* Thinking Question
> Ann Williams has multiple facial injuries, has both eyes patched, is breathing with a ventilator, and has been sedated. In what ways would you modify your techniques to facilitate communication with her?

THERAPEUTIC COMMUNICATION

Therapeutic versus Social Communication

The focus of therapeutic communication is on helping patients. Social communication involves equal disclosure of personal information and intimacy, and both parties enjoy equal opportunities for spontaneity. Therapeutic communication focuses on the patient but is planned and directed by the professional. During social exchanges, both participants seek to have personal needs met, whereas the needs of the patient are the focus of therapeutic communication. Therapeutic communication relies on patients' disclosures of personal and occasionally painful feelings with the professional at a calculated emotional distance, near enough to be involved but

objective enough to be helpful. In a social relationship, a friend may share feelings of anger and aggression toward a mutual friend with the expectation that the feelings will be kept confidential. In therapeutic communication, although confidentiality must be respected outside the treatment setting, a professional is obligated to share information within the treatment team. The nurse is a patient's advocate, not a patient's friend (see Chapter 10).

Therapeutic Use of Self

In psychiatric nursing, the nurse, using verbal and nonverbal communication, is the primary therapeutic agent with psychiatric patients (as compared with treatment procedures and physical interventions used by a medical-surgical nurse). The nurse's communication is a major vehicle that helps patients achieve productive emotional and behavioral outcomes. Use of self, use of medications, and use of the environments are the major components of psychotherapeutic management (see Chapter 2).

Therapeutic listening is an important component of the therapeutic use of self with patients and is crucial for getting to know patients as individuals, as well as their needs and concerns. Therapeutic listening has been described as being composed of the following attributes (Kemper, 1992):

THERAPEUTIC LISTENING ATTRIBUTES
- Being actively alert
- "Hearing" with all the senses
- Using eye contact
- Exhibiting an attending posture
- Ensuring concentration
- Being patient
- Displaying an openness to receive information
- Offering empathy and support
- Asking questions
- Assimilating verbal and nonverbal information
- Organizing, synthesizing, and interpreting information
- Validating and clarifying information
- Responding verbally and nonverbally to encourage patients to continue
- Summarizing important points
- Giving feedback appropriately

> ### *Critical* Thinking Question
> Select three or four of the previous behaviors and "communicate" with a friend. What difference did you see in the way in which your friend responds?

Therapeutic use of the self requires the sensitivity to recognize important cues and make decisions about the priority of these cues. Objectivity is the process of remaining open to as many aspects of patients, their problems, and potential solutions as possible. Nurses must not allow their own issues and biases to color interactions with patients and should avoid being "swept away" by patients' emotions and perceptions.

Communicating empathy is an essential skill of the nurse. Empathy is the ability to recognize and understand the patient's feelings and point of view objectively. Empathy is "communicated understanding" (Balzer Riley, 2000). Empathy, expressed verbally and nonverbally, conveys caring, compassion, and concern for patients but never implies that the nurse can fully experience patients' feelings. Empathy helps patients to be more accepting of their feelings and express them more readily. Potential barriers to empathy are time pressures, poor environment, and difficulties in communicating (Hope-Stone, Mills, 2001). (See Chapter 10 for more details about empathy.)

Being therapeutic includes being genuine and sincere as conveyed by congruent verbal and nonverbal behaviors, authenticity, and honesty (without total self-disclosure by the nurse). Patients must feel respected, valued, and accepted by the nurse, even when all of their behaviors are not tolerated. The nurse should not evaluate patients' beliefs, feelings, and behaviors as right or wrong; rather, the nurse helps patients evaluate the effects or consequences of these aspects. However, the nurse must also set limits on destructive behaviors to protect the integrity and dignity of patients, as well as the safety and rights of others.

Touching is a complex issue. The meaning of touch varies widely between cultures, individuals, and patients with different diagnoses. Touching a patient's hand or shoulder or giving a light hug can convey caring, empathy, support, and acceptance. Touching can also be viewed, however, as a violation of personal space or privacy, or it may be misinterpreted as a sexual gesture or an aggressive move. Therefore the use of touch with patients must be approached with caution. Patients' behaviors can give clues to the ability to tolerate and benefit from touch. For example, a patient who is unable to sit close to the nurse is less likely to want to be touched. A patient who is quite trusting of the nurse is more likely to accept being touched. A patient who is sexually preoccupied might misinterpret any type of touch. With many patients (particularly those who have been sexually or physically abused), asking about giving a gentle hug is appropriate: "Could you use a hug right now?" or "Would a hug help you feel better?"

THERAPEUTIC COMMUNICATION TECHNIQUES

Therapeutic techniques are a means of helping patients toward productive goals but are not goals in themselves. The communication techniques presented in Box 9-1 are arranged according to the steps of the nursing process that they tend to facilitate. Some techniques may be adequately versatile to be used in more than one step. Interactions with patients do not involve using all of these techniques sequentially. Moving among the steps of assessment, nursing diagnosis, and planning before reaching implementation and evaluation is common. Even during the implementation step, the nurse may realize that more analysis is needed and may thus return to the step of nursing diagnosis. Many nurse-patient interactions do not use the complete nursing process in a single session, but they always involve using therapeutic techniques. Occasionally, interactions have primarily a social or recreational focus rather than a problem-solving process, but these may still be beneficial to the patient. Every encounter with a patient can be therapeutic with or without full use of the nursing process (see Chapters 10 and 11).

> ### *Critical* Thinking Question
>
> Jack Riley was admitted with chronic paranoid schizophrenia. His only contact for years had been with his parents. In what way might various social and recreational activities be therapeutic for him?

COMMON CAUSES OF INTERFERENCE WITH THERAPEUTIC COMMUNICATION

In the same manner that therapeutic communication guides the patient toward goals, certain messages and behaviors interfere with reaching goals. Some behaviors occur frequently because of nervous mannerisms or are the result of social expectations in the therapeutic situation. The nurse must recognize and overcome any habitual communication problems that can interfere with effective therapeutic communication.

I Box 9-1 I Therapeutic Techniques to Facilitate the Nursing Process in Psychiatric Nursing

Assessment

Techniques fostering description

Offering self: Making self available and showing interest and concern

"I'll sit with you awhile."
"I'll stay with you."

Active listening: Paying close attention to verbal and nonverbal communications, patterns of thinking, feelings, and behaviors

Face the patient; maintain eye contact; be open, alert, and patient; respond appropriately.

Silence: Planned absence of verbal remarks to allow patients to think and say more

Maintain eye contact; convey interest and concern in facial expressions.

Empathy: Recognizing and acknowledging patients' feelings

"I can hear how painful it is for you to talk about this."

Questioning: Using open-ended questions to achieve relevance and depth in discussion

"Who?"
"What?"
"Where?"
"When?"
"What did you say?"
"What happened?"
"Tell me about it."

General leads: Using neutral expressions to encourage patients to continue talking

"Go on, I'm listening."
"I hear what you are saying."

Restating: Repeating the exact words of patients to remind them of what they said; to let them know they are heard

"You say you are going home soon."
"Your mother wasn't happy to see you?"

Verbalizing the implied: Rephrasing patients' words to highlight an underlying message

Patient: "There is nothing to do at home."
Nurse: "It sounds as if you might be bored at home."

Clarification: Asking patients to restate, elaborate, or give examples of ideas or feelings

"What do you mean by 'feeling sick inside'?"
"Give me an example of feeling 'lost.'"

Nursing Diagnosis

Techniques fostering analysis and conclusions

Making observations: Commenting on what is seen or heard to encourage discussion

"You seem restless."
"I noticed you had trouble making a decision about..."

Presenting reality: Offering a view of what is real and what is not without arguing with the patient

"I know the voices are real to you, but I don't hear them."
"I don't see it the same way."

Encouraging description of perceptions: Asking for patients' views of their situations

"What do you think is happening to you right now?"
"What do you think is your main problem?"

Voicing doubt: Expressing uncertainty about the reality of patients' perceptions and conclusions

"Is that the only way to interpret it?" "What other conclusion could there be?"

Placing an event in time or sequence: Asking for relationships among events

"When did you do this?"
"Then what happened?"
"What led up to...?"
"What is the connection between...?"

Encouraging comparisons: Asking for similarities and differences among feelings, behaviors, and events

"How does this compare to the last time?"
"What is different about your feelings today?"

Identifying themes: Asking patients to identify recurrent patterns in thoughts, feelings, and behaviors

"So what do you do each time you argue with your wife?"
"What feeling do you get when you see your father?"

Summarizing: Reviewing main points and conclusions

"Let's see, so far you have said..."

IBox 9–1I Therapeutic Techniques to Facilitate the Nursing Process in Psychiatric Nursing—cont'd

Techniques fostering interpretation of meaning and importance

Focusing: Pursuing a topic until its meaning or importance is clear

"Explain more about..."
"What bothers you about ...?"
"What happens when you feel this way?"

Interpreting: Providing a view of the meaning or importance of something

"It sounds as if this is very important to you."
"You seem to get in trouble when you..."

Encouraging evaluation: Asking for patients' views of the meaning or importance of something

"So what does all this mean to you?"
"How serious is this for you?"
"How important is it to change this behavior?"

Planning

Techniques fostering problem solving and decisions

Suggesting collaboration: Offering to help patients solve problems

"I can help you understand this better."
"Let's see if we can find an answer."

Encouraging goal setting: Asking patients to decide on the type of change needed

"What do you think needs to change?"
"What do you want to do differently?"

Giving information: Providing information that will help patients make better choices

"I can tell you about your medicines."
"There are self-help groups available."

Encouraging consideration of options: Asking patients to consider the pros and cons of possible options

"What would be the advantage of trying..."
"What might happen if you tried..."

Encouraging decisions: Asking patients to make a choice among options

"Which is the best alternative for you?"
"What would work best?"

Encouraging the formulation of a plan: Probing for step-by-step actions that will be needed

"What exactly will it take to carry out your plan?"
"What else do you need to do?"

Implementation

Techniques fostering the completion of plans

Testing out new behaviors:

1. Rehearsing: requesting a verbal description of what will be said or done

"Tell me exactly what you will say to your wife on Friday."

2. Role playing: practicing behaviors; the nurse plays a particular role

"I'll play your wife. What do you want to say to me?"

Supportive confrontation: Acknowledging the difficulty in changing, but pushing for action

"I know this isn't easy to do, but I think you can do it."
"It's hard but give it a try."

Limit setting: Discouraging nonproductive feelings and behaviors, and encouraging productive ones

"You're slipping into your aggressive tone again. Try it again..."
"That is a negative comment about yourself. Tell me something positive about yourself."

Feedback: Pointing out specific behaviors and giving impressions of reactions

"I thought you conveyed anger when you said..."
"When you said...I felt..."

Evaluation

Encouraging evaluation: Asking patients to evaluate their actions and the outcomes

"How well did it work when you tried...?
"What was your husband's reaction?"

Reinforcement: Giving feedback on positive behaviors

"This new approach worked for you. Keep it up."

Repeating steps of the nursing process if needed: Using the steps of the nursing process to get a description of what happened, the degree of success, and ideas for change

"What would help you do even better next time?"
"If things didn't go well, what do you want to do differently this time?"

Nurse's Fears and Feelings

Because therapeutic communication involves the use of self, many personal feelings are naturally evoked and can be disturbing. A nurse may easily develop a feeling of fear when communicating with individuals who are experiencing severe psychic or physical distress. Fear compromises therapeutic communication. The nurse may have concerns such as, "Could this be me someday?" or "My brother does this sometimes; does that mean he's crazy?" or "What if this patient gets angry with me?" Therapeutic communication relies on coming to terms with these types of issues. Individuals become patients because of serious difficulties in functioning, not because of an occasional dysfunctional behavior. The nurse should avoid personalizing the things patients say and do. Patients who abruptly end a conversation with a nurse are more likely responding to their own thoughts or anxieties than they would to something the nurse said. Nurses must understand their personal values, biases, and vulnerabilities. Nurses can benefit not only from analyzing the technique and content of interactions with patients, but also from analyzing their own feelings and reactions. (See Chapter 13 for further discussion on self-awareness.)

Occasionally, a nurse is afraid of harming patients by saying the "wrong thing." Patients do not fall apart or act out because of a nurse's single mistake, particularly when the nurse's overall attitude is positive and helpful; however, patients are sensitive to malicious intent and rejection. A mistake can actually become a therapeutic encounter because the nurse becomes a role model for the proper way to admit and apologize for an error. Many people, including psychiatric patients, have trouble recognizing and correcting mistakes with individuals who are significant to them. In many situations, a sincere apology, when warranted, can strengthen the relationship.

Another concern is invasion of privacy. Psychiatric nurses intensely investigate personal areas of patients' lives, such as values, beliefs, feelings, intimate relationships, and sexuality. The focus may also be on legally sensitive areas, such as incest, partner abuse, and drug use. Although patients must address these issues, they are not easy to discuss. The nurse enhances patients' abilities to be open and honest by explaining the need to know about a sensitive area, by asking questions in a kind and matter-of-fact manner, by conveying empathy, and by reiterating a desire to help.

Nurse's Lack of Knowledge and Insecurity

A lack of knowledge about psychiatric illnesses, defense mechanisms, medication responses, and the dynamics of behaviors and relationships causes insecurity and diminishes patients' confidence in the nurse. Patients are usually accepting, however, when the nurse is honest about not knowing an answer if the nurse is willing to find the answer.

In an attempt to achieve a sense of security, the nurse may assume a parental type of role toward the patient. Emrich (1989) reports that many staff-patient interactions are parental, that they maintain illness and are disconfirming. Parental responses can be a result of remarks that are consistently nurturing, critical, or condescending. Nurses occasionally exhibit one of these three patterns to decrease the feelings of insecurity in themselves; however, these responses must be avoided.

Inappropriate Responses

The nurse's response to messages should be based on assessment and knowledge of the situation, as well as the dynamics of patients' illnesses and problems. However, nurses may not always interact effectively. A nurse may withdraw from patients who are angrily cursing, rather than discussing the behavior. Nurses may get caught up in the unfounded fears and accusations of paranoid patients and thereby reinforce the symptoms. Distinguishing between fact and distortion in what patients say is often difficult, thus the nurse must avoid premature conclusions. For example, staff members do not believe a patient who says he wrote the theme song for a popular play. The patient finally brings in his original handwritten sheet music and the list of credits from the play's manuscript for the staff to see. Obtaining information from family members to validate information or waiting until medications help clear delusional thinking is occasionally helpful.

Nurses may be preoccupied with what they want to say next rather than with listening to patients. Overuse of one or two therapeutic skills, such as reflecting or restating, can stagnate communications when no movement toward analyzing and problem solving is evident. Giving advice to patients rather than helping them evaluate and choose their own solutions can also impede problem solving. False reassurances such as, "Everything will be all right" or "Things are bound to get better" are basically promises that the nurse cannot keep. Box 9-2 lists other responses and behaviors that are generally ineffective or inappropriate. Mistakes by the nurse can generally be corrected, explanations can be given, and damage to the relationship can be reversed. Patients usually evaluate nurses by an overall attitude of caring and concern rather than by a single inappropriate response.

Critical Thinking Question

What strategies you would use to be the patient's advocate rather than the patient's friend?

|Box 9-2| Ineffective Responses and Behaviors

Not listening
Looking too busy
Seeming uncomfortable with silence
Being opinionated
Avoiding sensitive topics
Arguing
Changing the subject
Being superficial
Having a closed posture
Ignoring the patient
Making false promises
Making sarcastic remarks
Talking too much
Not paying attention
Laughing nervously
Smiling inappropriately
Showing disapproval
Belittling feelings
Minimizing problems
Being defensive
Focusing on personal problems of the nurse
Using clichés
Making flippant remarks
Lying or being insincere

Key Concepts

1. Therapeutic techniques are skills to help people but are not goals in themselves.
2. Therapeutic communication occurs with a plan and a purpose, whereas social communication involves equal levels of intimacy, sharing, and the opportunity for spontaneity.
3. Therapeutic communication differs from social communication because the focus is on the patients rather than on a give-and-take experience.
4. Goals of psychiatric nursing are to understand patients, to ensure that patients understand the nurse, and to teach more effective communication skills.
5. Listening is a therapeutic communication technique that requires careful concentration to guide the conversation toward a goal.
6. Nurses are responsible for therapeutic communication and must recognize communication interferences that they may be causing.
7. Some common causes of interference to therapeutic communication are fear, lack of knowledge, insecurity, and inappropriate responses.

References

Balzer Riley J: *Communication in nursing,* St Louis, 2000, Mosby.

Dee V: Professionally speaking (on culturally specific body language), *J Psychosoc Nurs Ment Health Serv* 29(11):40, 1991.

Emrich K: Helping or hurting? Interacting in the psychiatric milieu, *J Psychosoc Nurs Ment Health Serv* 27(12):26, 1989.

Hope-Stone LD, Mills BJ: Developing empathy to improve patient care: a pilot study of cancer nurses, *Int J Palliat Nurs* 7(3):146, 2001.

Houston TK, Ehrenberger HE: The potential of consumer health informatics, *Semin Oncol Nurs* 17(1):41, 2001.

Kemper BJ: Therapeutic listening: developing the concept, *J Psychosoc Nurs Ment Health Serv* 30(7):21, 1992.

Mendyka BE: Exploring culture in nursing: a theory-driven practice, *Holist Nurs Pract* 15(1):32, 2000.

Simpson RL: High touch vs. high tech: rediscover the human element, *Nurs Manag* 30(6):33, 1999.

Suikkala A, Leino-Kilpi H: Nursing student-patient relationship: a view of the literature from 1984 to 1998, *J Adv Nurs* 33(1):42, 2001.

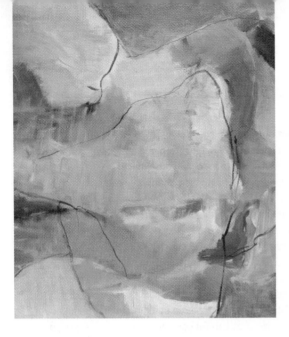

Chapter 10

Nurse-Patient Relationship

Lee H. Schwecke

Learning Objectives

After reading this chapter, you should be able to:

- Describe the meaning of being therapeutic.
- Describe the stages of a therapeutic nurse-patient relationship.
- Identify the major tasks of each stage of the nurse-patient relationship.
- Recognize verbal strategies in interacting with patients.

Hildegard Peplau defined nursing as "a significant, therapeutic, interpersonal process. Nursing is an educative instrument, a maturing force, that aims to promote forward movement of personality in the direction of creative, constructive, productive, personal, and community living" (Peplau, 1952). The nurse's relationship with patients consists of a series of goal-directed interactions. The nurse uses verbal and nonverbal communications to convey a willingness to listen, a genuine respect, a desire to help, and an understanding of patients as individuals with problems and needs (Klagsbrun, 2001). The nursing process (see Chapter 11) is the tool with which the nurse assesses patients' problems, elicits patient input, selects interventions, and evaluates the effectiveness of care. In psychiatric nursing, the nursing process is grounded in the knowledge of the nature of therapeutic relation-

ships, psychopharmacology, and milieu management, all of which are based on an understanding of concepts and processes of psychopathology. Developing the nurse-patient relationship is the first, and often the most pivotal, step in effective psychotherapeutic management (see Chapter 2).

THERAPEUTIC RELATIONSHIPS

Many factors influence the relationship between the nurse and the patient, and various therapeutic activities can be used within the relationship to facilitate successful patient outcomes. No theoretical model is effective with every patient, in every situation, or with every kind of problem. Even patients with the same psychiatric diagnosis will have somewhat different manifestations of symptoms depending on their history, current life situation, and emerging needs. Each person, including all patients, is a unique, worthwhile, holistic individual who is struggling with internal needs and external realities (Klagsbrun, 2001). The nurse should approach each patient individually by tailoring selected strategies to each patient's problems and needs.

Brief Therapeutic Relationships

Brief therapeutic relationships are not as formalized as therapy but are planned, patient centered, and goal directed. The nurse purposefully and carefully guides conversations with patients toward the exploration of problems, issues, and needs. The nurse then

Key Terms

Delusion False belief that is inconsistent with the individual's intelligence and culture and not amenable to reason, for example, the belief that one's body is inhabited by aliens.

Empathy Objective understanding of the way in which patients feel or perceive their situations; "putting yourself in their shoes."

Hallucination False sensory perception that is unrelated to external stimuli, for example, seeing things that are not there.

Psychomotor retardation Markedly slowed speech and body movements.

selects therapeutic strategies to facilitate awareness, decisions, changes, and comfort. Concern, compassion, and interest are demonstrated, while maintaining an objectivity that patients may lack. The nurse may share some personal data such as age, marital status, or title but should rarely disclose personal problems. Occasionally, a brief self-disclosure may help patients clarify specific issues, feel less vulnerable, or feel more "normal" (Deering, 1999). ("When I feel depressed, it's usually because I'm angry and not expressing it for some reason. What kinds of things do you get angry about ?" or "Sometimes I'm afraid to tell my husband something because I don't know how he will react. What is hard for you to talk about with your wife?") Therapeutic self-disclosure facilitates comfort, honesty, openness, and risk-taking but never burdens patients with the nurse's problems (Haddad, 2001).

Social versus Therapeutic Relationships

The nurse-patient relationship is not a social relationship (see Chapter 9). A social relationship involves companionship, mutual support, intimacy, and equal disclosure of personal information. Although the nurse may relate informally with patients, the maintenance of objectivity and goal-directedness is crucial. Patients, particularly those with a history of unsatisfying relationships, may misinterpret the nurse's interest and concern. Patients often ask (or wish to ask) the nurse to be a friend or to go out on a date. When this event occurs, reminding the patient of the nurse's role and taking the opportunity to discuss the need for friendship, love, and support becomes necessary; for example, "I real-

ize you would like to date. As a nurse I can help you find ways to form friendships that can offer you emotional support."

Collaboration

The nursing axiom of involving patients in their own care has relevance in psychiatric nursing. Patients have a right to make decisions about their care. When patients recognize their problems and needs, desire to change, and when they ask for assistance, the nurse is able to work with them on goals and plans. Collaboration generally produces more effective and enduring change than does coercion or simple compliance. Unfortunately, instances arise during which this collaboration is not possible, such as when patients have an obvious disturbance in their thought processes (as with severe hallucinations or delusions). Patients may be incapable of collaborating with the nurse in their care until these problems subside. Occasionally, the only goal to which a patient will agree is "to get out of the hospital." Even this goal, however, provides an opening for discussion of behavioral changes necessary before discharge can occur. Patients with chronic illnesses may be able to agree to only small changes. Unless the nurse is tolerant, flexible, and realistic, the patient may feel overwhelmed.

CLINICAL EXAMPLE

Jason Schmidy had four admissions in 3 years with a diagnosis of paranoid schizophrenia. During each admission, he had achieved new small goals. Initially, his suspicion was such that he talked only to his sister and refused medications "because they were poison." At the end of his second admission, he talked with staff members and agreed to monthly injections of a long-acting antipsychotic medication. During the third admission, he related that he enjoyed helping a neighbor in his garden. At Mr. Schmidy's last discharge, he expressed interest in attending a self-help group for chronically ill patients.

BEING THERAPEUTIC VERSUS PROVIDING THERAPY

The nurse's basic education provides the knowledge and skills for being therapeutic in encounters with patients; training as a clinical nurse specialist (CNS) or as a psychotherapist is not required. Psychotherapists and CNSs receive specialized training that may be focused on a particular therapeutic model that attempts to explain the causes of mental illness and offers specialized techniques for achieving desired outcomes. CNSs or psychotherapists are also interested in formalized, ongoing sessions that have a specified time, place, and length. These professionals are selective in their choice of patients and are restrictive in the sense that they have rules for conducting sessions.

In contrast, nurses who engage in therapeutic activities, particularly in an inpatient setting or outpatient program, recognize that each encounter with patients is part of an overall therapeutic picture: a therapeutic milieu. Patients discuss real problems and practical solutions, and they practice skills needed in real-life situations to enhance their functioning in the real community. Brief encounters offer an opportunity for patients to process feelings and thoughts as they occur. Validation and feedback from the nurse are available quickly. Many patients are unable to tolerate intense, ongoing therapy but can benefit from consistent therapeutic encounters with nurses, even when their hospitalization lasts only a few days or when attendance at an outpatient program is sporadic.

Informal or recreational encounters with patients (card games, craft classes, holiday parties) may be spontaneous but must be therapeutic. For example, the nurse might observe inappropriate social behaviors or a lack of social skills. Helping the patient develop appropriate social and verbal skills, test reality, and solicit feedback and support for new behaviors is then appropriate for the nurse. These informal activities also help patients reduce anxiety and body tension, develop a sense of competence, and take risks. Informal encounters are also opportunities for the nurse to demonstrate ways of handling situations: "Well, we didn't win this hand, but I'm enjoying the game anyway." "I've made that mistake before too. I can show you how to correct it." "Everyone has a right to his or her opinion. I'll listen to yours and then you can hear mine."

DEVELOPMENT OF A THERAPEUTIC RELATIONSHIP

Stages of the Nurse–Patient Relationship

When psychiatric care was provided primarily in long-term hospitals, Peplau believed that the nurse and the patient begin as strangers and move in stages to become collaborators in problem solving

(Forchuk et al, 2000). The stages in the nurse-patient relationship have been given various names by various authors, but Peplau's concepts remain valid. In the *stage of orientation,* patients feel needs and seek help. The nurse helps patients understand their problems and accept the help that is available. The nurse actively works to foster trust and to develop the relationship. In the *identification and exploration stage,* or *working stage,* clarification of perceptions and expectations about the relationship takes place. Problems and identification of tentative solutions are further defined. Patients become more motivated to take advantage of available resources to resolve problems. Patients may test the nurse and may fluctuate between dependence and independence. Peplau believed that the *resolution stage,* or *termination stage,* needs close attention to avoid destroying the benefits gained from the relationship. Focus is on the growth that occurred and on helping the patient develop self-responsibility for setting new goals. The entire relationship is viewed as promoting growth and as a learning experience for the nurse and for patients (Peplau, 1952).

Therapeutic relationships vary in depth, length, and focus. A brief therapeutic encounter may last only a few minutes, focusing on patients' *immediate needs, current feelings,* or *observed behaviors.* In a longer-term hospitalization or program, the relationship may last 1 to 3 months with regular meetings that focus on underlying causes of behaviors, developmental issues, or long-term problems. In an acute-care setting or outpatient program, patients relate to many nurses and staff members each day. In this situation, progress in the nurse-patient relationship is the responsibility of every nurse with whom the patient has contact. One nurse admits the patient to the unit or program and begins the relationship. Another nurse may discharge the patient and complete termination. Shift reports, team meetings, care plans, and progress notes help each nurse work with the patient toward the same goals.

In this era of brief hospitalization and time-limited outpatient care, the phases of the nurse-patient relationship are not a sequence of processes; rather, a matter of different emphases or goals. The nurse concentrates on nursing approaches of a particular phase, depending on the status and needs of individual patients. For example, approaches used in the orientation phase have priority when the patient is highly suspicious because a need exists to develop trust with the patient. For the patient with good insight and motivation, approaches in the working phase are most important because they concentrate on problem solving and change. If the patient is to be admitted for only 3 days, then approaches used in the termination phase are critical because of the need for formalizing plans for follow-up care and referrals to other services along the continuum of care (see Chapter 6).

Moving in and out of the three phases may depend on the patient's ability to cope with various issues (Gauthier, 2000). The patient may be ready to work on divorce issues but may not be able to process incest issues until more trust is established. Regardless of the phase of the relationship that is most appropriate at any given time, events can alter the patient's situation, necessitating a major change in the nurse-patient relationship. For example, if the patient experiences a crisis event, then the nurse must employ crisis intervention strategies. (See Chapter 12 for information on crisis issues and interventions.)

The knowledge and skills of the nurse may also affect which processes are emphasized. Less experienced nurses occasionally stay focused on orientation activities rather than on facilitating working interventions. Nurses in short-term settings or programs tend to move quickly and concentrate on the working and termination phase interventions.

Orientation stage

The orientation stage involves nurses learning about patients and their initial concerns and needs (Gauthier, 2000). Patients also learn about the roles of the nurse during this first stage. Patients are informed of the general purpose of talking with the nurse. The initial purpose may be stated as broadly as "identifying a problem on which you want to work," "helping you figure out what has been happening to you lately," or "getting to know what has been bothering you." After the problems become more evident, the nurse collaborates with patients to define more specific areas to pursue, for example, learning to be assertive or processing feelings about a divorce. Patients must realize that nurses cannot solve problems or make decisions for their patients. Rather, nurses help patients look at realistic options so that patients can make their own decisions.

In a longer-term outpatient relationship between the patient and the nurse, arrangements are made as to the time, length and frequency of the meetings. The session might be for 30 to 60 minutes once a week in a clinic or office or in the patient's home. Even in brief encounters in an outpatient setting or on an inpatient unit, nurses should be aware of the need for privacy and might suggest moving to an uncrowded area to talk. Helpful to patients is knowing the length of time the nurse can spend with them (usually 30 minutes or less) and that the relationship will end at the time of discharge or transfer to another level of care in the continuum of care.

Building trust

Regardless of the formality or length of the relationship, each nurse actively encourages patients to feel comfortable in the relationship. An effective connection is based on the patient and the nurse getting to know each other. The nurse conveys concern for and caring about the patient. Trustworthiness is built when the nurse is honest regarding intentions, is consistent, and keeps promises. Warmth, interest, and concern are conveyed with words and congruent body language. Clear, specific communications decrease confusion and suspiciousness. Confidentiality is explained in terms of patient information being shared *only* with the immediate unit or program staff and not with anyone outside of the treatment setting without the patient's consent (Wysoker, 2001). (See Chapter 4 for legal issues related to confidentiality.)

Many patients are afraid or unable to approach the nurses, thus reaching out and initiating conversations is important. Quiet, withdrawn patients are often overlooked because they cannot ask for assistance. An offer to listen and help conveys to patients that they are worthwhile individuals who are respected. Initially, the nurse is nonconfrontational by not openly challenging statements that the patient makes. Such a challenge would interfere with trust and with data collection. (Supportive confrontation is discussed in the working stage.)

Beginning assessment

The initial sessions, including intake interviews, provide an opportunity to begin an assessment of patients' needs, coping strategies, defense mechanisms, and adaptation styles. Patients' recurring thoughts, feelings, and behaviors are clues to problem areas. Assessing the degree of a patient's awareness of problems and the ability and motivation to change is important. Although assessment is ongoing and progresses over time, tentative goals are based on the most immediate needs or problems, for example, suicidal or homicidal thoughts, hallucinations, self-mutilation, or acting out. (For many facilities and programs, the initial care plan must be written within 24 hours of admission.)

Many opportunities are available between interviews (e.g., during activities, meals, free time with other patients, at medication times) to observe patients and their behaviors. The family may contribute information as well. Assessment tools may be used, such as a depression scale or personality test.

Managing emotions

At the time of admission to a unit or a program, patients typically experience painful thoughts and emotions such as fear, grief, anger, ambivalence, confusion, shame, embarrassment, or guilt. Patients are often afraid of losing control of themselves or of being viewed as weak for expressing their feelings. A way to keep feelings from escalating is to talk about them directly. Because patients are likely to try to conceal or minimize feelings, the nurse must be alert to indirect references, nonverbal cues, and voice tones. The nurse can then identify the feeling and ask for validation: "I sense that you are angry. What are you feeling right now?"

To cope effectively with feelings, particularly anger, the nurse should remember that the feeling is created not by the nurse but by some situation or significant person in the patient's life. A patient may displace anger onto the nurse at first. If supportively confronted about the anger, however, the patient is then more likely to recognize the real source of his or her emotions. Patients must understand that feelings are natural, but that the way they are expressed can cause a problem. Belittling or minimizing a patient's emotions is inappropriate, as is false reassurance, for example, saying, "Everything will be all right." In fact, patients may feel worse for a while as they begin to face their problems and feelings; thus such reassurance is dishonest, as well as inappropriate.

Empathy is an objective understanding of the way in which patients feel or see their situations.

Conveying empathy is a way of helping patients deal with emotional pain. Empathy comes from actively listening to patients' perspectives about their experiences (Walker, Alligood, 2001). Empathy can also convey a hope for improvement: "I hear how painful this is for you and would like to try to help you deal with the situation in a productive way." Sympathy, by contrast, is the nurse having the same feelings as the patient has, and objectivity is lost. Sympathy often leads to comforting, reassuring, or pitying patients. The outcome for patients is a sense of "poor me, I have a right to stay this way."

After patients are able to talk directly about emotions, the focus can be on coping more effectively with them. In the orientation stage, resolving the problem that created the feelings is not possible, but temporarily reducing the feelings to a tolerable level by using palliative coping mechanisms is possible (see Chapter 12). Explaining the experiences and feelings to an empathic listener helps, but when ventilation intensifies the feelings, distracting patients from that topic for a while may become necessary.

Adequate rest and nutrition reduce the impact of tension on the body. Physical exercise, meditation, imagery, and relaxation techniques also alleviate some of the tension that patients may feel (Folsom, 1999). Although these palliative mechanisms are less desirable than are adaptive ones in the long run, the goal at this stage is to prevent loss of control or total retreat from emotional pain.

Providing support

Support, similar to empathy, begins in the orientation stage and continues throughout the nurse-patient relationship. Support confirms patients' worth and rights as human beings and includes the nurse avoiding value judgments of patients (as bad, stupid, crazy, lazy), even when patients have made poor choices. Support acknowledges that no one is perfect, that making mistakes is human, and that learning from mistakes is beneficial. Support focuses realistically and concretely on patients' abilities and strengths; for example, the nurse would not say, "You're a good person," but rather, "I'm glad you were able to share your feelings in group today." Patients need recognition of their healthy actions and feelings. Patients' dependence is tolerated until they are capable of being more independent, but any independent actions are pointed out. Support includes realistic hope and promises, such as, "I don't have an answer right now, but I will work with you to find one."

Providing structure

A major strategy in the orientation stage is to provide structure for patients. When patients lose control of their thoughts, feelings, or behaviors, the nurse has the responsibility for taking temporary control. The action may mean offering an as-needed (prn) medication, directing patients to a quieter, less stimulating place, or staying with patients at a comfortable distance. If these measures are ineffective, seclusion or restraints may then be indicated (see Chapter 13). However, providing structure also includes decreasing the withdrawal and isolation of quiet, nonparticipating patients. Spending time with these patients, even in silence, is important. The nurse can also suggest activities such as watching television or taking a walk with the patient. A major facet of providing structure is *limit setting* (see Chapter 25). Decreasing or stopping dysfunctional behaviors is in the best interest of patients. The nurse accepts patients as human beings while discouraging self-defeating behaviors. Patients' rights and self-esteem need protection, but those of others who are around the patients need protection as well. Limit setting involves pointing out behaviors and their negative effect and suggesting alternative behaviors. For example, when a patient is self-deprecating, the nurse points out the negative comments, the way in which they affect the patient's self-esteem, and then suggests that the patient identify something positive about himself or herself.

Behaviors that typically require immediate intervention are verbal and physical aggression, self-destructive behaviors, setting fires, noncompliance with rules and medications, alcohol or drug abuse, manipulation of others, inappropriate touching of others, indecent exposure, attempts to leave the hospital without permission, and failure to eat or sleep. Continuous rumination over painful feelings or disturbed thought processes is nonproductive and self-perpetuating. The nurse first listens to the content and the process of negative feelings or thoughts long enough to understand the messages or themes they convey but then distracts the patient with more productive topics. Limit setting is a kind but firm strategy. "I know you are angry right now, but I'm hav-

ing trouble understanding the situation because of all the swearing; please stop" or "I realize these thoughts are really important to you, but there are other areas I need to know about so I can help you."

The transition from the orientation stage to the working stage is not smooth or firmly defined. Patients' anxiety may increase when they are working on issues, and they may return to more superficial matters for a while. Some patients with chronic illnesses or multiple hospitalizations may need more of a focus on orientation stage interventions because of their difficulty in forming relationships (Forchuk et al, 2000).

Critical Thinking Question

John Slider is suspicious, denying his illness, and hyperactive. What combination of nursing interventions would you use in working with him?

Working stage

When patients are ready, the work toward changing their thoughts, feelings, and behaviors can begin. However, change may not be the goal for some patients, particularly the chronically ill. Rather, stabilization with medications, reduction of symptoms, and development of supportive relationships are valid goals. For patients with chronic schizophrenia in particular, the ability to relate to someone is an important goal. Some patients may be hospitalized several times before they can accept the painful fact that they have a chronic illness and need ongoing treatment (McGorry, McConville, 2000). Most patients have sufficient awareness, motivation, and trust in the nurses to begin to explore problems, to identify possible solutions, and to test new behaviors (Gauthier, 2000).

Process of learning

Changing behavior is difficult. Peplau (1963) identified the process of learning as necessary for change. (See Chapter 9 for therapeutic techniques that facilitate learning.)

The first step, *observation,* is a prerequisite, because without awareness of a problem, motivation to change cannot exist. The nurse learns the extent to which patients understand their problems by asking for in-depth, detailed descriptions of situations, thoughts, feelings, and behaviors. The *analysis* step is then necessary to encourage accuracy in patients' conclusions about their problems. For a patient to describe the type and sequence of arguments she has with her husband is one process; to conclude that she is afraid of losing control over her husband is another. Even when patients are able to identify problems accurately, they may not automatically decide that their behavior is worth changing. The *interpretation* step leads to a decision that change is necessary and appropriate.

Problem solving is the crux of the *planning* step. Patients are guided in decisions about change, in developing and considering alternative solutions, and in formulating a method for carrying out the plan. The nurse does not give advice but helps patients solve their own problems. The nurse encourages short-term, realistic, and achievable daily goals.

The *testing-out* step involves trying the new behavior or solution in a safe environment first (e.g., with the nurse) and then in a real situation. The nurse asks patients to rehearse the things they will say and do in an upcoming situation: "Tell me what you will say to your daughter tomorrow." Practice allows the patient to obtain feedback and modify the plan. Role-playing is another way of practicing behaviors. Nurses play the roles of those with whom patients are having difficulty, and they assess the patients' communication and behavior patterns. This approach helps patients handle situations more effectively.

The objectives of the *evaluation* step are to assess the success of new behaviors or solutions to problems and to determine whether modification or a different approach is needed. The nurse provides feedback in a constructive manner and helps patients learn to ask for and use feedback appropriately. Effective behaviors are more likely to continue when their benefits are discussed and reinforcement is given. Destructive behaviors are more likely to be identified when patients are taught to evaluate the effects of their actions on themselves and others.

In-depth data collection

Nurses facilitate awareness, analysis, and interpretation through in-depth (but selective) exploration of issues and by identifying priority issues. Focusing on too many problems at once may overwhelm patients. The nurse directs the data collection and focuses on manageable and changeable issues, thereby helping patients make sense out of their confusion. Spending time and energy exploring an unchangeable problem is frustrating, both to patients and to the nurse, for example, rehashing what the patient *could have* done to prevent the divorce rather than focusing on activities he *can do* now to adjust to being single. In-depth data collection increases the nurse's knowledge of patients' needs, problems, and factors that can enhance or interfere with treatment. Nursing interventions can then be more individualized, using the patient's abilities and strengths. Assessments include estimating the tasks that can and cannot be accomplished during the expected length of care and identifying the types of referrals likely to be needed at the next level of treatment within the continuum of care.

Reality testing and cognitive restructuring

Reality testing is an important strategy in the analysis, interpretation, and planning steps. Reality testing helps patients see reality more clearly and objectively when distortions or inaccuracies were present in the past. Reality testing is not a matter of arguing with a patient's point of view; rather, it presents a new reality that allows the patient to consider another option. Reality testing is constructive, not destructive, feedback: "I know the voices seem real to you, but I don't hear any" or "You sound as if you think all men are alike; I don't see it that way."

The goal of reality testing is cognitive restructuring: helping patients cope with negative thoughts and beliefs and recognize other viewpoints that will help them come to more realistic conclusions. (Wells-Federman, Stuart-Shor, Webster, 2001). Patients might need to redefine the way in which they interpret a situation, or they may need to change their perception of another person's behavior. Patients may need to give up an irrational belief in favor of a more rational one, for example, changing from "I have to be perfect" to "It's OK to make mistakes; I can learn from them." This approach may also mean giving up an unrealistic goal for a more appropriate one. The redefinition may involve discovering that sadness is concealing anger.

Writing and journaling

Having patients write down their thoughts and feelings each day is often useful. This exercise can be a release for emotions and can facilitate a more objective analysis of issues (Wells-Federman, Stuart-Shor, Webster, 2001). The nurse asks patients to write a "homework assignment" between sessions, for example, making a list of their positive qualities and strengths. Patients might also write "letters" (that are *not* sent) to others with whom they are having problems (Day, 2001). In some instances, a letter may be reworked several times and the message eventually shared with the person to whom the patient is writing.

Supportive confrontation

Supportive confrontation is similar to reality testing but has a broader focus compared with specific perceptions, interpretations, or feelings. Supportive confrontation is aimed at contradictions, discrepancies, responsibility, accountability, independence, and behavioral change; it combines support with encouragement for constructive, productive action. The support acknowledges fears, pain, ambivalence, and the difficult process of change, while the confrontation includes hope and confidence that an action is possible.

- "Giving up alcohol is a scary idea, but in this program, you can get the information and support you need to do it."
- "I hear your reluctance, but taking the risk has much to offer."
- "We all like to be taken care of once in a while, but making our own decisions helps our self-esteem."

Supportive confrontation challenges patients to meet their own needs appropriately and to be accountable for their own feelings, behaviors, and decisions. Confrontation without support is generally perceived as an attack and is nonproductive. Confrontation is avoided because the patient often experiences this at home, school, or work.

Promoting change

In addition to problem solving and supportive confrontation, several other important strategies facilitate change as well. One strategy is to change the balance of the *risk-benefit ratio* because all change has a risk of failure. For example, change may mean the loss of a comfortable habit, the fear of rejection, or even the creation of new problems. The potential benefits may be growth, self-satisfaction, improved

relationships, and a healthier self-esteem. For everyone, change is more likely to occur when the risks are low and the potential for benefits is high. The nurse can help decrease risks by discussing ways to overcome them. Short-term and long-term benefits also need to be discussed. Change can be difficult, but several approaches increase the likelihood for success. For example:

1. Carefully considered rational decisions are more likely to result in healthy changes than are decisions that are hasty and emotional.
2. Patient-initiated change (with specific plans and actions) tends to be more successful than does change that others impose.
3. Practicing or rehearsing changes with the nurse builds confidence for trying new behaviors with others and increases success.
4. Support and acceptance of change by patients' friends and families encourage and help maintain the change.
5. Support groups can reinforce new behaviors.
6. Patients are likely to change when they are ready and motivated.
7. Pushing for change too quickly is frustrating for all concerned.

Teaching new skills

The desire to change is insufficient; the patient must know the proper way to change (Klagsbrun, 2001). For example, patients cannot change from being passive to being assertive if they do not understand the meaning or cannot site examples of assertiveness. Some patients may not have learned skills that a nurse takes for granted. Common skills that patients need to learn are relaxation; stress, conflict, and anger management techniques; assertiveness; problem-solving processes; symptom management; coping skills; stress reduction; and communication, social, and community living skills (Hogarty, 2000). Occasionally, skill training must begin at a basic, concrete level. One patient's first exercise was to approach another patient and read from his 3- × 5-inch card: "Hi, my name is Bill, and I'm from Greenfield. What's your name?" Skills are taught in small steps with frequent intermittent opportunities for practice and feedback. Again, homework assignments can be used; for example, the nurse might suggest that between sessions the patient practice a particular skill and report the results at the next session.

Termination stage

In acute inpatient settings and outpatient programs, the "work" and changes are rarely completed. Patients are discharged or transferred to another level of care, and nurses change units or jobs. However, strategies are available that facilitate a healthy closure of the relationship for both the patient and the nurse. If all the nurses involved with the patient are not available to discuss termination, then the nurse who is assigned to discharge or transfer the patient can implement the strategies.

Evaluation and summary of progress

The nurse guides discussions to help patients identify *for themselves* the specific changes in thoughts, feelings, and behaviors that have occurred. Even small steps toward long-term goals are discussed. Reinforcing changes in and strengths of patients is important. Areas or issues that need more work are outlined, cautioning patients to avoid trying to change everything at once. Patients are encouraged to set priorities for these issues and to establish reasonable time frames for action.

Synthesizing the outcomes

Synthesizing focuses on the more indirect outcomes of the nurse-patient relationship, such as more open communications or more appropriate expression of feelings. As a result of the relationship, patients often feel more comfortable with initiating interactions, making requests, and expressing opinions, even when these behaviors were not discussed during the nurse-patient encounters. Increased participation and socialization must be recognized as well. As the nurse points out the benefits from the relationship, patients are encouraged to form other relationships with future nurses, counselors, and new friends.

Referrals

For the problems that need continuing attention after discharge, referrals to appropriate resources are finalized (see Chapter 8). The resources provide support, foster treatment compliance, and promote continued growth. Receiving written discharge instructions that list medications, dosages, and times, as well as phone numbers, addresses, dates, and times of appointments and self-help meetings, is helpful for patients. Also important is assessing patients' ability to read these instructions; if they are unable to do so, then someone in the patient's support systems who can read the instructions should be found (Mason, 2001). If the patient speaks a language other than English, then the instructions can be translated into the patient's native language.

Discussion of termination

Regardless of the length, frequency of contact, or intensity of the nurse-patient relationship, discussing the participants' reactions to the relationship is important. Feelings may be positive, ambivalent, or negative and may vary in degree. Superficial relationships are likely to produce mild reactions. However, the relationship may mean more to the patient than it does to the nurse; therefore the loss of contact with the nurse may be significant to the patient. Patients may experience anger or fear related to losing the support and acceptance that the nurse provides. Some patients may avoid any discussion of termination. Nonetheless, the nurse should attempt to "make it official" by saying "good-bye" and stating his or her feelings about the relationship, for example, "I'm glad I had a chance to work with you." The nurse serves as a role model for the patient who is unable to discuss termination at the time. The feelings of the nurse are important and open for discussion (but not to the point of burdening the patient with the nurse's issues). Nurses may feel as though they are abandoning the patient, particularly when building trust was difficult for the patient.

Critical Thinking Question

What statements you would make to patients about your role and the role of the other nurses in the treatment of patients?

INTERACTIONS WITH SELECTED BEHAVIORS

The purpose of this section is to discuss interventions with selected behaviors that are appropriate in brief encounters with patients. The behaviors included here are ones the nurse may encounter with any patient, regardless of the patient's diagnosis. Longer-term interventions are discussed in the chapters dealing with psychiatric disorders. Certain problem behaviors, such as anger and withdrawal, have already been discussed.

Violent Behavior

Fear of violent behavior and of being injured is a concern with the few patients who do not respond to the verbal diffusing of anger or of those who feel extremely threatened (usually because of internal thought disturbances) by staff members. The following are a few precautions to take for protection:

- Stay out of striking distance (this also reduces the threat to the patient).
- Avoid touching patients without approval.
- Change the topic temporarily if a patient's behavior is escalating.
- Suggest "time out" for the patient in a quiet area with fewer stimuli.
- Sit by the patient's door (with the door open) until the patient is calmer.
- Avoid entering a room alone with a patient who is not in control of his or her behavior.
- Leave temporarily if the patient is agitated and asking to be left alone.
- Call for staff assistance if the patient is losing control.

Chapter 13 focuses on working with aggressive patients.

Hallucinations

The initial approach with patients who appear to be listening to or talking with "voices" is to comment on their behavior: "You look as if you are listening to something. What do you hear?" If the patient acknowledges hearing something the nurse cannot hear, the nurse can then say, "I don't hear anything. Tell me what you hear." The early assessment of hallucinations is based on the content of messages (Beck, Rector, 1998). The hallucinatory content often reveals the dynamics of the patient's illness and typically revolves around themes of powerlessness, hatred, guilt, or loneliness. After the content is known, focusing on the hallucinations is unnecessary; doing so might reinforce them: "I know the voices are important to you, but let's talk about your loneliness right now." The exception is with hallucinations that command patients to harm themselves or others or to do other destructive acts. Then the nurse should contract with patients to avoid acting on the commands they hear and to tell the staff.

Delusions

The initial approach with respect to delusions is clarification of meanings (Beck, Rector, 1998), for example, "Who do you think is trying to hurt you?" or "Tell me about this power you think you have." Similar to hallucinations, delusions are not discussed after the meanings are clarified. Arguing with a patient about delusions is ineffective, inappropriate, and may strengthen the patients' belief in them. The underlying themes reflected in the delusions are more appropriately addressed in interventions that help the patient who says she is a queen feel important in realistic ways. Careful monitoring is needed if the delusions might lead patients to harm themselves or others; for example, a patient does not want to eat because he believes all the food is poisoned.

Conflicting Values

Occasionally, nurses and patients encounter conflicts with their beliefs or values. Both participants can state their views in a discussion, but arguing is inappropriate. A better approach is to help patients examine the effects or outcomes of their beliefs on their lives, relationships, and happiness. For example, a patient may believe that she has the right to drink as much and as often as she wants because drinking is legal. Supportive confrontation can help her examine the effects of drinking on her marriage, job, health, and economic status.

Agreeing with every patient's beliefs, values, or behaviors is not necessary to be an effective nurse. Nurses must be aware of their own stance on issues and understand patients' points of view *as the patients see it*. Usually, patients need not change a belief or a behavior that is not causing problems for them or for others around them. Beliefs and behaviors that have positive effects need reinforcement.

Incoherent Speech Patterns

Disturbed thought processes are occasionally evident in speech; when these processes occur, the approach is to clarify the meaning of the communications. However, severely ill patients may be unable to be clearer, and repeated questions will only increase anxiety. Medications often decrease the anxiety and then clear the thought disturbances rather quickly. Until then, the nurse spends frequent, brief time with these patients (without pressuring or frustrating them), offers support, and builds trust.

Manipulation

Common manipulations are a means to gain attention, sympathy ("poor me"), control, and dependence (for others to take responsibility). Manipulation is not often recognized until it has already "worked." The nurse may then experience anger or embarrassment. The initial approach is to address that which is happening (or has happened): "I'm getting the feeling you would like me to tell you what to do. What scares you about this decision?" or "You are experiencing a lot of emotional pain and would like me to relieve it for you. Let's talk about what *you* can do to relieve it." Limit setting is useful with manipulative patients. A power struggle with the patient is useless. Helping patients to express their needs directly to others is more productive.

Crying

Unless crying is a manipulative gesture or is prolonged and unproductive, it should be allowed and even encouraged, verbally and nonverbally. By saying, "It's okay to cry" or quietly offering a tissue, the nurse gives patients permission to cry and relieve tension. Privacy should be provided. The nurse should be as quiet and unobtrusive as possible until the crying has ceased. The patient is then offered an opportunity to discuss the circumstance that precipitated the tears.

Sexual Innuendos or Inappropriate Touch

Patients generally stop these behaviors when asked to and are reminded that these actions are inappropriate. The nurse then discusses the underlying need. If the behaviors continue, then setting limits can be stronger: "I want to talk to you but not if you continue to touch me." "If you don't stop, I will have to leave and come back later." Pairing patients who act out sexually and have poor impulse control with staff members of the same sex may also help until these patients are further along in treatment. This strategy may be ineffective with homosexual patients.

Denial and Lack of Cooperation

Many reasons exist that cause patients to be uncooperative with the nurse in working toward treatment goals. A common reason is severe disturbances in thought processes (hallucinations, delusions, disorientation, and confusion) that interfere with patients' understanding the nature of the problems and the changes that are needed. With some patients, the disturbances are less evident, but denial of any problems remains, and insight into their problems and recognition of the need for treatment is lacking (McGorry, McConville, 2000). In fact, these patients

may be angry about being "forced" into treatment. Occasionally, a patient may admit to the need for help but disagree with the type of treatment offered. Other patients may be afraid of changing, even though they realize their behaviors are nonproductive or harmful. Listening, clarifying, and verbalizing thoughts that have been implied are appropriate for identifying the underlying causes of a lack of cooperation. Then to the extent possible, the causes, fears, and outcomes of patients' behaviors are discussed directly. "What are you afraid will happen if you have to give up alcohol as a way of avoiding your problem?" Trust is often an issue for these patients, thus measures to increase trust and a great deal of patience from the nurse will be needed.

Depressed Affect, Apathy, and Psychomotor Retardation

When patients express sadness, helplessness, hopelessness, lack of energy, or a negative attitude about everything, the nurse occasionally experiences sadness, helplessness, sympathy, or frustration. Patience, frequent contact, and empathy are more appropriate. Even when patients realize the change that must be made, they do not always have the energy to make the adjustment quickly. The nurse acknowledges feelings but discourages rumination: "You are so focused on your sadness that you are simply stuck. Come take a walk with me for a few minutes." Personal hygiene, nutrition, and a gradual increase in activities are encouraged. Major decisions are postponed until emotions subside and thinking is more logical.

Suspiciousness

When patients are suspicious, they may be afraid of everyone, everything, and every interaction around them. The nurse must therefore communicate clearly, simply, and congruently. Misinterpretations by patients are clarified, but arguments over differences in opinion are avoided. Rationales or explanations for rules, activities, occurrences, noises, and requests are offered regularly. Patients' participation is encouraged but not forced, thus increasing their fears is avoided.

Hyperactivity

Excessive physical and emotional activity of patients is upsetting to the staff, to other patients, and often to the hyperactive patients themselves. Even unintentionally, patients may harm themselves or others (see the previous discussion of violence). These patients should be in a quiet area with minimal auditory and visual stimulation. Physical activity such as walking or using a stationary bicycle may help to drain excess energy. The nurse must remain calm, speak slowly and softly, and respect patients' personal space. Directions are given in a kind, simple, but firm manner. Occasionally, a prn medication is required.

Transference

Transference involves the unconscious emotional reaction that patients have in a current situation that is actually based on previous, even childhood, relationships and experiences (Smith et al, 1997). For example, a patient perceives the nurse as acting the way his mother did, regardless of the way in which the nurse is truly acting. Transference may explain feelings that patients exhibit that do not fit in the current context of a situation or that are out of proportion to the situation. Common issues in transference are the wish to be taken care of, to have needs met by someone else, and to express unresolved emotions. Transference may be severe in the form of delusions, or they may be subtle, as in stereotyping all males as aggressive and all females as submissive. Transference can be positive if patients view the nurse as helpful and caring. Negative transference is more difficult with which to deal because of unpleasant emotions that interfere with treatment, such as anger and fear.

Nurses may experience transference reactions with patients, coworkers, and physicians. Guilt or anger about not helping a particular patient or anger toward a demanding physician may be an unconscious transference response. Countertransference (reactions based on the nurse's past experiences) (Smith et al, 1997) may occur in response to a patient's transference after the nurse-patient relationship is established. For example, when a patient criticizes the nurse, the nurse may relive feelings that were experienced in childhood, when a teacher criticized him or her in class. These feelings will interfere with the nurse's ability to be therapeutic. A reaction might lead to the nurse becoming sympathetic and unable to confront the patient appropri-

ately. Another reaction might lead to avoidance or rejection of the patient. In either case, the nurse's behavior is not therapeutic.

The first intervention is to recognize the transference or countertransference, which is difficult because of the unconscious processes involved. Coworkers are more likely than are others to recognize the phenomenon initially and give feedback to the nurse about it. After the reaction is recognized, the nurse can seek assistance in examining the countertransference issues. Nurses must examine their feelings, reactions, and behaviors before they will be able to interact more appropriately with patients (Eckroth-Bucher, 2001). The transference reactions of patients must also be examined gently but directly. Nurses must be open and clear about their genuine reactions when patients misperceive behavior. Nurses should also state actions that they can and cannot do to meet patients' needs. Limit setting is useful when patients act inappropriately toward the nurse. Redirection of needs to more appropriate people can also be a helpful intervention, for example, "I can't be your girlfriend, but let's talk about making new friends at home."

Key Concepts

1. To be therapeutic, the nurse uses verbal and nonverbal communications to convey a willingness to listen, genuine respect, a desire to help, and an understanding of the patient as a person with unique problems and needs.
2. The nurse-patient relationship is a series of goal-directed interactions that focus on the patient's thoughts, feelings, behaviors, and potential solutions to problems.
3. The nursing process is a tool with which the nurse assesses each patient's problems, selects and carries out specific interventions, and evaluates the effectiveness of care.
4. Each stage of the nurse-patient relationship (orientation, working, termination) involves specific tasks that are used according to the needs and problems of each patient.
5. Issues and patient behaviors that interfere with the progress of the nurse-patient relationship must be addressed by the nurse.

References

Beck AT, Rector NA: Cognitive therapy for schizophrenic patients, *The Harv Ment Health Lett* 15(6):4, 1998.

Day AL: The journal as a guide for the healing journey, *Nurs Clin North Am* 336(1):131, 2001.

Deering CG: To speak or not to speak? Self-disclosure with patients, *AJN* 99(1):34, 1999.

Eckroth-Bucher M: Philosophical basis and practice of self-awareness in psychiatric nursing, *J Psychosoc Nurs* 39(2):32, 2001.

Folsom D: Nursing the patient within, *AJN* 99(7):80, 1999.

Forchuk C et al: The developing nurse-client relationship: nurses' perspectives, *J Am Psychiatr Nurs Assoc* 6(1):3, 2000.

Gauthier PA: Use of Peplau's interpersonal relations model to counsel people with AIDS, *J Am Psychiatr Nurs Assoc* 6(4):119, 2000.

Haddad A: Ethics in action, *RN* 64(5):25, 2001.

Hogarty GE: Cognitive rehabilitation of schizophrenia, *Harv Ment Health Lett* 17(2):4, 2000.

Klagsbrun J: Listening and focusing: holistic health care tools for nurses, *Nurs Clin North Am* 36(1):115, 2001.

Mason DJ: Promoting health literacy, *AJN* 101(2):7, 2001.

McGorry PD, McConville SB: Insight in psychosis, *Harv Ment Health Lett* 17(5):3, 2000.

Peplau HE: A working definition of anxiety. In Burd SE, Marshall MA, editors: *Some clinical approaches to psychiatric nursing,* Toronto, 1963, Macmillan.

Peplau HE: *Interpersonal relations in nursing,* New York, 1952, Putnam and Sons.

Smith LL et al: Nurse-patient boundaries: crossing the line, *Am J Nurs* 97(12):26 1997.

Walker KM, Alligood MR: Empathy from a nursing perspective: moving beyond borrowed theory, *Arch Psychiatr Nurs* 15(3):140, 2001.

Wells-Federman CL, Stuart-Shor E, Webster A: Cognitive therapy: applications for health promotion, disease prevention, and disease management, *Nurs Clin North Am* 36(1):93, 2001.

Wysoker A: Legal and ethical considerations: confidentiality, *J Am Psychiatr Nurs Assoc* 7(2):57, 2001.

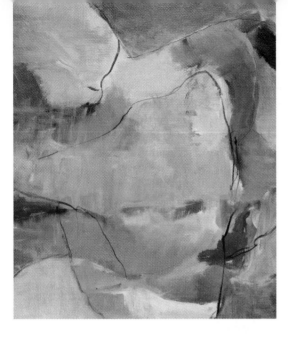

Chapter 11

Nursing Process

Lee H. Schwecke

Learning Objectives

After reading this chapter, you should be able to:

- Relate the nursing process to psychiatric nursing practice.
- Identify the components of an initial holistic patient assessment.
- Describe the components of the mental status examination.
- Describe the importance of writing a specific nursing diagnosis and care plan.

The use of the nursing process (Figure 11-1) has the same goal in psychiatric nursing as it has in other areas of nursing: patient-centered, goal-directed action that facilitates health promotion, primary prevention, treatment, and rehabilitation. Care is adapted to patients' unique needs. Individualized care begins with a detailed assessment.

ASSESSMENT

Initial Patient Assessment

This phase begins on admission to a unit or program with a nurse. Each psychiatric hospital, unit, clinic, and program has its own version of an intake or nursing assessment form. Box 11-1 provides a sample of the kind of information included in the initial assessment. Physiologic systems and medical problems are reviewed to identify the need for medical orders, special nursing care, or diets. Allergies, if any, are listed as well. Current medications with dosages, frequency, and time of last dose are important. The potential for withdrawal from medications or other drugs is a risk to be noted. Results from laboratory tests, physical examinations, x-ray examinations, and psychologic testing are other sources of data. Patient self-assessments, such as the "Geriatric Depression Scale" (see Appendix C), and patient perceptions of personal strengths, support systems, and resources are important factors to take into account.

The multidisciplinary team includes at least the nurse, psychiatrist, psychologist, social worker, pharmacist, and dietitian. The staff uses all information that team members collect to confirm the patient assessment, while minimizing the need for the patient to repeat information. Because most facilities use intake forms or checklists, the results of the interviews do not have to be written in narrative form. Summarization of the critical content as an admission note that is included in the progress notes may be expected.

Mental Status Examination

In psychiatric settings, an important component of patient assessment is the mental status examination

(MSE), which focuses on the patient's current state in terms of thoughts, feelings, and behaviors. The categories of the MSE help organize a summary of the information gathered during the initial patient

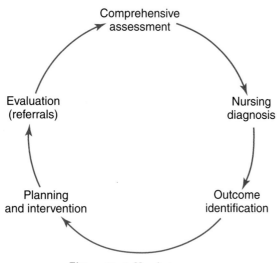

Figure 11-1 Nursing process.

| Box 11-1 | Initial Patient Assessment

- **Demographic data.** Full name, sex, age, date of birth, address, marital status, and family members' names and ages
- **Admission data.** Date and time of admission and type of admission (voluntary or committed)
- **Reason for admission.** Current problems as perceived by the patient; include stressors, difficulty with coping, developmental issues, "emergency behaviors" (suicidal or homicidal ideas and attempts, aggression, destructive behaviors, risk of escape), and family history
- **Previous psychiatric history.** Dates, inpatient or outpatient, reasons for and types of treatment and their effectiveness, current medications, and compliance
- **Current medical problems, and medications.**
- **Drug and alcohol use or abuse.** Amount, frequency, duration of past and present use of legal and illegal substances, and date and time of last use
- **Disturbances in patterns of daily living.** Sleep, intake, elimination, sexual activity, work, leisure, self-care, and hygiene
- **Culture and spirituality.** Ethnicity, beliefs, practices, and religious preference
- **Support systems.** Amount of contact, nature and quality of relationships, and availability of support

assessment. The information related to each of the categories includes the following:

- General appearance: type, condition, and appropriateness of clothing (for age, season, setting), grooming, cleanliness, physical condition, and posture
- Behaviors during the interview: Degree of cooperation, resistance, or evasiveness
- Social skills: friendliness, shyness, or withdrawal
- Amount and type of motor activity: psychomotor agitation or retardation, restlessness, tics, tremors, hypervigilance, or lack of activity
- Speech patterns: amount, rate, volume, tone pressure, mutism, slurring, or stuttering
- Degree of concentration and attention span
- Orientation: to time, place, person, and level of consciousness
- Memory: immediate recall, recent, remote, amnesia, and confabulation
- Intellectual functioning: educational level, use of language and knowledge, abstract versus concrete thinking (proverbs), and calculations (serial sevens)
- Affect: labile, blunted, flat, incongruent, or inappropriate affect
- Mood: specific moods expressed or observed—euphoria, depression, anxiety, anger, guilt, or fear
- Thought clarity: coherence, confusion, or vagueness
- Thought content: helplessness, hopelessness, worthlessness, suicidal thoughts or plans, homicidal thoughts or plans, suspiciousness, phobias, obsessions, compulsions, preoccupations, poverty of content, denial, hallucinations (auditory, visual, olfactory, gustatory, tactile) or delusions (of reference, influence, persecution, grandeur, religious, nihilistic, somatic)
- Thought processes reflected in speech: ambivalence, circumstantiality, tangentiality, thought blocking, loose associations, flight of ideas, perseveration, neologisms, or "word salad"
- Insight: degree of awareness of illness, behaviors, problems, and their causes
- Judgment: soundness of problem solving and decisions
- Motivation: degree of motivation for treatment

Some patients are too ill to participate in or complete the assessment interview. In these cases, objective data such as patient behaviors and reports by their family members are used. In some instances, information from staff in the outpatient setting that the patient attends will be available. During the initial assessment, behaviors can be described without knowing or identifying their causes, for example, anxiety level, degree of withdrawal, thought disturbances reflected in speech, voice tone, and general appearance. Causes and dynamics can be elicited later to form a strong basis for a treatment plan. A sample MSE is illustrated in Box 11-2.

On-Going Assessments

Even when the initial assessment is complete, each encounter with a patient involves a continuing assessment that may or may not be congruent with the initial assessment. No one acts or feels the same way 24 hours a day, 7 days a week. The ongoing assessment often involves an investigation of patients' statements and actions at the moment: "You have been sitting alone for a while. What have you been thinking about?" or "You mentioned being worried; what about?" When the nurse decides to investigate a patient's specific behavior, exploring the following may be valuable:

- Context or situation that precipitated the behavior
- Patient's thoughts at the time
- Patient's feelings then and now
- Whether the behavior makes sense in that context
- Whether the behavior was adaptive or dysfunctional
- Way in which this episode fits with the total picture of the patient
- Whether a change is needed

NURSING DIAGNOSIS

Nursing diagnoses are the identification of patients' problems based on conclusions about the dynamics evident in verbalizations and behaviors. Emergency behaviors (e.g., suicidal or homicidal ideas or attempts, aggression, destructive behaviors, risk of arson or escape) are given priority in establishing nursing diagnoses and in negotiating "no-harm contracts" with patients. Regardless of the format or style of nursing diagnosis in a particular setting, the diagnosis should be specific and point to a desired outcome for the patient. In this text, the North American Nursing Diagnosis Association (NANDA)

I Box 11-2 I Sample Mental Status Examination*

- **General appearance.** Dressed appropriately for season; clothes are clean but not pressed; hair is unwashed and uncombed; slouched shoulders; pale; blank expression
- **Behaviors during interview:**
  - **Cooperation-resistance-evasiveness.** Slow to respond but cooperative
  - **Social skills.** Withdrawn; no unusual habits; reduced socialization
- **Motor activity.** Slowed; crying at times; no tics or tremors noted
- **Speech patterns.** Amount is reduced with slowed rate and soft tone
- **Concentration-attention span.** Decreased concentration; easily distracted by stimuli; slight shortening of attention span
- **Orientation.** Aware of person, place, and time; responsive
- **Memory:**
  - **Immediate recall.** Remembers nurse's name.
  - **Recent.** Difficulty organizing sequence but mostly complete except for last week
  - **Remote.** Good detail on birth of children

- **Thought clarity.** Clear, coherent
- **Thought content.** Expressing helplessness, hopelessness, and suicidal thoughts without a plan; fears being alone; no evidence of hallucinations or delusions
- **Thought process.** No disturbances noted
- **Intellectual functioning.** College education evident in vocabulary; calculations and proverbs were not done; abstract thinking evident in discussion of love and fidelity
- **Affect.** Blunted
- **Mood.** Depressed; anxiety level is moderate; guilt and covert anger expressed
- **Insight.** Aware of problems in facing divorce but not yet able to describe factors leading to separation
- **Judgment.** No impairment until last 2 weeks when she became unable to make decisions, take action, or seek support
- **Motivation for treatment.** Wants help with depression, tiredness, and handling divorce; unable to state what type of help she needs

*Based on the Sample Process Recording (Table 11-1) on pages 114 and 115 and the Clinical Example on page 116.

|Table 11-1 | Sample Process Recording

Nurse introduces himself or herself and leads the way to the office, walking slowly but slightly ahead of the patient. The patient follows without looking at the nurse. In the office, the nurse sits in a chair at a desk and opens a folder of papers. The patient sits in a chair at the side of the desk, holding her purse with both hands on her lap.

NURSE		PATIENT		ANALYSIS	
Verbal	Nonverbal	Verbal	Nonverbal	Themes	Therapeutic Techniques
What do you prefer to be called, Mrs. Jarvis or Anita?	Has pen in hand, other hand is flat on desk; is looking at patient.	(pause) Anita	Is looking at floor.		Questioning, active listening
Anita, we will be better able to help you if we know more about you. What has happened in your life recently?	(Same as above.)	(pause) I couldn't get out of bed. (pause) I was so tired.	Is turning head slightly, still looking at the floor; is not smiling or frowning.	Content—describes fatigue and effects. Mood—sadness. Interaction—opens up with nurse.	Giving information, questioning
How long have you been feeling so tired?	Is writing and looking at patient.	I don't know. (pause) A week, I guess.	(Same as above.)	Content—unsure of time frames, marital separation, possible divorce.	Placing event in time or sequence, active listening
What happened a week ago? I can see this is difficult for you to talk about. (pause) What did he say when he left?	Leans toward patient. Moves tissue box. Looks at patient; both arms are on lap.	(pause) My husband (pause) left. That he was fed up. (pause) That he wanted a divorce.	Tears are in eyes; tries to open purse. Is nodding head; raises eyes slightly; is still not looking at the nurse. Starts to cry; gets tissue. Sobs occasionally.	Mood—sadness, guilt. Interaction—in conflict with husband, is more trusting of nurse.	Focusing Using empathy, and silence, questioning
What did you say to him?	Leans slightly toward patient. One arm is on lap, the other is on arm of chair.	I don't know. I don't remember. (pause) Maybe I asked him to stay.	Is crying quietly.	Content—difficulty describing situations, short-term memory disturbance.	Focusing, active listening
Then what happened?	(Same as above.)	It's all a blur, I think I cried all day.	(Same as above.)	Mood—sadness, guilt. Interactions—abandonment, loneliness.	Focusing

Nurse Verbal	Nurse Nonverbal	Patient Verbal	Patient Nonverbal	Analysis	Technique
Who did you talk to?	(Same as above.)	No one. (pause) My kids are married and gone. I just stayed in bed.	Is the same but crying less often.	Content—did not ask for help, avoidance of divorce issue. Mood—sadness. Interaction—perceived lack of support.	Focusing
When you were feeling so tired, did you have thoughts of killing yourself?	(Same as above.)	(pause) I was so scared of being alone. I thought I'd rather be dead.	Looks at nurse for the first time; both hands are in lap.	Content—aware of fears, suicidal ideation but no plan, difficulty with problem solving.	Questioning
How did you think about killing yourself?	(Same as above.)	I couldn't think of anything. I didn't know what to do.	Looks at floor again; fumbles in purse.	Mood—sadness, depression. Interaction—abandonment, lack of support, open with nurse.	Focusing
Are you still thinking about suicide?	Hands patient a tissue.	Not really. But (pause) I still wish I were dead. I don't know what to do.	Blows nose and then puts hands in lap; looks at the nurse.	Content—minimizing suicidal ideation but ambivalent, helplessness. Mood—sadness. Interaction—asking for help.	Focusing
While you are here, we are going to help you consider some options about what to do so you won't feel so alone and scared. (pause)	Leans forward. Looks at patient. Both hands on lap.	(silence)	Looks at floor; crying has stopped; looks at nurse.		Suggesting collaboration, verbalizing the implied, active listening
It will help us if I ask you some questions.	Turns back to papers. Is ready to write.	Okay.	Looks at nurse.		Giving information

diagnoses are used because they are the most widely accepted and commonly used nursing diagnoses. NANDA diagnoses suggest a statement that has three components:

1. Potential or actual problems
2. Contributing or etiologic factor
3. Defining characteristic or behavioral outcome

The statement is typically written as follows: (Problem) related to (contributing factor) as evidenced by (behavioral outcome), for example, "Anxiety, moderate, related to marital problems as evidenced by ineffective problem solving."

Actual or potential problems are identified from the list approved by NANDA (see Appendix B). Contributing or etiologic factors can include stressors, losses, past experiences, developmental issues, environmental circumstances, relationship issues, and self-perceptions. Defining characteristics or behavioral outcomes are the verbal and nonverbal cues that reflect the patient's actual or potential problems. These dysfunctional behaviors or cues are the focus of the nursing interventions—behaviors that it would be helpful to change. Being specific in describing the dysfunctional behaviors or cues is useful in giving direction for selecting desirable or adaptive behaviors identified in the patient's desired outcomes. Nursing diagnoses do not include medical diagnoses in any of the three parts.

OUTCOME IDENTIFICATION

A goal or outcome specifies an adaptive behavior to replace one that is dysfunctional. Expecting patients to change a negative self-image to a positive self-image during a short inpatient stay or outpatient program is unrealistic. A more realistic behavioral goal would be to ask patients to write a list of their strengths, abilities, or positive qualities. This goal is achievable and measurable. Short-term goals or outcomes are those achievable in perhaps 4 to 6 days for hospitalized patients and perhaps somewhat longer for patients in other settings. Long-term goals or outcomes relate to issues that require follow-up counseling after discharge to another type of service within the continuum of care. For example, a female patient's short-term goal may be to identify her fears about relationships with men. The longer-term goal is to practice ways of responding to potential dating situations thus her fears would decrease and enable her to handle these types of situations.

In establishing goals and outcomes *with* a patient, the nurse must understand the problems that the patient wants to address and the goals that the patient wants to achieve (Hansten, Washburn, 2001). Patient desires and motivation play a major role in attaining outcomes. Patient support systems and resources may also facilitate outcome achievement (Walden-McBride, McBride, 2000). Outcome achievement can also be used in evaluating the quality and effectiveness of nursing care (Oermann, Huber, 1999).

CLINICAL EXAMPLE

Anita Jarvis is a 46-year-old patient who is separated from her husband who asked for a divorce and left her 1 week ago. Her son and daughter brought Anita to the hospital after they visited her and found that she had not been getting out of bed to shower or eat. They reported that their mother stated that she wished she were dead. Anita admits to feeling suicidal but denies having any suicide plans. She has no history of medical or psychiatric illnesses and takes no medications. Anita stated that she stopped seeing her friend 1 month ago and does not want to do anything any more. She is not close to her parents who live out of state. She called the school in which she teaches 4 days ago and said she was sick. She admits to staying in bed "all the time" but sleeping only 3 to 4 hours a night. Anita was admitted to the hospital with an initial diagnosis of depression. Mrs. Jarvis and her situation are used in the chapter examples of a process recording (see Table 11-1 on pages 114 and 115), MSE (see Box 11-2 on page 113), progress note (Box 11-3), and Care Plan on page 119.

PLANNING AND INTERVENTION
Nursing Care Plans

Nursing staff, on units or in programs, often develop standardized care plans with expected outcomes for certain types of patient problems. These care plans may focus on psychiatric diagnoses (e.g., major depression) or more specific problems (e.g., self-mutilation). Standardized care plans may be called clinical pathways, critical pathways, or multidisciplinary care plans. The initial care plan may be updated at any time but begins with one or two behavior-oriented problems to be addressed immediately, for example, suicide, aggression, arson,

Box 11-3 | Progress Note Components

- **Subjective content.** The patient's statements about his or her own thoughts, feelings, behaviors, and problems
- **Objective data.** The nurse's observations or measurements, such as the patient's appearance, nonverbal behaviors, and vital signs
- **Analysis or conclusions.** The nurse's impressions of what the patient is experiencing or demonstrating in behavioral or descriptive terms (not medical diagnoses); defenses, mood, and issues are identified; depressed mood and paranoid ideas can be discussed, but "depression" and "paranoia" are not listed as illnesses; conclusions about changes (regression or progression) in the patient and medication responses are described
- **Plans.** Actions that the nurses or other team members can take to intervene with the problems described in the progress note

Sample Progress Note
Date and time: 11/10/02, 1600.
46-year-old white female voluntarily admitted to 3N, accompanied by son. Initial nursing assessment is complete.

S: Patient states she has been tired and in bed most of the day since husband left her a week ago. States she is unsure of what led to the separation and cannot face living alone. Has thoughts of suicide but no plan. "I still wish I were dead." Describes decrease in socialization and support. Saw one friend a month ago. Did not contact children about separation and is not close to family of origin. Verbalizes that she doesn't know what to do about impending divorce and being alone in the future.

O: Exhibits blunted, depressed affect, limited eye contact, slowed motor activity and speech. Cries occasionally. A "no-suicide contract" was signed and placed in chart.

A: Patient cannot describe her thoughts and feelings, but guilt, helplessness, and hopelessness are evident. Anger is barely evident at this point. Suicidal but lacks energy to plan. Support is available but not perceived as such.

P: 1. Approach and sit with patient frequently.
2. Encourage verbalization of feelings as tolerated in small doses.
3. Monitor energy level and suicidal ideation.
4. Initiate medications as ordered.
5. Encourage attendance at group meetings.

escape, withdrawal or isolation, delusions, hallucinations, impulsive or compulsive acts, suspiciousness, uncooperativeness, or altered thought processes. For example, a patient who has suicidal ideations (problem) would be expected to sign a "no-harm contract" (outcome) within 24 hours (time constraint) and to verbalize an absence of suicidal ideation (outcome) by day 3 of admission (time constraint). Related nursing interventions would include (1) a contract with the patient for safety, (2) removal of dangerous objects from the patient and the patient's room, and (3) assessment for suicidal ideation during every shift.

Given the current managed care climate, a goal of standardized care plans is to expedite treatment activities to achieve patient outcomes in a cost-effective manner (i.e., quickly). Nursing interventions focus particularly on "safety, structure, support, and symptom management" (Delaney, Pitula, Perraud, 2000). However, the nurse must remember that each patient is an individual, even when some of the patient's problems "fit" into a standardized plan. A patient's unique problems and needs must not be ignored when formulating the plan of care (Brenner, 2000).

Psychiatric nursing interventions involve few "hands-on" activities other than minor treatments, monitoring vital signs, and giving medications. Rather, the focus is on the verbal strategies discussed in this chapter and in Chapter 9 that are used to guide patients in solving problems for themselves and in achieving desired outcomes. Psychiatric nurses are primarily facilitators and educators. Solving problems and changing behaviors are never quite as easy as they sound. Patients may need help with developing specific and concrete plans for reaching their goals. For example, a patient may set a goal of finding a new apartment but needs assistance in locating rental options and in evaluating the pros and cons of each apartment option.

Progress Notes and Shift Reports

The style of charting progress notes (written or electronic) varies in each setting, but the components are basically the same: the patient's statements and the nurse's observations, analyses, and plans. Charting and shift reports are important ways of communicating with team members. These reports are also ways of evaluating the effectiveness of treatment plans and progress toward patient short-term and long-term outcomes (Hansten, Washburn, 2001). (Patients must also be kept informed of their progress toward their goals.) The nurse must remember that the entire chart is a legal document subject to review by peer review agencies, quality improvement staff, and accreditation bodies (Oermann, Huber, 1999). Box 11-3 details the components of a progress note and provides a sample note. Shift reports are a concise, focused, and abbreviated list of the items that are included in the progress notes.

EVALUATION

Patient Progress

The more realistic and measurable the goals are, the greater the likelihood is that patients and nurses will have a sense of progress. A major problem arises with evaluating care in psychiatric nursing when too much change is expected too soon. When the patient or nurse becomes aware of a lack of progress toward goals, evaluation should lead to reassessment. Using the nursing process leads to reformulation of the nursing diagnoses and the establishment of more realistic or appropriate outcomes. This concept is especially true in short-term settings in which patients are discharged before "all their problems are solved." Even when short-term goals are met, patients have other unsolved problems. If the short-term goals were related to learning better skills (e.g., communication, problem-solving, social skills), then patients are able to continue to progress after discharge.

Evaluating patient progress is important in determining patient referrals to other levels of care and supervision within the continuum of care (Gauthier, 2000) (see Chapter 6). In addition to evaluating the progress of patients, nurses evaluate the quality of their interventions and their professional behaviors.

Discharge Summaries

Many facilities and programs expect nurses to participate in writing transfer or discharge summaries and discharge instructions that will be given to patients. Summaries usually identify outcomes that the patient achieved and outcomes that must still be addressed. The following information is usually included in the discharge instructions: medication (including dosages and times), follow-up appointments (with dates and times), and referrals to other services along the continuum of care. As discussed in Chapter 10, assessing the patient's ability to read and understand the discharge instructions is important (Winslow, 2001).

Process Recordings

Peplau (1968) used process recordings in her writings to show applications of concepts and examples of interventions. The use of communication skills is emphasized as a means of helping patients learn and solve problems. Process recordings are tools for the nurse, particularly for the student nurse, to learn about working effectively with patients.

This method provides a means of assessing and analyzing communication skills, identifying patient themes, and evaluating the effectiveness of interventions (Festa et al, 2000). Audiotape or videotape recordings are more accurate compared with written reports but are not possible in most settings or with many patients. Written process recordings may begin with notes taken during the interview or may be totally assembled by recall afterward. A process recording is a record of an encounter with a patient that is as verbatim as possible. The recording generally includes the nonverbal behaviors of the nurse and the patient, as well as the verbal interaction.

Analysis of content, mood, and interaction themes (Gauthier, 2000) may be included next to each written statement or summarized at the end of the process recording. The process recording may be analyzed by the nurse or shared with a colleague who can give constructive feedback on problem areas and strategies for improvement. Videotaped nurse-patient clinical simulations can also be used (Festa et al, 2000). The recording is a learning tool, not an end in itself, which can be used periodically for professional growth. A sample written process recording of this chapter's "patient" is presented earlier in the chapter (see Table 11-1).

Critical Thinking Question

For the patient in this chapter (see Box 11-2, Box 11-3, and Care Plan), can you identify two additional nursing diagnoses, two short-term goals, two long-term goals, and four nursing interventions?

Care Plan

Name: Anita Jarvis _____   Admission Date: 11/10/01 _____

DSM-IV-TR Diagnosis: Depressive episode _____

Assessment | **Areas of strength:** Has family who cares; had good work record; has asked for help; is thinking abstractly.
Problems: Is unable to get out of bed and care for self; has suicidal thoughts but no plan; exhibits decreased socialization and support; impending divorce.

Diagnoses
- Risk, anxiety, moderate, for self-directed violence related to impending divorce as evidenced by a wish to be dead.
- Moderate anxiety related to fear of living alone as evidenced by expressed helplessness.
- Hopelessness related to lowered self-esteem as evidenced by not caring for self.

Outcomes

Short-term goals   *Date met*
- Patient will verbalize that she is no longer suicidal.   _____
- Patient will verbally express guilt and anger at husband and situation.   _____
- Patient will telephone friend, employer, and children for assistance.   _____

Long-term goals
- Patient will decide where to live after discharge.   _____
- Patient will verbalize confidence in ability to support self.   _____
- Patient will describe resources available to her.   _____

Planning/ Interventions
Nurse-patient relationship: Initial suicide precautions as a nursing measure; monitor energy level and suicidal ideas; offer support as feelings are expressed; reinforce strengths; compile list of resources.
Psychopharmacology: Fluoxetine 20 mg PO every morning.
Milieu management: Encourage patient to stay out of room; request patient attendance at grief and loss, self-esteem, assertiveness, problem-solving, and recreational groups.

Evaluation | Patient will stay with daughter after discharge; patient called employer and requested extended sick leave.

Referral | Patient made appointment for outpatient counseling; patient has information on divorce recovery group.

Key Concepts

1. The nursing process (a systematic approach to treatment) is relevant in psychiatric nursing practice.
2. The nursing process is a tool with which the nurse assesses each patient's problems, selects and carries out specific nursing interventions, and evaluates the effectiveness of these interventions on patient outcomes.
3. The initial patient assessment is holistic and includes data from all members of the multidisciplinary team.
4. Written patient assessments, care plans, and progress notes provide an important means of ensuring consistency and continuity of care.
5. Evaluation of patient progress is a foundation for discharge planning and for referrals to other services within the continuum of care.
6. Process recordings are learning tools that are used to facilitate professional growth.

References

Brenner P: The wisdom of our practice, *AJN* 100(10):99, 2000.
Delaney KR, Pitula CR, Perraud S: Psychiatric hospitalization and process description: what will nursing add, *J Psychosoc Nurs Ment Health Serv* 38(3):7, 2000.
Festa LM et al: Maximizing learning outcomes by videotaping, *J Psychosoc Nurs Ment Health Serv* 38(5):37, 2000.
Gauthier PA: Use of Peplau's interpersonal relations model to counsel people with AIDS, *J Am Psychiatr Nurs Assoc* 6(4):119, 2000.
Hansten R, Washburn M: Outcomes-based care delivery, *AJN* 101(2):24a, 2001.
Oermann MH, Huber D: Patient outcomes: a measure of nursing's value, *AJN* 99(9):40, 1999.
Peplau HE: Psychotherapeutic strategies, *Perspect Psychiatr Care* 6(6):264, 1968.
Walden-McBride DL, McBride JL: Listening for the patient's story, *J Psychosoc Nurs Ment Health Serv* 38(11):26, 2000.
Winslow EH: Patient education materials, *AJN* 101(10):33, 2001.

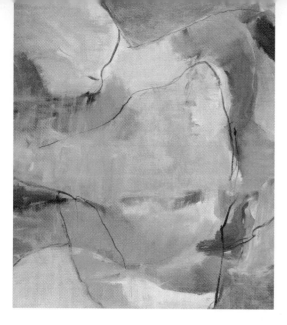

Anxiety, Coping, and Crisis

Lee H. Schwecke

Learning Objectives

After reading this chapter, you should be able to:
- Explain the relationships between anxiety and the neurochemical and physiologic responses to anxiety.
- Explain the relationships among anxiety, coping, and crisis.
- Identify common stressors that are likely to cause anxiety.
- Distinguish symptoms reflective of each of the four levels of anxiety.
- Match appropriate nursing interventions to each level of anxiety.
- Describe criteria for evaluating coping mechanisms.
- Identify differences among adaptive, palliative, maladaptive, and dysfunctional coping mechanisms.
- Describe characteristics and effects of crisis situations.
- Outline major crisis intervention goals and strategies.

nxiety in response to stress is inevitable in everyday life. The way in which individuals cope with anxiety and stress is important in understanding the quality with which individuals are functioning in their personal, social, and occupational roles. All of the theoretic models for working with psychiatric patients described in Chapter 3 address stress, anxiety, and coping either directly or indirectly. For nurses in any setting, including nonpsychiatric ones, understanding the nature of anxiety, its causes, the reasons that make it difficult to manage, and the way in which individuals normally cope with it is crucial (Figure 12-1).

COMMONLY PERCEIVED STRESSORS

The stressor that precipitates anxiety is whatever the individual perceives as a danger, a loss, or a threat to safety and security. The way in which individuals perceive an event depends on their background, needs, desires, self-concept, resources, knowledge, skills, personality traits, and maturity. For example, a skilled athlete might perceive a competitive event as an exciting challenge with a high probability of success. An athlete who is less skilled might perceive the same event as an overwhelming test with a high probability of failure. Each athlete, on the basis of his or her perception of the situation, will have different emotional and physical responses (i.e., a different level of anxiety) as a matter of course.

Commonalities exist among perceptions of what constitutes a threat, loss, or danger. Individuals typically feel anxious when they perceive a loss of or threat to the following:
1. Health or the ability to perform and function
2. Self-esteem or self-respect
3. Self-control

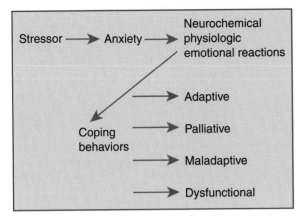

Figure 12-1 Process of anxiety.

4. Control or power over the individual's life
5. Status or prestige
6. Resources (emotional, physical, financial, spiritual, social, and cultural)
7. Loved ones
8. Freedom or independence
9. Needs, goals, desires, and expectations

Some threats or losses are external and visible to observers (objective); others are internal and less evident to observers (subjective). The perception of a threat or loss may not seem "valid" to others; perceptions can be inaccurate, misinterpreted, exaggerated, or unjustified. For example, the best friend of a person turns down an invitation to dinner, saying that she has to visit her grandmother who is ill. The best friend has always been honest, but doubts begin to mistakenly surface as to whether the friend really cares anymore.

Stressors may also be classified as maturational or situational. Maturational stressors are experiences that are expected as a part of normal processes of growth and development for most of the individuals in a given society (see Chapter 3). For example, in the United States, most individuals start school, leave school, develop relationships, become employed, support families, lose loved ones, and prepare for their own deaths. To varying degrees, these stressors can be anticipated, and plans can be made.

Situational stressors are less predictable, and specific actions are taken only when the threat is eminent or after the event has occurred. General precautions may be possible. For example, most individuals recognize that acute illnesses and accidents can happen; thus they purchase health, life, and

car insurance; but, they do not know exactly when, where, or how serious the illness or accident will be. Natural and man-made disasters, such as tornadoes, earthquakes, terrorist attacks, and explosions, fall into this category. Some situational stressors have early warning signs that an individual may ignore until the threat is more eminent or obvious, such as war, divorce, layoffs from work, and chronic illnesses.

RECURRING THEMES OF ANXIETY

Anxiety as a concept and process has been studied, defined, and described by many respected authors: Peplau (1952), Sullivan (1953), Lazarus (1966), Levitt (1967), Beck and Clark (1997), and Aguilera (1998). Anxiety is described as:

- A subjective experience that can be detected only by the objective behaviors that result from it
- Emotional pain
- Apprehension, fearfulness, or a sense of powerlessness resulting from a threat that is less visible or definable than is fear that has a visible object or trigger
- A warning sign of a perceived danger or threat

Diagnoses Related to Anxiety, Coping, and Crisis

NANDA*
Adjustment, Impaired
Anxiety
Breathing pattern, Ineffective
Communication, Impaired verbal
Coping, Ineffective family
Coping, Ineffective individual
Decisional conflict
Fear
Injury, Risk for
Post-trauma response
Powerlessness, Risk for
Role performance, ineffective
Self-esteem, Chronic low
Sensory/perceptual, Disturbed
Sleep pattern, Disturbed
Social interaction, Impaired
Social isolation
Spiritual distress
Thought processes, Disturbed
Violence, Risk for self-directed or Violence, Risk directed at others

*From North American Nursing Diagnosis Association: *NANDA nursing diagnoses: definitions and classifications,* Philadelphia, 2001, NANDA.

- An emotional response that triggers behaviors (automatic relief behaviors) aimed at eliminating the anxiety
- Alerting an individual to prepare for self-defense
- Occurring in degrees
- "Contagious": communicated from one person to another
- Part of a process, not an isolated phenomenon

GENERAL ETIOLOGY OF ANXIETY

Psychodynamic Theory

Freud viewed the ego as the part of the personality that develops defenses to help individuals to control or cope with anxiety (see Chapter 3). The need to control anxiety stems from conflicts between the id (instincts) and the superego (conscience) (Freud, 1936). Repression of feelings that are connected with early conflicts occurs.

Later in life, as conflicts are once again experienced, the defenses fail, and these feelings emerge, causing anxiety and discomfort. Freud (1936) viewed unrealistic or "neurotic" anxiety as the fear that instincts will cause the individual to do something that will result in punishment.

Interpersonal Theory

Sullivan (1953) examined interpersonal relations and the socialization process that are important to the way in which individuals feel about themselves. Sullivan saw individuals striving for security and relief from anxiety to protect their self-systems. In childhood, individuals take on the values of their parents and family to receive approval and to feel good about themselves. Later in life, a threat to the self is based on the way in which individuals perceive the danger or threat and on the way in which they were taught early in life to handle conflict. Because children are dependent on others for feelings of self-worth, they strive to gain approval to feel secure. The sense of self is based on the evaluations of others. Issues of dependency, control, security, and the related conflicts form the basis of handling anxiety. Parent-child conflicts change their form as the child matures, but the issues remain the same. For example, a 2-year-old child who resists getting dressed is trying to take control of his or her life to a small degree, but dependency and security requirements prevail. Years later, when the adolescent feels less dependent and more secure, the resistance to parental control becomes increasingly obvious and usually culminates in moving away from the family.

Biologic Theory

Selye (1956) found that the effects of stress might be observed by the objective measurement of structural and clinical changes in the body. Selye called these changes the general adaptation syndrome (see Chapter 3). More recent research on the effects of anxiety and the resulting neurochemical reactions has centered on the hypothalamic-pituitary-adrenal axis, the hypothalamic-pituitary-gonadal axis, and the limbic system-reward pathway. Major neurochemical changes identified include the following (Aguilera, 1998; Charney et al, 1993; Hoffart, Keene, 1998; Taylor et al, 2001; van der Kolk, Saporta, 1991; Williams, 1999):

- Increased regional norepinephrine turnover in the locus ceruleus, limbic regions, and cerebral cortex
- Increased corticotropin-releasing factor (CRF)
- Increased adrenocorticotropin hormone (ACTH) and corticosterone levels
- Increased dopamine release and metabolism in the prefrontal cortex and nucleus accumbens
- Increased endogenous opiate release
- Increased glucocorticoid levels
- Increased thyrotropin-releasing hormone (TRH)
- Increased thyroid-stimulating hormone (TSH)
- Increased peripheral sympathetic nervous system activity

Anxiety-related responses are critical for surviving and tolerating dangerous situations. The increased noradrenergic and dopaminergic system activity (leading to central nervous system [CNS] hyperarousal and hypervigilance) facilitate rapid behavioral reactions. Tolerating fear and pain associated with serious injuries is enhanced by increased release of the endogenous opiates (allowing emotional blunting and physical analgesia). Increased cortisol levels (resulting in metabolic activation) facilitate increased physical activity (Charney et al, 1993). However, the effectiveness of these responses fades if the individual is continuously exposed to the stressor (Clements, Turpin, 2000). This decrease in effectiveness is related to the alterations in the catacholamine and thyroid systems and the depressed immune system. These effects and a deficiency in serotonin may increase the risk of suicide (Jiwanlal, Weitzel, 2001).

If the "threshold set point" for anxiety is changed, then the individual becomes increasingly sensitive to subsequent stressors that more easily reactivate the anxiety-related response (Hoffart, Keene, 1998). This tendency is discussed in relation to acute stress disorder (ASD) and posttraumatic stress disorder (PTSD) in Chapter 31. A stress cycle can begin to occur in which physical and psychologic symptoms cause additional stress, negative thinking, and fears. These reactions lead to activation of the stress response again, resulting in increasingly severe or frequent symptoms or both. Eventually, other symptoms such as irritability, muscle tension, headaches, back pain, insomnia, gastrointestinal disturbances, and palpitations may develop (Hoffart, Keene, 1998; Soderstrom et al, 2000). In contrast, if the original stress is resolved, the body can return to normal (a relaxation response) through activation of the parasympathetic nervous system and the decreased activity in the hypothalamus and pituitary (Hoffart, Keene, 1998; Jech, 2001; Taylor et al, 2001; Williams, 1999).

LEVELS OF ANXIETY

To assess the way in which patients are responding to the feeling of anxiety that is generated by a stressor, the nurse should assess patients' perceptions of and reactions to the stressor (subjective). Another way of assessing the severity of responses to a stressor is to observe behaviors (objective). Table 12-1 describes the psychomotor, emotional, and cognitive symptoms of four levels of anxiety, as well as the nursing interventions for each level.

Even a moderate level of anxiety (+2) is uncomfortable and difficult to tolerate. As anxiety increases, a drive to relieve the anxiety as soon as possible develops. Selye's stress model included in Chapter 3 identifies stages of responses that result from the feeling of anxiety. More specific neurochemical and physiologic reactions have been described earlier in this chapter. Long-lasting high levels of anxiety (+3 and +4) are physically and emotionally draining to the extent that an individual will do almost anything to escape the pain, such as becoming ill (physically or emotionally) or even committing suicide, in rare instances. Fortunately, many less debilitating and more productive ways to cope with anxiety are available.

COPING WITH ANXIETY

Methods of coping with anxiety and the resulting neurochemical and physiologic reactions can be divided into four categories, according to the degree of effectiveness in decreasing anxiety or eliminating the source of anxiety, as described in Table 12-2.

Although *effectiveness* is the primary criterion for evaluating a coping method, *outcomes* must also be considered. Sometimes, coping reduces the anxiety and solves the problem but, at the same time, creates other significant problems. Stealing class notes from a friend may result in both an examination score of an "A" grade and permanent damage to the friendship. *Duration* and *frequency* of coping methods must be considered as well. Prolonged late-night studying may yield an "A" grade, but it may result in reduced resistance to a virus and an episode of influenza. Excessive studying may lead to a poorly balanced life of work, love, and play. Thus a coping method must be examined for its primary effectiveness and for its consequences on the patient's well-being and relationships.

A major role of psychiatric nurses is to help patients learn or regain highly effective coping strategies and avoid ineffective or destructive strategies, including most of the defense mechanisms. To accomplish this task, the nurse must identify the strategies that the patient knows and is using, those that the patient knows but is not using, and those that patient does not know. The nurse often assumes that patients know more about adaptive coping than they really do. The most common coping techniques taught and encouraged are:

- Problem solving
- Assertiveness
- Positive self-talk
- Stress and anger management
- Skills needed for communication and relationships
- Conflict resolution
- Time management
- Community living

Strategies* are also available for temporarily tolerating and decreasing the effects of anxiety, although these techniques do not directly manage the cause of the stress and anxiety. These strategies include:

- Visualization, guided imagery, and meditation: creating a safe, relaxing place, using some or all of the five senses, which enhances a sense of security and decreases tension and worry
- Concentrating on breathing and striving for slow, long, deep breathing

---

*Borgatti, 2000; Hoffart, Keene, 1998; Jech, 2001; Lyon, 2001; Nakao et al, 2001; Smoyak, 2001; Soderstrom et al, 2000.

| Table 12-1 | Levels of Anxiety

Levels of Anxiety and Interventions	SYMPTOMS		
	Psychomotor	Emotional	Cognitive
Mild +1			
Discuss source of anxiety (steps of learning)	Preparation of body for constructive action	Occasional slight irritability	Alertness
Problem solve	Slight muscle tension	Feeling challenged	Awareness of surroundings
Accept anxiety as natural; tolerate and benefit from it	Slight fidgeting	Confident	Concentration
	Energetic		Accurate perceptions
	Good eye contact	(Use of adaptive coping mechanisms)	Attentiveness
			Logical reasoning and problem-solving skills
Moderate +2			
Decrease anxiety—ventilation, crying, exercise, relaxation techniques	Preparation of body for protective action	Feeling uncomfortable, on edge, keyed up	Difficulty in concentrating
Refocus attention; relate feelings and behaviors to anxiety; then use problem-solving techniques; give oral medication, if needed	Moderate muscle tension	Motivated to decrease anxiety	Easily distracted, can focus with assistance
	Increased blood pressure, pulse, and respirations	Increased irritability	Circumstantiality
	Startle reflex	Decreased confidence	Tangentiality
	Slight perspiration		Loose associations
	Difficulty sitting still	(Use of palliative coping mechanisms)	Narrowed perceptions
	Repeated fidgeting		Decreased span of attention
	Periodic slow pacing		Misperception of stimuli
	Increased rate of speech		Tuning out of stimuli
	Sporadic eye contact		Problem solving and reasoning skills with effort or assistance
Severe +3			
Decrease anxiety, stimuli, and pressure	Preparation of body for "flight or fight"	Extreme discomfort	Distorted perceptions
Use kind, firm, simple directions	Extreme muscle tension	Feeling of dread	Difficulty focusing even with assistance
Use time out (seclusion)	Increased perspiration	Hypersensitivity	Flight of ideas
Give intramuscular medications, if needed	Continuous and rapid pacing	Defensiveness with threats and demands	Ineffective reasoning and problem solving skills
	Reflex responses		Disorientation
	Loud or rapid speech or both	(Use of maladaptive coping mechanisms)	Delusions and hallucinations, if prolonged
	Poor eye contact		Suicidal or homicidal ideations, if prolonged
	Somatic symptoms		
	Sleep disturbance		
Panic +4			
Guide firmly, or physically take control	Actual flight, fight, or immobilization	Feeling overwhelmed and out of control	Disorganized perceptions
Give intramuscular medication	Suicide attempts or violence	Rage	Disorganized or irrational reasoning and problem-solving
Order restraints, if needed	Depletion of body resources	Desperation	Neologisms
	Eyes fixed	Feeling totally drained	Clang associations
	Hysterical or mute		Word salad
	Incoherent	(Use of dysfunctional coping mechanisms)	Out of contact with reality
			Personality disorganization

Adapted from Longo D and Williams R: *Clinical practice in psychosocial nursing: assessment and intervention,* New York, 1986, Appleton-Century-Crofts; Peplau HE: *Interpersonal relations in nursing,* New York, 1952, GP Putnam's Sons; Selye H: *The stress of life,* New York, 1956, McGraw-Hill; Sullivan HS: *The psychiatric interview,* New York, 1954, WW Norton.

|Table 12-2| Coping with Anxiety

Type of Coping	Description	Common Use	Patient Example
Adaptive	Solves the problem that is causing the anxiety, so the anxiety is decreased. The patient is objective, rational, and productive.	Anxiety about an upcoming examination is reduced by studying effectively and passing the examination with a grade of A.	Anxiety about being discharged from the hospital is handled by writing down medications, dates and times of follow-up appointments, and self-help meetings in a calendar. The patient keeps appointments and attends two self-help meetings; takes medications and returns to work.
Palliative	Temporarily decreases the anxiety but does not solve the problem, so the anxiety eventually returns. Temporary relief allows the patient to return to problem solving.	Anxiety about the examination is temporarily reduced by jogging for half an hour. Effective studying is then possible and a grade of A is still achievable.	Anxiety about being discharged is handled by watching television in the evening. In the morning, the patient takes the discharge instructions written by the nurse and puts them in his pocket. He keeps his first follow-up appointment and attends one self-help meeting. He takes his medications and is able to return to work.
Maladaptive	Unsuccessful attempts to decrease the anxiety without attempting to solve the problem. The anxiety remains.	Anxiety about the examination is first ignored by going to a movie and then handled by frantically cramming for a few hours. A passing grade of C is obtained.	Anxiety about the discharge is handled by saying that he can remember all the appointments and meetings, and that the directions for the medications will be on the bottles. He misses the meetings and his appointment, but makes another appointment when called. He takes his AM and PM medication but forgets the noon dose all week. He goes to work but complains of being anxious all day.
Dysfunctional	Is not successful in reducing anxiety or solving the problem. Even minimal functioning becomes difficult, and new problems begin to develop.	Anxiety about the examination is first ignored by going out drinking with friends and then escaped by "passing out" for the night. A grade of F results and the course has to be repeated.	Anxiety about the discharge is handled by ignoring the nurse and starting an argument with another patient. When asked to take a "time out," the patient leaves the hospital without being discharged, and his bill is not paid by insurance. He does not get his prescriptions and is brought back to the hospital in 3 weeks.

- Relaxation training for decreasing tension and increasing muscle relaxation
- Engaging in stretching exercises, such as yoga
- Adopting a healthy lifestyle, such as a balanced diet, quality sleep, and exercise routine
- Decreasing unhealthy and self-destructive behaviors or coping, such as avoidance of issues
- Engaging in hobbies, noncompetitive activities that are fun, and laughter
- Spending time with caring, supportive, and optimistic people
- Reducing competing activities and commitments, when possible
- Using cognitive restructuring to decrease a negative view of self, others, problems, and life, replacing these with affirming, positive, and empowering thoughts
- Striving to increase a sense of self-confidence and mastery in solving problems
- Engaging in personal growth activities
- Listening to favorite calming and positive music

- Getting a massage (body, hands, and feet) with or without aromatherapy

Coping strategies take time to learn and use consistently. In a short-term hospitalization or program, the nurse begins the education process, but this should be continued in an after-care program. New skills need ongoing reinforcement until they become "habits." (See Chapter 31 for "Key Nursing Intervention to Reduce Anxiety" and "Key Nursing Interventions in Problem-Solving.")

CLINICAL EXAMPLE

Latasha was admitted to the hospital after a suicide attempt. She said that she was overwhelmed with problems and work, as well as with taking care of her aging parents in her home. "I just couldn't take any more stress. I'm not sleeping or eating right. I never have time for myself. My new boss is a demanding bitch who wants us to do all of her work for her." After affirming that she actually did not want to die, she agreed to make a list of the three most important stressors that she wanted to confront in the next 2 days. For each of these stressors, she identified a realistic goal and initial steps to take toward resolving the problems they cause, along with a reasonable time frame for accomplishing the goal. Latasha then listed three activities that might be put on hold. Latasha began practicing relaxation and visualization techniques to use periodically during the day and at bedtime to decrease body tension and anxiety. She agreed that she needed to resume her exercise routine and eating healthy meals while listening to her favorite music.

Critical Thinking Questions

What symptoms of each level of anxiety have you experienced at different times? Can you match these with various coping mechanisms you have used to deal with the anxiety levels?

RELATIONSHIP BETWEEN ANXIETY AND ILLNESS

Individuals feel increasing pain and discomfort as anxiety escalates from moderate to severe and then to panic levels. To feel better, these individuals may use behaviors and defense mechanisms to protect themselves. These behaviors are individualized. For instance, biologic and genetic endowments influence

reactions to stress. An individual is born with unique personality traits, predispositions, and physiologic and neurologic systems. If long-term palliative, maladaptive, or dysfunctional coping behaviors are displayed, then an anxiety-related disorder, a physiologic health problem, or even a psychosis may develop.

CRISIS

Any stressful event or hazardous situation has the potential for precipitating a crisis (Lindemann, 1956). The event or situation that comes at the end of a series of stressors may be "minor," making the situation more than the individual can handle (i.e., the proverbial "straw that breaks the camel's back"). A crisis differs from stress in that a crisis results in a period of severe disorganization resulting from the failure of individuals' usual coping mechanisms or the lack of usual resources or both. The feeling of being totally out of control and being unable to function on a daily basis is extremely disturbing and motivates patients to escape the pain (Caplan, 1961; Smith, 2000).

Individual Reactions

Anxiety generally rises to a severe or panic level during a crisis (see Table 12-1). Individuals feel a sense of overwhelming helplessness and hopelessness when nothing appears to be working (Smith, 2000); they may feel immobilized and either give up or keep trying the same, ineffective coping methods. An individual in a crisis needs and is generally receptive to help. During the period of disorganization, being dependent on others for guidance and assistance is a natural tendency. (Trust is less of an issue at this time.) The right kind of help at the right time generally enables individuals to overcome the problem, regain equilibrium, and return to normal. For individuals to learn new coping skills, develop new or improved relationships with others, and begin functioning better than they did before the crisis occurred is common. This tendency is the reason that a crisis is said to have growth-promoting potential (Aguilera, 1998).

The disorganization period of a crisis is distressing to the extent that it usually cannot be tolerated emotionally or physically for more than 4 to 6 weeks. If the right kind of help is unavailable and the crisis is not successfully resolved in that period, then the individual in crisis may likely become exhausted and physically ill, adopt dysfunctional coping patterns that manage the intense feelings without solving the problems (i.e., become emotionally ill), become violent, or attempt suicide to escape the pain. Dysfunctional patterns of coping tend to persist unless the individual seeks intensive counseling for a prolonged period. Intervening *during* the crisis to prevent the development of dysfunctional coping patterns rather than intervening *after* the crisis has occurred takes less time and is more effective.

> ### *Critical* Thinking Questions
>
> You are seeing a patient in an obstetrician's office. She complains of anxiety and lack of sleep for 2 weeks. What list of questions would you ask to assess her stressors, level of anxiety, and coping mechanisms? Can you list the type of intervention needed?

Strategies of Crisis Intervention

Crisis intervention is appropriate any time a crisis occurs for an individual in any setting. Strategies of crisis intervention are directed toward the immedi-ate cause of the anxiety and are aimed at bolstering emotional security and reestablishing equilibrium, rather than focusing on underlying issues and long-term resolutions (Aguilera, 1998). Table 12-3 compares the techniques used in crisis intervention and stress counseling. Crisis strategies begin with identifying the point at which the crisis began, in response to the stressor or series of stressors, and the resultant way in which the individual's life is being affected. The strengths, coping skills, resources, and support systems of the individual are assessed (Aguilera, 1998). Managing emotion and support are valuable parts of crisis intervention to prevent further decompensation, violence, or a suicide attempt (see Chapter 10, Chapter 13, and Chapter 29). Identifying irrational thought processes and providing supportive confrontation help move individuals to immediate decisions and actions to relieve immediate problems and the accompanying sense of helplessness. Alternative ways of coping are explored (Aguilera, 1998). Individuals may need kind but firm directions and assistance in finding and using external resources when they are feeling overwhelmed and immobilized.

|Table 12-3| Crisis and Suicide Intervention versus Stress Counseling

	Crisis and Suicide Intervention	Stress Counseling
Major focus	Immediate action Prevention of more decompensation Prevention of suicide/harm to others Resolution of crisis Restoration of functioning	Promoting growth Developing insight New coping
Content of sessions	Survival, safety, security Immediate action needed by client External resources needed Emotion management Immediate goals	Stressors Feelings Coping Internal resources Short and long goals
Counselor-client relationships	Intense and continuous over a short-time period (hours-days) Then 1-6 sessions for follow-up	Moderately intense and at regular intervals (1 hr/wk for 1-20 sessions)
Role of counselor	Supportive with confrontation Active, directive Gives commands, if needed Suggest adaptive coping strategies	Varies according to philosophy and style Facilitate problem solving Teach adaptive coping strategies
Significant others	Involve as soon as possible for continuous support, then sporadic follow-up Taught how to help and resources available	May or may not become involved in counseling or used for support
Other agencies	For rescue, longer term follow-up, and/or new support system	May or may not be used

Adapted from Admi H: Stress intervention: a model of stress inoculation training, *J Psychosoc Nurs* 35(8):37, 1997; Aguilera DC: *Crisis intervention: theory and methodology*, ed 8, St Louis, 1998, Mosby.

Working with an individual in crisis is demanding and intense for a short period, usually a few days to a few weeks. Therefore the nurse must involve other staff members and individuals' significant others who can help. These significant others are taught to help and to find resources if they lack knowledge. As the crisis subsides, support people and community resources are important for continued assistance, especially because the risk of suicide can persist for 2 to 3 months after the crisis has abated. This period is valuable for counseling that is aimed at learning or reinforcing adaptive coping strategies. With the trend of shorter hospital stays and patients being managed primarily in outpatient treatment settings, hospitalization is used primarily for crisis intervention. Patients are admitted only when they are unable to function (to meet their basic needs for food, clothing, and shelter) or are at risk of harming themselves or others. In these situations, the nurse uses crisis intervention strategies focused on providing physical safety, emotional security, and stabilization; thus the patient can be discharged as soon as possible. Although patients may be in crisis for 4 to 6 weeks, they are not hospitalized for this length of time. Therefore the nurse ideally collaborates with and makes referrals to an outpatient treatment facility or to other community resources.

CLINICAL EXAMPLE

Jalen, 19 years old, was admitted after an episode of acting out that involved breaking light fixtures and furniture in his room. His father called the police when he threatened to get his friend's gun and "kill everyone in sight." His father said Jalen was not sleeping well, was staying in his room too long, and was refusing to eat for the last 3 days since his best friend had been killed in a gang-related drive-by shooting. Jalen signed a "no-harm" contract. He refused to complete the admission interview but agreed to take an oral antianxiety medication. He went to sleep for 14 hours. After awakening, Jalen was tearful at times but still extremely angry. Jalen admitted he needed help to deal with the "senseless murder" of his friend. He chose to use a punching bag each time his anger got out of control. Afterward, he was able to talk about his sadness and guilt about not protecting his friend. Within 2 days, Jalen made a list of ways to deal with his anger and grief, including visiting his friend's family (because he had missed the funeral), seeing an outpatient counselor, and attending a meeting of the Survivors of Homicide support group.

Crisis intervention can be offered in a variety of ways. Walk-in crisis units or teams within a mental health center or mobile crisis teams who see individuals in their homes, in community clinics, or in emergency departments of hospitals are available. Many communities and mental health centers offer 24-hour telephone crisis (or hot) lines. Mobile disaster teams are often sent to areas in which natural or man-made tragedies have occurred, such as earthquakes, tornadoes, or the bombing of a building. These disaster teams may use one of several models for assisting individuals and groups of victims to debrief their experiences and deal with acute stress reactions in an effort to prevent PTSD (Everly, Flannery, Mitchell, 2000). These models are discussed in the Anxiety-Related Disorder chapter.

Key Concepts

1. A stressor is any event or circumstance that an individual perceives as a threat, loss, or danger.
2. Anxiety has been described in a variety of ways and can generate a variety of responses.
3. Based on Peplau's model, four levels of anxiety have been identified: mild, moderate, severe, and panic.
4. Nursing interventions vary according to the patient's level of anxiety.
5. Evaluating patients' adaptive, palliative, maladaptive, and dysfunctional coping mechanisms is crucial.
6. A crisis results in a period of severe disorganization resulting from the failure of individuals' usual coping mechanisms or the lack of usual resources or both.
7. Crisis intervention strategies concentrate on the immediate precipitant, as well as the individual's physical safety and emotional security.

References

Aguilera DC: *Crisis intervention: theory and methodology,* ed 8, St Louis, 1998, Mosby.

Beck AT, Clark DA: An information processing model of anxiety: automatic and strategic processing, *Behav Res Ther* 35(1):49, 1997.

Borgatti JC: Stressed for success, *Nursing Spectrum-Metro Edition* 24, Nov. 2000.

Caplan G: *An approach to community mental health,* New York, 1961, Grune & Stratton.

Charney DS et al: Psychobiologic mechanisms of post-traumatic stress disorder, *Arch Gen Psychiatry* 50(4):294, 1993.

Clements K, Turpin G: Life event exposure, physiological reactivity, and psychological strain, *J Behav Med* 23(1):73, 2000.

Everly GS Jr, Flannery RB, Mitchell JT: Critical incident stress management: a review of the literature, *Aggression and Violent Behavior* 5(1):23, 2000.

Freud S: *The problem of anxiety,* New York, 1936, WW Norton.

Hoffart MB, Keene EP: The benefits of visualization, *AJN* 98(12):44, 1998.

Jech AO: Calming the cognitively impaired, *Nursing Spectrum-Metro Edition* 30, Sept. 2001.

Jiwanlal SS, Weitzel C: The suicide myth, *RN* 64(1):33, 2001.

Lazarus RS: *Psychological stress and the coping process,* St Louis, 1966, McGraw-Hill.

Levitt E: *The psychology of anxiety,* Indianapolis, 1967, Bobbs-Merrill.

Lindemann E: The meaning of crisis in the individual and family, *Teachers College Record* 57:310, 1956.

Lyon BL: Strategies to enhance positive situational focusing skills, *Reflection Nurs Leadership* 36, third quarter, 2001.

Nakao M et al: Somatization and symptom reduction through a behavioral medicine intervention in a mind/body clinic, *Behav Med* 26(4):176, Winter 2001.

Peplau HE: *Interpersonal relations in nursing,* New York, 1952, GP Putnam's Sons.

Selye H: *The stress life,* St Louis, 1956, McGraw-Hill.

Smith DJ: Flight to Los Angeles: crisis at 30,000 feet, *J Psychosoc Nurs Ment Health Serv* 39(10):6, 2000.

Smoyak SA: The definition of the situation *is* the situation, *J Psychosoc Nurs Ment Health Serv* 39(2):6, 2001.

Soderstrom M et al: The relationship of hardiness, coping strategies, and perceived stress to symptoms of illness, *J Behav Med* 23(3):311, 2000.

Sullivan HS: *Interpersonal theory of psychiatry,* New York, 1953, WW Norton.

Taylor SE et al: Biobehavioral responses to stress in females: tend-and-befriend, not fight-or-flight, *Psychol Rev* 107(3):411, 2001.

van der Kolk BA, Saporta J: The biological response to psychic trauma: mechanisms and treatment of intrusion and numbing, *Anxiety Res* 4:199, 1991.

Williams RB: Social ties and health, *Harv Ment Health Lett* 15(10):4, 1999.

Chapter 13

Working with the Aggressive Patient

Lee H. Schwecke

Learning Objectives

After reading this chapter, you should be able to:

- Describe the differences among anger, aggression, passive aggression, and assertiveness.
- Recognize the developmental, individual, and stress models of aggression.
- Describe the five stages of the assault cycle.
- Explain the verbal nursing interventions for anger and nonviolent aggression.
- Match the external control interventions with the escalation and crisis phases of the assault cycle.
- Describe the nursing care of patients in seclusion and restraints.
- Explain the functions needed to support a staff victim of patient assault.

Anger is a normal human emotion that is crucial for individual growth and is a factor present in all relationships. When handled appropriately and expressed assertively (directly, without violating the rights of the self or others), anger is a positive creative force that leads to problem solving and productive change. When channeled inappropriately and expressed as verbal aggression (verbal attacks on others) or physical aggression, anger is a destructive and potentially life-threatening force. Physical aggression is also called assault, battery, or violence. Anger may be expressed indirectly as passive aggression (e.g., sarcasm, pouting), or it may be passively internalized and lead to unpleasant emotional and physical problems.

The focus of this chapter is on the individual patient's expressions of anger with the nursing staff and with other individuals in inpatient or outpatient psychiatric settings. However, it is important for nurses to recognize that anger and aggression occur in any setting, including emergency rooms, medical and surgical units, nursing homes, community-health settings, and clinics (Hospital Focus, 2001). Nonpsychiatric staff may be less familiar with anticipating, preventing, and managing aggression compared with psychiatric nursing staff members, who are trained in assessing and defusing anger and in safely managing aggressive behaviors.

RELATED CONCEPTS

Aggression

Everyone experiences feelings of anger, but aggressive displays of anger are considered socially inappropriate and are discouraged in American society. When adults in this culture aggressively express their anger toward someone, the recipient generally responds with fear, frustration, and avoidance of the aggressor, when possible. The recipient may also feel helpless, guilty, defensive, or angry. Occasionally, the recipient of anger may retaliate, seek revenge, or hold a grudge.

In its early stages, anger is healthy when expressed verbally and assertively to the person perceived as causing the anger. Visibly angry behaviors span a continuum from mild irritation and arguing, to verbal or physical abuse of the self or others, to uncontrolled violence (Table 13-1).

Externally expressed anger may lead to assault (any behavior that is physically or verbally aggressive and presents an immediate threat of physical injury to a person or property). Carrying out the threat of injury is defined as battery and includes actions such as hitting, kicking, pulling hair, throwing a chair, biting, and scratching, but does not include verbal abuse.

Nurses have the right, professionally and legally, to use physical restraint to prevent patients from injuring themselves and others. Nursing interventions are based on the principle of the least restrictive alternative meaning that the nurse will first try to set limits in a humane and least restrictive manner (such as talking and oral medications) to ensure the safety and security of patients and others. Physical restraint cannot be used unless eminent danger of physical injury exists (see discussion in Chapter 4).

Key Terms

Anger Normal emotional response to the perception of a frustration of desires or a threat to one's needs.

Assault Legally defined as any behavior that physically or verbally presents an immediate threat of physical injury to another individual.

Assertiveness Direct expression of feelings and needs in a way that respects the rights of others and the self.

Battery Inflicting physical injury on another individual.

Passive aggression Anger expressed indirectly through subtle and evasive ways.

Restraint Physical control of a patient to prevent injury to the patient, staff, and other patients.

Seclusion Process of placing a patient alone in a specially designed room for protection and close observation.

|Table 13-1| Expressions of Anger

TURNED OUTWARD		TURNED INWARD	
Overt Anger	Passive Aggression	Subjective	Objective
Verbalization of anger	Impatience	Feeling upset	Crying
Irritation	Pouting, sulking	Tension	Self-destructive behavior
Pacing with agitation	Frustration, annoyance	Unhappiness	Self-mutilation
Swearing	Tense facial expressions	Feeling hurt	Substance abuse
Hostility	Pessimism	Disappointment	Suicide
Contempt	Resentment	Guilt	
Clenched fists	Jealousy	Feelings of inferiority	
Insulting remarks	Bitterness	Low self-esteem	
Intimidation	Complaining	Sense of failure	
Bragging about violent acts	Deceptive sweetness	Humiliation	
Provoking behaviors	Unreasonableness	Somatic symptoms	
Sadistic acts	Intolerance	Feeling harassed	
Maliciousness	Resistance	Envy	
Verbal abuse	Cynicism, sarcasm	Feeling violated	
Temper tantrums	Stubbornness	Feeling alienated	
Violation of others' rights	Intentional forgetting	Feeling demoralized	
Screaming	Noncompliance	Feeling depressed	
Deviance	Procrastination	Resignation	
Rage	Antagonism	Powerlessness	
Argumentativeness	Belittling remarks	Helplessness	
Overt defiance	Fault-finding	Hopelessness	
Threats: words or weapons	Manipulation	Desperation	
Damage to property	Power struggles	Apathy	
Assault	Unfair teasing		
Rape	Sabotage of others		
Homicide	Domination		

In psychiatric settings, assault is never tolerated, but norms may allow controlled physical aggression, such as using a punching bag or foam bats or hitting a bed pillow, but would be stopped from damaging furniture or hitting others. If a patient hits a staff member, the staff member is not allowed to strike back, but the patient may then be restricted with seclusion or restraints. Nurses must be familiar with regulations that govern the use of seclusion and restraints in their own state.

Verbal Aggression or Abuse

Verbally aggressive attacks on others tend to have a repetitive pattern and are among the major warning signs of assault and battery. Verbal aggression tends to provoke unproductive counterreactions that seldom result in constructive solutions to problems. (Reactions tend to be the same as are the recipient's reactions to physical aggression previously described.)

Social norms influence the degree and amount of verbal aggression that are tolerated. At a sporting event, fans are allowed to scream, swear, and be verbally abusive, especially toward referees and umpires. The same behaviors toward an employer are not tolerated. A brother may verbally pick on his sister, but he stops the same behavior of a neighbor's child toward his sister. In psychiatric settings, the quiet mumbling or swearing by a patient with schizophrenia or an organic brain syndrome may be ignored. The louder swearing of a patient who is in contact with reality is not tolerated, especially if directed toward a patient who is unable to respond assertively. If two relatively competent patients are arguing, staff members might not intervene, except with brief suggestions, to allow patients the positive experience of conflict resolution. If one of those patients is less competent, staff members may stop the argument as soon as it begins.

Passive Aggression and Passivity

Passive-aggressive individuals express their anger indirectly and undermine others in a variety of subtle, evasive ways (see Table 13-1). They tend to deny the anger and its source, even when confronted about their behaviors, because they are afraid of rejection or punishment. A passive-aggressive person has difficulty discussing issues and maintaining a quality relationship; they are often inefficient in accomplishing tasks and frustrate those around them.

Passive individuals turn their anger inward (see Table 13-1), may be unaware of their underlying anger, and see themselves as good, kind, congenial, and helpful. They replace their anger with fear and indirectly damage, destroy, or avoid relationships and intimacy. Passive individuals are unable to say "no" and believe that others take advantage of them. Passive individuals waste energy and seldom achieve their goals, and they show signs of distress through low self-esteem, depression, substance abuse, physical illnesses, and suicide attempts.

Assertiveness

One of the widely accepted methods for replacing aggressive, passive-aggressive, and passive behaviors is healthy assertiveness—the direct expression of feelings and needs in a way that respects the rights of others and the self. Assertive individuals use their energy constructively to achieve goals and build productive relationships. Assertiveness training is aimed at teaching individuals the behavioral skills needed to interact successfully with others. Training uses a variety of behavior-modification techniques, such as relaxation training, homework assignments, and role-playing with feedback.

DEVELOPMENTAL VIEW OF AGGRESSION

Frequently, hostile individuals are described as being in "a rage"—a primitive, irrational, infantile response. Diffuse rage reactions are observed in an infant's loud, uncontrollable crying and screaming, profuse perspiration, difficulty in breathing (sometimes turning "blue"), and flailing of arms and legs. Children move from infantile rage to more focused "temper tantrums." With the development of impulse control and the maturing of coordination, children learn to focus unpleasant feelings on individuals, objects, or situations perceived to be responsible for their anger. By the early school-age years, or even earlier, children hit one another quite frequently (Smith, 1981).

Normally, preadolescents learn to restrict hitting each other and translate aggressive impulses to competitive sports, character assassinations, slander, sarcasm, practical jokes, and destructive gossip. By adolescence, fighting is controlled and purposeful. Group cooperation is emphasized in competitive, aggressive activities, accounting for the tendency of adolescent groups to deteriorate pathologically to gangs or cults (Smith, 1981).

As age increases, the ability to control impulses tends to increase, except in criminals, gang members, and psychiatric patients with certain diagnoses (described later in the chapter). Between the ages of 22 and 45 years, most expressions of aggression and fighting occur within the family, taking the form of spouse, older adult, and child abuse. After the age of 45 years, people appear to stop physical fighting until approximately the age of 70, when aging may result in diminished impulse control and cognitive impairment, and expressions of aggression again emerge as a problem (Smith, 1981).

Critical Thinking Question

In American culture, aggression toward family members often decreases after age 45 until age 70. What factors do you believe contribute to this temporary decrease in aggression?

ETIOLOGY OF AGGRESSION

Individual, Social-Psychologic, and Sociocultural Models

Individual models explain violence as a quality of being human and use biologically based explanations of aggression (Ollendick, 1996). Research continues to focus on areas of the limbic system, the frontal lobe, and the temporal lobe. The neurotransmitters—serotonin, gamma-aminobutyric acid (GABA), and dopamine—influence the expression or suppression of aggressive behaviors (see Chapter 5). Common problems related to aggression include[*]:

- Bifrontal head injuries, damage to the frontal and prefrontal cortex
- Damage to hippocampus, amygdala, and limbic system
- Temporal-parietal lobe dysfunctions
- Early dysfunctions of subcortical areas
- Alzheimer's disease
- Multiinfarct dementia
- Decreased serotonin, GABA, or acetylcholine
- Increased dopamine or norepinephrine
- Imbalances in hormone levels
- Alcohol and drug use or abuse
- Alcohol and drug withdrawal

- Nutritional deficiencies: tryptophan, thiamine, niacin, or lecithin
- Medication noncompliance

Social-psychologic models focus on the interaction of individuals with their social environment and locate the source of violence in interpersonal requirements and frustrations, such as chaotic families and forms of abuse (Teichner, Golden, 2000). Sociocultural models focus on social structures, norms, values, institutional organizations, and systems' operations to explain individual violence, such as gang activity, poverty, welfare, and availability of drugs and guns (Ollendick, 1996).

Stress Models

Stress models provide a useful framework for the nurse to understand and intervene when intense emotional reactions such as aggression, anxiety, panic, fear, and phobic attacks occur. Stress-driven aggression involves a chain of responses resulting from neurophysiologic actions and reactions known as general adaptation syndrome (GAS), which is explained in Chapter 3.

Assault Cycle

Smith's stress model (1981) includes the assault cycle with five stages of a predictable pattern or chain of aggressive responses to emotional or physical stress (Figure 13-1). Patients who are repeatedly assaultive exhibit behavior patterns that are ritualistic, stereotypical, and automatic. As the acuity of the aggressive response increases, a comparable decrease occurs in patients' problem-solving abilities, creativity, spontaneity, and behavioral options. Interventions in each stage of the cycle are discussed later in this chapter. The five-phase assault cycle adapted from Smith (1981) includes the following:

1. *Triggering phase.* The stress-producing event occurs, initiating the stress responses
2. *Escalation phase.* Responses represent escalating behaviors that indicate a movement toward the loss of control
3. *Crisis phase.* A period of emotional and physical crisis during which loss of control occurs
4. *Recovery phase.* A period of "cooling down" during which the person slows down and returns to normal responses
5. *Postcrisis depression phase.* A period during which the person attempts reconciliation with others

---

[*]Charney et al, 1993; Hawkins, Trobst, 2000; Ollendick, 1996; Teichner, Golden, 2000; Whitney, Jacobson, Gawrys, 1996.

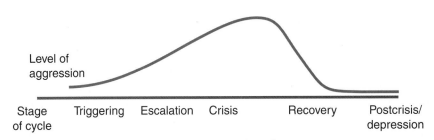

Figure 13-1 Assault cycle.

ASSESSING KEY VARIABLES OF AGGRESSION

Nurse (Self-Assessment)

Working with psychiatric patients who may "act out" requires nurses to be aware of their own aggressive impulses, the way in which they deal with their anger, and the methods they use to channel their anger into constructive, productive actions. Knowing the way in which nurses respond to patients who show anger, anxiety, fear, panic, and assaultive behaviors is important (Eckroth-Bucher, 2001). Nurses cannot defuse patients' anger or aggression when nurses themselves are in a similar state, and their anger may actually intensify the patients' emotions; additionally, nurses are ineffective if they withdraw from hostile patients.

When patients become aggressive, nurses may experience frustration, a feeling of professional inadequacy, or a sense of failure. Nurses may become overly controlling and stimulate power struggles with patients.

Some nurses believe their participation in physical control of acting-out patients damages the chances of developing or continuing a therapeutic relationship; in most cases, however, exactly the opposite is true. If patients' behaviors are viewed as a form of communication, then escalating anger should alert the staff to the fact that patients' inner controls are failing and that assistance is needed to regain impulse control. Nurses have the opportunity to convey to patients that help is available to regain control and deal more constructively with the stresses in the environment that caused the initial problems and hospitalization.

Environment (Milieu)

Variables in the milieu of a facility may contribute to the development and escalation of aggression: (1) an environment with excessive stimuli; (2) overcrowding and lack of sufficient space; (3) lack of resources for energy-draining activities, such as exercise equipment and sports areas; (4) patients' perceived lack of control of life and freedom; and (5) boredom resulting from a lack of structured and unstructured diversionary activities, such as movies, games, cards, calming music, crafts, television, and therapeutic and recreational reading materials (Allen, 2000; Corrigan, Yudofsky, Silver, 1993; Jech, 2001; Joseph-Kinselman et al, 1994).

Staff may need to guide patients in selecting appropriate activities. For example, watching television violence, including sexual aggression, may increase aggressiveness in some patients. Staffing must be sufficient for monitoring patients and supervising activities. Tolerance of a degree of pacing and smoking may reduce tension, but an excess of these activities may disturb other patients. Nurses can be instrumental in helping patients learn assertiveness, rage prevention, anger management, self awareness, social skills, cognitive restructuring, and positive coping behaviors (Allen, 2000; Corrigan, Yudofsky, Silver, 1993; Thomas, 2001).

The biases and attitudes of the staff, as well as the philosophies and policies of a facility, affect both the milieu and patients' behaviors. An overly controlled environment, such as excessive or unfair restriction of rights and privileges, may lead to aggression and rebellion. Reasonable yet flexible rules reduce the risk of power and control issues between staff and patients. Policies and rules can contribute to the structure, predictability, and consistency of the milieu (Allen, 2000; DeLacy, 2001).

Patient

Specific times occur when patients are more likely to become aggressive or assaultive: during admission, at change of shifts, at mealtimes, at visiting hours, during the evening, in elevators, during transportation to outside areas, and during periods of change. Hospitalization is a stress-producing situation that may escalate patients' anger, anxiety, and symptoms (Joseph-Kinselman et al, 1994). For example, paranoid patients may see the nursing staff as part of a plot to restrict them, while compulsive patients may become more stereotyped and rigid when they cannot repeat compulsive behavior.

Many aspects of admission are threatening and can undermine the little amount of impulse control that patients have. The admission process unavoidably involves focusing on emotionally charged issues, explaining rules and policies, personal searches, the removal or restricted use of personal items, physical examinations, and meeting unfamiliar professionals and patients (Joseph-Kinselman et al, 1994). Nurses must be sensitive to these stresses and integrate patients slowly into the unit. When patients have a history of assault or are currently agitated, delaying all but essential procedures and decreasing the stimuli and stress as much as possible are important.

Patients may be disruptive to each other, especially those who are hyperactive, intrusive, openly sexual, manipulative, threatening, or exhibiting bizarre behaviors. Staff members are responsible not only for helping these patients control their behaviors, but also for helping the other patients learn assertive responses for handling such situations.

Change is especially unnerving for patients who have dependency needs and shaky impulse control. Even positive changes in a patient's status may be experienced as a loss of support, care, and protection, for example, when a patient is transferred to a less restrictive unit or discharged back to the community. All physical moves, status changes, and changes in treatment, such as medications, should be carefully explained in advance. Rapid changes cause the most anxiety, and the nurse must convey support and confidence that the patient has the coping skills to deal with the event. Acting-out behavior is one way patients have of telling the staff that change is highly threatening. Fear of change may be the reason patients do not ask for more freedom, such as passes. Requests for more freedom may be a way of testing the staff.

Patients' admitting diagnoses and coexisting medical conditions may provide clues to potential aggression. Patients with a diagnosis of schizophrenia (especially paranoid), mania, substance abuse disorder, or an organic brain disorder have an increased incidence of aggression after admission. Patients with antisocial, passive-aggressive, and borderline traits may also have aggressive tendencies (Robinson, Littrel, Littrel, 1999). As previously mentioned, brain injury and brain dysfunction are medical problems that are especially associated with aggressive outbursts. Patients who suffer from intellectual or neurologic impairments that limit their abilities to communicate with or understand others are at high risk of assault.

Factors in patients' backgrounds that are particularly relevant in assessing for aggressive potential are a history of family (or cultural) violence, abuse, or gross disorganization (Ollendick, 1996). Other indicators are histories of truancy, setting fires, impulsivity, previous assaults, and destruction of property. A particularly relevant indicator is a specific threat of violence made within approximately 2 weeks before admission. This indicator is also related to a likelihood of being violent after discharge (Robinson, Littrel, Littrel, 1999).

Documentation in progress notes should include patients' habitual coping patterns and personal eccentricities. Specific examples of communications that alert staff to potential triggers of aggression include, "thinks all female nurses are going to be mean to him, like his mother"; "abuses men as his father abused him"; "gets upset whenever the female physician is here"; "is terrified whenever men are around." Other information includes the times and places patients appear to be especially vulnerable, such as during parental visits, in large groups, when alone with a staff member of the opposite sex, or when in the bathroom.

Some facilities have begun to present information in writing to patients and families about the possibility of using seclusion and restraints in the inpatient setting. This information includes rationales for using these procedures as safety precautions with risks and benefits, less restrictive alternatives that will be attempted first, and an explanation that these procedures will be ended as soon as the patient is safe from risk of self injury or risk of injuring others (Kozob, Skidmore, 2001a; Richman, 1998).

NURSING INTERVENTIONS FOR ANGER AND NONVIOLENT AGGRESSION

Three factors to consider in intervening with anger and nonviolent (or verbal) aggression are the *source* and the *target* of the patient's anger and the *likelihood of* escalation. For example, a patient may be angry about a situation or person outside the psychiatric setting but is directing her anger inward as depression or suicidal ideation. Another patient, angry at a situation or person outside, might show his anger as passive aggression and aim it at no one in particular. A third patient might express anger openly and loudly. In these instances, the anger is likely to be defused by directly discussing the situation each time the anger occurs.

In other situations, the possibility that the patient will lose control of the anger may increase. For example, a patient may be angry at a situation or person in the treatment setting; angry about an outside situation but displacing it onto the staff; threatening suicide with an available object; or responding to internal stimuli, such as hallucinations, delusions, or physiologic disruptions.

Nursing interventions in both escalating and nonescalating anger begin with an assessment at a safe distance. Chapter 10, on the nurse-patient relationship, describes normal precautions to take with any patient in a potentially unpredictable situation; for example, the nurse stays between the patient and an exit without blocking the exit and uses body language that is the least threatening to the patient. Warmth and empathy are essential, but a need for firm limit setting may also exist to help patients contain their behavior at a safe level (ED Nursing, 2001): "I want to talk, but put the ashtray down first" or "Stay here. I don't want you to leave the room."

If patients are less verbal, less direct, or overly controlling of their anger, the nurse must take an active, supportive, and directive role in facilitating ventilation and then problem solving. Initially, the nurse may have to point out specific behaviors and ask patients to explain the situation, for example, "I hear a lot of sarcastic remarks. What happened during your phone call?" or "You look so down right now. What are you thinking about?" Getting a full description of situations, thoughts, and feelings requires thorough questioning and patience. Patients who turn their anger inward should also be asked whether they are thinking about suicide.

The process of asking patients to describe their thoughts, feelings, and situations allows them to ventilate and diffuse some of the emotion. As the anger subsides, problem solving can focus on more effective ways of handling situations and feelings. Asking patients to assess their own potential for acting on

anger can be helpful: "How likely are you to try to hurt your wife when you are angry?" or "How serious are you about killing yourself?" The nurse may "contract" with patients to approach the staff and talk about their feelings each time they feel angry.

If the anger does not gradually diffuse during the assessment and ventilation processes, or if patients begin to become irrational and out of control, then interventions based on the assault cycle become necessary.

NURSING INTERVENTIONS BASED ON THE ASSAULT CYCLE

The goal of all interventions based on the assault cycle (Table 13-2) is to strengthen patients' control of feelings and impulses. Nurses should document attempts to use less restrictive measures (talking and oral as-needed [prn] medications, if ordered) before the more restrictive interventions of seclusion and restraints are used. Nurses should strive to achieve a balance between giving the least restrictive care and the restriction of rights to protect the patient and others, while providing quality care (APNA, 2001; Jones et al, 2000; Terpstra et al, 2001).

Patients' responses at each stress level and to each progressively restrictive intervention should be documented. Except in rapidly escalating situations, verbal strategies should be attempted before using physical interventions. Although interventions with patients who are potentially assaultive are unpleasant for nurses, studies show that some patients appreciate and want the staff to provide the external controls that are lacking and needed, such as seclusion (Jones et al, 2001). Calm, positive approaches convey to patients that they are expected to cope and that this attitude supports healthy functioning.

Triggering Phase

In the triggering phase, patients' responses are nonviolent and present no danger to others. The behavior reflects patients' usual coping and defense mechanisms. Importantly, the nurse must know the way in which patients perceive the nurse and the environment during the triggering phase and the likelihood that patients will act on these perceptions. If a patient's stressor is another individual in the immediate environment, the two patients can be separated and two nurses can talk with each patient individually to promote safe ventilation of emotions.

|Table 13-2 | Interventions Based on the Assault Cycle

Phase	Behaviors	Nursing Interventions
Triggering phase	Muscle tension, changes in voice quality, tapping of fingers, pacing, repeated verbalizations, noncompliance, restlessness, irritability, anxiety, suspiciousness, perspiration, tremors, glaring, changes in breathing	Convey empathic support. Encourage ventilation. Use clear, calm, simple statements. Ask patient to maintain control. Facilitate problem solving by discussing alternative solutions. If needed, ask the patient to go to a quiet area. Offer safe tension reduction and measures. If needed, offer oral medications (prn).
Escalation phase	Pale or flushed face, screaming, anger, swearing, agitation, hypersensitivity, threats, demands, readiness to retaliate, tautness, loss of reasoning ability, provocative behaviors, clenched fists	Take charge with calm, firm directions. Direct patient to a quiet room for "time out." Give oral medications (prn), if ordered. Ask the staff to be on stand-by at a distance. Prepare for a "show of determination" to take control.
Crisis phase	Loss of self-control, fighting, hitting, rage, kicking, scratching, throwing things	Use involuntary seclusion, restraints, or IM medications (prn), if ordered. Initiate intensive nursing care.
Recovery phase	Accusations, recriminations, lowering of voice, decreased body tension, change in conversational content, more normal responses, relaxation	Continue intensive nursing care. Process the incident with the staff and other patients. Assess patient and staff injuries. Evaluate patient's progress toward self-control.
Postcrisis depression phase	Crying, apologies, reconciliatory interactions, repression of assaultive feelings (which may later appear as hostility, passive aggression)	Process incident with patient. Discuss alternative solutions to the situation and feelings. Progressively reduce the degree of restraint and seclusion. Facilitate reentry to unit.

Adapted from Maier GJ: Managing threatening behavior: the role of talk up and talk down, *J Psychosoc Nurs Ment Health Serv* 34(6):25, 1996; Smith P: Empirically based models for viewing the dynamics of violence. In Babich K, editor: *Assessing patient violence in the health care setting*, Boulder, Colo, 1981, Western Interstate Commission for Higher Education; Stevenson S: Heading off violence with verbal de-escalation, *J Psychosoc Nurs Ment Health Serv* 29(9):6, 1991.

IM, Intramuscular; *prn*, according to circumstances.

To facilitate ventilation of anger, emphasis is on being supportive by using an empathic, nondirective, yet concerned technique. The nurse speaks softly in calm, clear, simple statements, avoiding any challenge to the patient. Aggressive, confrontational, or threatening approaches at this time usually result in escalation. Although ventilation is encouraged, patients are reminded to stay in control of themselves and to use relaxation techniques, such as deep breathing. Patients' loss of control is socially embarrassing for them and counterproductive, leaving them with feelings of vulnerability and loss of autonomy. To protect the dignity of patients and the rights and safety of others, patients can be asked to take a time out in their rooms or at least move to a quieter area; other patients may be asked to leave the scene (Kozob, Skidmore, 2001a). When the anger subsides, a problem-solving approach can begin to identify alternative solutions.

If, however, the ventilation has not been successful, the patients must be offered alternatives that allow them to express threatening emotions safely, while helping them regain control (ED Nursing, 2001). Popular approaches include journal writing, exercising, punching pillows, tearing up telephone books, pounding clay, or walking up and down the hall. Oral antianxiety or antipsychotic medications can also be given, if ordered (Kozob, Skidmore, 2001b).

CLINICAL EXAMPLE
John Henderson has been a patient on the unit for 3 days. While talking to his wife on the telephone, he becomes upset and raises his voice to her. The nurse calmly suggests that he tell his wife that he will con-

Continued

tinue their conversation later. He hangs up the telephone and starts pacing in the hallway. The nurse says, "Tell me what you are upset about." For 15 minutes, he describes the telephone conversation in detail, expresses anger toward his wife, and says he is afraid she will divorce him. As he visibly calms down, the nurse asks, "What would be most helpful in handling the situation with your wife?"

Escalation Phase

When verbalization and tension-reduction strategies fail and patients become irrational (e.g., they begin to swear, scream, threaten), the nurse must take control of the situation. For example, at a safe distance, the nurse calls the patient by name and states in a calm, firm manner that the patient's behaviors indicate a loss of control. The nurse does not threaten punishment or engage in power struggles, but offers help by taking charge on behalf of the patient, who is unable to do so at the time (ED Nursing, 2001; Kozob, Skidmore, 2001a, 2001b). The nurse avoids sudden movements and loud tones to prevent giving the appearance of an attack.

If the patient has orders for prn antianxiety or antipsychotic medications, an oral dose can be offered early in the escalation phase. If the oral dose is refused, or if the escalation is rapid, an intramuscular (IM) medication may be necessary, and the nurse may require help from other staff members. Among the oral antianxiety medications, lorazepam (Ativan) and alprazolam (Xanax) are often the drugs of choice because they take effect rapidly and have relatively few side effects. These medications may occasionally lower a patient's inhibitions and aggravate behaviors. Lorazepam may be given IM. Among the antipsychotic medications, the high-potency medications that can be given orally or IM—haloperidol (Haldol) and fluphenazine (Prolixin)—have less sedating qualities but help to decrease agitation (Corrigan, Yudofsky, Silver, 1993; Robinson, Littrel, Littrel, 1999).

Given the principle of the least restrictive alternative, a time out in a quiet room is first offered by the nurse in a kind but firm manner. If this measure is ineffective, then more restrictive measures may be instituted when the patient actually begins to lose control. Other staff members may be called to be on standby, but should initially try to remain out of the patient's view. When patients are potentially violent, their physical proximity to others is perceived as being much closer than it actually is, and they may feel threatened.

CLINICAL EXAMPLE

For the second time this shift, John Henderson is talking by telephone with his wife. He is now shouting, making threats, and demanding that she come to the hospital immediately. The nurse again asks him to end the call and talk about what is happening. As he describes this call, he gets more agitated and yells that he wants to go home immediately. The nurse calmly and firmly says, "I can hear how angry you are. (Pause.) You cannot go home now. (Pause.) I want you to go to your room and I will bring you an Ativan." Mr. Henderson does not respond immediately, but he stops yelling. The nurse says, "Please go to your room. I will get the Ativan." He goes to his room and slams the door. The nurse alerts other staff members as to the plans for Mr. Henderson. The nurse asks them to stay outside of his room until an assessment can be made as to whether a time out is going to be helpful for him and whether he is willing to take the medication.

The nurse who has been talking with the patient decides whether the patient is able to respond to directions in a reasonable time. If the patient does not respond to directions for self-control or to move to a quiet, safe place, the nurse then asks for staff assistance for a stronger "show of determination" to take control. This action involves having four to six staff members within sight of the patient, but at a greater distance from the patient than is the primary nurse; thus they do not appear ready to attack the patient. Frequently, when the patient becomes aware of the other staff members and is informed that the staff will take control (if the patient does not comply with directions), the patient is able to gain reasonable composure, cooperate with the nurse's request, take the medications, and go to a quieter room with or without staff escort (Kozob, Skidmore, 2001b), otherwise, the patient is usually close to entering the crisis phase.

Crisis Phase

The crisis phase is reached when the patient is approaching an attack on the environment, the self, other patients, or the staff. Verbal limits are ineffective, and external control by the staff is essential. In these emergency or crisis situations, immediate seclusion, restraint, or the administration of "stat" medications become necessary. The patient has the right to refuse medications, but staff may give it in the presence of a *significant* physical threat to others. These actions should be supported by emergency protocols that have been approved by the physicians and hospital, and the actions should be carefully and thoroughly documented in the patient's records (Haber, 2001).

Psychiatric emergencies must be dealt with in coordinated and organized ways, and the staff must have the opportunity to role-play their approach in advance of a crisis. All staff members should master self-protection techniques against behaviors such as kicking, hitting, and biting. Facilities usually provide aggression-management programs for staff members who are required to update these skills periodically, similarly to other emergency skills, such as cardiopulmonary resuscitation. Staff members who are well-trained in preventing and managing aggression are less likely to be victims of patient assaults.

Seclusion

Seclusion is the process of placing the patient alone in a specially designed, lockable room that is equipped with a security window or a camera for observation. Nurses usually make the decision to initiate and terminate the seclusion of patients according to the established protocols and are almost always involved in the care of patients during seclusion. The principle of seclusion is *containment*: restricting patients so they do not hurt themselves or others, decreasing stimulation, and increasing intensive nursing care. Agitation and disruptive or inappropriate sexual behaviors are other reasons for seclusion. Seclusion may be viewed as a preventative strategy to *avoid* aggressive assaults, as well as a responsive action. Time out, closer supervision, quiet interactions, and medication are therapeutically effective when used appropriately for brief periods.

The degree of seclusion depends on the patient's current status. The patient, who is able to choose time out voluntarily, especially if that patient is already taking regular medication, may stay voluntarily in his or her room without a locked door. This degree of seclusion may be relatively brief. The less cooperative patient may be escorted by two staff members, without bodily contact, to a seclusion room that contains only a bed (bolted to the floor) and a mattress. This kind of room decreases stimuli, protects the patient from injury, prevents destruction of property, and provides for the patient's privacy. The security window or camera allows observation of the patient, and the door, lockable from the outside, keeps the patient from leaving the room. Dangerous articles (for example, belts, sharp objects such as pens and keys, shoes, and eyeglasses) are taken away from the patient.

Restraint

The staff must take immediate action when assaults occur. Six to eight staff members (including hospital security officers, if insufficient unit staff members are available) are needed to *safely* control a patient and ensure that no injuries to the staff, the patient, or other patients on the unit will occur. The number of staff needed should not be underestimated because of the size, age, or sex of the patient. Some agencies include patients' previous athletic interests and accomplishments, such as weight lifting and black belts in karate, on the admission form.

Details of restraint procedures are not described here, but a general outline is presented. To prepare for control of a patient, staff members remove their own glasses, rings, earrings, pens, watches, keys, and anything else that might cause injury to the patient or to the staff. Furniture and objects that can be used as weapons are removed from the area (Robinson, Littrel, Littrel, 1999). One staff member becomes the team leader to organize and direct the planned, coordinated approach, while the original staff member continues talking with the patient. At least one staff member gets the other patients to a safe place and stays with them.

The team approaches the patient calmly, in a show of force or determination, to take control. The patient is told that the team is here to help, will not hurt the patient, and will not allow the patient to hurt anyone. Two team members approach from each side and take control of the patient's arms. Simultaneously, three other staff members quickly take control of the patient's legs and head so that the patient can be carried to the room or held on the floor until a bed is brought to the patient. Physical contact is protective and defensive, not aggressive. One staff member brings the restraint cuffs, opens doors, and moves obstacles. A nurse prepares the IM medication (or calls to get an order if no routine prn order exists). Once in the seclusion room, the patient is usually placed on the bed on his or her back. Four or more staff members hold the patient's extremities and head securely without hyperextending the patient's joints. Wrist and ankle restraints are applied to all four extremities and secured to the frame of the bed. The patient's arms are tied in a position at the side, not above the head. The restraints are tight enough to inhibit slipping out of them but not tight enough to interfere with circulation. The patient is to be free of all belongings that the patient might use to cause harm to self or others. A waist restraint, a restraint between the ankles, or a restraint blanket (or any combination of these) is applied *only* if the patient is at risk of injury because of fighting the restraints. Before staff members leave, the patient is checked for injuries and observed for the ability to move safely in the restraints. Medications may be administered at this time.

Within 1 hour, an order to restrain the patient must be obtained, and a physician must perform a face-to-face evaluation of the patient. Federal, state, and hospital regulations or policies govern the extent to which the patient must be evaluated by the nurse and physician for the need to continue the restraints, by the physician in a face-to-face examination, and in the progress notes by the nurse and physician (Kozob, Skidmore, 2001b).

Critical Thinking Question

A visitor to the unit begins to hit a patient. How would you handle this situation?

Care of patients in seclusion or restraints

When a patient is placed in seclusion or restraints, intensive nursing care is instituted. The patient is continuously observed directly or by video monitor. Other patients are not allowed to be near a restrained patient. The patient's mental status, response to and side effects of medications, hydration, nutrition, elimination, range of motion, vital signs, and hygiene are monitored. Immediate attention to any injuries resulting from the incident or from the restraints is critical and requires documentation. Every 1 to 2 hours, with two staff members present, the restraints

are removed one at a time, for 10 minutes each, to allow range-of-motion activities. Change of position and skin care is also important. Restricting visitors, telephone calls, and diversional materials, such as radios and magazines, reduces stimuli; however, regular staff contact decreases the patient's sense of isolation and loneliness.

Recovery and Depression Phase

In this phase, patients are assured that they are not being punished while in seclusion and that they will be allowed back in the milieu as soon as possible. Patients must be assisted in relaxing, sleeping, and benefiting from these phases of cooling down and reconciliation. The time patients are in restraints or seclusion should be a supportive, restorative time. Otherwise, patients may remain afraid, frustrated, and angry, possibly leading to future aggression.

After patients are calm and in control, they are encouraged to discuss the circumstance during which they lost control, as well as alternatives for handling similar situations in the future (Kozob, Skidmore, 2001a).

Patients are ready to be released from restraints when they show signs of self-control, decreased anxiety and agitation, a stabilized mood, increased attention span, reality orientation, and sound judgment. Patients may be kept in the seclusion room a brief time to assess the reaction to release from the restraints. Patients need assistance to reenter the unit with as little fear and embarrassment as possible. The nurse should make efforts to help other patients accept these patients back into the unit.

Immediately after a patient is secluded and restrained, the staff should meet, ensure that no staff injuries occurred, evaluate the way in which they handled the situation, and give each other mutual support and feedback. Feelings and attitudes are discussed, along with suggestions for improved use of procedures. These debriefing meetings provide the unit staff with ongoing, in-service opportunities to monitor their reactions, as well as augment their skills. Careful documentation of patients' behaviors before, during, and after the incident and a rationale for physical control interventions, seclusion, and restraint are essential legal protections for the staff. Documentation may be recorded as "incident reports" and should be written after everyone concerned has calmed down. Staff perceptions are compared for accuracy. Documentation is descriptive, sequential, organized, and specific about what was seen, heard, and felt; what was said and by whom; who was notified; and what actions were taken and are to be taken. The request for and granting of a physician's order for seclusion and restraint are also recorded.

Other patients' reactions to restraint and seclusion situations should be openly discussed and explored in a special meeting with staff. Patients must have the opportunity to share their concerns, reactions, and fears of losing control. Other patients must be told that staff members are providing control and care until the patient who has lost control regains it.

Critical Thinking Question

Why is it important for other patients to share their opinions and reactions to the seclusion and restraint of another patient?

STAFF MEMBERS AS VICTIMS OF ASSAULT

Most incidents of patient outbursts of anger do not result in restraint procedures; but when they occur, the process is always difficult for the staff and patient. The staff and the patient are understandably drained physically and emotionally. The process of debriefing and recovery is complicated when a staff member has been injured.

Being injured by a patient is similar emotionally to being a victim of crime (Chapter 41). This type of occurrence can destroy the staff member's sense of trust in others and sense of control of his or her life and can result in a loss of self-esteem. The staff member often expresses feelings of guilt, being vulnerable, irritable, depressed, and anxious; experiences nightmares, grief, and symptoms of posttraumatic stress disorder (PTSD); and is afraid of the patient who caused the injury. The assault may be minimized and feelings may even be denied if emotional support and debriefing are not provided after the medical examination and treatment are completed. If the injured staff member is away from work for a period, the rest of the staff may be unaware that their emotions have subsided much more than did those of their injured colleague. To ensure that the staff victim achieves emotional resolution of the incident, some facilities have developed a formalized process of follow-up. A peer support program that understands the dynamics of assault and the common responses of victims is important. Supportive interventions should be available to the person who was injured (Poster, 1996; Whitney, Jacobson, Gawrys, 1996). The needs of the victim determine the frequency and number of meetings. A counselor may facilitate meetings between the victim and staff and between the victim and the assaultive patient to facilitate the victim's return to work. Victims are encouraged to share their feelings with family or significant others. The goal of this process is to facilitate emotional resolution, help the person remain productive, and decrease the chance of resignation and development of PTSD (Poster, 1996; Whitney, Jacobson, Gawrys, 1996). Whether staff members who are assaulted by patients can or should take legal action against the patient is being currently debated (Poster, 1996).

Key Concepts

1. Anger is a normal human emotion that may be expressed assertively, passively, passive-aggressively, and aggressively.
2. Verbal and physical aggression, especially assault and battery, require safe, immediate interventions based on the principle of the least restrictive alternative.
3. The individual, social-psychologic, and stress models of aggression offer explanations for the development of aggression.
4. Factors regarding the nurse, the environment, and the patient affect the development and expression of anger.
5. The assault cycle describes the predictable phases of aggression: triggering, escalation, crisis, recovery, and depression.
6. Nursing interventions with anger and nonviolent aggression concentrate on ventilation to defuse the anger and then on problem solving to identify ways of appropriately handling the causes of the anger.
7. Tension reduction, medications, physical control, seclusion, or restraints become necessary in the escalation and crisis phases of the assault cycle.
8. Patients in seclusion and restraints require intensive physical and emotional nursing care.
9. Staff members who are injured by a patient may require assistance in recovering.

References

Allen JJ: Seclusion and restraint of children: a literature review, *J Child Adolescent Psychiatr Nurs* 13(4):159, 2000.

APNA: American psychiatric nurses association position statement on the use of seclusion and restraint, *J Am Psychiatr Nurs Assoc* 7(4):130, 2001.

Charney DS et al: Psychobiological mechanisms of posttraumatic stress disorder, *Arch Gen Psychiatry* 50(4):294, 1993.

Corrigan PW, Yudofsky SC, Silver JM: Pharmacological and behavioral treatments for aggressive psychiatric inpatients, *Hosp Community Psychiatry* 44(2):125, 1993.

Delacy LC: Seclusion and restraint standards: a platform for creating safety for patients and staff, *J Am Psychiatr Nurs Assoc* 7(4):99, 2001.

Eckroth-Bucher M: Philosophical basis and practice of self-awareness in psychiatric nursing, *J Psychosoc Nurs* 39(2): 2001.

ED Nursing: Let agitated patients know they have choices, *RN* 64(8):24, 2001.

Haber J: APNA plays a leadership role in shaping mental health policy related to seclusion and restraint, *J Am Psychiatr Nurs Assoc* 7(4):134, 2001.

Hawkins KA, Trobst KK: Frontal lobe dysfunction and aggression: conceptual issues and research findings, *Aggression and Violent Behavior* 5(2):147, 2000.

Hospital Focus: Let agitated patients know they have choices, *RN* 64(8):24hf1, 2001.

Hospital Focus: When a patient turns violent, *RN* 64(5):32hf2, 2001.

Jech AO: Calming the cognitively impaired, *Nursing Spectrum* metro ed:30, September 2001.

Jones J et al: Psychiatric inpatients' experience of nursing observation, *J Psychosoc Nurs* 38(12):10, 2000.

Joseph-Kinselman A et al: Clients' perceptions of involuntary hospitalization, *J Psychosoc Nurs Ment Health Serv* 32(2):28, 1994.

Kozob ML, Skidmore R: Seclusion and restraint: understanding recent changes, *J Psychosoc Nurs* 39(3):25, 2001a.

Kozob ML, Skidmore R: Least to most restrictive interventions, *J Psychosoc Nurs* 39(3):32, 2001b.

Maier GJ: Managing threatening behavior: the role of talk up and talk down, *J Psychosoc Nurs Ment Health Serv* 34(6):25, 1996.

Ollendick TH: Violence in youth: where do we go from here? Behavior therapy's approach, *Behav Ther* 27:485, 1996.

Poster EC: A multinational study of psychiatric nursing staffs' beliefs and concerns about work safety and patient assault, *Arch Psychiatr Nurs* 10(6):365, 1996.

Richman D: To restrain or not to restrain? *RN* 61(7):55, 1998.

Robinson L, Littrel SH, Littrel K: Managing aggression in schizophrenia, *J Am Psychiatr Nurs Assoc* 5(2):s9, 1999.

Smith P: Empirically based models for viewing the dynamics of violence. In Babich K, editor: *Assessing patient violence in the health care setting,* Boulder, Colo, 1981, Western Interstate Commission for Higher Education.

Stevenson S: Heading off violence with verbal de-escalation, *J Psychosoc Nurs Ment Health Serv* 29(9):6, 1991.

Teichner G, Golden CJ: The relationship of neuropsychological impairment to conduct disorder in adolescence, *Aggression and Violent Behavior* 5(6):509, 2000.

Terpstra TL et al: Nursing staff's attitude toward seclusion and restraint, *J Psychosoc Nurs* 39(5):20, 2001.

Thomas SP: Teaching healthy anger management, *Perspect Psychiatr Care* 37(2):41, 2001.

Whitney GA, Jacobson GA, Gawrys MT: The impact of violence in the health care setting upon nursing education, *J Nurs Educ* 35(5):211, 1996.

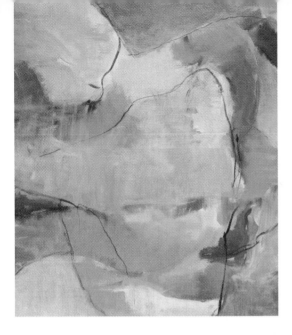

Chapter 14

Working with Groups of Patients

Carol E. Bostrom

Learning Objectives

After reading this chapter, you should be able to:
- Describe specific therapeutic benefits of groups.
- Identify the major purpose of each type of group.
- Explain the value of co-leadership of groups.
- Recognize qualities that the nurse leader of groups should have.
- Identify intervention strategies for specific group situations.

Working with groups of patients is an integral component of both inpatient and outpatient psychiatric care. Nursing has 24-hour accountability for patient care on the inpatient psychiatric unit and is responsible for leading patient groups. This responsibility dictates economic use of nursing personnel; hence working with groups of patients addresses manpower concerns, while providing a proven therapeutic intervention. Similarly, working with groups in the community or outpatient arena has increased because of brief inpatient psychiatric hospitalization and the demand of managed care for the least expensive, most effective care, in addition to increased use of less-restrictive nontraditional treatment in settings outside of the hospital (Farkas-Cameron, 1998).

Patients with mental illnesses face problems in their daily living similar to anyone else but with the complication of symptoms of mental illness. Although mental illness interferes with the way patients are able to cope with their problems, conflicts, and interpersonal relationships, patients have the capacity to learn techniques to cope and negotiate life's problems. Groups deal with current "here-and-now" issues and stressors whether patients are in or out of the hospital. Patients gain awareness and knowledge about their behaviors and the way in which those behaviors impede communication and coping; they become aware of alternatives that help them make better decisions and choices. On inpatient units and in community settings, nurses lead numerous educational and skill-development groups. Nurses also lead groups for patients' families to teach them about mental illness and to help them cope with the mentally ill family member. This chapter is dedicated to answering two questions:

1. Given a patient population that has serious interpersonal and cognitive disturbances, how does group work benefit the individual?
2. What can the nurse realistically expect to accomplish through formal and informal group work with patients?

Because inpatient groups typically have short-term, goal-oriented sessions and are composed of acutely ill patients, nurses must have relevant information for developing group strategies. Benefits of groups, types of groups, and leadership of groups are addressed to provide this information. Because working effectively with groups of patients is inextricably related to milieu management, the nurse is encouraged to read the chapters on milieu.

BENEFITS OF GROUPS

Benefits that patients receive from any group experience include the following:

- Patients gain knowledge about ways to relate to and communicate with others (Yalom, 1995).
- Patients gain acceptance, reassurance, and support from their peers and the group leader.
- Patients gain feelings of hopefulness and a sense of power regarding their ability to help themselves and others in the group.
- Patients are provided the opportunity to *test out* new behaviors with others during their treatment.
- Patients can share their feelings, problems, concerns, and ideas with others in a safe and structured environment.
- Patients' strengths that can enhance self-esteem are affirmed and further developed.
- Patients experience a sense of importance and an increased sense of worth.

These benefits may occur at different times for individual patients and in different group situations. Each group, depending on its goal or purpose, may focus on one particular outcome. For example, an activity group for art may focus on acceptance; no matter what the patients paint, the patients will be accepted and praised for their work.

THERAPEUTIC FACTORS

Irvin Yalom has described 11 "therapeutic factors" that help patients, regardless of the therapeutic group (Box 14-1). Patients experience certain factors or benefits, depending on the type of group in which they participate, and factors that the patients as individuals deem to be beneficial and important to them. Yalom originally related the therapeutic factors to psychotherapy groups but has developed their application to brief, one-time-only groups along the continuum of care. The meaning of these therapeutic factors and their significance to patients are important for the nurse to understand. The nurse who understands the ways groups help patients will be more likely to initiate, lead, and participate in formal and informal groups. Nurses do not make therapeutic factors happen, but they facilitate the development and occurrence of these factors for patients.

TYPES OF GROUPS

Making the inpatient group a positive, beneficial experience for patients is of primary importance (Yalom, 1995). Patients must believe that they have gained something for themselves during their hospitalization. A positive inpatient group experience favorably predisposes patients to seek treatment on an outpatient basis. After discharge, follow-up care in the community is the setting in which the majority of ongoing treatment occurs.

|Box 14-1| Yalom's Therapeutic Factors

- Instillation of hope. Patients receive hope from observing others who have benefited from the group experience.
- Universality. Patients experience relief in knowing that they are not alone and unique but that others experience similar problems, feelings, and concerns.
- Imparting of information. Patients learn or are provided information about areas related to their needs.
- Altruism. Patients experience themselves as helpful or useful to others.
- Corrective recapitulation of primary family group. Patients review previous dysfunctional family patterns and learn that these patterns can be changed to effectively meet their present needs.
- Development of socializing techniques. Patients are taught appropriate social skills.
- Imitative behavior. Patients selectively model healthy behaviors of the leader and other group members.
- Catharsis. Patients are not only allowed to express feelings but are also taught ways to express them appropriately.
- Existential factors. Patients share feelings about "ultimate concerns" of existence, such as death or isolation, and learn to accept that a limit to their control of these issues exists.
- Cohesiveness. Patients experience feelings of being accepted, valued, and part of a group experience.
- Interpersonal learning. Patients learn the ways in which their behaviors affect others and more appropriate ways of relating in the supportive atmosphere of the group.

From Yalom I: *The theory and practice of group psychotherapy*, ed 4, New York, 1995, Basic Books.

Numerous types of groups can be offered in both inpatient and outpatient settings: support, activity, education, problem solving, and therapy. Self-help or special-problem groups and multiple-family or couple groups are also available in some treatment settings.

SUPPORT GROUPS

The very nature of nursing implies support. The nurse supports patients in therapeutic interactions. Support means accepting, empathizing, and showing concern while listening and talking with patients. The nurse focuses on responding to patients' needs. The nurse's presence, interest, and encouragement facilitate the expression of patients' feelings and concerns. The nurse is then instrumental in helping patients cope with their feelings and situations. Support is useful in many types of group situations.

The support group is a maintenance group; its purpose is to reinforce or maintain existing strengths and behaviors of patients, rather than to confront or change behaviors or defenses. Patients in a support group can be acutely or chronically ill. Group members may need a great deal of reassurance and emotional support during their hospitalization. These patients also need to reduce their anxiety to mild or moderate levels.

The reality-orientation group is an example of a support group frequently found in inpatient settings. Patients who exhibit confusion and short attention spans resulting from some psychopathologic factor can benefit from this type of group. The nurse must provide an atmosphere of safety and security because these patients may be frightened, unsure, anxious, uncomfortable, and isolated. The reality-orientation group can assist patients with decreasing isolation and increasing self-esteem. Focusing on "the here and now" provides a framework with structure, social support, and reality testing. The nurse as leader of this group facilitates orientation to time, person and place, rules and routines of the unit, and behavioral expectations, including some limit setting. Feeling valued, respected, and important as human beings is a feeling these patients may not have experienced in a while.

ACTIVITY GROUPS

Activity groups use a variety of techniques to facilitate self-expression, interaction, and acceptance of self and others (McGarr, Prince, 1998). For example, some groups may use art or music to motivate patients to interact and promote socialization. Withdrawn, depressed, and regressed patients benefit from these groups because these individuals have experienced isolation and lack interpersonal relationships. The general goals of these groups are to help patients increase self-esteem, openness, and the expression of feelings and decrease isolation. When interpersonal communication increases, focus on the activity per se decreases. The activity is a vehicle or means to facilitate self-expression of both positive and negative feelings in a creative way, patient interaction, and fun or enjoyment. Table 14-1 describes two types of activity groups.

EDUCATION GROUPS

Nurses who work in inpatient and outpatient settings lead groups to teach patients and their families a variety of content and skills. Typical groups deal with medication, the dynamics and management of illness, problem solving, stress management, social skills, interpersonal skills, and relapse prevention. The reduction in inpatient hospitalization has increased the need for patients to learn skills that help them manage their illnesses and their lives in the community.

Table 14-2 illustrates an example of educational groups that can be used in a community mental health center for groups of patients and families. Ses-

| Table 14-1 | Activity Groups

Type	Nurse's Purpose or Role	Examples
Recreation	Provide opportunity for fun and relieve tension. Enable patients to experience sense of participation, acceptance, and accomplishment.	Indoor-outdoor sports, field trips, exercise groups, and games
Creative expression	Facilitate expression of feelings, communication with others, and socialization. Allow for creativity, self-expression, and praise for accomplishments.	Arts and crafts, activities of daily living, art, poetry, music, dance, and pet therapy

|Table 14-2| Education Groups

Type	Nurse's Purpose or Role	Examples
Psychoeducation	Teach patients and families content related to dynamics of illness, symptoms of illness, signs of relapse, management of illness, and dealing with crises.	Addiction processes, coping with symptoms, management of moods, causes and treatments of illnesses, relapse prevention, community resources
Medication	Dispense medications. Assess symptoms and side effects. Explain type and purpose of medication, dosage, therapeutic effects and side effects. Support adherence to medication regimens and to prevent relapse.	Groups based on category of medications (e.g., antipsychotics vs antidepressants, intramuscular vs oral)
Problem solving	Help identify and describe current problems; discuss and develop solutions and their effects; decide on an alternative method and how to try it. Evaluate and choose another method, if necessary.	Milieu issues, conflict resolution, job concerns, relationship issues, discharge planning
Stress management	Teach and facilitate adaptive coping behaviors.	Life-style balance and management, relaxation training, tension-reduction strategies, and anger management
Social skills	Teach, develop, and practice skills to enhance interactions with others. Focus on realistic, day-to-day patient needs.	Assertiveness training, handling social interactions (e.g., meeting new people, going on interviews, negotiating the return of a purchase)

sions may vary in length but typically include an hour for content presentation and discussion. An example might be a weekly session for patients with bipolar disorder. Another example might be a weekly social skills group for patients with schizophrenia. Patients from a variety of health care settings identified having a nurse teach about the illness, medications, treatments, and staying healthy as areas indicative of quality nursing care (Oermann, Templin, 2000). Nurses must collaborate with patients in treatment planning and developing educational programs based on the patients' needs and interests. A study conducted by Payson, Wheeler, and Wellington (1998) found that patients are interested primarily in medication and side effects, obtaining necessary care from the mental health system, and learning ways to solve problems. The nurse's expertise, empathy, and support help patients learn that they themselves can successfully take care of their illnesses and themselves.

Nurses also provide psychoeducational programs for families of mentally ill individuals. Families are interested in the content on illnesses, medication benefits and side effects, communication with the ill family member, ways to manage crisis situations

with patients, and ways to negotiate with the mental health system and managed care to have needs met. Families benefit not only from the information they receive in groups but also from the high level of support that these groups provide. The benefits that families receive from group participation are similar to the patient benefits discussed earlier. Additionally, families experience less anger and improved relationships with family members as they learn new family communication skills. Families also learn about available sources along the continuum of care and look to the nurse as an advocate and expert in helping them arrange for needed services.

THERAPY GROUPS

Therapy groups help patients develop an understanding of and insight into their feelings, behaviors, and roles in relationships. Some groups assist patients in changing behaviors and developing healthier responses to others. For therapy groups to be most beneficial, patients must have a desire to develop awareness of their problems and be motivated and willing to change. Table 14-3 lists examples of therapy groups.

|Table 14-3| Therapy Groups

Type	Nurse's Purpose or Role	Examples
Insight-oriented	Facilitate an understanding of how individuals affect and are affected by others. Assist in examining role-relationship issues. Help develop healthier ways to handle feelings and response to others.	Process groups, survivors groups, self-esteem groups
Psychodrama	Achieve intense emotional release and insight through acting out intrapersonal and interpersonal conflicts. Help patients improvise their roles in specific situations or with a script or play. Provide support and discussion after the drama.	Psychodrama, but may be called by other names
Sociodrama	Focus on solutions and insight into role communication. Reenact specific social roles. Give feedback and role play alternative methods of communication. (Examples of roles are parent-child, worker-boss, and teacher-student.)	Sociodrama, also considered a form of psychodrama

SELF-HELP OR SPECIAL PROBLEM GROUPS

Problem-Centered Groups

Numerous groups focus on helping individuals with special problems, for example, child abuse, anorexia and bulimia, and diabetes. These groups are homogeneous, meaning that all group members share the same problem. Members feel accepted and understood by the group and are therefore more willing to share concerns and ask questions. Information is shared along with personal feelings and difficulties. Members assist each other with helpful strategies; they do not feel alone or isolated but learn that others with the same problem or need are coping effectively. The nurse who leads special problem groups is interested, knowledgeable, and skilled in working with patients with specific problems.

Traditional Self-Help Groups

Traditional self-help groups are also homogeneous but are not professionally organized and led. Self-help groups are organized and led by group members who share a similar problem. Self-help is based on the belief that an individual with a problem can be truly understood and helped only by others who have the same problem. Millions of people participate in hundreds of self-help groups. In some groups, such as Alcoholics Anonymous, individual 24-hour support is available. Members of self-help groups understand each other's lifestyles and needs, help each other solve problems and cope with stress, and confront each other about dysfunctional behaviors.

Professionals may be invited to a self-help group for a specific purpose, such as providing an educational program. Nurses commonly refer individuals to self-help groups and must therefore be knowledgeable about the self-help groups in their area. Interested individuals can call their local mental health organization for information about the availability of groups such as the Alliance for the Mentally Ill, Recovery Incorporated, and Incest Survivors Anonymous.

> **Critical Thinking Question**
>
> A patient is extremely depressed and nearly mute. Which combination of groups would you encourage this patient to attend?

GROUP LEADERSHIP

Group leadership functions range from the formal to the informal. The inpatient psychiatric nurse may engage in spontaneous, informal interactions with a group of patients in a card game or participate formally in a planned, structured group session in a special setting. An informal card game provides the nurse with an opportunity for therapeutic interpersonal interaction, socialization, and role-modeling behavior. Another example might be responding to medication questions that arise in small informal groups; the nurse reinforces compliance with medication and attempts to alleviate anxiety or concerns. These informal, spontaneous interventions with groups of patients occur repeatedly during the course of a day on an inpatient unit.

Brief clinical group encounters are also known as fluid groups. Fluid groups allow the nurse to facilitate interpersonal competencies and learning in informal, around-the-clock contacts with patients in the inpatient milieu (Echternacht, 2001).

Although degrees of formality and types of patients vary, the nurse invariably uses group leadership skills to meet patients' needs in the therapeutic milieu. As managers and providers of patient care (24 hours a day), nurses intervene with groups of patients. Consequently, nurses must use effective communication skills to interact with groups of patients (described later in this chapter).

Nurses on inpatient units should be aware of factors that influence the clinical setting. Short-stay inpatient hospitalization affects group work in many ways. For example, short hospitalizations create a rapid turnover of patients in groups; thus expecting a high level of trust and cohesion to develop is unrealistic. Patients may also have an assortment of serious illnesses. The nurse must quickly assess the mental status of patients to determine the length of time necessary before patients can enter groups or whether they can tolerate a group at all. The nurse also assesses the appropriate placement of patients in specific groups based on the level of functioning and the ability to tolerate particular groups. Charting patient progress in the group is an important nursing responsibility for both therapeutic and legal reasons.

Similarly, in outpatient care and in the community, nurses must consider realistic factors that impinge on treatment. Patients may be limited to a specific number of visits because of payment providers, or participation in day-treatment or substance-related programs may be limited to a specific number of days during the course of a year.

Confidentiality must be explained to group participants; that is, patients must understand that what is said or takes place in the group setting must remain private. However, statements within group sessions may be shared with staff members or the treatment team because of their responsibility for patient care. Personal information is of course shared in the group and should not leave the unit or care facility. In reality, group confidentiality can be difficult to ensure because trust and cohesion may not be fully developed. Content or what is learned in group settings, such as medication, can be shared outside of the treatment setting.

CO-LEADERSHIP

An important factor to consider about group leadership, particularly on the inpatient unit, is that nurses have days off and may rotate shifts. Therefore the presence of a co-leader can lend consistency to the group and directly support its structure and purpose. Co-leaders can complement each other and learn from each other; they collaborate and share responsibility for the group. If the group is large, charting and communicating information to other staff members can be expedited. Additionally, one leader may observe something in the group that the other leader may not notice. Co-leadership provides patients with examples of the proper way to relate to another person with respect. A co-leader may be a professional from another discipline, and having a man and a woman as co-leaders may occasionally help. In the community, the nurse may be the only leader of groups for patients and families.

PHYSICAL SETTING

Physical arrangements are important considerations in creating an atmosphere that is conducive to group work. Finding adequate space or a private room is often difficult but is nevertheless important to ensure privacy and a quiet atmosphere. Adequate lighting, comfortable temperature, ample seating, and proper equipment also contribute to successful group function. Forming a circle of chairs allows patients to see each other and indicates an expectation that patients will relate to leaders and other group members. Chairs in rows may be appropriate for a didactic group. A blackboard, a dry marker board, a projector, or a video recorder may be necessary. Handouts or printed materials may be used for patients and families.

FORMAL GROUPS

Nurse leaders must be active, structured, and empathetic. Because of time constraints, leaders cannot afford to be nondirective or to allow the group to be free floating. The nurse must be goal directed and focus on the here and now in each inpatient or outpatient group session. The nurse assesses the needs of the patients and formulates a realistic goal for that session. Each session should be treated as a separate entity, with the patient feeling that something positive was attained during the group session (Yalom, 1995). The formal group should meet for approximately 1 hour. The leader succinctly states the group's purpose at the beginning of the session, and most of the session is spent on the work to be accomplished. Patients generally prefer leaders who provide the group "with an active structure" (Yalom, 1995). The final 5 to 10 minutes is used to summarize and close the session. The summary should have a positive focus and include information that the patients have learned or gained from the group. The leader gives positive feedback to the group regarding progress during the session.

Patients are expected to arrive at the group session on time. Depending on the patient's level of functioning, the group leader may gather the members of the group and walk with them into the meeting room. Smoking and refreshments are not permitted during group sessions. Patients remain for the entire group session, if possible. The group leader may permit patients to pace or leave the room and then return when they are able. The inability to sit still for an extended period may be the result of anxiety or drug side effects (usually akathisia). The decision to exclude patients from the group should be made carefully. The nurse may exclude patients who are acutely manic, disoriented, and too psychotic to benefit from group therapy, or those who will disrupt the group. Patients who are hostile and verbally threatening are also not appropriate candidates for group sessions.

INTERVENTIONS

Basic interventions for groups are based on facilitative communication techniques (see Chapter 9). Nurses use these skills with patients individually and within groups. Nurses who facilitate group interactions on a therapeutic level enable patients to share feelings and problems. Some basic communication skills that are useful for nurse leaders are listed in Table 14-4. These skills are not unique to the group setting; they are skills that nurses use on a daily basis. These general interventions are therapeutic, regardless of the type of group. The use of positive feedback helps patients in their attempt to use new skills. For example, in an attempt to use a particular assertiveness skill, the patient goes off on a tangent. The nurse may say, "You have done well, Mr. Johnson. When you gave us the example of saying to your boss, 'I need to talk with you about my work schedule,' you used

an excellent example of 'I' statements." The nurse chooses to repeat the portion of Mr. Johnson's statement that is realistic and is a correct example of an "I" statement for emphasis and clarity. As a result, the patient feels a sense of accomplishment and increased self-esteem.

For the group experience to be successful, the nurse leader must recognize and manage process and content areas (Rindner, 2000). The combination of teaching didactic material (psychoeducation) along with managing process issues requires knowledge and skill. The structure of the group session must include a balance between content to be taught and group process for the group experience to be beneficial.

Dominant Patient

The dominant patient monopolizes the entire group session to the extent that other patients may believe that they do not have the opportunity to participate. The nurse employs gatekeeping functions to offer all patients the opportunity to contribute to the group. For example, the nurse can say, "Miss Benson, you are doing well in contributing to our session today, but I would like to hear what others are thinking about at this time." This intervention can forestall monopolization of the group by a single patient without putting her down, while giving others the opportunity to express themselves. The other patients in the group may be unable to handle this patient or may be too afraid. If the group leader is afraid or cannot control the patient, the integrity of the group is compromised.

Uninvolved Patient

The uninvolved patient presents another challenge to the nurse leader. The patient may be quiet because of anxiety or fear. Patients with chronic schizophrenia find relating in group sessions difficult and threatening. The nurse can say, "It is hard to talk about ourselves in the group, but I know that everyone here has something to share that can help someone else." The nurse recognizes that patients are mistrustful and anxious but relates the message that each individual is important and capable of helping another.

Some patients who are uninvolved in the group may believe themselves to be at a higher level of functioning than the other members. These patients

|Table 14-4| Communication Skills: Eliciting, Qualifying, and Clarifying Communication

Techniques of the Leader(s)	Group Member Response	Outcome
1. Giving information: "My purpose in offering this group experience is..."	Further validates his assumptions: "How is this going to happen?"	Leader(s) and member(s) enter into a dialogue in which member(s) get more information to make decisions and build trust in group experience.
2. Seeking clarification: "Did you say you were upset with John because he said that?"	May try to restate his thoughts or feelings: "Yes, I guess I was upset."	Member becomes aware that he was not clear and learns to identify thoughts and feelings more precisely, at the same time taking responsibility for them.
3. Encouraging description and exploration (delving further into communication or experiences): "How did you feel when Joann said that to you?"	Elaborates on his message: "I was angry."	Member deals in greater depth with an experience in the group and again takes responsibility for his reactions. (This example also places events in time or in sequence lending further perspective to group events.)
4. Presenting reality: "Would other members think Joann was unstable if they interviewed her for a job? You don't appear shaky to me."	Listens and considers other possibilities.	Member compares perception of self with others' perceptions of him.
5. Seeking consensual validation (seeking mutual understanding of what is being communicated): "Did I understand you to say that you feel better now than you did last week?"	Further clarification: "Well, yes, I'm better than last week but not as good as I'd like to be."	Group and leader(s) learn how member views his progress and in which way they should receive his evaluation of himself.
6. Focusing (identifying a single topic to concentrate on): "Maybe we could identify one problem you have and talk more about that."	Channels thinking: Members may think of the most puzzling problem they have.	Group and leader(s) identify specific topics they can resolve before the meeting ends. They increase their understanding of one problem before jumping to others.

From Van Servellen G: *Group and family therapy,* St Louis, 1983, Mosby.

may believe that they are not as sick as the others, do not belong in the group, and will not benefit from the session. The nurse leader may give attention to these members by giving them a job to perform for the group, for example, arranging chairs for the session. Respect and recognition by the nurse is therapeutic for these patients because they will believe that they can contribute to group.

Critical Thinking Question

During a group session on problem solving, a patient states, "I learn more by listening." How and why would you involve this patient in the group discussion?

Hostile Patient

Hostility may mask a patient's fear, self-anger, or unresolved anger toward others. To help this patient appropriately verbalize feelings of anger, the nurse can say, "Mrs. Robinson, you sound angry today. What happened?" or "Tell us about it." The nurse directly confronts the patient in a supportive manner and attempts to help the patient deal with her feelings. Allowing verbal or nonverbal hostility to continue jeopardizes the progress of the group session. Unchecked hostility causes discomfort and uneasiness and impairs the ability of other patients to attend to the group's work. Patients may also mistakenly interpret anger as being directed toward them.

|Table 14-4| Communication Skills: Eliciting, Qualifying, and Clarifying Communication—cont'd

Techniques of the Leader(s)	Group Member Response	Outcome
7. Encouraging comparison (asking members to compare and contrast their experiences with others in the group): "How did the rest of the group handle this problem?"	Group members share their experiences as they relate to the topic.	Leader(s) and members gain greater insight into their commonalities and differences and learn from one another alternative ways of responding to problems.
8. Making observations: "You look more comfortable now, John, than you did at the beginning of the meeting." *or* "The group has been silent for the last 5 minutes."	Group members have something to respond to: "I feel more at ease now." *or* "I think we are quiet because we are bored."	Group members and leader(s) place attention on significant events and can elaborate on their meanings.
9. Giving recognition or acknowledging: "John, you are new to the group. Perhaps we can introduce ourselves."	Feels acknowledged and included: "Yes, I'm John, and I came here because.... "	Members view specific instances as important, and the leaders reinforce the behavior or event they choose to notice—in this case, the desire to come to group.
10. Accepting (not necessarily agreeing with but receiving communication with openness): "Yes, I hear you say that you don't know if you want to be in the group or not."	Feels heard and understood without fear of attack.	Members learn that even "nonacceptable" attitudes can be talked about, and perhaps any thought is not so horrible that they cannot share it.
11. Encouraging evaluation (asking the group as a whole or individual members to judge their experiences): "When Marilyn gives you support, do you feel better?" *or* "How did we do in helping Joann with her problem?"	Members reflect on progress made: "Not exactly, because I don't know if I can trust her to be honest." *or* "It was hard. I'd like to know from her."	The criteria for success become clearer to members, and new directions may be formulated as a result of the discussion.
12. Summarizing (encapsulating in a few sentences what has occurred): "The group discussed several issues and problems today—they were...."	Members recall significant points events and close off consideration of new or extraneous topics.	Members and leader(s) place in perspective, identifying salient points of a group session. Such a summary can lead to a better understanding of group process.

These group interventions will help the nurse develop as a group leader. Patients quickly recognize the group leader's empathy, understanding, and respect for each patient as caring behaviors. Even though some patients make only minimal progress toward their individual treatment goals, interacting with the nurse who possesses these traits can increase the patients' feelings of worth as human beings.

Critical Thinking Question

A member of the group states, "This group is a waste of time. I don't get anything out of it." Which communication skills would you use in this situation?

Key Concepts

1. The psychiatric nurse interacts and intervenes with patients and families in informal groups, as well as in formally structured sessions in inpatient and community settings.
2. Patients benefit from group experiences by gaining acceptance, hopefulness, and support from others. Through mutual sharing of feelings and problems, patients learn the way in which their communication methods and behaviors interfere with relationships. Their strengths are reinforced and accumulated.
3. Families of the mentally ill benefit from the information and support they receive in a group.

4. Nurse leaders must be active, empathetic, goal directed, and deal with the here and now in each group session.

5. Various types of groups exist in inpatient and outpatient settings to benefit the acutely and chronically ill. Typical types are support, motivation, education and problem solving, therapy, and self-help or special problem groups. Support and educational groups exist for families of mentally ill patients.

6. Nurses use facilitative communication techniques and role-modeling behaviors as group leaders.

7. The nurse leader structures the group session by attending to content and process issues.

8. The nurse leader intervenes therapeutically with dominating, uninvolved, and hostile patients.

References

Echternacht M: Fluid group: concept and clinical application in the therapeutic milieu, *J Psychiatr Nurs Assoc* 7(2):39, 2001.

Farkas-Cameron M: Inpatient group therapy in a managed health care environment: application to clinical nursing practice, *J Psychiatr Nurs Assoc* 4(5):145, 1998.

McGarry T, Prince M: Implementation of groups for creative expression on a psychiatric inpatient unit, *J Psychosoc Nurs* 36(3):19, 1998.

Oermann M, Templin T: Important attributes of quality health care: consumer perspectives, *J Nurs Scholarship* 332(2):167, 2000.

Payson A, Wheeler K, Wellington T: Health teaching needs of clients with serious and persistent mental illness: client and provider perspectives, *J Psychosoc Nurs* 36(2):32, 1998.

Rindner E: Combined: group process-psychoeducation model for psychiatric clients and their families, *J Psychosoc Nurs* 38(9):34, 2000.

Van Servellen G: *Group and family therapy,* St Louis, 1983, Mosby.

Yalom I: *The theory and practice of group psychotherapy,* ed 4, New York, 1995, Basic Books.

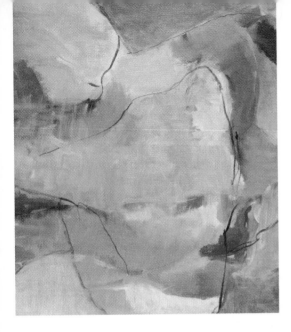

Chapter 15

Working with the Family

Sandra J. Wood

Throughout history, the family unit has functioned to perpetuate society. The family is the institution into which ideally children are born and in which they grow up and receive affection, education, and cultural beliefs and values. Because the family has a long-term and significant effect on each individual, it becomes a focus of mental health care. Families are intimately involved with their mentally ill members and are affected by the illness of their family member, thus including family members enhances the positive effects of that involvement. Over the years, many changes have occurred in family structure and function, but the ability of the family to adapt to societal changes is precisely what the family must have to remain as the primary unit of childrearing and the touchstone of most people's lives (Johnson, 1995).

This chapter presents characteristics of families, the effects of mental illness on families, and issues of working with families in various settings. The emphasis in this chapter is on understanding and assessing families as a basis for brief therapeutic interactions, family conferences, education, support, and referrals.

DEFINITION OF FAMILY

The family, which had been defined as two or more related people living together who have a commitment to each other, has undergone major changes in adapting to modern life. Whereas, two generations ago, the extended family predominated, and one generation ago, the nuclear family was the norm, now, single-parent families and blended or stepfamilies are common in the United States (Johnson, 1995). Unrelated individuals may also choose to live together and assume the functions of a family.

FAMILY TASKS

Although families with one or more children continue to perform the eight basic tasks of family life defined by Duvall and Miller (1985), theses tasks are performed differently and may be shared with other societal institutions, such as schools and churches. The following list of the basic tasks of family life illustrates the alterations in the ways families have managed these tasks in today's society.

1. *Physical maintenance and safety.* This task remains important in the care of children and

ill or infirmed family members, such as older adults, but the function is now shared with schools, day-care centers, retirement centers, and nursing homes to a greater extent than it was in the past.

2. *Allocation of resources.* This function can be affected by outside resources, such as Medicaid, Medicare, and child support payments to a greater degree than it was in the past. If the number of these resources is increased or decreased, the quality of life of family members can be affected. For example, if a child support decree is changed to give more money to children, educational opportunities not previously possible may become available to the family. If federal allocations for Medicare are reduced, low-income seniors will have to decrease spending and forego food or medicine to pay the rent.

3. *Division of labor.* This task is much less gender based than it was in the past and often involves outside resources, such as cleaning services to clean the house while family members work at other jobs. An entire sector of the current economy (the service sector) is now devoted to work that was previously managed by family members.

4. *Socialization of family members.* This function is still performed primarily in the family; but because families are different, socialization may be significantly more complicated than it was in the past. For example, with a blended family, two sets of parents, as well as several more grandparents, may be available to socialize children. This change can lead to an enrichment of the child's life or confusion if the values of the various adults are significantly different. Socialization of children is also shared much earlier now compared with the past, with the rise of out-of-home care for infants and young children.

5. *Reproduction and release of family members.* Although reproduction still involves a sperm and an egg, the advent of artificial insemination enables this function to be carried out differently in some cases. Families still release members when they reach adulthood, but this release may be postponed because of pursuit of higher education or may involve a "boomerang" effect when grown children return home to live after having lived on their own.

6. *Maintenance of order, authority, and decision making.* Although this function is maintained in the family, new family forms make the task increasingly complex. In a family in which divorce and remarriage have occurred, the authority and decision making may be shared among several adults in more than one household. If the adults do not communicate and negotiate the rules when decisions are made, everyone can suffer. In any case, the task is more difficult than it was in a nuclear family.

7. *Placement of members in the larger society.* Families continue to perform this function, but because of increasing numbers of working parents, the need for day care, and the ubiquitous nature of various forms of media in our daily lives, contacts with the outside world occur early with less shielding of children from society. Children now become aware of events, often tragic, that occur in distant cities or even in other countries but do not have the knowledge or perspective to fully understand the events. The explosion of the space shuttle Challenger and the destruction of the World Trade Centers and Pentagon, viewed live by many children in classrooms and homes across the nation, are good examples of the lack of shielding of children from the tragedy in today's world.

8. *Maintenance of bonds of affection and provision of stability, values, and family cohesion.* Some would argue that current difficulties in the "normal" family have eroded the quality of family functioning in this area of family life. However, others would point to the many families who are successfully managing these tasks despite the complexities of separation, divorce, remarriage, and blended families. For example, in many families, parents or adult parental figures share custody of their children and are both able to play significant roles in their children's everyday lives. Whatever the family configuration, this function remains an important task for families to perform.

FAMILY CHARACTERISTICS

The nurturing of individuals as they grow and develop is a primary function of the family. The goal of these efforts is the achievement of autonomy, as a well-functioning, healthy adult (Johnson, 1995). Development from an infant, who is dependent on others for all of his or her needs, to a young adult with a positive self-concept, problem-solving skills, and appreciation of and ability to reach out to others is a lengthy, complicated process. By providing needed guidance, support, and values, parents facilitate this process. However, parents are also burdened with external stressors that can range from heavy job demands to care for an aging relative. Although families have deficits and weaknesses, they also possess strengths and abilities that can be used in overcoming the deficits. The nursing student should recognize that, in most cases, families are trying to do the best job possible with the skills and resources available to them.

Healthy families demonstrate several characteristics that enable them to function effectively. Families are *open systems* that seek assistance from outside resources, when necessary, rather than having closed, rigid boundaries. *Clear and congruent communication* among family members is noted. *Shared power* is observed between parents, if more than one parent is part of the family. Appropriate *autonomy* of family members consistent with the member's developmental level is encouraged. *Feelings are expressed openly,* and family interactions, for the most part, have a *warm, caring tone.* The family *negotiates the performance of tasks* by involving all members in decisions, to the extent appropriate. *Values are instilled by the parent or parents* and subscribed to by all family members (Johnson, 1995).

These characteristics provide the basis for the family to cope effectively with internal pressures, such as the illness of a member, or external pressures, such as the loss of a job by a parent. During times of stress, a family may experience disruption in one or more of the aforementioned characteristics; however, the retention of other characteristics and the support of caregivers and the extended family can enable the family to "weather" the disruption and remain resilient. When a father loses his job because of company downsizing, he may initially resent the fact that his wife changes her employment from part-time to full-time to meet family expenses. He may assume that he no longer shares the power in the family. The couple may argue about the role of the husband-father in the family. However, if the family's cohesion and the happiness of its members are valued, the crisis can be resolved such that the husband-father retains his shared authority in the family. For example, he can involve the family in his decision to return to school to prepare for a new career that will be more fulfilling for him and provide more stability for the entire family.

STAGES OF FAMILY DEVELOPMENT

Duvall and Miller (1985) defined stages of family development based on the people and events involved in a family at different periods of life. Initially, the single individual marries and becomes part of a "beginning family" (a couple). If children enter the family, the stage changes to the "early childbearing family" when the oldest child is no more than $2^1/_2$ years old, and the family concentrates on incorporating the children into the family. When children reach the age of $2^1/_2$ years, they are likely to attend preschool, if they have not already been in day care, and the parents' focus shifts to introducing them to the outside world while maintaining control of their contacts with others, that is, "families with preschool children." As the oldest child enters elementary school—"families with school children"—parents must accept increased contact of their children with the outside world and must focus on education, as well as socialization. "Families with teenagers" have the oldest child encountering increasing independence and planning for the future, as the child negotiates high school and work or college. After the oldest child reaches the end of the teenage years, plans are made for the child to begin a life on his or her own—"launching center families"—followed by "families in mid-life," in which the couple readjusts to life without children—"the empty nest." In the final stage, "families in retirement," the couple deals with issues of adjusting to retirement, becoming grandparents, and facing eventual death of spouse and friends (Duvall, Miller, 1985).

The aforementioned stages still apply to contemporary families, but with some differences when compared with families in the past. Changes in the configuration of the family (e.g., single parenting, blended families) have complicated this assessment. Parents who were previously dealing with one or two stages of family development may be propelled into later stages by the addition of step-children and will often be dealing with more stages than they faced before the divorce or remarriage. Furthermore, the addition of children by the birth of a child from the new union can mean that the blended family will be dealing with children in all stages of family development, from birth to young adulthood. Nurturing an infant while simultaneously guiding an adolescent to maturity and self-reliance require different parenting skills. Knowledge of appropriate behavior at each developmental level of childhood and providing sufficient external supports are important to the success of parenting in these situations.

EFFECTS OF MENTAL ILLNESS ON THE FAMILY

Mental illness is a particularly stressful event in a family's life. The diagnosis of a mental illness in a family member can elicit feelings of guilt over possible genetic transmission of the disease to the family member by parents, concern over the prognosis and course of the disease, worry among other family members that they may become mentally ill, and shame or embarrassment in the family about the way in which people outside the family will view the family and the ill member. Besides the feelings engendered in family members by the diagnosis, the ill member may display unusual or dangerous behavior, such as making suicidal or homicidal threats. The family must deal with the behavior of the ill member, as well as with agencies and institutions that are available to assist the ill family member. Law enforcement agencies, courts, social service agencies, schools, hospitals, clinics, and churches are among the many agencies with differing rules and procedures that the mentally ill person and family must negotiate. These agencies may need to be consulted in the process of obtaining needed care, or contacts may come about as a result of behavior related to the family member's mental illness. For example, the mentally ill family member may feel that the neighbor is planning to harm him or her and, as a result, may make a threat against the neighbor. This action will bring the local law enforcement agency and possibly the courts into contact with the family, as

well as mental health agencies, and perhaps a hospital when the person who is making the threat is revealed as mentally ill. Issues that may surface as a result of a family member's mental illness include:

- Medication compliance and presence and treatment of side effects of medication
- Lack of energy to complete activities of daily living (ADLs)
- Social isolation, avoidance of contact with others
- Acting out behaviors, particularly threatening or paranoid behavior
- Mood swings
- Denial of illness, lack of appropriate reasoning or judgment about ADLs
- Inappropriate or incomprehensible communication
- Persistence of dangerous behavior (e.g., drug or alcohol abuse)
- Manipulation of others to achieve desired goals

When a family member is diagnosed as mentally ill, the family must deal with grief issues. These issues include the loss of individual functioning and the loss of family functioning because of the illness of the mentally ill member. Income may be lost if the family member was a wage earner. Stress on the ill member and other family members can increase and affect school or work performance of all members of the family. Stigma from inside or outside the family related to being mentally ill can affect the ill individual and other family members. The future of both the individual and the family may also be jeopardized. The diagnosis of a mental illness can break apart a family, as when a spouse can no longer live with and subject children to an alcoholic partner, or it can bring family members together. Kay Redfield Jameson, a professor of psychiatry who also has manic-depressive illness, speaks of her mother in her autobiography, *An Unquiet Mind* (1995) in the following terms: "She could not have known how difficult it would be to deal with madness: had no preparation for what to do with madness—none of us did—but, consistent with her ability to love and her native will, she handled it with empathy and intelligence" (Jameson, 1995, p. 19). Nurses should offer this type of empathy to mentally ill patients and families with whom they come into contact. By giving empathy and support to patients and families, the nurse can empower them to be in control of the mental illness that affects them. This empowerment will help them manage their illness, thus preventing or minimizing complications as much as possible. The National Alliance for the Mentally Ill (NAMI) available at http://www.nami.org and other groups such as local and national mental health associations effectively advocate for the rights of patients and their families. These groups provide information about the effectiveness of various treatments, the risks and benefits of specific treatments, the cost-benefit ratio of specific services, the availability of services such as mutual support groups, and assistance in negotiating the insurance and mental health systems and other bureaucratic mazes in the government and social services sectors.

REASONS FOR SEEKING FAMILY TREATMENT

As stated previously, the mental illness of a family member can cause the entire family to seek treatment. Other causes for seeking treatment include:

- Situational crises, such as loss of job, legal troubles, and divorce
- Developmental crises, such as children starting school or the oldest or youngest child leaving home
- Relationship problems and conflicts, such as abuse of one or more family members
- Conflicts between families of origin and current family (family of marriage)
- Addition of family members through remarriage, adoption, and foster care
- Family conflicts over treatment when a family member has another type of illness
- Custody conflicts and issues
- Family exploitation of an ill family member
- Family confrontation or conflict with caregivers

FAMILY REACTION TO TREATMENT

When a family seeks treatment for any of the problems previously listed or for other problems, the nurse must listen to all parties involved and withhold judgment until all points of view have been examined. The nurse and other caregivers must refrain from giving the impression that the family caused the problems of an individual member or that the ill individual is responsible for the problems that the family is experiencing. Family members who become emotionally ill may not be the sickest members of the family. "Scapegoating" the ill family member as the cause of all family problems may be tempting but is inaccurate. Often, the ill family member is the one who is most sensitive to the disruptions in family life and most desirous of obtaining help to overcome the problem. The nurse can ameliorate some of the scapegoating that may be occurring in a family by consulting directly with the patient, as well as other family members. The nurse can offer the patient positive reinforcement about the patient's willingness to engage in the treatment process. Even if the patient is only minimally cooperative with treatment, positive reinforcement can serve to improve the patient's cooperation and boost his or her self-esteem.

FAMILY REACTIONS TO PSYCHIATRIC HOSPITALIZATION

When a family member is hospitalized in a psychiatric facility, patients and families react in various ways. Relief may be felt among family members and, at times, by the patient. The patient may desire help and agree to be admitted, or the patient may want help but refuse to be admitted to an inpatient facility. The patient may not want others to know about the admission because of fear concerning the reaction of family and friends. The family may wish for the patient to be admitted, either because of family member's difficulty in coping with the patient's bizarre behavior or concern about the safety of the patient or others related to suicidal or homicidal threats or actions. When the ill individual must be involuntarily committed to a facility, conflicting emotions can arise on the part of the family. The family may want the person admitted, but not agree with the coercion used to force the patient into admission.

The frequent admissions that may become common in chronic mental illness may cause the family to experience "burnout." When stress in the family is high, the family may wish that the mentally ill family member is admitted to provide relief for the family system. Admission may be helpful to the entire family if the treatment provided meets the current safety and security needs of the patient and family. However, if a family wishes to hospitalize a patient for his or her problems when only the family unit is experiencing difficulties, then the patient is made to feel responsible for the entire family health and is further burdened beyond the stress of his or her illness. Family therapy may be indicated for all or some of the members of the family (Merrell, 2001).

Psychiatric admissions in which abuse or assault is discovered within the family are problematic for caregivers, patients, and others in the family. Abused members may experience relief that the "secret" has finally been revealed but may also experience anger, rejection, or humiliation from exposure of abuse. Fear about the future, fear of retribution, or fear of legal consequences of the abuse may be the concern of family members who have been victimized by another family member. Ensuring the safety of abused family members is necessary for them to confront the pain and suffering caused by the abuse.

The nurse must evaluate the patient and family's reasons for seeking treatment whenever a family seeks care. The nurse must also assess the reactions of the patient and family to care. The nurse must suspend negative judgment concerning the patient and family's motivation for and response to treatment and offer the patient and family support and guidance as they negotiate the care system.

BRIEF NURSING INTERACTIONS WITH FAMILIES VERSUS FAMILY THERAPY

Nurses spend considerable time with patients and families and are in an ideal position to be therapeutic in interactions with them. Most nurses operate within a scope of practice that involves patient and family support and education. Family therapy is not within the area of practice of generalist nurses. Providing family therapy requires specialized education or certification and practice beyond the basic nursing educational level. Nurses who function as family therapists are generally prepared at the level of a Master's or Doctoral degree in psychiatric nursing. All nurses, however, can be therapeutic in their interactions with families and individual patients; they can be empathetic to patients and their families, educate them about their disease and any medications they are taking, assist them in managing their illness, and inform and assist them in accessing the mental health care systems needed to obtain appropriate treatment. Current short hospital stays make the educational and support aspects of family care even more important than it was in the past.

SKILLS FOR WORKING WITH THE FAMILY

To work constructively with patients and their families, the nurse must possess important abilities: self-knowledge; ability to assess; ability to communicate therapeutically; spirituality; ability to collaborate with patients, families, and other caregivers; and ability to provide appropriate referrals to patients and families.

Self-Knowledge Skills

The nurse must recognize and accept his or her own values, beliefs, biases, and behaviors. The nurse must avoid allowing personal concerns to mix with the problems of patients and families. Coping effectively with the nurse's own personal problems through the use of adaptive stress-management techniques, such as regular exercise, healthy eating, strong support and nurturance from friends and family, should help the nurse prepare to assist patients and families in learning better coping techniques and overcoming their problems.

Assessment Skills

The nurse should refrain from perceiving one family member or an entire family as problematic. The interactions among all family members are the raw material for family problem solving. The nurse must become the family's partner in assessment and decision making for the family to "own" and be invested in problem solving (Johnson, Wright, Ketring, 2002). A family assessment guide (Box 15-1) can help the nurse obtain information about the family and the problem or problems for which they seek assistance. The nurse and family base their problem solving on family strengths and resources rather than family deficits. Individual and family strengths are used to overcome deficits so that the family sees themselves as capable of change rather than as being at the mercy of their circumstances and problems. Additionally, by participating in the assessment of the problems, the family learns valuable skills that can be used in managing future problems that the family might face. For example, the parent who has been distracted and overburdened by work deadlines and whose child acts out as a result of the parent's neglect of his or her needs often feels guilty about the situation. If the nurse recognizes the

Box 15-1 | Family Assessment Guidelines—
Possible Questions to Ask

I. Family Membership and Development
- "Tell me about the members of your immediate (nuclear) family, including ages and gender (male or female)."
- "What other relatives do you have? How are they involved with your immediate family?"

II. Family Strengths and Needs
- "What do you think is a strength of your family?"
- "What do you see as something you dislike about your family?"

III. Family Coping
- "Describe a problem that your family has dealt with successfully."
- "What helped you to successfully deal with this problem?"

IV. Family Problem Identification
- "What is your perception of the current family problem?"
- "How do you think the current problem should be resolved?"

V. Family Use of Resources
- "What resources or agencies have you used in the past in dealing with this type of problem?"
- "What does your family do to stay healthy? What does your family do to treat or control illness?"
- "What type of help would you like from me [the nurse] in resolving the current problem?"

parent's guilt as a sign of concern for the child, the guilt can be turned into action to help alleviate the problem and the parent's guilt. The nurse can help the parent reorder priorities and set necessary limits at work. The nurse might say, "You seem overwhelmed by the demands made on you at work and at home." If the parent validates that the nurse has perceived the situation correctly, the nurse can offer an insight such as, "It seems to me that your son may be feeling your stress and acting out as a result." Questions such as, "What is your assessment of your home and work responsibilities?" and "What are you not doing that you would like to do?" might assist the parent in problem analysis. Depending on the parent's response, the nurse might suggest that the parent set more limits on her time at work and home, while maintaining priorities, such as spending time with the child daily. A solution might involve limiting work projects to avoid bringing

work home from the office and asking other family members to help with household chores to create sufficient time each day for a short bedtime story. Even a shared bedtime story is better for children compared with receiving no attention because of a parent's busy schedule. How much better would it be for the nurse to form an alliance with the parent rather than to decry their lack of involvement with their children and approach the parent in such a way that the parent's guilt and alienation from the nurse is increased?

Therapeutic Communication Skills

Therapeutic interactions should be based on the nurse's understanding that families are generally functioning as well as they can, in view of their available resources and abilities; that families are capable of solving their problems with the guidance and support of caregivers; that all families have strengths that can be applied to the solving of their problems; that placing blame does nothing to solve the family's problems and serves only to diminish the self esteem of family members and the family as a whole; and that family members act out frustration or pain when they are unable to face their problems directly. Therapeutic interviewing skills include the ability to display respect for all family members and an ability to be nonjudgmental about the family, its members, and the problems they face. The nurse's observational skills are important when interacting with members of the family. The nurse should observe the behavior and words of all family members and consider the ways in which members relate to each other and to the nurse, rather than focusing on the actions of one individual (the patient) alone. The nurse must consider all available information, its relevance, and impact before arriving at conclusions about a family. If conclusions are drawn too quickly and with too little information, the solution is not likely to be effective, which may discourage the family from seeking help in the future when they encounter family problems.

Family Education Skills

Through education, the nurse can serve as a support to families in both treating and preventing mental health problems. For at-risk families, preventive education can enhance functioning and prevent the occurrence of mental health problems. Nardi (1999) demonstrates that a parenting education program such as Systematic Training for Effective Parenting (STEP) can diminish the use of harsh discipline, promote parent-child attachment, and encourage parents in a low-income, high-violence geographic area to play with their children. By seeking input from participants and reinforcing their contributions, the nurse builds family confidence and supplies needed information. Nurses, who have always been a source of information for patients and families, can promote a "therapeutic partnership" by acting as a family educator. Wilson and Hobbs (1999) describe this type of nursing role with newly diagnosed psychotic patients and their families. The nurse explains the disorder and the symptoms so frightening to patients and their families to ease the shock and distress that occurs when patients begin to act and talk in strange ways. This role involves partnership-advocacy of the family with the treatment team and community, reinforcement of family strengths, and facilitation of transition to postdischarge rehabilitation. Programs of family education, such as those recounted by Wilson and Hobbs (1999), are similar to the rehabilitation programs that patients and family members receive in medical settings after a family member experiences stroke or heart attack.

These educational programs can give patients and families the information needed to be knowledgeable consumers of mental health care, who can manage their chronic mental illness, as well as a patient and family with another medical problem (e.g., diabetes) can manage the care needed to effectively cope with their chronic illness. Effective education of patients and families requires knowledge of learning styles and the ability to present information in a variety of ways, such as through writing, pictures, and stories. The best educators adapt the information to the patient and family's preferred method of learning. For example, if the nurse must educate a family whose members have a low level of formal education, pamphlets written at an elementary school reading level with pictures to illustrate important information would be helpful. The proliferation of information on the Internet provides rich educational resources for the nurse and family, although the nurse must evaluate the quality of the information and determine whether the information comes from reliable sources and is accurate.

Spiritual Skills

Family members appreciate having caregivers who show respect for all members of the family. By demonstrating caring, empathy, support, patience, and hope, the nurse facilitates care and provides a spiritual dimension to treatment, which enriches interventions implemented (Sperry, 2000). Because of their close and frequent contact with patients and families, nurses are adept at providing spiritual care by partnering with the patient and family, sharing their pain and joy, and respecting the values and beliefs of the patient and family. The nurse must recognize and respect the spiritual values and customs of patients and their families (Sperry, 2000). If a family's spiritual beliefs conflict with the prescribed treatment, the nurse should accommodate the beliefs whenever possible, unless doing so would hinder the patient's care. The nurse, other caregivers, and the patient and family must collaborate on the cost-benefit ratio of accommodating the family beliefs versus the needed medical treatment and decide the best action in view of the conflict of values and beliefs. When possible, the conflict should be resolved in a manner that accommodates both viewpoints.

Collaboration Skills

The nurse must work effectively with colleagues in providing care for families and helping families reach their goals. Nurses collaborate with multidisciplinary teams and agencies to advocate for patients and to achieve positive family outcomes.

Collaboration skills are identified in an article by McDaniel and Campbell (1996). The skills that nurses need when working with families and other agencies include the following:

- Recognize and value one's own contributions to professional collaboration.
- Value the contributions of other professionals working with the family.
- Value the involvement of families in problem identification and problem solving.
- Recognize the ability of the family to both learn from and teach professionals about their problems.
- Value available resources and learn to use them wisely.
- Believe that all families should have access to health care and strive to help them obtain the care they need.

- Share responsibility and power in providing families with the best possible care.
- Provide leadership, when appropriate, but also be prepared to assist other caregivers when they are in a leadership position regarding the family's problems.
- Be sensitive to issues of spirituality, race, culture, values, and beliefs of families and caregivers, and respond effectively when conflicts surface.

Skills for Referrals and Family Support

Referrals can be helpful when working with families whose needs are unmet. The nurse must have the knowledge and skills to support families as they enter the health care system to ensure that they can receive the assistance they require for the specific problems they are experiencing. The nurse must also be knowledgeable about the resources to which he or she refers families. The referral is most effective when the patient and family know where to go, whom to meet, the reason for the referral, and what to expect when they get there. If the nurse merely gives the patient and family the name and address of a facility or support person, the chance that the patient and family will follow up is decreased. The family may not know how to get to the site, they may be afraid that the treatment will be harmful or costly, or they may fear that the ill family member will be taken away from them and hospitalized. The extra effort made by the nurse to personalize and individualize a referral will pay dividends in better continuity of care and better mental health for the entire family.

APPLICATION OF THE NURSING PROCESS TO THE FAMILY

Assessment

Assessments include the following:
- Family characteristics in both the family of origin and the present family
- Developmental stage of the family at the present time
- Family's accomplishment of developmental and everyday tasks
- Patient and family's reasons for seeking treatment and reactions to hospitalization or care
- Effects of mental illness on the family
- Family strengths

- Family's understanding and coping skills for managing the patient's illness and behaviors
- Other health problems of family members or significant others

The assessment process begins within the context of the nurse-patient-family relationship. Assessment provides the nurse, patient, and family an opportunity to discuss the way in which problems are viewed. Questions may be asked when the patient and the family are together, when only some family members are present, or when only the patient is available.

Patients who seek treatment may live with their intact family of origin, a parent who has remarried, adoptive parents, foster parents, other relatives, a spouse or significant other, or in a residential setting. The nurse must consider living arrangements and the person or persons involved in treatment. Although patients may not live with their family of origin, present problems may be an extension of problems that began with the original family. Alternatively, individual problems may not stem from the family of origin.

An assessment should also consider other health problems within the family that may be a result of dealing with the mentally ill member or those that may impinge on care given to the mentally ill member. Vaddadi (1996) reported that a caregiver's subjective and objective financial and personal burdens were significant predictors of physical and emotional health problems in the caregiver.

Families cope in different ways when dealing with a family member with a mental illness. Doornbos' research findings (1997) identifies effective coping methods—assuming facilitative attitudes; relying on faith; increasing knowledge of illness; attending support groups; gaining support of family, friends, and professionals; and distancing self from the client when necessary. Rose (1996) suggests that the stage of family development is related to the perception of stressors and identification of coping methods. In the two studies examined by Yamshita and Forsyth (1998), four similarities were found among families successfully coping with a family member's mental illness:

1. An acceptance of the diagnosis of mental illness is necessary.
2. Information about the disease is needed.
3. A return to normal family functioning helps the family and patient cope and signals further acceptance of the ill family member.

4. The family's openness with friends and co-workers enables them to gain needed support and to promote acceptance of people with mental illness in their community (Yamashita, Forsyth, 1998).

A family assessment guideline can assist the nurse to think of the family as a system when conducting a family assessment. Examples of the type of questions the nurse may wish to ask during a family assessment are contained in Box 15-1. The questions are designed as triggers to help the family "tell their story," rather than respond to standardized questions that might not reflect the family's problems and concerns. Through nurse-guided discussions, families can be actively engaged in decision making regarding health priorities (Yamashita, Forsyth, 1998). Theoretical and conceptual perspectives incorporated into this family assessment include general systems theory (Bertalanffy, 1968) and family developmental theory (Duvall, Miller, 1985) described earlier in the chapter.

Critical Thinking Questions

What family-oriented theories and approaches would you use with a family who is having difficulty adjusting to the increasing dependence of an older adult member who has physical and psychologic impairments and is becoming less able to function independently but who resents being dependent on other family members? What referrals might you make as part of treatment?

Nursing Diagnosis

Based on the family assessment, the nurse develops priority nursing diagnoses, such as those listed in Box 15-2. These nursing diagnoses help define the problems that the family is facing and thus provide a foundation for outcome identification.

Outcome Identification

Based on the family assessment, the nurse works with patients and their families to establish goals to be accomplished during treatment. These goals may be individual goals for a specific family member, goals for the family as a whole, or both. Referrals for family therapy may be necessary if supportive interventions fail to provide a resolution of family difficulties.

Extremely troubled families may be encountered in psychiatric treatment and require referral to fam-

---

| Box 15-2 | Selected Nursing Diagnoses Related to Family Nursing |

Impaired verbal communication
Ineffective family therapeutic regime management
Impaired social interaction
Decisional conflict
Social isolation
Health-seeking behaviors
Ineffective role performance
Diversional activity deficit
Impaired parenting
Impaired home-maintenance management
Risk for impaired parenting
Hopelessness
Sexual dysfunction
Powerlessness
Family processes: interrupted
Knowledge deficient
Parental role conflict
Dysfunctional grieving
Family processes: alcoholism, dysfunctional
Relocation stress syndrome
Ineffective sexuality patterns
Readiness for enhanced family coping
Readiness for enhanced sexuality patterns
Caregiver role strain
Spiritual distress
Risk for caregiver role strain
Impaired adjustment
Posttrauma response
Defensive coping
Anxiety
Ineffective denial
Fear
Potential for violence
Ineffective family coping: disabling or compromised

From the North American Nursing Diagnosis Association: *NANDA nursing diagnoses: definitions and classifications,* Philadelphia, 2001, The Association.

---

ily therapy. These families' problems often extend to their environment. Because of this circumstance, other agencies may need to be involved, or they may be already involved at the time of initial contact. When establishing goals with these families, the nurse must consider the way in which these agencies will be involved in the treatment process. Agency contact may focus on economic issues, protection for one or more family members, reporting of abuse to a state agency, contacts with police, or actions of a court order. The nurse can assist these families in finding helpful resources and arranging

Key Nursing Interventions | for Working with Families

- Provide respect, empathy, support, and acceptance to patients and families.
- Advocate for patients and families in their interactions with other providers, institutions, and organizations.
- Help families build patients' self-esteem, yet be realistic in their expectations of the patient, themselves, and others.
- Facilitate resolution of normal developmental problems.
- Help the family learn more adaptive coping skills, thereby preventing future disruptions in family functioning.
- Provide referrals to support groups and resources for families that are experiencing normal developmental issues of family life, as well as families that are dealing with more serious crises.
- Empower the family by teaching problem-solving, limit-setting, and conflict-resolution skills.
- Help families validate, clarify, negotiate, and communicate feelings appropriately.
- Assist families in recognizing and coping with abuse issues to maintain safety of all family members.

- Offer feedback to patients and families concerning their progress in dealing with their problems.
- Negotiate role flexibility with patients and their families in response to family needs.
- Provide support for families through referral to brief, problem-focused groups.
- Be honest with patients and families if abuse must be reported.
- Teach communications and parenting skills.
- Teach families about the causes, manifestations, and treatment of psychiatric illnesses.
- Teach about the desired and side effects of medications and symptoms to be reported to prevent relapse.
- Teach and role model the management of difficult behaviors of patients.
- Include the patient and family in goal setting and treatment planning.

for services. These services may include social welfare agencies, churches, emergency food services, voluntary agencies, support groups, hospices, community health services, and psychiatric home-care services. Additional resources for families include the following:

- Al-Anon/Al-a-Teen
- Alcoholics Anonymous
- Families Anonymous
- Narcotics Anonymous
- NAMI and NAMI-CAN (Child/Adolescent Network)
- Parents Anonymous
- Alzheimer's Association
- State and national mental health associations

Planning and Implementation

The skills needed for therapeutic conversations have already been specified in this text. Other interventions that the nurse may use when working with patients and their families individually and in groups are listed in the box entitled, "Key Nursing Interventions for Working with Families." Through the process of understanding the family's viewpoint concerning living with a mentally ill member, the nurse can develop interventions that are "relevant, timely, and specific to the needs of the family" (Saunders, 1997, p. 12).

EVALUATION

Outcomes of working with patients and their families can be measured by determining whether treatment goals have been met and whether patients and families have developed solutions for present problems. Periodically throughout treatment, the nurse and family must evaluate their progress toward the resolution of the family's problems. When appropriate, the nurse can assist patients and families in reformulating goals and creating posttreatment goals toward which the family can work after the patient's discharge from an inpatient unit or outpatient program.

Additionally, recent research (Ascher-Svanum et al, 1997) indicates that interventions should include family education. These findings indicate that families want information concerning their relative's illness and treatment, and patients want to understand their illness and learn effective ways to cope with it. Discussion of this topic and examples of education of families are included earlier in this chapter.

Key Concepts

1. The nurse who works with families sees many types of contemporary families.
2. Difficulties in accomplishing family tasks and developmental stages reflect the complexities and issues of modern life in a family.

3. The family of origin influences the communication skills, self-esteem, and coping skills that a person brings to the present family; however, healthy skills can be developed, even if they are deficient when a person begins his or her own family.
4. Individuals who seek help for their individual problem often assist the family to function more effectively.
5. The nurse must assess a family's function and then refer the family to the most appropriate resource for intervention.
6. The nursing process with families requires that the nurse possess self-knowledge skills, assessment skills, therapeutic communication skills, spiritual skills, collaboration skills, and skills regarding referrals and family support.

References

Ascher-Svanum H et al: Educational needs of families of mentally ill adults, *Psychiatr Serv* 48(8):1072, 1997.

Bertalanffy L: *General systems theory: foundation, development, applications,* New York, 1968, Braziller.

Doornbos MM: The problems and coping methods of caregivers of young adults with mental illness, *J Psychosoc Nurs Ment Health Serv* 35(9):22, 1997.

Duvall E, Miller B: *Marriage and family development,* ed 6, New York, 1985, Harper & Row.

Jameson KR: *An unquiet mind,* New York, 1995, Vintage Books Alfred Knopf.

Johnson BS, editor: *Child, adolescent, and family psychiatric nursing,* Philadelphia, 1995, Lippincott.

Johnson LN, Wright DW, Ketring SA: The therapeutic alliance in home-based family therapy, *J Marital Fam Ther* 28(1):93, 2002.

McDaniel S, Campbell T: Training for collaborative family health-care, *Fam Syst Health* 14(2):147, 1996.

Merrell J: Social support for victims of domestic violence, *J Psychosoc Nurs* 39(11):30, 2001.

Nardi DA: Parenting education as family support for low-income families of young children, *J Psychosoc Nurs* 37:7, 1999.

North American Nursing Diagnosis Association: *NANDA nursing diagnoses: definitions and classifications,* 2001, Philadelphia, 2001, NANDA.

Rose LE: Families of psychiatric patients: a critical review and future research directions, *Arch Psychiatr Nurs* 10:67, 1996.

Saunders J: Symbolic interaction issues for families living with severe mental illness, *J Psychosoc Nurs Ment Health Serv* 35(6):8, 1997.

Sperry L: Spirituality and psychiatry: incorporating the spiritual dimension into clinical practice, *Psychiatr Ann* 3(8):518, 2000.

Vaddadi K: Stress of caregiving for the chronically mentally ill, *Psychiatr Ann* 26(12):766, 1996.

Walsh F: Conceptualization of normal family processes. In Walsh F, editor: *Normal family processes,* ed 2, New York, 1993, Guilford.

Wilson JH, Hobbs H: The family educator: a professional resource for families, *J Psychosoc Nurs Ment Health Serv* 37(6):22, 1999.

Yamashita M, Forsyth DM: Family coping with mental illness: an aggregate from two studies, Canada and United States, *J Am Psych Nurs Assoc* 4(1):1, 1998.

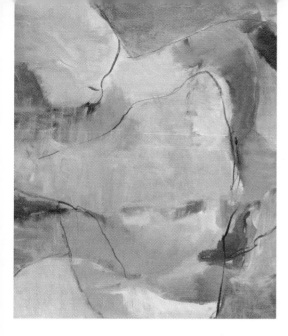

Chapter 16

Cultural Competence in Psychiatric Nursing

Barbara Jones Warren

Learning Objectives

After reading this chapter, you should be able to:

- Understand the importance of cultural variables on health and health care.
- Describe the components of cultural competence.
- Describe the factors involved in patients' and nurses' cultural perspectives.
- Articulate the differences in and the importance of worldview.

- Explain the way in which incorporation of cultural competence can enhance psychiatric nursing clinical excellence.
- Analyze the symptomatology suggestive of culture-bound syndromes.
- Apply understanding of ethnopharmacology as it might relate to a specific drug and a specific ethnic group.

INTRODUCTION

Culture is a critical component of patients' lives that affects their health care attitudes and actions as well as their ability to understand and use the interventions that psychiatric nurses develop (Campinha-Bacote, 1998; Warren, 2000, 1999). *Culture* is the internal and external manifestation of a person, group, or community's learned and shared values, beliefs, and norms that are used to help individuals function in life and understand and interpret life occurrences (Leininger, 1995). The cultural perspectives and patterns of both the nurse and the patient influence the nurse-patient interaction. These perspectives and patterns also affect a patient's level of mental health. For example, a patient's behaviors may be labeled as *pathologic* if a nurse misinterprets the patient's "normal" or culturally relevant beliefs and

health care actions (Warren, 2000). Furthermore, a patient labeled as *noncompliant* may not be receiving culturally competent care (Purnell, Paulanka, 1998). The purpose of this chapter is to explain the role of the nurse and relationship of culture and cultural competence as they relate to psychiatric nursing.

Importance of Cultural Competence

Cultural competence is the process whereby the nurse proficiently develops cultural awareness, knowledge, and skills to promote effective health care. A culturally competent psychiatric nurse not only possesses knowledge about the process of cultural competence, but also incorporates the process into interactions with peers, students, patients, families, and communities. The use of cultural competence, in conjunction with the psychotherapeutic manage-

Key Terms

Acupressure Meridians are stimulated by use of pressure to restore balance.

Acupuncture Meridians are stimulated to restore balance through the use of needles.

Analytic worldview Values detail to time, individuality, possessions.

Community worldview Community needs and concerns are more important than individual ones. Quiet respectful communication is valued, as well as mediation and reading as a learning style.

Cultural competence The process whereby the nurse has developed cultural awareness, knowledge, sensitivity, and skills to promote effective and quality health care for patients.

Cultural diversity The variety of cultural groupings. These groups may include age, gender, socioeconomic status, religion, race, and ethnicity.

Cultural negotiation The nurse's ability to work within a patient's cultural belief system to develop culturally appropriate interventions.

Cultural preservation The nurse's ability to acknowledge, value, and accept a patient's cultural beliefs.

Cultural repatterning The nurse's ability to incorporate cultural preservation and negotiation to identify patient needs, develop expected outcomes, and evaluate outcome plans.

Culture The internal and external manifestation of an individual, a group, or a community's beliefs, values, and norms that are used as premises for everyday life and functioning.

Culture awareness The process whereby the nurse acknowledges his or her cultural biases and recognizes that other individuals, groups, or communities have their unique cultural similarities and differences.

Cupping An alternative, cultural, and medical treatment approach that uses a small glass or cup to conduct the moxibustion treatment.

Ecologic worldview Based in the belief that interconnectedness between an individual and the earth exists and that people have a responsibility to take care of the earth.

Ethnopharmacology The study of pharmacogenetic, pharmacodynamic, and pharmacokinetic influences based on different ethnic, racial, and cultural groups.

Hot or cold treatments Cultural or medical approaches that maintain or return a person to a state of wellness. These approaches do not refer to the temperature of a treatment; rather, they refer to the fact that a specific, defined approach is appropriate for each state of wellness or illness.

Meridians Lines in a body that are representative of psychologic or physical body functions. Cultural healers stimulate meridians and release harmful toxins or illness-producing spirits through the use of alternative treatment approaches, such as moxibustion, cupping, coining, or skin scraping.

Moxibustion An alternative, cultural, medical treatment approach that uses moxi and heat to release illness-producing spirits from a person's body, mind, or spirit.

Natural cause of illness The belief that everyone and everything in the world is interrelated and that a disruption of this connectedness causes illness or disease.

Relational worldview Grounded in the belief in spirituality and the significance of relationships and interactions between individuals.

Scientific cause of illness The belief that specific concrete explanations exist for every illness and disease. This explanation involves the entrance of pathogens, such as viruses, bacteria, and germs into the body.

Unnatural cause of illness The belief that outside forces, such as a spell or hex being cast on the sick person, is the cause or source of the illness or disease.

---

ment model, can enhance clinical excellence and promote recovery for psychiatric patients. Research on the use of culturally competent mental health strategies indicates that cultural competence is key to patients' recovery process (Anthony, 1993; Lutz, Warren, 2000; Warren, 2000).

Culture and Psychiatric Nursing

The Surgeon General's report on mental health emphasizes the need for culturally competent mental health care (U.S. Department of Health and Human Services [USDHHS], 1999). Nurses provide services to a multitude of patients from diverse cultures. *Cultural diversity* may encompass areas such as age, gender, socioeconomic status, religion, race, ethnicity, mental illness, and physically challenging conditions (Andrews, Boyle, 1999; Campinha-Bacote, 1998; Comas-Diaz, Green, 1994; Giger, Davidhizar, 1999; Leininger, 1995; Spector, 2000). The *Diagnostic and Statistical Manual of Mental Disorders-IV-Text Revision*

(DSM-IV-TR) has incorporated additional information regarding specific cultural features for each diagnostic category and includes an appendix entitled, "Outline for Cultural Formulation and Glossary of Culture-Bound Syndromes" (American Psychiatric Association [APA], 2000, pp. 897-903).

Barriers to Culturally Competent Care

A growing knowledge and research base indicates that patients' adherence to treatment increases when cultural needs are incorporated into health care planning (APA, 2000; USDHHS, 1999). Because nurses are often the gatekeepers for health care systems, knowledge of cultural factors related to psychiatric care is important.

The most common barrier to the delivery of culturally competent nursing care involves miscommunication between nurses and patients. A nurse may lack knowledge and sensitivity regarding a patient's cultural beliefs and practices; hence the nurse may not recognize the importance and value of these beliefs to the patient as they relate to health care practices. Similarly, patients may be unaware of the nurse's cultural perspectives and misinterpret health care recommendations from the nurse (Diala et al, 2000). Consequently, to facilitate successful relationships with their patients, the nurse must understand his or her own cultural beliefs and values and the way in which these beliefs and values influence patient care. This cultural awareness facilitates the psychotherapeutic relationship and the nursing process (Quander, 2001).

Critical Thinking Question

Mr. Hoy, a 40-year-old African-American man, comes into the medical clinic for his 6-month check-up. The nurse who assesses him notices there is no information in his chart regarding cultural issues. How would she gather this information?

Another barrier to culturally competent care results from failure to assess the patient's cultural perspective. A variety of clinical cultural assessment tools and models are available for assessing cultural perspective. Some of these tools may be found in Tables 16-1 through 16-4 (Berlin, Fowkes, 1982; Bloch, 1983; Hicks et al, 2001; Warren, Campinha-Bacote, Munoz, 1994).

| Table 16-1 | European-American Worldview |
Component	Perspective
Cultural value	Value is placed on the member or object or on the attainment of the object.
Knowledge base	Knowledge is acquired according to the proof of the existence of anything; that is, the ability of an individual to see, hear, touch, taste, or smell it.
Logic	Dichotomous mode of reasoning used.
Relationship	Relationships are developed, based on the perceived need for them.

| Table 16-2 | African, African-American, Hispanic, and Arabic Worldview |
Component	Perspective
Cultural value	Value is placed on the development and maintenance of interpersonal relationships.
Knowledge base	Knowledge bases are developed through the use of the affective or feeling senses.
Logic	Reasoning ability is based on the union of opposites.
Relationship	Development of interpersonal relationships is based on the fact that all relationships are interrelated across all continua.

| Table 16-3 | Asian, Asian-American, and Polynesian Worldview |
Component	Perspective
Cultural value	Value is placed on the balance within member-group interactions.
Knowledge base	Knowledge bases are developed in striving for transcendence of the mind and body.
Logic	Reasoning ability is based on the fact that the mind and body can exist independent of the physical world.
Relationship	Development of relationships is grounded in the thought that everyone and everything in the physical and spiritual worlds are related.

|Table 16-4| Native-American Worldview

Component	Perspective
Cultural value	Value is placed in the context of a person's relationship to a Greater or Supreme Being.
Knowledge base	Knowledge bases are developed on the basis of a person's understanding of an individual's relationship with the Greater or Supreme Being.
Logic	Reasoning ability is grounded in the belief that every person is innately good and has no evil within.
Relationship	Development of relationships with another person, group, or community is grounded in the idea that the Greater or Supreme Being is in every person; hence, all persons should be valued.

Finally, barriers to culturally competent nursing care are primarily grounded in differences between nurses and patients' cultural worldviews. These differences increase the miscommunication and thus negatively affect the nurse-patient relationship and interaction.

Cultural Etiology of Illness and Disease

Nurses' and patients' health care actions and beliefs are generally formulated by three factors: their definition of health, their perception of the way in which illness occurs, and their cultural worldview (Carter, 1995; Herrera, Lawson, Sramek, 1999). Nurses and patients may define *health* quite differently.

Closely connected to a nurse or patient's definition of health is his or her belief in the way in which illness and disease occur. The nurse or patient may believe that illness and disease are created by natural, unnatural, or scientific causes. For example, a person who believes in the concept of *natural cause* of illness or disease believes that everyone and everything in the world is interrelated and that a disruption of this connectedness (e.g., a tornado) causes an illness or disease (Giger, Davidhizar, 1999; Spector, 2000). Conversely, nurses or patients may believe that *unnatural* or outside forces create illness and disease. An individual may believe that another person enlists the services of a magician, witch, ghost, or supernatural being to cast a spell or hex on them. Finally, nurses or patients may believe in the *scientific* cause of illness: specific, concrete explana-

tions exist for every illness and disease (i.e., the entrance of pathogens such as viruses, bacteria, and germs into the body) (Campinha-Bacote, 1998; Warren, 1999). The scientific model is the typical model taught in most Western-culture schools of nursing. However, many non-Western cultures acknowledge and teach health care providers the importance of the natural and unnatural causes of illness.

Patients' health care beliefs and actions are related not only to the way in which health, illness, and the cause of illness is defined but also to individual worldviews. There are four primary worldviews: analytic, relational, community, and ecologic. This primary worldview is often the one that individuals express or are comfortable with when they are with family, significant others, or during stressful times. Many individuals use a mixture of the four worldviews or adopt another worldview when they are in other environments, such as work or business settings. The nurse's failure to understand the patient's primary worldview may negatively affect the nurse-patient relationship and impede successful interventions and mental health outcomes. Overarching worldviews that can be associated with ethnic populations are presented in Tables 16-1 through 16-4.

Critical Thinking Question

Mr. Hernandez is admitted to the emergency department with complaints of headache, nausea, and vomiting. He states that he has had these symptoms for 3 days and believes that he was "hexed" by someone at work who was angry with him. The nurse conducts a complete assessment of the patient, which validates the presence of his symptoms. The physician concurs with the assessment and diagnoses a common viral infection that is currently affecting many people. The physician prescribes medication and tells the patient to rest and follow-up with his family physician. Mr. Hernandez states that he goes to a faith healer and will see him after leaving the hospital. How should the nurse handle informing Mr. Hernandez about his symptoms and supporting the prescribed treatment protocol?

Four Worldviews

A person who expresses the *analytic worldview* values detail to time, individuality, and possessions. A person with this view also prefers to learn through written, hands-on, and visual resources. The *relation-*

al *worldview* is grounded in a belief in spirituality and the significance of relationships and interactions between and among individuals. The preferred learning style is through verbal communication. An individual who expresses the *community worldview* believes that community needs and concerns are more important than are individual ones. Quiet, respectful communication, as well as meditation and reading, are valued as a learning style. The *ecologic worldview* is based on a belief that a form of inter-connectedness exists between human beings and the earth and that individuals have a responsibility to take care of the earth. Learning is accomplished through quiet observation and contemplation, and conversation is minimized.

Worldviews form the basis for the expression of culturally bound mental health and wellness issues. For example, a patient or nurse using an *analytic* worldview perspective might espouse specific detail to time, calculations, individuality, and the importance of acquiring material objects. Being on time for appointments, immediately getting to the purpose of a health visit, and using printed pamphlets and books for health education are valued. Nurses and other health care professionals must be extremely accurate and precise when providing care for these patients. The example of individuality and valuing material goods are often embodied in traditional American society's values, beliefs, and actions.

The individual with a *relational* worldview values the development of interactions and relationships, usually prefers learning through verbal communication, and views spirituality as an important context for living life. These individuals may want to "chat" for a moment before getting to the heart of the health visit. These patients may desire the involvement of relatives, friends, or spiritual and religious advisors during the health visit or during the nurse's development of the nursing process. The relational view may be observed in certain individuals from African-American, Latino and Latina, or Hispanic cultures (Plummer, 1996; Warren, 1999).

Individuals with a *community* view value the importance and needs of the community over the individual. People with this view often use meditation and contemplation techniques. A patient with this view is respectful and polite regarding health care advice and may not want to question a nurse or physician. This reticence may occur even if the

patient does not understand the nurse's recommendation. People from some of the Asian cultural groups often embody these philosophies (Warren, 1999).

Finally, a patient or nurse with an *ecologic* worldview values an interconnectedness with other people and the universe, takes responsibility for others and the world, and feels a need to maintain peace and tranquility. These individuals prefer a quiet, restful approach in interactions with others. Conversation is respectful, concise, and often kept to a minimum. Individuals from some of the indigenous or Native-American cultures may embrace this worldview.

Critical Thinking Questions

Why is it important for nurses to understand worldview perspectives for themselves and their patients? What are some questions that a psychiatric nurse might ask to discover a patient's world perspective?

CULTURE-BOUND MENTAL HEALTH ISSUES

Culture-bound syndromes are reoccurring patterns of behavior that create disturbing experiences for individuals (APA, 2000). These behaviors may or may not be congruent with symptomatology presented in the DSM-IV-TR for various diagnostic categories. However, because these behaviors can be culturally based, nurses must be aware of the symptoms to assess accurately patients who are from racially and ethnically diverse cultures.

People from racially and ethnically diverse cultures often use culturally specific language to describe mental distress they experience (Ross, 2001). One of these examples involves the description of depressive symptoms and the actual symptomatology (Baker, 2001; Delahanty et al, 2001; Pouissaint, Alexander, 2000). Native Americans may state they are "having heart pain" or are "heartbroken" when they experience depressive symptomatology (Warren, 1999). A person of Hispanic descent may say that his or her "soul was lost" *[susto]* because of another person's ability to cause a frightening experience or to place an "evil eye" *[mal ojo]* on them (APA, 2000; Campinha-Bacote, 1998). Someone who is experiencing a lost soul may be lethargic, have appetite and sleep changes, and have multiple physical complaints. Because good health is contingent on the restoration of a person's equilibrium, an ill person may initially consult a healer or root doctor to help break the spell of the evil eye and return the lost soul (Giger, Davidhizar, 1999). Traditional Western health care may be the last resource that the person contacts. Nurses must be knowledgeable about and sensitive to these beliefs.

People from diverse cultural groups often describe psychotic symptomatology differently. Individuals from Malaya and Laos use the term *running amok.* People from certain Native-American nations may use the term *ghost sickness.* African- and Appalachian-American individuals may say a *spell* has been cast on them. A more inclusive description of culture-bound syndromes may be located in Appendix I of the DSM-IV-TR (APA, 2000).

CLINICAL EXAMPLE

Pete is a 23-year-old white man with a history of paranoid delusions and congruent auditory hallucinations. He is estranged from his mother and father, who raised him in a religious culture then interpreted his psychotic manifestations as demon possession. Both his parents and his pastor believe Pete's sinfulness is the cause of his behavior. With a certain level of insight, Pete states, "I don't blame them no more. They're just ignorant people."

The assessment of possible culture-bound syndromes and the cultural expression of psychiatric symptomatology must be part of the psychotherapeutic and nursing processes. This additional assessment may provide important knowledge that the nurse must have to provide culturally competent services for patients.

ALTERNATIVE THERAPIES

People from racially and ethnically diverse groups often use alternative therapies. These treatments might include the use of acupuncture, acupressure, nutritional therapies, skin scraping, moxibustion, and cupping. Acupressure and acupuncture use linear and circular lines throughout the body, known as *meridians,* which are stimulated to restore balance through the use of needles *(acupuncture)* or pressure *(acupressure)* (Giger, Davidhizar, 1999). *Nutritional*

therapies may include the use of certain foods or herbs. *Skin scraping* or *coining, moxibustion,* and *cupping* are used to restore balance by bringing heat to the skin surface, which allows the release of the toxin or evil spirit from the affected body area (Giger, Davidhizar, 1999). In the case of skin scraping or coining, a person, generally a healer in the community, uses a coin and briskly rubs or scrapes the skin surface. In moxibustion, a cotton ball containing a substance known as moxa is ignited with a match in a small glass or cup, which is then placed on the skin above a meridian. The belief is that the illness or evil is released from a person's body when heat is generated within the meridians. Skin abrasions and contusions, often occurring on the skin as a result of skin scraping or coining, moxibustion, or cupping, may provide a climate for infection.

Certain cultural groups (e.g., Hispanic, South American) believe certain liquids, foods, or medicines must be taken in balance to restore health (Kuhn, 1999). A medicine might be labeled as being *hot* and might need to be taken in conjunction with a *cold* liquid or food to be effective. The terms hot and cold have nothing to do with temperature but are indicative of the way in which the substance reacts within the body to restore equilibrium.

ETHNOPHARMACOLOGY

Ethnopharmacology is the study of pharmacogenetic, pharmacodynamic, and pharmacokinetic influences based on different ethnic, racial, and cultural groups (Herrera, Lawson, Sramek, 1999; Warren, 1999). Culturally competent care is enhanced when this growing area of cultural knowledge is incorporated into patient care.

Individuals react to pharmacologic interventions based on their normal biologic makeup, environmental influences, and cultural influences (Herrera, Lawson, Sramek, 1999; Keltner, Folks, 2001). Specific ethnic, racial, and cultural differences affect a patient's medication options and dose requirements.

Metabolism variation is most often cited as the cause of cross-ethnic differences in response to medications. Herrera and associates (1999) indicate that individuals from certain racial and ethnic groups have a genetically based pharmacokinetic variation, which causes them to be fast or slow metabolizers. Drugs may accumulate in a patient's body when medications are metabolized too slowly. For example, people of Asian (~50%) and Native-American descent are more sensitive to the effects of alcohol than are those from other ethnic racial cultures. This sensitivity is based on their relative deficiency of aldehyde dehydrogenase, resulting in slowed metabolism of the highly toxic intermediate product, acetylaldehyde (Herrera, Lawson, Sramek, 1999). Symptoms include a reddened flush to the neck and face, tachycardia, and a burning sensation in the stomach.

Most psychotropic drugs are metabolized by the cytochrome P450 system (Ruiz, 2000). Basically, only two of the cytochrome P450 enzymes (see Chapter 18 for this discussion) appear to have extensive cross-ethnic variability: 2D6 and 2C19. Substrates of these enzymes (again see Chapter 18) would be metabolized more slowly (poor metabolizers) in a certain percentage of each of these cultural groups (Keltner, Folks, 2001). For example:

Ethnic Group	Percentage of 2D6-Poor Metabolizers	Percentage of 2C19-Poor Metabolizers
African Americans	~2%	~19%
Caucasians	3%-9%	2.5%-6.7%
Hispanics	1.0%-4.5%	~5%
Native Americans	0	~21%
East Asians	0.0%-2.4%	17%-22%

Other enzymes also substantially vary across ethnic groups. For example, alcohol dehydrogenase, aldehyde dehydrogenase, butylcholinesterase catechol-O-methyltransferase, dopamine beta-hydroxylase, and monoamine oxidase all have interethnic and intraethnic variabilities of expression.

ROLE OF THE NURSE

Nurses should not only use the process of cultural competence within their practice settings, but also help others to understand the need for culturally competent health care. One of the skills every nurse must develop is the ability to integrate cultural factors in the health assessment.

Cultural Assessment Issues

Nurses must include some basic elements within their cultural assessments of patients. These elements include communication, orientation, nutrition, family relationships, health beliefs, education, spiritual or religious, and biologic or physiologic elements. Table 16-5 provides a handy assessment sheet to consider when evaluating culturally relevant information.

Questions and observations relative to cultural issues must be smoothly and sensitively incorporated into the nursing assessment process; to ensure that the nurse does not appear rude or intrusive. Including someone from the patient's community or from the same cultural background during the assessment interview may also be appropriate. Cultural preservation, cultural negotiation, and cultural repatterning are other culturally competent techniques that nurses may use during assessment and in-care planning.

Cultural preservation is the nurse's ability to acknowledge, value, and accept a patient's cultural beliefs. *Cultural negotiation* is the nurse's ability to work within a patient's cultural belief system to develop culturally appropriate interventions. *Cultural repatterning* is the nurse's ability to incorporate cultural preservation and negotiation to identify patient needs, develop expected outcomes, and evaluate outcome plans (Leininger, 1995). The case study and critical thinking questions, located at the end of this chapter, provide examples of the way in which these three techniques may be incorporated into the care of a patient.

SUMMARY

Cultural competence is an important component of effective psychiatric nursing. Important components for the development of culturally competent nursing care include the nurse's understanding of the concepts of a worldview, culture-bound syndromes, ethnopharmacology, and the nurse's role in assessing patients for cultural variables that may affect patient care.

ITable 16-5 I Cultural Assessment Worksheet

Assessment Area	Questions or Areas of Inquiry
Communication	1. Do you speak any foreign languages? 2. Is English your first language? 3. Does the patient speak English fluently? 4. Does the patient prefer an interpreter? 5. Does the patient believe appropriate touching is acceptable? 6. Are there ethnic behaviors that the patient uses?
Orientation	1. How long have you lived where you now live? 2. Where were you born? 3. With which ethnic, racial, or cultural group do you identify yourself? 4. How closely do you follow the traditional values, beliefs, and practices of your self-identified group? 5. What are the patient's thoughts on the following: human nature, development of knowledge, work ethic, relationship with nature?
Nutrition	1. Do you have certain foods you prefer? 2. What kind of foods do you eat when you are ill? 3. Do you avoid certain foods because of your beliefs?
Significant others and family	1. Who do you consider as important to you? 2. Is there anyone you would like for me to contact or not contact while you are here for treatment? 3. How are decisions made in your home environment? 4. In your home, what are the roles for children, women, and men? 5. What are some of the social customs or practices that you do at home? 6. Share with me three of your most important values.
Health	1. What brought you here for treatment today? 2. What do you think will help you feel better or get well? 3. Have you used treatments in the past that were helpful for you? 4. What type of treatments don't you like or feel comfortable receiving? 5. Is there something you think I can assist you with to help you improve? 6. Who do you usually go to for help or treatment when you are ill? 7. What do you think causes physical and mental problems?
Education	1. How do you prefer to learn new things and tasks (e.g., reading, watching television or videos, talking with someone)? 2. How have you received your education (e.g., in school, by self instruction)? 3. How would you prefer to pay for your treatment?
Spirituality and religion	1. Do you consider yourself spiritual or religious? If so, what does that mean to you? 2. Do you have a religious preference? 3. Are there certain individuals you like to talk with regarding your spiritual, religious beliefs, or health care; or are there practices that you like to participate in?
Biology and physiology	1. Do you have any specific health problems or disease conditions in your family of origin? 2. Are there certain medications, herbs, or therapies that you avoid because they make you ill? 3. Are there specific skin, hair, grooming, or health care needs that you prefer? 4. Are you taking any medications now? (Include an examination of vitamin, nutritional, and herbal approaches.) 5. How many cigarettes do you smoke every day? 6. How many glasses of wine do you drink per week? 7. How many cans or bottles of coke, root beer, or beer do you drink per week? 8. How many cups of tea or coffee or both do you drink every day? 9. Are there any other beverages you drink every day? 10. How many bars or pieces of chocolate do you eat every day?

Warren BJ, Campinha-Bacote J, Munoz C: *Cultural assessment worksheet*, Columbus, Ohio, 1994, Authors.

Key Concepts

1. Culture is the manifestation of an individual, group, or community's beliefs, values, and norms that are used for everyday life functioning.

2. Cultural competence is the process whereby the nurse develops cultural awareness, knowledge, and skills to promote effective health care for patients.

3. Cultural diversity refers to the unique differences in areas such as age, gender, socioeconomic status, religion, race, and ethnicity.

4. A person's worldview is a perspective of the way in which people function, interact, and behave everyday.

5. Barriers to culturally competent care include miscommunication, failure to assess for a cultural perspective, and differences in worldview.

6. Illness can be viewed as resulting from natural, unnatural, or scientific (i.e., explainable) causes.

7. Four worldviews include the analytic, relational, community, and ecologic worldviews.

8. Culture-bound syndromes are reoccurring patterns of behavior that create disturbing experiences for persons.

9. Patients from non-Western cultures may use acupuncture, acupressure, nutritional therapies (e.g., herbal remedies), skin scraping, moxibustion, and cupping to treat illness.

10. Ethnopharmacology is the study of culture-related factors that can affect drug therapy.

11. An important nursing role is the incorporation of cultural knowledge into addressing health and health care.

References

American Psychiatric Association: *Diagnostic and statistical manual of mental disorders-IV-Text Revision [DSM-IV-TR]*, ed 4, Washington, DC, 2000, APA.

Andrews MM, Boyle JS: *Transcultural concepts in nursing care,* ed 3, Philadelphia, 1999, Lippincott.

Anthony WA: Recovery from mental illness: the guiding vision of the mental health services in the 1990's, *Psychiatr Rehabil J* 2(3):17, 1993.

Baker FM: Diagnosing depression in African Americans, *Community Ment Health J* 37(1):31, 2001.

Berlin J, Fowkes W: A teaching framework for cross-cultural health, *West J Med* 139(6):934, 1982.

Bloch B: Bloch's assessment guide for ethnic/cultural variations. In Orque M, Monry L, editors: *A multicultural approach,* St Louis, 1983, Mosby.

Campinha-Bacote J: *The process of cultural competence in health care: a culturally competent model of care,* ed 3, Wyoming, Ohio, 1998, Transcultural C.A.R.E. Associates.

Carter RT: *The influence of race and racial identity in psychotherapy: toward a racially inclusive model,* New York, 1995, Wiley & Sons.

Comas-Diaz L, Green B: *Women of color: integrating ethnic and gender identities in psychotherapy,* New York, 1994, Guilford.

Delahanty J et al: Differences in rates of depression in schizophrenia by race, *Schizophr Bull* 27(1):29, 2001.

Diala C et al: Racial/ethnic differences in attitudes toward professional mental health care and the use of services, *Am J Public Health* 91(5):805, 2001.

Giger JN, Davidhizar RE: *Transcultural nursing: assessment and intervention* ed 3, St Louis, 1999, Mosby.

Herrera JM, Lawson WB, Sramek JJ: *Cross cultural psychiatry,* New York, 1999, Wiley & Sons.

Hicks PL et al: *Creating a culturally competent mental health system: consolidated culturalogical assessment tools.* Columbus, Ohio, 2001, Ohio Department of Mental Health.

Keltner NL, Folks DG: *Psychotropic drugs,* ed 3, St Louis, 2001, Mosby.

Kuhn MA: *Complementary therapies for health care providers,* Philadelphia, 1999, Lippincott-Williams & Wilkins.

Leininger M: *Transcultural nursing: concepts, theories and practices,* New York, 1995, McGraw-Hill.

Lutz W, Warren BJ: A consumer-oriented practice model for psychiatric mental-health nursing, *Arch Psychiatr Nurs* 14(3):117, 2000.

Plummer P: Developing culturally responsive psychosocial rehabilitative programs for African Americans, *Psychiatr Rehabil J* 19(4):38, 1996.

Pouissant AF, Alexander A: *Lay my burden down: unraveling suicide and the mental health crisis among African Americans,* Boston, 2000, Beacon Press.

Purnell L, Paulanka P: Purnell's model for cultural competence. In Purnell L, Paulanka P, editors: *Transcultural health care: a culturally competent approach,* Philadelphia, 1998, FA Davis.

Quander L: Let's talk: answers to your questions about cultural competency, *HIV Impact* 7, Winter, 2001.

Ross H: Office of Minority Health publishes final standards for cultural and linguistic competence, *Closing the Gap* 1, February/March, 2001.

Ruiz P: *Ethnicity and psychopharmacology,* Washington, DC, 2000, American Psychiatric Press.

Spector R: *Cultural diversity in health & illness,* ed 5, Upper Saddle River, NJ, 2000, Prentice Hall Health.

U.S. Department of Health and Human Services, Public Health Service: *Mental health: a report of the Surgeon General,* 1999. [WWW document]. URL http://www.surgeongeneral.gov/library/mentalhealth.html

Warren BJ: Cultural competence in psychiatric nursing: an interlocking paradigm approach. In Keltner NL, Schwecke LH, Bostrom CE, editors: *Psychiatric nursing,* St Louis, 1999, Mosby.

Warren BJ: Point of view: a best practice process for psychiatric mental health nursing, *J Am Psychiatr Nurs Assoc* 6(4):135, 2000.

Warren BJ, Campinha-Bacote J, Munoz C: *Cultural assessment worksheet,* Columbus, Ohio, 1994, Authors.

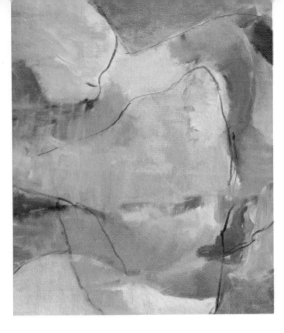

Chapter 17

Spirituality

Gordon I. G. Pugh

Learning Objectives

After reading this chapter, you should be able to:

- Describe two general uses of the term "spirituality."
- Identify the four largest "religious groups" in the United States.
- Explain three helpful theoretical constructs regarding spirituality.
- Discuss and evaluate benefits and concerns of including spiritual care in patients' treatment.
- Discuss two aspects of spirituality in mental health patients.

- Be familiar with the *Diagnostic and Statistical Manual of Mental Disorders, 4th edition, Text Revision* (DSM-IV-TR) and the North American Nursing Diagnosis Association (NANDA) diagnoses of spiritual care issues.
- Practice spiritually sensitive things to say to bereaved individuals (and know what things to avoid saying).
- Convey four stories about the way in which spirituality can be understood.
- Know how and when to make a referral to a spiritual care professional.

One criticism of some psychologic theories is that they are "psychology without the psyche, and this suits people who think they have no spiritual needs or aspirations. But here both doctor and patient deceive themselves.... In a word, they do not give enough meaning to life, and it is only meaning that liberates" (Jung, 1984, p. 198).

The previous chapter, in discussing issues of cultural diversity, mentions being aware of patients' spiritual concerns or spirituality. The North American Nursing Diagnosis Association (NANDA) and the American Psychological Association's *Diagnostic and Statistical Manual,* fourth edition, text revised, (DSM-IV-TR) also have categories for spiritual concerns. When people hear the term *spirituality,* they frequently infer a certain understanding of the term's meaning that is most often based on their own experience. In the United States, the most common understandings of spirituality are tied to people's experiences of religion. These experiences with particular religions can be both positive and negative. People hold to these opinions about spirituality quite tenaciously. In 2001 the majority of religious adherents (~80%) identify with a monotheistic religion (Adherents, 2002). Hence, the language used in this text will be familiar to the majority of nurses and their patients. It should be noted that approximately 13% of Americans identify themselves as nonreligious or secular (Table 17-1).

Key Terms

Agnostic One who is uncertain about whether God exists (Greek, *a* meaning "no" and *gnosis* meaning "knowledge").

Atheist One who believes God does not exist (Greek, *a* meaning "no" and *theos* meaning "God").

Creed A set formula that states the religious and spiritual beliefs of a community of faith (Latin, *credo* meaning "I trust" or "believe").

Existentialism A philosophy that emphasizes the individual's ability and responsibility to make one's existence meaningful by making choices in the face of life's deep pain and uncertainty.

Faith Traditionally, the creed to which one assents within one's religious community, but the term can be used more broadly to describe one's total life view, religious or not.

Humanist One who emphasizes people rather than the other parts of the observable world, or religion.

Professional health care chaplain Also known as a spiritual care professional, one who has extensive postgraduate clinical training to offer spiritual care within a health care organization (see Box 17-4).

Religion Defined structures, rituals, beliefs, and values through which communities frequently attend to spiritual concerns.

Smudging A common sacred rite of purification and cleansing practiced by many Native-American nations. The practice includes the burning of cedar and sage for the purpose of fanning smoke with an eagle feather over or near the patient; it is viewed as purifying the spirit and preparing the patient for a difficult spiritual journey such as illness or death, as well as being used for other spiritual rituals.

Soul The nonphysical, transcendent part of human beings involving one's mind and will.

Spirituality An awareness of relationships with all creation, an appreciation of presence and purpose that goes beyond the five senses and the physical world, and includes a sense of meaning and belonging; it can be inclusive of religion.

Theist One who believes in God, without necessarily conforming to a particular set of religious beliefs. Based on Greek word *theos,* meaning "God."

Table 17-1 U.S. Religious Affiliations—2002*

Religion	1990 Estimated Adult Population	2001 Estimated Adult Population	Percentage of U.S. Population (2000)	Percentage of Change (1990–2000)
Christianity	151,225,000	159,030,000	76.5%	+5%
Nonreligious; secular	13,116,000	27,539,000	13.2%	+110%
Judaism	3,137,000	2,831,000	1.3%	−10%
Islam	527,000	1,104,000	0.5%	+109%
Buddhism	401,000	1,082,000	0.5%	+170%
Agnostic	1,186,000	991,000	0.5%	−16%
Atheist	—	902,000	0.4%	—
Hinduism	227,000	766,000	0.4%	+237%
Unitarian Universalist	502,000	629,000	0.3%	+25%

*Unlike some countries, the United States does not include a question about religion in its census and has not for over 50 years. Religious adherents statistics in the United States are obtained from surveys and organizational reporting.
From http://www.adherents.com/rel_USA.html. Accessed 4/3/02.

In the past, the term *spirituality* was understood by most Americans to be roughly equivalent to overt religious expressions. Today, however, the term is understood more broadly than it was in the past. Even among people who identify themselves as belonging to a particular religion (or subgroup within a religion), diverse (and divergent) expressions of spirituality exist. The term has taken on a variety of meanings, particularly in light of postmodern culture (Box 17-1).

TOWARD A DEFINITION OF SPIRITUALITY

Psychiatry Based on Greek Psyche (the Soul)

The word psychiatry comes from two Greek words, *psyche* (soul) and *iatreia* (healing), thus healing of the soul. *Psyche* has a variety of meanings: the breath of life, the seat of feelings and emotions, and the part of humans that transcends the earthly. Spirituality

| Box 17-1 | Fulghum's Story

"Do you believe in God, Mr. Fulghum?" (The journalist interviewing me has shifted scale suddenly from the details of dailiness to the definition of the Divine.)

"No, but I do believe in Howard."

"Howard? You believe in Howard?"

"It all has to do with my mother's maiden name."

"Your mother's maiden name..."

"Was Howard. She came from a big Memphis clan that was pretty close and was referred to as the Howard Family. As a small child, I thought of myself as a member of the Howard Family."

"Howard was a name that was important to me from early on in my life. What happened was that I got packed off to Sunday School at around age four and the first thing I learned was the Lord's Prayer, which begins 'Our Father, which art in heaven, Hallowed be Thy name.' And what I heard was, 'Our Father, which art in heaven, HOWARD be Thy name.' And since little kids tend to mutter prayers anyhow, nobody realized what I was saying, so I went right on believing that God's name was Howard. And believing I was a member of His family—the Howards. Since I was told that my grandfather had died and gone to heaven, God and my grandfather got all mixed up in my mind as one and the same. When I knelt beside my bed each night and prayed, 'I thought about my grandfather and what a big shot he was.' I went on to bed feeling pretty well connected to the universe for a long, long time. It was a Howard Family Enterprise."

"I thought it for so long that even when I passed through all the stages of skepticism, disbelief, revision, and confusion—somewhere in my mind I still believed in

Howard. Because at the heart of that childhood image there is no alienation. I *belonged* to the whole big scheme of things. I lived and worked and had my being in the family store."

"In some cultures if a man says, 'I am God,' he will get shunned or even locked up as crazy. In some other cultures if a man says, 'I am God,' people will say, 'What took you so long to find out?' If you say you pray and talk to God, we will think of you as religious. If you say God talks to you, we will think of you as looney."

"I'm not sure I understand."

"Consider it this way. It makes a big difference if you think of God as transcendent or immanent; as up there somewhere or present here."

"Yes."

"Howard is a transcendent image of God. The God of childhood...up there, somewhere else, separate from us...transcendent. On the other hand, if God is immanent, then there is no place God is not, and I am not separate from God. Hence, no boundaries between God and me."

There was a long silence between us. The journalist smiled. I smiled. She changed the subject. None of this discussion about Howard appeared in her article. I understand. Some things are hard to write about...hard to think about...hard to sort out. Maybe when she asked the first question, I should have just said, "Yes." As a favor to her. But the truth is I haven't finished thinking about God, and the God of my childhood and the God of my middle age are all mixed up with the God of the wisdom that may yet come to me in my later years. Howard would understand.

From *UH-OH* by Robert Fulghum, ©1991 by Robert Fulghum. Used by permission of Villard Books, a division of Random House, Inc.

means the things beyond mere biologic existence. Spiritual things are considered when advanced directives and quality of life issues are considered.

Common Understandings of Spirituality

The variety of ways in which the word spirit is used underscores an important problem in understanding what is meant by spirituality. This ambiguity has existed for a long time and continues today. People talk of having school spirit, of the spirit of the times, of raising someone's spirits, of a spirit of cooperation, of a sweet spirit, of the Holy Spirit, of distilled spirits, of evil spirits, and of mineral spirits. When people talk of spirituality, not surprisingly, definitions are personalized, nebulous, and subjective. Falardeau (1997) writes, "Several authors have attempted to define spirituality, but no complete

definition seems to be accepted universally" (p. 133).

Most people will agree, however, that spirit means something not material and that which gives life, depth, and meaning to existence (Jung, 1980). Common understandings of spirituality have to do with making sense of life; with hopes, plans, and fears; with things that people value; with the way in which individuals relate to others; and with issues of meaning and belonging. The word spirituality is generally used in two ways. The first sees the human spirit as inextricably tied with a transcendent source, or Higher Power, and is often expressed within the individual's religious community. The second use seeks to distinguish itself from a religious perspective by emphasizing aspects of the human spirit and its relationship to other human spirits.

Spirituality in relation to a transcendent spirit (theistic view)

The first view is exemplified in the Judeo-Christian tradition's creation story. In short, God constructs the world, including human beings. God molds dirt to form and breathes life into a human being; thus it becomes "a living soul." The first understanding therefore is that human lives are inspired (literally, breathed into) by a Supreme Being. This view is often marked by a sense of gratitude for basic existence. Although this view is theistic, that is, it includes a concept of God, it is not necessarily an exclusively religious view.

Spirituality in relation to human spirit (humanistic view)

Jung also considered the second general understanding of the word spirituality, describing spirituality as "the sum total of intellectual and cultural possessions...." (Jung, 1980, p. 208). This understanding includes the way in which people attempt to bring meaning in their lives in secular ways, apart from a religious community or from traditional understandings of God. The emphasis is on the human spirit. These two understandings (theistic and humanistic) are not necessarily mutually exclusive; however, the latter understanding deemphasizes (and sometimes completely rejects) the theistic approach. This understanding emphasizes not a transcendent source but self-transcendence in particular.

Clinical Understanding

N.S. Xavier (1987), a clinical psychiatrist, makes a similar distinction between spirituality and religion and offers a useful vocabulary from his psychiatric experience between "healthy spirituality" and "sick religiosity." People who generalize institutional religion (e.g., church, synagogue, mosque) as only negative have often had some painful, dehumanizing experience at the hands of those who practice sick religiosity. William James (1958) says that this sick religiosity comes from a lack of balance. Xavier (1987) says that sick religiosity is also marked by a "lack of openness to other possibilities, a sense of exclusiveness and absolutism." Xavier recognizes, however, that many religious expressions are healthy. This reminder is especially important to his fellow psychiatrists who appear to see a greater amount of

Box 17-2 | Why Do So Many Psychiatric Patients Have Religious Ideations?

Stephen Mann, director of pastoral care at Johns Hopkins hospital says, "It's simple. When any person is in distress, he or she has spiritual needs. When someone experiences medical problems to the degree that requires hospitalization, that person is in distress, manifests spiritual concerns, and needs spiritual care." The same is true of the psychiatric patient, he says. These common spiritual needs, however, are expressed through the prism of the patient's diagnosis and within the religious-spiritual context of the patient's culture. R. P. Rao, assistant clinical professor of psychiatry at the University of Alabama Medical School concurs. He says that these patients have a "deep unanswered need inside for connection with some form of essence." People who suffer from disease, whether mental or physical, "are looking for something higher or greater" than themselves.

Mann S: *Personal communication with the author,* 2001.

psychopathology characterized by manifestations of sick religiosity than would presumably be found in the general population (Box 17-2).

Other Especially Helpful Understandings for the Psychiatric Nurse

Having explored a basic definition of spirituality as that part of the human being that is not merely physical and learning the two general views (a theistic approach and a humanistic approach), some meaningful theoretical constructs are called for. The author has found the following theoretical constructs, or models, to be especially helpful in understanding the way in which spiritual concerns are demonstrated.

Construct 1: Making meaning through freedom to choose

The first model is derived from a notable psychiatrist's reflection on his own experience of intense suffering. Viktor Frankl, a psychiatrist, was a prisoner in the Nazi concentration camps of Dachau and Auschwitz during World War II. His understanding of meaning in the face of brutality is based on the philosophy of existentialism. Frankl recognized that, although we cannot always choose the circumstances within which individuals find themselves, people always have a choice, at least in the attitudes they have toward their experiences. This view was forged in the midst of the helplessness he witnessed at the death camps. Prisoners who had no desire to live first gave up hope, then life. Prisoners who did not exchange their cigarettes for food, for example, "were those who had lost the will to live and wanted to 'enjoy' their last days" (Frankl, 1984). Many of the prisoners who found a reason to live, however, maintained hope and were able to survive.

Frankl's primary emphasis is on finding meaning in a person's life, beginning with the question of who the person is. Frankl believes that an individual cannot directly search for his or her identity. To do so would be a futile effort. Human beings find meaning when they commit themselves to something beyond themselves, to a cause greater than themselves. A person must still decide what sort of something outside the individual is worth living for. Obviously, a risk of choosing badly, of making a commitment to an unworthy cause, is present. However, without this risk, no freedom would exist. In contemplating the meaning of existence and trying to live out this meaning, Frankl says that a connection is established between the way in which a person constructs meaning and the person's mental health. In other words, people who have something to live for outside of themselves experience better mental health.

Construct 2: Higher power, higher purpose, higher principles

The second helpful model comes from the clinical reflections of another psychiatrist, N.S. Xavier (1987), who makes the distinction between healthy spirituality and sick religiosity. Xavier likes the distinction Alcoholics Anonymous (AA) makes between religion and spirituality. AA asserts belief in "a power greater than ourselves" that can restore the alcoholic to sanity. AA calls this power "God as we understood God" or a "Higher Power." Xavier spent his childhood in the state of Kerala in South India, where Hinduism, Christianity, and Islam, as well as other religions, have peacefully coexisted for centuries. His discussion of the psychopathology of sick religiosity from a cross-cultural perspective is especially insightful. Three essential by-products of mature, healthy spirituality, Xavier says, are *courage, love,* and *wisdom.*

Xavier (1994) has seized on AA's wording of Higher Power and expanded that understanding, saying that spiritual maturity is marked, quite simply, by three higher things: higher power, higher purpose, and higher principles.

Higher power

Spiritually mature people know healthy ego boundaries; they display a humility that comes from an inner strength in being comfortable with who they are. Thus spiritually mature people see themselves as part of something bigger than they are, before which or to whom they are responsible.

Higher purpose

Spiritually mature people understand that life has meaning and that their individual lives have a purpose in the grand scheme of the universe; thus they can experience deep satisfaction in living out their responsibilities *vis-à-vis* their higher power.

Higher principles

Understanding that a higher power exists, a source of life to which or to whom they give gratitude, and understanding that each individual's life has meaning within the context of responsibility to a higher power, spiritually mature people seek to live their lives by ethical standards that incorporate these values and ideals. Xavier finds this view mentally healthy.

Construct 3: Acknowledging a presence that orders the world

The third helpful model will look at a simplified form of Loder's (1989) research into the relationship between theology and psychiatric theory. James E. Loder is a professor at Princeton Theological Seminary who specializes in interdisciplinary studies combining theology and science, especially the human sciences and psychology. Loder says that early developmental experiences set the stage for later spiritual dynamics within the individual. In the biblical languages, the words for "face" also mean "presence." At the age of 3 months, infants begin to recognize faces. The most important face, at least insofar as the development of trust is considered, is the primary caregiver, typically the mother. The primal response to this presence is a smile. At this point in the infant's development, a concept of time has yet to develop. By the age of 9 months, the child will understand that times occur when the mother is not present and will experience anxiety at her absence, because the mother meets the child's basic needs. For the 3- to 6-month-old child (who has not yet developed a sense of time or absence), these basic needs are met by one whose presence is always assumed, who loves unconditionally (or at least appears to), and who orders the child's whole world. The child experiences no shame when gazing at this face.

Loder describes the way in which the child's burgeoning capacity to trust is strengthened by the presence (face) of this nurturing person. The infant's experiences are thus a model for the adult's search for spiritual fulfillment. Loder writes, "I suggest that what is established in the original face-to-face interaction is the child's sense of personhood and a universal prototype of the Divine Presence" (1989, p. 163). Loder also contends that the spiritual search that many people later experience is connected with the desire to experience in a new way the nature of being "given a place in the cosmos, confirmed as a self, and addressed by the presence of a loving other" (p. 166). Loder's model can be useful in helping deal with the spiritual issues of abandonment and shame.

Frankl's search for meaning in the midst of suffering, Xavier's distinction between sick religiosity and healthy spirituality, as well as Loder's notion that nurture in infancy provides a prototype for later seeking and recognizing connection with a presence that orders one's world have all been examined. These three perspectives are meant to provide the nurse with ways of looking at patients as spiritual beings and helping to see their spiritual struggles and concerns from more than one perspective.

IS SPIRITUALITY A LEGITIMATE CONCERN OF PSYCHIATRIC NURSES?

Professional Evidence Supporting the Importance of Spiritual Care

Aside from the implicit importance of that which gives meaning and principles to guide human lives, other reasons exist as to the importance of addressing issues of spirituality within the health care setting. Nursing, medical, and accrediting groups recognize this importance. For example, the NANDA nursing diagnoses include "Spiritual distress," "Spiritual distress, Risk for" and "Spiritual well-being, Readiness for enhanced." The DSM-IV-TR has a diagnostic category dedicated to a "Religious or Spiritual Problem" (see DSM-IV-TR and NANDA Box). Furthermore, the Canadian Council on Health Services Accreditation as quoted by VandeCreek and Burton

---

DSM-IV-TR and NANDA   Religious or Spiritual Problem

This category can be used when the focus of clinical attention is a religious or spiritual problem. Examples include distressing experiences that involve loss or questioning of faith, problems associated with conversion to a new faith, or questioning of spiritual values that may not necessarily be related to an organized church or religious institution.[1]

Spiritual Distress (Distress of the Human Spirit)

Definition
Disruption in the life principle which pervades a person's entire being and which integrates and transcends one's biological and psychosocial nature.

Defining Characteristics
Expresses concern with meaning of life or death and belief systems; anger toward God; questions meaning of suffering; verbalizes inner conflict about beliefs; verbalizes concern about relationship with deity; questions meaning of own existence; unable to participate in usual religious practices; seeks spiritual assistance; questions moral and ethical implications of therapeutic regimen; gallows humor; displacement of anger toward religious representatives; description of nightmares and sleep disturbances; alteration in behavior and mood evidenced by anger, crying, withdrawal, preoccupation, anxiety, hostility, apathy, and so forth.

Related Factors
Separation from religious and cultural ties; challenged belief and value system (e.g., resulting from moral and ethical implications of therapy, intense suffering).

Potential for Enhanced Spiritual Well-Being[2]

Definition
Spiritual well-being is the process of an individual's developing and unfolding of mystery through harmonious interconnectedness that springs from inner strengths.

Defining Characteristics
Inner strengths: a sense of awareness, self-consciousness, sacred source, unifying force, inner core, and transcendence; *unfolding mystery:* one's experience about life's purpose and meaning, mystery, uncertainty, and struggles; *harmonious interconnectedness:* relatedness, connectedness, harmony with self, others, higher power or God, and the environment.

---

[1]American Psychological Association: *Diagnostic and Statistical Manual,* ed 4, text revised, Washington, DC, 2000, APA.
[2]North American Nursing Diagnosis Association: *Nursing diagnoses: definitions and classifications 1999-2000,* Philadelphia, 1999, NANDA.

(2001, p. 3) states, "When developing the service plan, the team considers the client's physical, mental, spiritual, and emotional needs. The team respects the clients' cultural and religious beliefs and enables them to carry out their usual cultural or religious practices as appropriate." The Joint Commission on the Accreditation of Healthcare Organizations (JCAHO, 1998) maintains that patients have a basic right to care that respects their cultural, psychosocial, and spiritual values. Worth noting is that for both of these accreditation groups, the spiritual aspect is viewed as unique and separate from the cultural, mental, emotional, psychosocial, and religious aspects.

The nurse must remember that, although many people identify themselves as part of a religious tradition, "evidence suggests that…the percentage of people with a deep, transforming, lived-out [religious] faith is far smaller than the overall percentage of religious belief would seem to indicate" (Gallup Organization, 2001). Barrett, Kurian, and Johnson (2001) found a similar phenomenon by showing the number of "unaffiliated" Christians as 15.8%. Hence, having a broader view of spirituality than reported by religious affiliation can be especially helpful and can serve the patient well (Box 17-3).

| Box 17-3 | Ojibway Indian Smudging in an Intensive Care Unit |

Mike McLemore, an elder of the Native American Ojibway Nation, gives the reminder that many Native Americans count themselves as adherents of Christianity, yet they continue to practice what he calls "the traditional ways." He relates the story of being called on to perform a smudging in an intensive care unit. With his smudge pot and eagle feather, he entered the unit, as requested by the patient. The nurses, seeing the smoke, were understandably concerned; their lack of knowledge about the patient's spiritual practices may have proved to be a problem. They may have made lots of assumptions based on the fact that the patient listed her religious affiliation as Catholic. The nurses were, however, open to helping address the patient's spiritual needs. When the elder explained the spiritual significance of the healing ritual and told the nurses of its importance to the patient (and assured them that there was no open flame!), the nurses allowed him to provide the cultural and spiritual practice that the patient requested.

McLemore M: *Personal communication with the author*, 2001.

Clinical Attention to Spiritual Concerns

Despite the declared validity of spirituality, spiritual concerns are rarely the focus of clinical attention. Given the importance of patients' spirituality, and its declared recognition by health care professionals from a clinical perspective, an individual might think that spirituality is often a focus of clinical attention. This notion does not appear to be the case, however. One study found that 60% of adolescent psychiatric inpatients reported that they had never been asked about their religious or spiritual beliefs by any mental health professional (other than the chaplain) (Grossoehme, 2001). Grossoehme makes the following observation concerning the disparity between the professed importance of spiritual care and the actual treatment that psychiatric patients generally receive: "A study of the relationship between psychiatrists' religious beliefs and their practice documented that the majority of them believe spirituality to be an area with which psychiatrists may appropriately be concerned. However, over half of the psychiatrists in that study inquired about their patients' religious beliefs 'occasionally' or even less frequently; those that did assess this area generally did not have any interventions based upon their findings" (p. 139).

Community clergy are frequently not prepared to address the spiritual needs of psychiatric patients. Möller (1999) reported on an adult group of psychiatric inpatients from widely diverse religious backgrounds, discovering that only 12.3% of participants reported receiving any spiritual care during an inpatient psychiatric hospitalization. Patients' heartbreaking stories centered around fumbling attempts of community clergy, which were offensive and which proved to do more harm than good. Only 12.5% of these patients (1.5% of the total group) reported a positive experience with community clergy. Despite the paucity of spiritual care that these patients were offered, Möller says that 40% of people with mental illness call on their religious leaders. Participants describe significant resistance on the part of the hospital staff when they have tried to talk about spiritual concerns. The staff labeled these desires as religious delusions. Some facilities have even removed bibles from the patients' rooms after these conversations.

One community minister (anonymous, 2001) reported praying with a Muslim family member and further reported being surprised when the family member was offended. "But I've been praying in the name of Jesus all of my life!" the minister said. Stories abound of well-meaning clergy who tell psychotic patients to resist the devil, that people who commit suicide automatically go to hell, or that their illness has come about because of a lack of piety or faith. It is no wonder, then, that people want to make a distinction between sick religiosity and healthy spirituality and that mental health professionals are hesitant to call on clergy.

Given staff concerns about psychiatric patients' religious delusions, and given patient reports that they desire competent pastoral care (in addition to the fact that JCAHO considers spiritual care as a fundamental patient right), that a clinically trained professional chaplain be an integral component of the health care team makes sense (Box 17-4). Psychiatric health care settings do a terrible disservice to patients when they leave "untrained and insensitive clergy to provide pastoral care" (Post, Whitehouse, 1999).

Box 17-4 Making a Referral to a Professional Chaplain

1. Definition of a professional chaplain. Over 10,000 professional chaplains serve in North America, from Catholic, Jewish, Muslim, Protestant, and other traditions. When religious beliefs and practices are tightly interwoven with cultural contexts, professional chaplains constitute a powerful reminder of the healing, sustaining, guiding, and reconciling power of religious faith.

   What is required of a professional chaplain? Graduate theological education; endorsement by a faith group; 1 year of postgraduate clinical pastoral training; demonstrated clinical competency; annual continuing education; adherence to a code of ethics for health care chaplains; and professional growth in competencies demonstrated in peer review.

   What do professional chaplains do? Serve as a member of the interdisciplinary health care team; reach across faith group boundaries; do not proselytize; seek to protect patients in their institutions from being confronted by other, unwelcome, forms of spiritual intrusion; participate in interdisciplinary education regarding the interface of religion and spirituality with medical care; point to human value aspects of institutional policies and behaviors; interpret and analyze multifaith and multicultural traditions as they influence clinical services; offer patients, family members, and staff an emotionally and spiritually "safe" professional from whom they can seek counsel or guidance; and establish and maintain important relationships with community clergy.

2. When to consult a professional chaplain. When patients, family members, or staff need time-tested spiritual resources that help them focus on transcendent meaning, purpose, and value; when a religious or spiritual leader is needed to fill the special requirements involved in intense medical environments, when local religious leaders cannot, (such as when patient confidentiality is considered, especially with minors, substance abusers, and psychiatric patients); when one of these people needs someone who can take the time to listen; when people ask spiritually relevant questions; when a patients' religious or cultural requirements appear to be in conflict with institutional policy; when someone is being proselytized by an unwelcome intrusion; when the institution fails to consider the human value aspects of care; when a new diagnosis is made; when a more in-depth spiritual assessment or intervention is needed; when an ethical consultation is needed; and when a crisis, death, or impending death occurs.

3. *How to consult a professional chaplain.* Depending on the structure of the hospital, contacting a chaplain, if one is available in the institution, can be performed in a variety of ways. One way is to ask the nursing supervisor or hospital operator. Asking to meet a chaplain can be helpful if the patient has not already met him or her. The nurse generally spends more time with a given patient than anyone else in a health care setting. The nurse's being attuned to spiritual needs and communicating these to the spiritual care provider of the patient's choice (within the policies and procedures of the institution) is vitally important to the spiritual care of patients.

   If the chaplain is a part of the health care team, the nurse may sometimes make a referral without asking the patient. An important point to remember, however, is that patients have a right to decline pastoral services. It is best not to say to the patient such statements as, "You don't want me to call the chaplain, do you?" A better way to approach the patient is to say, "Have you met our Chaplain, Terry Smith? I have found her to be really helpful with people who are asking these kinds of questions [or who are going through these kinds of difficult times]. May I call her for you?"

Information adapted from VandeCreek and Burton: *Professional chaplaincy: its role and importance in healthcare,* 2001. http://www.healthcarechaplaincy.org/publications/publications/white_paper_05.22.01/index.html

Evidence of Clinical Benefits of Healthy Spirituality

Wallace and Forman (1998) studied the relationship between religion and health among adolescents. Although most research of adolescents' religious practices describes their religion as a "social control" against deviant behavior, these researchers examined the secondary benefits of religious practice as a primary factor that effects tendencies to engage in dangerous (or at-risk) behaviors. The study notes that strongly religious high school seniors tend to begin sexual activity later and have fewer sexual partners, are less likely to be involved in drug use, and are less given to interpersonal violence compared with less religious students. The preventative health issues related to these avoidance behaviors are obvious. These religiously oriented adolescents benefit not only from the deterrent aspects of negative lifestyle choices, but also are more apt as a group to engage in behaviors that promote health, such as eating more healthily, exercising more regularly, and getting adequate sleep, the study says.

Harris and associates (1999) recount that cardiac patients who were prayed for experienced "a measurable improvement in the medical outcomes." The authors also cite a 6-month trial of "distant healing" in which patients with Acquired Immune Deficiency Syndrome who were prayed for experienced "statistically significant benefits." Ellison and Levin (1998) maintain, "Contrary to the assertions of critics, who base their claims primarily on anecdotal accounts of religion's pathological effects, systematic reviews of the research literature over the years have consistently reported that aspects of religious involvement are associated with desirable mental health outcomes" (p. 702). These associations might exist because of lifestyle practices of highly religious people as a group or possibly that the practice of a person's spirituality through religious practices "may lead to the experience or expression of certain emotions that, through psychoneuroimmunologic or neuroendocrine pathways, could affect physiological parameters" (p. 708). Ellison and Levin maintain that these practices "may lead to positive emotions such as forgiveness, contentment, and love, as well as to negative emotions such as guilt and fear" (p. 708). The authors caution that "overinterpretation" of the data "must be discouraged to eliminate unrealistic assumptions" about the connections between spirituality and health (pp. 712-713).

Additionally, clear is that some beliefs, those which Xavier (1987) identifies with sick religiosity, are correlated with increased risk for mortality. A study reported at the annual meeting of the American Psychological Association in Washington, D.C. identifies three beliefs that increase risk of death by 19% to 28% (*Spirituality & Health,* 2001): (1) Feeling separated from God, (2) feeling unloved by God, or (3) attributing illness to the devil. This view illustrates the importance of health care professionals being attentive to patients' spiritual concerns.

Although evidence of the clinical benefits of addressing spirituality is growing, some researchers raise the concern that improved medical outcomes do not mean that prescribing spiritual practices will bring about a specific healing function in a given patient. Sloan, Bagiella, and Powell (1999) fear that some patients may feel that "illness is the result of insufficient faith." This view may reflect the very "overinterpretation" against which Ellison and Levin (1998) caution.

Chamberlain and Hall (2000) give a similar caveat. The comprehensive research of Chamberlain and Hall documents over 300 published scientific studies that have examined Christianity, Judaism, Islam, and Hinduism. The majority of studies show that beliefs and practices of these religions appear to have a positive influence on depression, anxiety, suicide rates, and promotion of a healthy lifestyle. Other researchers find a weak connection or none at all, explaining that prescribing religious activities to achieve health benefits assumes too strong of a cause-and-effect relationship and might therefore be ineffective in these cases.

The author of this chapter recommends that patients with these types of concerns should be referred to a clinically trained spiritual care professional and that this person should be part of an interdisciplinary health care team (see Box 17-4).

HEALTH CARE APPLICATIONS

Not Everyone Agrees that Spirituality is a Valid or Realistic Nursing Concern

VandeCreek (2001) reports that, although many health care professionals want to engage in spiritual care and assessment, most are simply too overwhelmed to do so (Box 17-5). VandeCreek (2001) cites a 1998 survey completed by readers of the

American Journal of Nursing. VandeCreek contends that the survey demonstrates that nurses have little time or energy to conduct meaningful spiritual assessments or to provide spiritual care. The reasons he cites include more patients, more cross-training responsibilities, higher patient acuity, more work-related injuries, unexpected readmission of patients, workplace violence, family complaints, and medication errors. These nurses report decreased continuity of care, time to comfort and talk to patients, time to provide basic nursing care, and time to teach patients and their families. Of the nurses surveyed, 57% answered "No" when asked if the quality of health care they provide met their professional standards. These are serious considerations to ponder.

Suffering and Illness Elicit Crises

In the wake of people's worry and confusion following the terrorist attacks of September 11, 2001 in New York City and Washington, D.C., as well as the downed flight in Pennsylvania, many Americans began realizing how short, precious, and unpredictable life can be. The number of new wills and life insurance policies has reportedly surged as a result. A major life crisis such as facing an individual's own mortality is among the most difficult points in a person's life. Suffering, distress, illness, and death can induce an existential urgency that causes people to consider their own mortality. However, although this type of crisis may be common, it virtually always comes unexpectedly. At these critical life junctures, people have the opportunity to become more acutely aware of and interested in issues of meaning and their place in the world (Box 17-6).

Suffering Physical Distress and Death

Physical suffering, such as that which often accompanies terminal or chronic illness, can lead to a realization of life's brevity. People with severe back pain who have had multiple surgeries with little pain relief, sometimes report being ready to die. Patients who battle terminal illness frequently take great spiritual comfort in the words of St. Paul, "I have fought the good fight"; or of the Koheleth (i.e., the preacher) in Ecclesiastes, "For everything there is a season and a time for every purpose under heaven" including "a time to die"; or in the hymn "Amazing Grace." This hymn, written in 1779, remains so popular that journalist Bill Moyers has made a television documentary about it and its powerful words: "Through many dangers, toils and snares I have already come; 'Tis grace has brought me safe thus far and grace will lead me home."

People who have not experienced a physical disability are sometimes called merely "the temporarily abled" (Little, 2001), clearly suggesting that everyone will eventually become disabled in some way. Many patients who grow up with cystic fibrosis form close friendships with one another during their long and frequent hospitalizations. For these individuals, seeing these friends die as they grow into adolescence and young adulthood becomes common. By the age of 15 years, these patients often make life and death decisions for themselves, such as whether to consent to a lung transplant. For many people, these experiences of death, and decisions about their own health care, raise spiritual questions that they have been considering for as long as they can remember.

Dying patients report that they find value in praying and coming to peace with God. In fact, "coming to peace with God and pain control were nearly identical in importance for [dying] patients and bereaved family members" (Steinhauser et al, 2000).

Death and other tragedies, and their accompanying grief, can arouse symptoms of depression and other profound spiritual crises in patients, family members, and health care professionals. The nurse's first experience with the death of a patient can be sad, disturbing, sacred, and beautiful at the same time. Most people, however, do not have much experience with the dying; their first encounter can be frightening. The experience with death can leave them feeling inadequate, even speechless. In

|Box 17-6| A Story of Spirituality in a Pediatric Setting

Reverend Doreen M. Duley is coordinator of pastoral care at Children's Hospital in Birmingham, Alabama. A board-certified chaplain and pediatric chaplain, she relates the following story:

"Tracy" was a 7-year-old boy with leukemia who was completing a 3-year cycle of treatment and was now in remission. He was going to another state, north of the hospital, for a bone marrow transplant. The health care staff worked with Tracy's mother to help make arrangements and to prepare for being away from home for 3 months. Tracy was an active part of his faith community, and had a keen sense of spirituality. He loved the Power Rangers; they were his favorite toys.

The day before Tracy was supposed to leave the state to go "up north" for the bone marrow transplant, his hospital room was a flurry of activity. Lots of last-minute preparations for air travel and treatment were being finalized with the physicians, nurses, social workers, and others on the team. Chaplain Duley took Tracy out of the room so as not to disrupt the preparations but also to assess his own understanding of the treatment that Tracy was about to undertake.

Tracy and the chaplain went to play and to talk next to a large picture window overlooking the surrounding city below. Tracy had his Power Ranger toys with him. "Tomorrow is a big day for you," the chaplain said. "What's going to happen?" Tracy responded: "I'm going to fly up *really high,* higher even than this," he explained looking out the window at the ground below. "Higher than I've ever been before." This was the way he interpreted what he had heard about his first ride in an airplane.

"And then what?" the chaplain asked.

"Then I fall into a deep, deep pit, lower than the ground—real far down," Tracy answered. This is the way he understood that which he had heard about his counts going so low and the way he would be "down" emotionally and physically. Tracy would be sicker than he had ever been before, close to death because of the virtual erasure of his immune system.

"What will happen then?"

"I don't know."

"How will you get out?"

"A Power Ranger will get me. It will be a Power Ranger, dressed in white, but not *this* one (as he showed her his white Power Ranger). It will be a different one. It will come and get me, bring me back to my mom, and I'm going to be OK."

"Do you know the Power Ranger's name?"

"Maybe Jesus? I think it is. It's Jesus."

When Tracy and the chaplain returned, Tracy's mother was frightened. She had pulled away from her faith of origin and was afraid that she had not taught him enough of her religious tradition. She was concerned that Tracy did not understand the journey he was about to undertake. "I think he does understand," the chaplain said and explained what Tracy had told her.

Duley DM: *Personal communication with the author,* 2001.

our own efforts at making meaning of someone else's tragedy, we may say things that are inappropriate. The nurse's efforts at making sense of a tragedy can be vastly different from that of others touched by this type of calamity. Most people genuinely want to be helpful, but in the chaos of their emotions and in coming face-to-face with the realization that they, too, will die one day, they can say things that are amazingly insensitive. Even nurses, known for their deep commitment to care for the sick and injured, can be at a loss and can make inappropriate statements. Because the fear of death raises deeply spiritual issues, not only for the dying and their loved ones who might seek psychiatric assistance but also for health care professionals, a reminder of things not to say and some guidelines about what things can be truly helpful are provided. Although a grieving person may make meaning of a loved one's injury, illness, or death with a statement such as those found in Box 17-7, any conclusion must belong to one experiencing the grief and not to the one attempting to provide comfort. Of special note is the use of religious language in many of these efforts at creating meaning from the death experience.

Serious illness can also present loved ones with equally difficult dilemmas that bring about questions of meaning. Religious activities are important coping mechanisms for African-American caregivers of older adult patients. Post and Whitehouse (1999) believe that religious practice has a bearing on reducing rates of depression, noting that depression is especially marked among caregivers of patients with Alzheimer's disease (AD). Individuals who suffer from AD often find comfort in the religious rituals they recall from their youth, such as reciting prayers or songs from their own religious tradition.

Critical Thinking Question

Psychiatric patients describe concrete thinking during a psychotic episode. How can these patients be open to spiritual care when spiritual language is by nature symbolic?

INTERSECTION OF SPIRITUALITY AND MENTAL OR EMOTIONAL DISTRESS

Mental illness is a distressing factor that can give rise to important spiritual questions. Jung (1984) asserts, "A neurosis must be understood, ultimately, as the suffering of a soul which has not discovered its meaning" (pp. 198-199). Oates (1978) recounts that some influential religious figures in the history of the Christian tradition experienced symptoms of clinical depression. Examples include St. Augustine, Martin Luther, John Bunyan, Jonathan Edwards, and Henry Emerson Fosdick. Oates (1978) asserts that suicide is ultimately a spiritual question, because the question is not ultimately whether to believe in the existence of God but rather to accept our own humanity.

Oates (1978) identifies the way in which aspects of schizophrenia affect the patient's spiritual care. The incapacity to symbolize, that is, the patient's concrete thinking, can cause special problems, because "religious language is symbolic by nature." Oates relates the story of a schizophrenic patient who decompensated while at a Pentecostal religious gathering. "She was terrified at the thought of Jesus 'entering her heart.' To her this was a literal invasion of her body" (p. 146).

Möller's (1999) participants report being especially frustrated by their concrete thinking and with clergy's lack of understanding of this phenomenon. To a psychotic patient, a prayer such as, "Hold Susan close" might be less than therapeutic.

Oates (1978) discusses the incapacity to accept human limitations of the body, noting that the patient's history often includes "dreadfully distorted" religious teaching and a "wretched exploitation of the body." Oates further discusses the incapacity for commitment and blunted affect, as well as ascetic tendencies, that is, the way people separate themselves from the world. Some people separate themselves for religious reasons, as in the case of certain hermits, but this phenomenon can also exist among

the mentally ill. Oates says that, although religion can be a common theme in hallucinations and delusions and that these vary among cultures, the diminished capacity for trust tends to be consistent cross-culturally. This trust is built on consistently demonstrated, genuinely compassionate behavior on the part on the caregiver. Patients report that they want most of all for their spiritual care provider to be authentic, caring, and respectful and to speak slowly and in concrete terms.

|Box 17-7| Dos and Don'ts in a Death Situation

What Not to Say

Grieving family members have offered this partial list of wrong and right things to say. As ridiculously inappropriate as these look in print, a great many people who want to offer comfort (including health care professionals who should know better) frequently make discounting or patronizing statements such as these:
"I know how you feel."
"It is time to get on with your life."
"God needed her (more than you did) [or God needed another angel in heaven, or another flower in his garden]."
"He was in the wrong place at the wrong time."
"It must have been his time."
"God won't put on you any more than you can bear."
"You can always find someone worse off than yourself."
"Someday we'll understand why."
"It was God's will."
"You can (or still do) have other children [in event of miscarriage, stillbirth, loss of child]."
"It was for the best."
"Good will come out of this."
"Don't feel that way."
"Be strong."

What to Say or Do (especially for the health care professional)

A heart-felt "I'm so sorry."
"They did everything they could to save him."
"It's harder than most people think."
"I'm here for you" [and then *be available*].
"What questions do you have?" [Or, in some cultures, it is better to ask, "What concerns can I answer for you?"]
Be sure to answer all questions honestly.
Listen carefully. Ask questions. Check out all your assumptions.

Adapted from Reverend James Woodson (speech), 4/25/2001, Thanatology workshop, University of Alabama, and author's interview with Melissa Wallace of Mercy Medical Hospice Grief Group, Mobile, Ala, September 2001 (personal communication with the author).

How Can the Nurse Assess and Intervene in a Realistic Way?

The issue of trust is at the core of providing quality spiritual care. Möller (1999) says that her group of psychiatric inpatients cited a primary need for their spiritual advisor, imam, pastor, or rabbi not to abandon them. Patients with no formal religious affiliation strongly wanted at least to be asked whether they had a religious preference and wanted the nurse to contact a member from the group they identified. Möller found four essential spiritual themes that arose, namely, the patients' desire for:

1. Comfort
2. Companionship
3. Conversation
4. Consolation

Many spiritual assessment tools of different lengths and complexity are available from a variety of disciplines. Among the simplest and easiest to use is this "Spiritual Self Test" provided by Children's Health System (2001). The instructions are simply to answer yes or no.

1. I have close friends with whom I feel secure.
2. I have a purpose in life that gives my life meaning.
3. Tomorrow can be as good as, or better than, today.
4. I make choices each day that positively affect my life.
5. I often risk being honest with my feelings and thoughts.
6. I experience life as sacred, giving me rules that guide my life.
7. I am forgiven and forgiving of myself and others.

Any "no" answer can be an opportunity for further exploration of the spiritual issues involved.

FINAL THOUGHT

It has been said that the professional's best friend is a Rolodex; that is, knowing one's strengths and limitations, as well as the proper time to refer to someone else, is an important mark of personal and professional maturity.

This author's hope is that patients' spiritual concerns will continue to receive attention and that health care professionals will make the patient's spiritual considerations an important adjunct to conventional therapies.

Critical Thinking Question

Why do you think so many people want to draw a distinction between religion and spirituality?

Key Concepts

1. It is generally understood that spirituality is a major component to mental health and psychiatric care.
2. Spirituality is more broadly defined today in the postmodern culture than it was in the past.
3. At its most basic, spirituality has to do with making sense of life; with hopes, plans, and fears; with things that people value; with the way in which individuals relate to others; and with issues of meaning and belonging.
4. There are two basic views of spirituality: (1) Transcendent view. Life is ordered and given meaning by a source greater than humankind. (2) Humanistic view. Life is ordered and given meaning by humankind.
5. The chapter discusses three different models for clinical application: (1) making meaning through freedom to choose; (2) higher power, higher purpose, higher principles; and (3) acknowledging a presence that orders the world.
6. NANDA, DSM-IV-TR, JCAHO, and the Canadian Council on Health Services Accreditation all recognize the importance of and encourage a spiritual component to nursing care.
7. Some nurses and other professionals believe that nurses are not prepared to provide in-depth spiritual care.
8. Although often discussed by clinicians, spiritual care remains a neglected component of psychiatric care. Nurses should not be afraid of patients' desires to discuss these issues.
9. There is evidence of the clinical benefits of a healthy spirituality.
10. There is evidence of harmful consequences of "sick" religiosity.
11. A clinically trained spiritual care professional should be part of the health care team.
12. Patients suffering physical distress and facing death often find comfort in the transcendent view of spirituality, although these issues can arouse a sense of discomfort for health care providers.

13. Patients suffering from psychiatric disorders frequently present conditions with spiritual themes.
14. Nurses can provide comfort, companionship, conversation, and consolation.
15. Nurses can use a spiritual assessment tool to help patients explore spiritual issues. A brief tool is included in the text and many facilities have their own approach to spiritual assessment.

References

Adherents, 2002. www.adherents.com/rel_usa.html. Accessed 4/3/02.

American Psychological Association: *Diagnostic and Statistical Manual,* ed 4, text revised, Washington, DC, 2000, APA.

Anonymous: *Personal communication with the author,* 2001.

Barrett DB, Kurian GT, Johnson TM: The world by countries: religionists, churches, ministries. In *World Christian encyclopedia: a comparative survey of churches and religions in the modern world,* Oxford, Eng, 2001, Oxford University Press.

Chamberlain TJ, Hall CA: *Realized religion: research on the relationship between religion and health,* Radnor, Penn, 2000, Templeton Foundation Press.

Children's Health System: *Spiritual self test,* Birmingham, Ala, 2001. URL http://www.chsys.org/simon/simon.htm

Ellison CG, Levin JS: The religion-health connection: evidence, theory, and future directions, *Health Educ Behav* 25(6):700, 1998.

Falardeau M: Intervenir auprès des personnes souffrant de dépression en tenant compte de la dimension spirituelle, *La Revue Canadienne D'Ergothérapie* 64(3):128, 1997. (English translation in this text by the chapter's author, Gordon Pugh.)

Frankl VE: *Man's search for meaning,* New York, 1984, Touchstone.

Frankl VE: *Psychotherapy and existentialism,* New York, 1967, Washington Square Press.

Gallup Organization: *Easter season finds a religious nation,* April 13, 2001. URL www.gallup.com/poll/releases/pr010413.asp. Accessed 9/01/01.

Grossoehme DH: Self-reported value of spiritual issues among adolescent psychiatric inpatients, *J Pastoral Care* 55(2):139, 2001.

Harris WS et al: A randomized, controlled trial of the effects of remote, intercessory prayer on outcomes in patients admitted to the coronary care unit, *Arch Int Med* 159:2273, 1999.

James W: *The varieties of religious experience,* New York, 1958, New American Library.

The Joint Commission on the Accreditation of Healthcare Organizations: CAMH Refreshed Core, January, RI1, 1998.

Jung CG: *Psychology and Western religion,* translated by RFC Hull, New York, 1984, Princeton University Press.

Jung CG: *The Archetypes and the Collective Unconscious,* translated by RFC Hull, New York, 1980, Princeton University Press and Bollingen Foundation.

Little TH: *Personal communication with the author,* 2001.

Loder JE: *The transforming moment,* Colorado Springs, Colo, 1989, Helmers & Howard.

Möller MD: Meeting spiritual needs on an inpatient unit, *J Psychosoc Nurs* 37(11):5, 1999.

North American Nursing Diagnosis Association: *Nursing diagnoses: definitions and classifications 1999-2000,* Philadelphia, 1999, NANDA.

Oates WE: *The religious care of the psychiatric patient,* Philadelphia, 1978, Westminster Press.

Post SG, Whitehouse PJ: Spirituality, religion and Alzheimer's disease, *J Health Care Chaplain* 8(1-2):45, 1999.

Sloan RP, Bagiella E, Powell T: Religion, spirituality, and medicine, *Lancet* 353:664, 1999.

Spirituality and Health: Beliefs that make you sick, 3(4):16, 2001. Presented at the annual meeting of the American Psychological Association in Washington, DC, August, 2000.

Steinhauser KE et al: Factors considered important at the end of life by patients, family, physicians, and other care providers, *JAMA* 284(19):2476, 2000.

VandeCreek L: Spiritual assessment and care by nurses? *The APC News* 4(2):18, 2001.

VandeCreek L, Burton L, editors: *Professional chaplaincy: its role and importance in healthcare,* 2001, The Association for Clinical Pastoral Education, The Association of Professional Chaplains, The Canadian Association for Pastoral Practice and Education, The National Association of Catholic Chaplains, The National Association of Jewish Chaplains.
http://www.healthcarechaplaincy.org/publications/publications/white_paper_05.22.01/ index.html

Wallace JM, Forman TA: Religion's role in promoting health and reducing risk among American youth, *Health Educ Behav* 25(6):721, 1998.

Xavier NS: *Personal communication with the author,* 1994.

Xavier NS: *The two faces of religion: a psychiatrist's view,* Tuscaloosa, Ala, 1987, Portals Press.

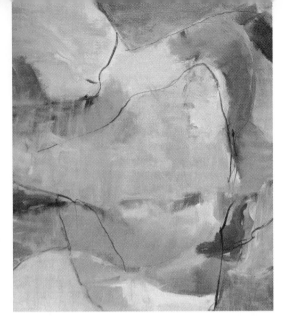

Chapter **18**

Introduction to Psychotropic Drugs

Norman L. Keltner

Learning Objectives

After reading this chapter, you should be able to:
- Define the role of psychopharmacology in psychotherapeutic management.
- Identify the nurse's responsibilities in administering psychotropic drugs.
- Describe pharmacokinetic and pharmacodynamic processes as they relate to clinical practice.
- Describe the function and inactivation of neurotransmitters.
- Discuss the function of the blood-brain barrier and the significance of lipid solubility.
- State the benefits of teaching patients about psychotropic drugs.
- Describe common reasons psychiatric patients may not comply with prescribed drug regimens.

"Telling me that I have a brain disease and that I should take medications does not solve my problems."

Riffer NW: It's a brain disease, *Psychiatr Serv* 48(6):773, 1997.

The United States is a drug-taking society. People take all kinds of drugs: drugs to sleep, drugs to wake up, drugs to fight infections, drugs to lower blood pressure, drugs to lower cholesterol, drugs to lose weight. People take drugs for all kinds of reasons. People take prescription drugs, over-the-counter drugs, legal drugs, and illegal drugs. Drugs, drugs, drugs! Drugs are taken to fix things, including mental and emotional problems.

Among these drugs are those that treat delusions and hallucinations (antipsychotics), slow down runaway thinking (mood stabilizers or antimanic agents), improve mood (antidepressants), calm nerves (anti-anxiety drugs), improve thinking (drugs for Alzheimer's disease), and even drugs to correct problems caused by some of the drugs just listed (e.g., antiparkinson drugs).

The introductory quote from Dr. Riffer, when coupled with the pejorative tone of the opening paragraph, would suggest a negative view of psychotropic drugs by the authors of this text. Nothing can be further from the truth. In fact, no other psychiatric nursing textbook has historically emphasized the importance of these agents more than has this text. Nonetheless, the following points must be made:

1. Psychotropic drugs are not always effective.
2. Not every patient needs psychotropic drugs.
3. Even when psychotropic drugs are effective, best outcomes typically occur when other interventions (e.g., counseling, therapy) are co-administered.

Key Terms

Axon The part of a neuron that transmits impulses away from the cell body.

Blood-brain barrier A barrier that guards the brain from fluctuations in body chemistry; it regulates the amount of and speed with which substances in the blood enter the brain.

Dendrites The part of the neuron that transmits impulses toward the cell body.

Lipid solubility The ability of a substance to dissolve in fat (and pass through lipid membranes).

Neurotransmitters Chemical substances in the nervous system that facilitate the transmission of nerve impulses across synapses between neurons.

Noncompliance Failure to take medication as prescribed.

Precursor Something that precedes. Tyrosine is a precursor to dopamine in the synthesis of dopamine in the body.

Substrate A substance on which an enzyme acts. Monoamines are substrates of MOA.

Synapse The microscopic space between two neurons.

Vesicle Storage sac at the synaptic terminal.

4. Psychotropic agents can be used (by both patients and clinicians) to avoid the hard work of "getting better."

5. Many psychotropic drugs have significant or even life-threatening side effects or drug interactions or both.

6. Unfortunately, "finding" the right drug regimen is often a trial-and-error exercise.

Ideally, psychotropic drugs should be prescribed based on an accurate diagnosis and then taken until an acceptable mental or emotional state can be maintained. At this point, the patient can hopefully be withdrawn from the medication and then proceed with his or her life. Unfortunately, this scenario does not always occur. Some individuals recover and never need medications again, others become dependent on psychotropic agents to function thus finding it difficult to "quit," and still others may need the chemistry-correcting properties of these drugs for the remainder of their lives. Tragically, some individuals, especially those referred to as the severely or chronically mentally ill, may improve enough to warrant drug continuation but never improving enough to be functionally independent.

In Chapter 1, a brief historical review of the development of psychotropic drugs is presented. Box 18-1 outlines a summary of significant points

Box 18-1 | Significant Points in the Evolution of Psychotropic Drugs

1930s	Sternbach first synthesizes benzodiazepines.
1948	Rapport, Green, and Page isolate "serotonin" from beef serum.
1949	John Cade, an Australian psychiatrist, reports on the efficacy of lithium in mania.
1949	The U.S. Food and Drug Administration bans lithium because of deaths of patients with cardiac disease.
1951	Chlorpromazine is developed as a nonsedating antihistamine. Laborit and others report diminished surgical anxiety in conscious patients.
1952	Iproniazid, a derivative of the antituberculosis agent isoniazid, is identified as a monoamine oxidase inhibitor (MAOI).
1953	Bein isolates reserpine from rauwolfia. Reserpine, effective in treating psychosis, causes severe depression related to depletion of norepinephrine.
1954	Lehman publishes the first American article on chlorpromazine in the *Archives of Neurology and Psychiatry*.
1955	Researchers alter the molecular structure of chlorpromazine, developing new antipsychotic agents (e.g., haloperidol, fluphenazine).
1957	The first papers appear on MAOIs as antidepressants.
1957	Haloperidol (Haldol) is developed.
1958	Kuhn publishes the first article on tricyclic antidepressants in the *American Journal of Psychiatry*.
1960	Harris presents the first paper on the effectiveness of benzodiazepines in *The Journal of the American Medical Association*.
1970	The ban on lithium is lifted in the United States.
1980s	A new class of antidepressants, selective serotonin reuptake inhibitors (SSRIs), is developed.
1980s	The antiepileptic drugs carbamazepine and valproate are reported to have mood-stabilizing properties.
1990s	Clozapine (Clozaril) and risperidone (Risperdal), the first truly new antipsychotic agents in 40 years, are released in the United States.
1990s	Drugs used to treat patients with Alzheimer's disease are made available.

From Ayd FJ: The early history of modern psychopharmacology, *Neuropsychopharmacol* 5(2):71, 1991; Kuhn R: The treatment of depressive states with G 22355 (impramine hydrochloride), *Am Psychiatry* 115(5):459, 1958; Rifkin A: Extrapyramidal side effects: a historical perspective, *J Clin Psychiatry* 48(9):3, 1987.

in the evolution of psychopharmacology. A careful reading of this summary reveals that antipsychotics, antidepressants, and antimanic agents were all developed before 1960. Although many related drugs were eventually synthesized from the prototypes of each class, the "clones" were remarkably similar to the original. However, in the last decade or so, several substantially different kinds of drugs have emerged. Clozapine (Clozaril) and other atypical antipsychotic medications are different from the traditional antipsychotics (see Chapter 20); and selective serotonin reuptake inhibitors (e.g., Prozac) and other new antidepressants (e.g., Effexor) are quite different from the earlier antidepressants (see Chapter 21). Finally, new drugs in the treatment of Alzheimer's disease (e.g., Cognex, Aricept, Exelon) are providing hope and encouragement to many patients and families plagued by this illness. These examples point to the continual effort by clinicians and researchers to address effectively the mental, emotional, and addictive disorders afflicting approximately 25% of Americans. These exciting new developments in psychopharmacology should challenge every nurse to understand psychopharmacologic concepts and apply them to practice.

NURSING RESPONSIBILITIES

Psychopharmacology is the second component of the psychotherapeutic management model (see Chapter 2 to review model if needed). The effectiveness of treatment with antipsychotic, antidepressant, antimanic, and antianxiety drugs is well established (Table 18-1). These drugs have enabled millions of individuals to live increasingly satisfying and productive lives. The least restrictive alternative

| Table 18-1 | Success of Treatment for Selected Mental Disorders |

Disorder	Percentage of Patients Demonstrating Some Improvement
Panic disorder	80%
Bipolar disorder	80%
Major Depression	65%
Schizophrenia	60%
Obsessive compulsive disorder	60%

From: A *Journal of Psychiatric Nursing* summarization of National Institutes of Health data, *J Psychosoc Nurs Ment Health Serv* 35[6]:5, 1997. Treatment can include all treatment modalities.

or environment, a concept that captures the community mental health effort to allow individuals to live their lives in an unrestrictive atmosphere, has evolved, in large part, as a result of the impact of these drugs.

Because nursing provides 24-hour care (i.e., inpatient care), the nurse is responsible for assessing drug side effects, evaluating desired effects, and applying preventative care to reduce potential problems. Additionally, the nurse usually makes decisions concerning as-needed (prn) medications. The nurse must therefore understand key dimensions of psychotropic drug use. Box 18-2 outlines nursing responsibilities for psychotropic drug administration based on the American Nurses' Association's (ANA) guidelines on psychopharmacology.

Each chapter in Unit Four provides a discussion of pharmacologic effects (desired effects), pharmacokinetics (i.e., absorption, distribution, metabolism, excretion), administration, side effects (undesired effects), and drug interactions. Equally important, a discussion of nursing implications emphasizes nursing interventions related to therapeutic versus toxic drug levels, use during pregnancy, use for older adults, side effects, interactions, and teaching patients.

| Box 18-2 | Objectives from the American Nurses' Association Guidelines on Psychopharmacology |

The psychiatric mental health nurse can:
1. Describe psychopharmacologic agents based on similarities and differences
2. Discuss actions of psychopharmacologic agents from global responses to cellular responses
3. Differentiate psychiatric symptoms from medication side effects
4. Apply basic principles of pharmacokinetics and pharmacodynamics
5. Identify appropriate use of psychopharmacologic agents in special populations
6. Involve clients and their families
7. Identify factors that may prevent the active involvement of clients in their care
8. Describe appropriate nonpsychopharmacologic interventions
9. Discuss the use of standardized rating scales
10. Demonstrate the knowledge necessary to develop psychopharmacologic education and treatment plans

Adapted from Laraia MT et al: *Psychiatric mental health nursing psychopharmacology project*, Washington, DC, 1994, ANA.

Understanding psychopharmacology involves more than memorizing facts. Now, memorization is not a "dirty" word. Some basics of pharmacology must be memorized; but the nurse who tries to get by on memorization alone is a medication error waiting to happen. Because of our strong belief in the importance of nurses' (and nursing students') understanding of the basics of psychopharmacology, several important concepts will be reviewed. These concepts are:

- Pharmacokinetics
- Pharmacodynamics
- Blood-brain barrier
- Neurons and neurotransmitters
- Receptors

This chapter will conclude with a few general strategies for helping patients and families understand important parameters of psychotropic drug use. Drug-specific patient-teaching content is presented in each chapter.

Critical Thinking Questions

Some nurses may have little knowledge about some drugs they administer. Do you consider this unethical, unprofessional, unsafe, or simply a reality of the nursing profession? Because no one can know every drug, what basic information should a nurse know before giving medication?

PHARMACOKINETICS

Pharmacokinetics is defined as the effects the body has on a drug. The four aspects of pharmacokinetics are the following:

- *Absorption,* or getting the drug into the bloodstream
- *Distribution,* or getting the drug from the bloodstream to the tissues and organs
- *Metabolism,* or breaking the drug down into an inactive and typically water-soluble form
- *Excretion,* or getting the drug out of the body

Absorption

Drugs taken orally must get out of the gastrointestinal (GI) tract and into the bloodstream to have an effect. For a drug to get out of the GI tract, the drug molecule must pass through the stomach or small intestinal wall into blood vessels. Molecules pass through cell membranes (which are composed of a phospholipid bilayer) in three ways:

1. Small molecules can fit through pores or channels in the membrane.
2. Some drug molecules have special transport systems to ferry them across the membrane.
3. Lipid-soluble drugs (and most drugs are lipophilic) can pass through phospholipid membranes.

Only a percentage of an oral drug reaches systemic circulation, whereas approximately 100% of a drug given intravenously reaches systemic circulation. The percentage to reach systemic circulation is said to be a drug's bioavailability. Bioavailability is only a fraction of the dose for many drugs given orally because of incomplete absorption and first-pass metabolism. First-pass metabolism is the enzymatic breakdown of drugs before they reach systemic circulation. First-pass metabolism occurs during passage through the *gut wall* and in a presystemic hepatic exposure. The latter occurs because the capillaries in the GI tract do not behave as do most capillaries (i.e., dumping into venules) but rather connect with hepatic portal veins, shunting drugs through the *liver* before reaching the general system. Some drugs are substantially metabolized in this manner. For instance, buspirone (BuSpar), an antianxiety drug, has a bioavailability of 1% to 4%, which means that the majority of this drug is metabolized before it gets into general circulation. If by some mechanism the first pass through the liver can be eliminated for buspirone, its dose would have to be dramatically reduced.

Clinical relevance: only absorbed drugs can have an effect. Drugs with high first-pass metabolism and low bioavailability after oral ingestion must be significantly reduced in dose levels if given intramuscularly or intravenously.

Distribution

Distribution is the process of the body getting the drug out of the bloodstream and to tissues and organs. If a psychotropic drug cannot leave the bloodstream, then it cannot have a therapeutic effect. Lipid-soluble molecules can penetrate capillary membranes as easily as they can penetrate other cell membranes. However, water-soluble (or polar) molecules also leave circulation because of significant gaps between the cells of the capillary wall. Essentially, because molecules are innately active, water-soluble molecules "bounce around" inside the capillary until they hit a gap and move into extracellular fluid. Another distribution issue involves protein binding. Most drugs bind to plasma proteins (mostly albumin) to some degree or another.

For example:

Familiar Psychotropic Drugs	Protein Binding (%)
Valium	98
Elavil	97
Ativan	92
Depakote	92
Demerol	56
Effexor	23

Protein binding is important because molecules that are bound to proteins cannot leave circulation—the protein is simply too large to pass through the gaps. Hence protein bound drugs do not have a pharmacologic effect, cannot be metabolized, and cannot be excreted. Specifically, Valium, which has a calming (or anxiolytic) effect, produces its results because of the 2% or so of active drug. Other drugs that can reduce Valium's protein binding to 96% would literally double its effect.

Clinical relevance. Effects, both desired and undesired, of highly protein-bound drugs result from the activity of the few free drug molecules in circulation. Drug combinations that compete for binding sites have the potential of causing significant increases in the free or active drug.

Metabolism

Metabolism is the process by which the body breaks down a drug molecule. Most drugs are metabolized to inactive and water-soluble states in preparation for excretion from the body in the urine. An important point to note is that not all drugs are broken down into inactive forms, nor are all drugs converted into water-soluble particles, nor are all drugs eliminated via the renal system. More detailed descriptions of metabolism can be found in a general pharmacology text.

Most metabolism occurs in the liver, but it is not the only site; some metabolic activity occurs in the kidneys, the lungs, the GI tract, and the plasma. Enzymes facilitate the metabolic processes and are said to be catalysts because they provoke yet are unaffected by the biochemical reaction. An enzyme is much larger (perhaps one hundred times larger) compared with the drug molecule and is configured in such a way that only those molecules matching that specific configuration (i.e., the enzyme's substrates) can be metabolized (Keltner, Zielinski, Hardin, 2001). A single enzyme performs its metabolic task over and over and, in the case of cholinesterase, metabolizes 5000 molecules of acetylcholine per cholinesterase molecule per second (Purves et al, 1997).

Two enzyme systems of particular importance to nurses who give psychotropic drugs must be mentioned here: the monoamine oxidase system and the cytochrome P450 system. The monoamine oxidase (MAO) system metabolizes monoamines, which include dopamine, norepinephrine, and serotonin. The other system, cytochrome P450, breaks down most psychotropic drugs.

Monoamine oxidase system

MAO is the enzyme that rapidly inactivates monoamines (e.g., serotonin, dopamine, norepinephrine) and slowly metabolizes noncatecholamines (e.g., ephedrine, phenylephrine). MAO is located in the liver, intestinal wall, and in the central nervous system (CNS) in the terminals of neurons containing serotonin, norepinephrine, or dopamine. In the liver, MAO inactivates tyramine, which is found in many foods, and the biogenic amines found in some drugs. When liver MAO is prevented from metabolizing these amines, serious sympathetic effects can develop. MAO is present in two forms: MAO-A, which inactivates norepinephrine and serotonin, and MAO-B, which inactivates dopamine. Some psychotropic drugs inhibit both MAO-A and MAO-B and are rightly described as *nonselective* MAO inhibitors. A few drugs are highly selective and inhibit either MAO-A or MAO-B. These agents are described as *selective* MAO inhibitors. Monoamine inhibitors are discussed in Chapter 21.

Cytochrome P450 enzyme system

Beyond being involved in the metabolism of psychotropic drugs, the P450 system is said to be the point at which the majority of drug interactions occur (Cozza, Armstrong, 2001). Box 18-3 presents a list of psychotropic drugs that are substrates for these enzymes and a broad list of inhibitors.

IBox 18-3I Psychotropic Substrates and General Inhibitors of Selected P450 Enzymes

2D6 Substrates	2D6 Inhibitors	3A4 Substrates	3A4 Inhibitors
Antidepressants	paroxetine	*Antidepressants*	nefazodone
Some tricyclic antidepressants (e.g., desipramine, nortriptyline)	fluoxetine	amitriptyline	fluvoxamine
venlafaxine	fluphenazine	imipramine	sertraline (> 100 mg)
fluoxetine	sertraline (> 100 mg)	clomipramine	cimetidine
paroxetine	quinidine	sertraline	diltiazem
trazodone	haloperidol	mirtazapine	verapamil
mirtazapine	cimetidine	nefazodone	ketoconazole
Antipsychotics	thioridazine	bupropion	erythromycin
thioridazine	amitriptyline		fluoxetine
risperidone	oral contraceptives	*Antipsychotics*	progestagens
haloperidol	clomipramine	clozapine	grapefruit juice
clozapine	desipramine	haloperidol	paroxetine
		quetiapine	

1A2 Substrates — **1A2 Inhibitors**

Antidepressants: amitriptyline, imipramine, fluvoxamine, mirtazapine, clomipramine

Antipsychotics: clozapine, haloperidol, olanzapine, phenothiazines

Other drugs: caffeine, tacrine

1A2 Inhibitors: fluvoxamine, fluoroquinolines, beta-estradiol, ciprofloxacin, erythromycin, grapefruit juice

Benzodiazepines: alprazolam, diazepam

Psychotropic Drug Inhibitors of 2C9: fluoxetine, fluvoxamine, paroxetine, sertraline

2C19 Substrates — *Antidepressants*: amitriptyline, citalopram, clomipramine, imipramine, moclobemide

2C19 Inhibitors: fluvoxamine, fluoxetine, paroxetine

Keltner NL, Folks DG: *Psychotropic drugs,* ed 3, St Louis, 2001, Mosby.

The cytochrome P450 enzyme (P450 enzyme) system has been traditionally referred to as the hepatic microsomal enzyme system (Lehne, 2001). This complex name can be broken down as follows: *cyto* stands for microsomal vesicles, the *P* stands for pigmentation (because the enzymes contain red-pigmented heme), and the *450* refers to the wavelength in nanometers at which light absorption occurs (Cozza, Armstrong, 2001). Although this much information is probably more than is necessary, the foregoing is included for two reasons: (1) this is the same system that older texts refer to as

hepatic microsomal system, and (2) it outlines the reasoning behind an otherwise intimidating name.

P450 enzymes contain 12 families, with over 40 individual enzymes found in humans (Lehne, 2001). Six enzymes account for approximately 90% of P450 enzymes in humans: 1A2, 3A4, 2C9, 2C19, 2D6, and 2E1 (Cozza, Armstrong, 2001). These enzymes are sometimes referred to as *isoenzymes* or *isozymes.* This text will use only the more generic but equally accurate term, *enzymes.*

Clinical relevance. Most drugs must be metabolized to an inactive and water-soluble form to be excreted from the system. Conditions (e.g., liver disease, kidney disease) or drug combinations that inhibit metabolism can lead to significant, and even deadly, results.

Critical Thinking Questions

As stated, most psychotropic drug interactions occur as a result of the effects on the P450 system. If an inhibitor of the P450 3A4 enzyme is to be given (e.g., Serzone, grapefruit juice), which psychotropic drugs will be affected? What is the effect? (Refer to Box 18-3 to answer this question.)

Half-life of drugs

The half-life of a drug is the amount of time required for 50% of the drug to disappear from the body. If drug X has a half-life of 4 hours, then 50% of the drug will be out of the system in 4 hours. In another 4 hours, only 25% of the original dose will remain. It will not matter whether the patient took 100 mg or 300 mg; the amount of drug in the body will decrease by 50% every 4 hours. This action is referred to as linear kinetics, and most drugs follow this pattern. This rule has exceptions, most notably alcohol, in which only a set amount of the drug is metabolized in a given period, regardless of the amount ingested (i.e., nonlinear kinetics). If the nurse gives the same drug dose (e.g., 100 mg) at the same time (e.g., three times a day [tid]), a steady state is achieved in four to five half-lives. When discontinuing a drug, four to five half-lives are required to eliminate 95% of the drug. This period is referred to as the washout period.

Critical Thinking Questions

Prozac has a half-life of approximately 10 days or longer (including its active metabolite). How long is the washout period? If a drug known to interact with Prozac is to be given, how long should the interval be between stopping Prozac and beginning the new drug? If replacing another drug with Prozac, would the time interval between drugs be the same?

Excretion

The kidney excretes most drugs, but other routes of excretion exist, such as breast milk, bile, feces, saliva, sweat, and the lungs. Factors that can affect excretion include kidney disease, age, and drug competition for active tubular transport.

Clinical relevance. Drugs that are not adequately excreted (e.g., kidney disease), particularly drugs excreted unchanged (i.e., drugs that are not metabolized, such as lithium and amphetamines), have a more pronounced effect compared with drugs that are excreted.

PHARMACODYNAMICS

Pharmacodynamics is the effect a drug has on the body. The two global responses to drugs are the desired effects and side, or adverse, effects. Drugs that activate receptors are termed agonists, and drugs that block receptors are named antagonists. Some psychotropic drugs are agonists, while many others are antagonists. Pharmacodynamic effects of particular interest to this discussion are downregulation of receptors and pharmacodynamic tolerance.

Downregulation

Downregulation of receptors is an important concept primarily because chronic exposure to certain psychotropic drugs causes receptors to change. For example, consistent use of antidepressants causes postsynaptic receptors to decrease in number. Because this downregulation occurs at about the same time that the antidepressant effect develops (approximately 2 to 4 weeks), it is thought that reduction in postsynaptic receptors may provide a better explanation for mood elevation than do increases in neurotransmitters.

Pharmacodynamic Tolerance

Pharmacodynamic tolerance is a term used to describe a reduction in receptor sensitivity. A good example is the chronic drinker of alcohol. When the newspaper reports a person driving a car with a blood alcohol level (BAL) of 0.35, the story is likely about a case of pharmacodynamic tolerance. This person's receptors are no longer responding to the ethanol in the way a "normal" person's receptors would respond. Although at first glance, this idea may appear appealing, it really is not. Tolerance to BALs that can cause deadly respiratory depression does not occur. Hence a person who is "functioning" at an elevated BAL can drink only a little more and die.

Clinical relevance. Knowledge of downregulatory functions helps the nurse explain the lag time between initiating drug therapy and clinical improvement. Knowledge of pharmacodynamic tolerance aids in teaching patients and families about drug tolerance to some effects but lack of tolerance at slightly higher doses to some lethal effects.

BLOOD-BRAIN BARRIER

The blood-brain barrier is also an important concept for understanding psychotropic drug activity. The brain, more than other organs of the body, requires a constant internal milieu. Whereas other parts of the body experience fluctuations in body chemistry, even small changes in the brain produce serious problems. The brain is protected from fluctuations by the blood-brain barrier. This barrier regulates the amount and speed of substances in the blood entering the brain. Water, carbon dioxide, and oxygen readily cross the barrier; other substances are excluded from the brain.

The blood-brain barrier has three dimensions: an anatomic dimension, a physiologic dimension, and a metabolic dimension. The anatomic dimension is the structure of the capillaries that supply blood to the brain and prevent many molecules from "slipping" through. There are no gaps!

The physiologic dimension is a chemical and transport system that recognizes and then allows certain molecules into the brain. Lipid solubility is the most important of the chemical properties that determine whether a molecule will pass through the blood-brain barrier. Highly lipid-soluble substances pass the blood-brain barrier with relative ease. Highly water-soluble substances penetrate this barrier slowly and in insignificant amounts. Nicotine, ethanol, heroin, caffeine, and diazepam (Valium) are examples of highly lipid-soluble substances. This characteristic is clinically significant because only drugs that can pass through this barrier in significant amounts are effective in treating a psychiatric or medical disorder of the brain. Certain nonlipid-soluble substances such as glucose, which is the brain's primary energy source, and essential amino acids, which are needed for the synthesis of neurotransmitters, are required for normal brain function. Special transport systems carry these essential substances across the blood-brain barrier.

The metabolic barrier prevents molecules from entering the brain by enzymatic action within the endothelial lining of the brain capillaries. For example, levodopa can pass the blood-brain barrier, but much of it is reduced to dopamine before it can pass completely through the capillary wall into the brain. The metabolic product, dopamine, does not readily pass this barrier, thus illustrating the third way the brain protect humans from substances in peripheral circulation.

Understanding the blood-brain barrier helps the nurse accurately conceptualize, administer, and monitor drug therapy, as well as understand addiction with highly lipid-soluble substances such as alcohol and heroin. A comparison of systemic penicillin and dopamine serves as an example for understanding this important principle. For instance, if penicillin were the only antibiotic available (which was true at one time), large doses would then be needed for a CNS infection because this water-soluble drug does not pass the blood-brain barrier easily. When a large dose of penicillin is given, only a fraction of that dose enters the brain. Most of the penicillin stays in the peripheral system, which does not cause alarm because penicillin has relatively few adverse effects. On the other hand, dopamine (and many other drugs) has many adverse effects on the body. The dose needed to penetrate the blood-brain barrier and thus adequately affect the brain (a central effect) is so large that it would have serious adverse effects on the rest of the body (e.g., cardiac stimulation, a peripheral effect).

Dopamine

Activation
Positive symptoms of schizophrenia
Psychoses
Dyskinesias
Hallucinations
Delusions
Nausea
Vomiting
Addictive behaviors
Sexual function enhancement

Antagonism
Antipsychotic effect for positive symptoms of schizophrenia
Negative symptoms of schizophrenia
Temperature dysregulation
Antiemetic effect
Parkinson's and related disorder
Dystonias
Akathisias
Cognitive problems
Sexual dysfunction
Neuroendocrine dysregulation
Depression, anhedonia
Lack of energy, motivation

NEURONS AND NEUROTRANSMITTERS

Nerve cells, or neurons, comprise the basic unit of the nervous system. Nerve cells are designed to receive and give information. Dendrites are the projections from the neuron that receive information and transmit it to the cell body. Axons send information from the nerve cell to the dendrites, axons, or cell bodies of other neurons. Axons of one cell are separated from the dendrites, axons, or cell body of another by a microscopic space known as a synapse (Figure 18-1). Figure 18-2 depicts the relationships among neurotransmitters, neurons, and psychotropic drugs.

Information, in the form of an electrochemical excitation, is communicated between cells in a specific manner. An electrochemical impulse runs from the cell body through the axon to the presynaptic terminal. Neurotransmitters are stimulated and released from the presynaptic terminal into the synaptic cleft and combine with the postsynaptic receptors on the dendrites of the neuron, evoking a neuronal response. Lest the student be misled, neurons are not strung throughout the brain end on end. The neuronal system is highly complex, with some neurons receiving input from thousands of other neurons. Furthermore, the arborization or branching of dendrites continues into late adolescence and early adulthood. It is when most of these connections are finally complete that we are who truly emerges.

Neurotransmitters are synthesized from natural precursors (e.g., amino acids) in the body (Box 18-4). These precursors are extracted from the bloodstream and synthesized in the cell into neurotransmitters. Neurotransmitters are stored in storage vesicles in the presynaptic terminals of the cell. Neurotransmitters come in many forms, and they combine with specific receptors. For instance, the neurotransmitter norepinephrine combines with a norepinephrine receptor. After norepinephrine electrochemically stimulates the norepinephrine receptor, information is transmitted from the dendritic outgrowth to the cell body, which, in turn, communicates to the next neuron, and so on. After it is in the synaptic cleft, the neurotransmitter can, until it is inactivated, continue to stimulate the postsynaptic receptor. Neurotransmitters are inactivated in two ways: they are metabolized by enzymes, or, more often, they are taken back into the presynaptic storage vesicles (referred to as reuptake) or into surrounding glial cells. Knowledge of this inactivation process has facilitated the evolution of psychopharmacology. The most important neurotransmitters for psychiatric nursing students to understand are presented in Box 18-5 and 18-6.

Box 18-4 | Four Categories of Neurotransmitters*

Monoamines
Dopamine (a catecholamine)
Norepinephrine (a catecholamine)
Serotonin (an indolamine)

Cholinergic
Acetylcholine

Amino acids
Gamma-aminobutyric acid (GABA)

Peptide
Enkephalins

*See Table 5-1 for greater detail.

Box 18-5 | Most Important Neurotransmitters for Psychiatric Nursing Students to Know*

Psychotropic drugs work by affecting neurotransmitter systems. The authors believe the foundation for understanding psychotropic drugs rests on knowledge of only five neurotransmitters. Although a great deal is to be learned, the authors are satisfied that understanding the way psychotropic drugs affect acetylcholine, dopamine, gamma-aminobutyric acid (GABA), norepinephrine, and serotonin is the starting point. As the following chapters will discuss:
- Acetylcholine is important in conceptualizing the pathology and treatment of Alzheimer's disease and parkinsonism.
- Dopamine is important in conceptualizing the pathology and treatment of schizophrenia and parkinsonism.
- GABA is important in conceptualizing the pathology and treatment of anxiety.
- Norepinephrine is important in conceptualizing the pathology and treatment of mania and depression.
- Serotonin is important in conceptualizing the pathology and treatment of mania and depression.

*Box 18-6 illustrates the relationship between these neurotransmitters and specific mental disorders.

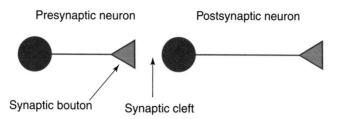

Figure 18-1 Two-neuron chain shows the presynaptic and postsynaptic neurons interconnected by a synapse. The synapse is composed of a synaptic bouton *(triangle)* or presynaptic terminal, the synaptic cleft, and the postsynaptic membrane, which, in this instance, is the dendrite or cell body *(circle)* of the postsynaptic neuron. (From Keltner N, Folks D: *Psychotropic drugs,* St Louis, 1997, Mosby.)

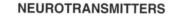

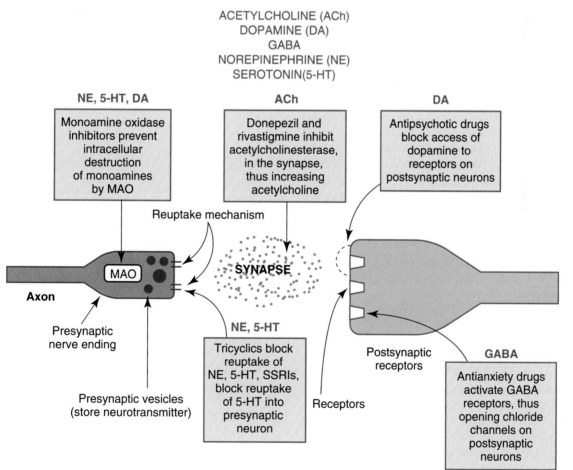

Figure 18-2 Explanation of the way psychotropic drugs affect the five major neurotransmitters. (Adapted from Stuart G, Sundeen S: *Principles and practice of psychiatric nursing,* ed 5, St Louis, 1995, Mosby.)

| Box 18-6 | Neurotransmitters and Related Mental Disorders*

Neurotransmitter-Related State	Mental Disorder
Increase in dopamine	Schizophrenia
Decrease in norepinephrine	Depression
Decrease in serotonin	Depression
Decrease in acetylcholine	Alzheimer's disease
Decrease in GABA	Anxiety

*The authors realize this explanation is overly simplistic, but the box nevertheless serves to convey the basic neurotransmitter theories for the related mental disorder.

RECEPTORS

Receptors are proteins on cell surfaces that respond to endogenous ligands or to drug molecules. A ligand is a transmitter substance or molecule that "fits" and evokes a response from a receptor. Examples of ligands include drugs, neurotransmitters, hormones, prostaglandins, and leukotrienes. Receptors are configured such that only precisely shaped molecules are able to fit and subsequently cause or prevent a response. For example, the neurotransmitter serotonin fits serotonin receptors, but acetylcholine molecules do not fit serotonin receptors.

Four primary receptor processes exist (Lehne, 2001). The two most commonly addressed processes in psychopharmacology literature are the ligand-gated ion channel or first-messenger process and the G protein-coupled or second-messenger process. When the ligand-gated receptor is activated, an ion channel such as a sodium, calcium, or chloride channel opens, and the respective ion flows through into the cell. Depending on the ion, this action causes cell depolarization (the cell fires) or hyperpolarization (cell firing slows down, or the cell does not fire). The process is extremely rapid, usually occurring within milliseconds. Acetylcholine (for nicotinic receptors only), gamma aminobutyric acid (GABA), glycine, and glutamate use the first-messenger system. The G protein-coupled receptor is a more complex process—a biologic cascade of intracellular reactions develops—and is slower compared with the first-messenger system (Piercey, 1998). Norepinephrine, serotonin, dopamine, acetylcholine (for muscarinic receptors only), and peptides couple with G protein or second-messenger receptors. Consequences of selected-receptor activation or antagonism are found in Box 18-7.

| Box 18-7 | Results of Activation or Antagonism of Selected Receptors

Serotonin Activation	Serotonin Antagonism
Antidepressant effect	Depression
Anxiety	Dysthymia
Migraine headaches	Suicidality
Nausea	Aggressiveness
Vomiting	Obsessive thinking
Other GI disturbances	Sleep-wake cycle disruption
Sexual dysfunction	Pain
Decrease in penile erection capability	Compulsive behavior
Reduced appetite and weight loss	Anxiety
Insomnia	Migraine headaches
Movement disorders	Panic
Temperature dysregulation	
Psychotic thinking (e.g., hallucinations)	

Acetylcholine Activation	Acetylcholine Antagonism
Pupil contraction	Dilated pupil
Decreased heart rate	Increased heart rate
Constriction of bronchi	Dilation of bronchi
Increased respiratory secretions	Decreased respiratory secretions
Increased voiding	Decreased voiding
Salivation	Dry mouth
Increased gastric secretions	Decreased gastric secretions
Increased defecation	Constipation
Sweating	Decreased sweating
Enhancement of cognitive processes	Cognitive slowing

Norepinephrine Activation	Norepinephrine Antagonism
Antidepressant effect	Depressive effect
Vasoconstriction (alpha-1)	Vasodilation (alpha-1 antagonism)
Increased heart rate (beta-1)	Decreased heart rate (beta blocker)
Bronchial dilation	Sexual dysfunction
Other physical effects	Other physical effects

Adapted from: Keltner NL, Zielinski AL, Hardin MS: Drugs used for cognitive symptoms of Alzheimer's disease, *Perspect Psychiatr Care* 37(1):31, 2001; Keltner NL, Hogan B, Guy DM: Dopaminergic and serotonergic receptor function in the CNS, *Perspect Psychiatr Care* 37(2):65, 2001; Keltner NL et al: Adrenergic, cholinergic, GABAergic, and glutaminergic receptor function in the CNS, *Perspect Psychiatr Care* 37(4):140, 2001.

Psychotropic drugs can affect neurotransmitters in several ways:

1. Prevent metabolism (e.g., some antidepressants and drugs for Alzheimer's disease)
2. Prevent reuptake (e.g., selective serotonin reuptake inhibitor [SSRIs] and other antidepressants)
3. Block postsynaptic receptors (antagonists) (e.g., antipsychotic drugs)
4. Activate or block autoreceptors (see discussion on autoreceptors later in this chapter)
5. Block calcium channels (calcium channel blockers are occasionally used in psychiatry)

The following list of terms relate to receptors that are defined to facilitate understanding of information presented in the drug chapters (Keltner, 2000; Keltner, Hogan, Guy, 2001).

Receptor antagonism. Receptor antagonism is the process in which receptor function is compromised related to blocking of that receptor by a psychotropic drug. Antagonists prevent the endogenous ligand from activating the receptor.

Receptor agonist. Receptor agonist is a drug that fits and activates the receptor in the same manner as does the naturally occurring ligand.

Autoreceptors. Autoreceptors are the feedback mechanism that neurons use to increase or decrease the release of a neurotransmitter; they are typically, but not always, found on the presynaptic neuron. Autoreceptor agonists "tell" the neuron that enough of the neurotransmitter is present hence a decrease in the release of the neurotransmitter occurs. Autoreceptor antagonists tell the receptor to release more of the neurotransmitter.

Receptor affinity. Receptor affinity is the attraction or strength of attraction between neurotransmitters and receptors.

Receptor life cycle. Receptors are continually being formed and continually breaking down. The life cycle of the average receptor is short (Lehne, 2001).

Receptor modulation. Some neurotransmitters do not have a direct effect but modify (or modulate) the effect of another neurotransmitter. The following scenario may help in the understanding of receptor modulation. The reader should picture, if possible, one neuron (#1) "synapsing" with the synaptic terminal of a presynaptic neuron (#2), which is synapsing in the traditional way with a third neuron (#3).

Neuron #1 influences the release of neurotransmitter from #2, which then will affect the amount of neurotransmitter released into the synapse between #2 and #3. Neuron #1 is modulating neuron #2.

PATIENT EDUCATION

The importance of patient and family education cannot be overemphasized. Historically, many psychiatric patients and their families demonstrated little understanding of their medications. Although the emphasis on education has partially remedied this problem, teaching about these potent drugs will always be a nursing priority. Furthermore, many rehospitalizations are related to patients' nonadherence to medication schedules. As knowledge deficits are removed, better compliance can be anticipated.

Despite a certain risk associated with discussing medications and side effects with patients, nurses have a professional duty to do so with knowledge and sensitivity, that is, with balance. The nurse may frighten patients with too much or inappropriate information. Good professional judgment is important, including teaching patients about what effects are visible, what can be felt, and what the possibilities are of becoming drug-dependent. The nurse should also emphasize regular checkups and tests. Specific areas of education include:

1. Discussion of side effects:
   - Side effects can directly affect the patient's willingness to adhere to the drug regimen; for example, the selective serotonin reuptake inhibitors, such as Zoloft, are known to reduce libido and sexual functioning. Of course, these drugs indirectly affect spouses as well.
   - Side effects can cause medical problems or even cause death.
   - Some drugs cause patients to experience emotional flattening, thus "dulling" responses to the environment, counseling, and family.
   - Some drugs cause cognitive slowing.
   - The nurse should always inquire about the patient's response to a drug, both therapeutic responses and adverse responses.
2. Discussion of safety issues:
   - Does the patient take the drug as prescribed?
   - Does the patient and family know which effects should be reported to the nurse or physician?

- Because some drugs, such as tricyclic antidepressants, have a narrow therapeutic index, thoughts of self-harm must be explored.
- Does the drug have potential for abuse or dependence?
- Can the drug be discontinued abruptly without effect? Patients should know that many drugs must be tapered gradually.
- Because many psychotropic drugs cause sedation or drowsiness, discussions concerning use of hazardous machinery, driving, and so forth must be reviewed.

3. Attitudes of patient and nurse about medications:
   - Because many patients and families believe that the use of medications is a sign of weakness or lack of faith in God, the nurse must explore these issues.
   - Some nurses do not really "believe" in psychotropic medications either. These nurses must examine their own views and perhaps work in areas of nursing that do not involve psychotropic drugs.
   - For patients and families who are resistant to the use of psychotropic agents, the nurse must discuss the potential ramifications of noncompliance.
   - Issues of dependence and long-term medication use must be discussed.
   - Because many patients and families do not want to become "addicted," the nurse must point out the specific addiction potential of any specific drug. Most psychotropic drugs are not addicting.

4. Drug interactions:
   - Patients and families must be taught to discuss the addition of over-the-counter drugs, alcohol, and illegal drugs to the current prescribed drugs.
   - Patients who meet with more than one clinician must make potential prescribing professionals aware of all drugs that are currently being taken.

5. Instructions for older adult patients or children of older adult patients. Because older individuals have a different pharmacokinetic profile than do younger adults, special instructions concerning side effects, and drug-drug interactions, should be tailored for this population.

6. Instructions for pregnant or breast-feeding patients. because pregnant or breast-feeding patients have special risks associated with psychotropic drug therapy, special instructions should be tailored for these individuals.

Teaching patients about their medications enables them to be mature participants in their own care and to decrease undesirable side effects. Furthermore, effective teaching can reduce noncompliance, or the failure to take medications as prescribed. Box 18-8 lists common reasons patients give for not taking their medication as prescribed. Each chapter in this unit outlines patient education issues specific to each class of drugs discussed.

| **Box 18-8** | Common Reasons for Patients Not Taking Medication as Prescribed |

Sexual dysfunction
Specific side effects—dry mouth, insomnia, sleepiness
Other side effects
Emotional dulling
Cognitive slowing
Denial of need
Fear of becoming "addicted"
Religious reasons
Interference with work
Inability to use alcohol or other recreational drugs
Pregnancy
Illness (suspiciousness, delusion of conspiracy)

Critical Thinking Question

In this chapter, the author states that the nurse should use balance when giving information to a patient about a drug. What is the balance between arousing unneeded apprehension in a patient who is vulnerable to suggestion (i.e., giving "complete" information) and treating that adult patient as a child (i.e., withholding information to "protect" the patient)? Obviously, in your role as student and later as nurse, you would not want to do either.

Key Concepts

1. Psychopharmacology is the second component of psychotherapeutic management. Psychotropic drugs have enabled millions of people to live more productive lives in the least restrictive alternative or environment.

2. Nurses assess for drug side effects, evaluate desired effects, and make decisions about prn medications, thus nurses must understand general principles of psychopharmacology and have specific knowledge concerning frequently used psychotropic drugs.

3. Pharmacokinetic processes include the absorption, distribution, metabolism, and excretion of drugs.

4. Absorption is the process by which drugs get out of the GI tract into the bloodstream.

5. Bioavailability is the percentage of a drug that reaches systemic circulation.

6. Distribution refers to the process of drug molecules leaving the bloodstream to reach tissues and organs. Drugs that do not leave the bloodstream cannot have a psychiatric effect.

7. Lipid solubility is a property that affects both absorption and distribution. Highly lipid-soluble drugs easily penetrate the blood-brain barrier.

8. Protein binding, that is, the propensity of a drug to bind to serum proteins, also affects drug distribution. Drugs bound to serum proteins cannot leave the bloodstream.

9. Metabolism is the process by which the body breaks down a drug so as to remove the drug from the body.

10. The liver is the site of most drug metabolism.

11. The two major enzyme systems associated with psychotropic drugs include the MOA system and the cytochrome P450 system.

12. An individual enzyme breaks down thousands of drug molecules per second.

13. The P450 system is mentioned often in today's psychotropic drug literature. Older texts refer to the P450 system as the hepatic microsomal enzyme system.

14. Most drug-drug interactions are related to interference with the P450 system.

15. The half-life of a drug is the length of time required for the body to remove 50% of the original dose. If a single dose of a drug is given and the drug has a half-life of 4 hours, 50% of the drug will remain in the body after 4 hours, 25% of the drug will remain after 8 hours, and 12.5% of the drug will remain after 12 hours.

16. Excretion is the removal of drug from the body through the kidneys via the urine.

17. Pharmacodynamics involves the effects of the drug on the body.

18. Drug effects are typically categorized as desired effects or side effects.

19. Downregulation of a receptor refers to a decrease in receptor numbers.

20. Pharmacodynamic tolerance is a state in which receptors become less sensitive to agonists.

21. Highly lipid-soluble drugs such as ethanol, heroin, and diazepam (Valium) pass the blood-brain barrier with ease. This characteristic partially accounts for the widespread abuse of these drugs.

22. Only drugs that pass the blood-brain barrier can affect the CNS. Consequently, these agents are useful in the treatment of mental disorders but can also cause drug dependence.

23. Neurotransmitters, which are neurochemical substances in the brain, evoke a neuronal response, are synthesized by cytoplasmic enzymes, and are typically stored in storage vesicles in the presynaptic terminals of the neuron.

24. Because both neurotransmitter deficiency (e.g., norepinephrine and serotonin in depression) and excess (e.g., dopamine in schizophrenia) are related to mental disorders, psychotropic drugs are effective because they cause an increase or decrease in the brain's ability to use a specific neurotransmitter.

25. Receptors are proteins on the cell surface that respond to specific ligands.

26. Two receptor processes most important for psychiatric nurses to understand are the first-messenger system and the second-messenger system.

27. The first-messenger system causes a cellular response when a ligand couples with the receptor, which, in turn, immediately opens an ion channel.

28. The second-messenger system is more complex compared with the first-messenger system. The initial ligand-receptor coupling initiates a series of events that culminate in a neuronal response.

29. The blood-brain barrier protects the brain from the physiologic fluctuations that the body experiences and regulates the amount of substances entering the brain and the speed with which they enter.

30. Teaching patients can decrease the incidence of side effects while increasing compliance with the drug regimen. The nurse should use good clinical judgment when deciding what to share with patients and their families.

References

Cozza KL, Armstrong SC: *The cytochrome P450 system*, Washington, DC, 2001, American Psychiatric Publishing.

Keltner NL: Neuroreceptor function and psychopharmacologic response, *Issues Ment Health Nurs* 21:31, 2000.

Keltner NL, Folks DG: *Psychotropic drugs*, ed 3, St Louis, 2001, Mosby.

Keltner NL, Hogan B, Guy DM: Dopaminergic and serotonergic receptor function in the CNS, *Perspect Psychiatr Care* 37(2):6568, 2001.

Keltner NL, Zielinski AL, Hardin MS: Drugs used for cognitive symptoms of Alzheimer's disease, *Perspect Psychiatr Care* 37(1):31, 2001.

Keltner NL et al: Adrenergic, cholinergic, GABAergic, and glutaminergic receptor function in the CNS, *Perspect Psychiatr Care* 37(4):140, 2001.

Laraia MT et al: *Psychiatric mental health nursing psychopharmacology project,* Washington, DC, 1994, ANA.

Lehne RA: *Pharmacology for nursing care,* Philadelphia, 2001, WB Saunders.

Piercey MF: Pharmacology of pramipexole, a dopamine D3-preferring agonist useful in treating Parkinson's disease, *Clin Neuropharmacol* 21:141, 1998.

Purves D et al: *Neuroscience,* Sunderland, Mass, 1997, Sinauer Associates.

Stuart G, Sundeen S: *Principles and practice of psychiatric nursing,* ed 5, St Louis, 1995, Mosby.

Bibliography

Cozza KL, Armstrong SC: *The cytochrome P450 system,* Washington, DC, 2001, American Psychiatric Publishing.

Keltner NL, Folks DG: *Psychotropic drugs,* ed 3, St Louis, 2001, Mosby.

Lehne RA: *Pharmacology for nursing care,* Philadelphia, 2001, WB Saunders.

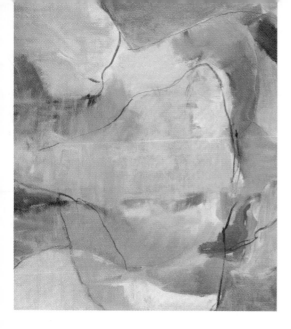

Chapter **19**

Antiparkinson Drugs

Norman L. Keltner

After reading this chapter, you should be able to:

- Differentiate between Parkinson's disease and parkinsonism.
- Discuss the causes and symptoms of parkinsonism.
- Identify the two neurotransmitters primarily associated with Parkinson's disease.
- Describe the biochemical relationship between Parkinson's disease and extrapyramidal side effects.
- Discuss side effects of antiparkinson drugs.

PARKINSON'S DISEASE AND EXTRAPYRAMIDAL SIDE EFFECTS

Extrapyramidal side effects (EPSEs) are serious and sometimes dangerous complications of treating people with psychotropic drugs. Antipsychotic agents typically cause these adverse responses (see Chapter 20), but other drugs can also produce EPSEs. EPSEs are the result of the same biochemical alterations that are found in Parkinson's disease (Keltner, Folks, 2001).

Parkinson's disease (PD) is a progressive, chronic, degenerative disease of unknown cause that involves the area of the brain called the extrapyramidal system. A well-regulated extrapyramidal system is needed for normal coordination of involuntary movement, which, in turn, supports voluntary movement. For example, when a person walks down the street,

a host of involuntary movements facilitate the voluntary movements associated with walking. PD is characterized by four cardinal symptoms: tremors, bradykinesia, rigidity, and postural instability (Pennachio, 2000). A balance of two neurotransmitters, acetylcholine (ACh) and dopamine, is required for normal function of the extrapyramidal system. The four primary symptoms and other associated symptoms (e.g., difficulty in swallowing, drooling, weight loss, choking, impaired breathing, urinary retention, constipation) occur when these two neurotransmitters are out of balance.

Critical Thinking Question

How are the associated or secondary symptoms linked to the primary symptoms?

Dopamine is synthesized in the midbrain by pigmented cells in an area called the substantia nigra (i.e., black substance). Cell bodies are located in the substantia nigra, and their axons project to the basal ganglia (a major component of the extrapyramidal system), where they release dopamine, which, in turn, activates dopamine receptors. This pathway, from the midbrain to the basal ganglia, is known as the nigrostriatal tract. In PD, the pigmented neurons of the substantia nigra lose their pigmentation, indicating a decline in dopamine production. A deficiency in dopamine and a subsequent decrease in dopa-

Key Terms

Akathisia Motor restlessness generally expressed as the inability to sit still. Akathisia is an EPSE.

Akinesia Absence of movement. Akinesia is an EPSE.

Anticholinergic effect An effect caused by drugs that block ACh receptors. Common anticholinergic effects include dry mouth and blurred vision. (See the anticholinergic side effects table on page 209 for more symptoms.)

Basal ganglia Subcortical structures, including the caudate nucleus, putamen, and globus pallidus, that fine-tune involuntary movement.

Bradykinesia Slow or retarded movement.

Dyskinesia Abnormal voluntary skeletal muscle movement usually producing a jerky motion. Dyskinesia is an EPSE.

Dysphagia Difficulty in swallowing.

Dystonia Sustained, twisted contractions of muscles that control posture, gait, or ocular movement. Dystonia is an EPSE.

EPSEs Side effects caused by drugs that block dopamine in the extrapyramidal system, thus creating a dopamine-ACh imbalance. EPSEs include akathisia, akinesia, dyskinesia, dystonia, drug-induced parkinsonism, and NMS.

Extrapyramidal system Outside the pyramidal (voluntary) tract; coordinates involuntary movements that support voluntary movement.

Neuroleptic drug Another term for antipsychotic drug.

Oculogyric crisis Involuntary tonic muscle spasms of the eye in which the eye usually rolls upward in a fixed stare. Antipsychotic drugs can cause this extremely frightening dystonic reaction.

Parkinsonism Causes of the disease are known, such as brain injury, antipsychotic drugs, carbon monoxide.

Parkinson's disease Also known as idiopathic parkinsonism, PD is a disease in which the cause is unknown; presents pathologically by a loss of dopaminergic neurons in the substantia nigra and clinically by a variety of motor and nonmotor signs and symptoms.

Substantia nigra Literally, black substance; a pigmented area of the midbrain where dopamine is synthesized.

Tardive dyskinesia Literally, a late-appearing dyskinesia; usually affects the muscles of the mouth and face and rarely the trunk. Signs include lip smacking, grinding of teeth, and a rolling or protruding tongue. The side effects can be irreversible.

mine transmission to the basal ganglia result in an imbalance with ACh in the basal ganglia. The basal ganglia are shown in Figure 19-1 in what is referred to as a coronal cut of the brain (a cut that runs from side to side). Figure 19-2 provides a good example of depigmentation occurring in PD by comparing the substantia nigra and locus ceruleus (where norepinephrine is synthesized) of a young man with those of an older man without PD (on the right) and an older man with PD (on the left). This figure clearly illustrates normal aging that results in a loss of pigmented neurons and that PD dramatically accelerates the process (Keltner et al, 1998).

EPSEs are also caused by an imbalance between ACh and dopamine (Figure 19-3 helps visualize this relationship); however, with one important difference. Whereas PD is related to neurodegeneration of the substantia nigra at the beginning of the dopamine tracts, EPSEs are caused by blockade of dopamine receptors in the basal ganglia at the end of the dopamine tracts.

PD is treated with antiparkinson agents that increase dopamine (or dopaminergics), such as Sinemet and levodopa or with anticholinergic agents (e.g., benztropine [Cogentin]) or both. EPSEs are treated only with anticholinergics because psychosis

is thought to be related to an increase in dopamine levels. To give a dopamine-enhancing drug to a patient suffering from schizophrenia might cause psychotic symptoms to increase (Table 19-1). Box 19-1 provides a handy list of both dopaminergic and anticholinergic agents.

Critical Thinking Question

What is the connection between PD and schizophrenia from a neurotransmitter perspective? (Hint: You may need to look at the next chapter.)

Table 19-1 Psychiatric Side Effects of Dopaminergics*

Drugs	Psychiatric Side Effects*
Amantadine	Confusion, hallucinations
Levodopa	Delusions
Pergolide	Paranoid ideation
Selegiline	Depression
Sinemet	Agitation
	Anxiety
	Euphoria

*Common to most of these drugs.

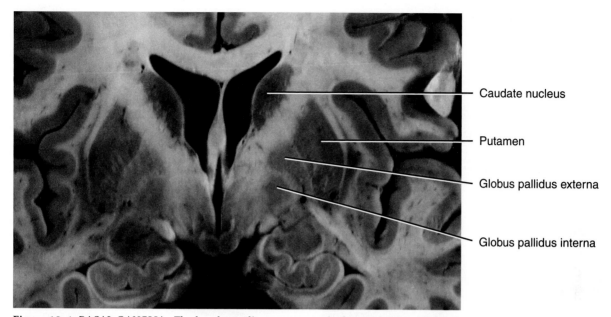

Figure 19-1 BASAL GANGLIA. The basal ganglia are composed of several subcortical (below the surface of the outer brain gray matter [or cortex]) nuclei, including the caudate nucleus, the putamen, and the globus pallidus. The globus pallidus can be further divided into the globus pallidus externa and the globus pallidus interna. (Courtesy Richard E. Powers, Director, Brain Resource Program, University of Alabama at Birmingham.)

Caudate nucleus

Putamen

Globus pallidus externa

Globus pallidus interna

I Box 19-1 I Antiparkinson Drugs

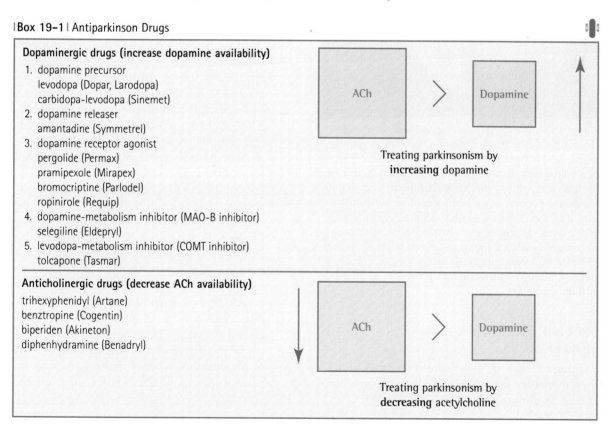

Dopaminergic drugs (increase dopamine availability)
1. dopamine precursor
   levodopa (Dopar, Larodopa)
   carbidopa-levodopa (Sinemet)
2. dopamine releaser
   amantadine (Symmetrel)
3. dopamine receptor agonist
   pergolide (Permax)
   pramipexole (Mirapex)
   bromocriptine (Parlodel)
   ropinirole (Requip)
4. dopamine-metabolism inhibitor (MAO-B inhibitor)
   selegiline (Eldepryl)
5. levodopa-metabolism inhibitor (COMT inhibitor)
   tolcapone (Tasmar)

ACh > Dopamine

Treating parkinsonism by
increasing dopamine

Anticholinergic drugs (decrease ACh availability)
trihexyphenidyl (Artane)
benztropine (Cogentin)
biperiden (Akineton)
diphenhydramine (Benadryl)

ACh > Dopamine

Treating parkinsonism by
decreasing acetylcholine

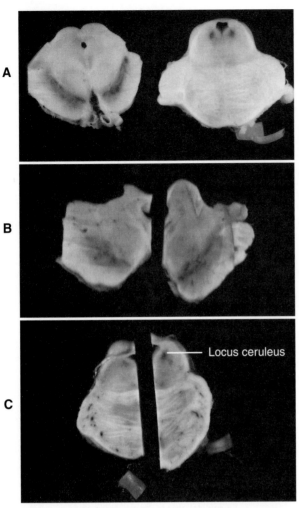

Figure 19-2 The effects of aging and disease on catecholamine centers in the brainstem. **A,** Normal pigment in the substantia nigra *(left)* and locus ceruleus *(right)* of a young man. **B,** Mild age-related loss of pigment in the brainstem of a normal individual *(right)* and loss of pigmented neurons in the brainstem of an individual with Parkinson's disease *(left).* **C,** Mild depigmentation of the locus ceruleus (site of norepinephrine synthesis) in an aged individual *(right)* and severe depigmentation in Parkinson's disease *(left).* (Courtesy Richard E. Powers, Director, Brain Resource Program, University of Alabama at Birmingham.)

SPECIFIC EXTRAPYRAMIDAL SIDE EFFECTS

Although EPSEs are biochemically related to PD, they are not the same as PD. EPSEs are divided into at least six distinct areas (Keltner, Folks, 2001).

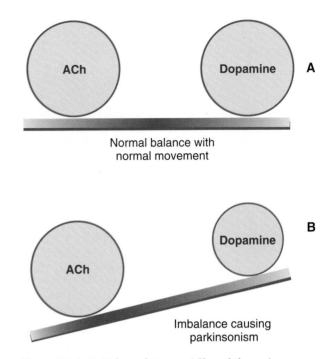

Figure 19-3 A, Balance between ACh and dopamine resulting in normal movement. **B,** Imbalance (too little dopamine) results in movement disorder.

- *Akathisia.* Akathisia is a subjective feeling of restlessness that elicits restless legs, jittery feelings, and nervous energy. Akathisia is the most common EPSE and responds poorly to treatment. Approximately 25% of patients taking traditional antipsychotics will develop akathisia. This side effect typically occurs early in treatment.
- *Akinesia.* Akinesia refers to an absence of movement, but a slowed movement (i.e., bradykinesia) is more likely. Symptoms include weakness, fatigue, painful muscles, and anergia. Akinesia responds to anticholinergics.
- *Dystonia.* Dystonias are abnormal postures that are caused by involuntary muscle spasms. Symptoms manifest as sustained, twisted, and contracted positioning of the limbs, trunk, neck, or mouth. Dystonias tend to appear early in treatment (within 3 days or so) and respond to anticholinergic drugs. These agents must occasionally be given parenterally because of the gravity of the situation. Types of dystonias include:
  - Torticollis—contracted positioning of the neck

- Oculogyric crisis—contracted positioning of the eyes upward
- Writer's cramp—fatigue spasms affecting a hand
- Laryngeal-pharyngeal constriction (potentially life threatening)

- *Drug-induced parkinsonism.* The cardinal symptoms of PD include tremors, bradykinesia, and rigidity. Approximately 20% of patients receiving traditional antipsychotics develop these symptoms, typically early in treatment.
- *Tardive dyskinesia (TD).* Tardive means "late appearing." This EPSE tends to develop after 6 months or so of antipsychotic therapy. It is not the dopamine-ACh imbalance *per se* that causes tardive dyskinesia; as a result, anticholinergics are not administered for treatment. In fact, anticholinergics typically worsen tardive dyskinesia. Chronic use of antipsychotics is thought to cause dopamine receptors in the basal ganglia to become hypersensitive. Symptoms are bothersome and can be embarrassing. Typical symptoms include tongue writhing, tongue protrusion, teeth grinding, and lip smacking. TD stops with sleep. Although TD movements can be suppressed willfully for a short time, they soon reappear. Up to 35% of individuals undergoing chronic traditional antipsychotic therapy will develop TD. Many times, TD is irreversible. No satisfactory pharmacologic response has been developed at this time; however, the atypical antipsychotic clozapine has been used with some success (Bassitt, Louza Neto, 1998; Casey, 1998).
- Neuroleptic malignant syndrome (NMS). NMS is a potentially lethal side effect of antipsychotic agents. Less than 1% of patients taking antipsychotics will develop this problem, but 5% to 20% of those untreated will die (Pelonero, Levenson, Pandurangi, 1998). The incidence was much greater in the past, but careful scrutiny of patients by nurses and physicians has reduced both incidence and mortality. Cardinal symptoms include hyperthermia, rigidity, and autonomic dysfunction. NMS can be treated with muscle relaxants (e.g., dantrolene) and with centrally acting dopaminergics (e.g., bromocriptine).

DRUGS TO TREAT EXTRAPYRAMIDAL SIDE EFFECTS

Anticholinergic drugs are used to treat EPSEs and work by restoring the imbalance caused by antipsychotic drugs. As noted in this chapter and in Chapter 20, antipsychotic agents block (or antagonize) dopamine receptors. This dopamine-receptor antagonism causes a man-made or iatrogenic parkinsonian-like syndrome—the aforementioned EPSEs. However, restoring the balance with a dopaminergic is inappropriate because, as the chapter on schizophrenia emphasizes, the most compelling hypothesis for schizophrenia is the presence of excessive amounts of dopamine. Hence anticholinergics (drugs that block ACh receptors) are used to restore the balance (Box 19-2).

The following outline is repetitive but may be helpful:

1. Individuals with schizophrenia have excessive amounts of dopamine.
2. Antipsychotic agents (particularly those referred to as high-potency antipsychotics) block dopamine receptors.
3. When dopamine is blocked, a drug-induced parkinsonism can develop.
4. An antiparkinson drug is needed to "fix" the problem that antipsychotics create.
5. If dopaminergic antiparkinson drugs are given, schizophrenia may worsen. (See Table 19-1 for psychiatric side effects of dopaminergics.)
6. Hence anticholinergic drugs are given to restore ACh-dopamine balance.

Several anticholinergic drugs are available to treat EPSEs. These drugs' site of action for relieving EPSEs is the central nervous system (CNS). They also have pronounced peripheral effects. The prototype drug for this class of drugs is atropine but is not used to treat EPSEs. Atropine is most commonly used to reduce aspiration during surgery. Benztropine (Cogentin) and trihexyphenidyl (Artane) are much more likely to be used to alleviate EPSEs. Atropine is twice as potent as benztropine and five times as potent as is trihexyphenidyl on a milligram-per-milligram basis. Benztropine is the most commonly prescribed anticholinergic for EPSEs. The relative anticholinergic potency of selected psychotropic drugs is found in Table 19-2. (See Box 19-3 for the adult dosages of anticholinergics.)

| Box 19-2 | Model for Drug-Induced Parkinsonism

Clinical Manifestation	**Theoretical Understanding**	**Intervention**	**Possible Effect of Intervention**
1. Positive symptoms of schizophrenia	2. Increased levels of dopamine	3. Antipsychotic drug(s) (dopamine antagonists) given	4. Improvement of psychotic symptoms and possible development of EPSEs
5. EPSEs (e.g., parkinsonism, akathisia)	6. A drug-induced imbalance between ACh and dopamine has occurred	7. Add anticholinergic drug to treatment regimen	8. Continued improvement in psychotic symptoms and amelioration of EPSEs (restored balance between dopamine and ACh)

Source: From Keltner NL et al: *Psychobiological foundations of psychiatric care,* St Louis, 1998, Mosby.

| Table 19-2 | Anticholinergic Effect of Frequently Prescribed Psychotropic Drugs Compared with Benztropine (Cogentin)

Drug	Equivalent (in mg)	Typical Use
atropine	0.5	Given before surgery
benztropine (Cogentin)	1.0	Antiparkinson
trihexyphenidyl (Artane)	2.5	Antiparkinson
biperiden (Akineton)	1.0	Antiparkinson
amitriptyline (Elavil)	10.0	Antidepressant
doxepin (Sinequan)	30.0	Antidepressant
nortriptyline (Pamelor)	60.0	Antidepressant
imipramine (Tofranil)	75.0	Antidepressant
desipramine (Norpramin)	150.0	Antidepressant
amoxapine (Asendin)	600.0	Antidepressant
clozapine (Clozaril)	15.0	Antipsychotic
thioridazine (Mellaril)	50.0	Antipsychotic
chlorpromazine (Thorazine)	370.0	Antipsychotic
diphenhydramine (Benadryl)	50.0	Antihistamine

According to this table, 50 mg of thioridazine has the same anticholinergic effect as does 1 mg of benztropine.
Adapted from de Leon J et al: A pilot effort to determine benztropine equivalents of anticholinergic medications, *Hosp Community Psychiatry* 45(6):606, 1994.

Pharmacologic Effects (Desired Effects)

Primarily, anticholinergic drugs inhibit ACh, thus preventing its stimulation of the cholinergic excitatory pathways. These drugs may also inhibit reuptake of dopamine. Of course, both of these effects contribute to the restoration of the ACh-dopamine balance. Anticholinergics are used alone in the treatment of EPSEs.

Treating drug-induced extrapyramidal side effects

Antipsychotic drugs block dopamine receptors, frequently causing EPSEs. Many of the symptoms associated with "naturally" occurring PD—tremors, rigidity, and bradykinesia—are present in drug-induced parkinsonism, along with related symptoms such as akathisia, dystonic reactions, and dyskinesias. Blockade or depletion of dopamine in the basal ganglia or the nigrostriatal tract produces EPSEs. High-potency antipsychotic agents such as haloperidol cause EPSEs more often than do low-potency agents. Additionally, several nonneuroleptic drugs, including certain antidepressants, antiemetics, and lithium, cause EPSEs (Blair, Dauner, 1993). These symptoms contribute to the discomfort, anxiety, and frustration of this already troubled population and are major contributors to noncompliance. Patients taking antipsychotic drugs can experience a gradual or sudden onset of EPSEs.

Side Effects

Anticholinergic drugs produce both CNS and peripheral nervous system (PNS) side effects, which are listed in the anticholinergics side effects box. CNS effects include confusion, agitation, dizziness, drowsiness, and disturbances in behavior. Because the cholinergic system contributes to memory and learning, anticholinergic drugs affect these cognitive functions as well (Keltner, Zielinski, Hardin, 2001). Ingesting drugs with anticholinergic properties can often explain recent changes in cognition among older adults.

PNS anticholinergic effects such as dry mouth, blurred vision, nausea, and nervousness occur in 30% to 50% of these patients. Peripheral anticholinergic side effects result basically from blocking the parasympathetic system (a cholinergic [ACh] system) (Table 19-3). For instance, blurred vision results from pupils that dilate because of the blocking of ACh receptors of the third cranial nerve (oculomotor nerve). The third cranial nerve constricts the

pupil; when it is blocked, the pupil dilates. Dry mouth results when cranial nerves VII and IX (facial and glossopharyngeal) are blocked from causing salivation. Decreased tearing is related to cranial nerve VII. Although these problems are annoying, they are not typically major health hazards. On the other hand, when cranial nerve X (vagus nerve) is blocked, tachycardia can occur and cause serious problems. The sinoatrial (SA) node has a rhythm of 100 to 120 impulses per minute. The reason that hearts do not beat this fast is because the parasympathetic system provides a braking action. When anticholinergic drugs are given, part of the brake is removed, which can result in major problems, particularly for older individuals. Constipation, a problem with parkinsonism patients because of rigidity, can be worsened by anticholinergics as well. Urinary hesitance and retention and decreased sweating are other PNS effects. Interestingly, patients who drool or perspire excessively may welcome dry mouth and decreased sweating.

Nursing Implication for Anticholinergic Drugs
Therapeutic versus toxic dose levels

Therapeutic ranges are found in Box 19-3. Doses above this range can cause toxic effects. Overdose may result in CNS hyperstimulation (confusion, excitement, hyperpyrexia, agitation, disorientation, delirium, or hallucinations) or CNS depression (drowsiness, sedation, or coma). The cardiovascular, urinary, and gastrointestinal systems are particularly involved. The eyes are also affected. High fevers are the result of the CNS effects of anticholinergics and their ability to decrease sweating.

Table 19-3	Anticholingeric Effect on Cranial Nerves with Parasympathetic Functions	
Cranial Nerve	Parasympathetic Function	Anticholingeric Effect
III	Constricts pupils	Mydriasis (dilates pupils), blurred vision
	Alters shape of lens	Impairs accommodation
VII	Salivation	Dry mouth
	Lacrimation	Decreased tearing
	Nasal mucous secretion	Dry nasal passage
IX	Salivation	Dry mouth
	Nasal mucous secretion	Dry nasal passage
X	Slows heart rate	Tachycardia
	Promotes peristalsis	Slows peristalsis; constipation
	Constricts bronchi	Dilates bronchi

Box 19-3	Anticholinergic Drug Dosages for EPSEs*	
benztropine (Cogentin)	1-4 mg, qd or bid, PO or IM or IV *For acute dystonic reactions:* 1-2 mg IM, then 1-2 mg PO bid
biperiden (Akineton)	2 mg qd or tid
trihexyphenidyl (Artane)	Start with 1 mg daily and increase Usual dose range of 5-15 mg/day

*Dosages for adults.

Side Effects and Nursing Interventions for Anticholinergics

Side Effects	Interventions
Peripheral nervous system effects	
Dry mouth	Offer sugarless hard candy and chewing gum; encourage frequent rinses; take medication before meals.
Nasal congestion	Recommend over-the-counter nasal decongestant, if approved by physician.
Urinary hesitation	Introduce running water, privacy, warm water over perineum.
Urinary retention	Catheterize for residual fluids; encourage frequent voiding.
Blurred vision, photophobia	Provide reassurance (normal vision typically returns in a few weeks); encourage sunglasses, advise caution when driving (tolerance develops).
Constipation	Give laxatives, as ordered; encourage diet with roughage; recommend 2500 to 3000 ml of water per day.
Mydriasis	If eye pain develops, undiagnosed narrow-angle glaucoma—may be the cause; immediate attention is warranted.
Orthostatic hypotension	Request patient to get out of bed slowly, to sit on the edge of the bed a short while, and rise slowly.
Sedation	Help patient get up early and to get the day started.
Decreased sweating	Decreased sweating can lead to fever; take temperature; if fever occurs, reduce body temperature (e.g., sponge baths).
Temperature	Advise limited strenuous activity; encourage patient to wear appropriate clothing.
Central nervous system effects of antipsychotics	
Akathisia	Be patient and reassure patient who is "jittery" that you understand the need to move and that appropriate drug interventions can help differentiate akathisia and agitation. Because akathisia is the chief cause of noncompliance with antipsychotic regimens, switching to a different class of antipsychotic drug may be necessary to achieve compliance. Anticholinergics help reduce the intensity of akathisia.
Dystonias	If a severe reaction (e.g., oculogyric crisis, torticollis) occurs, give antiparkinson drug (e.g., benztropine [Cogentin]) or antihistamine (e.g., diphenhydramine [Benadryl]) immediately, as needed; offer reassurance. If an order for intramuscular administration has not been written, call the physician at once to obtain the order. When an order for an antiparkinson drug is warranted for less severe dystonias, notify the physician.
Drug-induced parkinsonism	Assess for the major parkinsonism symptoms: tremors, rigidity, and bradykinesia; report to physician. Antiparkinson drugs will probably be indicated.
Tardive dyskinesia	Assess for signs by using the abnormal inventory movement scale. Drug holidays may help prevent tardive dyskinesia. Anticholinergic agents will worsen tardive dyskinesia; therefore question their indiscriminate prophylactic use.

Use during pregnancy

Anticholinergics should be used cautiously during pregnancy. Theoretically, these drugs will decrease milk flow during lactation.

Use in older adults

As this chapter and a number of other chapters in this text have emphasized, older individuals are particularly sensitive to anticholinergic agents. Cognitive, cardiovascular, and gastrointestinal side effects are more pronounced in this age group compared with the younger population. Older men with prostatic enlargement can have these difficulties exacerbated with the use of these agents.

Side effect interventions

Numerous annoying side effects are associated with anticholinergic drugs (see the anticholinergics side effects box). Several nondrug alternatives to help the patient are listed in this table.

Interactions with anticholinergic drugs

The nurse should alert the patient to the dangers of over-the-counter drugs and other prescription drugs that intensify the atropine-like effects of centrally acting anticholinergics. Several important interactions follow:

- Amantadine: a dopaminergic antiparkinson drug that has anticholinergic properties as well
- Chlorpromazine: additive anticholinergic effect
- Monoamine oxidase inhibitors: additive anticholinergic effect
- Antihistamines: additive anticholinergic effect
- Antiarrhythmic drugs: additive anticholinergic effect

Other interactions include an intensification of sedative effects when combined with CNS depressants and a decrease in absorption when combined with antacids and antidiarrheal drugs.

Teaching patients

In addition to teaching appropriate information about side effects, the nurse should also emphasize certain points. The patient and family should be advised of the following:

- Avoid discontinuing these drugs abruptly. Tapering off over a 1-week period is advised.
- Avoid driving or other hazardous activities until tolerance develops and drowsiness and blurred vision diminish.

- Avoid over-the-counter medications (e.g., cough and cold preparations) that have anticholinergic or antihistamine properties; alcohol, which will exacerbate CNS depression; and antacids, which will interfere with absorption of anticholinergics.

Selected Anticholinergic Drugs

Benztropine (Cogentin)

Benztropine is used to treat all parkinsonian-like disorders, including drug-induced EPSEs. Benztropine, which is the most frequently prescribed anticholinergic antiparkinson drug, is usually given orally at a dose of 1 to 4 mg a day; it can be given intramuscularly (1 to 2 mg) for noncompliant psychotic patients and intramuscularly or intravenously (1 to 2 mg) for acute dystonic reactions. Benztropine causes greater and longer-lasting sedation than does trihexyphenidyl; when given at bedtime, the sedation effect may be desirable.

Biperiden (Akineton)

Biperiden is used adjunctively in all parkinsonian-like disorders, including drug-induced EPSEs. Typically, 2 mg one to three times daily is given for EPSEs. For acute symptoms, 2 mg is given intramuscularly or intravenously every 30 minutes as needed (prn) (up to 8 mg in 24 hours).

Diphenhydramine (Benadryl)

Diphenhydramine, the prototype antihistamine, is effective for most parkinsonian-like disorders. The usual dose is 25 to 50 mg, three to four times daily. Diphenhydramine can cause considerable sedation in some individuals and little in others and is considerably less potent than is benztropine (see Table 19-2).

Trihexyphenidyl (Artane)

Trihexyphenidyl, which was the first anticholinergic used extensively for EPSEs, is usually initiated at 1 to 2 mg per day up to a maximum of 5 to 15 mg per day. Trihexyphenidyl is not available in a parenteral form; thus its use for acute dystonias is limited.

Critical Thinking Question

The rate-limiting step in the "natural" synthesis of dopamine is the availability of the enzyme tyrosine hydroxylase that converts tyrosine to levodopa (or L-dopa or dopa). How does this fact determine what is given to increase dopamine in the patient with PD?

Key Concepts

1. PD is related to degeneration of the substantia nigra, the dopamine-generating portion of the brain; however, the cause is unknown.
2. Normal muscle activity requires a balance between dopamine and ACh; consequently, a dopamine deficiency is responsible for symptoms of PD.
3. The four primary symptoms associated with PD include tremors, bradykinesia, rigidity, and postural instability.
4. Secondary symptoms of PD (i.e., difficult swallowing, respiratory problems, constipation) are a result of the primary symptoms.
5. Drug treatment of PD is based on reestablishing a balance between dopamine and ACh.
6. Reestablishing this balance involves three basic approaches: using dopaminergic drugs to increase dopamine levels, using anticholinergic drugs to decrease ACh levels, or a combination of these approaches.
7. Major anticholinergic antiparkinson drugs include benztropine (Cogentin) and trihexyphenidyl (Artane).
8. Anticholinergic drugs are used to treat EPSEs.
9. EPSEs are caused by a drug-induced imbalance of ACh and dopamine.
10. Anticholinergic agents help restore the balance.
11. Dopaminergic drugs are inappropriate for use because they may theoretically worsen the psychosis by adding more dopamine.
12. Anticholinergic drugs have many side effects. Older individuals are particularly sensitive to these side effects.

Case Study

A 25-year-old woman who is taking an antipsychotic drug (haloperidol) starts to experience psychomotor slowing as she walks down the hallway of the hospital. Before she reaches the end of the hall, she requires assistance. Within 2 minutes of sitting down, her neck becomes rigidly hyperextended, and the eyes roll upward in a fixed stare. Her breathing becomes labored because of the position of her neck, and she is frightened. Because she is also delusional, what this frightening side effect of her medication represents to her is difficult to imagine. Benztropine (Cogentin), 2 mg, is given intramuscularly then repeated in 15 minutes because she did not respond as quickly as was hoped. Within another 5 minutes, she was back to her "normal" self.

References

Bassitt DP, Louza Neto MR: Clozapine efficacy in tardive dyskinesia in schizophrenic patients, *Eur Arch Psychiatry Clin Neurosci* 248(4):209, 1998.

Blair DT, Dauner A: Nonneuroleptic etiologies of extrapyramidal symptoms, *Clin Nurs Specialist* 7(4):225, 1993.

Casey DE: Effects of clozapine therapy in schizophrenic individuals at risk for tardive dyskinesia, *J Clin Psychiatry* 59(suppl 3):31, 1998.

de Leon J et al: A pilot effort to determine benztropine equivalents of anticholinergic medications, *Hosp Community Psychiatry* 45(6):606, 1994.

Forman L: Medication: reasons and interventions for noncompliance, *J Psychosoc Nurs Ment Health Serv* 31(10):23, 1993.

Keltner NL: Neuroreceptor function and psychopharmacological response, *Issues Ment Health Nurs* 21:31, 2000.

Keltner NL et al: *Psychobiological foundations of psychiatric care,* St Louis, 1998, Mosby.

Keltner NL, Folks DG: *Psychotropic drugs,* ed 3, Philadelphia, 2001, Mosby.

Keltner NL, Zielinski AL, Hardin MS: Drugs used for cognitive symptoms of Alzheimer's disease, *Perspect Psychiatr Care* 37(1):31, 2001.

Lang ET, Fahn S: Assessment of Parkinson's disease. In Munsat TL, editor: *Quantification of neurologic deficit,* London, 1989, Buttersworth.

Pelonero AL, Levenson JL, Pandurangi AK: Neuroleptic malignant syndrome: a review. *Psychiatr Serv* 49(9):1163, 1998.

Pennachio DL: Parkinson's disease: progress along the continuum of care, *Patient Care Nurs Pract* 3(2):26, 2000.

Bibliography

Agid Y: Parkinson's disease: pathophysiology, *Lancet* 337:1321, 1991.

Keltner NL: Neuroreceptor function and psychopharmacological response, *Issues Ment Health Nurs* 21:31, 2000.

Keltner NL, Folks DG: *Psychotropic drugs,* ed 3, Philadelphia, 2001, Mosby.

Lehne RA: Pharmacology for nursing care, ed 4, Philadelphia, 2001, WB Saunders.

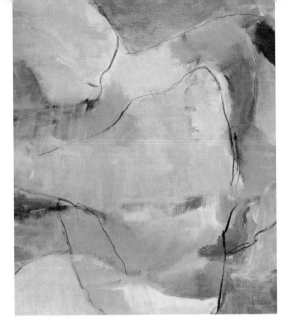

Chapter 20

Antipsychotic Drugs

Norman L. Keltner; Regina Mims

Learning Objectives

After reading this chapter, you should be able to:

- Explain the concept of neurotransmitters, specifically dopamine, in relation to psychosis.
- Identify the clinical uses of antipsychotic drugs.
- Recognize differences between high-potency and low-potency traditional antipsychotic drugs.
- Identify a representative high-potency, low-potency, and atypical antipsychotic drug, including the specific side effects and interactions of each drug.

- Describe signs and symptoms associated with extrapyramidal side effects.
- Describe potential interactions of antipsychotic drugs.
- Discuss implications for teaching patients about antipsychotic drugs.

Antipsychotic or neuroleptic drugs are used to treat schizophrenia and other psychoses. Additionally, various other manifestations of mental illness are amenable to these agents. Traditional antipsychotic drugs are most effective for treating acute psychoses and the agitation associated with mania and other mental disturbances. Newer atypical agents such as clozapine (Clozaril), risperidone (Risperdal), olanzapine (Zyprexa), quetiapine (Seroquel), and ziprasidone (Geodon) appear to be effective in the treatment of more chronic forms of psychoses as well. Other uses of antipsychotics, such as antiemetics and those used in the treatment of hiccoughs, will not be addressed in this book.

Antipsychotics were discovered "accidentally" circa 1950. A French scientist was hoping to develop a new antihistamine and in the process formulated chlorpromazine, which was initially used to calm presurgery jitters but was soon found to possess antipsychotic properties. Chlorpromazine (Thorazine) is considered the first antipsychotic drug.

Before the introduction and acceptance of chlorpromazine and the many related drugs, hundreds of thousands of patients with severe psychiatric disturbances were hospitalized under poor conditions in some instances. These patients were isolated, physically restrained, and occasionally subjected to psychosurgery (lobotomy). The treatments rarely

Antipsychotic Drugs for Schizophrenia and Other Psychoses

Indications	Mechanism of Action	Major Side Effects	Overdose Potential
Hallucinations, delusions, agitation, blunted affect, bizarre thinking, social withdrawal, and paranoid thinking	Efficacy probably related to their ability to block dopamine and other neurotransmitter receptors	Extrapyramidal side effects; anticholinergic, antiadrenergic, endocrine, and cardiac effects	Overdoses are seldom fatal and treatment is supportive

Key Terms

Akathisia Motor restlessness generally expressed as the inability to sit still. Akathisia is an EPSE.

Anticholinergic effect An effect caused by drugs that block ACh receptors. Common anticholinergic effects include dry mouth and blurred vision.

Basal ganglia Subcortical structures that fine-tune involuntary movement.

Bradykinesia Slow or retarded movement.

Dyskinesia Abnormal voluntary skeletal muscle movement, usually producing a jerky motion. Dyskinesia is an EPSE but is probably related to dopamine receptor sensitivity rather than to dopamine receptor blockade.

Dysphagia Difficulty in swallowing.

Dystonia Sustained, twisted contractions of muscles that control posture, gait, or ocular movement. Dystonia is an EPSE.

Extrapyramidal side effects (EPSEs) Side effects caused by drugs that block dopamine, thus creating a dopamine-ACh imbalance. EPSEs include akathisia, akinesia, dyskinesia, dystonia, drug-induced parkinsonism, and NMS.

Extrapyramidal system Outside the pyramidal (voluntary) tract. Coordinates involuntary movements that support voluntary movement.

Neuroleptic drug Another term for antipsychotic drug.

Oculogyric crisis Involuntary tonic muscle spasms of the eye in which the eye usually rolls upward in a fixed stare, which is a frightening dystonic reaction caused by antipsychotic drugs.

Tardive dyskinesia (TD) Literally, a late-appearing dyskinesia; usually affects the muscles of the mouth and face. Signs include lip smacking, grinding of teeth, and a rolling or protruding tongue. This side effect may be irreversible.

Ventral tegmental area (VTA) Another site of dopamine synthesis. Also located in midbrain near the substantia nigra. The VTA is not pigmented.

restored patients to a state that enabled them to function productively or to interact in a reasonably normal way with others.

Although all the hopes for antipsychotic drugs have not been realized, these drugs have had a dramatic impact on psychiatric care. The use of antipsychotic drugs by the psychiatric community resulted in the abandonment of most early and ineffective treatments, and long-term hospitalizations fell from more than 500,000 in 1955 to approximately 70,000 today. A more complete review of the history of these drugs can be found in Keltner and Folks (2001).

The drugs discussed in this chapter are generally called antipsychotic agents, but historically they have also been referred to as major tranquilizers, ataractics (drugs that produce calmness or serenity), and neuroleptics (because they can produce neurologic symptoms).

CLASSIFICATION SYSTEMS

Antipsychotic drugs are generally conceptualized in three overlapping ways. The first and most accurate classification system is based on chemical class, as listed in Table 20-1. These drugs have diverse chemical properties, but they all effectively reduce various psychiatric symptoms. The type, intensity, and frequency of side effects vary among these drugs because of the differences in chemical class. Therefore when a drug is "not working," it should be substituted with a drug of a different class.

The second classification of antipsychotic drugs is based on potency (Box 20-1). Classification based on potency is a less "scientific" approach than classification by chemical class, but it has gathered support because of its clinical utility. Essentially, the effects of traditional antipsychotics are related to the blockade of a specific type of dopamine receptor D_2. Clinical

|Table 20-1| Major Traditional and Atypical Antipsychotic Drugs

Drug	Usual Adult Maintenance Range (mg/day)	Rate of EPSEs	Rate of Anticholinergic Effects	Rate of Orthostasis	Rate of Sedation	Rate of Weight Gain
Traditional Antipsychotic Drugs						
High-Potency Antipsychotic Drugs						
fluphenazine (Prolixin)	0.5-40.0	High	Low	Low	Low	Low
haloperidol (Haldol)	1-15	High	Low	Low	Low	Low
thiothixene (Navane)	5-40	High	Low	Low	Moderate	Moderate
trifluoperazine (Stelazine)	5-40	High	Low	Moderate	Low	Low
Moderate-Potency Antipsychotic Drugs						
loxapine (Loxitane)	20-250	Moderate	Low	Moderate	Moderate	Low
molindone (Moban)	15-225	Moderate	Moderate	Low	Low	Low
Low-Potency Antipsychotic Drugs						
chlorpromazine (Thorazine)	200-1000	Moderate	Moderate	High	Moderate	High
thioridazine (Mellaril)	200-800	Low	High	High	High	High
chlorprothixene (Taractan)	75-600	Moderate	Moderate	Moderate	High	Moderate
Atypical Antipsychotic Drugs						
clozapine (Clozaril)	75-900	Low	High	High	High	High
risperidone (Risperdal)	0.5-6.0	Low*	Low	Moderate	Moderate	Moderate
olanzapine (Zyprexa)	5-20	Low	Moderate	Low	High	High
quetiapine (Seroquel)	75-750	Low	Low	Moderate	Moderate	Moderate
ziprasidone (Geodon)	40-160	Low	Low	Low	Low	Low

EPSEs, Extrapyramidal side effects.
*However, EPSEs develop at high doses.

effectiveness occurs when 60% to 70% of these receptors are blocked. For instance, approximately 100 mg of chlorpromazine (Thorazine) is required to achieve the same clinical effect as 2 mg of haloperidol (Haldol). This classification system is not as "clean" as is the chemical classification system. A few drugs, such as loxapine, molindone, and perphenazine, do not fall comfortably into either high- or low-potency groups. Nonetheless, this dichotomy is clinically significant because low-potency drugs tend to cause more intense anticholinergic effects (e.g., dry mouth, blurred vision) and antiadrenergic effects (e.g., orthostatic hypotension), whereas high-potency drugs cause more extrapyramidal side effects (EPSEs). Knowing this difference prepares the nurse for the most obvious set of side effects. Table 20-1 illustrates that, as a general rule, drugs with increased anticholinergic effects produce decreased EPSEs. Table 20-2 outlines the theoretical effects of specific receptor blockade.

The third means of categorizing these drugs is based on "typicality." That is, drugs developed between 1950 and 1990 are considered traditional or

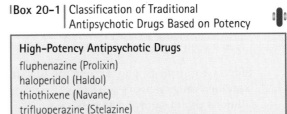

|Box 20-1| Classification of Traditional Antipsychotic Drugs Based on Potency

High-Potency Antipsychotic Drugs
fluphenazine (Prolixin)
haloperidol (Haldol)
thiothixene (Navane)
trifluoperazine (Stelazine)

Moderate-Potency Antipsychotic Drugs
loxapine (Loxitane)
molindone (Moban)

Low-Potency Antipsychotic Drugs
chlorpromazine (Thorazine)
chlorprothixene (Taractan)
thioridazine (Mellaril)

typical antipsychotics. The newer agents, which will be discussed later in this chapter, are referred to as atypical because of the following characteristics (Jibson, Tandon, 1998; Keltner, Coffeen, Johnson, 2000a):

1. Reduced or no risk for EPSEs
2. Increased effectiveness in treating negative or cognitive symptoms or both

| Table 20-2 | Theoretical Effects of Receptor Blockade

Receptor	Putative Effects
D_1, D_5	?Antipsychotic effects
D_2	Mesolimbic tract: antipsychotic effect (all antipsychotic drugs antagonize D_2)
	Nigrostriatal tract: EPSEs
	Tuberoinfundibular tract: prolactin elevation
	Mesocortical tract: may cause secondary negative symptoms (symptoms caused by antipsychotic drugs themselves)
D_3	?Antipsychotic effect on negative symptoms
D_4	?Antipsychotic effect on positive symptoms
5-HT1	?May cause mood and/or cognitive symptoms
5-HT2A	?Antipsychotic effect on negative symptoms
5-HT2C	Weight gain
5-HT3	?Nausea
M*	Can restore ACh-dopamine balance for EPSEs
	Anticholinergic side effects
H_1	Sedation, orthostasis, weight gain
Alpha-1	Orthostasis, dizziness, sedation
Alpha-2	Sexual dysfunction
	?Antidepressant effect
GABA	Lowers seizure threshold

*M = cholinergic muscarinic receptors
From Bezchlibnyk-Butler, Jeffries, 1997; Jibson, Tandon, 1998; Keltner, Hogan, Guy, 2001; Keltner, 2000.

3. Efficacy for patients who are unresponsive to traditional antipsychotics
4. Minimal risk of tardive dyskinesia
5. Absence of prolactin elevation and the associated side effects

Atypical antipsychotics are much more effective than are typical agents in modifying negative symptoms of schizophrenia. Table 20-3 presents a brief synopsis of positive and negative symptoms.

NEUROCHEMICAL THEORY OF SCHIZOPHRENIA

The neurochemical theory affords the best explanation for the effectiveness of antipsychotic agents. The neurochemical theory states that increased levels of dopamine in the limbic area of the brain cause schizophrenia and psychotic symptoms (e.g., hallucinations, delusions). Because antipsychotic drugs are dopamine blockers, it follows that their effectiveness

| Table 20-3 | Positive and Negative Symptoms of Schizophrenia

Symptom Category	Symptoms
Positive (Type I)	
Prognosis: good	Abnormal thought form
Precipitating factors: yes	Agitation, tension
Onset: acute	Associational disturbances
Sensorium: dreamlike quality	Bizarre behavior
Intellectual impairment: none	Conceptual disorganization
	Delusions
Pathophysiology: D_2 hyperactivity	Excitement
	Feelings of persecution
Pathoanatomy: VBRs may be normal	Grandiosity
	Hallucinations
Response to typical neuroleptics: fair to good	Hostility
	Ideas of reference
	Illusions
Effect of levodopa: increases symptoms	Insomnia
	Suspiciousness
Negative (Type II)	
Prognosis: poor	Alogia
Onset: chronic	Anergia
Family history: more than type I	Anhedonia
	Asocial behavior
Sensorium: clear	Attention deficits
Intellectual impairment: yes	Avolition
	Blunted affect
Pathophysiology: possibly hypodopaminergic, decreased CBF	Communication difficulties
	Difficulty with abstractions
Pathoanatomy: increased VBRs, other changes	Passive social withdrawal
	Poor grooming and hygiene
Response to typical neuroleptics: varies	Poor rapport
	Poverty of speech
Response to atypical neuroleptics: better	
Effect of levodopa: minimal	

From Harris D, Keltner NL: Medication management. In Worley NK, editor: *Mental health in the community*, St Louis, 1997, Mosby.
CBF, Cerebral blood flow; *VBRs*, ventricular brain ratios.

can be attributed to this dopamine-blocking activity. Furthermore, this theory of schizophrenia is supported by clinical observations and clinical research, both of which demonstrate that high doses of levodopa and amphetamines can produce schizophrenic symptoms. These drugs increase dopamine levels.

This explanation, however, does not answer all of the questions surrounding the issue, most specifically those regarding negative symptoms. Figure 20-1 provides additional useful information. As shown in

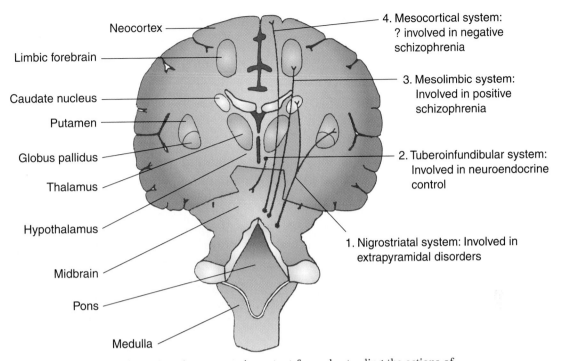

Figure 20-1 Four dopaminergic tracts are important for understanding the actions of antipsychotic drugs. *1,* Nigrostriatal system: when antipsychotic drugs antagonize this system, a pseudoparkinsonism or extrapyramidal effect occurs. *2,* Tuberoinfundibular system: when antipsychotic drugs antagonize this system, the dopamine inhibition of the pituitary hormone prolactin is lifted and can lead to gynecomastia and galactorrhea. *3,* Mesolimbic system: when antipsychotic drugs antagonize this system, a decrease in the symptoms of schizophrenia occurs (primarily positive symptoms). This particular effect makes these drugs antipsychotic. *4,* Mesocortical system: when antipsychotic drugs antagonize this system, the disorder can worsen in some patients. Atypical antipsychotics are thought to antagonize serotonin receptors in the cortex that, in turn, liberate dopamine there; that is, theories suggest that a mesocortical hypodopaminergic state may contribute to negative symptoms. Much remains to be understood about the role, if any, of the mesocortical dopaminergic tract in schizophrenia. (From Roberts GW, Leigh PN, Weinberger DR: *Neuropsychiatric disorders,* London, 1993, Wolfe Publishing.)

this figure, the brain has four major dopaminergic tracts. Dopamine is synthesized primarily in the substantia nigra and ventral tegmental area and is delivered to "distant" sites via dopaminergic tracts. To fully appreciate the complexity of psychopharmacologic treatment of schizophrenia, the student must recognize the existence of dopamine-dependent areas of the brain that communicate with dopamine-synthesizing areas (substantia nigra and ventral tegmental areas in the midbrain) via different neuronal tracts.

Tract 1. The *nigrostriatal tract* is involved in movement. Antipsychotic blockade can cause EPSEs.

Tract 2. The *tuberoinfundibular tract* modulates pituitary function. Antipsychotic blockade can lead to elevation in prolactin levels.

Tract 3. The *mesolimbic tract* is involved in emotional and sensory processes. Antipsychotic blockade normalizes these processes in individuals with schizophrenia.

Tract 4. The *mesocortical tract* is involved in cognitive processes. Antipsychotic blockade can intensify cognitive problems, while blockade of serotonin 5-HT2 receptors (by atypical agents) are thought to liberate dopamine and thus improve cognitive processes.

The ultimate antipsychotic agent may be one that blocks dopamine receptors in the mesolimbic area (decreasing hallucinations and delusions) and blocks serotonin 5-HT2 receptors, thus liberating dopamine in the mesocortical area (treating negative schizophrenia), while not obstructing the function of the nigrostriatal tract (that is, not causing EPSEs) or blocking receptors in the tuberoinfundibular tract (i.e., not elevating prolactin levels).

PHARMACOLOGIC EFFECTS (DESIRED EFFECTS)

Chlorpromazine and the other antipsychotic drugs are used primarily to treat psychotic disorders, specifically, schizophrenia and other chronic mental illness. Psychosis is a phenomenon of brain activity; therefore the sought-after effects of these drugs occur in the central nervous system (CNS). Tolerance to an antipsychotic effect is uncommon.

Central Nervous System Effects

CNS effects include sedation, emotional quieting, and psychomotor slowing, all of which explain the reasons that these drugs were once generally referred to as "major tranquilizers." Emotional quieting enables the patient to take advantage of other forms of therapeutic intervention, for example, the therapeutic nurse-patient relationship and the well-managed milieu.

Sedation decreases insomnia, a frequent complaint of psychotic patients. Whether this characteristic is a result of the sedating effect itself or of being "freed" from disturbing thoughts (or a combination of the two) is not fully understood. Not all antipsychotic drugs are significantly sedating. High-potency drugs are less sedating than are low-potency drugs. For example, haloperidol (Haldol) and fluphenazine (Prolixin) are not particularly sedating but are quite effective. The conclusion that the effectiveness of antipsychotic agents results from more than their tranquilizing qualities alone is reasonable.

Psychiatric Symptoms Modified by Antipsychotic Drugs

Antipsychotic drugs are most effective in treating what have been called the "positive" symptoms of schizophrenia (see Table 20-3). Positive symptoms include hallucinations and delusions. Symptoms that are less responsive to antipsychotic drugs, or "negative" symptoms, include those developed over an extended period, such as a flattened affect, verbal paucity, and a lack of drive or goal-directed activity. Referring once again to Figure 20-1, the student can infer that positive symptoms arise from too much dopamine in the limbic area (hyperactive mesolimbic tract) and that negative symptoms arise from too little dopamine in the cortex (hypoactive mesocortical tract). It stands to reason then that antipsychotic drugs that are dopamine antagonists are better at decreasing the effect of dopamine in the limbic area than they are at increasing the effect of dopamine in the cerebral cortex. Ultimately, improvement in objective and subjective or positive and negative symptoms is the measurement of progress. Psychotic symptoms associated with other mental disorders such as mania and cognitive disorders also improve with these drugs.

Alterations of perception

As a rule, the more bizarre the behavior is of a person experiencing psychotic symptoms (the more positive symptoms), the more likely that an antipsychotic drug will be beneficial. Hallucinations and illusions are reduced with these drugs. Even when the symptoms are not fully eradicated, antipsychotic drugs may enable the person to understand that hallucinations and illusions are not real, which is an improvement.

Alterations of thought

Antipsychotic drugs improve reasoning, decrease ambivalence, and decrease delusions. Because clouded reasoning, ambivalence, and delusional thoughts are frustrating and, at times, frightening, antipsychotic agents can free the patient to think more clearly and communicate better with others.

Alterations of activity

Individuals with schizophrenia are often hyperactive because of their internal turmoil and, perhaps, their neurochemical state. Antipsychotic drugs slow psychomotor activity. Low-potency drugs, such as chlorpromazine, are sedating and may be used for agitated and combative individuals.

Alterations in consciousness

Mental clouding and confusion are anxiety-producing symptoms associated with psychosis. Some mental health professionals believe these disorders are the most disabling. Antipsychotic drugs are effective in decreasing confusion and clouding.

Alterations in personal relationships

Patients with schizophrenia often have histories of social withdrawal and may have few, if any, close personal relationships. If relationships with family members exist, they are often strained. Individuals with schizophrenia may invest little effort in their appearance and may not be particularly careful about their behaviors. The combination of introspection, rumination, and self-focused speech produces ineffective communication patterns that reinforce isolation and alienation. In the give-and-take of society, individuals with schizophrenia often have little to give and, as a result, are basically socially unattractive to most people. Antipsychotic drugs enable patients to become less focused on themselves and more focused on others. The socially damaging, self-absorptive thinking experienced by patients with schizophrenia may be a result of the considerable energy they must expend to maintain some degree of equilibrium in the face of psychologic turmoil, which is similar to the way many people give less attention to their appearance or behavior during an illness. Antipsychotic drugs reduce the inner turmoil, freeing psychic energy for normal interpersonal relationships and for the therapeutic nurse-patient relationship.

Critical Thinking Question

If the positive symptoms of schizophrenia are caused by excessive bioavailability of dopamine, and if antipsychotic drugs are effective because they are dopamine antagonists, and if decreased dopamine levels contribute to EPSEs, then why do not all patients who are receiving antipsychotic drugs develop EPSEs? (Hint: review the four major dopaminergic tracts in the brain.)

Alterations of affect

Affective flattening, inappropriateness, and lability are affective symptoms sometimes associated with schizophrenia, and they often respond to antipsychotic drugs. However, a flat affect is a cardinal symptom of negative schizophrenia and may respond only to an atypical antipsychotic drug.

PHARMACOKINETICS

A pharmacokinetic discussion of each antipsychotic agent would be prohibitive. Rather, an overview of pharmacokinetics for traditional antipsychotics will

be presented. Atypical drugs will be discussed separately, and an overview of their pharmacokinetic properties will be addressed at that point.

Absorption for these drugs is variable. Peak plasma levels are seen in 1 to 6 hours. A tranquilizing effect occurs within an hour or so after ingestion. Antipsychotic effects are often observed within a few weeks with improvement continuing for up to 6 to 8 weeks or more. These drugs accumulate in fatty tissue and are released slowly, which may explain the reason that patients who abruptly stop taking their medications may continue to experience an antipsychotic effect for a while. This slow release from fatty stores may also account for noncompliance, because the patient who stops taking this medication does not experience an immediate return of symptoms. The following clinical example probably represents this phenomenon.

CLINICAL EXAMPLE

Bob, a 48-year-old military veteran with a long history of mental illness, has been taking chlorpromazine for 20 years. Over that time, the nursing staff at the Veterans' Administration hospital has gotten to know Bob well because he periodically requires hospital-based intervention. One day, Bob calls the nursing office on the psychiatric floor and tells the nurse that he believes that he can conquer his problems by using "mind over matter." He is going to stop all psychotropic medications. Bob appears to do quite well for a couple of weeks, causing some of the nursing staff to wonder about the new approach. At the end of 3 weeks, Bob is brought to the hospital in a highly disturbed psychotic state. His medication is reinstituted, and Bob's delusional thoughts subside.

Antipsychotics are highly bound (91% to 99%) plasma proteins. Physiologic changes that even slightly disrupt this level of protein-binding action may increase the percentage of free drug and potentially have a greater effect. As with most highly protein bound drugs, a greater effect may occur in older adults (who have a decline in serum proteins). Antipsychotics are metabolized in the liver by the P450 system. Half-lives are from 10 to 30 hours. Impaired hepatic function extends the half-life and effect of these drugs.

Although many traditional antipsychotic drugs are available, little documentation exists that one drug is more effective compared with another. Some patients, for example, respond to chlorpromazine, and some respond to haloperidol. Therefore the choice of antipsychotic drug is usually based on the prescriber's preference and experience, the likelihood that a certain drug will be helpful (e.g., based on the patient's previous response to a certain drug), and an educated guess about the chance of drug-induced side effects. The last factor can be used therapeutically. For instance, a patient might benefit from a drug that has a sedating effect.

Most antipsychotic drugs are available in oral and parenteral forms. Oral administration is the preferred route for a variety of reasons, including the fact that patients generally prefer this route. Tablets, however, have consistently created a problem because they are so easy to "cheek." "Cheeking" occurs when patients place the tablet to one side of the mouth and pretend to have swallowed it. Noncompliance is thought to be the single most important cause of symptom exacerbation and rehospitalization. Psychiatric patients may not want to take their medication for several reasons, including the admission of illness that taking medication may imply, paranoid fears of poisoning, or unpleasant reactions or side effects. Many inpatient units use liquid forms of antipsychotic drugs to counteract noncompliant tendencies. Liquids or concentrates usually have an unpleasant taste and should be diluted.

Parenteral drugs are usually used to treat acutely disturbed individuals or patients who represent significant compliance risks. Long-acting injectable forms are available and require injection every 2 to 4 weeks or longer. These long-acting injections are particularly beneficial for outpatients or patients who are noncompliant.

1. fluphenazine (Prolixin) decanoate
   - Usual dose range: 12.5 to 50.0 mg intramuscularly (IM)
   - Usual duration: 2 to 3 weeks
2. haloperidol (Haldol) decanoate
   - Usual dose range: 50 to 300 mg IM
   - Usual duration: 3 to 4 weeks

When a patient does not respond to antipsychotic drug therapy, the nurse's assessment of the patient may be quite helpful to the prescriber. Three principles should be kept in mind when assessing a patient's response and the possibility of changing drugs. The nurse should assess for the following:

1. Is the patient actually taking the drug?
2. Has the drug been given a fair trial (usually 3 to 6 weeks)?
3. If a change of medication is indicated, is the new agent from a different chemical class? Drugs within a class act similarly and offer no therapeutic advantage.

SIDE EFFECTS

Antipsychotic drugs produce numerous side effects because of peripheral nervous system (PNS) and CNS actions (see Table 20-1 and Box 20-2). Side effects resulting from PNS autonomic blocking (i.e., anticholinergic, antiadrenergic) actions are more likely to be caused by low-potency forms, such as chlorpromazine. EPSEs are more likely to be caused by high-potency drugs, such as haloperidol.

Anticholinergic Effects

PNS anticholinergic effects are a result of the blocking of cranial nerves (CN) with parasympathetic components. For example:
- CNIII: Oculomotor nerve blockade results in mydriasis (resulting in blurred vision) and impaired accommodation.
- CNVII: Facial nerve blockade results in dry mouth, decreased tearing, and dry nasal passage.
- CNIX: Glossopharyngeal nerve blockade results in dry mouth and dry nasal passage.
- CNX: Vagus nerve blockade results in tachycardia, constipation, and urinary hesitation.

Mydriasis can cause an increase in intraocular pressure that can aggravate narrow-angle glaucoma. Patients with a history of glaucoma or prostatic hypertrophy are not ordinarily placed on highly anticholinergic drugs. Cardiovascular disease should be carefully evaluated before being given these drugs. Antipsychotic drugs have caused sudden death related to arrhythmias and decreased cardiac output.

Antiadrenergic Effects

Hypotension is the major antiadrenergic effect of antipsychotic drugs. The blocking of alpha-1 receptors is the primary cause of hypotension. Blocking these sympathetic receptors on peripheral blood vessels prevents these vessels from responding (constricting) automatically to changes in position. Hypotension occurs most often in older adults. Hypotension often occurs when the individual stands or changes positions suddenly (orthostatic hypotension); thus precautions against falls must be instituted. In a healthy, younger person, accommodation usually occurs within 2 weeks; however, many patients cannot tolerate orthostatic hypotension for that long. Hypotension also causes a reflex tachycardia that can, in turn, cause gen-

eral cardiovascular inefficiency. A reflex tachycardia is, by definition, tachycardia that automatically occurs as an adaptive function to compensate for lower extremity vasodilation. Antipsychotic drugs are prescribed cautiously for individuals with severe hypotension, heart failure, or a history of arrhythmias.

Cardiac Effects

A growing concern among clinicians prescribing antipsychotics is that these drugs have a potential for lengthening the QT interval. Lengthening the QT interval can be associated with a fatal paroxysmal arrhythmia known as torsades de pointes (Welch, Chue, 2000). Because of this concern, electrocardiogram monitoring is becoming increasingly important.

Extrapyramidal Side Effects

The following formula traces the events that lead to rehospitalization.

EPSEs → noncompliance → relapse → rehospitalization

Hence preventing or minimizing EPSEs whenever possible is important. Estimates suggest that between 60% and 90% of all patients receiving antipsychotic medications have EPSEs (American Psychiatric Association, 1997) and, in turn, EPSEs may account for up to 50% of readmissions (Blair, Dauner, 1993). Abnormal involuntary movement disorders develop because of drug-induced imbalances between two major neurotransmitters, dopamine and acetylcholine (ACh), in specific parts of the brain. High-potency antipsychotic drugs such as haloperidol often lead to this imbalance. EPSEs can be grouped as follows: akathisia, akinesia, dystonias, tardive dyskinesia, drug-induced parkinsonism, and neuroleptic malignant syndrome. Tardive dyskinesia, a late-appearing dyskinesia, can be irreversible. Guidelines for minimizing EPSEs are found in Box 20-3.

|Box 20-2| Major Adverse Responses to Antipsychotic Drugs in Summary

Neuroleptic Malignant Syndrome (NMS)

Cause: A hypodopaminergic state
Offending agents: Typically, high-potency antipsychotics

Signs and symptoms:

Altered levels of consciousness
Autonomic hyperactivity
Hyperreflexia
Hyperthermia (up to 108)
Intense sweating
Rigidity
Elevated enzymes
Rhabdomyolysis—leading to acute myoglobinuric renal
     failure

Anticholinergic Side Effects

Cause: Blockade of cholinergic receptors (muscarinic receptors)
Offending agents: Anticholinergic drugs such as the low-potency antipsychotics and anticholinergic antiparkinson drugs

Signs and symptoms:

Blurred vision
Constipation
Decreased sweating
Diminished lacrimation
Dry mouth
Mydriasis
Tachycardia
Urinary hesitancy

EPSEs

Cause: Hypodopaminergic state
Offending agents: Typically, high-potency antipsychotics

Signs and symptoms:

Akathisia
Akinesia
Dystonia
Drug-induced parkinsonism
Tardive dyskinesia*

*Tardive dyskinesia is thought to be related to dopamine hypersensitivity rather than to the actual hypodopaminergic state.

|Box 20-3| Guidelines for Minimizing EPSEs

1. Antipsychotic drugs should not be used for nonapproved indications; for example, they should not be used to treat simple anxiety.
2. The dose for certain groups should be limited. Older adults, for instance, are especially susceptible to hypotension and TD.
3. As is the case with all drugs, but especially because of the apparent dose-EPSE relationship, the lowest effective dose of an antipsychotic drug should be given.

Akathisia

Akathisia is a subjective feeling of restlessness demonstrated by restless legs, jittery feelings, and nervous energy. Akathisia is the most common EPSE and responds poorly to treatment. Approximately 25% of patients taking traditional antipsychotics will develop akathisia. This side effect typically occurs early in treatment.

CLINICAL EXAMPLE
During a group therapy session in a state public hospital, Bill continually stands up and cannot sit down for long. The moment the group leader instructs Bill to sit down, he does so but immediately stands up again. The group leader misinterprets Bill's behavior as defiance. This misinterpretation escalates into a confrontation that culminates when Bill is forcibly restrained and given a prn injection of an antipsychotic agent.

Had the group leader been more aware of EPSEs, akathisia would have been suspected and further recognized that an antipsychotic would only make the patient worse.

Akinesia

Akinesia refers to an absence of movement; however, a slowed movement (i.e., bradykinesia) is more likely. Symptoms include weakness, fatigue, painful muscles, and anergia. Akinesia responds to anticholinergics.

Critical Thinking Question

The chapter states that low-potency antipsychotic drugs have fewer EPSEs than do high-potency drugs. Why might this be true? (Hint: The answer may be related to the type of effects that are more prominent with low-potency drugs and the kind of drugs that are used to treat EPSEs.)

Dystonia

Dystonias are abnormal postures that are caused by involuntary muscle spasms. Dystonias elicit a sustained, twisted, and contracted positioning of the limbs, trunk, neck, or mouth. Dystonias tend to appear early in treatment (within 3 days or so). Types of dystonias include:

- Torticollis—contracted positioning of the neck
- Oculogyric crisis—contracted positioning of the eyes upward
- Writer's cramp—fatigue spasms affecting a hand

- Laryngeal-pharyngeal constriction (potentially life threatening)

Dystonias respond to anticholinergic drugs, which must occasionally be given parenterally because of the gravity of the situation.

Drug-induced parkinsonism

The cardinal symptoms of Parkinson's disease (PD) include tremors, bradykinesia, and rigidity. Approximately 20% of patients receiving traditional antipsychotics develop these symptoms, typically early in treatment.

Tardive dyskinesia

Tardive means "late appearing." Tardive dyskinesia (TD) is an EPSE that tends to develop after approximately 6 months of antipsychotic therapy and is not caused by the dopamine-ACh imbalance *per se*; consequently, anticholinergics are ineffective. In fact, anticholinergics typically worsen the symptoms of TD. Chronic use of antipsychotics is thought to cause dopamine receptors in the basal ganglia to become hypersensitive. Symptoms are bothersome and can be embarrassing. Typical symptoms include tongue writhing, tongue protrusion, teeth grinding, and lip smacking. The symptoms stop with sleep. Though TD movements can be suppressed willfully for a short time, they will eventually reappear. Up to 35% of individuals on chronic traditional antipsychotic therapy will develop TD. Many times, TD is irreversible. No satisfactory pharmacologic response has been developed at this time; however, the atypical antipsychotic clozapine has been used with some success (Bassitt, Louza-Neto, 1998; Casey, 1998).

Neuroleptic malignant syndrome

Neuroleptic malignant syndrome (NMS) is a potentially lethal side effect of antipsychotic agents. Less than 1% of patients taking antipsychotics will develop this problem, but 5% to 20% of those will die without treatment (Pelonero et al, 1998). The incidence was much greater in the past, but careful scrutiny of patients by nurses and physicians has reduced both incidence and mortality. NMS occurs most often when high-potency antipsychotic drugs are prescribed. Haloperidol (Haldol) is frequently cited as the causative neuroleptic. NMS is not related to toxic drug levels and may occur after only a few doses. Typically, onset is from 3 to 9 days after initiation of an antipsychotic (Kline et al, 1989). NMS shares some symptoms with other EPSEs, including muscular rigidity, tremors, impaired ventilations, muteness, altered consciousness, and autonomic hyperactivity. Perhaps the cardinal symptom is high body temperature. Temperatures as high as 108° F (42.2° C) have been reported, although temperatures are more likely to be 101° to 103° F. Because an increased temperature is the chief sign of NMS, the nurse should monitor temperatures closely.

Dantrolene (Dantrium) and bromocriptine (Parlodel) are the drugs of choice for treating NMS and should be continued for 8 to 12 days after improvement. Antipsychotics should not be reinstituted for at least 2 weeks after complete resolution of NMS symptoms.

Endocrine Side Effects

Traditional antipsychotics elevate prolactin levels. Dopamine inhibits prolactin, and when dopamine receptors are blocked, prolactin levels rise. A number of bothersome side effects occur because of chronic prolactin elevation (Box 20-4).

Other Side Effects

Other side effects that may occur in patients taking antipsychotic drugs include hyperglycemia, jaundice, blood dyscrasias, susceptibility to hyperthermia, sun-sensitive skin (sunburn), nasal congestion, and wheezing. A non-EPSE CNS effect is memory loss. Because the cholinergic system is implicated in memory and learning, anticholinergic drugs and low-potency antipsychotic drugs may play a role in this cognitive symptom. Clozapine (Clozaril) causes agranulocytosis in 1% of patients and is potentially fatal. Agranulocytosis will be discussed later in this chapter.

NURSING IMPLICATIONS

Therapeutic versus Toxic Levels

Overdoses of antipsychotic drugs are seldom fatal, and treatment is supportive (e.g., gastric lavage to empty the stomach). Overdose can cause severe CNS depression (somnolence to coma), hypotension, and

EPSEs. Restlessness or agitation, convulsions (antipsychotic drugs lower the seizure threshold), hyperthermia, increased anticholinergic symptoms, and arrhythmias are other indicators of an overdose.

Use during Pregnancy

Antipsychotics pose few risks during pregnancy; nonetheless, they should be avoided during the first trimester (Richards, Musser, Gershon, 1999). These drugs readily pass the placental barrier, reach significant levels in the fetus, and have been documented to cause EPSEs in some newborns (Arana, Hyman, 1991).

When possible, antipsychotic drugs should be discontinued to reduce the risk of transient neonatal toxicity (Cohen, 1989).

Use in Older Adults

Because older individuals have decreased hepatic metabolism capability, reducing the dose in this age group is prudent. Furthermore, age-related nigrostriatal and cholinergic degeneration cause pharmacodynamic responses that are more intense than are those experienced by younger individuals. Older adults are also at higher risk for TD (Byne et al, 1998; Jeste et al, 1999; Woerner et al, 1998). For example, older patients have a more robust response than do younger people to the dopaminergic and cholinergic antagonism of these agents. Hence both extrapyramidal and anticholinergic effects can be heightened. Dosages equivalent to 0.5 to 2.0 mg of haloperidol (Haldol) daily are typically adequate.

Side Effects

PNS anticholinergic and antiadrenergic effects of antipsychotic drugs are troublesome but are not always as serious or as disturbing to the patient as are CNS EPSEs. The nurse can provide several specific interventions to ameliorate side effects or to prevent serious consequences (see the antipsychotic drugs side effects boxes).

Interactions

Antipsychotic drugs interact with many other drugs. Because these interactions can be serious, the nurse must review offending agents and then advise the family and patient accordingly. CNS depressants such as alcohol, antihistamines, antianxiety drugs, antidepressants, barbiturates, meperidine, and morphine have additive effects that can cause profound CNS depression.

| Box 20-4 | Consequences of Chronic Prolactin Elevation |

Sexual dysfunction
Menstrual dysfunction
Galactorrhea (seepage from breast, even in men)
Gynecomastia (enlarged breast in either sex)

Peripheral Nervous System Effects and Nursing Interventions | for Antipsychotic Drugs

Side Effects	Interventions
Peripheral Nervous System Effects	
Constipation	Encourage high dietary fiber and increased water intake; give laxatives as ordered.
Decreased sweating	Avoid exposure to extreme heat if possible.
Dry mouth	Advise patient to take sips of water frequently; provide sugarless hard candies, sugarless gum, and mouth rinses.
Nasal congestion	Give over-the-counter nasal decongestant if approved by physician.
Blurred vision	Advise patient to avoid potentially dangerous tasks. Reassure patient that normal vision typically returns in a few weeks, when tolerance to this side effect develops. Pilocarpine eye drops can be used on a short-term basis.
Mydriasis	Advise patient to report eye pain immediately.
Photophobia	Advise patient to wear sunglasses outdoors.
Hypotension or orthostatic hypotension	Ask patient to get out of bed or chair slowly. Patient should sit on the side of the bed for 1 full minute while dangling feet, then slowly rise. If hypotension is a problem, measure blood pressure before each dose is given. Observe to see whether a change to another antipsychotic agent is indicated.
Tachycardia	Tachycardia is usually a reflex response to hypotension. When intervention for hypotension (previously described) is effective, reflex tachycardia usually decreases.
Urinary retention	Encourage frequent voiding and voiding whenever the urge is present. Catheterize for residual fluids. Ask patient to monitor urine output and report output to nurse. Older men with benign prostatic hypertrophy are particularly susceptible to urinary retention.
Urinary hesitation	Provide privacy, run water in the sink, or run warm water over the perineum.
Sedation	Help patient get up early and get the day started.
Weight gain	Help patient order an appropriate diet; diet pills should not be taken.
CNS Side Effects and Nursing Interventions for Antipsychotic Drugs	
Akathisia	Be patient and reassure patient who is "jittery" that you understand the need to move. Appropriate drug interventions can help differentiate akathisia from agitation. Because akathisia is the chief cause of noncompliance with antipsychotic regimens, switching to a different class of antipsychotic drug may be necessary to achieve compliance.
Dystonias	If a severe reaction such as oculogyric crisis or torticollis occurs, give antiparkinson drug (e.g., benztropine [Cogentin]) or antihistamine (e.g., diphenhydramine [Benadryl]) immediately, as needed, and offer reassurance. More than likely, an order for IM administration will not have been written, therefore call the physician at once to obtain the order. For less severe dystonias, notify the physician when an order for an antiparkinson drug is warranted.
Drug-induced parkinsonism	Assess for three major parkinsonism symptoms (tremors, rigidity, and bradykinesia). Antiparkinson drugs will probably be indicated.
TD	Assess for signs by using the abnormal inventory movement scale (see Appendix D). Anticholinergic agents will worsen TD.
NMS	Be alert for this potentially fatal side effect. Routinely take temperatures and encourage adequate water intake among all patients on a regimen of antipsychotic drugs; routinely assess for rigidity, tremor, and similar symptoms.
Seizures	Seizures occur in approximately 1% of patients receiving antipsychotic drug treatment. Clozapine causes an even higher rate, up to 5% of patients taking 600 to 900 mg/day. If a seizure occurs, discontinuing antipsychotic may be necessary.

CNS, Central nervous system; *NMS*, neuroleptic malignant syndrome; *TD*, tardive dyskinesia.

Prescription drugs

The nurse should review prescriptions to serve as a safety net for the prescriber who might make an inadvertent error. This safety measure is also important because nurses often act as case managers or advocates for the patients who are seeing many caregivers and receiving prescriptions from multiple providers.

Nonprescription drugs

Many nonprescription drugs have potentially harmful interactive effects with antipsychotic drugs. CNS depressants such as alcohol, cold and influenza agents, and sleep aids can have additive effects. Other drugs decrease the effect of antipsychotics. For instance, antacids decrease absorption of antipsychotic drugs. Table 20-4 provides a list of some of the important interactions between antipsychotic and other drugs.

Teaching Patients

Teaching patients is an important dimension of nursing care for patients who are taking antipsychotic drugs. The nurse should use discretion in selecting the content of educational sessions because some patients have a tendency to become anxious about potential side effects. The nurse should focus on symptoms that can be seen or felt. The patient should be given a simply written description of drug benefits and side effects with instructions on ways to cope with the side effects. Having this information in a written format helps the patient and family feel more in control and therefore act as collaborators in treatment.

In addition to the education issues already mentioned, the patient and family should be taught the following:

- Avoid immersion in hot water because hypotension may occur, causing falls.

Table 20-4	Adverse Interactions of Antipsychotics with Other Drugs
Drug	Effect of Interaction
Amoxapine, fluoxetine	Increased EPSEs
Amphetamines	Decreased antipsychotic effect
Anticholinergic/ antiparkinson drugs	Increased anticholinergic effect; delayed onset of the effects of oral doses of antipsychotics; potentially increased risk of hyperthermia
Barbiturates, nonbarbiturate hypnotics	All cause respiratory depression and increase sedation; all decrease antipsychotic serum levels; hypotension
Benzodiazepines	Increased sedation; respiratory depression with lorazepam and loxapine
Beta-adrenergic blocking agents (e.g., propranolol)	Effects of either or both drugs increased
Cigarette smoking	Decreased serum levels of some antipsychotic drugs
Cimetidine	Chlorpromazine absorption decreased; increased sedation with chlorpromazine
Diazoxide	Can cause severe hyperglycemia
Dopaminergic antiparkinson drugs (e.g., levodopa)	Antagonizes the antipsychotic effect
Guanethidine	Control of hypertension is decreased
Insulin, oral hypoglycemics	Control of diabetes is weakened
L-dopa	Decreased antiparkinson effect of L-dopa; may exacerbate psychosis
Lithium	Decreases antipsychotic effect; lithium toxicity may be masked by antiemetic effect of antipsychotic drugs; increases EPSEs
Narcotics	Hypotension with chlorpromazine and meperidine; increased sedation; hypotension augmented; respiratory depression augmented
Phenytoin	May increase phenytoin toxicity; decreased antipsychotic blood serum levels
Trazodone	Additive hypotension with phenothiazines
Tricyclics	Possible ventricular arrhythmias with thioridazine; possible increased blood serum levels of both; hypotension; sedation; anticholinergic effect; increased risk of seizures

From Keltner NL, Folks DG: *Psychotropic drugs*, ed 3, St Louis, 2001, Mosby.

- Avoid abrupt withdrawal of medication because EPSEs can occur.
- Use a sunscreen to prevent sunburn and use a maximum strength variety when sunbathing.
- Take the drug as prescribed. Noncompliance is the leading cause of the return of symptoms and a leading cause of readmission (Forman, 1993).
- Immediately report signs of a sore throat, malaise, fever, or bleeding. These signs may indicate a blood dyscrasia.
- Dress appropriately in hot weather and drink plenty of water to avoid heatstroke.

Critical Thinking Questions

Clozapine remains an expensive drug and can cause fatal agranulocytosis. It is easy to say that everyone who needs clozapine should have it. Focus on the population who is most resistant to traditional drugs, as well as to the compliance problems among this population. Consider a delivery system for getting this drug to the people who need it. How can this goal be accomplished? What role can nursing play in the solution to this problem?

TRADITIONAL DRUGS BY CHEMICAL CLASS (INTRODUCED IN 1950)

This section of the chapter provides additional details about the traditional antipsychotics. Traditional antipsychotics account for only 2.9% of market sales dollars and about 20% of prescriptions (IMS, 2002). These drugs are arranged according to chemical class; however, as mentioned, thinking of them in terms of high versus low potency has more clinical utility. Although a great deal of attention is directed toward the newer atypical antipsychotics, the assumption that the older, more traditional medications are no longer useful would be incorrect. Haloperidol, for instance, is by far the most frequently prescribed traditional drug and is highly effective (IMS, 2002). Furthermore, economic considerations alone dictate that older, less-expensive drugs continue to be prescribed. For example, a month's supply of haloperidol costs less than $20, while a month's supply of olanzapine (Zyprexa) costs several hundred dollars.

Phenothiazines: Chlorpromazine, Thioridazine, Fluphenazine, Trifluoperazine

Phenothiazines are divided into three chemical subclasses: the aliphatics (chlorpromazine comes from this subclass), the piperidines (Mellaril comes from this subclass), and the piperazines (Prolixin and Stelazine come from this subclass). Within each subclass, some drugs are seldom prescribed. Only the agents that are somewhat commonly used are discussed in this text.

Chlorpromazine (Thorazine)

Chlorpromazine was the first antipsychotic developed. Chlorpromazine, available in an injection form, is a low-potency agent and thus provokes anticholinergic and antiadrenergic effects.

Thioridazine (Mellaril)

Thioridazine (Mellaril) is almost as old as is chlorpromazine and was the best-selling antipsychotic in the United States at one time (Wysowski, Baum, 1989). Some patients tend to respond to thioridazine better than they do to other drugs. Thioridazine is also used for the short-term treatment of marked depression accompanied by anxiety in adult patients, and for agitation, anxiety, depressed mood, tension, sleep disturbances, fears, and other symptoms in geriatric patients. Thioridazine has been therapeutic in children with severe behavioral problems marked by combativeness. This drug has a maximum upper limit of 800 mg per day because of the possibility of pigmentary retinopathy, which decreases visual acuity, impairs night vision, and is characterized by pigment deposits on the fundus.

Fluphenazine (Prolixin)

Fluphenazine (Prolixin), a high-potency antipsychotic, is commonly prescribed and considered to be an effective medication. Fluphenazine decanoate (Prolixin Decanoate), the long-acting form, is beneficial for patients who do not comply with a daily oral medication regimen. This injection can be given every 2 to 3 weeks.

Trifluoperazine (Stelazine)

Trifluoperazine (Stelazine) is prescribed relatively often. This drug is indicated for excessive anxiety, tension, and agitation, as well as for psychotic manifestations.

Butyrophenone: Haloperidol

Haloperidol (Haldol) is a high-potency drug (2 mg of haloperidol is equivalent to 100 mg of chlorpromazine) that tends to cause more EPSEs and fewer anticholinergic side effects than do the low-potency drugs. Haloperidol accounts for about 7% of all antipsychotic drugs prescribed (IMS, 2002) and is used extensively in older adults (because of fewer anticholinergic effects) and in pediatric psychiatry (see Chapter 42 for pediatric implications).

A problem of ongoing concern to psychiatric nurses is the threat of aggressive behavior of psychiatric patients. Chemical restraint, an unfortunate choice of words for describing psychopharmacologic intervention of this kind, is a means of relieving a patient of distressing symptoms that lead to aggressive behavior. Parenteral haloperidol alone or in combination with the benzodiazepine, lorazepam (Ativan), is an excellent approach to helping patients stay in control. These two agents can be drawn up in the same syringe and administered as a single injection.

Haloperidol decanoate, which is a long-acting form and can be given at 2- to 4-week (or longer) intervals, is particularly beneficial for individuals who struggle with compliance.

Thioxanthenes: Chlorprothixene and Thiothixene

Chlorprothixene (Taractan) and thiothixene (Navane) have different potencies. Chlorprothixene is similar in potency to that of chlorpromazine. Thiothixene is similar to haloperidol in potency. Thiothixene is prescribed more often than is chlorprothixene.

Dibenzoxazepine: Loxapine

Loxapine (Loxitane) is a moderately potent antipsychotic (approximately 10 times as potent as chlorpromazine), thus the generalizations associated with the high- versus low-potency categorizations are not as helpful. Table 20-1 reveals severe EPSEs, moderate orthostasis and sedation, and low anticholinergic side effects. Loxapine is available in capsule, concentrate, and parenteral forms. The concentrate is reportedly quite unpleasant and should be diluted with orange juice.

Loxapine is known to antagonize 5-HT2 receptors, thus fitting the profile of the atypical agents. Accordingly, loxapine is associated with better outcomes for refractory and negative type schizophrenia (Kapur et al, 1997).

Dihydroindolone: Molindone

Molindone (Moban) is also a moderate-potency drug and is approximately 10 times as potent as chlorpromazine (see Table 20-1). Molindone is used exclusively for the treatment of psychosis and provokes heavy menstruation in previously amenorrheal women.

ATYPICAL ANTIPSYCHOTICS (INTRODUCED IN 1990)

Chlorpromazine, the first antipsychotic, was developed circa 1950. Atypical agents were not marketed until 1990. During this 40-year period, hundreds of antipsychotic formulations were developed, although the drugs were not terribly different; they were all traditional or typical. Atypical antipsychotics are atypical because they work differently than do the traditional drugs and have a greater effect on negative symptoms. As previously noted and repeated here, these drugs have the following features that make them "atypical":

1. Reduced or no risk for EPSEs
2. Increased effectiveness in treating negative or cognitive symptoms or both
3. Efficacy for patients who are unresponsive to traditional antipsychotics
4. Minimal risk of TD
5. Absence of prolactin elevation and the associated side effects

Point 2 is thought to be produced by the blockade of serotonin 5-HT2 receptors, which putatively liberates dopamine in the cortex. The reasoning is as follows: if negative schizophrenia is related to reductions in dopamine in the cortex, and if atypical antipsychotics increase dopamine levels in the cortex, then this serotonin receptor-blocking property is potentially therapeutic. Whether this action is the exact mechanism is unclear (Lieberman, Tasman, 2000). Because of laboratory findings and clinical improvements, these drugs are also being described in the literature as serotonin-dopamine antagonists (SDAs). In the 12 years since their introduction, atypical drugs have totally dominated the market. Atypical antipsychotic drugs account for 97% of market sales (in dollars) and over 80% of prescriptions written (IMS, 2002). The first atypical agent to be marketed was clozapine.

Clozapine (Clozaril)

Clozapine, which was released to the retail market in 1990, was the first truly new antipsychotic agent to be introduced in the United States in 40 years. Clozapine has been referred to as the "gold standard" in the management of refractory schizophrenia (Oyemumi, 1999). Although clozapine had been used in Europe and China for some time, it was not approved in America because of the seriousness of a major side effect, agranulocytosis (i.e., an absolute neutrophil count [ANC] of less than 500/mm^3 [Novartis, 2000]). Because of this, clozapine is indicated only after severely mentally ill patients with schizophrenia have failed to respond to other antipsychotic drugs. The following summary underscores the severity of his adverse effect:

> In Finland, during the months of June and July of 1975, 9 out of 18 patients who developed clozapine-induced agranulocytosis died (Idanpaan-Heikkila et al, 1975). This alarming event sent shudders through the psychiatric community, thus clozapine was not approved in the United States for another 15 years. By the mid-1980s, studies revealed a more optimistic picture of this drug tempered by a still too high excessive morbidity rate of 1% to 2% for agranulocytosis and a mortality rate of approximately one third for those developing this blood dyscrasia (Keltner, 1997b). Currently, investigations infer a slightly lower morbidity rate of less than 1%. The mortality rate has significantly declined as well (Alvin, Lieberman, 1994). When deaths related to agranulocytosis occur, they tend to occur early in treatment (Micromedex, 2002).

In the previous discussion of the way in which antipsychotic agents work, it was noted that traditional antipsychotic drugs antagonize or block dopamine D_2 receptors. Clozapine has greater affinity for blocking dopamine D_4 and serotonin (5-HT2) receptors than it does for D_2 and other dopamine receptors (see Table 20-2). This difference in receptor affinity helps to explain the reason that clozapine was called the first truly new antipsychotic in 40 years. Nonetheless, it is still not clear if this "different" combination of receptor antagonism accounts for clozapine's effectiveness.

Clozapine also antagonizes cholinergic, alpha-1, alpha-2, and histamine H_1 receptors. As demonstrated from comparing clozapine's receptor-antagonism profile with Table 20-2, clozapine causes significant anticholinergic effects, orthostasis, sexual dysfunction, sedation, and weight gain. Sexual dysfunction and weight gain are particularly troublesome and, of course, have social implications.

Clozapine has a half-life of 4 to 12 hours, allowing once-per-day dosing. Clozapine is also 97% bound to serum proteins and is primarily metabolized by P450 1A2 and by 2D6 to a lesser extent. Nonmedical substances can affect clozapine serum levels; for example, cigarette smoking induces 1A2, causing a decreased level of clozapine (Keltner, Coffeen, Johnson, 2000a)

Critical Thinking Questions

How can traditional antipsychotic drugs have a 20% share of prescriptions written but only a 2.9% share of market sales (in dollars)? How can it be said that olanzapine has the highest market sales (in dollars) while it is said that risperidone has the most prescriptions written?

CLINICAL EXAMPLE

Fred White is a 37-year-old man who has struggled with schizophrenia since late adolescence. Because his illness was not manageable at times, he experienced several short hospitalizations. He was eventually placed involuntarily in the state hospital and was living there in 1990 when clozapine became available. After 4 months of taking clozapine, Fred was discharged from the state hospital. After 3 years, Fred's WBC count began to drop, and he was withdrawn from clozapine and placed on large doses of haloperidol. He was hospitalized "locally" on several occasions, and then, as a "last-ditch effort," the psychiatrist rechallenged Fred with clozapine after gaining approval from the manufacturer. Fred improved again but was hospitalized several months later for a decreased WBC count. Fred's presenting symptoms were sore throat (to the extent that he gave up eating and had trouble speaking), malaise, and a high temperature (103° F). He was withdrawn from clozapine again, never to be rechallenged. Today (2002), Fred remains in the state hospital.

|Box 20-5| Protocols for Clozapine Therapy

1. If baseline white blood cell (WBC) count is less than 3500/mm^3, do not start clozapine.
2. Once started, monitor the WBC count weekly.
3. If WBC levels are normal for 6 months, monitor WBC level once every other week.
4. If WBC levels drop below 3000/mm^3, or the absolute neutrophil count (ANC) is below 1500/mm^3, clozapine should be discontinued. Monitoring the WBC count and ANC should be performed daily.
5. If no sign of infection is present, clozapine therapy can be resumed once the WBC count is higher than 3000/mm^3 and the ANC is higher than 1500/mm^3.
6. If the WBC count drops below 2000/mm^3 and the ANC is below 1000/mm^3, clozapine should be permanently discontinued.

Klasco RK, editor: *USP DI® Drug information for the healthcare professional,* 2000, MICROMEDEX, Greenwood Village, Colo.

Agranulocytosis is clinically defined as an ANC below 500/mm^3 and may be caused by bone marrow suppression (Box 20-5). Because of its life-threatening potential, the manufacturer of Clozaril requires that the manufacturer or its representative closely monitor patients. Patients with an acceptable white blood count are monitored weekly for the first 6 months and then every other week thereafter.

Clozapine is associated with several other important side effects, including dose-related seizures and sialorrhea (excessive salivation). In clinical testing, up to 5% of patients who took 600 to 900 mg of clozapine per day experienced seizures. Sialorrhea occurred in 31% of the patients. Some patients carry paper cups to hold excessive saliva. Myocarditis is another significant side effect. Patients should be instructed to report dyspnea, fever, chest pain, palpitation, tachycardia, and other symptoms of heart failure immediately. Fatal overdoses (e.g., >2500 mg) have been associated with clozapine (Keck, McElroy, 2002).

Risperidone (Risperdal)

Risperidone, approved in 1994, is the most frequently prescribed antipsychotic (IMS, 2002) and is atypical yet different from clozapine. Risperidone has a greater affinity for dopamine D_2 receptors and a similar antagonism of serotonin 5-HT2 receptors compared with clozapine; thus risperidone theoretically has a favorable receptor profile for both positive and negative schizophrenia (Keltner, 1995).

Risperidone's lack of serious side effects make it a well-tolerated drug as well. Risperidone has little affinity for muscarinic (i.e., cholinergic) receptors, thus anticholinergic side effects are minimized (see Table 20-1). Nor does risperidone appear to cause agranulocytosis, EPSEs, TD, or NMS. Moreover, risperidone appears to be a safe drug, with patients surviving amounts many times higher than therapeutic doses (Brown et al, 1993). Nonetheless, risperidone significantly blocks alpha-1 and histamine H-1 receptors, resulting in orthostatic hypotension and sedation and appetite stimulation, respectively. Other side effects include insomnia (in some patients), agitation, headache, anxiety, and rhinitis.

Risperidone is readily absorbed from the gastrointestinal tract and can be given with meals. Its metabolite, 9-hydroxyrisperidone, is active. Its half-life with the active metabolite is approximately 24 hours. It is metabolized by P450 2D6 and 3A4 enzymes (Keck, McElroy, 2002). If given with other drugs metabolized by 2D6, risperidone's plasma levels increase.

A long-acting, intramuscular version (Risperdal Consta), when approved, will be the first atypical antipsychotic drug available in this formulation (www.psychiatry24x7.com. Accessed 2/15/02).

Olanzapine (Zyprexa)

Olanzapine (Zyprexa), which was released into the market in 1996, is comparable to risperidone in efficacy and side effect profile, and does not cause agranulocytosis. Olanzapine is the highest selling antipsychotic, accounting for 46% of market sales (IMS, 2002). Olanzapine blocks 5-HT2, D_2, D_1, and D_4 receptors significantly (Keltner, Coffeen, Johnson, 2000b). Olanzapine also has high affinity for cholinergic, H_1, and alpha-1 receptors, resulting in anticholinergic effects, sedation, weight gain, and orthostasis (Ganguli, 1999; Sussman, Ginsberg, 1999; Wirshing et al, 1999). Olanzapine has a broad affinity for several neurotransmitter systems now thought to be implicated in schizophrenia (Tollefson, 1997). Additionally, olanzapine appears to demonstrate regionally specific activity in the brain. Olanzapine modulates mesolimbic function without a significant effect on the extrapyramidal system (Tollefson, 1997). Moreover, olanzapine normalizes N-methyl-D-aspartate (NMDA) receptor function in the glutaminergic system, thus blocking some signs and symptoms associated with schizophrenia. Olanzapine has a favorable side effect profile, with few incidents of EPSEs. Early clinical studies indicate its efficacy in the treatment of both positive and negative symptoms. Olanzapine causes considerable weight gain in some patients, but co-administration of nizatidine (Axid) appears to reduce this tendency (NAMI, 2001).

Olanzapine has proven effective in treating acute mania (Keck, McElroy, 2002; Tohen et al, 1999) and is the only atypical FDA-approved drug for monotherapy for bipolar disorder. Pharmacokinetically, olanzapine has a relatively long half-life of 30 hours, is suitable for once-per-day dosing, and has few significant interactions. It is 93% bound to plasma proteins and metabolized via the P4501A2 and 2D6 pathways. An intramuscular formulation is available.

The following clinical example illustrates the way olanzapine has made a significant difference in one man's life.

CLINICAL EXAMPLE

Bill, a man in his early 30s, was first diagnosed with schizophrenia when he was 19 years of age. He experienced a sudden onset and was hospitalized locally five times in 6 months. In the early 90s, he was admitted to the state hospital; clozapine was prescribed within a few weeks, and he responded favorably. Bill was discharged from the hospital after 5 months to a day-treatment program and did well in that program while on a regimen of clozapine. As protocols required, he was monitored for blood work on a weekly basis and after several years experienced a drop in his WBC count. Clozapine therapy was discontinued, and olanzapine therapy was started. Bill is doing well with olanzapine. His parents have described him as being as well or better than he was before he became ill. After years in the day-treatment program and only a few months on olanzapine therapy, he was discharged and now lives on his own.

Quetiapine (Seroquel)

Quetiapine (Seroquel) was made available in 1997. Quetiapine, similar to clozapine, has a lower affinity for dopamine D_2 receptors than it does for serotonin 5-HT2 receptors (McManus et al, 1999). Quetiapine has little affinity for muscarinic cholinergic receptors, therefore few anticholinergic side effects are expected. However, quetiapine antagonizes alpha-1 receptors, which leads to orthostatic hypotension, and H-1, which leads to sedation and appetite stim-

ulation. Clinically, quetiapine is effective for both positive and negative symptoms, it provokes few EPSEs, it does not significantly increase serum prolactin levels, and it appears to improve elements of cognitive function.

Quetiapine is rapidly absorbed by the body and is 83% bound to serum proteins. Quetiapine is metabolized in the liver to more than 20 metabolites with a small amount excreted unchanged, can be given with or without food, and has a low potential for interactions with other drugs. Current formulations must be titrated slowly over a 4- to 5-day period. Anecdotal reports suggest that the effective dose range is higher than manufacturer's recommendations.

Ziprasidone (Geodon)

Ziprasidone, which is the newest atypical antipsychotic, has been found effective for both positive and negative schizophrenia (Blin, 1999). Ziprasidone acts on several neurotransmitter systems (Tandon, 1997), has a high affinity for 5-HT2 receptors and for dopamine D_2 receptors, moderately blocks the reuptake of serotonin and norepinephrine, and is an agonist for the serotonin 5-HT1A receptor. These pharmacologic properties suggest a drug that has the potential to ameliorate depression and anxiety, which are commonly associated with schizophrenia (Keck, Strakowski, McElroy, 2000). Ziprasidone causes few EPSEs, few anticholinergic side effects, and mild antihistaminic effects. Common side effects include nausea, dyspepsia, abdominal pain, constipation, somnolence, insomnia, and coryzal symptoms.

Ziprasidone appears to cause less weight gain than some other atypical agents (www.plsgroup.com. Accessed 3/16/02). Ziprasidone has been linked to potential cardiac problems related to lengthening the QT interval. Studies indicate a low potential for drug-drug interactions. An intramuscular form is in development. Absorption is increased when ziprasidone is given with food. Ziprasidone is highly bound to serum protein (99%) and has a half-life of about 7 hours (Keck, McElroy, 2002).

Critical Thinking Question

Perhaps you are caring for a person who needs medication but will not take it; for example, a patient with paranoid delusions might truly believe that you are poisoning her with the antipsychotic drug. What are your legal and ethical grounds for nursing care in this situation?

NEXT GENERATION OF ANTIPSYCHOTIC DRUGS

A new drug, aripiprazole, is expected to be available in late 2002 when the Food and Drug Administration approval is gained. Aripiprazole is referred to as a dopamine-system stabilizer (DSS). DSSs are thought to balance the dopamine systems (i.e., increase dopamine in brain areas in which dopamine is deficient and decrease dopamine in brain areas where dopamine is overactive). Aripiprazole accomplishes this because it is a partial dopamine agonist: activating where lower dopamine tone exists and inhibiting at brain sites with high dopaminergic tone (Stahl, 2001). Clinical studies suggest a very good side effect profile.

Critical Thinking Question

Some clinicians believe that, unless a patient has some level of EPSEs, the patient is not receiving enough medication. What might the rationale be for this view?

Key Concepts

1. The dopamine hypothesis of schizophrenia states that an excessive level of dopamine in the brain causes schizophrenia.
2. Antipsychotic drugs block dopamine receptors, reducing the effect of excessive availability of dopamine in the brain.
3. Antipsychotic drugs are classified in three ways that are based on chemical class, on potency, and on "typicality."
4. Desired effects of antipsychotic drugs include sedation, emotional quieting, psychomotor slowing, and the alleviation of major symptoms of schizophrenia (i.e., alterations in perceptions, thoughts, consciousness, interpersonal relationships, affect).
5. Anticholinergic side effects (e.g., dry mouth, blurred vision, constipation) and EPSEs, including akathisia, akinesia, dystonic reactions, drug-induced parkinsonism, and TD, are the major categories of side effects associated with antipsychotic drugs.
6. High-potency antipsychotic drugs, such as haloperidol (Haldol) and fluphenazine (Prolixin), tend to cause more EPSEs. Low-potency antipsychotic drugs, such as chlorpromazine (Thorazine) and thioridazine (Mellaril), tend to cause more anticholinergic side effects.

7. NMS is a serious adverse effect of antipsychotic drugs (primarily high-potency drugs).
8. Overdoses of antipsychotic drugs are seldom fatal.
9. Antipsychotic drugs interact with other CNS depressants such as alcohol, meperidine (Demerol), and morphine, thereby increasing CNS depression.
10. Patient teaching should focus on recognizing side effects and on avoiding CNS depressants.
11. The nurse should routinely assess for NMS by taking the patient's temperature and evaluating for rigidity and tremors.
12. Clozapine (Clozaril), introduced in 1990, was the first truly new antipsychotic drug in 40 years.
13. Clozapine has a greater affinity for dopamine D_1, D_4, and serotonin 5-HT$_2$ receptors, produces few EPSEs, and has had remarkable success in treatment-resistant patients.
14. Clozapine causes agranulocytosis, a potentially fatal illness, and is relatively expensive.
15. The other atypical antipsychotics are promising drugs in the treatment of schizophrenia and do not cause the life-threatening illness, agranulocytosis, associated with clozapine.
16. Weight gain can be a particularly troublesome side effect of atypical agents.

References

Alvin JM, Lieberman JA: Agranulocytosis: incidence and risk factors, *J Clin Psychiatry* 55(suppl B):137, 1994.

American Psychiatric Association: *Practice guidelines for the treatment of patients with schizophrenia,* Washington, DC, 1997, APA.

Arana GW, Hyman SE: *Handbook of psychiatric drug therapy,* ed 2, Boston, 1991, Little Brown.

Bassitt DP, Louza-Neto MR: Clozapine efficacy in tardive dyskinesia in schizophrenic patients, *Eur Arch Psychiatry Clin Neurosci* 248(4):209, 1998.

Blair DT, Dauner A: Nonneuroleptic etiologies of extrapyramidal symptoms, *Clin Nurs Specialist* 7(4):225, 1993.

Blin O: A comparative review of new antipsychotics, *Can J Psychiatry* 44:235, 1999.

Brown K et al: Overdose of risperidone, *Ann Emerg Med* 22(12):140, 1993.

Byne W et al: Tardive dyskinesia in a chronically institutionalized population of elderly schizophrenic patients: prevalence and association with cognitive impairment, *Int J Geriatr Psychiatry* 13(7):473, 1998.

Casey DE: Effects of clozapine therapy in schizophrenic individuals at risk for tardive dyskinesia, *J Clin Psychiatry* 59(suppl 3):31, 1998.

Cohen LS: Psychopharmacology: psychotropic drug use in pregnancy, *Hosp Community Psychiatry* 40:566, 1989.

Forman L: Medication: reasons and interventions for noncompliance, *J Psychosoc Nurs Ment Health Serv* 31(10):23, 1993.

Ganguli R: Newer antipsychotics versus older neuroleptics. Is weight gain still a problem? *Ther Adv Psychoses* 6:8, July, 1999.

Harris D, Keltner NL: Medication management. In Worley NK, editor: *Mental health in the community,* St Louis, 1997, Mosby.

Idanpaan-Heikkila J et al: Clozapine and agranulocytosis, *Lancet* 2:611, 1975. (letter).

IMS: *Antipsychotic market sales,* 2002, IMS.

Jeste DV et al: Conventional vs newer antipsychotics in elderly patients, *Am J Geriatr Psychiatry* 7(1):70, 1999.

Jibson MD, Tandon R: New atypical antipsychotic medications, *J Psychiatr Res* 32:215, 1998.

Kapur A et al: PET evidence that loxapine is an equipotent blocker of 5-HT2 and D$_2$ receptors: implications for the therapeutics of schizophrenia, *Am J Psychiatry* 14(11):1525, 1997.

Keck PE, McElroy SL: Clinical pharmacodynamics and pharmacokinetics of antimanic and mood-stabilizing medications, *J Clin Psychiatry* 63(suppl 4):3, 2002.

Keck PE, Pope HG, McElroy SL: Declining frequency of neuroleptic malignant syndrome in a hospital population, *Am J Psychiatry* 148:880, 1991.

Keck P, Strakowski S, McElroy S: The efficacy of atypical antipsychotics in the treatment of depressive symptoms, hostility, and suicidality in patients with schizophrenia, *J Clin Psychiatry* 61(suppl 3):4, 2000.

Keltner NL: Catastrophic consequences secondary to psychotropic drugs. Part I, *J Psychosoc Nurs Ment Health Serv* 35(4):41, 1997a.

Keltner NL: Catastrophic consequences secondary to psychotropic drugs. Part II, *J Psychosoc Nurs Ment Health Serv* 35(5):48, 1997b.

Keltner NL: Neuroreceptor function and psychopharmacologic response, *Issues in Mental Health Nursing* 21:31, 2000.

Keltner NL: Risperidone: the search for a better antipsychotic, *Perspect Psychiatr Care* 31(1):30, 1995.

Keltner NL, Coffeen H, Johnson JE: Atypical antipsychotics: part I, *Perspect Psychiatr Care* 36(4):139, 2000b.

Keltner NL, Coffeen H, Johnson JE: Atypical antipsychotics: part II, *Perspect Psychiatr Care* 36(3):101, 2000a.

Keltner NL, Folks DG: *Psychotropic drugs,* St Louis, 2001, Mosby.

Keltner NL, Hogan B, Guy DM: Dopaminergic and serotonergic receptor function in the CNS, *Perspect Psychiatr Care* 37(2):65, 2001.

Kline S et al: Serotonin syndrome versus neuroleptic malignant syndrome as a cause of death, *Clin Pharmacol* 8:510, 1989.

Land W, Salzman C: Risperidone: a novel antipsychotic medication, *Hosp Community Psychiatry* 45(5):434, 1994.

Lieberman JA, Tasman A: *Psychiatric drugs,* Philadelphia, 2000, WB Saunders.

McManus DQ et al: Quetiapine, a novel antipsychotic: experience in elderly patients with psychotic disorders, *J Clin Psychiatry* 60:292:1999.

Micromedex: *Drug information for the health care professional,* Englewood, Colo, 2002, author.

NAMI: Things to watch, *Advocate,* Summer 2001, p. 18.

Novartis: *Clozaril,* East Hanover, NJ, 2002, The author.

Oyemumi LK: Does lithium have a role in the prevention and management of clozapine-induced granulocytopenia? *Psychiatr Ann* 29:597, 1999.

Pelonero AL, Levenson JL, Pandurangi AK: Neuroleptic malignant syndrome: a review, *Psychiatr Serv* 49(9):1163, 1998.

Persing JS: Neuroleptic malignant syndrome: an overview, *S D J Med* 47(2):51, 1994.

Richards SS, Musser WS, Gershon S: *Maintenance pharmacotherapies for neuropsychiatric disorders,* Philadelphia, 1999, Brunner/Mazel.

Roberts GW, Leigh PN, Weinberger DR: *Neuropsychiatric disorders,* London, 1993, Wolfe Publishing.

Seeman P, Van Tol HH: Dopamine receptor pharmacology, *Trends Pharmacol Sci* 57(7):264, 1994.

Shalev A, Hermesh H, Munitz H: Mortality from neuroleptic malignant syndrome, *J Clin Psychiatry* 50(1):18, 1989.

Stahl SM: Dopamine system stabilizers, aripiprazole, and the next generation of antipsychotics: part I, "Goldilocks" actions at dopamine receptors, *J Clin Psychiatry* 62(11):841, 2001.

Sussman N, Ginsberg D: Effects of psychotropic drugs on weight gain, *Psychiatr Ann* 29:580, 1999.

Tandon R: Ziprasidone (Zeldox), *The decade of the brain* 8(3):13, 1997.

Tohen M et al: Olanzapine versus placebo in the treatment of acute mania, *Am J Psychiatry* 156:702, 1999.

Tollefson GD: Olanzapine (Zyprexa), *The Decade of the Brain* 8(3):7, 1997.

Welch R, Chue P: Antipsychotic agents and QT change, *J Psychiatry Neurosci* 25(2):154, 2000.

Wirshing DA et al: Novel antipsychotics: comparison of weight gain liabilities, *J Clin Psychiatry* 60:358, 1999.

Woerner MG et al: Prospective study of tardive dyskinesia in the elderly: rates and risk factors, *Am J Psychiatry* 155(11):1521, 1998.

Wysowski DK, Baum C: Antipsychotic drug use in the United States, 1976-1985, *Arch Gen Psychiatry* 46:929, 1989.

Web Sites

www.pskgroup.com: *Geodon better tolerated than Zyprexa in schizophrenia and schizoaffective disorders.* Accessed 3/16/02.

www.psychiatry24x7.com: *New data suggest long-term efficacy of risperidone.* Accessed 2/15/02.

Bibliography

Ayd FJ: The early history of modern psychopharmacology, *Neuropsychopharmacol* 5(2):71, 1991.

Bezchlibnyk-Butler KZ, Jeffries JJ: *Clinical handbook of psychotropic drugs,* Seattle, 1997, Hogrefe & Huber.

Fuller MA, Sajatovic M: Psychotropic drug information handbook, ed 3, Cleveland, 2002, American Pharmaceutical Association.

Keltner NL, Folks DG: *Psychotropic drugs,* St Louis, 2001, Mosby.

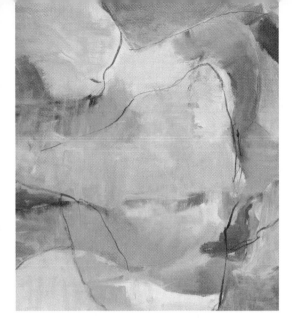

Chapter **21**

Antidepressant Drugs

Norman L. Keltner

Learning Objectives

After reading this chapter, you should be able to:
- Understand neurobiologic concepts of depression.
- Describe the differences among the three major classes of antidepressant drugs: tricyclic antidepressants, selective serotonin reuptake inhibitors, and monoamine oxidase inhibitors.
- Explain the mechanism of action of antidepressant drugs including the novel antidepressants.
- Discuss side effects of antidepressant drugs.
- Identify therapeutic versus toxic levels of tricyclic antidepressants and monoamine oxidase inhibitors.
- Describe potential interactions of antidepressant drugs.
- Discuss the implications of teaching patients about antidepressant drugs.

Antidepressants are used in the treatment of depressive and other disorders. This chapter will focus on the psychopharmacologic classes of drugs used to treat depression (Box 21-1). Complete discussion of depressive disorders is found in Chapter 29.

BIOCHEMICAL THEORY OF DEPRESSION

A number of theories exist concerning the cause of depression, but the efficacy of antidepressants is best understood from a neurochemical perspective that had its genesis 50 years ago. In the early 1950s Bein isolated reserpine from rauwolfia serpentina, a naturally occurring medicinal agent that had been used to treat hypertension (Ayd, 1991). Reserpine was found to have additional value in the treatment of psychosis, but some patients developed profound depres-

sion and became suicidal. The researchers related this action of reserpine to norepinephrine depletion. From this early linking of neurotransmitter depletion to depression, scientists began conceptualizing pharmacologic interventions. The crucial step in the development of antidepressant drugs was the synthesizing of agents that would increase the intrasynaptic availability of certain neurotransmitters, such as norepinephrine, serotonin, and possibly dopamine (Anand, Charney, 2000; Hirshfeld, 2000). A complementary view suggests that changes in receptors may be an important aspect of antidepressant activity. This point is bolstered by the observation that antidepressants require 2 to 4 weeks for a clinical response. Elevations in these neurotransmitters occur within a day of treatment initiation, whereas receptor changes take approximately 2 to 4 weeks.

233

| Treatment of Depression with Antidepressant Drugs

Indications	Mechanisms of Action	Major Side Effects	Overdose Effects
Depression • Apathy • Loss of energy • Worthlessness • Inappropriate guilt • Suicidal ideation Some antidepressants used to treat: • OCD • Panic disorder • Anxiety disorders	Increase levels of norepinephrine and serotonin	TCAs • Anticholinergic • Cardiac • Antiadrenergic • Sedation SSRIs • Sexual dysfunction • Gastrointestinal effects MAOIs • CNS hyperstimulation • Hypotension • Anticholinergic	TCAs • Overdose can be lethal SSRIs • Low potential for overdose MAOIs • Overdose can be lethal

CNS, Central nervous system; *MAOIs*, monoamine oxidase inhibitors; *OCD*, obsessive-compulsive disorder; *SSRIs*, selective serotonin reuptake inhibitors; *TCAs*, tricyclic antidepressants.

| Box 21-1 | Antidepressant Drugs Based on Traditional Classifications

Selective Serotonin Reuptake Inhibitors

citalopram (Celexa)
fluoxetine (Prozac)
fluvoxamine (Luvox)
paroxetine (Paxil)
sertraline (Zoloft)

Novel Antidepressants

bupropion (Wellbutrin, Zyban)
mirtazapine (Remeron)
nefazodone (Serzone)
reboxetine (Vestra)
trazodone (Desyrel)
venlafaxine (Effexor)

Tricyclic and Related Nonselective Cyclic Antidepressant Drugs

amitriptyline (Elavil)
amoxapine (Asendin)
desipramine (Norpramin)
doxepin (Sinequan)
imipramine (Tofranil)
maprotiline (Ludiomil)
nortriptyline (Aventyl, Pamelor)
protriptyline (Vivactil)
trimipramine (Surmontil)

Monoamine Oxidase Inhibitors

moclobemide (Manerix)
phenelzine (Nardil)
tranylcypromine (Parnate)

Psychopharmacologic treatment is based on the restoration of normal levels of these neurotransmitters. Available antidepressants achieve this goal in eight different ways (Bezchlibnyk-Butler, Jeffries, 1997; Keltner, 2000; Stahl, 1998). Although the following list may appear complex, understanding these eight mechanisms will provide a firm grasp on the way antidepressants work.

1. *Selective serotonin reuptake inhibition.* Selective serotonin reuptake inhibitors (SSRIs) selectively block the uptake of serotonin. These drugs are first-line agents for treatment of depression. SSRIs are effective and have a good side effect profile. Unfortunately, SSRIs cause significant sexual dysfunction and gastrointestinal symptoms.

2. *Selective dopamine reuptake inhibition.* Bupropion (Wellbutrin, Zyban) is the only drug in this category and is unique in two ways: it is the only antidepressant that inhibits dopamine uptake and the only one that does not affect serotonin systems. Bupropion also inhibits norepinephrine uptake and is considered a novel antidepressant.

3. *Selective norepinephrine reuptake inhibition.* Reboxetine is a new drug that selectively blocks the reuptake of norepinephrine and is considered a novel antidepressant.

4. *Variable inhibition of serotonin, norepinephrine, and dopamine uptake.* Venlafaxine (Effexor) is the only drug in this category; its inhibition activ-

Key Terms

Anticholinergic effect An effect caused by drugs that block acetylcholine receptors. Common anticholinergic effects include dry mouth, blurred vision, constipation, and urinary hesitancy.

Depression Mood disturbance characterized by feelings of sadness, despair, apathy, and discouragement caused by loss in the person's life or by neurobiologic imbalance of neurotransmitters.

Dysthymia A chronic mood disturbance characterized by a depressed mood that lasts for at least 2 years.

Monoamine oxidase An enzyme that metabolizes monoamines such as dopamine, norepinephrine, and serotonin.

Monoamines Neurotransmitters such as dopamine, norepinephrine, and serotonin.

Monoamine Oxidase Inhibitors (MAOIs) Antidepressant drugs that increase certain neurotransmitters by interfering with their metabolism.

Suicide Self-inflicted death.

Tyramine A substance derived from the amino acid, tyrosine, and found in many common foods such as aged cheeses, yogurt, and avocados (see Box 21-5). Tyramine-rich foods can cause a hypertensive crisis in a person being treated with MAOIs.

Tyrosine An amino acid that is the precursor to levodopa, dopamine, norepinephrine, and epinephrine.

Box 21-2 Antidepressant Treatment Strategies

First line agents—SSRIs, Novel antidepressants
Second line agents—TCAs
Third line agents—MAOIs, ECT

5-HT3, it produces no gastrointestinal symptoms associated with the SSRIs. Mirtazapine is considered a novel antidepressant.

7. *Nonselective inhibition of norepinephrine and serotonin.* The tricyclic antidepressants (TCAs) block the reuptake of both norepinephrine and serotonin. Some TCAs are more potent norepinephrine-uptake inhibitors and some are more potent serotonin-uptake inhibitors. Because of their nonselectivity, TCAs cause many side effects. Until the development of the SSRIs, the TCAs were the gold standard for treatment of depression.

8. *Blocking enzymatic breakdown.* The monoamine oxidase inhibitors (MAOIs) are the only antidepressants that inhibit neurotransmitter breakdown as the primary mechanism of action.

It should be noted that all but the eighth mechanism work by blocking the reuptake of neurotransmitters (Figure 21-1).

Antidepressants are not always indicated when individuals report being depressed (e.g., grief); however, when antidepressants are indicated, approximately 70% of patients respond to treatment. Technically, treatment response means the patient has experienced a 50% decline in depression severity (Gumnick, Nemeroff, 2000). These drugs do not cure depression, but long-term use has been successful in reducing symptoms. Most relapses are associated with patient-initiated tapering off or discontinuance.

TCAs have been around for some time and are still the first choice of some clinicians. However, SSRIs and the so-called novel antidepressants (Box 21-2) are the first-line agents selected by many prescribers for several reasons that are discussed later in this chapter. MAOIs are usually the last choice because of their serious side effects. Another effective treatment approach, electroconvulsive therapy (ECT), is discussed in Chapter 39. Obviously, consideration of various forms of psychotherapy and other psychotherapeutic interventions is always indicated.

---

ity is dose dependent. At lower doses, venlafaxine inhibits serotonin uptake, and as the dose level is increased, the other neurotransmitters' uptake is blocked as well. Venlafaxine is considered a novel antidepressant.

5. *Serotonin reuptake inhibition with 5-HT2 antagonism.* Nefazodone (Serzone) is similar to the SSRIs in that it selectively inhibits serotonin uptake but has the added advantage of antagonizing 5-HT2 receptors—the receptors thought to mediate sexual dysfunction, anxiety, and insomnia. Nefazodone is considered a novel antidepressant.

6. *Alpha-2 antagonism with 5-HT2 and 5-HT3 antagonism.* Mirtazapine (Remeron) increases the availability of both serotonin and norepinephrine by its antagonism of alpha-2 autoreceptors. This antagonism triggers the feedback system to increase norepinephrine and serotonin activity. By blocking 5-HT2 receptors, mirtazapine does not have the side effects associated with this receptor, and by blocking

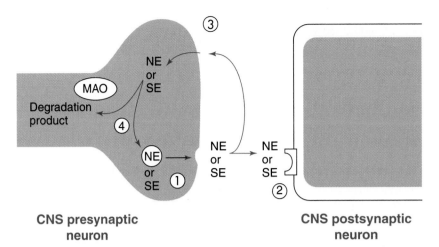

Figure 21-1 Depression results from an amine (e.g., norepinephrine, serotonin) concentration that is too low to activate sufficient receptors; mania results from overabundance of amines acting at receptors. Biogenic amine theory of depression is applied to actions of antidepressant drugs, tricyclic antidepressants (TCAs), selective serotonin reuptake inhibitors (SSRIs), and monoamine oxidase inhibitors (MAOIs), and to the action of lithium, which is used to treat mania. *1,* Lithium inhibits release of norepinephrine and serotonin; *2,* TCAs and MAOIs increase receptor sensitivity to norepinephrine and serotonin; *3,* TCAs block reuptake of norepinephrine and serotonin; SSRIs block reuptake of serotonin. Lithium enhances reuptake of norepinephrine and serotonin; *4,* MAOIs prevent degradation of norepinephrine and serotonin. *NE,* Norepinephrine; *SE,* serotonin. (From Clark J, Queener S, Karb V: *Pharmacologic basis of nursing practice,* ed 4, St Louis, 1993, Mosby.)

SELECTIVE SEROTONIN REUPTAKE INHIBITORS

SSRIs are effective antidepressants that have fewer side effects than do TCAs and MAOIs and are first-choice drugs for treatment of depression (Table 21-1, pages 238 and 239). These newer agents have fewer anticholinergic, cardiovascular, and sedating side effects. Fluoxetine (Prozac) was the first SSRI marketed in the United States. Stories of near-miraculous recoveries were followed by reports of major problems associated with this drug. Early anecdotal information, coupled with some research findings, associated fluoxetine with suicidal and homicidal behaviors. Subsequent studies indicate that fluoxetine is an effective antidepressant and that suicidal patients taking this drug (as well as other antidepressants) should be closely monitored as they become energized by fluoxetine's *activating properties.*

Critical Thinking Question

Examine Table 21-1 on pages 238 and 239. What are the factors that make SSRIs so appealing?

Pharmacologic Effect (Desired Effect)

The antidepressant effect of SSRIs is thought to be linked to their inhibition of serotonin reuptake in neurons. These drugs do not bind significantly to histaminic, cholinergic, dopaminergic, or adrenergic receptors, thus reducing many of the side effects that plague people who are taking TCAs.

Pharmacokinetics

SSRIs are absorbed in the gastrointestinal (GI) tract. Peak plasma levels are achieved for most of these drugs between 4 and 6 hours. SSRIs are metabolized in the liver and have relatively long serum half-lives. The long half-lives allow once-a-day dosing schedules. Both fluoxetine and sertraline have active metabolites that significantly extend their half-lives.

Side Effects

As previously noted, the SSRIs have relatively few anticholinergic, antihistaminic, or antiadrenergic effects; thus they do not cause the same intensity of side effects associated with TCAs. Dry mouth, blurred vision, sedation, and cardiovascular symptoms are not as common with these agents as with the TCAs; however, these side effects do occur. However, GI symptoms such as nausea, diarrhea, loose stools, and weight loss are relatively common. It is thought that activation of 5-HT3 receptors by the elevated levels of serotonin causes these GI symptoms.

Central nervous system (CNS) effects include headache, dizziness, tremors, anxiety, insomnia, decreased libido, ejaculatory delay, and decreased orgasm. Up to one third of patients prescribed SSRIs experience sexual dysfunction. Anxiety, insomnia, and sexual dysfunction are thought to be related to serotonin 5-HT2 receptor activation. Anecdotal reports from some practitioners suggest as many as 70% suffer some aspect of sexual dysfunction. Obviously, for many individuals, sexual dysfunction is a major factor in decisions about compliance. Nonetheless, because of the overall less-severe side-effect profile, SSRIs are frequently prescribed.

Interactions

SSRIs interact with several drugs (Table 21-2, page 240), and some of these interactions are related to SSRI inhibition of the P450 enzyme system. Combining SSRIs and MAOIs have proven to be fatal. This phenomenon is called the serotonin syndrome, which is discussed in Box 21-3.

Nursing Implications

Therapeutic versus toxic drug levels

SSRIs have a low potential for overdose. Even high doses have not resulted in fatalities. Toxic symptoms include nausea, vomiting, tremor, myoclonus, and irritability. Treatment is symptomatic and supportive.

Use during pregnancy

SSRIs are pregnancy category B drugs (meaning that risks to the fetus have not been established). However, these drugs should be avoided during the first trimester as a prudent precaution. The long half-lives of fluoxetine and sertraline may also be significant factors in treating the pregnant patient.

Use in older adults

SSRIs are safe for use in older adults because of the good side-effect profile of these drugs. As with most medications, SSRI dose levels should be reduced in older adults. However, older adults' potential for weight loss must be monitored. The half-life of paroxetine (Paxil) increases two or three times in older adults, thus extra precautions are warranted.

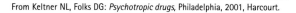

| Box 21-3 | Serotonin Syndrome

Serotonin syndrome is likely to occur if SSRI combined with the following:
- MAOIs—phenelzine, tranylcypromine
- MAOIs (selective)—selegiline, moclobemide
- Tryptophan-serotonin precursor
- St. John's wort

Signs and symptoms of serotonin syndrome (most to least frequent):
- Mental status changes, including confusion or hypomania
- Restlessness or agitation
- Myoclonus
- Hyperreflexia
- Diaphoresis
- Shivering (or shaking chills)
- Tremor
- Diarrhea, abdominal cramps, nausea
- Ataxia or incoordination
- Headaches

From Keltner NL, Folks DG: *Psychotropic drugs*, Philadelphia, 2001, Harcourt.

Sources of Drug Interactions in SSRIs and Novel Antidepressants

Competition for Protein Binding

SSRIs are highly bound to proteins, and when given with other highly bound drugs (e.g., TCAs) they compete for binding sites. This results in displacement from protein binding sites and a consequent increase in free (i.e., unbound) molecules.

Inhibition of Cytochrome P450 Enzymes

SSRIs and some novel antidepressants inhibit cytochrome P450 hepatic enzymes. Drugs metabolized by P450 enzymes can have their metabolic process slowed if given with SSRIs or nefazodone, thus leading to increased serum levels.

Individual Selective Serotonin Reuptake Inhibitors

Citalopram

Citalopram (Celexa) is the newest SSRI. Because of its pharmacologic profile (i.e., its weaker inhibition of P450 enzymes compared with other SSRIs), citalopram has fewer serious drug-drug interactions.

Fluoxetine

Fluoxetine (Prozac, Sarafem) was the first SSRI developed and is frequently prescribed. Beyond the more typical uses of fluoxetine, it is approved for the

| Table 21-1 | Comprehensive Table of Antidepressants: Dosage and Pharmacokinetics; Specificity for NT Reuptake; Receptor Antagonism; and Side-Effect Profile

	DOSAGES AND PHARMACOKINETICS			SPECIFICITY FOR NT REUPTAKE		
	Daily Dosage/ Range (mg)	Half-Life* (hrs)	Protein Binding (%)	NE	5-HT	DA
Tricyclic and related cyclic antidepressants						
amitriptyline (Elavil)	75-300	31-46	97	1	3	1
amoxapine (Asendin)	100-300	8-30	92	3	1	1
clomipramine (Anafranil)	75-300	19-37	97	1	4	1
desipramine (Norpramin)	75-300	12-24	90-95	5	1	1
doxepin (Sinequan)	75-300	8-24	90	1	2	1
imipramine (Tofranil)	75-300	11-25	89-95	2	3	1
maprotiline (Ludiomil)	25-225	27-58	88	2	1	1
nortriptyline (Pamelor, Aventyl)	50-150	18-44	92	3	2	1
protriptyline (Vivactil)	10-60	67-89	92	5	2	1
trimipramine (Surmontil)	75-300	7-30	95	1	1	1
Selective serotonin reuptake inhibitors (SSRIs)						
citalopram (Celexa)	10-60	35	80	1	3	1
fluoxetine (Prozac)	10-80	48-216	95	0	3	1
fluvoxamine (Luvox)	50-300	15-19	80	0	4	1
paroxetine (Paxil)	10-60	3-21	95	1	5	1
sertraline (Zoloft)	25-200	26-98	98	0	4	2
Novel antidepressants						
bupropion (Wellbutrin)	150-450	8-15	80	0/1	0	2
mirtazapine (Remeron)	7.5-45.0	20-40	85	1	1	0
nefazodone (Serzone)	100-600	2-4	99	0	3	1
trazodone (Desyrel)	150-600	4-9	89-95	0	2	1
venlafaxine (Effexor)	75-225	5-11	25	2	3	1
Monoamine oxidase inhibitors (MAOIs)						
Irreversible MAOIs						
phenelzine (Nardil)	30-90	2-3	—	—	—	—
tranylcypromine (Parnate)	20-60	2-3	—	—	—	—
Reversible inhibitor of MAO-A (RIMA)						
moclobemide (Manerix)	300-600	1-3	50	—	—	—

*With active metabolite.
†Scale for receptor antagonism specificity: *1*, low; *5*, high.
‡Percentage of patients experiencing side effects: *S*, <2%; *X*, >2%; *XX*, >10%; *XXX*, >30% (Bezchlibnyk-Butler and Jeffries, 1997).
NT, Neurotransmitter; *NE*, norepinephrine; *5-HT*, serotonin; *DA*, dopamine; *ACh*, acetylcholine; *H₁*, histamine; *alpha-1*, alpha adrenergic; *OH*, orthostatic hypotension.

treatment of bulimia and premenstrual dysphoric disorder (under the trade name Sarafem). Unapproved uses include pain management and smoking cessation (Bezchlibnyk-Butler, Jeffries, 1997). Fluoxetine has a long half-life of up to 9 days or more (including its active metabolite). Drugs that have a high probability for serious interactions (e.g., MAOIs) will need to be withheld for up to 5 weeks as fluoxetine is washing out of the system. Prozac is now available in once weekly formulation for long-term treatment of depression. This formulation contains a special delayed-release coating.

Fluvoxamine

Fluvoxamine (Luvox) is specifically approved for the treatment of obsessive-compulsive disorder (OCD). Fluvoxamine does not have an active metabolite and has a side-effect profile similar to that of other SSRIs.

RECEPTOR ANTAGONISM[†]			SIDE-EFFECT PROFILE (%)[†]					
ACh	H$_1$	Alpha-1	OH	Dry Mouth	Insomnia	Sedation	Seizures	Sexual Dysfunction
3	4	3	XX	XXX	X	XXX	S	X
2	3	3	XX	XXX	XX	XX	S	–
3	3	3	XX	XXX	XX	X	S	XXX
2	2	2	X	XX	XX	XX	S	X
3	5	3	XX	XXX	XX	XXX	S	X
3	3	3	XXX	XXX	XX	XX	S	XXX
2	4	3	X	XXX	S	XX	X	S
2	3	3	X	XX	S	X	S	X
3	3	2	XX	XX	XX	S	S	S
1	5	3	XX	XX	X	XXX	S	–
–	2	1	XX	XX	XX	XX	S	X
1	1	1	XX	XX	XX	XX	S	XXX
1	–	1	XX	XX	XX	XX	S	XXX
2	1	2	XX	XX	XX	XX	S	XXX
2	1	1	XX	XX	XX	XX	S	XX
1	1	1	X	XX	XX	X	X	S
1	5	2	X	XX	XX	XXX	S	X
1	1	3	XX	XX	XX	XX	S	S
–	2	3	XX	XX	XX	XXX	S	S
–	–	–	XX	XX	XX	XX	S	X
2	2	2	XX	XXX	XX	XX	S	XXX
2	2	2	XX	XX	XX	XX	–	X
2	1	2	XX	XX	XX	XX	S	S

Paroxetine

Paroxetine (Paxil) is a potent serotonin reuptake blocker and is approved for the treatment of panic attacks. Because its metabolites are not active, paroxetine has a shorter half-life and poses fewer problems than other SSRIs should the need arise to discontinue it. The most common side effect is nausea, but this effect rarely leads to dose reduction or drug discontinuation. Paroxetine has also been shown to be effective for the prevention of depressive relapse (Nemeroff, 1993). Similar to the other SSRIs, paroxetine can be given on a once-a-day basis; and similar to sertraline, paroxetine delays or inhibits orgasm.

Sertraline

Sertraline (Zoloft) is a widely marketed SSRI and was the second drug of this class to be used in the

| Table 21-2 | Significant Drug Interactions with SSRIs |

Drug	Effect of Interaction
Irreversible MAOIs	AVOID; this combination can be fatal (i.e., serotonin syndrome)
Lithium	Increased lithium levels, increased serotonergic effect
Antipsychotics	Increased EPSEs
Benzodiazepines	Increased benzodiazepine half-life
TCAs	Increased TCA serum levels → toxicity
	Displacement of TCAs from serum proteins → toxicity
Carbamazepine, phenytoin	Increased anticonvulsant serum levels

United States. Sertraline, too, can be given once a day, morning or evening, with or without food. Sertraline may delay or totally inhibit ejaculation in men and orgasm in women. Orgasmic ability returns 2 to 3 days after drug cessation.

Novel Antidepressants

Bupropion

Bupropion (Wellbutrin, Zyban)—a selective dopamine reuptake inhibitor (SDRI)—is unique in two ways: (1) it is the only antidepressant with dopamine uptake inhibition as a major mechanism of action, and (2) it does not affect serotonin systems. Bupropion has a good side-effect profile. Clinical tests indicate that orthostatic hypotension, cardiovascular conduction problems, anticholinergic effects, and daytime sedation are minimal with bupropion compared with other antidepressants. On the other hand, agitation is not uncommon because, like fluoxetine and desipramine, bupropion is an *activating* antidepressant.

Bupropion is contraindicated for patients with seizure disorders, and it lowers the seizure threshold for all patients (particularly at doses above 450 mg/day). Bupropion is thought to be more likely than are other antidepressants to cause seizures. Patients who are suffering from bulimia or anorexia should not be given bupropion because of its tendency to cause weight loss. Bupropion should not be given in combination with MAOIs, fluoxetine, or dopaminergic drugs (e.g., levodopa). Finally, bupropion has proven to be an effective replacement for,

or as an addition to, SSRIs when these drugs cause sex-related problems (e.g., decreased libido). In a general sense, it can be said that dopamine enhances sexuality (dopamine yea!!) and serotonin tends to inhibit sexual functioning (serotonin boo!!). Because bupropion increases intrasynaptic dopamine, it offsets SSRI-mediated sexual inhibition and is prescribed in low doses along with SSRIs for this reason (Keltner, 2000). Bupropion has a narrow therapeutic index but has far less lethal effects than do TCAs or MAOIs. Under the trade name Zyban, bupropion is marketed as a smoking-cessation agent. It is thought that dopamine counters the craving associated with nicotine withdrawal for smokers who have quit or who want to quit.

Reboxetine

Reboxetine (Vestra)—a selective norepinephrine reuptake inhibitor (NRI)—is a new antidepressant that selectively inhibits the reuptake of norepinephrine. It is the only antidepressant in this category. Some clinicians believe that severely depressed patients, in particular, benefit from agents that include a noradrenergic component (Frazer, 2000; Möller, 2000). Reboxetine has a half-life of 12 to 24 hours and is metabolized by P450 3A4 enzymes but does not interfere with this enzyme's activity at normal doses. Reboxetine has a low potential for drug interactions, though 3A4 inhibitors such as nefazodone may increase reboxetine plasma levels. Common side effects include typical anticholinergic effects. The starting dose for reboxetine is 4 mg twice daily with a maximum dose of 10 mg per day.

Venlafaxine

Venlafaxine (Effexor) is structurally unrelated to any currently marketed antidepressant. Venlafaxine is classified as a selective serotonin norepinephrine reuptake inhibitor (SNRI) (Stahl, 1998). Venlafaxine appears to combine the best qualities of TCAs and SSRIs in that it inhibits the reuptake of both norepinephrine and serotonin as do the TCAs and, like the SSRIs, does not bind significantly to muscarinic, histaminergic, or adrenergic receptors. Theoretically, few anticholinergic, antihistaminic, or antiadrenergic side effects should occur. Elevation in blood pressure has occurred in some patients, especially at higher dosages (e.g., 300 mg/day or more). Venlafaxine has a lower potential for drug interaction than do other antidepressants and does not exaggerate the effects of alcohol. Venlafaxine may be effective in treating SSRI-induced sexual dysfunction, OCD, and panic disorders.

Nefazodone and trazodone

Nefazodone (Serzone) and trazodone (Desyrel) are classified as serotonin reuptake inhibitors-receptor 5-HT2 blockers. Nefazodone is a first-line agent for depression and is chemically related to trazodone but is not associated with the same level of orthostatic hypotension and certain other cardiovascular effects as is trazodone. Nefazodone also does not have the same potential for priapism as does trazodone. Nefazodone is similar to the SSRIs in that it selectively inhibits the uptake of serotonin into presynaptic terminals but has the added advantage of antagonizing 5-HT2 receptors—receptors thought to mediate sexual dysfunction, anxiety, and insomnia (Keltner, 2000). This pharmacologic effect provides the advantages of SSRIs without their most troubling side effect. 5-HT2 antagonism probably causes an antimigraine effect as well, and it may be beneficial in difficult cases of schizophrenia mixed with depression (review Chapter 20, if needed, for role of 5-HT2 in schizophrenia).

Nefazodone has a good side-effect profile and does not cause insomnia, sexual dysfunction, or nervousness. However, it does now have the black box warning related to life-threatening hepatic failure (Bristol-Myers Squibb, 2002). Nefazodone is also a potent inhibitor of the P450 enzyme system, thus drugs that are metabolized by this system will have their plasma levels increased if given with nefazodone. Nefazodone has a relatively wide therapeutic index.

Trazodone enhances serotonin but not norepinephrine. Trazodone is seldom prescribed as an antidepressant anymore. It has almost no anticholinergic effects and few cardiac effects. Trazodone is a sedating drug and is often prescribed for sleep in nondepressed individuals. Trazodone's absorption is increased by 20% if it is taken immediately after a light meal. One unusual adverse reaction to this drug is *priapism* (i.e., prolonged penile erection). Surgical intervention has been required in a significant percentage of affected men. If priapism occurs, the nurse should stop the medication and notify the prescriber.

Mirtazapine

Mirtazapine (Remeron)—an alpha-2 antagonist with 5-HT2 and 5-HT3 antagonism—is the newest antidepressant and is approved for major depression only. Mirtazapine's pharmacologic effect is different from that of other antidepressants: it selectively blocks alpha-2 autoreceptors, which increases norepinephrine and serotonin by using the presynaptic feedback system; that is, blockade of alpha-2 autoreceptors signals the need for more of these neurotransmitters. Mirtazapine has a moderately high protein binding (85%) and a relatively long half-life (20 to 40 hours). Mirtazapine is not accompanied by the anticholinergic and alpha-1 antagonism associated with TCAs. Related to its antihistaminic effects, sedation is reported in over 20% of patients taking mirtazapine, and weight gain occurs in approximately 10% of patients (Bezchlibnyk-Butler, Jeffries, 1997). An increase in serum cholesterol occurs in some patients. Mirtazapine's uniqueness is attributable to its antagonism of both 5-HT2 (i.e., reducing sexual dysfunction, anxiety, and insomnia) and 5-HT3 (i.e., reducing GI distress). (Other side effects can be found in Table 21-1.) Remeron is available in an orally dissolvable form under the trade name Remeron SolTab. It dissolves on the tongue in approximately 30 seconds. Remeron SolTab is the only dissolvable antidepressant currently available.

TRICYCLIC ANTIDEPRESSANTS
Pharmacologic Effects (Desired Effects)

Theoretically, the serum level of monoamines (i.e., norepinephrine, serotonin) in the depressed person is so low that achieving a normal mood is impossible. TCAs block the reuptake of these released neurotransmitters, thereby increasing the intrasynaptic levels and alleviating the symptoms of depression.

Because reuptake terminates normal neurotransmitter activity, this "blocking" causes greater neurotransmitter availability and thus prolongs their stimulating action. As noted, clinical studies have shown that this specific effect occurs quickly; yet a lag period of 2 to 4 weeks occurs before an antidepressant effect is experienced.

TCAs can be categorized further as secondary amines or tertiary amines. Drugs that tend to increase the availability of norepinephrine more than serotonin are termed secondary amines, and drugs that tend to increase serotonin availability more than nor-epinephrine are called tertiary amines. This refinement of TCAs is not used consistently in the clinical setting. but it should be noted that secondary amines produce fewer side effects in older adults (Smith, Buckwalter, 1992).

Secondary amines (enhance norepinephrine more)	Tertiary amines (enhance serotonin more)
Amoxapine	Amitriptyline
Desipramine	Doxepin
Nortriptyline	Imipramine
Protriptyline	

Clomipramine (Anafranil), although a strong potentiator of serotonin, is not typically prescribed for depression but is a drug of choice for OCD.

Other therapeutic effects of tricyclic antidepressants

Sedation is a therapeutic effect of these drugs, because depressed patients commonly experience insomnia and agitation. Tolerance to sedation usually develops.

Lethargy is a common symptom of depression. Some TCAs, which are described as *"activating antidepressants,"* may alleviate lethargy.

Improved appetite is another effect of TCAs. Loss of appetite and a consequent loss of weight are symptoms of depression. This effect is probably related to the TCAs antihistaminic effect but may be related to improved mood. Unfortunately, weight gain can be significant and may contribute to a new set of problems.

Anxiety reduction is another positive effect of TCAs.

Urinary hesitancy, though definitely problematic for many patients, can be used therapeutically for childhood enuresis.

Pharmacokinetics and Dosing

TCAs are absorbed well from the GI tract and are usually given orally (PO). TCAs are metabolized in the liver, and some metabolites have antidepressant effects (e.g., desipramine is a metabolite of imipramine; nortriptyline is a metabolite of amitriptyline).

Peak plasma concentrations are reached in 2 to 4 hours on average; however, because of a significant first pass through the liver, only about 30% to 70% of an oral dose reaches the bloodstream (DeVane, 1986). TCAs are highly bound to plasma proteins (e.g., amitriptyline, 97%) hence their effects are the result of a small fraction of free drug. Even a small increase in free drug is potentially serious. Individuals with diminished liver function (e.g., older adults, children, alcoholics, individuals with a history of hepatitis) or those with decreased plasma protein levels (e.g., older adults) may be at special risk of elevated serum levels. People over the age of 55 are often started at one half the regular adult dose.

The relatively long half-lives of these drugs usually allow once-per-day dosing schedules. A steady state is typically reached in approximately 5 days. These drugs are initiated at low doses and increased every 3 to 5 days until the patient becomes intolerant of side effects.

All TCAs appear to be equally effective. Table 21-1 captures several important treatment parameters of antidepressants.

Side Effects

Patients taking TCAs experience undesirable side effects of both the peripheral nervous system (PNS) and the CNS. Tertiary amines have more frequent and more severe side effects than do the secondary amines or the other non-MAOI antidepressants (Gomez, Gomez, 1992).

Peripheral side effects

Anticholinergic effects

Anticholinergic effects on the peripheral autonomic nervous system range from annoying to dangerous. Dry mouth is common but not dangerous. Visual disturbances include blurred vision, dry eyes, and photosensitivity resulting from mydriasis (pupil dilation). These symptoms, too, are more annoying than they are dangerous. However, mydriatic action can precipitate an acute attack of glaucoma, particularly in individuals with undiagnosed narrow-angle glaucoma.

Other anticholinergic side effects include slowing of the GI tract that leads to constipation and slowing of bladder function that leads to urinary hesitancy or retention. Older adults are most susceptible to these side effects, and older men with benign prostatic hypertrophy are at a special risk for bladder problems. Anhidrosis (decreased sweating) impairs body cooling.

Cardiac effects

Anticholinergic effects on the cardiovascular system are common enough to warrant serious consideration. Essentially, the parasympathetic system serves as a "brake" for the heart and, when this system is blocked by anticholinergics, the brake is released, and the heart speeds up. Tachycardias and arrhythmias can lead to myocardial infarction. TCAs can also have a quinidine-like effect that delays conduction. In susceptible patients, this effect can lead to heart block. Patients with a history of heart problems must be carefully evaluated. Amitriptyline (Elavil) is considered the most cardiotoxic antidepressant and, with its high levels of sedation, anticholinergic activity, and orthostatic hypotension, is a less desirable drug in older adults (Gomez, Gomez, 1992).

Children have shown troublesome cardiovascular responses to TCAs (notably desipramine) that warrant serious consideration. Since these concerns were first noted, several deaths have occurred in children taking these drugs. In each case, sudden death, usually associated with physical activity, was the cause. The serum level may be almost 50% higher in children than it is in adults at the same dose (Bezchlibnyk-Butler, Jeffries, 1997). Children receiving these drugs must be monitored carefully (Biederman et al, 1989; Fletcher et al, 1993).

Antiadrenergic effects

These drugs also block alpha-1 adrenergic receptors on peripheral blood vessels and inhibit the body's natural vasoconstricting reaction when a person stands. A pooling of blood occurs in the lower extremities, leading to inadequate cerebral perfusion. The heart responds with a reflex tachycardia to help the body adapt. Dimming of vision, dizziness, and fainting cause a sense of loss of control and can lead to falls and serious injury. Box 21-4 provides a reference for orthostatic hypotension, a significant and disabling side effect of both antidepressant and antipsychotic drugs. Healthy individuals, however, frequently accommodate cardiovascularly, and this side effect diminishes within a few weeks. Patients with a history of heart problems must be carefully evaluated and closely monitored.

| Box 21-4 | Orthostatic Hypotension (OH) Caused by Antidepressant and Antipsychotic Drugs

Definition	On standing, the patient will experience: • Systolic blood pressure: a drop of 10-25 mm Hg • Diastolic blood pressure: a drop of 5-10 mm Hg • Heart rate: an increase of 5-20 beats/min
OH in the older adult	20% of patients >65 50% of patients >75 20% of falls attributed to OH
Risk factors	Age 65 or older Dehydration Recent immobility Fluid loss (i.e., diarrhea) Diuretics Cardiac medications
Interventions	Regularly monitor OH vital signs Caffeine Sodium chloride tablets Teach the patient to rise slowly, dangle feet before standing Teach the patient that OH is worse in the morning Teach the importance of adequate fluids Teach the patient to avoid hot showers and baths Teach the patient that symptoms decrease with time Support stockings

Adapted from McCarthy P, Snyder JC: Orthostatic hypotension: a potential side effect of psychiatric medications, *J Psychosoc Nurs Ment Health Serv* 30(8):3, 1992.

Central nervous system side effects

Sedation

Sedation is a common side effect and can be helpful because insomnia is a frequent symptom of depression. Sedation occurs because of histamine H1 antagonism.

Cognitive or psychiatric effects

Cognitive CNS effects include confusion, disorientation, delusions, agitation, hallucinations, and lowering of the seizure threshold. Blockade of cholinergic receptors accounts for many of these symptoms. These psychiatric side effects may be found in a significant number of patients treated with TCAs. The effects usually occur when serum TCA levels are elevated and most often affect older adult patients. TCAs may aggravate an existing dementia or may mimic dementia. Other potential CNS effects include anxiety, insomnia, nightmares, ataxia, and tremors. Some patients report nightmares so terrifying that they avoid sleep, even though they are sleep-deprived.

Suicide

A clear association exists between suicide and depression. In fact, most of those who commit suicide are found to have demonstrated characteristics of depression. Consequently, considerable evidence exists to support treating depressed individuals who are suicidal with antidepressants. Paradoxically, however, antidepressants can *energize* patients who have been too depressed to act on their suicidal thoughts. Therefore depressed individuals who are suicidal warrant special nursing consideration after antidepressant therapy is initiated. Activating antidepressants such as desipramine and fluoxetine may increase the likelihood of energizing a patient in this manner. Furthermore, as will be discussed later, TCAs, for the most part, are highly toxic, which means that the very drugs a patient is taking to treat depression can be used to overdose and die. TCAs account for nearly 7% of all deaths from intentional drug overdose (Zimmermann, 1997).

Trazodone, bupropion, nefazodone, and mirtazapine have a lower potential for lethal overdose than TCAs; thus these drugs may be better suited for actively suicidal patients.

Critical Thinking Question

Many people who are depressed are also suicidal. Antidepressants are effective in the treatment of depression but can also contribute to suicidal risk. In what way do each of the following variables contribute to suicide?
a. Lag time
b. Narrow therapeutic index
c. Energizing effect of some antidepressants
d. Serious interactions, particularly with MAOIs

Interactions

TCAs are metabolized primarily by P450 enzymes 2D6, 1A2, and 3A4. Several serious drug interactions occur with TCAs when drugs affecting these

same enzymes are used. Other problematic interactions may also occur. Table 21-3 outlines significant interactions.

Central nervous system depression

Increased CNS depression may occur when TCAs are taken with CNS depressants such as alcohol, anticonvulsants, antipsychotics, benzodiazepines, sedatives, and some antihypertensives (e.g., beta blockers, reserpine).

Cardiovascular and hypertensive effects

Cardiovascular arrhythmias or hypertension can occur when sympathomimetic drugs are given with TCAs. Because TCAs block the reuptake of norepinephrine, sympathomimetic agents cause an increase in norepinephrine in the synaptic cleft. Interactants to avoid include norepinephrine, dopamine, ephedrine, and phenylpropanolamine

Table 21-3	Drug Interactions with Tricyclic Antidepressants
Drug	**Effect of Interaction**
Cimetidine	Increased TCA serum levels
MAOIs	Hyperpyrexia, excitability, muscular rigidity, convulsions, fatal hypertensive crisis, mania
Sympathomimetics	Cardiac arrhythmias, hypertension
Clonidine, guanethidine	Decreased antihypertensive effect, decreased antidepressant effect
Warfarin	Increased bleeding
Barbiturates, carbamazepine, phenytoin	Decreased TCA effect
Antipsychotics	Increased extrapyramidal side effects (EPSEs), sedation, hypotension; risk of seizures; anticholinergic effect
Procainamide, quinidine	Prolongation of cardiac conduction
Anticholinergics	Increased anticholinergic effect
L-dopa	Increased agitation, tremor, and rigidity
Alcohol, anticonvulsants, benzodiazepines	Increased sedation

From Keltner NL, Folks GE: *Psychotropic drugs*, ed 3, St Louis, 2001, Mosby.

(found in many over-the-counter stimulants). MAOIs are almost always avoided. Severe reactions, including high fever, seizures, and a fatal hypertensive crisis, can occur. MAOIs are not usually prescribed unless TCAs have failed. When changing to MAOIs, the patient *must discontinue TCAs for 14 days* before the new drug is given.

TCAs block alpha-adrenergic receptors, thus compromising the effectiveness of many antihypertensives to control hypertension.

Additive anticholinergic effects

Additive anticholinergic effects can occur when TCAs are given with other anticholinergic drugs, including antipsychotic drugs, atropine, scopolamine, antiparkinson drugs, and antihistamines. Older adult patients are especially susceptible. All the PNS and CNS anticholinergic effects mentioned earlier in this chapter can be worsened.

Nursing Implications
Therapeutic versus toxic blood levels

TCAs do not produce euphoria and are not addicting; therefore the potential for abuse is not great. Overdose, however, is a real issue. TCA overdose accounts for approximately 7% of all deaths from intentional overdose (Zimmermann, 1997). The difference between a therapeutic dose and a lethal dose is small. Only three times the maximum therapeutic dose (see Table 21-1) can be lethal (Bezchlibnyk-Butler, Jeffries, 1997). For this reason, outpatients who are at risk for suicide are frequently restricted to a 7-day supply.

Toxic blood levels may result in sedation, ataxia, agitation, stupor, coma, respiratory depression, and convulsions. Exaggeration of side effects previously mentioned can also occur. Cardiovascular reactions can occur suddenly and cause acute heart failure, even several days after the overdose. Lengthening of the QRS complex (normal is 0.08 to 0.11) to greater than 0.12 is a danger sign (Bezchlibnyk-Butler, Jeffries, 1997). Furthermore, cardiovascular reactions can be "delayed"; that is, they can occur after "recovery" from overdose. For these reasons, all antidepressant overdoses should be considered serious, and the patient should be admitted to a hospital for monitoring.

The nurse should be aware of several assessment and intervention strategies when a toxic level of TCAs is suspected (see the TCA nursing interventions box).

Use during pregnancy

These drugs have not been clearly found to cause teratogenic effects but should be avoided in the first trimester. Because depressive symptoms, such as loss of appetite, can interfere with fetal development by preventing adequate fetal weight gain, antidepressants should be prescribed cautiously to pregnant women. Antidepressants are typically placed in FDA pregnancy categories B or C. During pregnancy, TCAs with low anticholinergic effects (e.g., nortriptyline, desipramine) are preferred to those with high anticholinergic effects. TCAs must be tapered off before delivery to avoid transient perinatal toxicity (Cohen, 1989). Approximately 1% of a mother's dose is excreted in breast milk (Bezchlibnyk-Butler, Jeffries, 1997).

Use in older adults

TCAs should be given in reduced doses to older adult patients. The maxim "start low and go slow" is particularly true for this population. The secondary amines (i.e., desipramine, nortriptyline, protriptyline) are preferred. Side effects previously mentioned such as cardiovascular effects, orthostatic hypotension, cognitive impairment, and all peripheral anticholinergic effects are more pronounced in this age group.

Key Nursing Interventions   for TCA Overdose

- Monitor blood pressure, heart rate and rhythm, and respirations.
- Maintain patent airway.
- ECG is recommended.
- Cathartics or gastric lavage with activated charcoal *to prevent further drug absorption* (for up to 24 hours).

- The antidote for severe TCA poisoning (anticholinergic toxicity) is physostigmine (Antilirium), an acetylcholinesterase inhibitor *(inhibits the breakdown of acetylcholine)*. Should be given only in patients with life-threatening symptoms (e.g., coma, convulsions) because of risk associated with physostigmine use.

Side Effects and Nursing Interventions | for Antidepressants

Side Effects	Interventions
Peripheral nervous system	
Dry mouth	Advise frequent sips of water, hard candies, sugarless gum.
Mydriasis	Advise wearing of sunglasses outdoors.
Diminished lacrimation	Suggest artificial tears.
Blurred vision	Caution about driving and potential for falls. Usually subsides in 1 to 2 weeks. The patient should remove objects in the house that might be tripped over (e.g., throw rugs, small tables).
Eye pain	Advise patient to report eye pain immediately, as it may indicate an acute glaucoma attack. All elderly persons should be screened for glaucoma before treatment with TCAs is initiated.
Urinary hesitancy/retention	Monitor fluid intake. Patient should be told to avoid putting off urinating. Catheterization may be needed.
Constipation	Monitor fluid and food intake. Urge patient to heed the urge to defecate. A high-fiber diet and large amounts of water (2500 to 3000 ml/day) are helpful.
Anhidrosis	Decreased sweating can lead to increased body temperature. Adequate fluids, appropriate clothing, and sensible exercise should be stressed.
Cardiovascular effects	TCAs are contraindicated during the recovery phase of myocardial infarction.
Orthostatic hypotension	See Box 21-4.
Central nervous system	
Sedation	Caution patient about driving.
Delirium or mania	Discontinue the drug and call the physician.
Suicidal patients	Observe patients closely since antidepressants may increase energy for suicide.

Side effects

Selected side effects and appropriate nursing interventions are listed in the side effects box.

Interactions

The nurse should be aware of the interactants mentioned in Table 21-2. As a general rule, individuals who are taking TCAs should avoid certain types of drugs, both prescribed and over-the-counter drugs:

- Drugs that have anticholinergic properties
- Drugs that depress the CNS
- Drugs that stimulate the CNS
- MAOIs (deaths have occurred)

A history of hypersensitivity to TCAs precludes their use. Because TCAs lower the seizure threshold, concomitant use of ECT should be considered only after careful evaluation.

Teaching patients

The nurse should discuss side effects and several important principles with patients and their families:

- A "lag period" of 2 to 4 weeks occurs before full therapeutic effects are experienced.
- Certain drugs must be avoided, including over-the-counter preparations.
- Abrupt discontinuation can cause nausea, headache, and malaise.
- Eye pain must be reported immediately, particularly in older adults, in which undiagnosed narrow-angle glaucoma can lead to an emergency situation.
- Some side effects will lessen after patients adjust to the medication.

Individual Tricyclic Antidepressants

The following are brief descriptive statements about TCAs. Only unique features of usage and side effects are mentioned here. Uses and side effects that are common to all of the drugs are not discussed nor is information that can be gleaned from tables in this chapter.

Amitriptyline

Amitriptyline (Elavil) is prescribed often but, because of its side-effect profile, is not a first-choice agent for older adults (Nakra, Grossberg, 1990). Amitriptyline is highly anticholinergic and one of the most sedating and cardiotoxic antidepressants. Amitriptyline is available in parenteral form and in a fixed-dose combination with the antipsychotic perphenazine (this combination is named Triavil).

Amoxapine

Amoxapine (Asendin), a secondary amine, is a metabolite of the antipsychotic drug loxapine and blocks dopamine receptors. As might be expected, amoxapine can cause side effects typically associated with neuroleptics (e.g., extrapyramidal side effects [EPSEs], tardive dyskinesia). Because of its potential to cause tardive dyskinesia, amoxapine should be avoided in older adults if possible (Gomez, Gomez, 1992). Amoxapine may be beneficial for patients who are both psychotic and depressed.

Desipramine

Desipramine (Norpramin) is a secondary amine and a metabolite of imipramine. Some clinicians believe desipramine to be a good choice for older adults who are depressed and are known to be sensitive to anticholinergic side effects because desipramine has relatively minor anticholinergic effects. Desipramine is an *activating antidepressant* and thus may be advantageous for apathetic, lethargic, and hypersomnic patients. Because of its aforementioned effects on cardiovascular systems of children, desipramine should be used with care in this age group. Desipramine is particularly therapeutic in the treatment of panic attacks and dysthymia (Bezchlibnyk-Butler, Jeffries, 1997).

Doxepin

Doxepin (Sinequan), which enhances the effects of serotonin, is sedating, has anticholinergic activity, and causes relatively high antianxiety effects. Doxepin has few cardiovascular effects, but orthostatic hypotension and weight gain occur in over 10% of

patients taking this drug. Doxepin may have antiulcer properties.

Imipramine

Imipramine (Tofranil) is the oldest TCA. None of the newer antidepressants have proven to be more effective. Imipramine pamoate (Tofranil-PM) is available in a single bedtime dose for adults. Imipramine, because of its anticholinergic properties, has proven effective in the treatment of childhood enuresis. Imipramine is used in the treatment of panic disorder as well. Imipramine should be used with care in children because of its cardiovascular effects.

Maprotiline

Maprotiline (Ludiomil) primarily enhances the effects of norepinephrine, has anticholinergic effects, and is sedating. Maprotiline produces a strong antianxiety effect and may be indicated in patients who present with anxiety. Maprotiline is well tolerated and poses little cardiovascular risk.

Nortriptyline

Nortriptyline (Aventyl, Pamelor), a secondary amine TCA, is preferred for individuals with a history of unfavorable responses to antidepressants because it has a good side-effect profile. Nortriptyline has a decreased tendency to cause orthostatic hypotension, so it is a good choice for older adult patients, for patients who are beset by dizziness, or for those who have a tendency to fall. Because nortriptyline is somewhat sedating and has a good side-effect profile, it is often prescribed for older adult patients who are depressed and who are agitated and suffering from insomnia. Nortriptyline is a metabolite of the tertiary amine, amitriptyline.

Protriptyline

Protriptyline (Vivactil) is a secondary amine that enhances the effects of norepinephrine much more than it does serotonin. Protriptyline produces greater incidence of tachycardia, cardiovascular problems, and orthostatic hypotension because of its *stimulating* effects. Because some depressed patients experience hypersomnia instead of insomnia, protriptyline may enable these individuals to reduce their amount of sleep. Protriptyline has significant anticholinergic effects.

MONOAMINE OXIDASE INHIBITORS

MAOIs, the third major class of antidepressants, are usually administered to hospitalized patients or to individuals who can be closely supervised. In the early 1950s, a derivative of the tuberculosis drug isoniazid was developed and was found to have mood-elevating properties (Ayd, 1991). The derivative worked by inhibiting monoamine oxidase. Better MAOIs were soon synthesized. Two of these drugs (phenelzine [Nardil] and tranylcypromine [Parnate]) have survived the test of time and are still used; they are referred to as *irreversible nonselective inhibitors* of both monoamine oxidase-A (MAO-A) and monoamine oxidase-B (MAO-B). Moclobemide (Manerix), a new MAOI, is a reversible selective inhibitor of MAO-A (or a RIMA only).

The older, irreversible MAOIs are almost always prescribed after other antidepressants have failed because of the serious adverse reactions to these drugs, especially life-threatening hypertension. However, some clinicians believe MAOIs are particularly effective in treating atypical depression (e.g., hypersomnia, excessive eating). Nonetheless, MAOIs are seldom prescribed.

Moclobemide does not seem to interact with tyramine-containing foods, therefore it lacks the serious side effects of the older MAOIs.

Pharmacologic Effects (Desired Effects)

MAOIs block monoamine oxidase, a major enzyme involved in the metabolic decomposition and inactivation of norepinephrine, serotonin, and dopamine. This enzyme inhibition lasts for 10 days in the irreversible MAOIs and 24 hours in moclobemide. The enzyme inhibition increases the levels of these neurotransmitters in the PNS and the CNS. According to the neurochemical theory of depression, depressed individuals have lower than normal amounts of these neurotransmitters available. MAOIs help to achieve the normal amounts by slowing the deactivation of these amines. This action is in contrast to the TCAs, which help achieve normal amounts by preventing the reuptake of amines by the neurons. Approximately 2 to 4 weeks is required for the antidepressant effect of MAOIs to occur; however, as is the case with the TCAs, the inhibition of monoamine oxidase occurs right away. This characteristic suggests that factors other than low levels of specific neurotransmitters are involved in depression.

Absorption, Distribution, Administration

MAOIs are well absorbed from the GI tract and are given PO; they are metabolized in the liver. Because monoamine oxidase does not decline with age, MAOIs do not present the same age-related risks associated with other drugs.

Moclobemide has a high first-pass metabolism. Age does not affect moclobemide's pharmacokinetic activities; it has modest protein binding (50%), a half-life of 1 to 3 hours, and is metabolized by P450 2D6 and 2C19 (Cozza, Armstrong, 2001).

Side Effects

MAOIs cause CNS, cardiovascular, and anticholinergic side effects. Serious, life-threatening reactions can occur when irreversible MAOIs interact with certain drugs or foods (see the following discussion on interactions).

Because MAOIs increase the availability of biogenic amines in the brain, CNS hyperstimulation may occur, causing agitation, acute anxiety attacks, restlessness, insomnia, and euphoria. In individuals thought to have quiescent schizophrenia (an unrecognized, latent form), full schizophrenic episodes have erupted. Hypomania (which is less severe compared with full mania) is a more common effect.

Hypotension is a common cardiovascular effect, resulting from the slowdown in the release of norepinephrine. Unlike the effect of TCAs, a reflex tachycardia does not occur, because other adrenergic nerves also experience the slowed release of norepinephrine, and the heart does not reflexively speed up. Hypotension, combined with failure of a compensatory increased heart rate, can lead to heart failure.

MAOIs can cause anticholinergic effects, such as dry mouth, blurred vision, urinary hesitancy, and constipation. Hepatic and hematologic dysfunctions can occur and, although rare, are potentially serious. Blood counts and liver function tests should be obtained before therapy begins.

Interactions

MAOIs have a number of serious interactions. Potentially lethal interactants include both drugs and foods.

Drug-drug interactions

The nurse should be aware of several types of drug interactions (Table 21-4):
- Those that cause hypertension (including hypertensive crisis)

| Table 21-4 | Significant Drug Interactions with Irreversible Nonselective MAOIs* |

Drugs	Effect of Interaction
Anticholinergic drugs	Compound anticholinergic response
Anesthetics (general)	Deepen CNS depression
Antihypertensive (diuretics, beta-blockers, hydralazine)	Cause hypotension
CNS depressants	Intensify CNS depression
Guanethidine, methyldopa, reserpine	Produce severe hypertension
Sympathomimetics (mixed and indirect acting): amphetamines, methylphenidate, dopamine, phenylpropanolamine (in many over-the-counter hay fever, cold, and diet medications)	Precipitate hypertensive crisis, cardiac stimulation, arrhythmias, cerebrovascular hemorrhage
Sympathomimetics (direct-acting): epinephrine, norepinephrine, isoproterenol; less likely to cause problems	Theoretically should not produce a reaction but caution is recommended
Serotonergic drugs (e.g., SSRIs)	Avoid. This combination can be fatal.

*Less severe interaction with these drugs also occur with the RIMA, moclobemide.

- Those that cause severe anticholinergic responses
- Those that can cause profound CNS depression

Sympathomimetic drugs are classified as direct-acting, indirect-acting, and mixed-acting (having both direct and indirect properties) drugs. Indirect-acting and mixed-acting sympathomimetics cause serious and sometimes fatal hypertension. Direct-acting sympathomimetics add new norepinephrine to the body, whereas indirect-acting sympathomimetics release existing norepinephrine from the neurons. Because MAOIs increase the amount of stored norepinephrine in the PNS, a potential exists for indirect-acting and mixed-acting sympathomimetics to release relatively large amounts of norepinephrine. Therefore avoiding these interacting drugs is crucial. Even small amounts can trigger a hypertensive crisis. Typical indirect-acting and mixed-acting sympathomimetics include amphetamines, cocaine, methylphenidate (Ritalin), dopa-

mine, mephentermine, and ephedrine. Over-the-counter weight-loss and stimulant products contain phenylephrine, phenylpropanolamine, and pseudo-ephedrine, which are mixed- or indirect-acting sympathomimetics. Direct-acting sympathomimetics such as norepinephrine, epinephrine, and isoproterenol, theoretically, should not trigger the release of existing norepinephrine. Moclobemide should not be combined with the irreversible MAOIs or with narcotics. Finally, MAOIs should not be given in combination with TCAs, except in unusually refractory cases, and never in combination with SSRIs.

The initial symptoms of hypertensive crisis are palpitation, tightness in the chest, stiff neck, and a throbbing, radiating headache. Extremely high blood pressure with elevation of the heart rate is common. Cardiovascular consequences have included myocardial infarction, cerebral hemorrhage, myocardial ischemia, and arrhythmias. Diaphoresis and pupillary dilation are also prominent signs.

Anticholinergic effects can be severe if other anticholinergic drugs are given with MAOIs. Typical anticholinergic side effects can be reviewed in the discussion of TCA side effects.

Finally, because MAOIs "inhibit" monoamine oxidase in the liver, some drugs, particularly CNS depressants, are not rapidly metabolized in the liver and create serum levels high enough to seriously depress the CNS.

Meperidine (Demerol) is specifically contraindicated. A marked potentiation of these drugs can occur, and deaths are documented. Hypotensive drugs are also enhanced by MAOIs. The nurse should be aware that MAOI inhibition continues for up to 10 days after tranylcypromine and phenelzine are discontinued. In other words, the potential for serious interactions continues for some time after MAOIs are discontinued.

Critical Thinking Questions

Bill took some amphetamines while taking an MAOI. Will these drugs interact? If so, what will happen? If not, why not?

Food-drug interactions

Food-drug interactions center on the amine tyramine, a decarboxylation product of tyrosine, the precursor to dopamine, norepinephrine, and epi-

Box 21-5 | Tyramine-Rich Foods to Avoid with MAOIs

Alcoholic beverages
Beer and ale
Chianti and sherry wine
Alcohol-free beer

Dairy products
All mature cheese: cheddar, blue, brie, mozzarella
Sour cream
Yogurt

Fruits and vegetables
Avocados
Bananas
Fava beans
Canned figs

Meats
Bologna
Chicken liver
Fish, dried
Liver
Meat tenderizer
Pickled herring
Salami
Sausage

Other foods
Caffeinated coffee, colas, tea (large amounts)
Chocolate
Licorice
Sauerkraut
Soy sauce
Yeast

nephrine. Tyramine is found in many foods commonly consumed in the North American diet (Box 21-5). Aged cheese, bananas, salami, and coffee are a few foods containing tyramine that must be avoided by the patient. In fact, all high-protein foods that have undergone protein breakdown by aging, fermentation, pickling, or smoking should be avoided. Hypertension and hypertensive crisis can develop from this food-drug combination.

Nursing Implications

Therapeutic versus toxic drug levels

An intensification of the effects already discussed occurs with overdose. A lethal dose of MAOIs is only 6 to 10 times the daily dose (see Table 21-1

for dosages). Careful monitoring when these medications are given is important. "Cheeking" and hoarding of these drugs can be disastrous. If MAOI overdose is indicated, the nurse should know the following:

- Emesis and gastric lavage may be helpful if performed early.
- Monitoring of vital signs is important.
- External cooling is warranted if high fever occurs.
- Hypotension should be treated in the standard manner.

Use during pregnancy

MAOIs should be avoided during the first trimester. Later use in the pregnancy is justified only when the anticipated benefit outweighs the potential risk to the fetus.

Use in older adults

MAOIs may be effective in older patients because monoamine oxidase activity increases with age (Bezchlibnyk-Butler, Jeffries, 1997). Precautions for orthostatic hypotension should, however, be observed in this age group.

Side effects

The nurse should be familiar with the common side effects of MAOIs and the appropriate nursing interventions (see the MAOIs side effects box).

Interactions and contraindications

The nurse must understand that drug-drug and food-drug interactions are serious and potentially fatal. The nurse should also know the following:

- Sympathomimetic drugs should not be combined with MAOIs.
- Foods containing tyramine must not be ingested by the patient who is taking MAOIs.

MAOIs are contraindicated in patients:

- With a history of stroke or cardiovascular disease
- With a pheochromocytoma, a tumor that secretes pressor substances (i.e., substances producing a rise in blood pressure)
- Undergoing elective surgery (because of the hypotensive potential of combining MAOIs and anesthesia)

MAOIs should not be given in combination with:

Side Effects and Nursing Interventions | for MAOIs

Side Effects	Interventions
CNS hyperstimulation	Reassure the patient. Assess for developing psychosis, hypomania, or seizures. If symptoms warrant, withhold the drug and notify the physician.
Hypotension	Monitor blood pressure frequently and intervene to prevent falls and injuries; having patient lie down may help return blood pressure to normal.
Anticholinergic effects	See antidepressant side effects for appropriate nursing interventions.
Hepatic and hematological dysfunction	Blood counts and liver function tests should be performed. If dysfunction is apparent, MAOI should be discontinued.

- Other MAOIs
- TCAs or SSRIs
- Meperidine (Demerol)

Hypertensive crisis is a major concern. If it occurs, then the nurse should:

- Discontinue MAOIs and contact the physician.
- Know that therapy to reduce the blood pressure is warranted and that phentolamine (Regitine), an alpha-adrenergic blocker, is the appropriate drug (Bezchlibnyk-Butler, Jeffries, 1997).
- Monitor vital signs.
- Have the patient walk (which will lower blood pressure somewhat).
- Manage fever by external cooling.
- Institute supportive nursing care as indicated.

Teaching patients

The nurse must be persistent in teaching patients and their families about MAOIs and their side effects. Although most of these drugs are administered in a closely supervised setting, the nurse is nonetheless responsible for educating patients. Because patients taking MAOIs can experience serious reactions to certain other drugs and foods, the nurse must clearly convey this information.

- Therapeutic effects are achieved within 2 to 4 weeks.
- Driving must be avoided if the patient is drowsy.
- Certain over-the-counter drugs should be avoided, and all of the patient's health-care providers should be aware that the patient is taking an MAOI.
- High-tyramine foods should be avoided.
- Headaches, palpitations, and stiff neck should be reported immediately.

Irreversible Monoamine Oxidase Inhibitors

Two irreversible MAOIs are used in the treatment of depression.

Phenelzine

Phenelzine (Nardil) has been found to be most effective in depressed individuals who are clinically characterized as "atypical." Phenelzine is the most sedating MAOI and has also been used as a deterrent to cocaine abuse and for panic attacks.

Tranylcypromine

Tranylcypromine (Parnate) appears most effective for severe reactive or endogenous depression. Tranylcypromine is the most stimulating MAOI and is contraindicated in patients over 60 years of age. Because of severe hypertension leading to death in some patients, the FDA banned tranylcypromine in 1961. Sharp protests by influential psychiatrists eventually led to a reversal of the FDA position (Ayd, 1991).

Reversible Inhibitor of MAO-A: Moclobemide

Moclobemide (Manerix), which is a new class of MAOI, is selective in that it inhibits only the A type of monoamine oxidase. Moclobemide's inhibition lasts only 24 hours versus 10 days for the older MAOIs; thus it is considered reversible. Age or renal function does not affect dosing. Though moclobemide does not have the classic and significant reactions to tyramine-containing foods that phenelzine and tranylcypromine have, it is still recommended that moclobemide be taken after meals to reduce potential tyramine-related responses (Bernstein, 1995; Bezchlibnyk-Butler, Jeffries, 1997). Moclobemide causes minimal hypotension, excitation, and sexual effects (Keltner, Folks, 2001).

Key Concepts

1. According to the neurochemical theory, depression is the result of a decreased availability of the neurotransmitters norepinephrine, serotonin, and possibly dopamine in the brain.

2. The three major classes of antidepressants are SSRIs, TCAs, and MAOIs. An additional major group of agents that cannot be easily categorized are known as novel antidepressants.

3. SSRIs and TCAs block the reuptake of neurotransmitters back into the nerve ending, thereby increasing their availability.

4. MAOIs slow the breakdown of these neurotransmitters by inhibiting the enzyme, monoamine oxidase, thereby increasing the availability of these neurotransmitters.

5. SSRIs have fewer anticholinergic, antihistaminic, antidopaminergic, and antiadrenergic side effects than do TCAs.

6. SSRIs are first-choice drugs for the treatment of depression.

7. SSRIs are highly bound to serum proteins and can displace other protein-bound drugs.

8. All SSRIs affect cytochrome P450 metabolizing enzymes and affect the metabolism of other drugs metabolized by this system.

9. Newer novel antidepressants include bupropion, reboxetine, venlafaxine, nefazodone, and mirtazapine. These agents are first-line agents in the treatment of depression.

10. Common side effects of TCAs (dry mouth, blurred vision, constipation, and tachycardia) are associated with their anticholinergic properties.

11. Because TCAs have a narrow therapeutic index, amounts even slightly greater than therapeutic doses can be fatal. TCAs account for approximately 7% of all deaths from intentional overdose.

12. Patients should be taught about the "lag time" of 2 to 4 weeks that is required for a full therapeutic effect to be experienced with TCAs.

13. MAOIs can cause central (stimulation), cardiovascular (hypotension), and anticholinergic system side effects.

14. Traditional irreversible nonselective MAOIs interact with several foods that contain tyramine (e.g., aged cheese, bananas, salami) and with indirect- and mixed-acting sympathomimetic drugs (e.g., amphetamines, methylphenidate [Ritalin]) to cause hypertensive crisis. Reversible inhibitors of MAO-A (RIMAs) appear to have minimal interactions with foods containing tyramine.

15. MAOIs have a lag time of approximately 2 to 4 weeks.

References

Anand A, Charney NS: Norepinephrine dysfunction in depression, *J Clin Psychiatry* 61(suppl 10):16, 2000.

Ayd FJ: The early history of modern psychopharmacology, *Neuropsychopharmacol* 5(2):71, 1991.

Bernstein JG: *Handbook of drug therapy in psychiatry,* ed 3, St Louis, 1995, Mosby.

Bezchlibnyk-Butler KZ, Jeffries JJ: *Clinical handbook of psychotropic drugs,* Seattle, 1997, Hogrefe and Huber Publishers.

Biederman J et al: A double-blind placebo-controlled study of desipramine in the treatment of ADD. II. Serum drug levels and cardiovascular findings, *J Am Acad Child Adolesc Psychiatry* 28(6):903, 1989.

Bristol-Meyers Squibb: Serzone, www.bms.com. Assessed 5/28/02.

Cohen LS: Psychotropic drug use in pregnancy, *Hosp Community Psychiatry* 40:566, 1989.

Cozza KL, Armstrong SC: *The cytochrome P450 system,* Washington, DC, 2001, American Psychiatric Publishing.

DeVane CL: Cyclic antidepressants. In Evans WE, Schentag JJ, Jusko WJ, editors: *Applied pharmacokinetics: principles of therapeutic drug monitoring,* Spokane, Wash, 1986, Applied Therapeutics.

Fletcher SE et al: Prospective study of ECG effects of imipramine in children, *J Pediatr* 12(4):652, 1993.

Frazer A: Norepinephrine involvement in antidepressant action, *J. Clin Psychiatry* 61(suppl 10):25, 2000.

Gelenberg AJ: The MAOI diet, *Biol Ther Psychiatry Newslett* 21(2):1, 1998.

Gomez GE, Gomez EA: The use of antidepressants with elderly patients, *J Psychosoc Nurs Ment Health Serv* 30(11):21, 1992.

Gumnick JF, Nemeroff CB: Problems with currently available antidepressants, *J Clin Psychiatry* 61(suppl 6): 5, 2000.

Hirshfeld RMA: History and evolution of the monoamine hypothesis of depression, *J Clin Psychiatry* 61(suppl 1):4, 2000.

Jenike MA: *Handbook of geriatric psychopharmacology,* Littleton, Mass, 1985, John Wright-PSG.

Keltner NL: Mechanisms of antidepressant action: in brief, *Perspect Psychiatr Care* 36(2):69, 2000.

Keltner NL, Folks DG: *Psychotropic drugs,* Philadelphia, 2001, Harcourt.

Meador-Woodruff JH: Psychiatric side effects of tricyclic antidepressants, *Hosp Community Psychiatry* 41:84, 1990.

Möller H-J: Are all antidepressants the same? *J Clin Psychiatry* 61(suppl 6):24, 2000.

Nakra BRS, Grossberg GT: Mood disorders. In Bienenfeld D, editor: *Verwoerdt's clinical geropsychiatry,* Baltimore, 1990, Williams & Wilkins.

Nemeroff CB: Paroxetine: an overview of the efficacy and safety of a new selective serotonin reuptake inhibitor in the treatment of depression, *J Clin Psychopharmacol* 13(6)(suppl 2):10, 1993.

News: A steep price to pay, *J Psychosoc Nurs Ment Health Serv* 36(5):10, 1998.

Shelton RC: Psychopharmacology: pharmacotherapy of panic disorder, *Hosp Community Psychiatry* 44(8):725, 1993.

Smith M, Buckwalter KC: Medication management, antidepressant drugs, and the elderly: an overview, *J Psychosoc Nurs Ment Health Serv* 30(10):30, 1992.

Stahl SM: Basic psychopharmacology of antidepressants, Part I: antidepressants have seven distinct mechanisms of action, *J Clin Psychiatry* 59(suppl 4):5, 1998.

Zimmermann PG: Tricyclic antidepressant overdose, *Am J Nurs* 97(10):39, 1997.

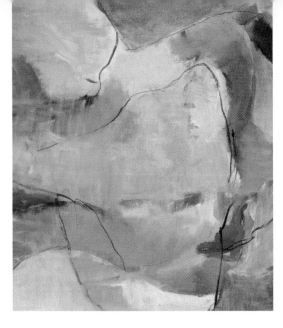

Chapter 22

Antimanic Drugs

Norman L. Keltner

Learning Objectives

After reading this chapter, you should be able to:

- Understand neurobiologic concepts of bipolar disorder.
- Explain the mechanism of action of antimanic drugs.
- Discuss the side effects of antimanic drugs.
- Identify therapeutic versus toxic serum levels of lithium.
- Describe potential interactions of antimanic drugs.
- Discuss the implications of teaching patients about antimanic drugs.

"Lithium has a unique and pivotal position in psychopharmacology. It preceded the introduction of chlorpromazine into psychiatry and in fact fired the first barrage that initiated the modern era of psychopharmacology"

(Soares, Gershon, 2000, p. 16).

Antimanic drugs are used in the treatment of mood disorders. In conceptualizing a "mood continuum," depression (dysphoria) is placed on one end and elation (euphoria or mania) on the other. Although these extremes in emotions are seemingly opposite, they are related, as previously noted. This chapter will focus on the psychopharmacologic classes of drugs used to treat bipolar disorders, the antimanic drugs (Box 22-1). Box 22-2 lists the typical signs and symptoms associated with bipolar disorder. A complete discussion of bipolar disorder is found in Chapter 30.

LITHIUM

Lithium, a naturally occurring element, is not much different from sodium. The differences, however, are significant enough to make lithium useful in treating manic depression. Lithium was discovered in 1817 by Arfwedson, who named it after the Greek word for stone. Lithium was touted as a cure for epilepsy, gout, and other problems. In 1949 an Australian, John Cade, reported his research in the *Medical Journal of Australia,* showing lithium to be effective in the treatment of manic depression. Of the manic patients he treated, 6 out of 6 demonstrated considerable improvement (Soares, Gershon, 2000). Lithium's effect was so pronounced that Cade (1949) called the illness a "lithium deficiency disease" (McIntyre et al, 2001, p. 322). In that same year, the March 12 issue of *The Journal of the American Medical Association* reported two accounts of fatal lithium poisoning in cardiac patients who were given lithium chloride as a salt substitute. These deaths sounded the death knell for lithium in this country (Ayd, 1991). Fears of lithium were compounded by a lack of interest on the part of drug companies. As a natural element, lithium is not patentable, and, consequently, a drug company might have invested research funds only to have another pharmaceutical company legally use the findings (Ayd, 1991). Lithium was not made available in the United States until 1970.

Lithium is now used for the treatment and prophylaxis of the manic phase of manic-depressive ill-

| Antimanic Drugs in the Treatment of Bipolar Disorder

Indications	Mechanisms of Action	Major Side Effects	Overdose
Acute mania Long term control or prophylaxis of bipolar disorder Augmentation of antidepressant therapy for nonbipolar depression	Alters neuronal conductances, leading to decreased release of neurotransmitters	*Lithium:* GI upset, fine postural tremor, anorexia, general weakness *Valproates:* GI upset, weight gain, transient hair loss, thrombocytopenia *Carbamazepine:* GI upset, sedation, anemia, leukopenia	*Lithium:* Has narrow therapeutic index (0.6-1.2 mEq/L) over 1.5 mEq/L is toxic *Valproates:* Restlessness, visual hallucinations are typical but deaths and coma have occurred *Carbamazepine:* Neuromuscular disturbances, irregular breathing, respiratory depression

Key Terms

Bipolar disorder A mood disorder that is characterized by one episode of manic behavior, with or without a history of episodes of depression.
Mania A condition characterized by a mood that is elevated, expansive, or irritable.

ness. At one time, 80% to 90% of patients responded to lithium, but now only approximately 50% seem to respond (Surgeon General, 1999). It is not clear why fewer patients with bipolar disorders are responding to this drug today. Additionally, a growing body of clinical research supports its use as an antidepressant, for augmentation with antidepressants in refractory depression, and for other disorders.

Pharmacologic Effects (Desired Effects)

Although the precise way that lithium achieves its normalizing effect on mania is unknown (Phiel, Klein, 2001), theories suggest that the lithium ion substitutes for the sodium ion in neurons. It has been said that the body cannot distinguish lithium from sodium. This exchange compromises the ability of the neurons to release, inactivate, and respond to neurotransmitters and facilitates the reuptake of norepinephrine and serotonin into presynaptic terminals. Figure 22-1 illustrates the basic mechanisms of action for lithium. Although this explanation simplifies what is thought to occur, it does capture the "bottom line." Lenox and Hahn (2000), after an in-depth review of lithium's mechanism of action, reduce its effect to,

| Box 22-1 | Antimanic Drugs and Dosages

Carbamazepine. Initial doses of 250 mg two or three times a day, titrated slowly to achieve serum level of 8 to 12 µg/ml
  Lithium carbonate. 600 mg three times a day; maintenance dose 300 mg three or four times a day
  Valproates. Start with 750 mg/day in divided doses; increase daily dose by 250 to 500 mg every 3 days
  Olanzapine. 15 to 45 mg/day

| Box 22-2 | Signs and Symptoms of Bipolar Disorder-Mania

Elevated mood
Increase in activities
Flight of ideas
Racing thoughts
Inflated self-esteem
Decreased need for sleep
Agitation
More talkative than is usual
Pacing, hand wringing
Extreme restlessness
Unintentional weight gain
Loses temper often
Significant irresponsible behavior
Increased goal-directed activities (e.g., sexual, social)
Impaired excessive involvement in pleasurable activities with high potential for painful consequences
Delusions
Hallucinations

What Goes Wrong in Bipolar Disorder

What is known about bipolar disorder is that individuals have specific signs and symptoms (e.g., elevated mood, grandiosity, irritability, insomnia, anorexia). What is not known is exactly what causes this disorder to happen. Thus the question remains, "What goes wrong in bipolar disorder?" El-Mallakh (1996) proposes a convincing model for the pathology of bipolar disorder, suggesting that a disruption in ion regulation is the cause. Ion regulation is important for normal mood. A key part of ion regulation is the sodium (Na) and potassium (K) activated adenosine triphosphatase (ATPase) pump. As this chapter will explore, bipolar depression and mania are related, and this model proposes a biochemical explanation.

According to this model, both bipolar depression and mania result from a decrease in Na,K-ATPase activity. As activity declines, neuronal membranes become irritable, requiring fewer stimuli to provoke cell firing. Furthermore, as Na accumulates intracellularly because of this faulty "pumping action," hyperpolarizing functions of inhibitory neurotransmitters (e.g., gamma-aminobutyric acid [GABA])

are diminished. Additionally, because neurotransmitter release is calcium dependent, the presynaptic terminals may release more neurotransmitter because of a related deficiency in Na-dependent calcium efflux.* All of these factors contribute to increased neurotransmitter release and firing—or mania.

However, the very term bipolar means two poles—the pole of mania and the pole of depression. These two poles are related. As the Na,K-ATPase pump continues to decrease in activity, neuronal irritability reaches a point that less stimulation triggers depolarization. The neuron fires more easily, but the action potential loses amplitude. Hence, this loss of amplitude causes calcium channels* to decrease their activity and a subsequent reduction in neurotransmitter release. In a nutshell, mania is the first disorder to occur when ion dysregulation occurs, but as the Na,K-ATPase pump becomes more dysfunctional, the depressive side of bipolar disorder develops. Catatonia may be the ultimate expression of ionic dysregulation (El-Mallakh, 1996).

Note to students: Calcium also enters the presynaptic terminal via voltage-regulated channels that are driven by the amplitude of the action potential. The amplitude is directly related to the amount of calcium entering the cell.

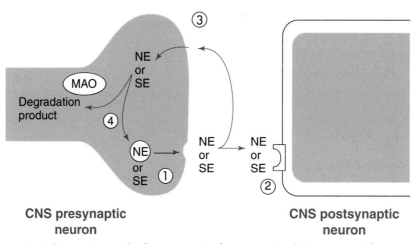

CNS presynaptic neuron

CNS postsynaptic neuron

Figure 22-1 Depression results from an amine (e.g., norepinephrine, serotonin) concentration that is too low to activate sufficient receptors; mania results from overabundance of amines acting at receptors. Biogenic amine theory of depression is applied to actions of antidepressant drugs, tricyclic antidepressants (TCAs), selective serotonin reuptake inhibitors (SSRIs), and monoamine oxidase inhibitors (MAOIs), and to the action of lithium, which is used to treat mania. *1,* Lithium inhibits release of norepinephrine and serotonin; *2,* TCAs and MAOIs increase receptor sensitivity to norepinephrine and serotonin; *3,* TCAs block reuptake of norepinephrine and serotonin; SSRIs block reuptake of serotonin. Lithium enhances reuptake of norepinephrine and serotonin; *4,* MAOIs prevent degradation of norepinephrine and serotonin. *NE,* Norepinephrine; *SE,* serotonin. (From Clark J, Queener S, Karb V: *Pharmacologic basis of nursing practice,* ed 4, St Louis, 1993, Mosby.)

"...the ability of the monovalent cation to uniquely alter signaling in critical regions of the brain" (p. 5).

Using El-Mallakh's (1996) model as an explanatory guide, the previous paragraph can be expanded. Lithium can substitute for sodium, thus normalizing Na,K-ATPase pump activity, and it increases the number of sodium pumps. The net effect is a decrease in intracellular sodium (creating a higher threshold for cell depolarization). Apparently, lithium also accelerates calcium removal from the neuronal terminal, thus normalizing calcium-dependent neurotransmitter release. The overall effect is a reduction in neurotransmitter release. If bipolar depression is viewed as a more severe manifestation of ion imbalance compared with mania, then it follows that lithium can be effective for bipolar depression as well.

Pharmacokinetics

Lithium is well absorbed from the gastrointestinal (GI) tract and is therefore given orally (PO) in tablets, capsules, or concentrate. Peak blood levels are reached in 1 to 3 hours. The kidneys excrete more than 95% of the amount ingested unchanged. Lithium is not metabolized. Hence renal disease lengthens the half-life, necessitating a reduction in dose. Lithium's typical plasma half-life is approximately 24 hours. The absorption and excretion of lithium and sodium are closely linked. Lithium is reabsorbed with sodium in the proximal tubule. Diuretics, particularly those affecting the loop of Henle and the distal tubule, lead to increased retention of lithium (Horne, Heitz, Swearingen, 1991; Trimble, 1996). If dietary sodium intake increases, plasma lithium levels will likely drop as lithium is excreted more rapidly. Conversely, if sodium in the diet decreases, or if sodium is lost in ways other than through the kidneys (e.g., sweating, diarrhea), lithium levels increase. These considerations are important because a therapeutic serum level of lithium is not much lower than a toxic serum level. Diet and activity levels should not change abruptly (Table 22-1).

Lithium is effective in about 50% of cases (Surgeon General, 1999); however, 7 to 10 days is required to achieve a clinical response. Lithium dosage is based on both clinical response and serum lithium levels. The typical dosage for acute mania is 600 mg three times per day, which usually produces a serum level of 1.0 to 1.5 mEq/L. Desirable maintenance blood levels are 0.6 to 1.2 mEq/L and can be maintained on 900 to 1200 mg per day. Blood levels over 1.5 mEq/L can be toxic.

Side Effects

Lithium's side effects are linked to serum blood levels. Blood levels over 1.5 mEq/L can be considered toxic. Common side effects are nausea, dry mouth, diarrhea, and thirst. Drowsiness, mild hand tremor, polyuria, weight gain, a bloated feeling, sleeplessness, and lightheadedness are other relatively common side effects. Polyuria and polydipsia occur in approximately 70% of patients taking lithium (Martin, 1993). These effects occur at therapeutic levels but usually cease after the sixth week. However, these same side effects increase in severity at toxic serum levels.

Side effects unrelated to serum levels include weight gain, a metallic taste, headache, edema of the hands and ankles, and pruritus. Even at therapeutic levels, lithium can affect thyroid gland function. Approximately 3% of patients develop hypothyroidism. Some patients may require a thyroid hormone. Lithium may also impair the mental or physical abilities required for driving.

Lithium is generally contraindicated in people with cardiovascular disease. Lithium may also harm the fetus and is a U.S. Food and Drug Administration (FDA) category D drug (evidence of fetal risk has been established). Adverse reactions to toxic blood levels are discussed later. Lithium therapy is contraindicated for individuals with renal disease; if lithium is necessary, close supervision of these patients is recommended. Lithium-induced renal insufficiency (creatinine level consistently over 2 mg/100 ml) is

| Table 22-1 | Pharmacokinetics of Antimanic Agents

Drug	Absorption	Protein Binding	Active Metabolites	Half-Life
Lithium	100%	0%	None	24 hours
Depakote	100%	Up to 95%	Many	6-16 hours
Olanzapine	>99%	93%	None	30 hours

Adapted from Keck PE: Pharmacokinetics and pharmacodynamics of antimanic and mood-stabilizing agents, *J Clin Psychiatry Visuals* 4(1):1, 2002.

apparently uncommon (Gitlin, 1993). However, polyuria and diabetes insipidus are present in 12% to 20% of patients taking lithium (Martin, 1993). Nephrogenic diabetes insipidus is caused by inhibition of the action of antidiuretic hormone (ADH) on the distal tubule and collecting duct cells. When ADH is blocked, the patient experiences polyuria (defined as urinating in excess of 3 L per day). The following clinical example highlights nephrogenic diabetes insipidus and the attempts to treat it.

Critical Thinking Question

If a person taking lithium suffers from serious diarrhea, what will happen to the person's serum level?

CLINICAL EXAMPLE

Mr. Jones, a 67-year-old man on the geropsychiatric unit, drinks approximately 4 L of water per day. He urinates more than 3 L per day. His creatinine level is 2 mg/dL. Mr. Jones is diagnosed with nephrogenic diabetes insipidus related to long-term lithium treatment. His potassium level is 3 mEq/L. He complains of shakiness, tremors, weakness, and general malaise. He is on daily fluid balance profiles. Treatment follows a stepwise approach:

1. Lithium is discontinued.
2. Potassium supplement is started.
3. Amiloride (Midamor) is begun to enhance ADH activity.

Interactions

Familiarity with the drugs that can elevate lithium serum levels is essential. Diuretics (except acetazolamide) decrease lithium excretion and thereby elevate serum lithium levels. Indomethacin and other nonsteroidal antiinflammatory drugs reduce renal elimination of lithium, thereby increasing serum lithium levels. Switching to a low-salt diet after treatment begins also elevates serum lithium levels.

Some drugs decrease serum lithium levels and pose the problem of inadequate treatment and symptom exacerbation. Drugs that increase lithium excretion include acetazolamide (Diamox), caffeine, and alcohol.

Combining lithium with antipsychotic drugs or benzodiazepines is not uncommon. These drugs are ordered with lithium because of lithium's clinical-

response lag time of 1 to 2 weeks. Antipsychotic agents are prescribed to produce a neuroleptic effect until the lithium produces a clinical response. A potential problem with this combination is that the antiemetic properties of the antipsychotic mask early signs of lithium toxicity—nausea and vomiting. A second concern centers on the specific combination of lithium and haloperidol. Some studies report a significantly higher percentage of neurotoxicity with this combination.

Lithium also prolongs the paralyzing effect of neuromuscular blocking agents given before surgery and electroconvulsive therapy (ECT). Apnea and oxygen deprivation can be avoided if appropriate steps are taken (e.g., extra oxygenation).

Nursing Implications
Therapeutic versus toxic drug levels

Therapeutic serum lithium levels are 0.6 to 1.2 mEq/L. The optimal maintenance level is approximately 0.8 mEq/L (McIntyre et al, 2001). Serum levels above 1.5 mEq/L can cause adverse reactions. Typically, the higher serum levels correspond directly to the severity of the reaction. Mild-to-moderate toxic reactions occur at levels from 1.5 to 2.0 mEq/L, and moderate to severe reactions occur at 2.0 to 3.0 mEq/L. Diarrhea, vomiting, drowsiness, muscular weakness, and lack of coordination can be early signs of lithium toxicity. At higher levels (i.e., 2.0 to 3.0 mEq/L), ataxia, giddiness, tinnitus, blurred vision, and large output of dilute urine may be observed. At serum levels above 3 mEq/L, multiple organs and organ systems may be involved, leading to coma and death (Sugarman, 1984). Levels above 4 mEq/L are associated with poor outcomes. Serum levels should be monitored and not allowed to exceed 2 mEq/L.

No antidote is available for lithium poisoning. Discontinuing the drug may be enough when supportive nursing care is available. Gastric lavage has been used successfully. Parenteral normal saline may provide enough volume and sodium to prevent major problems for serum levels below 2.5 mEq/L. For severe lithium poisoning, forced diuresis or hemodialysis may be needed.

Use during pregnancy

Treating bipolar disorder during pregnancy is difficult. There are no good drug treatment alternatives. Cessation of lithium during pregnancy is suggested

Key Nursing Interventions for Patients Taking Lithium

- Prepare the patient for expected side effects without instilling anxiety.
- Discuss the side effects that should subside (e.g., nausea, dry mouth, diarrhea, thirst, mild hand tremor, weight gain, bloatedness, insomnia, light-headedness).
- Identify the side effects that require immediate notification of the physician (e.g., vomiting, severe tremor, sedation, muscle weakness, vertigo).

- Suggest taking lithium with meals to reduce nausea.
- Suggest drinking 10 to 12 glasses of water per day to reduce thirst and maintain normal fluid balance.
- Advise the patient to elevate feet to relieve ankle edema.
- Advise the patient to maintain a consistent dietary Na intake, but to increase Na if a major increase in perspiration occurs.

because of fetal cardiovascular malformation when lithium is taken in the first trimester and of neonatal toxicity if taken thereafter. The occurrence of major congenital abnormalities for lithium-taking mothers is 4% to 12% and 2% to 4% for pregnant women taking the anticonvulsant alternatives. The risk of congenital abnormalities in the general population is 2% to 4% (Fact Sheet, 1998). Lithium is present in breast milk at 30% to 100% of mother's serum level; therefore postnatal treatment also poses problems (Bezchlibnyk-Butler, Jeffries, 1997).

Use in older adults

Older adult patients can benefit from lithium; but, because of the severity of side effects and adverse reactions, these patients must be assessed for renal function and dietary history. Most of the lithium-induced reactions are more likely in this age group. Serum levels of 0.4 to 0.8 mEq/L are appropriate for older patients.

Side effects

Because lithium has a narrow therapeutic index, serum lithium levels should be determined frequently. Daily levels are not uncommon in some acute treatment units. After the patient is stabilized, monthly or even less frequent serum level determinations are usually adequate. Blood levels are usually drawn before the first dose in the morning (usually 8 to 14 hours after the last dose). However, the nurse should not rely on laboratory tests alone and should continue clinical evaluation of the patient. (See the lithium nursing interventions box.)

Interactions

The nurse should help patients understand the basic mechanisms affecting serum lithium levels. Drug interactions that increase or decrease serum levels

should be reviewed. The nurse must impress on all patients the necessity for alerting all other health care providers to the lithium treatment, even though some patients may be reluctant to do so.

Teaching patients

The nurse should teach patients and their families the following:

- Symptoms of minor toxicity, which include vomiting, diarrhea, drowsiness, muscular weakness, and lack of coordination
- Symptoms of major toxicity, which include giddiness, tinnitus, blurred vision, and dilute urine
- Side effects associated with lithium and the proper time to notify the physician (Box 22-3 provides a complete list of patient guidelines for taking lithium.)
- To avoid conception, because lithium may harm the fetus
- To avoid driving until stabilized on the lithium

Critical Thinking Question

Johnny is a good basketball player. He is 23 years of age and is taking lithium. Because Johnny perspires a great deal on the days he plays (approximately four times per week), his nurse is concerned about his serum levels being consistent. What is this nurse considering?

ALTERNATIVES TO LITHIUM: VALPROATES, CARBAMAZEPINE, AND OLANZAPINE

Although lithium is often the first drug prescribed for bipolar disorder, only about 50% of patients respond to it today (Surgeon General, 1999). Approximately 80% of all individuals diagnosed with bipolar disorder will have one or more subse-

|Box 22-3| Patient Guidelines for Taking Lithium

To achieve a therapeutic effect and prevent lithium toxicity, patients taking lithium should be advised of the following:
1. Lithium must be taken on a regular basis, preferably at the same time daily. For example, a patient taking lithium on a three-times-daily schedule, and who forgets a dose, should wait until the next scheduled time to take the lithium, but should not take twice the amount at that time, because lithium toxicity could occur.
2. When lithium treatment is initiated, mild side effects such as a fine hand tremor, increased thirst and urination, nausea, anorexia, and diarrhea or constipation may develop. Most of the mild side effects are transient and do not represent lithium toxicity. Additionally, in some patients taking lithium, some foods such as celery and butter fat will have an unappealing taste.
3. Serious side effects of lithium that necessitate its discontinuance include vomiting, extreme hand tremor, seda-
tion, muscle weakness, and vertigo. The prescribing physician should be notified immediately if any of these side effects occur.
4. Lithium and Na are eliminated from the body through the kidneys. An increase in salt intake increases lithium elimination, and a decrease in salt intake decreases lithium elimination. Thus the patient must maintain a balanced diet and salt intake. The patient should consult with the prescribing physician before making any dietary alterations.
5. Various situations can require an adjustment in the amount of lithium administered to a patient, for example, the addition of a new medication to the patient's drug regimen, a new diet, or an illness with fever or excessive sweating.
6. For determination of lithium levels, blood should be drawn in the morning approximately 8 to 12 hours after the last dose was taken.

quent bouts with the disorder (Sanger et al, 2001). Because of the seriousness of bipolar disorder, researchers have diligently sought alternatives for patients who do not respond to lithium (Table 22-2). Antiepileptics alternatives include the valproates (including three formulations), carbamazepine (Tegretol), and other antiseizure drugs. A more recently approved alternative is the atypical antipsychotic olanzapine (Zyprexa).

Valproates

Valproic acid (Depakene), sodium valproate (Depacon), and divalproex sodium (Depakote) have been used since the 1960s as antiepileptic agents. In 1995 these drugs were approved for treatment of mania and are considered first-line agents. Valproates appear to be particularly effective for patients with a rapid-cycling variant of bipolar disorder and for those with mania secondary to a general medical condition (Lennkh, Simhandl, 2000).

Advantages of the valproates are a rapid onset, the fact that they can be used initially without attempting lithium, and they are well tolerated with little effect on cognition. Disadvantages include transient hair loss, weight gain, tremors, GI upset, and dose-related thrombocytopenia.

Bioavailability is approximately 100% with up to 95% protein binding. The drug can be replaced at binding sites by other drugs such as carbamazepine or warfarin, causing toxic effects. Valproates have a

How Valproates Work

Although the precise nature of the valproates' action is not known, three or four mechanisms may be responsible for their antimanic effect.
1. An increase in GABA by either decreasing GABA metabolism or reducing its uptake
2. An increased postsynaptic response to GABA
3. An increase in the resting membrane potential (the membrane is less irritable)
4. Suppression of calcium influx through specific calcium channels (Keltner, Folks, 2001)

half-life of 6 to 16 hours and reach steady state in 2 to 5 days. The drug is initially given at 250 mg two to three times per day and titrated upward at 250 to 500 mg every three days. Therapeutic serum levels are from 50 to 100 µg/ml or the levels consistent with its antiepileptic effects.

Carbamazepine

Carbamazepine (Tegretol) is effective for most patients who do not respond to lithium or the valproates; it also has a faster onset of action compared with lithium. Patients who are more likely to be unresponsive to lithium and who, in turn, do respond to carbamazepine, are patients with a rapidly cycling bipolar episode. Carbamazepine may, at times, be given in combination with lithium. It is thought that the effectiveness of carbamazepine may

|Table 22-2| Agents Used to Treat Bipolar Disorder

Lithium	Eskalith, Lithane
Antiepileptic agents	carbamazepine (Tegretol)
	valproates
	valproic acid (Depakene)
	sodium valproate (Depacon)
	divalproex sodium (Depakote)
	gabapentin (Neurontin)
	lamotrigine (Lamictal)
	topiramate (Topamax)
Atypical antipsychotics	olanzapine (Zyprexa)
	clozapine (Clozaril)
	risperidone (Risperdal)
	quetiapine (Seroquel)
	ziprasidone (Geodon)

be related to its inhibition of "kindling" activity in the brain. In other words, just as kindling in the fireplace is the first step in building a fire, so it is thought that some abnormal brain activities begin as "kindling" and spread. A cup of water can dowse the fire from kindling but is ineffective in the control of a raging fire. The concept of kindling is used to explain seizure activity in the brain. Carbamazepine's probable mechanism of action is related to normalizing sodium-channel activity (and sodium influx), thus increasing the threshold of stimulation needed for cell firing. Carbamazepine's therapeutic antimanic serum levels are 8 to 12 μg/ml.

Although generally well tolerated, side effects include nausea, anorexia, and occasional vomiting. Sedation and drowsiness are other relatively common side effects. The most serious potential side effect of carbamazepine is agranulocytosis. Complete blood counts should be performed weekly when this drug treatment is initiated.

Significant drug interactions with carbamazepine include antibiotics, other anticonvulsants, lithium, calcium-channel blockers, and angiotensin-converting enzyme (ACE) inhibitors. Drugs that inhibit the P450 3A4 enzyme such as nefazodone and the SSRIs can cause toxic effects (Cozza, Armstrong, 2001).

Olanzapine

Olanzapine (Zyprexa) is the newest drug approved for treatment of bipolar disorder. Studies have shown that olanzapine controls mania and acts as a mood stabilizer (Price, 2000; Sanger et al, 2001). This particular pharmacologic profile may reduce the risk of precipitating a depression after treatment for acute mania. The dose for olanzapine is 15 to 45 mg per day.

Other Agents Used in the Treatment of Bipolar Disorder

Several benzodiazepines (e.g., clonazepam [Klonopin], lorazepam [Ativan]), the atypical antipsychotics clozapine (Clozaril), risperidone (Risperdal), and quetiapine (Seroquel); and other antiepileptics such as gabapentin (Neurontin), lamotrigine (Lamictal), and topiramate (Topamax) have all been used with some success in treating bipolar disorder (Keck, McElroy, 2002).

Key Concepts

1. Lithium is a naturally occurring element that has been the mainstay of bipolar disorder treatment for over 50 years.
2. Other first-line agents used to treat bipolar disorder are valproate, carbamazepine, and olanzapine.
3. Lithium alters intracellular conductance, and valproates and carbamazepine affect GABA receptors.
4. Clinically therapeutic serum levels of lithium are 0.6 to 1.2 mEq/L; at higher serum levels, serious or even fatal reactions occur.
5. Common side effects of lithium include nausea, dry mouth, diarrhea, thirst, and mild hand tremor.
6. Lithium has a narrow therapeutic index and a lag time of 7 to 10 days.
7. Valproates are effective and are relatively well tolerated.
8. Valproates have a rapid onset of action.
9. Carbamazepine has a more rapid onset compared with lithium and is generally well tolerated.
10. Olanzapine controls mania and acts as a mood stabilizer, thus preventing a depressive event after the acute mania subsides.

References

Ayd FJ: The early history of modern psychopharmacology, *Neuropsychopharmacol* 5(2):71, 1991.

Bezchlibnyk-Butler KZ, Jeffries JJ: *Clinical handbook of psychotropic drugs,* Seattle, 1997, Hogrefe and Huber Publishers.

Cade JF: Lithium salts in the treatment of psychotic excitement, *Med J Aust* 36:349, 1949.

Clark J, Queener S, Karb V: *Pharmacologic basis of nursing practice,* ed 4, St Louis, 1993, Mosby.

Cohen LS: Psychotropic drug use in pregnancy, *Hosp Community Psychiatry* 40:566, 1989.

Cozza KL, Armstrong SC: *The cytochrome P450 system,* Washington, DC, 2001, American Psychiatric Publishing.

Dunner DL, Fieve RR: Clinical factors in lithium carbonate prophylaxis failure, *Arch Gen Psychiatry* 30:229, 1974.

El-Mallakh RS: *Lithium: actions and mechanisms,* Washington, DC, 1996, American Psychiatric Publishers.

Fact Sheet: Taking mood stabilizers during childbearing years, *NAMI Advocate* 19(4):16, 1998.

Gitlin MJ: Lithium-induced renal insufficiency, *J Clin Psychopharmacol* 13(4):276, 1993.

Horne MM, Heitz UE, Swearingen PL: *Fluid and electrolyte balance,* St Louis, 1991, Mosby.

Keck PE: Pharmacokinetics and pharmacodynamics of antimanic and mood-stabilizing agents, *J Clin Psychiatry Visuals* 4(1):1, 2002.

Keck PE Jr, McElroy SL: Clinical pharmacodynamics and pharmacokinetics of antimanic and mood-stabilizing medications, *J Clin Psychiatry* 63(suppl 4):3, 2002.

Keltner NL, Folks DG: *Psychotropic drugs,* St Louis, 2001, Mosby.

Lennkh C, Simhandl C: Current aspects of valproate in bipolar disorder, *Inter Clin of Psychopharmacol* 15(1):1, 2000.

Lenox RH, Hahn C-G: Overview of the mechanism of action of lithium in the brain: fifty-year update, *J Clin Psychiatry* 61(suppl 6):5, 2000.

Martin A: Clinical management of lithium-induced polyuria, *Hosp Community Psychiatry* 44(5):427, 1993.

McIntyre RS et al: Lithium revisited, *Can J Psychiatry* 46(5):322, 2001.

Phiel CJ, Klein PS: Molecular targets of lithium action, *Ann Rev Pharmacol Toxicol* 41:789, 2001.

Price PL: Olanzapine to treat the acute mania of bipolar disorder, *S D J Med* 53(12):523, 2000.

Sanger TM et al: Long-term olanzapine therapy in the treatment of bipolar I disorder: an open-label continuation phase study, *J Clin Psychiatry* 62(4):273, 2001.

Soares JC, Gershon S: The psychopharmacologic specificity of the lithium ion: origins and trajectory, *J Clin Psychiatry* 61(suppl 9):16, 2000.

Sugarman JR: Management of lithium intoxication, *Fam Pract* 18:237, 1984.

Surgeon General: *Mental health: a report from the Surgeon General,* Washington, DC, 1999, Department of Health and Human Services.

Trimble MR: *Biological psychiatry,* New York, 1996, John Wiley and Sons.

Watsky EJ, Salzman C: Psychotropic drug interactions, *Hosp Community Psychiatry* 42(3):247, 1991.

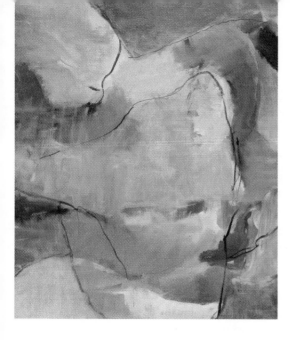

Chapter 23

Antianxiety Drugs

Norman L. Keltner

Learning Objectives

After reading this chapter, you should be able to:

- Describe the differences between benzodiazepines and buspirone.
- Identify when benzodiazepines are indicated.
- Discuss the side effects of benzodiazepines.
- Identify benzodiazepines appropriate for older adults.
- Identify the specific antidote for benzodiazepine overdose.

- Describe potential drug interactions with benzodiazepines, particularly with central nervous system depressants such as alcohol.
- Discuss the implications for teaching patients about antianxiety drugs.

People have been seeking relief from anxiety since the beginning of recorded history. Alcohol is the oldest drug used to reduce anxiety and has been used by countless millions to self-medicate fears, phobias, and "nerves." From biblical times through the present, men and women have taken alcohol to calm down, to forget, and to escape reality. Alcohol is still the most often self-prescribed anxiolytic. However, individuals who drink alcohol for these reasons have found it to be a two-edged sword—with relief has come abuse, dependence, assorted other problems, and even more anxiety.

In recent times, other drugs have been developed to alleviate anxiety. In the early 1900s, bromo seltzers were advertised as having anxiolytic properties, but problems surfaced with bromide dependency, and bromo seltzers had to be withdrawn from the market (Harvey, 1985). In the 1930s and 1940s, barbiturates were heralded as having potential to treat anxiety, but they too were found to have many adverse effects, including seizures, dependence, addiction, and withdrawal.

The first drug specifically for treating anxiety was meprobamate (Miltown, Equanil), developed in 1955 (Ayd, 1991). This drug, with its ability to calm nerves, to blur the reality of stressors, and, in general, to make people feel better, was a national sensation. Ayd (1991) describes the impact of meprobamate as follows:

> In the months thereafter the demand for Miltown, a name derived from the New Jersey town in which Wallace Laboratories manufactured meprobamate, far exceeded that for any drug previously marketed in the United States. For a time Milton

Antianxiety Agents in the Treatment of Anxiety

Indications	Mechanism of Action	Major Side Effects	Overdose
• Chronic anxiety • Time limited response to crisis • Presurgery jitters • Panic disorder	Benzodiazepines • Enhance the inhibiting influence of GABA	Benzodiazepines • Oversedation • Memory impairment • Paradoxical excitement • Emotional blunting • CNS depression • Drowsiness • Fatigue • Mental impairment	Benzodiazepines • Benzodiazepines alone do not cause deaths from overdose • Benzodiazepines mixed with CNS depressants can be lethal

CNS, Central nervous system; *GABA,* gamma-aminobutyric acid.

Key Terms

Abuse Excessive use of a substance that differs from societal norms.

Anxiety Feeling of apprehension, uncertainty, or tension.

Anxiolytic Antianxiety drug.

Dependence State in which a drug user must take a usual or increasing dose of a drug to prevent the onset of abstinence symptoms or withdrawal. The drug user must take the drug to feel "normal."

Disinhibition State in which a person is unable to suppress urges or statements that may be socially unacceptable (e.g., telling a dirty joke in an inappropriate situation, making sexual comments to the employer's wife).

Tolerance Need for increasing amounts of a substance to achieve the same effects. Pharmacokinetic tolerance results when the drug is metabolized more rapidly. Pharmacodynamic tolerance occurs when more of the drug is required at the receptor sites to achieve the same effect.

Withdrawal Physical signs and symptoms that occur when the addictive substance is reduced or withheld; also referred to as *abstinence syndromes.*

Berle was renamed Miltown Berle, magicians pulled Miltown instead of rabbits from their magical hats, and newspaper and national coverage of this drug was unprecedented. (p. 71)

This reception probably says far more about the American psyche than it does about the efficacy of meprobamate. Obviously, the nation was ready for a drug to buffer the stressors of a busy society. For several years, meprobamate was a widely prescribed medication, but similar to alcohol, bromo seltzer, and barbiturates, problems surfaced. Individuals using meprobamate were subject to abuse, tolerance, and lethal overdose. Its appeal as an antianxiety agent

began to diminish. Fortunately, waiting in the wings were new agents to calm the trembling hands of a nation besieged with anxiety.

Before the 1950s were over, another class of antianxiety drugs was developed: the benzodiazepines. These drugs had advantages over barbiturates in that they were less likely to be abused and were safer when overdoses occurred (Hollister, 1994). Though first synthesized in the 1930s, benzodiazepines were not discovered to have a psychiatric effect until the late 1950s. Ayd (1991) outlines the nearly serendipitous nature of the development of chlordiazepoxide (Librium), the first benzodiazepine. After nearly 40 benzodiazepine derivatives had been synthesized and found lacking in therapeutic qualities, the last one was laid aside only to be tested 20 years later. During that testing, psychotropic properties were noted. The first written report of those properties was published by Harris in the *Journal of the American Medical Association* in 1960. Eventually, several thousand benzodiazepine derivatives would be synthesized, including familiar drugs such as diazepam (Valium), lorazepam (Ativan), alprazolam (Xanax), oxazepam (Serax), and clonazepam (Klonopin). However, these drugs too are linked to significant problems. Benzodiazepines were (and continue to be) abused, they induced tolerance, and they were implicated in lethal overdoses (though always when combined with other drugs). In a recent report, over 10% of American adults admitted using benzodiazepines in the previous year, with a significant number of long term users reporting dependence (Ashton, 2000).

Clinical researchers and drug manufacturers continue to search for the perfect antianxiety drug, the drug that will ameliorate anxiety without significant adverse effects. A nonbenzodiazepine antianxiety agent that is widely marketed is buspirone (BuSpar).

Buspirone apparently does not have the potential for abuse, dependency, and withdrawal that is associated with the benzodiazepines. A large group of unrelated drugs appear to have antianxiety properties, or at least have been found useful in the treatment of specific anxiety-like syndromes. Examples of drugs with antianxiety properties include some beta blockers (e.g., propranolol), antihistamines, monoamine oxidase inhibitors (MAOIs), tricyclic antidepressants (TCAs), selective serotonin reuptake inhibitors (SSRIs), phenothiazines, hydroxyzine (Vistaril), and opioids. Finally, a host of potentially new antianxiety drugs are currently being tested.

BENZODIAZEPINES

Quite a few benzodiazepines are on the market, and they vary considerably in potency (e.g., 0.5 mg of alprazolam [Xanax] is roughly equivalent to 5 mg of diazepam [Valium]), in half-life (e.g., 2 to 6 hours for lorazepam [Ativan] and up to 100 hours or more for chlorazepate [Tranxene] and flurazepam [Dalmane]), and in duration of effect (e.g., triazolam [Halcion] is short acting, and diazepam is long acting).

Historically, antianxiety agents have been referred to as anxiolytics or minor tranquilizers. The major class of antianxiety drugs is benzodiazepines; these drugs are used most often to treat anxiety. Benzodiazepines are widely used by both psychiatric and general-medicine patients. Major indications for benzodiazepines include chronic anxiety, time-limited treatment for crisis, presurgery nervousness, and panic disorder.

Anxiety is a subjective experience that can be observed by others (Box 23-1). The anxious person feels excessively alert, is easily startled, is restless, talks too much, visually scans the environment, has tremors, and may have dilated pupils. Although many people use these drugs as needed (prn), benzodiazepines generally should not be taken for the stresses of everyday living. Benzodiazepines have no therapeutic value in the treatment of psychosis.

How Benzodiazepines Work

Benzodiazepines enhance the effects of the inhibitory neurotransmitter gamma-aminobutyric acid (GABA). GABA attaches to GABA receptors, which trigger the opening of chloride channels. Chloride has a hyperpolarizing effect on the neuron, which makes the neuron less responsive to excitatory neurons such as norepinephrine, serotonin, and dopa-

| Box 23-1 | Psychologic Symptoms of Anxiety

Patient may be:
- Anxious
- Apprehensive
- Compulsive
- Fearful
- Experiencing feelings of dread
- Irritable
- Intolerant
- Nervous
- Overconcerned
- Panicky
- Phobic
- Preoccupied
- Experiencing repetitive in motor activities
- Feeling threatened
- Wound up
- Sensitive to shame
- Worried

mine. The overall effect is one of slowing down or halting neuronal firing (Ashton, 2000). Neuronal inhibition is important. Inhibition is as important to brain function as the brake is to the operation of a car. Driving a car without brakes risks being involved in a runaway accident. A brain without the inhibition of GABA can produce thought acceleration, autonomic dysfunction, excessive anxiety, panic, or even seizure activity—or to stretch the analogy—a runaway brain (Keltner et al, 2001; Sterling, 2001). Benzodiazepines "help" GABA tone down or inhibit the anxiety response to stressors.

GABA is a product of a product of the Krebs cycle and is synthesized by the decarboxylation of glutamate (i.e., the acid group of the amino acid glutamate is taken off), an amino acid produced from the Krebs cycle.

GABA receptors are located on approximately 40% of all neurons (Keltner, 2000; Sugerman, 2001). GABA receptors are composed of five subunits, and, on a particular receptor complex, these subunits can be arranged in any number of configurations (Seighart, 1995). The composition of these subunits determines the functional characteristics of the receptor (Low et al, 2001). Because of these unique configurations, some GABA receptors are selective for specific ligands (molecules that bind to and evoke a response from the receptor). Specific subunit configurations exist for benzodiazepines—a benzodiazepine receptor site. When they attach to these receptor types, benzodiazepines enhance the effects of GABA. Benzodiazepine effects are dependent on endogenous GABA, and these drugs are inactive in the absence of GABA. In other words, the level of endogenous GABA limits the effect of benzodiazepine. Barbiturates, on the other hand, both enhance GABA and mimic GABA. Hence barbiturates can cause profound central nervous system (CNS) depression and even death in overdose (Lehne, 2001; Williams, Akabas, 2000)

Pharmacologic Effect (Desired Effect)

Benzodiazepines have a generally depressing effect on the CNS, including the limbic system, the thalamus, the hypothalamus, and the reticular activating system (through which incoming sensory information is funneled). Benzodiazepines have five major effects that are used for therapeutic purposes (Ashton, 2000). Benzodiazepines are used therapeutically as:

1. Anxiolytics
2. Hypnotics
3. Muscle relaxants
4. Anticonvulsants
5. Amnesics

Because benzodiazepines depress the reticular activating system, incoming stimuli are muted and evoke less reaction. To illustrate the concept of *muting,* two symptoms will be highlighted: hyperalertness and environmental scanning. The anxious person uses these defensive reactions to guard against an environment perceived to be threatening. The "stressed out" person might overreact to being startled because the body's system is on alert. As the antianxiety agent "decreases" environmental input, a general relaxing of the anxious posture takes place.

These drugs can cause several levels of CNS depression, from sedation to anesthesia. Benzodiazepines accomplish this task by sedating the patient and depressing the inhibitory neurons affecting arousal. The latter effect causes a state of disinhibition, or loosening of inner impediments to conduct. Disinhibition results in feelings of euphoria and excitement that, in turn, can lead to poor judgment. The natural restraint that minimizes social blunders is depressed.

To visualize the potential allure of benzodiazepines, one might imagine a tension continuum, with anxiety on one end and a carefree sense of being on the other. Benzodiazepines have the potential to move the anxious person from the agony of the anxiety end to the relaxed feeling of the carefree end. In therapeutic doses, this degree of shift from anxiety to disinhibition is not gained or sought, but because of the possibility of reaching a carefree zone, benzodiazepines have become drugs of abuse (Schedule IV; see Appendix G). Furthermore, many polysubstance abusers also use benzodiazepines because of the drug's ability to increase the high of other drugs.

The inhibiting effect of benzodiazepines also accounts for their anticonvulsive activity. Intravenous diazepam (Valium) and lorazepam (Ativan) are first-line agents for status epilepticus, and clonazepam (Klonopin) is regularly prescribed orally as an anticonvulsant.

Paradoxical reactions to benzodiazepines

A significant number of individuals (up to 29% in some studies) have a paradoxical reaction to benzodiazepines (Gutierrez et al, 2001). These symptoms include agitation, emotional lability, and occasionally rage. Children, older adults, patients with poor impulse control, and individuals with organic brain syndrome are most at risk.

Pharmacokinetics

Benzodiazepines are readily absorbed after oral ingestion; however, intramuscular administration produces slow and inconsistent absorption for most of these drugs (lorazepam [Ativan] is an exception). The benzodiazepines are highly lipid soluble and therefore readily cross the blood-brain barrier. The benzodiazepines are metabolized by the liver but do not significantly induce their own hepatic metabolism compared with barbiturates, and they are excreted in the urine. The active metabolites can exert an effect for up to 10 days. In fact, a convenient way of categorizing benzodiazepines is to divide them into those with short half-lives (20 hours or less) and those with long half-lives (more than 20 hours). Of the selected benzodiazepines with short half-lives listed in Table 23-1, lorazepam (Ativan), oxazepam (Serax), and temazepam (Restoril) are preferable for use in older adults. Clorazepate (Tranxene), chlordiazepoxide (Librium), and diazepam (Valium) have long half-lives and hence have extended duration of action. Accordingly, these drugs are not suited for use in older patients.

However, looking at half-lives alone is misleading. An important factor in half-life determination over time is the metabolic process that each benzodiazepine undergoes. Most benzodiazepines are oxidized in the liver to active metabolites; but because hepatic function and volume change with age, the liver becomes less efficient at metabolizing these drugs over a lifetime. For instance, the half-life of diazepam is approximately 20 hours in a young man but stretches to 80 hours in a man 80 years of age. On the other hand, a few benzodiazepines rely on conjugation with glucuronic acid to form inactive metabolites (Keltner, Folks, 2001). This process is not significantly affected by the aging process. These benzodiazepines are lorazepam, oxazepam, and temazepam. Because the half-lives of these drugs remain fairly stable over the life span, and because these drugs have no active metabolites, they are better suited for use in older adults.

Because hepatic metabolism is the primary mechanism for drug disposition, drugs that interfere with liver metabolism (e.g., alcohol) dangerously compound the effect of benzodiazepines.

Table 23-1 presents information on these drugs, including duration of effect, the usual adult daily dose, equivalent dose, elimination half-life, anxiolytic effect, and sedative effect.

> ### *Critical* Thinking Question
>
> Why is it preferable to give a benzodiazepine with a shorter half-life to older adult patients?

Side Effects

Commonly, CNS side effects such as drowsiness, fatigue, and decreased coordination are exhibited. A certain mental impairment and slowing of reflexes also occurs. Less frequently, confusion, depression, and headache may be present. Peripheral nervous system (PNS) effects include occasional constipation, double vision, hypotension, incontinence, and urinary retention. Benzodiazepines can exacerbate narrow-angle glaucoma. Older adults with impaired liver or renal function and individuals who are debilitated experience increased side effects and, consequently, should receive a decreased amount of these drugs (see nursing interventions box and discussion of pharmacokinetics).

Dependence, Withdrawal, and Tolerance

Beyond these undesired effects are the triple problems of dependence, withdrawal, and tolerance.

| Table 23-1 | Anxiety Drugs: Usual Daily Dose, Equivalent Dose, Half-Life, Anxiolytic Effect, Sedative Effect

Anxiety Drug	Usual Daily Dose (mg/day)	Equivalent Dose (mg)	Half-Life (hr)	Anxiolytic Effect	Sedative Effect
Benzodiazepine					
Short-acting	triazolam (Halcion) 0.125-0.500	0.25	1.5-5.5	X	XXX
Intermediate	alprazolam (Xanax) 0.75-4.00*	0.50	12-15	XX	X
Intermediate	halazepam (Paxipam) 60-160*	40.00	14-100†	XX	—
Intermediate	lorazepam (Ativan) 2-6* (P)	1.00	10-20	XXX	XX
Intermediate	oxazepam (Serax) 30-60	15.00	5-20	XX	X
Intermediate	temazepam (Restoril) 10-60	10.00	10-15	X	XXX
Long-acting	chlordiazepoxide (Librium) 15-100* (P)	25.00	5-30†	XX	—
Long-acting	clonazepam (Klonopin) 0.5-10.0*	0.25	18-60†	XX	X
Long-acting	clorazepate (Tranxene) 7.5-60.0*	10.00	30-100†	XX	—
Long-acting	diazepam (Valium) 4-40* (P)	5.00	20-80†	XXX	XX
Long-acting	flurazepam (Dalmane) 15-30	15.00	3-150†	X	XXX
Long-acting	prazepam (Centrax) 20-40*	10.00	30-100†	XX	—
Long-acting	quazepam (Doral) 7.5-30.0*	7.50	30-150†	X	XXX
Nonbenzodiazepine	buspirone (BuSpar) 15-40*	n/a	2-11†	XXX	—

Adapted from Bezchlibnyk-Butler KZ, Jeffries JJ: *Clinical handbook of psychotropic drugs,* ed 7, Seattle, 1997, Hogrefe & Huber; Lieberman JA, Tasman A: *Psychiatric drugs,* St Louis, 2000, WB Saunders; Keltner NL, Folks DG, *Psychotropic drugs,* St Louis, 2001, Mosby.
*Given in divided doses.
†With active metabolites.
P, Parenteral form available.

| Table 23-2 | Symptoms Emerging after Withdrawal from Benzodiazepines

Neurologic	Gastrointestinal	Psychiatric	Other
Convulsions	Nausea	Anxiety	Tachycardia
Insomnia	Vomiting	Irritability	Sweating
Light-headedness	Diarrhea	Cognitive	
Involuntary movements	Weight loss	Memory impairment	
Headache	Decreased appetite	Depression	
Weakness		Confusion	

Dependence

Dependence can be defined as a state in which the body functions "normally" when the drug is present. The body, in turn, functions "abnormally" when the drug is absent. Dependence can develop within a few weeks or months of regular use. When benzodiazepine is withdrawn from the dependent person, symptoms such as agitation, tremor, irritability, insomnia, vomiting, sweating, and even convulsions may be experienced. Ashton (2000) has described three types of benzodiazepine dependence:

1. *Therapeutic dose dependence.* These individuals take the drug as prescribed but develop a "need" for the drug; they have "outgrown" the original reason for taking the drug but now "need" the drug to get through the day; and they are in regular contact with their physician about the drug and want their prescriptions filled right on time. If taking a short-acting benzodiazepine, these individuals become anxious between doses.

2. *Prescribed high-dose dependent.* These individuals are still taking prescribed benzodiazepines but have talked their doctor into escalating the dose. Sometimes, these individuals are receiving prescriptions from more than one clinician. This person may also use alcohol to enhance the effect.

3. *Recreational benzodiazepine abuse.* These individuals use benzodiazepines outside the traditional medical system. Benzodiazepines are often used to enhance the effects of other abused substances. Typically, the amount of drug used is significantly greater than the amount prescribed for medicinal purposes. For example, a high-end dose of diazepam is 40 mg per day (see Table 23-1). Recreational abusers often ingest 100 mg daily. Some abusers take benzodiazepines intravenously.

Withdrawal

Abrupt withdrawal from benzodiazepines can cause troublesome to serious effects. For example, agitation, tremor, irritability, insomnia, vomiting, sweating, convulsions, and even psychotic episodes have occurred. Thus gradual tapering of the dose is imperative. Because GABA is an inhibitory neurotransmitter, releasing the "inhibition" results in a "taking off the brake" phenomenon. Because long-term use of benzodiazepines reduces the number of GABA receptors, an abrupt discontinuation of these drugs leaves the brain unable to fulfill inhibitory functions (Ashton, 2000). Hence the adverse effects previously mentioned occur. The tapering or withdrawal process is highly individual and can take up to a year or more in some heavily dependent individuals. Table 23-2 provides a more complete list of withdrawal symptoms.

Tolerance

Tolerance to the effects of benzodiazepines occurs, hence individuals need an increasing amount of the drug to achieve the same effect. Tolerance to sedation develops fairly quickly (within weeks), while tolerance to antianxiety effects occurs somewhat slowly (over a few months). Anticonvulsive tolerance also develops slowly, thus use of benzodiazepines for epilepsy is probably ill advised for most patients. Cognitive and memory effects appear to continue throughout the use of these agents (Ashton, 2000). In review, tolerance develops to some of the desired effects of benzodiazepines (i.e., hypnotic, anxiolytic, anticonvulsive effects), although tolerance does not appear to develop to the unwanted effects of cognitive and memory deficits.

Interactions

Benzodiazepines are CNS depressants and interact *additively* with other CNS depressants. Alcohol,

Table 23-3 | Major Interactions with Benzodiazepines

Interactant	Interaction
Alcohol and other CNS depressants	Increased sedation, CNS depression
Antacids	Impaired absorption rate of benzodiazepine
Disulfiram (Antabuse) and cimetidine (Tagamet)	Increase the plasma level of benzodiazepines that are oxidized
Nefazodone (Serzone)	Inhibits metabolism of alprazolam and triazolam
Phenytoin	Increased anticonvulsant serum level
TCAs	Increased sedation, confusion, impaired motor function
MAOIs	CNS depression
Succinylcholine	Decreased neuromuscular blockade

CNS, Central nervous system; *TCAs*, tricyclic antidepressants; *MAOIs*, monoamine oxidase inhibitors.

TCAs, nefazodone (Serzone), opioids, antipsychotics, and antihistamines increase the sedative effects of benzodiazepines. Further, the common refreshment, grapefruit juice, can also cause problems because it inhibits the cytochrome P450 3A4 enzyme, thus extending the life of several benzodiazepines (Keltner, Opara, 2002). Table 23-3 lists major interactants for the benzodiazepines.

Nursing Implications

Therapeutic versus toxic drug levels

Benzodiazepines taken alone are relatively safe drugs. Overdoses hundreds of times higher than a therapeutic dose have been reported without resulting in death. However, if benzodiazepines are combined with other drugs, such as alcohol, then effects can be fatal. Signs and symptoms of overdose include somnolence, confusion, coma, diminished reflexes, and hypotension. Effective treatment begins with emptying the stomach by induced vomiting and gastric lavage, followed by activated charcoal. The nurse should monitor blood pressure, pulse, and respirations and provide supportive care as indicated. Hypotension can be treated with levarterenol (Levophed). Physostigmine is a potent antidote for acute diazepam poisoning and can be effective for respiratory depression associated with diazepam overdose (Ciraulo et al, 1989). Dialysis has limited value.

Benzodiazepine-receptor antagonist

Flumazenil (Romazicon) blocks the benzodiazepine-binding site on the GABA receptor. Flumazenil selectively blocks benzodiazepine receptors but does not block adrenergic or cholinergic receptors. Because flumazenil does not stimulate the CNS and does not block other receptors, it can be given when benzodiazepine overdose is suspected without fear of unexpected interactions. However, if severe cyclic (e.g., tricyclic) antidepressant toxicity is present, flumazenil should be withheld until the toxicity is abated (*United States Pharmacopeia*, 2001). A response to flumazenil typically occurs within 30 to 60 seconds. Two important considerations when giving flumazenil are that it does not speed the metabolism or excretion of benzodiazepines and that it has a short duration of action. These considerations present a clinical management problem. If the patient responds to flumazenil, then benzodiazepines are present, but because flumazenil does not speed metabolism and has a short duration of action, the patient may "recover" only to return to a "pre-flumazenil" state. This problem requires constant vigilance by the nurse and repeated doses of flumazenil as the body eliminates the benzodiazepine from the system. Furthermore, flumazenil may not reverse benzodiazepine-induced respiratory depression and can precipitate seizures (Lehne, 2001).

Use during pregnancy

The association of benzodiazepine use and fetal abnormalities is not supported (Cohen, 1989). Some concern exists that benzodiazepines may be associated with cleft lip and cleft palate in the first trimester, but the evidence is inconclusive. Even these inconclusive findings might warrant discontinuance during pregnancy. Benzodiazepines are also known to enter breast milk thus nursing mothers should not use these drugs. However, if the drug cannot be discontinued without exacerbation of symptoms, then tapering to the lowest possible dose is desirable.

Side Effects and Nursing Interventions | for Benzodiazepines

Side Effects	Interventions
Dry mouth	Advise rinsing mouth with water often, eating sugarless hard candies, and chewing sugarless gum.
Ataxia	Provide assistance with ambulation.
Dizziness, drowsiness	Assist with ambulation and with getting in and out of bed. Caution about driving.
Nausea	Take with food.
Withdrawal symptoms (increased anxiety, influenza-like symptoms, tremors)	Contact prescriber.

Use in older adults

As has been mentioned in the pharmacokinetic discussion, specific benzodiazepines are acceptable for use in older adults, but most are not recommended. This dichotomy is based on metabolic processes. Lorazepam (Ativan) and oxazepam (Serax) are considered to be the best benzodiazepines for older individuals. Temazepam (Restoril) and, occasionally, alprazolam (Xanax) are also used in this age group. The other benzodiazepines, including diazepam (Valium) and chlordiazepoxide (Librium), have extended half-lives and active metabolites and should not be routinely prescribed for older patients.

Side effects

The most common side effects are related to sedation and mental alertness. The patient should be cautioned about driving or operating hazardous machinery. Tolerance to sedation quickly develops. Blood pressure should be monitored routinely, and a 20 mm Hg drop of the systolic level while the patient is standing warrants withholding the drug and notifying the physician. (See the above box titled, "Side Effects and Nursing Interventions for Benzodiazepines" for other side effects and interventions.)

Interactions

Benzodiazepines interact with a number of CNS depressants. The nurse should explain this characteristic carefully to patients who are taking benzodiazepines. A high percentage of psychiatric patients abuse drugs, thus a real potential exists for deadly combinations. Also probable is that these patients will develop a cross-tolerance to hepatic-metabolized drugs. For instance, individuals who develop a tolerance to alcohol have an increased tolerance to

Use of Benzodiazepines (BZs) for Anxiety in Older Adults

Good BZs	BZs to Avoid
Lorazepam (Ativan)	Diazepam (Valium)
Oxazepam (Serax)	Chlordiazepoxide (Librium)

diazepam but not when alcohol and diazepam are taken together. Hearing a patient who is experienced in taking diazepam speak with disdain about typical doses is not uncommon; for example, "Ten mg of Valium doesn't even touch me!" Although diazepam alone may not "touch" these patients, diazepam combined with alcohol *will*. The nurse should remind these patients that if they mix diazepam with alcohol, they might die.

Teaching patients

Patient education is important because benzodiazepines have tremendous potential for abuse or misuse. Consequently, teaching patients and their families about these drugs is important. The nurse should teach the following:

- Benzodiazepines are not intended for the minor stresses of everyday life.
- Over-the-counter drugs may enhance the actions of benzodiazepines.
- Certain herbal preparations such as kava and valerian cause an additive effect.
- Driving should be avoided until tolerance develops.
- The prescribed dose should not be exceeded.
- Alcohol and other CNS depressants exacerbate the effects of benzodiazepines.
- Hypersensitivity to one benzodiazepine may mean hypersensitivity to another.
- These drugs should not be stopped abruptly.

Specific Benzodiazepines

Alprazolam

Alprazolam (Xanax) is particularly useful for generalized anxiety, adjustment disorders, panic disorder, and anxiety associated with depression (Shelton, 1993). Alprazolam is also prescribed as an antitremor agent. Alprazolam has been criticized for its potential to cause addiction and dependence and for reports of alprazolam-induced violent or aggressive behavior (Glod, 1992; Shelton, 1993). Little risk exists of accumulation of alprazolam during repeated dosing. Alprazolam is available in an oral solution.

Chlordiazepoxide

Chlordiazepoxide (Librium) is prescribed for anxiety disorders, the relief of the symptoms of anxiety, and acute alcohol withdrawal. Chlordiazepoxide is absorbed well orally. Additionally, chlordiazepoxide can be used as an antitremor agent. Parenteral chlordiazepoxide is used as an antipanic agent. Accumulation occurs with this drug. An intramuscular formulation is available and should be administered deeply.

Clonazepam

Clonazepam (Klonopin) is used most often as an anticonvulsant but also has clinical utility in the treatment of panic disorder. Clonazepam alone or as an adjunct is useful in the treatment of Lennox-Gastaut syndrome (a *petit mal* variant) and akinetic, absence, and myoclonic seizures. Patients taking clonazepam long term should be slowly tapered off this drug because evidence suggests that abrupt withdrawal can precipitate status epilepticus (Shelton, 1993). Clonazepam is also used for benzodiazepine withdrawal (Keltner, Folks, 2001). Animal models indicate the potential for congenital abnormalities if used during pregnancy.

Clorazepate

Clorazepate (Tranxene) is used to treat anxiety and acute alcohol withdrawal and as an adjunct in the treatment of partial seizures. Clorazepate has some use as an anticonvulsant. Accumulation occurs after repeated dosing. An extended release form is available.

Diazepam

Diazepam (Valium) is an often-prescribed antianxiety agent that has multiple uses related to its CNS-depressing effect. Besides anxiety disorders and short-term relief from symptoms of anxiety, diazepam is used preoperatively to relieve presurgery "jitters," for skeletal muscle spasms (e.g., lower back pain), as a drug of choice for status epilepticus, and as an adjunct for endoscopic procedures. Additionally, diazepam may be useful for symptomatic relief of alcohol withdrawal. Parenteral, emulsive, and rectal forms are available.

Lorazepam

Lorazepam (Ativan) is used to treat anxiety disorders and also has uses as an antitremor agent, an antipanic agent, as an anticonvulsant (parenteral only), and as an antiemetic for chemotherapy cancer patients. The metabolites of lorazepam are inactive, thus the effects of this drug do not persist. Patients with impaired liver function can handle this drug better than they can most other benzodiazepines because lorazepam is metabolized to inactive metabolites. Lorazepam is recommended for use in older patients when a benzodiazepine is indicated.

Oxazepam

Oxazepam (Serax) is similar to lorazepam in that its metabolite is inactive, and it is metabolized by conjugative reaction. Thus the drug is effective for a relatively short time (24 hours) and is suitable for individuals with liver disorders and for older adults. Oxazepam is used for anxiety associated with depression and relief from acute alcohol withdrawal.

Buspirone

Buspirone (BuSpar) is not a benzodiazepine and does not bind to benzodiazepine recognition sites but probably acts as a serotonin agonist (the same neurotransmitter implicated in depression). Considerable interest exists in buspirone because it differs from benzodiazepines in several important ways:

- Is not sedating
- Is not a drug that causes a "high" thus has almost no abuse potential
- Has no cross-tolerance with sedatives or alcohol
- Takes 1 to 6 weeks to be effective
- Does not produce dependence, withdrawal, or tolerance
- Does not cause muscle relaxation

Buspirone's effects help distinguish anxiety control from the sedative and euphoric actions of older benzodiazepines. Buspirone is particularly effective in reducing symptoms of worry, apprehension, difficulties with concentration and cognition, and irritability. Buspirone does not depress the CNS, and its lack of a sedative effect make buspirone less attractive for abuse. Because it has no abuse potential, buspirone is not a controlled substance.

Buspirone provides relief from anxiety within 7 to 10 days, but maximal therapeutic gain is not achieved until 3 to 6 weeks of treatment. Buspirone has a half-life of 2 to 11 hours (includes active metabolite), thus it is usually given in divided doses. Buspirone is extensively metabolized after the first pass; as little as 1% to 4% becomes bioavailable. Foods increase its bioavailability by decreasing first-pass metabolism. Side effects include dizziness, nausea, headache, nervousness, light-headedness, and excitement.

Buspirone is a remarkably safe drug. No deaths have been reported from taking buspirone alone. Dosages as high as 2400 mg per day have been taken without major side effects (Keltner, Folks, 2001). No data is available on the use of buspirone during pregnancy.

Buspirone produces few drug interactions, but haloperidol and MAOIs have been reported to cause some adverse effects when co-administered.

The reader should note that when switching from a benzodiazepine to buspirone, buspirone must not be substituted immediately for the benzodiazepine. Because of dissimilarities in their pharmacologic properties, the benzodiazepines must be tapered while the buspirone is initiated.

OTHER DRUGS WITH ANTIANXIETY PROPERTIES

Propranolol

Propranolol (Inderal) is a beta blocker that effectively interrupts the physiologic responses of anxiety related to social phobia. Propranolol is less effective than are the benzodiazepines but is relatively safe and has little abuse potential. Most side effects are transient and mild. However, bradycardia, light-headedness, and heart block have occurred.

Clomipramine

Clomipramine (Anafranil) is a TCA that is effective for obsessive-compulsive disorder (OCD) at a dose of approximately 100 to 150 mg per day. Clomipramine is a serotonin reuptake inhibitor (SRI), although it is not as potent as are the more traditional SSRIs. The major central side effects of clomipramine include headache (52% of patients), reduced libido (21%), nervousness (18%), myoclonus

(13%), and increased appetite (10%). Peripheral effects include dry mouth, constipation, and ejaculation failure (42%), erectile dysfunction (20%), and weight gain (Keltner, Folks, 2001).

Other Tricyclic Antidepressants

Imipramine (Tofranil) in higher dosages has proven to be effective for panic-anxiety attacks. Desipramine (Norpramin), at higher doses and for longer trial periods, has also proven effective. Trazodone (Desyrel) has antianxiety properties. Trazodone has a highly sedative quality and is often prescribed for individuals who are experiencing anxiety, particularly older adults, to facilitate sleep.

SELECTIVE SEROTONIN REUPTAKE INHIBITORS

SSRIs are prescribed for OCD, panic attacks, and phobias. SSRIs are considered first-line approaches to OCD (Table 23-4). Specifically, fluoxetine (Prozac), fluvoxamine (Luvox), paroxetine (Paxil), and sertraline (Zoloft) are approved for treatment of this disorder. SSRIs may be the most effective, as well as the safest, agents for the prophylaxis and long-term treatment of panic attacks (Black et al, 1993). GABA receptors are thought to be involved in the pathophysiology of panic disorders. Theories suggest that the overwhelming anxiety associated with panic may stem from abnormal serotonin transmission (Sterling, 2001). Saito (2001) believes that SSRI effectiveness in panic and other anxiety disorders can be partially explained by serotonin's role in upregulating GABA transmission in the prefrontal cortex.

Venlafaxine

Venlafaxine is approved for generalized anxiety. Doses at the higher range are thought to be more effective possibly because of the increased norepinephrine reuptake inhibition at that range.

Table 23-5 outlines pharmacologic interventions for specific anxiety disorders.

Flunitrazepam: A Benzodiazepine Associated with Date Rape

Flunitrazepam (Rohypnol) is a benzodiazepine that has been used in date rape. Flunitrazepam tablets are also known as roofies, rophies, roche, roaches, and ruffies (Taylor, Donoghue, 2001). Flunitrazepam will be covered in the Substance Abuse chapter, but a brief mention will be made here as well.

| Table 23-4 | Antidepressants Indicated for Anxiety

Agent	Class	Dose Range (mg/day)	Comment (FDA Approval)
clomipramine (Anafranil)	TCA	100-250	Approved for OCD; 250 mg is the maximum dose because of increased risk of seizures
fluvoxamine (Luvox)	SSRI	100-300	Approved for OCD
paroxetine (Paxil)	SSRI	40-60	Approved for panic, OCD, and social anxiety
sertraline (Zoloft)	SSRI	50-200	Approved for panic, OCD (adults and children), and PTSD
venlafaxine (Effexor XR)	SNRI	75-225	Approved for generalized anxiety; 150- and 225-mg doses are superior (possibly because of more potent norepinephrine reuptake blockade)
fluoxetine (Prozac)	SSRI	20-80	Approved for OCD

FDA, U.S. Food and Drug Administration; *OCD*, obsessive compulsive disorder; *PTSD*, posttraumatic stress disorder; *SNRI*, selective serotonin norepinephrine reuptake inhibitor; *SSRI*, selective serotonin reuptake inhibitor; *TCA*, tricyclic antidepressant.
From: Keltner NL, Folks DG: *Psychotropic drugs*, St Louis, 2001, Mosby.

| Table 23-5 | Pharmacologic Interventions for Specific Anxiety Disorders

Disorder	Pharmacologic Treatment
Panic disorder	
Exhibited as discrete and intense period of anxiety, apprehension, and distress Associated symptoms include palpitations, sweating, trembling, and dyspnea	SSRIs are perhaps the safest for long-term and prophylaxic doses: gradual titration to sertraline 50 mg qd or paroxetine 40 mg qd have proven to be minimum effective doses. Benzodiazepines. Clonazepam (average dose 1.5 mg per day) and alprazolam (average dose 3 mg per day) can provide more immediate relief. TCAs. Same dose as that used in treating depressive syndromes, but dose level should be carefully titrated because of the risk of a paradoxical effect.
Phobic disorder	
Agoraphobia	
Fear of being away from home or in situations in which escape is inhibited	Alprazolam at the relatively high dose of 3 to 6 mg per day has proven effective. TCAs. Dose is typically between 150 and 200 mg per day. SSRIs and highly serotonergic TCAs (e.g., clomipramine, amitriptyline, trazodone) are effective for agoraphobia.
Social phobia	
Persistent fears of situations in which the person is exposed to the scrutiny of others (e.g., stage fright)	Beta blockers are often taken in combination with antidepressant or benzodiazepine; propranolol 10 to 20 mg tid or qid. Benzodiazepines alone or in combination with antidepressants. Clonazepam 0.5 mg bid. SSRIs. Low doses initially.
Obsessive compulsive disorder	
Obsessions, compulsions, or both	Clomipramine 100 to 200 mg per day. Fluvoxamine 200 to 300 mg per day. Other SSRIs. Gabapentin (Neurontin) titrated to 1800 to 2400 mg per day.

bid, Twice a day; *qid*, four times a day; *SSRIs*, selective serotonin reuptake inhibitors; *TCAs*, tricyclic antidepressants; *tid*, three times a day.

Flunitrazepam is manufactured in 0.5- to 1.0-mg tablets and, until recently, was tasteless, odorless, and undetectable if dissolved in water (Taylor, Donoghue, 2001). Flunitrazepam would often be slipped into the alcoholic drink of a young woman who would then become intoxicated. A notable side effect is amnesia. Young women would be given this drug and then be unable to remember what had happened the night before. Flunitrazepam is not sold in the United States but is routinely smuggled into the country.

What are some approaches to dealing with anxiety without drugs?

In the introductory paragraphs to this chapter, a review of historic data reflects this nation's passion for solutions to our anxieties and fears. What is happening in this society to contribute to this desire? Do you think this characteristic is unique to America?

Case Study

John is a 32-year-old man with a history of panic disorder with agoraphobia. He reports being a happy-go-lucky boy until the age of 12 when he experienced extremely traumatic physical abuse by a stepfather. His stepfather beat and ridiculed John for not fighting back. John reports becoming more and more reclusive and anxious, and a successful school year deteriorated into failing grades. John states that he reached the point that he hated going to school, but once he was at school, he dreaded going home. He felt confined at school, particularly when he was not allowed to select his own seat at the rear of the class. Over and over, John experienced what he can now describe as panic attacks at school. Class tests would push him to the point of a near "nervous breakdown." Nonetheless, John persevered for a while. John was anxious at school and fearful at home. He had a miserable life, and he spiraled downward until he gave up on school in the tenth grade. Though John believes he had the talent to be a "white collar" professional, his work life has been a series of day-laborer jobs. John has been prescribed alprazolam (Xanax), 1 mg twice a day and sertraline (Zoloft) 200 mg per day.

Key Concepts

1. Antianxiety agents are the most commonly prescribed psychotropic drugs, and benzodiazepines are the most commonly prescribed class of antianxiety agents.
2. Diazepam (Valium) is the prototype benzodiazepine; however, other benzodiazepines, particularly alprazolam (Xanax) and lorazepam (Ativan), are now used extensively.
3. Antianxiety drugs have four basic clinical uses: for treating people with chronic anxiety, for time-limited periods in people going through crises, for presurgery nervousness, and for the treatment of panic disorder.
4. Antianxiety drugs achieve their effect by depressing the CNS, particularly the reticular activating system, where they mute incoming stimuli.
5. The ability to mute incoming stimuli gives benzodiazepines a great potential for abuse.
6. Benzodiazepines can cause a physical dependence and produce a withdrawal syndrome. Discontinuance should be tapered gradually.
7. Side effects of the benzodiazepines include drowsiness, fatigue, ataxia, and other peripheral and central effects; however, tolerance to side effects occurs.
8. Benzodiazepines are relatively safe drugs when taken alone but can be deadly if mixed with other CNS depressants (e.g., alcohol).
9. Benzodiazepines that ultimately rely on conjugation with glucuronic acid to inactive metabolites are more appropriate for older adults (e.g., lorazepam [Ativan] and oxazepam [Serax]).
10. Buspirone is a nonbenzodiazepine and has gained extensive use for the treatment of anxiety. Buspirone differs from the benzodiazepines in the following ways:
    - It is not sedating.
    - It is not a drug that causes a "high" thus it has almost no abuse potential.
    - It has no cross-tolerance with sedatives or alcohol.
    - It takes 1 to 6 weeks to be effective.
    - It does not produce dependence, withdrawal, or tolerance.
    - It does not cause muscle relaxation.
11. Buspirone is a relatively safe drug that interacts with few other drugs.

References

Ashton CH: *Benzodiazepines: how they work & how to withdraw,* Newcastle, UK, 2000, University of Newcastle.

Ayd FJ: The early history of modern psychopharmacology, *Neuropsychopharmacology* 5(2):71, 1991.

Beeber LS: Treatment of anxiety, *J Psychosoc Nurs Ment Health Serv* 27:42, 1989.

Bezchlibnyk-Butler KZ, Jeffries JJ: *Clinical handbook of psychotropic drugs,* ed 7, Seattle, 1997, Hogrefe & Huber.

Black DW et al: A comparison of fluvoxamine, cognitive therapy, and placebo in the treatment of panic disorder, *Arch Gen Psychiatry* 50:44, 1993.

Carey KB: Emerging treatment guidelines for mentally ill chemical abusers, *Hosp Community Psychiatry* 40:341, 1989.

Ciraulo DA et al: *Drug interactions in psychiatry,* Baltimore, 1989, Williams & Wilkins.

Cohen LS: Psychotropic drug use in pregnancy, *Hosp Community Psychiatry* 40:566, 1989.

Glod CA: Xanax: pros and cons, *J Psychosoc Nurs Ment Health Serv* 30(6):36, 1992.

Gutierrez MA, Roper JM, Hahn P: Paradoxical reactions to benzodiazepines, *AJN* 101(7):34, 2001.

Harvey SC: Hypnotics and sedatives. In Gilman AG, Goodman LS, Rall TW, editors: *The pharmacological basis of therapeutics,* ed 7, New York, 1985, Macmillan.

Hollister LE: New psychotherapeutic drugs, *J Clin Psychopharmacol* 14(1):50, 1994.

Keltner NL: Neuroreceptor function and psychopharmacologic response, *Issues in Mental Health Nursing* 21:31, 2000.

Keltner NL, Folks DG: *Psychotropic drugs,* St Louis, 2001, Mosby.

Keltner NL, Opara I: Psychotropic drug interactions with grapefruit juice, *Perspect Psychiatr Care* 38(1):31, 2002.

Keltner NL et al: Adrenergic, cholinergic, GABAergic, and glutaminergic receptor function in the CNS, *Perspectives in Psychiatric Care* 37(23):45, 2001.

Lehne RA: *Pharmacology for nursing care,* Philadelphia, 2001, WB Saunders.

Lieberman JA, Tasman A: *Psychiatric drugs,* St Louis, 2000, WB Saunders.

Low K et al: Molecular and neuronal substrate for the selective attenuation of anxiety, 2001. [On-line] http://usm.maine.edupsy/broida/366/anxietyattenuation.html Downloaded 2/8/01.

Lydiard RB, Roy-Byrne PP, Ballinger JC: Recent advances in the psychopharmacological treatment of anxiety disorders, *Hosp Community Psychiatry* 39:1157, 1988.

Saito T: GABA circuitry and the implications for psychiatric and neurologic disorders. XXIInd Congress of the Collegium Internationale Neuro-Psychopharmacologicum, 2001. [On-line] http://www.medscape.com/medscape/cno/2000/CINP/Story.cfm?story_id=1511. Downloaded 2/08/01.

Seighart W: Structure and pharmacology of gamma-aminobutyric acid-A receptor subtypes, *Pharmacologic Rev* 47:181, 1995.

Shelton RC: Pharmacotherapy of panic disorder, *Hosp Community Psychiatry* 44(8):725, 1993.

Sterling L: Pharmacologic review of SSRIs in panic disorder, *Clinician Reviews Supplement,* 2001. [On-line] http://www.medscape.com/CPG/ClinReviews/1999/TherSpot/c03ts.02.ster/c03ts.o2.ster-01.html. Downloaded 2/08/01

Sugerman RA: Functional neuroanatomy. In Keltner NL, Folks DG, editors: *Psychotropic drugs,* ed 3, St Louis, 2001, Mosby.

Taylor B, Donoghue J: Club drugs—its effects on our youth, *The Alabama Nurse* 28(2):20, 2001.

United States Pharmacopeia: *Drug information for the health care professional,* Englewood, Colo, 2001, Micromedex.

Watsky EJ, Salzman C: Psychotropic drug interactions, *Hosp Community Psychiatry* 42(3):247, 1991.

Williams DB, Akabas MH: Benzodiazepines induce a conformational change in the region of gamma-aminobutyric acid type A receptor alpha (1) subunit M3 membrane spanning segment, *Mol Pharmacol* 58:1129, 2000.

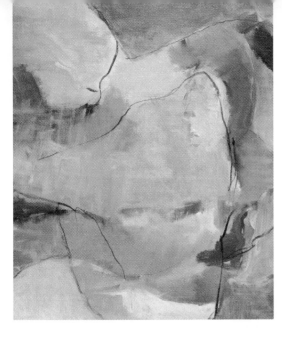

Chapter 24

Introduction to Milieu Management

Norman L. Keltner; Beverly K. Hogan

Learning Objectives

After reading this chapter, you should be able to:

- Define and describe the terms therapeutic milieu, therapeutic community, and therapeutic environment.
- Describe the goal of milieu management in the care of psychiatric patients.
- Identify the elements of the therapeutic milieu.
- Discuss several ways in which nurses can influence the therapeutic milieu.

Note to Students: Political, economic, and other forces have resulted in a health care system that changes quickly. These forces dictate the setting in which care takes place. Although hospitals used to employ the majority of psychiatric nurses, a great number of psychiatric nurses are currently practicing in community settings. As the struggle to define a system of mental health care continues, treatment settings will be diverse; however, treatment principles remain the same when they are guided by the nurse's focus on assisting patients in coping with problems caused by their illness. The treatment environment is affected by variables such as length of stay, patient population, and nature and goals of the treatment program. Notwithstanding these constraints, the nurse's involvement in creating a caring environment ultimately determines the overall atmosphere of the treatment setting. This role is true in any specialty area, but is the focus of psychiatric nursing and thus the essence of these chapters.

The purpose of a therapeutic environment is to help patients recover from psychiatric problems. The environment *always* affects the patient's treatment. Therapeutic environment and therapeutic milieu are used interchangeably to describe the atmosphere of a psychiatric unit. Therapeutic milieu, by the strictest definition, implies a formalized treatment modality, as described later in this chapter under *"history of milieu therapy."* Therapeutic environment is the preferred term of the authors thus encompassing even those treatment environments claiming not to use milieu therapy. In the opinion of the authors, all treatment environments constitute a milieu, therapeutic or nontherapeutic. To say that one is not using milieu principles is to acknowledge neglect of a significant responsibility of psychiatric nursing.

In the sections that follow, a history of the concept of milieu therapy is presented, followed by a discussion of the essential components of a therapeutic environment.

HISTORICAL OVERVIEW

Concepts related to milieu management were originally applied only to inpatient settings. The discussion in this section will therefore focus on milieu as it applies to hospital inpatient settings.

For many years, custodial care was the norm in inpatient settings. Custodial care does not necessarily mean cruel or neglectful care; rather, it refers to a *mind-set* in which nursing interventions focused

Key Terms

Acceptance Allowance of respect for individuality.

Balance Process of encouraging independent behavior within a treatment environment that fosters dependency.

Community meeting Meeting that occurs within the therapeutic milieu during which joint problem solving by community members is encouraged.

Feedback Articulation of one's perception of what another person has said or meant; this process requires at least two people.

Here-and-now focus Assisting patients to understand the way in which their current behaviors influence daily living.

Independence Taking actions for one's behalf rather than asking others to do so.

Individual responsibility Owning ones tasks, needs, feelings, and thoughts and taking action to address these responsibilities and needs.

Limit setting Holding people to established norms with the intent of assisting them to function more constructively and effectively.

Milieu management Purposeful manipulation of the environment to promote a therapeutic atmosphere.

Milieu therapy The use of any care environment to promote optimal functioning of a group or an individual.

Nonviolence Solving conflictual situations by methods other than verbal or physical aggression.

Norm Expected behavior for a given therapeutic setting.

Openness Atmosphere in which people are free to express their thoughts and feelings without fear of ridicule or censure.

Personal control Exerting limits on one's own impulses to act in a manner that is contrary to one's best interests, treatment goals, or personal needs.

Physical and emotional security Feeling safe from emotional, verbal, and physical assault.

Privacy Allowance of physical and emotional space for self and others.

Respect for the individual Acknowledgment and allowance of the rights of others to be unique.

Therapeutic milieu Context in which treatment occurs.

exclusively on meeting safety and physical needs. Even these basic goals were sometimes not reached. In a "better," usually private institution, custodial care was provided 23 hours of the day with 1 hour per day spent with a therapist. Less than 5% of the day was spent in a *therapeutic* situation!

Custodial care was a paternalistic system in which the staff "knew best" what the patient needed. Few attempts were made to "allow" the patient to participate in his or her own treatment.

Critical Thinking Questions

In what ways are the concepts of *norms* and *limit setting* similar? How are they different?

After World War II, several individuals began to be concerned about this "waste" of potentially therapeutic time. Stanton and Schwartz (1954) noted the discrepancy between "what could be and what was" in the hospital. They believed a better yield from hospitalization might be realized if all dimensions of care were focused on therapeutic benefits.

The most notable figure of this time was Maxwell Jones. In 1953, Jones wrote his landmark book, *The Therapeutic Community,* in which he described the benefits of an environment that was therapeutic in and of itself. Jones proposed patient involvement in decision-making, daily group meetings (i.e., therapeutic community) about the day-to-day living aspects of the unit, patient participation in planning ward activities, and the concept of patient self-responsibility.

Just as the therapeutic environment was realized as a legitimate psychiatric treatment modality, other forces converged to direct energies away from milieu therapy. (See Chapter 1 for a more detailed recounting of these events.) Psychopharmacology, concern for patients' rights, and reactions to conditions of institutional care started the community mental health movement. These forces worked against a basic underpinning of milieu therapy: hospital care for patients.

The pendulum has swung back toward *therapeutic milieu* as an important treatment modality in community-based care programs. This approach is consistent with shorter inpatient stays and a shifting of illness management to community treatment settings.

Historically, the term *therapeutic milieu* refers to a broad conceptual approach in which all aspects of the environment were channeled to provide a therapeutic environment for patients. The idea was that the milieu can be therapeutic "in and of itself" (Jones, 1953) and can be applied in many settings.

Therapeutic community, on the other hand, has been considered a concept restricted to the inpatient setting in which a patient-led government establishes and enforces community rules. Over the years, the distinction between therapeutic milieu and therapeutic community has all but disappeared, and the terms are now often used synonymously. Regardless of the term used to describe the context in which milieu principles are used, interventions are successful only when the environment is effectively managed. *Milieu management,* then, is a descriptive term that implies the need for purposeful activity by the nursing staff to develop a *therapeutic environment.*

Traditionally, the hospital has been the only setting thought to be appropriate for milieu concerns. Today, however, psychiatric nurses expend energies on developing a therapeutic environment in residential programs and in home care management, as well as in the hospital setting. Appropriate management of the environment, regardless of the setting, is an important aspect of patient care. Peplau (1995) notes that movement of psychiatric nurses into community practice settings provides opportunities to facilitate a therapeutic environment, whether it is in a private family home, group home, or among homeless people.

Nursing's History and the Therapeutic Milieu

Florence Nightingale recognized nursing's responsibility for creating and controlling patients' milieu. In the inpatient setting, psychiatric nursing has 24-hour responsibility for patient care. No other discipline provides this on-site, around-the-clock care. Patients and nurses all benefit from a therapeutic environment. Patients benefit because the use of many resources, including interpersonal interactions, psychotropic drugs, and the environment, keeps the focus on their recovery. Nurses benefit because staff relationships and patient care issues are "in the open."

Creating and maintaining a therapeutic environment is a *core function* of psychiatric nursing. The treatment environment may occur in a hospital setting, such as a short inpatient stay on a psychiatric unit or a slightly longer stay in a state mental hospital. More likely, treatment will occur in a variety of community-based settings, such as:

- Residential care homes (i.e., group homes)
- Partial hospitalization
- Day-treatment programs

- Patients' home
- Homeless shelters

The treatment environment may even be a mobile health care unit visiting "homeless patients" in whatever environment they are found. Again, regardless of the treatment setting, an environment is available in which treatment occurs, and manipulation of this environment can be used for good or can be counterproductive.

Because nurses are responsible for managing the treatment environment, the nurse must thoroughly comprehend its components and the essential ingredients required for creating an environment conducive to recovery. The treatment environment affects patient satisfaction with treatment, rates of dropout from treatment, and adaptation in the community (Timko, Moos, 1998).

The milieu, like the therapeutic relationship, is designed to provide a "corrective" learning experience that enables the patient to recover. All interactions are considered potentially therapeutic and are organized around the established treatment goals of the individual patients. Distortions, conflicts, and inappropriate behavior are dealt with in the here-and-now of each interaction. Interactions are opportunities to reinforce treatment objectives.

Working effectively in a milieu is a true challenge for psychiatric nursing. So many conflicting and confounding variables affect the milieu that the nurse must actively work (i.e., expend mental and physical energy) to make the treatment environment therapeutic.

As previously noted, *milieu management* is the purposeful use of all interpersonal and environmental forces to enhance mental health. What Talbot and Miller (1966) wrote over 30 years ago remains true: "An ideal psychiatric hospital is not merely a sanctuary, a cotton-padded milieu that emphasizes the fragility, the incompetence, the helplessness, the bizarreness of patients. Rather it should reflect a sane society by permitting the optimal use of the intact ego capacities through its social organization, its social supports, and its community values" (p. 165).

CLINICAL EXAMPLE
South of Birmingham in a rural area of the state is a day-treatment program for chronically mentally ill individuals. The day-treatment program is housed in a large rustic building in which individuals with chronic mental disorders attend educational and therapy sessions during

the day, 5 days a week. Within easy walking distance are two group homes. Emphasis is placed on developing a therapeutic milieu at both the day-treatment center and the group home. Trained staff members structure the days and evenings at the group homes.

GOAL OF MILIEU MANAGEMENT

The goal of milieu management, regardless of setting, is to organize all interpersonal and environmental forces toward developing an atmosphere that facilitates the patient's growth, rehabilitation, and restoration of health. The effectiveness of milieu therapy is judged by its effectiveness during every 24-hour period. This concept suggests that all members of the health care team are responsible for understanding and maintaining the therapeutic environment.

Ineffective milieus are often characterized by an overabundance of television watching. Hillbrand, Waite, and Young (1998) describe this as a "default" activity and wonder about the effect of indiscriminate television watching on patients whose condition renders them vulnerable to its negative effects.

Patients will be no more active in the treatment environment than are the nurses. Nurses must be available, flexible, and willing to help patients develop coping and problem-solving skills if the benefits of therapeutic environment are to be realized.

ELEMENTS OF THE EFFECTIVE MILIEU

For the milieu to be effectively managed, six environmental elements must be present:

- Safety
- Structure
- Norms
- Limit setting
- Balance
- Environmental modification

Safety

Safety implies freedom from danger or harm. Safety trumps other concerns in the therapeutic environment and encompasses freedom from *both* psychologic and physical harm. In the therapeutic environment, safety of all members of the environment is equally important.

Protection from psychologic harm is provided by norms that do not permit undue confrontation of one patient by another or excessive confrontation of patients by others. Restricting visitors, including family members who are known to disparage patients, may also protect patients.

Patients who experience severe anxiety may suffer unnecessarily if staff members do not intervene. Interventions to decrease anxiety and promote a feeling of psychologic safety may include giving psychotropic medications, assuring patients that a staff member will stay with them, and providing these patients with a nonstimulating environment.

Freedom from physical harm is also important. Developing unit norms that do not permit physical violence by any community member ensures safety. Policies and procedures for control of aggression are necessary. Some institutions use "time-out" rooms (the patient's room or a designated but isolated spot on the unit) to which patients who are acting in a threatening way are directed to go until they are in control. At times, patients must be physically restrained with leather restraints or secluded in a seclusion room until they are more in control. Whenever patients are restrained or secluded, they must be told that they are not being punished, but rather, that external controls are being used until they are able to regain control. Consider the following clinical problem.

CLINICAL EXAMPLE

In response to hearing voices, a patient named Tim hits one of the staff nurses. Tim agrees to walk to the seclusion room. At that time, he is given an intramuscular dose of an ordered medication to help control his agitation. Tim is told that the medication is to help him relax and that he will be kept in seclusion until he indicates, and staff members agree, that he can control his behavior. A staff member is either assigned to stay with Tim to reaffirm that he is not being punished or reassures him of frequent observation and attention to the patients' safety, comfort, and physical care needs. The message to the patient is that the staff are concerned that patients on the unit remain safe.

The student should note that although this scenario is realistic, giving the as-needed (prn) medication after the hitting incident occurred is somewhat in opposition to the principles presented in Chapter 13. The conceptualization of aggression presented there (the assault cycle) suggests that the time to medicate be during the escalation phase, *not* after the crisis has occurred.

Structure

Structure refers to the physical environment, regulations, and daily schedule of classes and groups provided in a treatment setting. Establishing therapeutic community meetings, exercise and recreation activity groups, social skills groups, and a number of other therapeutic activities provides structure. Groups in which patients share problems and triumphs are also part of the therapeutic environment.

The design of the unit is an important aspect of the structure. Adequate space, areas for socializing and receiving visitors, telephones, and areas for privacy are all required elements of a therapeutic environment. Because seclusion rooms are often necessary, their design, location, and furnishings must maintain both safety and dignity. Furnishings, the color of the walls, and so on all communicate facility philosophy to the patients, their families, and the staff. While considering "structure," the student should ask, "What is it about a given dimension of unit structure that makes it therapeutic?"

Norms

Norms are specific expectations of behavior that pervade the setting; they are intended to promote community living through behaviors that are socially acceptable. For instance, a common norm is that violent behavior is not permitted. A norm of nonviolence provides for physical and emotional security. The following clinical example illustrates the way that a norm of nonviolence would be implemented.

CLINICAL EXAMPLE
John is angry with another patient and is threatening him with bodily harm. The nurse intervenes by firmly directing John to go to his room. The nurse stays with John and encourages him to talk about what he is feeling rather than to act on his feelings.

Deescalating a patient avoids potentially violent encounters and provides patients with an opportunity to examine the circumstance that generated the anger and the way they might more effectively resolve the issue.

Other norms focus on the level of personal control. For example, patients may be required to take psychotropic drugs. However, the time at which they take the medication may be negotiable. The same is true for other aspects of treatment. This type of environment creates a norm of personal choice within reason. Other norms focus on openness, giving and receiving feedback, respect for the patient, privacy, acceptance, independence, and individual responsibility. All these norms attempt to build a climate of universality or shared experience. (Box 24-1 lists the common norms for psychiatric treatment environments.)

Limit Setting

Limit setting is important in inpatient settings, as well as other settings, and is related to norms. Limits should be set on acting-out behavior, such as self-destructive acts, physical aggressiveness, sexual behavior, lack of compliance, use of alcohol or illicit drugs, use of over-the-counter drugs, and elopement (running away). If patients are likely to engage in any of these behaviors, then discussing the behavior with the patient in an anticipatory fashion is important, rather than waiting until after the fact. These discussions reinforce the *norm* of making rules and expectations clear and also encourage the milieu concept of responsibility for self.

Critical Thinking Question

In this chapter, *balance* is defined as "... the process of gradually allowing independent behavior in a dependent situation." What is meant by a *dependent situation*?

Closely related to limit setting are rules. Box 24-2 lists important inpatient rules on a psychiatric unit.

Balance

Balance is also an important concept but is difficult to describe and does not lend itself to a concrete list of rules. Perhaps more than any other dimension of

---

Box 24-1 | Unit Norms on an Inpatient Psychiatric Unit

- Acceptance
- Feedback
- Independence
- Individual responsibility
- Nonviolence
- Openness
- Personal control
- Physical and emotional security
- Privacy
- Respect for the individual

Mary, who is attending a partial hospital day program, is very anxious and approaches the nurses' station every 10 minutes, asking to talk with a staff member. Staff members are concerned that they may be encouraging Mary to be too dependent by talking with her each time she approaches. The staff jointly decides to set limits on Mary by telling her that a staff member will meet with her once every 4 hours for a 15-minute period. This approach encourages the patient to limit her demands on others and also to meet some of her own needs between the times she meets with a staff member.

milieu management, balance represents the "art" of nursing. Balance is the process of gradually allowing independent behaviors in a dependent situation. Independence is gained in increments because too much independence may overwhelm the patient. Examples best illustrate this point.

In the case of a self-destructive patient, the nurse attempts to balance the patient's (and the nurse's) need for safety (a dependency-creating approach) with the patient's need for self-control and independence. Another example is patients who are very religious. The nurse may have to balance the patients' rights to religious expression with the need for treatment. For patients to refuse medication on religious grounds is somewhat common, even though they are frankly psychotic. Religion may also be out of balance when the religiously preoccupied patient forces sermons on other patients. These types of unsolicited discourses are a violation of other patients' rights to privacy, choice, and protection from the symptom expression of other patients.

The skillful use of balance comes with an understanding of ethical concerns, legal issues, and psychopathologic factors.

Environmental Modification

Through *environmental modification,* the nurse can facilitate the development of a therapeutic environment and communicate worth to the patient. Physical arrangements, safety issues, and orientation features, when addressed, can create an atmosphere in which patients are enabled to maximize their strengths. Ongoing review of environmental norms, rules, and regulations is an important aspect of milieu modification. Flexibility in maintaining a therapeutic environment is accomplished by ongoing evaluation of its effectiveness. The following example of environmental modification also makes reference to a unit norm, illustrating the way in which components of the therapeutic environment interact.

Critical Thinking Question

A 16-year-old boy with a diagnosis of bipolar disorder has been admitted to the adolescent unit of a psychiatric hospital because of recent fighting at school and threatening his parents at home. How might the use of therapeutic milieu assist this patient changing his behaviors?

CLINICAL EXAMPLE
A unit norm requires that the television be turned off at 10:00 PM on weeknights. During a morning community meeting, several residents of the home indicate that a special television program, of interest to patients, is scheduled to air from 10:00 PM until midnight. A joint decision by staff and patients is made to permit the residents to watch this special show. Temporarily modifying the norm promotes autonomy and allows for individuality, while keeping the basic structure intact.

Box 24-2 | Important Inpatient Rules

Social Rules
- Abides by rules regarding smoking and handling matches
- Does not interrupt conversations
- Does not intrude into areas designated off-limits by staff
- Listens attentively when others talk in meetings
- Does not dress in a sexually revealing manner
- Uses telephone with consideration for others
- Eats at designated places and times
- Uses television and stereo with consideration for others
- Abides by rules regarding visitors

Therapeutic Rules
- Acknowledges the need for treatment
- Accepts the need for hospitalization
- Participates in individual therapy
- Attends individual therapy as scheduled
- Seeks out staff to help control psychotic or illness-related behavior
- Actively participates in setting therapeutic goals for self
- Examines own progress realistically when considering changes
- Participates in family therapy and group conferences

From Morrison EF: Determining social and therapeutic rules for psychiatric inpatients, *Hospital & Community Psychiatry* 38:994, 1987.

ROLES OF THE PSYCHOTHERAPEUTIC MANAGER

Milieu management requires nurses to serve in multiple roles. Some of these roles include:

- Working individually with patients
- Leading groups
- Participating in community meetings
- Coordinating medical care (with physicians)
- Dispensing routine medications and making decisions concerning prn medications
- Making discharge arrangements
- Working with families in a variety of health care settings

Additionally, nurses provide leadership in interdisciplinary team meetings and are the professionals who most often implement team decisions.

Teaching is also an important role for nurses who are involved in the therapeutic milieu. Nurses actively engage in teaching patients and their families about the therapeutic use of medications, as well as about the possible side effects. Medication compliance is a major factor in preventing recidivism and often in maintaining a patient in the community.

Critical Thinking Questions

Review Box 24-3 *On Being Sane in Insane Places.* What were the things that were wrong on the inpatient unit? How should this be corrected to facilitate a therapeutic environment?

| Box 24-3 | On Being Sane in Insane Places

Rosenhan wondered whether the "sane" could be distinguished from the "insane." He selected eight pseudopatients (people who pretended to be mentally ill) and instructed them to attempt to gain admission to public mental hospitals. The task was much easier than anyone had anticipated. Twelve hospitals in five states were used. The pseudopatient group consisted of a graduate student in psychology, three psychologists (including Rosenhan himself), a pediatrician, a psychiatrist, a painter, and a housewife; three were women and five were men. No one in the hospital knew of the deception.

The pseudopatients were trained to do the following:

1. Call the hospital and make an appointment.
2. On arriving at the hospital, pseudopatients were to tell the psychiatrist that they had been hearing voices.
3. On being asked to describe the voices, all were to say that they were not sure but did remember the words "empty," "hollow," and "thud."
4. Other than giving this false information and false information about their names, occupations, and employers, they were, from that point forward, to be truthful and "normal."
5. Immediately on admission, the pseudopatients were instructed to cease simulating abnormal behavior and to behave "normally."
6. When asked how they were doing, the pseudopatients were trained to respond "fine" and to inform the staff that they were no longer experiencing problems.

Despite behaving normally, the staff discovered none of the pseudopatients. However, approximately 25% of the other patients made comments about the pseudopatients' "sanity," and a few even guessed that the pseudopatients were doing some kind of undercover work. Rosenhan noted reluctance by the staff to see mental health in their patients. He stated, "Having once been labeled schizophrenic, there is nothing the pseudopatients can do to overcome the tag." Pseudopatient histories were written to support their diagnosis. In other words, psychiatrists saw problems that had never existed.

The pseudopatients were also asked to write down their observations. At first, elaborate precautions were followed to avoid detection; however, they were soon jotting down observations in front of the staff. The pseudopatients had discovered that no one was paying any attention to them.

Another part of the experiment was to determine the amount of time that was spent with patients. The time was difficult to measure, so a proxy behavior was substituted: time the nurses spent outside of the nurses' station. Nursing attendants had the highest percentage of time outside the station (11.3%). Rosenhan found it impossible to measure the time registered nurses spend outside of the nurses' station because it occurred so infrequently. Psychiatrists were even worse because they hid behind closed office doors; at least the patients were able to see the nurses. Rosenhan concluded, "Those with the most power have least to do with patients, and those with the least power are most involved with them."

Rosenhan decries the powerlessness and the depersonalization experienced by the pseudopatients. He remembered the way in which he was frequently awakened in the hospital at which he was admitted: "Come on you, [obscene profanity], out of bed."

The pseudopatients were hospitalized on average for 19 days before they were deemed well enough for discharge. The range of stays was from 7 to 52 days.

From Rosenhan DL: On being sane in insane places, *Science* 179:250, 1973.

Key Concepts

1. Milieu management is the purposeful use of all interpersonal and environmental forces to enhance the mental health of psychiatric patients through the development of a therapeutic environment.
2. When nursing has 24-hour accountability for patient care, nurses have the major responsibility for shaping the therapeutic environment.
3. Historically, nurses provided only custodial care; but after World War II, Maxwell Jones (1953) and others conceptualized an environment in which all aspects of the psychiatric patient's day would be used to promote mental health.
4. Nurses gained more influence over the care of patients as the result of this emphasis on the environment. However, just as milieu therapy was gaining acceptance as a viable treatment form, other forces converged and eventually changed the locus of psychiatric treatment from a therapeutic inpatient setting to a community mental health setting.
5. The effective use of milieu management in other settings is currently being reconsidered as psychiatric nursing leaders look for more effective ways to treat individuals with mental disorders.
6. The effectively managed milieu is composed of six elements: (1) safety, (2) structure, (3) norms, (4) limit setting, (5) balance, and (6) environmental modification.
7. Concepts of the well-managed milieu are increasingly being applied to care settings other than inpatient units.

References

Hillbrand M, Waite BM, Young JL: Restricting TV access by forensic patients, *Psychiatr Serv* 49(1): 107, 1998.
Jones M: *The therapeutic community,* New York, 1953, Basic Books.
Morrison EF: Determining social and therapeutic rules for psychiatric inpatients, *Hosp Community Psychiatry* 38:994, 1987.
Peplau HE: Some unresolved issues in the era of biopsychosocial nursing, *J Am Psychiatr Nurs Assoc* 1(3):92, 1995.
Rosenhan DL: On being sane in insane places, *Science* 179:250, 1973.
Stanton A, Schwartz M: *The mental hospital,* New York, 1954, Basic Books.
Talbot E, Miller SC: The struggle to create a sane society in the psychiatric hospital, *Psychiatry* 29:165, 1966.
Timko C, Moos RH: Outcomes of the treatment climate in psychiatric and substance abuse programs, *J Clin Psychol* 54(8):1137, 1998.

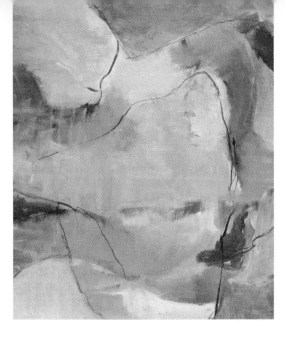

Chapter 25

Variables Affecting the Therapeutic Environment

Beverly K. Hogan

Learning Objectives

After reading this chapter, you should be able to:

- Identify variables affecting creation and maintenance of a therapeutic environment.
- Describe the influence of staff relationships on the treatment environment.
- Describe the importance of nursing management to the treatment environment.
- Describe the impact nurses have on the therapeutic environment.
- Understand the implications of the Joint Commission on Accreditation of Healthcare Organizations (JCAHO) guidelines for a therapeutic environment.

In Chapter 24, milieu management was presented as a process of establishing safety, structure, norms, limit setting, balance, and environmental modification. Variables influencing the creation and maintenance of the therapeutic environment will be explored in this chapter.

INFLUENCE OF STAFF RELATIONSHIPS ON THE TREATMENT ENVIRONMENT

The treatment environment includes the physical layout of the unit and, most importantly, the relationships among staff members and between patients and staff. As is the case with all relationships, the potential for conflict, strained relationships, and dissatisfaction exists. Conflict and disgruntled attitudes permeate the atmosphere of a treatment environment and interfere with the development of a therapeutic environment. Most people can identify with a *particular feeling* they get when walking into a social setting, business, or health care setting. The feeling may be one of tension, stirring the desire to *get away* as soon as possible, or it might be a *good atmosphere,* leaving one with a positive feeling about being there. The latter is sought in creating a therapeutic environment. If one were to examine factors in the environment that make it positive, factors such as how well people get along, whether people smile, and welcoming comments and gestures would likely be present. On the other hand, chronic conflict among staff members creates more of the "can't wait to get away from there" feeling.

Nurses are keenly aware of the impact of good relationships with colleagues and recognize that this ultimately affects the treatment environment (Cleary, Edwards, 1999). Staff members who are unable to cope with conflict are *less effective* in their interactions with patients. Conflict is more likely in treatment environments characterized by an explicit hierarchy, which overrides collaboration and communication among staff (Simms, 1999). In such environments, a parental style of communication is prevalent (Cleary, Edwards, 1999).

Key Terms

Aggression Verbal or physical expressions of anger aimed at hurting others.

Bureaucracy Excessive rules and structure that get in the way of efficient, responsive, and creative nursing care solutions.

Burnout Spiraling process of decreased effectiveness.

Clinical supervision Formal meeting between psychiatric nursing peers whose purpose is to provide a place for nurses caring for patients to examine attitudes, reactions, and conflicts with patients on the unit and to find new ways of approaching patient problems.

Co-morbidity Simultaneous existence of medical and psychiatric problems, each complicating the other.

Conflict Differing perspectives among staff or patients regarding various aspects of treatment.

Consumer Patient in treatment for psychiatric services.

Model of care Philosophy of causative and curative factors of mental illness that drives the nature of the care activities offered.

Nurse-patient interaction Purposeful use of the relationship between patient and nurse for achieving patient treatment goals.

Teamwork Staff working together to achieve agreed on goals for the unit and for patient care.

Therapeutic environment Growth-promoting atmosphere created in a treatment setting, which is chiefly influenced by relationships among staff and between staff, patients, and visitors. Physical structure and amenities are also an influence.

The model of care in a given treatment facility dictates the kind of psychiatric treatment offered. Usually, the psychiatrist, as head of the treatment team, sets the tone for treatment based on their theoretical model of care. Some psychiatrists have a purely medical focus and minimize the value of psychosocially oriented interventions. Because nurses are educated to provide holistic care, conflict can erupt in a setting that marginalizes psychosocial intervention. Unresolved conflict about treatment approaches is not conducive to effective, consistent interventions.

Nurses *trapped* in a model of care divergent from their belief system or their theoretical model of care find this unresolved conceptual conflict adversely affects the care they provide. For instance, milieu therapy may conflict greatly with a purely medical model of care. In a pure medical model, the use of medications and other biologically based interventions are seen as the solution, with psychosocial care given little importance. Chronic dissonance about the care being provided is one factor leading to burnout and low morale of the nursing staff.

Burnout deteriorates the nurse's ability to be effective on a psychiatric unit. Burned out staff members score high on scales measuring feelings of being *emotionally burdened,* and they tend to *overinterpret* patient care failures as their *fault.* This tendency leads to a spiraling process of decreased effectiveness in nurse-patient interactions at all levels. Some of

the manifestations of burnout on a psychiatric unit are low morale, passivity, avoidance, disinterest, chronic complaining, and negative, hostile reactions to others (Schreiber, Lutzen, 2000). This negativity precludes the development of a therapeutic relationship and erodes the therapeutic treatment environment. Walking onto a unit in which burnout is a problem leaves one with a very negative impression.

The reader is encouraged to review the summary of the classic article "On Being Sane in Insane Places" in Chapter 24, Box 24-3. Notably in this excerpt, the "pseudopatients" went unnoticed while making written observations for the "study" because so little attention was paid to them. In fact, the pseudopatients had difficulty recording a percentage of time nurses spent with patients because it occurred so infrequently. The pseudopatients described feeling depersonalized and powerless; they even reported being called demoralizing names by the staff. Certainly, most people would agree that fellow human beings should not be treated in this manner; treating patients who have presented for psychiatric help in this manner is morally incomprehensible. Patients should certainly expect the treatment environment to be less toxic than the environment from which they came.

If maintaining good relationships among staff is already a difficult task, it is certainly complicated by the day-to-day stresses of dealing with patients with behavioral problems. Patients in a public psychiatric hospital are among the sickest, with limitless needs, poor insight, frequent readmissions, few placement alternatives, and sometimes, violent behavior. Stressors such as these take their toll on the nurse. Seen by outsiders as inappropriate, humor is a method frequently used in stressful occupations to help relieve the anxiety, fear, or horror of coping with the nature of stressful work (Sayre 2001).

Sayre (2001) studied the use of humor by mental health professionals in psychiatry, categorized humor into types ranging from whimsical to sarcastic or hostile, and examined its influence on patient care. Although whimsical humor (defined as *playful,* poking of fun) was generally accepted as a way of coping with stress, humor that falls on the sarcastic (defined as intentional hurt with mocking ridicule) and hostile end of the scale tended to erode professional competence and morale, ultimately affecting patient care. When interactions between staff and patients were perceived as more stressful, staff tended to engage in more of the *sarcastic* variety of humor. Under the veil of sarcasm, feelings of anger and a discounting or vengeance for the target of sarcastic humor was evident. The use of sarcastic humor, in particular, creates a kind of nontherapeutic distancing, thereby interfering with successful development of a therapeutic relationship with patients. This type of humor is so commonplace in the media that recognizing its antitherapeutic effects may be difficult. Although nurses in Sayre's study used sarcastic humor about patients quite often, they rarely ridiculed the misfortune of patients directly. One can only guess how long it might be before patients, too, become the recipients of such humor. Although sarcasm and burnout are understandable responses to underlying distress within nurses' work environments, it is neither acceptable nor effective interpersonal behavior in a health care environment. On the positive side, Sayre found openness among staff facilitated increased work satisfaction and teamwork. Healthy work relationships can have conflict, but the commitment of staff to resolve it allows a therapeutic environment to develop. This level of commitment is consistent with the Code of Behavior for professional nursing practice as defined by the American Nurses' Association (ANA, 1997).

Critical Thinking Question

How would you use the principles learned in this chapter or course to deal with a coworker who constantly complains and gossips about other co-workers?

IMPACT OF MANAGEMENT PRACTICES AND ORGANIZATIONAL STRUCTURE ON THE TREATMENT ENVIRONMENT

Aside from dealing with conflictual staff relationships, dealing with bureaucracy is seen by nurses as a major impediment to their effectiveness (Boey, 1999). Staff requires administrative and management support to deliver the care required on a psychiatric unit (Smith, 1998). As representatives of the *model of care* of an agency, management influences the practice of nursing. Stated another way, nursing practice can only be as effective as management allows. It is difficult to imagine that nursing management would engage in practices that restrict the practice of *good* nursing care, however, it does occur. Several studies have documented the influence of management on nursing morale and implementation of care (Boey, 1999; Brekke et al, 1997; Graham, 2001; Lutzen, 1998; Schreiber, Lutzen, 2000; Smith, 1998). Nurses cannot practice the art and science of their profession unless management establishes structures that support and reinforce good nursing care.

Institutional restraints and bureaucracy affect the caring ethic of nurses. Upholding the standards of professional nursing practice is greatly influenced by the support of management. In a nonsupportive, oppressive atmosphere, nurses face sanctions for "doing the right thing." These sanctions come from peers, or worse, from management. In a study of *moral survival strategies* practiced by nurses in these environments, Lutzen (1998) found management practices to be a significant influence. Nurses become demoralized when they do not have appropriate support to practice nursing. This type of oppression is harmful not only to the patient, but also to the nurse (Schreiber, Lutzen, 2000).

Organizational structures that are rigid and characterized by a high need for efficiency interfere with nursing care. An *excessively rigid* focus on rules and efficiency diminishes the ability to focus on the patient as an individual. The goals of psychiatric nursing can become eclipsed by the practical considerations of *surviving* in such an environment. Patients refer to staff members who are more concerned with rules, efficiency, and order as "institutionalized," a term originally coined by professionals to describe patients with the same characteristics.

Lack of positive reinforcement and being held accountable for impossible to meet care objectives with dwindling resources erode the morale and professional competence of nurses (Sayre, 2001). In studies examining strategies for reducing burnout and dissatisfaction in nurses, most researchers conclude that effective management actions can alleviate many of the problems.

> ### *Critical* Thinking Question
> What might you do, other than transfer or resign, should you find yourself in a work environment in which management is unsupportive of nursing staff?

NURSING'S CONTRIBUTION TO THE TREATMENT ENVIRONMENT

Nurses perceive their roles as essential to effective management of the treatment environment (Cleary, 1999). Studies measuring patient satisfaction with treatment show a strong correlation with the quality of the nursing staff. Like it or not, nurses are seen as responsible for creating the environment of care within a given nursing unit (Baker, 2000).

The way in which nurses enforce rules and norms in a treatment environment affects the nurse-patient relationship and the therapeutic environment. Excessive focus on rules and efficiency may be seen as necessary and desirable to some staff but is harmful to patients. Abrupt dismissal of the patients' perspective occurs when rules and regulations have a stronger focus than do individualized patient care and creativity among the nursing staff.

> ### *Critical* Thinking Questions
> What are the advantages of openness and feedback on a psychiatric unit? Can you think of any drawbacks? Are the nurses "open" on the unit where you have clinicals?

CLINICAL EXAMPLE
The unit routine dictates that patients take a bath in the morning and take medications at 8:00 AM. A patient recently admitted involuntarily angrily refuses both. The nurse talks with the patient and offers a choice about when to take a bath. The nurse also learns that the patient usually takes medications later in the morning. The nurse negotiates with the treatment team and pharmacy department to change the times of the patient's scheduled medication.

Nurses also influence the therapeutic environment through communicating and developing nurse-patient relationships. Staff-patient interactions influence the patient's overall perception of treatment.

When patients have a choice about terminating treatment, the effectiveness of interpersonal relationships with staff is an important consideration in their decision to discontinue treatment. For instance, one study demonstrated a relationship between dropout rates in substance abuse treatment facilities and the interpersonal environment (Timko, Moos, 1998).

Mental health nursing is founded on interpersonal interactions and therapeutic use of self as an essential aspect of care (Cleary, 1999). Nurses must be able to engineer the environment so that therapeutic interaction can occur.

The article excerpt, "On Being Sane in Insane Places" (see Box 24-3), notes that nurses spent little time interacting with patients. More recent studies document that less than one half of the nurses' time is spent in direct patient contact, with the percentage of time devoted to potentially therapeutic interaction slightly less than 7% (Whittington, McLaughlin, 2000). Other studies find that patients spend the majority of their time alone, and although they understand the nurse's time constraints, patients regret the lack of time available to spend with them (Cleary, 1999).

Patients interpret this lack of attention as a dismissal or minimization of their symptoms and problems. Cleary (1999) found that patient dissatisfaction with nursing care is related to the quality and time that nurses spend with them. Patients valued nurses who dealt with problem patients, an important function of the nurse in creating safety as noted in the previous chapter. If nurses were simply available, if they greeted the patients by name and made time to spend with them, patients viewed nurses as valuable.

In environments where the need to be efficient supercedes the interpersonal relationship focus, patients suffer. The low percentages of interaction in a nursing specialty in which interaction is a primary treatment modality demands attention.

> ### *Critical* Thinking Question
> How would you ensure good nurse-patient interaction within a unit?

Some studies relate the quality of interaction to the nurses' stress levels. High stress levels among staff contribute to burnout. Evers and colleagues (2001) found that staff reporting high levels of emotional exhaustion tended to have cold, callused treatment attitudes.

One factor that minimizes vulnerability to burnout is having a sense of meaning in one's work. Being able to clearly define one's role contributes to a greater sense of meaning in nursing (Graham, 2001). In a descriptive, exploratory study of the way nurses define their role, nurses delineated their chief aim as promoting a positive self-concept in patients by exploring their *lived experiences* through the nurse-patient relationship.

Nurses have published both research and anecdotal details of their successes in implementing an improved therapeutic environment in psychiatric care settings. Improvement in patient functioning has been documented as a result of implementing these changes (Baker, 2000; Smith, Gross, Roberts, 1996). Nurses deliver interventions for a variety of behavior disturbances, including hallucinations and delusions. Studies demonstrate that these interventions are superior to medication alone.

PHYSICAL LAYOUT OF THE UNIT

One can surmise a lot about a unit by the way it is physically arranged. Units without places to sit and talk privately say a lot about the way the unit will be "run" (Cleary, Edwards, 1999). Inaccessible nursing stations with locked doors also send messages to patients. On the other hand, a unit with an attractive décor, access to amenities as needed, and accessible staff communicate a very different message.

JCAHO ENVIRONMENT OF CARE ISSUES

Environment of care standards requires that facilities be designed and constructed to ensure that the environment is safe and accessible and that the facility is routinely evaluated for ongoing effectiveness of providing care. Additionally, the facility must establish a social environment that supports its basic philosophy; and finally, it must establish and enforce a nonsmoking policy throughout the institution. (Box 25-1 lists the environment of care standards on inpatient psychiatric units.) Standards for managing the environment of care are outlined and described in detail in the JCAHO's *Comprehensive Accreditation Manual for Hospitals* (2001). The goal of management of the environment is "to provide a safe, functional, supportive, and effective environment for patients, staff members, and other individuals in the hospital" (p. EC-1). These standards also apply to outpatient clinics and counseling centers.

| **Box 25-1 | JCAHO Environment of Care Standards**

Environmental safety is attained through:
- On-going assessment and maintenance of all equipment
- Hazard surveillance
- Reporting and investigation of safety issues
- Monitoring of safety management techniques and procedures
- Orientation programs that address safety issues

A health care facility ensures the security of all people through:
- Mechanisms for addressing security issues
- Provision of appropriate identification for all staff, patients, and visitors
- Security orientation programs
- Mechanisms for handling emergencies
- Mechanisms for interacting with the media

The social environment must provide:
- Space for storage of grooming and hygiene articles
- Closet and drawer space for personal property
- Clothing that is suitable for clinical conditions

The physical setting must provide:
- Adequate privacy to insure respect for patients
- Door locks consistent with program goals
- Availability of telephones that allow for private conversations
- Sleeping rooms with doors for privacy unless clinically contraindicated
- Furnishings suitable to the population served
- Access to the outdoors unless contraindicated for therapeutic reasons

DEALING WITH AGGRESSION AND VIOLENCE

Probably the greatest concern students have about psychiatric nursing involves the potential for violence. Safety is an essential component of the therapeutic environment. To the extent that nursing staff is competent in managing potential aggression (and is adequately staffed), aggression on a psychiatric unit is managed by prevention and early intervention (see Chapter 13 for detailed discussion of the aggressive patient). This prevention—early intervention approach to potential aggression—is required to maintain the feeling of safety to everyone within the unit.

The importance of an adequate assessment of the patient and the treatment environment cannot be overemphasized when it comes to being prepared to address issues of potential aggression and violence. Recognition of a number of risk factors can help the nurse anticipate potential problems with violence and respond accordingly (see Chapter 13 for a further discussion of violence on inpatient psychiatric units).

One variable affecting the risk of aggression is staff attitude. A study of attitudinal variables and risk of being targeted for patient aggression found that a higher risk exists for staff with more authoritarian attitudes, an external locus of control (looking outside themselves for blame rather that looking within [i.e., self-reflection]), and a high degree of anxiety (Ray, Subich, 1998).

Dealing with aggressive behavior is stressful. However, having the perception of competence to deal with aggression or violence or both can lessen stress. Research shows that nurses trained in physical and verbal intervention techniques for dealing with aggression have greater confidence (Evers, Tomic, Brouwers, 2001).

Restraints and seclusion are sometimes required to control aggression that is unresponsive to less restrictive alternatives. The use of restraints as an intervention to control patient behavior creates distress for nurses (Johnson, 1998). Restraining patients restricts the person and requires the nurse to act against the patient's wishes. Studies show actions such as these greatly reduce the patients' trust and therefore interfere with the nurse's ability to develop a therapeutic relationship. Johnson found that *most patients* feel scarred and angry about being restrained. A slightly lower percentage of patients experienced restraints as helpful. Often times, struggle over rules is the precipitating factor leading to a patient being restrained. Rules on a psychiatric unit are intended for safety, not for a control battle. Nonetheless, restraints are *sometimes* the only available mechanism for controlling a patient's behavior that cannot be deescalated.

Johnson and Hauser (2001) studied the practices of expert nurses in dealing with the potentially aggressive patient. (The methods of effectively calming the aggressive patient are noted in Box 25-2.) Expert nurses were able to use their skills to find a way to *connect with the patient* and interpret patient behavior within the context and knowledge of a patient's pathology. Understanding the patient's experience is considered a crucial factor in establishing a "less aggressive milieu."

| **Box 25-2** | Interventions Used by Expert Nurses in Deescalating Patients |

- Separate the patient from others and away from the "center" of the milieu.
- Listen.
- Empathize.
- Use a calm voice.
- Be aware of body language.
- Set clear and specific limits.
- Allow the patient to verbalize.
- Show respect for patients and interest in their well being.
- Try to connect and stay connected with the patient.
- Point out the problematic behavior and state what will happen if it continues.
- Offer alternatives and choices rather than giving ultimatums.
- Do not argue with the patient.
- Use a "show of force" judiciously.

From Johnson M, Hauser P: The practices of expert psychiatric nurses: accompanying the patient to a calmer interpersonal space, *Issues Ment Health Nurs* 22:651, 2001. Taylor & Francis Ltd., website: http://www.tandf.co.uk/journals

The necessity of staff-patient interaction cannot be overemphasized. Nurses cannot know what is occurring on the unit if they spend most of their time in the nursing station. Additionally, nursing students are likely to feel less fearful when interacting with patients if they see staff doing so.

DEALING WITH INPATIENT SUICIDAL BEHAVIOR

One of the most frequently reported distressing events on a psychiatric unit is dealing with suicidal behavior. In fact, among a group of forensic psychiatric nurses, dealing with suicidal patients ranked higher than dealing with aggressive behavior (Coffey, 1999). Clinical supervision is discussed later in this chapter as a resource for nurses in psychiatry when dealing with stressful patient situations such as suicidal behavior. (See Box 25-3 for JCAHO tips on preventing inpatient suicides.)

CONSUMERS AND ADVOCATES ON THE PSYCHIATRIC UNIT

In response to a system that has failed at meeting the needs of the chronically mentally ill and has a history of patient right violations, the consumer movement has emerged as a highly active and present voice for recovery from mental illness (Center for Mental Health Services, 1999). Consumers serve on

| Box 25-3 | JCAHO Tips for Preventing Inpatient Suicides

Environmental issues that mitigate inpatient suicides include the following:
- Breakaway bars, rods, showerheads, safety rails, low flush toilets-weight tested for safety
- Adequate visualization of high risk areas
- Monitoring use of equipment
- Complete assessment of risk at admission and thereafter
- Standardized assessments with test possessing known psychometric properties
- Orientation, training, competency review, credentialing, and staffing levels
- Continuity of care on transfer
- Appropriate unit assignment
- Checking for contraband on admission
- Observation at frequency prescribed by risk
- Engagement of family, friends in process
- Identification of high-risk populations
- Prescribed checklists used for observations
- Use of standard vocabulary for communicating
- Consideration of staff assignment, including consideration of circadian rhythms, workloads, and time pressures
- Same personnel providing care should perform reviews and make quality improvement on errors
- Provisions for shift change
- Using medications to treat conditions that contribute to risk
- Pacts not useful

boards of mental health care facilities and are often invited, if not mandated to be a part of the review process for an agency receiving state funds.

Dialogue among patients (consumers) has provided important feedback to professionals about the experiences and needs of individuals with a mental illness. Patients report that they do not like being labeled; they conceptualize themselves as a *person with a mental illness* rather than a mentally ill patient (Center for Mental Health Services, 1999). Increasingly, consumers are making a presence within treatment programs for the purpose of increasing staff sensitivity to the patients' perspective. In the *Surgeon General's Report,* better outcomes for patients are noted with the use of consumers in psychosocial rehabilitation programs (Satcher, 2001).

Patients often have excessive dependency and no connection to the community in which they will live and cope with their illness. Consumers bring a recovery perspective that offers hope and support for inte-

grating into the community. For example, consumer-run psychosocial rehabilitation drop-in centers may have staff available for crisis intervention, but the focus is on consumers helping each other attain mutual goals of recovery (Brekke et al, 1997).

IMPACT OF MANAGED CARE

Managed care in psychiatry and the resulting cuts in the numbers of professional nurses leads to "unmanaged care." The cost-efficient, driven managed care approach forces quick amelioration of symptoms in inpatient units and a rapid return to the community for less expensive treatment (Satcher, 2001). Forces such as these necessarily change the model of care to crisis management from individualized care and leave little time for the development of therapeutic relationships and psychosocial interventions. Lacking time to plan care, nurses find themselves responding only to emerging crises. Patients learn quickly that getting the nurses' attention requires a crisis.

The acuity and rapid turnover in psychiatric units make the task of developing and maintaining a therapeutic environment difficult. Some research suggest a correlation between longer stays of first-episode psychosis and better long-term adjustment (Wirt, 1999). In past years, longer inpatient stays were not uncommon, but the inpatient psychiatric units of today have high turnover and acuity rates. Patients are often quite ill when admitted to an inpatient psychiatric unit as a result of insurance and managed care restrictions on admissions. Additionally, many psychiatric patients have co-morbid medical conditions that further increase the acuity on the unit, leaving less time for psychosocial intervention.

Lack of improvement in the patient's functioning at discharge, an overreliance on medications, and inadequate time to assess and diagnose patients adequately cause serious disturbances in the purported goal of developing a therapeutic relationship (Grinfeld, 2000).

Therapists struggle to document goals and outcomes of their interventions (Shultis, 1999). Certainly, there should be some evidence that interventions are useful and outcome-driven care is potentially one positive aspect of managed care's impact on treatment. As is the case with most things, a balance is in order; outcomes need to be demonstrated through documentation, and nurses need appropriate levels of staffing and resources to achieve these outcomes.

TREATMENT ENVIRONMENT AND PATIENTS WITH SCHIZOPHRENIA

The more impaired the patient is, the more important the therapeutic environment becomes (Smith, Gross, Roberts, 1996). Patients with schizophrenia suffer from impairment in attention, information processing, learning, and memory (Timko, Moos, 1998; Smith, Gross, Roberts, 1996). Patients with schizophrenia are known to be sensitive to interactions with others, especially interactions characterized by hostility and criticism. Research in this area has generally focused on relapse rates for patients in a family environment with high degrees of criticism and hostility; however, nurses can also develop these characteristics (Baker, 2000). Patients often cope with these environments by withdrawing. Rigid, understimulating (or overstimulating), impersonal environments have negative impact on patients suffering from schizophrenia. Studies show that patients want environments that are supportive, organized, and have some structure, but not overly rigid (Melia, Moran, Mason, 1999).

It is likely that patients need a different environment, depending on where they are on the continuum of illness (Smith, Gross, Roberts, 1996). Nurses must engineer the environment to accommodate the needs of many different patient problems. This task can be accomplished only when the nurse is *out among the patients* and aware of the many dynamics that occur on psychiatric units.

CLINICAL SUPERVISION

Clinical supervision is an important aspect of the therapeutic environment. The purpose of clinical supervision is to provide a place for nurses caring for patients to examine attitudes, reactions, and conflicts with patients on the unit and to find new ways of approaching patient problems. This goal requires a commitment by the nurse to a process of self-awareness, openness, and receptiveness to feedback. Providing a structured time for this important process ensures that it will occur. Studies have demonstrated an improvement in staff cohesiveness, morale, and creativity (Berg, Hallberg, 1999). Activities such as these also help nurses develop sensitivity to the patient. The importance of understanding the patients' distress and providing supportive interpersonal communication has remained unchallenged even in an era of biologic psychiatry (Reynolds, Scott, 1999).

Critical Thinking Question

How do you think the treatment environment affects the physical and emotional recovery of patients in nonpsychiatric treatment settings?

Note to Students: A number of variables affecting the therapeutic environment of a psychiatric unit have been presented in this chapter. Although the interpersonal environment is not necessarily the primary focus on other units, these same variables affect the environment in which all nursing care takes place. Thus it behooves the student to take note of these factors, because it will certainly advance your value to the patients you care for in any setting.

Key Concepts

1. Teamwork in psychiatry is essential in maintaining a therapeutic environment. Staff members must be able to work together and resolve any conflicts that arise. Failure to do so adversely affects the treatment environment.
2. The theoretical model of care adopted by a health care facility affects the kind of nursing care provided.
3. Staff burnout negatively affects patient care and the therapeutic environment.
4. Management plays an extremely important role in the kind of care nurses are empowered to deliver.
5. Nurses cannot assess the environment from the nursing station. Interaction with patients is an important part of a therapeutic environment.
6. JCAHO mandates that psychiatric facilities invest resources in developing a therapeutic environment.
7. Maintaining safety on the psychiatric unit requires staff members who feel competent to manage aggressive behavior. This goal can be accomplished through specific training sessions. Attitude is also important, and an authoritarian attitude is associated with a greater likelihood of assaults on staff.
8. The consumer movement has influenced treatment settings by providing feedback to staff about the patients' perspective on the treatment environment.
9. Managed care has led to sicker patients with a more rapid turnover in census, which creates stress for the staff and patients.
10. The use of clinical supervision for nursing staff can be a tool to facilitate improved staff cohesion, morale, and ability to maintain therapeutic relationships with patients.

References

American Nurses Association: *Code for nurses with interpretive statements,* Kansas City, Mo, 1997, APA.

Baillie L: How nurses view emotional involvement with patients, *Nursing Times* 92(9):35, 1996.

Baker JA: Developing psychosocial care for acute psychiatric wards, *J Psychiatr Ment Health Nurs* 7(2):95, 2000.

Berg A, Hallberg IR: Effects of systematic clinical supervision on psychiatric nurses sense of coherence, creativity, work-related strain, job satisfaction and view of the effects of clinical supervision: a pre-post test design, *J Psychosoc Ment Health Serv* 6:371, 1999.

Blair DT: Where assault begins, *J Psychosoc Ment Health Serv* 30(6):4, 1992 (letter, reply).

Boey KW: Distressed and stress resistant nurses, *Issues Ment Health Nurs* 20(1):33, 1999.

Brekke J et al: The impact of service characteristics on functional outcomes from community support programs for persons with schizophrenia, *J Consult Clin Psychol* 65(3):464, 1997.

Center for Mental Health Services, Substance Abuse and Mental Health Services Administration, U.S. Department of Health and Human Services: Consumers and psychiatric-mental health nurses in dialogue July 26-27, 1999, Willard Inter-Continental Hotel, Washington, DC. Available at: http://www.mentalhealth.org/publications/allpubs/Cs00-0015/Cs000015.htm

Cleary M, Edwards C: Something always comes up: nurse-patient interaction in an acute psychiatric setting, *J Psychiatr Ment Health Nurs* 6(6):469, 1999.

Coffey M: Stress and burnout in forensic community psychiatric nursing: an investigation of its causes and effects, *J Psychiatric Ment Health Nurs* 6(6):433, 1999.

Evers W, Tomic W, Brouwers A: Effects of aggressive behavior and perceived self-efficacy on burnout among staff of homes for the elderly, *Issues Ment Health Nurs* 22(4):439, 2001.

Graham IW: Seeking a clarification of meaning: a phenomenological interpretation of the craft of mental health nursing, *J Psychiatr Nurs Ment Health Serv* 8:335, 2001.

Grinfeld MJ: Managed care for public mental health yields mixed results, *Psychiatric Times* 17(4):32, 2000.

Johnson ME: Being restrained: a study of power & powerlessness, *Issues Ment Health Nurs* 19:191, 1998.

Johnson ME, Hauser PM: The practices of expert psychiatric nurses: accompanying the patient to a calmer interpersonal space, *Issues Ment Health Nurs* 22:651, 2001.

Joint Commission on Accreditation of Healthcare Organizations: *Comprehensive accreditation manual for hospitals,* Chicago, 2001, JCAHO..

Lutzen K: Subtle coercion in psychiatric practice, *J Psychiatr Ment Health Nurs* 5(2):101, 1998.

Melia P, Moran T, Mason T: Triumvirate nursing for personality disordered patients: crossing the boundaries safely, *J Psychiatr Ment Health Nurs.* 6(1):15, 1999 Feb.

Ray CL, Subich LM: Staff assaults and injuries in a psychiatric hospital as a function of three attitudinal variables, *Issues Ment Health Nurs* 19(3):277, 1998.

Reynolds WJ, Scott B: Empathy: a crucial component of the helping relationship, *J Psychiatr Ment Health Nurs* 6(5):363, 1999.

Satcher D: Mental Health: A Report of the Surgeon General, 2001. Available at: http://www.surgeongeneral.gov/library/mentalhealth/home.html.

Sayre J: The use of aberrant medical humor by psychiatric nursing staff, *Issues Ment Health Nurs* 22:669, 2001.

Schreiber R, Lutzen K: Revisiting nursing in a nontherapeutic environment, *Issues Ment Health Nurs* 21(3):257, 2000.

Shultis CL: Music therapy for inpatient psychiatric care in the 1990s, *Psychiatric Times* February 16(2):46, 1999.

Simms C: Don't become a causality in the war of words, *Nursing* 29(12):48, 1999.

Smith J, Gross C, Roberts J: The evolution of a therapeutic environment for patients with long-term illness as measured by The Ward Atmosphere Scale, *J Psychiatr Ment Health Nurs* 5(4):349, 1996.

Smith R: Rehab rounds: implementing psychosocial rehabilitation with long-term patients in a public psychiatric hospital, *Psychiatr Serv* 49:593, 1998.

Timko C, Moos RH: Outcomes of the treatment climate in psychiatric and substance abuse programs, *J Clin Psychol* 54(8):1137, 1998.

Whittington D, McLaughlin C: Finding time for patients: an exploration of nurses' time allocation in an acute psychiatric setting, *J Psychiatr Ment Health Nurs* 7(3):259, 2000.

Wirt GL: Causes of institutionalism: patient and staff perspectives, *Issues Ment Health Nurs* 20(3):259, 1999.

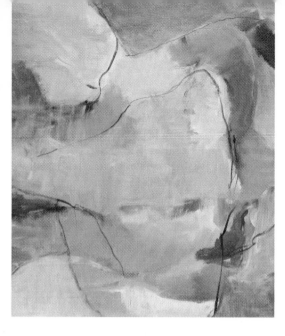

Therapeutic Environment in Different Treatment Settings

Beverly K. Hogan; Norman L. Keltner

Learning Objectives

After reading this chapter, you should be able to:

- Describe the treatment environment of inpatient psychiatric settings including:
  - Open adult units
  - Adolescent psychiatric units
  - Medical psychiatric units
  - Acute or intensive psychiatric units
  - Substance abuse units
  - Dual diagnosis units
  - Geropsychiatric units
- State psychiatric hospitals
- State forensic psychiatric hospitals
- Describe the treatment environment of community psychiatric settings including:
  - Outpatient mental health clinics
  - Day treatment facilities
  - Residential care facilities
  - Mobile mental health clinics
  - Home psychiatric care

In the preceding two chapters, discussion focused on the characteristics and variables of a therapeutic environment. The purpose was to define the structure of the treatment environment and factors that enhance or detract from its goals. In this chapter, emphasis is placed on the setting of the therapeutic environment.

INPATIENT SETTINGS

Milieu therapy, as initially described by Maxwell Jones (1953), was designed for inpatient settings. Most inpatient settings have a forum for discussing patient treatment and milieu issues. One such forum is the team meeting. Psychiatrists, psychologists, psy-

chiatric social workers, pharmacists, occupational therapists, recreational therapists, and psychiatric nurses all provide input about treatment issues. The team meeting is an excellent opportunity to enhance collegial relationships with other mental health professionals. In the team meeting, the nurses provide patient assessment data and observations about the treatment environment (Boxes 26-1 and 26-2). The many changes engendered by managed care, including cutting of resources, has led many participants to be concerned about the increasingly "undemocratic" manner in which team meetings are conducted (Barker, Walker, 2000) and therefore about the potential for devaluing of the team concept.

The following section focuses on the unique aspects of various inpatient treatment settings of varying degrees of restrictiveness.

Critical Thinking Question

What is it about a treatment setting that defines its degree of restrictiveness? (Hint: What is it that is being restricted?)

Therapeutic Activities in the Inpatient Setting

Before discussing the unique aspects of treatment environments, it is helpful to have a general idea of the types of therapeutic activities typically offered in a psychiatric setting. As the various settings are described in this chapter, particular differences in the nature and scope of these therapeutic activities are addressed. See Box 26-2 for a typical inpatient schedule, which includes treatment activities offered by each of the following disciplines.

Occupational therapy

Occupational therapists (OTs) are typically educated at the baccalaureate level, although many employed in psychiatry have earned master's degrees. OTs are concerned with functional capacities of patients as they affect their capacity to work and perform tasks of daily living. OTs assist patients in mastering the skills needed for self-care, work, and play. Occupational therapy (OT) uses the activities of everyday living to help people with mental disabilities achieve maximal functioning and independence at home, in the workplace, or both (Box 26-3). Unknowledgeable ob-

servers may minimize the therapeutic value of OT by making references to "arts and crafts" classes; however, these arts and crafts classes are skillfully selected based on the OTs' functional assessment of the patients' deficits and strengths. For example, certain arts and crafts may be selected for their value in improving the patient's attention span and concentration. (See Box 26-1 for a sample of a treatment plan.)

Recreational therapy

The use of leisure time is an important intervention for psychiatric patients. Recreational therapists (RTs) assist patients in finding leisure interests that will enable the patients to learn to balance work and play. RTs complete a bachelor's or master's degree program in therapeutic recreation; however, wide variability exists in the level of training of RTs employed at various facilities. RTs are skilled at assessing patient leisure needs and formulating individualized plans of care. Learning to make time for pleasure and fun can be therapeutic for individuals dealing with the stress of a mental illness.

Exercise therapy

The benefits of exercise in modulating mood and well being are well documented. As patients become withdrawn, their motivation to exercise decreases. Exercise groups counter this tendency to a degree. Exercise therapy is especially important on a psychiatric unit because it helps channel energies of anxiety or agitation into more appropriate outlets. The level of training or education varies greatly in treatment settings. Ideally, exercise therapists have an educational background incorporating the principles of exercise physiology and its therapeutic application to clinical settings. Exercise therapists also develop individualized plans of care on treatment plans (see Box 26-1).

Patient education

Educating patients regarding symptom recognition and management is essential if the patient is to maintain stability outside the treatment environment. Sometimes, the term psychoeducational group is used to refer to educating patients about psychiatric illness management. Psychoeducational efforts are based on empirical evidence that understanding mental illness helps patients and their families cope more positively with the illness. Numerous studies demonstrate the value of psychoeducation

| Box 26-1 | Sample Interdisciplinary Treatment Plan

Patient Strengths   **Limitations**

_____   _____

_____   _____

_____   _____

_____   _____

Support System:

Name: _____   Phone Number: _____

DSM IV Diagnoses:

Axis I _____

Axis II _____

Axis III _____

Axis IV _____

Axis V _____

Discharge Plan: _____

_____

_____

_____

Problem #1	Goal or Measurable Outcome	Intervention	Evaluation	Signature
Time imbalance between work and leisure activity	State leisure interests	Explore leisure interests		
	Name barriers to participation in leisure	Reinitiate leisure activities		
	Participate in leisure activity in unit			
Impaired ability to concentrate	Read for 30 minutes and complete assigned tasks	Engage in activities and tasks for progressively increased time periods		
Physical inactivity	Participate in exercise therapy	Attend exercise therapy daily		
	State benefits of exercise	Instruct regarding benefits of exercise		
Spiritual distress	Participate in spirituality group	Attend spirituality group twice weekly		
	Decrease subjective distress	Explore beliefs and relationship to distress		

|Box 26-2| Sample Treatment Schedule

	Monday through Friday	Saturday and Sunday
7:00-8:00	Breakfast	Breakfast
8:00-8:45	Community meeting	Community meeting
9:00-9:45	Patient education	Patient education
10:00-11:00	Meet with treatment team	Physician rounds
11:00-12:00	Occupational therapy	Free time
12:00-1:00	Lunch	Lunch
1:00-2:00	Group therapy	Visiting hours
2:30-3:30	Exercise therapy	Exercise therapy
4:00-5:00	Free time	Spirituality group
5:00-6:00	Dinner	Dinner
6:00-7:00	Visiting hours	Visiting hours
7:00-8:00	Recreational therapy	Recreational therapy
8:30-9:00	Relaxation group	Free time

|Box 26-3| Psychoeducational Topics

- Medication self-management
- Symptom self-management
- Recreation for leisure
- Grooming and self-care
- Money management
- Finding employment
- Food preparation
- Personal effectiveness

|Box 26-4| Examples of Topics for Psychoeducational Groups

- Recognizing signs of relapse
- Using public transportation
- Talking with your therapist-case worker-psychiatrist
- Coping with stress
- Managing your medications
- Coping with symptoms
- Knowing when to call your physician
- Getting along with family members
- Returning to work

groups in improving quality of life, preventing relapse, and altering negative family reactions (Dixon, Adams, Lucksted, 2000; Herz, 2000; Motlova, 2000; Pekkala, Merinder, 2000; Schimmel-Spreeuw, Linssen, Heeren, 2000). Studies generally, but not always, show a high degree of patient satisfaction with such programs (Dowrick et al, 2000). The psychoeducation content rated most helpful by patients is information about diagnosis and medications (Ascher-Svanum et al, 2001). This finding supports studies demonstrating increased compliance rates in patients participating in medication—focused psychoeducational groups. Clinicians who took time and energy to implement these kinds of programs transformed their treatment environments from custodial to rehabilitative (Smith, 1998). Because families often assume much of the care burden for chronically ill patients, their inclusion in psychoeducational groups is essential. (Box 26-4 offers an example of topics that are appropriate for psychoeducational groups.)

Group therapy

Group therapy may be conducted by psychiatric nurses, psychiatric clinical nurse specialists, psychologists, psychiatric residents, licensed professional counselors, or licensed psychiatric social workers. Group therapy is a kind of therapeutic environment of its own because it uses the principles of therapeutic environments: openness, giving and receiving feedback, respect for the patient, privacy, acceptance, independence, and individual responsibility. In general, it can be said that the purpose of group therapy is to facilitate awareness and insight about one's behavior and to develop plans for change or coping. (See Chapter 14 for a full discussion of therapeutic groups.)

Spirituality groups

Although spiritual groups are not consistently offered in psychiatric treatment settings, it is likely that the Joint Commission on Accreditation of Healthcare Organizations (JCAHO) will soon specifically mandate formal attention to the spiritual needs of patients. The JCAHO already has standards requiring the assessment and interdisciplinary planning for the spiritual concerns and needs of patients. A chaplain or other mental health treatment team professional conducts these groups; the focus of these groups is usually on topics such as forgiveness, grieving, finding meaning in life, and like topics. Patients vary in their response to these groups, but the potential for enhancing treatment is available to patients choosing to participate.

Therapeutic groups related to living skills

Some mental illnesses, such as schizophrenia and Alzheimer's disease, result in an impairment that works against developing meaningful relationships. Still other mental illnesses have as a characteristic symptom the withdrawal from others. Social skills groups help psychiatric patients learn, practice, and develop skills for dealing with people in social situations. Skills training might focus on appropriate dress, grooming, or table manners. More advanced efforts address appropriate social and interpersonal verbal skills, for example, meeting new people, initiating conversations, and interviewing for a job.

The opportunity to try out new skills and make mistakes in a safe environment is crucial to learning. Feedback helps patients assess their progress in improving or acquiring social skills development.

Therapeutic Community

The therapeutic community meeting consists of all patients, staff, and students in the treatment setting. The community meeting is a regular meeting that all staff and patients attend for the purpose of welcoming new patients, reviewing milieu rules, and making general announcements about the day's activities. The community meeting also serves as a forum for patients to voice their opinions about the treatment environment, to receive feedback from staff and other patients, and to initiate discussions of community or individual concerns.

A community constitution is a formal, written document providing the basis for the therapeutic community. The constitution includes definitions, objectives, meetings, responsibilities of patients who are elected as officers, officer approval or removal procedures, and community response to infractions. A written community constitution is not used in all milieu environments, but it is especially appropriate in environments with longer lengths of stay.

Community meetings can also be used to plan activities, such as program picnics or social gatherings. The community meeting provides a forum for exploring the problems of community living. Conflicts between patients or between patients and staff are frequent concerns. Common patient-patient conflicts involve the control of the television, generational issues (e.g., the radio is played too loudly, type of music), and personal hygiene (e.g., someone is not bathing regularly).

Patient-staff conflicts are more delicate; but in the effective community meeting, they can be handled skillfully. Common conflicts between patients and staff include issues related to the way in which staff act or fail to act with patients. Community meetings are not forums for discussing individual treatment needs and issues of patients; rather, they serve to address the day-to-day aspects of being in the treatment environment. (See Chapter 24 for further discussion of the milieu concept of balance.) The skilled group leader will direct patients to discuss personal issues with an appropriate staff person following the community meeting.

Some units include a step system as part of the therapeutic community. A step system is a process by which inpatients gain privileges and responsibilities based on their progress. New patients and acutely disturbed patients in the hospital are typically assigned to the most restrictive level, sometimes designated on the medical orders as "Unit Status" or "No OFF unit privileges." Each agency has specific codes or names that are defined in unit policies or rules. Through various efforts, individual patients can earn privileges and responsibilities leading to discharge status. A step system serves to motivate patients and provides content for community meetings. In recent years, legislation has reduced the number of privileges that can be withheld, and step programs have lost some of their therapeutic appeal.

Open Adult Psychiatric Unit

The open adult psychiatric unit is probably the least restrictive of all inpatient psychiatric units; it is the treatment setting of choice for patients with less severe symptoms and some degree of self-control over their symptoms. Patients appropriate for the open unit include those with the full range of psychiatric disorders; however, the patient on the open unit is generally able to participate in the therapeutic activities and is not actively suicidal (i.e., does not have a definite plan of action for suicide). Most units have admission criteria detailing appropriate patients for the specific treatment milieu on a unit. Physicians and nurses sometimes have conflict over the physician's decision to admit a patient who does not meet the designated criteria. These conflicts are sometimes worked out through discussion and negotiation between the nurse and physician but may require intervention by administration or management. Although patients on the open unit may be able to control their symptoms within the "safety" of the inpatient environment, they are not "well"; rather, they have active psychiatric symptoms that interfere with their daily functioning outside the hospital.

Activities on the open psychiatric unit tend to focus on developing insight into problems surrounding admission and on problem-solving strategies. Less severe symptoms enable the use of more verbal or talk therapies. Generally, patients on the open unit are more amenable to and cooperative with therapeutic activities.

CLINICAL EXAMPLE

Mary is a 37-year-old Caucasian woman who has had severe panic attacks and depression off and on since her early 20s. Mary takes Klonopin 0.5 mg twice daily and Paxil 40 mg four times daily for the panic disorder and depression. A recent series of stressors involving her work and marriage precipitated this admission. Mary is married to a man with an alcohol problem and a pattern of irresponsibility related to family finances. Mary works two jobs to make ends meet; one boss is very demanding, frequently giving her last-minute projects at the end of the work day with a deadline for the following morning. Recently, Mary has started having panic attacks as she is driving to work. Yesterday, she experienced an especially severe panic attack and pulled over on the side of the road and started crying. After seeing her psychiatrist, she was admitted for medication management and inpatient therapy. In OT, Mary practices relaxation and cognitive behavioral exercises to help her deal with the panic attacks in various situations, such as driving. The RT works with Mary on finding time for activities she once enjoyed, such as camping and reading novels. During group therapy sessions, Mary works on her problem of taking care of others while neglecting her own needs. The

nurse works with Mary to reinforce all of these therapeutic activities and also identifies problem areas with the patient to explore in their one-to-one therapeutic interactions.

Critical Thinking Question

Physicians and nurses traditionally get along very well in psychiatry. Why might this be true?

Critical Thinking Question

What are the major contributing factors to the trend for hospitalized psychiatric patients to be more medically ill now than they were in the past?

Intensive or Acute Care Psychiatric Units (Locked Units)

The goal of an acute psychiatric unit is to provide rapid amelioration of symptoms (Surgeon General, 2000). Patients on an acute, locked psychiatric unit usually meet the criteria for an involuntary admission, even if they are admitted voluntarily. Patient acuity tends to be quite high with the need for close supervision and intervention by nursing staff. Therapeutic activities tend to focus more on managing acute symptoms and improving ability to function on the unit. The high turnover and intensity of care required by patients in an acute psychiatric unit create a stressful environment. Unless action is taken to assist the staff in dealing with this high-stress environment, the staff will suffer professionally and personally. It is therefore incumbent on management to provide a forum for dealing with work-related stress.

CLINICAL EXAMPLE

John is a 23-year-old Caucasian man who barricaded himself in his family's home and called the FBI to report that his parents were aliens infiltrating the city government. Although John had not been overtly violent, he had a rifle in his possession and reportedly aimed it at his father. The county sheriff brought John to the emergency room for a psychiatric evaluation. John agreed to be admitted to the psychiatric unit where he would be "safe" from the alien invasion. John's parents were contacted and agreed to file a petition for involuntary evaluation and treatment in case John should decide to leave against medical advice. John attends group therapy with other patients on the unit and is confronted by his peers about having a mental illness. John also attends psychoeducational groups to learn about the signs and symptoms of mental illness. One-to-one interactions with John's nurse focus on dealing with other patients on the unit and ways to deal with the resulting anxiety. The nurse also reinforces teaching about mental illness and medication management. John refuses to participate in the other therapies at this time. As John's illness is better controlled and he begins to develop insight, John will work with the OT to determine the activities that will help him with his trouble concentrating.

Child-Adolescent Inpatient Unit

It has been said many times, "Children are not little adults." The child-adolescent unit must meet specific age-appropriate criteria in terms of the physical environment and the treatment activities offered. (See Chapter 42 for further discussion of the child-adolescent population.)

Although it is widely accepted that the milieu of the adolescent psychiatric unit is important, little research has been conducted into the nature, construction, maintenance, and function of the milieu, especially with regard to how the unit affects treatment outcomes (Geanellos, 2000).

A number of traditional views about adolescent psychiatric nursing are now being reconsidered. For instance, in the past, separating parents from their child during a psychiatric admission was considered essential; this action often communicated that the parent was part of the problem. This approach has shifted in an entirely different direction in that it is now realized that nurse-parent relationships are essential to the treatment process for the child or adolescent patient.

Another shift concerns the frequently used "time-out" intervention (Delaney, 1999). The original intent of time-out was to remove the patient from potential reinforcers for inappropriate behavior. Because it is an effective and easily learned intervention, staff tends to rely on time-out as an intervention for any behavioral problem that occurs. For instance, if a patient breaks a unit rule, he or she might be sent to his or her room for time-out. In contrast, a patient who is receiving a lot of attention from peers for his or her rebellious remarks might also be sent to his or her room for time-out. The former is an action intending to apply negative sanctions to the inappropriate behavior (punish), whereas the latter is a direct effort to remove the source of reward for inappropriate behavior (operant shaping). The purpose of a time-out must be clearly in mind; otherwise, the potential for it becoming a form of punishment is great. The need for more active and innovative strategies for dealing with the complex problems presented by today's child adolescent psychiatric patient is clear. For example, cognitive behavioral approaches for dealing with aggressive behavior through skills training groups and reinforcement of appropriate behavior have been effective in reducing aggressive behavior in adolescents (Snyder, 1999).

Another important aspect of the interpersonal environment on the child-adolescent unit is the interactions among patients. Quite easily, peers can unduly influence each other, especially in the case of adolescent patients who are seeking to establish their own identities. Potentially, patients can learn some self-defeating behavior patterns from each other. Hence, part of the nurses' role in developing a therapeutic environment within a child-adolescent unit is the monitoring of peer relationships and intervening as conditions warrant.

Consistency of staff is important in any psychiatric setting and is especially important on the child-adolescent unit. Adolescents and children who have grown up entirely in foster care or residential care settings may have difficulty establishing relationships and may have developed a number of defenses counterproductive to forming relationships with others. Nurses can intervene by being consistent and trustworthy. Nurses who have not successfully mastered the developmental tasks of childhood and adolescence themselves will have great difficulty working on a child-adolescent psychiatric unit.

CLINICAL EXAMPLE

Kisha is an 8-year-old African-American girl who has been getting into trouble at school for fighting. Kisha

Continued

has also been running away from home and setting fires at neighbor's houses. Kisha talks with the nurse about difficulties with peers at school and how she feels sad all the time. Kisha participates in group therapy by discussing her behavior with peers and getting feedback about the way she interacts with others. Kisha works with the OT to complete projects she chooses, even though other patients on the unit are making fun of her. During community meetings, treatment team members and peers point out to Kisha how she has improved since being in the hospital and participating in the unit treatment activities.

Medical Psychiatric Units

In recent years, there has been a resurgence in the recognition of the interrelationship between mind and body. At least 50% of patients admitted to hospitals have co-morbid medical and psychiatric problems (Kathol, 1998). Psychiatric co-morbidity increases the length of stay for the hospitalized medically ill psychiatric patient (Wancata et al, 2001). Likewise, the medical patient with a psychiatric condition poses a challenge to the traditional medical unit and can be quite disruptive to the unit routine. A medical unit lacks the necessary physical and safety characteristics important for patients with a psychiatric problem. Similarly, the psychiatric patient with medical problems may not receive adequate attention to their co-morbid medical condition if the staff members do not actively maintain their medical nursing skills. Medical equipment on a traditional psychiatric unit can also pose a challenge in terms of availability and safety. Although the majority of these co-morbid cases require only a straightforward consideration of factors in care planning, at least 10% of patients require simultaneous specialty care of both conditions.

The high percentage of chronically mentally ill patients with coexisting medical problems and the high prevalence of medical disorders among chronically mentally ill patients has led to the creation of specialized units addressing both problems simultaneously. These units, called *integrated medicine-psychiatric units,* can yield significant savings for the hospital and improve outcomes for patients with psychiatric-medical co-morbidity. Understandably, the focus of therapeutic activities will depend on the nature of the medical infirmity.

CLINICAL EXAMPLE
Marvin is a 47-year-old African-American man with a history of bipolar affective disorder, diabetes, and congestive heart failure. He was brought to the emergency room with a blood sugar of 700 µg/ml, severe dehydration, and cardiac arrhythmia. Marvin had stopped taking his medications recently because he believed he was able to handle his problems on his own. He has been walking the streets and preaching to people in fast-food restaurants. Last night, the McDonald's store manager found Marvin babbling and acting "drunk." The manager called the police, who then escorted Marvin to the local emergency room. Typically, Marvin's diabetes is difficult to control. After Marvin was rehydrated and his blood sugar stabilized, Marvin was admitted to the integrated medical-psychiatric unit for close observation of his medical status and simultaneous participation in treatment activities for his mental illness. Marvin attends a psychoeducational group with several other patients who have also had problems with medication compliance and exacerbation of serious medical problems. Once Marvin is stabilized medically, he will continue to participate in other treatment activities.

Substance Abuse Units

Although substance abuse treatment requires a specialized, controlled environment for optimal recovery, it is still fairly common for patients with substance abuse problems to undergo initial evaluation and detoxification on an open or closed psychiatric unit. Therapeutic activities on a substance abuse unit include rigorous patient education, sensitization groups, and confrontive feedback sessions. Traditionally, substance abuse treatment approaches tend to be more confrontive because of the severity of denial. (See Chapter 35 for further discussion of the patient with substance-related problems.)

CLINICAL EXAMPLE
Sara is a 42-year-old Caucasian woman who has been drinking alcohol excessively and taking Xanax for about 3 years now. Sara's withdrawal symptoms were managed on the open psychiatric unit, after which Sara was transferred to the substance abuse unit. On the substance abuse unit, Sara attends educational sessions about addiction, alcoholism, and dealing with unhealthy relationships. Sara also attends group thera-

py in which she talks about a number of underlying, unattended feelings of grief about her mother's death. As Sara progresses through treatment, she will participate in a number of therapy groups aimed at helping her avoid relapse after discharge.

Dual Diagnosis Units

More than 50% of patients in mental health treatment settings have a coexisting substance-related disorder. Likewise, more than 50% of patients in substance abuse treatment settings have a coexisting psychiatric disorder (Minkoff, 2001). Some hospitals and free-standing psychiatric facilities (not attached to a general hospital) find a dual diagnosis unit to be better able to meet the unique needs of this population (Timko, Moos, 1998). The treatment approach on the dual diagnosis unit balances the confrontive and supportive approach. (See Chapter 36 for a discussion of treatment issues of the dually diagnosed patient.)

CLINICAL EXAMPLE

Several months after discharge from the substance abuse unit, Sara was diagnosed with panic disorder. Sara relapsed from her commitment to drug and alcohol abstinence and became very depressed. She was admitted to the dual diagnosis unit for simultaneous management of both disorders. Sara will participate in therapeutic activities with other patients who are dually diagnosed.

Geropsychiatric Units

Population demographics reflect an increasing aging population. Patients on a geropsychiatric unit have complex medical, psychologic, and social needs. A number of differences in the treatment environment are dictated by these multicomplex needs. In particular, the physical structure of the geropsychiatric unit must be designed with special consideration for safety issues and cognition limitations. For example, physical space must be less cluttered to address safety, and it should be free of unnecessary noise to counter the vulnerability of older patients' to sensory overstimulation. A smaller unit size with fewer patients has been shown to improve interaction not only among patients, but also between patients and staff (Teresi, Holmes, Ory, 2000; Day, Carreon, Stump, 2000).

Older patients, especially those with dementia, may have difficulty navigating the hospital environment without environmental cues. Environmental cues include large orientation boards on which the date, time, and location of daily events are posted; clearly marked names or graphic images (e.g., bathroom, bedrooms with patients' names on the doors); and color-coding different locations. Just as children are not little adults, geriatric patients are not just chronologically older adults. Older patients are likely to have co-morbid medical conditions that may affect mobility, balance, and vision. Increased lighting is needed to counter diminished vision of the older adult. Confusion and disorientation can be exacerbated or helped by environmental interventions.

Falls are of great concern on the geropsychiatric unit, and many of the medications prescribed in this setting may increase the risk of falls.

A patient with dementia needs a different environment than the older patient who is cognitively intact. For example, bathing is considered one of the most stressful events associated with dementia. Design accommodations should include features that maximize the patient's autonomy and independence. Bathrooms should be large enough to accommodate the need for others to assist the patient.

The importance of the environment for the geropsychiatric patient is evident by the increasing numbers of studies on facility design and planning. These studies show an association between the environmental design of the unit and patients' level of improvement on variables such as self-care, agitation, and mood. Interestingly, nurses identify their greatest challenge in caring for patients with dementia is not cognitive impairment, but, rather, it is dealing with agitated behavior (Keatinge et al, 2000). Group therapy, for those able to participate may involve issues such as grief and loss. For less cognitively functional patients, group therapy may involve orientation, memory enhancement, and reminiscence activities in a more structured format.

CLINICAL EXAMPLE

Ms. Jones is an 82-year-old Hispanic woman who was admitted to the geriatric psychiatric unit for increasing confusion and wandering behavior at home. Ms. Jones is diagnosed with Alzheimer's disease and is started on Aricept. The OT works with Ms. Jones to complete her bathing and dressing with minimal assis-

Continued

tance. The nurse works closely with Ms. Jones and her family members to identify triggers to episodes of agitation and strategies for dealing with these episodes. The nurse has noticed that Ms. Jones does very well at dinnertime if her favorite song from her teenage years is played.

State Psychiatric Hospitals

The primary difference in the treatment environment between a state hospital setting and other facilities is based on the length of stay, greater degree of restrictiveness, and the need to prepare patients for community placement.

CLINICAL EXAMPLE

Marvin, who was previously an inpatient on the medical psychiatric unit in a private hospital, continued to be uncooperative with his treatment. An involuntary commitment hearing was held, and Marvin was admitted to the state psychiatric hospital for further treatment. Marvin currently receives many of the same treatments he received at the private facility; however, the state hospital has greater focus on developing insight, improving compliance, and preparing to live back in the community than does the private short-stay inpatient facility.

State Forensic Psychiatric Hospitals

The forensic psychiatric unit or hospital is the most restrictive of all treatment environments. Similar to a prison, a forensic psychiatric hospital is a secure environment, with strict rules and regulations to ensure safety and security. The building is designed for maximal security to prevent patients from escaping. The primary difference between a prison and a forensic psychiatric unit is that the focus of a prison is control, whereas forensic hospitals focus on treatment. The kinds of patients admitted to a forensic unit include those with court-ordered psychiatric assessments, pre-sentence defendants, and defendants found "not guilty by reason of insanity" by the court.

CLINICAL EXAMPLE

Sam is a 22-year-old Caucasian man who was transferred to the state forensic psychiatric hospital from jail after his recent court case in which he was found not guilty of embezzlement by reason of insanity. Sam embezzled several million dollars from his employer's accounts because he thought his boss was Satan and was planning to use the money to destroy all the men in America. At the forensic hospital, Sam can participate in all the usual treatment activities of a psychiatric hospital while being more closely supervised to avoid any further acting out of his delusional ideas.

COMMUNITY TREATMENT SETTINGS

Once restricted to inpatient settings, the concept of therapeutic community is being applied to the care of patients living in the community. Currently, much of psychiatric care takes place in group homes, partial or day hospitals, or through support offered to patients and their family members through home health visits. Once a patient is discharged from the hospital to a community setting, safety takes on different characteristics. Ongoing assessments must be done to ensure that patients are able to manage outpatient care. For example, a patient preoccupied with internal stimuli (i.e., hallucinations) might be at risk for walking into traffic when leaving a day program. He or she therefore may need to be escorted home to his or her family. When patients are cared for in the community, there is less control over factors outside the immediate treatment environment; therefore, nurses make thorough assessments and clinical judgments about patient progress. This next section will focus on the unique aspects of community treatment.

DAY TREATMENT, PARTIAL HOSPITALIZATION, AND RESIDENTIAL TREATMENT HOMES

Preparing patient's to live in the community requires the teaching of social and independent living skills (Umansky et al, 1999).

A metaanalysis of psychosocial skills training indicates a moderate-to-strong correlation relationship to fewer patient symptoms and better functioning (Dilk, Bond, 1996). When psychosocial skills training targets vocational and social skills, a consistent benefit has been demonstrated in most studies (Dilk, Bond, 1996). By targeting specific areas of functioning, it is possible to achieve positive patient outcomes (Brekke et al, 1997). The importance of research such as this is its ability to demonstrate a positive treatment effect above that of medication alone.

Settings that combine intense programming with increased patient-staff contact are found to be most efficacious. Program for Assertive Client Treatment (PACT) teams are examples of professionals working as a unit to intervene before patient problems require hospitalization. PACT teams are in wide use today and are recognized as an important means for delivering psychiatric mental health care in the community (Essock, Kontos, 1995; McFarlane et al, 1996). Another major change in health care delivery is the ever-increasing use of advanced-practice psychiatric nurses to both prescribe and evaluate patients' responses to psychotropic drugs (Kaas et al, 1998). The presence of advanced-practice psychiatric nurses in the community also aids in keeping patients at home, in group homes, or attending day programs. See Chapter 8 for further discussion of community-based care.

Note to Students: *These chapters have given an overview of the concept of the treatment environment. Regardless of the clinical setting (e.g., psychiatric, medical, pediatric), the atmosphere and care provided is affected by the variables discussed in this chapter.*

Key Concepts

1. Milieu therapy was originally designed for the inpatient setting but has increasingly been used in other settings (e.g. mental health clinics), especially in the community.
2. A variety of health care professionals are involved in the treatment milieu of a psychiatric facility, including physicians, nurses, psychologists, social workers, chaplains, occupational therapists, recreational therapists, and exercise therapists.
3. All members of the treatment team and patients attend therapeutic community meetings to welcome new patients, review milieu rules, and make general announcements about the day's activities. (Note: Not all units have therapeutic community meetings.)
4. A variety of treatment activities is used within psychiatric units, such as group therapy, recreational therapy, exercise therapy, spirituality groups, and patient education.
5. The open psychiatric unit is the least restrictive inpatient treatment environment. Generally, patients on the open unit require less "close" supervision and can actively take responsibility for their treatment.
6. Patients in an acute, locked psychiatric unit are often admitted involuntarily and tend to need close supervision and intervention by nursing staff.
7. A special focus of the child-adolescent psychiatric unit is the interpersonal relationships among patients.
8. Medical psychiatric units are specialty psychiatric environments that address the needs of chronically medically ill patients with coexisting psychiatric problems.
9. Therapeutic activities on a substance abuse unit tend to use confrontation more often because of the extensive use of denial within this patient population.
10. Patients with both a substance abuse problem and a psychiatric diagnosis can be treated on dual diagnosis units, which balance the confrontive and supportive approaches.
11. Geropsychiatric units address specialized needs of the older adult, including environmental modifications necessary for sensory losses and other safety factors.
12. The primary difference in the treatment environment of a state hospital setting is the length of stay and the focus on preparing patients for community placement.
13. A forensic psychiatric unit (or hospital) is the most restrictive of all treatment environments.
14. Today, significant levels of psychiatric care takes place in group homes, partial and day hospitals, and other community settings.
15. Preparing patients to live in the community requires the treatment emphasis on social skills, independent living skills, and prevention of rehospitalization and relapse.

References

Ascher-Svanum H et al: Patient education about schizophrenia: initial expectations and later satisfaction, *Issues Ment Health Nurs* 22:325, 2001.

Baker JA: Developing psychosocial care for acute psychiatric wards, *J Psychiatr Ment Health Nurs* 7(2):95, 2000.

Barker PJ, Walker L: Nurses' perceptions of multidisciplinary teamwork in acute psychiatric settings, *J Psychosoc Nurs Ment Health Serv* 7:539, 2000.

Brekke J et al: The impact of service characteristics on functional outcomes from community support programs for persons with schizophrenia, *J Consult Clin Psychol* 65(3):464, 1997.

Cleary M, Edwards C: "Something always comes up": nurse-patient interaction in an acute psychiatric setting, *J Psychiatr Ment Health Nurs* 6(6):469, 1999.

Day K, Carreon D, Stump C: The therapeutic design of environments for patients with dementia: a review of the empirical research, *Gerontologist* 40(4):397, 2000.

Delaney K: Time-out: an overused and misused milieu intervention, *J Child Adolesc Psychiatr Nurs* 12(2):53, 1999.

Dilk M, Bond G: Meta-analytic evaluation of skills training research for individuals with severe mental illness, *J Consult Clin Psychol* 64(6):1337, 1996.

Dixon L, Adams C, Lucksted A: Update on family psychoeducation for schizophrenia, *Schizophr Bull* 26(1):5, 2000.

Dowrick C et al: Problem solving treatment and group psychoeducation for depression: multicentre randomized controlled trial. Outcomes of Depression International Network (ODIN) Group, *BMJ* 321(7274):1450, 2000.

Essock SM, Kontos N: Implementing assertive community treatment teams, *Psychiatr Serv* 46(7):679, 1995.

Geanellos R: The milieu and milieu therapy in adolescent mental health nursing, *Int J Psychiatr Nurs Res* 5(3):638, 2000.

Herz MI et al: A program for relapse prevention in schizophrenia: a controlled study, *Arch Gen Psychiatry* 57(3):277, 2000.

Jones M: *The therapeutic community,* New York, 1953, Basic Books.

Kaas MJ, Markley JM: A national perspective on prescriptive authority for advanced practice psychiatric nurses, *J Am Psychiatr Nurs Assoc* 4(6):190, 1998.

Kathol R: Integrated medicine and psychiatry treatment programs, *Med Psychiatry* 1:10, 1998.

Keatinge D et al: The manifestation and nursing management of agitation in institutionalized residents with dementia, *Int J Nurs Pract* 6(1):16, 2000.

McFarlane WR et al: A comparison of two levels of family-aide assertive community treatment, *Psychiatr Serv* 47(7):744, 1996.

Melia P, Moran T, Mason T: Triumvirate nursing for personality disorder patients: crossing the boundaries safely, *J Psychiatr Ment Health Nurs* 6(1):15-20, 1999.

Minkoff K: Best practices. Developing standards of care for individuals with co-occurring psychiatric and substance use disorders, *Psychiatr Serv* 52(5):597, 2001 May.

Motlova L: Psychoeducation as an indispensable complement to pharmacotherapy in schizophrenia, *Pharmacopsychiatry* 33(suppl 1):47, 2000.

Pekkala E, Merinder L: Psychoeducation for schizophrenia, *Cochrane Database Syst Rev* (4):CD002831, 2000.

Schimmel-Spreeuw A, Linssen AC, Heeren TJ: Coping with depression and anxiety: preliminary results of a standardized course for elderly depressed women, *Int Psychogeriatr* 12(1):77, 2000.

Smith R: Rehab rounds: implementing psychosocial rehabilitation with long-term patients in a public psychiatric hospital, *Psychiatr Serv* 49:593, 1998.

Snyder K, Kymissis P, Kessler K: Anger management for adolescents: efficacy of brief group therapy, *J Am Acad Child Adol Psychiatry* 38(11):1409, 1999.

Surgeon General: *Mental health: a report of the Surgeon General,* Washington, DC, 1999, Department of Health and Human Services.

Teresi J, Holmes D, Ory M: The therapeutic design of environments for people with dementia: further reflections and recent findings form the national institute on aging, *Gerontologist* 40(4):417, 2000.

Timko C, Moos RH: Outcomes of the treatment climate in psychiatric and substance abuse programs, *J Clin Psychol* 54(8):1137, 1998.

Umansky R et al: A school for mental health inpatient preparation for reinsertion in the community, *Int J Psychosoc Rehabil* 3(8):526, 1999.

Wancata J et al: Does psychiatric co-morbidity increase the length of stay in medical, surgical and gynecological departments? *Gen Hosp Psychiatry* 23(1):8, 2001.

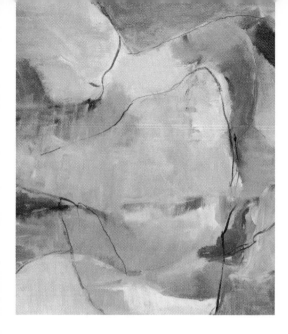

Chapter 27

Introduction
to Psychopathology

Norman L. Keltner

Learning Objectives

After reading this chapter, you should be able to:

- Describe the extent of mental illness in the United States.
- Identify the most common mental disorders in the United States.
- List the three requirements for understanding psychopathology.
- Describe several guidelines applicable to all aspects of psychotherapeutic management.

"Psychoanalysis took a while to conquer the United States, but once it did, after the Second World War, its dominance was unquestioned, and its arrogance breathtaking. Schizophrenia, autism, and numerous other disorders were blamed on the mother, with no evidence, just utter certainty."

Acocella, 2000, p. 114

According to the Surgeon General's (1999) report on mental health, 20% of the U.S. population is affected by mental disorders during a given year. When the full spectrum of mental, emotional, and addictive disorders are included, it is thought that 25% or more of Americans suffer each year (Surgeon General, 1999; Regier et al, 1993; *News,* 1997). As seen in the table titled, "12-Month Prevalence Rate of Mental Disorders in the United States," anxiety disorders are the most prevalent, followed by mood disorders (collectively), alcohol disorders, and major depression. This table, also found in Chapter 1 and in each chapter in this unit, lists prevalence rates for a 12-month period (Regier et al, 1993). Lifetime incidence of these disorders is slightly higher (Kessler et al, 1994). Table 27-1 provides the data for lifetime prevalence rates for the most common mental and chemical-abuse disorders. It is important to note that many individuals have a co-morbid status; for example, they may be depressed, anxious, and abuse a chemical or have some other combination of disorders. Therefore psychiatric morbidity is quite concentrated, with approximately 17% of the population having a history of three or more co-morbid disorders (Kessler et al, 1994). Most of these individuals do not seek professional help. Kessler (1994) found that less than 60% of people with a lifetime disorder, and less than 80% of those with a recent disorder, seek professional help. This factor suggests a great reservoir of unmet mental health needs in the United States.

Critical Thinking Questions

You are in this course to learn about caring for psychiatric patients. Do you believe people with mental disorders can become completely well? If not, can you justify the necessity of this course?

12-Month Prevalence Rate of Mental Disorders in the United States

Diagnosis	Percentage of Population Over 17 Years of Age	Number of People
Anxiety disorders	12.6	20,034,000
Phobia disorders*	10.9	17,331,333
Mood disorders	9.5	15,143,000
Alcohol disorders	7.4	11,766,000
Major depression†	5.0	7,950,000
Drug disorders	3.1	4,929,000
Cognitive impairment	2.7	4,293,000
Obsessive-compulsive disorder	2.1	3,339,000
Antisocial disorder	1.5	2,385,000
Panic disorders*	1.3	2,067,000
Bipolar disorder†	1.2	1,908,000
Schizophrenia	1.1	1,749,000
Somatization	0.2	365,000

*Also calculated in anxiety statistics.
†Also calculated in mood disorders statistics.
From Regier DA et al: The de facto U.S mental and addictive disorders service system: epidemiological catchment area prospective, 1-year prevalence rates of disorders and services, *Arch Gen Psychiatry* 50:85, 1993; Surgeon General: *Mental health: a report from the Surgeon General*, 1999, Washington DC, Department of Health and Human Services.

| Table 27-1 | Lifetime Prevalence Rates for Mental Disorders in the United States

Disorder	Lifetime Rate Prevalence (%)
Anxiety disorders (all)	24.9
Panic disorder	3.5
Agoraphobia with panic disorder	5.3
Social phobia	13.3
Simple phobia	11.3
Generalized anxiety disorder	5.1
Mood disorders (all)	19.3
Major depressive disorder	17.1
Bipolar disorder	1.6
Dysthymia	6.4
Chemical-abuse disorder (all)	26.6
Alcohol abuse without dependence	9.4
Alcohol dependence	14.1
Drug abuse without dependence	4.4
Drug dependence	7.5
Schizophrenia and other psychoses	0.7
Antisocial personality disorder	3.5
Any mental or chemical abuse disorder	48.0

Adapted from Kessler RC et al: Lifetime and 12-month prevalence of DSM-III-R psychiatric disorders in the United States, *Arch Gen Psychiatry* 51:8, 1994.

Key Terms

Etiology Study of the causes of diseases, including both direct and predisposing causes.
Incidence New cases of a condition, which occurs during a specified time.
National Institute of Mental Health Government organization within the National Institutes of Health concerned with mental health issues in the United States.
Nature argument Etiology is related to biology.
Nurture argument Etiology is related to upbringing, life events, or other stressors.
Prevalence Cases (both new and existing) of a condition observed at a point in time.
Psychopathology Systematic study of mental disorders.

The incidence of psychopathology is high, and nurses' understanding of psychopathology is basic to effective psychotherapeutic management of mental disorders. Understanding psychopathology requires that knowledge be organized, operational definitions be formed, and criteria for diagnosis be developed. Several diagnostic systems have been developed, but this text will present criteria from *The Diagnostic and*

Statistical Manual of Mental Disorders (DSM), which is published by the American Psychiatric Association (APA) and is the official diagnostic manual in use in the United States. The current version, DSM-IV-TR (APA, 2001), is the sixth version since DSM was first published in 1952 (DSM-I, DSM-II, DSM-III, DSM-III-R, DSM-IV, and DSM-IV-TR). Because diagnostic consistency among clinicians is so important, psychiatric experts are continually evaluating and updating criteria for this manual. All chapters in this unit are developed around DSM criteria that convey important concepts related to each mental disorder discussed. Because people are more than their symptoms, and successful treatment demands an assessment beyond the presenting disorder, the DSM involves evaluation on several axes. Five axes have been identified:

1. Axis I. Clinical disorders (e.g., schizophrenia, bipolar disorder)
2. Axis II. Personality disorders (e.g., paranoid personality disorder, narcissistic personality disorder), mental retardation

3. Axis III. General medical conditions (that are potentially relevant to understanding the mental disorder) (e.g., neoplasms, endocrine disorders)
4. Axis IV. Psychosocial and environmental problems (e.g., educational, housing)
5. Axis V. Global assessment of functioning (e.g., rating of psychologic, social, and occupational functioning on a "mental-health" scale [0 to 100])

In addition, each chapter presents a discussion of common behaviors, etiologic issues, and psychotherapeutic management strategies.

BEHAVIOR

Patients' behaviors are presented to help the student identify behavioral phenomena. Some behaviors can be observed directly (objective assessment or signs), whereas the patient must report other behaviors (subjective or symptoms). Knowledge of these signs and symptoms helps the nurse anticipate and plan appropriate interventions.

ETIOLOGY

For many years, psychiatric clinicians have typically fallen into one of two etiologic camps: those who believe that mental disorders arise from *nature* (organic, biologic, genetic) and those who believe that mental disorders arise from *nurture* (psychodynamic, functional, environmental stressors, early life experiences). In recent years, most clinicians have come to recognize that both views provide valuable insights into the complexities of the human mind. In fact, research suggests that some life experiences (i.e., nurture) actually change biology (i.e., nature), thus underscoring a more holistic view of mental illness. Threads of the "nature versus nurture" argument (or the "biologic versus psychodynamic" argument) are presented in discussions of etiology; however, the overriding theme of this unit is the recognition of the unifying symptoms that point to the contributions of each etiologic factor.

PSYCHOTHERAPEUTIC MANAGEMENT

Sections on psychotherapeutic management in each chapter draw on the general intervention strategies presented in Units Three through Five to develop appropriate interventions for each disorder. In addition, a case study and a related nursing care plan (see

sample care plan on page 308) are presented for each disorder. The following rules provide relevant guidelines for all aspects of psychotherapeutic management:
- Provide support for patients
- Strengthen patients' self-esteem
- Treat patients as adults
- Prevent failure or embarrassment
- Treat patients as individuals
- Provide reality testing
- Handle hostility therapeutically
- Be calm and matter-of-fact about norms and limits

NURSES NEED TO UNDERSTAND PSYCHOPATHOLOGY

"Life was hell in that private hospital. I was heavily medicated, and the staff treated me with indignity. They watched me constantly, even while I was relieving myself and showering. I was permitted only to sit, smoke cigarettes, and play cards with other patients. By the time of my discharge four months later, I had been stripped of my self-esteem. I had lost my confidence; I could not perform even the simplest of tasks." (Jacqueline Chapman, MS, MFCC, former mental patient, 1997)

Nurses cannot gain a true understanding of patients with mental disorders until they understand mental disorders. Psychiatric nursing is more than warm, caring feelings about patients. Although being affirming and kind are wonderful attributes in daily life, more is required of the effective psychiatric nurse. This "more" is based on an understanding of psychopathology.

> ### *Critical* Thinking Questions
> The biologic versus psychodynamic argument has gone on for a long time. Why is it important to be open to both points of view? Although you may not have used the same words, you probably had a bias one way or the other before you started nursing school. What was your bias?

The psychiatric nurse can no more effectively plan and provide psychiatric care without an understanding of psychopathology than can the medical-surgical nurse plan and provide care without an understanding of pathophysiology. In this unit the author has provided a discussion of psychopathology for each disorder. The authors of this text have included chapters on the following mental disorders

▌Care Plan

Name: _____   Admission Date: _____

DSM-IV-TR Diagnosis: _____

Assessment   **Areas of strength:** _____

              Problems: _____

Diagnoses   _____

              _____

              _____

Outcomes   *Short-term goals:*   *Date met*

              _____   _____

              _____   _____

              _____   _____

              Long-term goals:

              _____   _____

              _____   _____

              _____   _____

Planning/   **Nurse–patient relationship:** _____
Interventions
              _____

              Psychopharmacology: _____

              _____

              Milieu management: _____

              _____

              _____

Evaluation   _____

              _____

Referrals   _____

              _____

using the language of the DSM-IV-TR: schizophrenia, mood disorders, anxiety-related disorders, cognitive disorders, personality disorders, sexual disorders, substance-related disorders, dual diagnosis, and eating disorders.

▌Key Concepts

1. According to the Surgeon General, 25% or more Americans suffer from some type of mental or addictive disorder in any given 12-month period.

2. Anxiety disorders are the most common category of mental disorder, followed by mood disorders (collectively), and alcohol disorders.

3. Understanding psychopathology is fundamental to effective psychotherapeutic management. Understanding psychopathology requires organizing knowledge, operationally defining terms, and developing criteria for diagnosis.

4. The DSM-IV-TR (APA, 2001) is the official diagnostic system used in American psychiatry and is emphasized in this textbook.

5. Etiologic explanations of mental disorders can be broadly placed under one of two categories: biologic (nature or organic causes) and psychologic (nurture, psychodynamic, or functional causes).

6. Guidelines appropriate for all aspects of psychiatric care include supportive care, strengthening self-esteem, preventing failure or embarrassment, treating patients as individuals, reinforcing reality, and handling patients' hostility calmly and matter-of-factly.

References

Acocella, J: The empty couch, *The New Yorker,* May, p 112, 2000.

American Psychiatric Association: *Diagnostic and statistical manual of mental disorders, text revision,* ed 4, Washington, DC, 2001, APA.

British Columbia Schizophrenia Society: Schizophrenia: Youth's greatest disabler. *BCSS* 6(1):11, 2000.

Chapman J: The social safety net in recovery from psychosis: a therapist's story, *Psychiatr Serv* 48(10):1257, 1997.

Deegan PE: Recovering our sense of value after being labeled mentally ill, *J Psychosoc Nurs Ment Health Serv* 31(4):7, 1993.

Huxley NA, Rendall M, Sederer L: Psychosocial treatments in schizophrenia: a review of the past 20 years, *J Nerv Men Dis* 188(4):187, 2000.

Ichikawa J, Meltzer HY: Relationship between dopaminergic and serotonergic neuronal activity in the frontal cortex and the action of typical and atypical antipsychotic drugs, *Eur Arch Psychiatry Clin Neurosci* 249 (Suppl 4):IV90, 2001.

Kaplan HI, Saddock BJ: *Comprehensive textbook of psychiatry/IV,* ed 6, Baltimore, 1995, Williams and Wilkins.

Keck PE, Strakowski SM, McElroy SL: The efficacy of atypical antipsychotics in the treatment of depressive symptoms, hostility, and suicidality in patients with schizophrenia, *J Clin Psychiatry* 61(suppl 3):4, 2000.

Kessler RC et al: Lifetime and 12-month prevalence of DSM-III-R psychiatric disorders in the United States, *Arch Gen Psychiatry* 51:8, 1994.

Kolb LC, Brodie HKH: *Modern clinical psychiatry,* Philadelphia, 1982, WB Saunders.

McGrath J, Emmerson WB: Fortnightly review: treatment of schizophrenia, *BMJ* 319(7216):1045, 1999.

News: Key messages of mental health month, *J Psychosoc Nurs Ment Health Serv* 35(5):9, 1997.

Regier DA et al: The de facto US mental and addictive disorders service system: epidemiologic catchment area prospective 1-year prevalence rates of disorders and services, *Arch Gen Psychiatry* 50:85, 1993.

Surgeon General: *Mental health: a report from the Surgeon General,* Washington, DC, 1999, Department of Health & Human Services.

Talan J: Schizophrenia fight leads experts to a retrovirus, *The brain in the news,* January-May (Special Issue):1, 2001.

Yamada S: *The role of serotonin in schizophrenia,* www.medscape.com/medscape/cno/2000/CINP/Story.cfm?story_id=1497. Accessed 4/19/01.

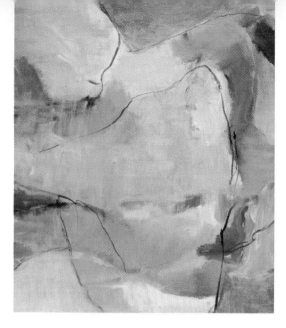

Chapter 28

Schizophrenia and Other Psychoses

Norman L. Keltner

Learning Objectives

After reading this chapter, you should be able to:
- Define the term schizophrenia.
- Describe the major historic figures, events, and theories that have contributed to the current understanding of schizophrenia.
- Identify Bleuler's four As.
- Recognize *The Diagnostic and Statistical Manual of Mental Disorders-Fourth Edition-Text Revision* (DSM-IV-TR) criteria and terminology for schizophrenia.
- Differentiate and describe DSM-IV-TR subtypes, and type I and type II subtypes.
- Recognize and describe objective and subjective symptoms of schizophrenia.
- Identify biologic explanations for schizophrenia.
- Describe two theoretical psychodynamic explanations for schizophrenia.
- Develop a nursing care plan for patients with schizophrenia.
- Identify the major drugs used in the treatment of schizophrenia, their mechanisms of action, their target symptoms, and their major side effects.
- Evaluate the effectiveness of nursing interventions for patients with schizophrenia.

There are three inescapable "facts" about schizophrenia that should be taken into account by any effort to explain it: first, the very high probability that it will become clinically apparent in late adolescence or early adulthood; second, the role of "stress" in onset and relapse; and third, the therapeutic efficacy of neuroleptic drugs.

Weinberger, 1987, p. 660

Psychosis is a disruptive mental state in which an individual struggles to distinguish the external world from internally generated perceptions. An impaired ability to relate to others complicates this state. Common symptoms of psychosis include hallucinations, delusions, and difficulty with thought organization. Psychosis can be present in schizo-phrenia, acute mania, depression, drug intoxication, dementia, and delirium. Schizophrenia is one of the most common causes of psychosis.

SCHIZOPHRENIA

Although many laypeople are quite sophisticated medically, it is not uncommon to hear the word schizophrenia defined as "split personality." By split personality, people mean something akin to a "Jekyll and Hyde" experience or a multiple personality disorder. This popular depiction does not begin to portray schizophrenia. Schizophrenia is not characterized by a changing personality; it is characterized by a deteriorating personality. Therefore this popular notion of a dramatic personality

Key Terms

Ambivalence Simultaneous opposite feelings (e.g., love and hate); often expressed as approach-avoidance behavior.

Anergia Absence of energy.

Anhedonia The inability to experience pleasure.

Apathy Lack of feeling, concern, interest, or emotion.

Autism Preoccupation with the self with little concern for external reality; a self-made private world of the patient with schizophrenia.

Avolition Lack of motivation.

Blocking Interruption of thoughts due to psychologic factors.

Catatonia Immobility as a result of psychologic causes.

Clanging associations Use of rhyming words.

Concrete thinking Use of literal meaning without the ability to consider abstract meaning (e.g., "Don't cry over spilt milk" might be interpreted as "because the milk is dirty").

Delusions Fixed, false beliefs of importance to the individual, which are resistant to reason or fact.

Double-blind Conflicting demands by significant individuals in a patient's life; unable to meet both demands, the patient is doomed to fail.

Echolalia Repetition of words heard.

Echopraxia Repetitive, meaningless movement.

Flight of ideas Rapid process in which a patient's speech changes abruptly from topic to topic based on superficial or chance associations.

Hallucinations False sensory perception unrelated to external stimuli (e.g., seeing things that are not there).

Hebephrenia Outdated schizophrenic subtype characterized by silliness, delusions, hallucinations, and regression.

Ideas of reference Belief that some events have a special meaning (e.g., people laughing near the patient are perceived as laughing at the patient).

Illusion Misinterpretation of a real sensory stimulus.

Loose association Thinking characterized by speech in which ideas shift from one subject to another that is unrelated.

Mutism Refusal to speak.

Negativism Motiveless resistance to all instruction.

Neologism Word or expression invented by the patient.

Paranoia Extreme suspiciousness of others and their actions.

Premorbid State before the onset of a disorder.

Psychosis Inability to recognize reality, complicated by a severe thought disorder and the inability to relate to others.

Religiosity Preoccupation with religious ideas or content.

Stereotypy Persistent repetition of senseless acts or words.

Withdrawal Behaviors designed to avoid interacting with others.

Word salad Randomized set of words without logical connection.

12-Month Prevalence Rate of Mental Disorders in the United States

Diagnosis	Percentage of Population Over 17 Years of Age	Number of People
Anxiety disorders	12.6	20,034,000
Phobia disorders*	10.9	17,331,000
Mood disorders	9.5	15,143,000
Alcohol disorders	7.4	11,766,000
Major depression†	5.0	7,950,000
Drug disorders	3.1	4,929,000
Cognitive impairment	2.7	4,293,000
Obsessive-compulsive disorder	2.1	3,339,000
Antisocial disorder	1.5	2,385,000
Panic disorders*	1.3	2,067,000
Bipolar disorder†	1.2	1,908,000
Schizophrenia	1.1	1,749,000
Somatization	0.2	365,000

*Also calculated in anxiety statistics.
†Also calculated in mood disorders statistics.
From Regier DA et al: The de facto U.S. mental and addictive disorders service system: epidemiological catchment area prospective, 1-year prevalence rates of disorders and services, *Arch Gen Psychiatry* 50:85, 1993; Surgeon General: *Mental health: a report from the Surgeon General*, 1999, Washington DC, Department of Health and Human Services.

change comes far short of capturing the devastating effect that schizophrenia has on the life of a person and the person's family. Simply stated, schizophrenia is one of the most profoundly disabling illnesses, mental or physical, the nurse will ever encounter.

Schizophrenia is a diagnostic term used to describe a major psychotic disorder characterized by disturbances in:

- Perception (e.g., hallucinations)
- Thought processes (e.g., thought derailment [or loose associations])
- Reality testing (e.g., delusions)
- Feeling (e.g., flat or inappropriate affect)
- Behavior (e.g., catatonia [(i.e., motoric immobility)]
- Attention (e.g., inability to concentrate)
- Motivation (e.g., avolition [cannot initiate or persist in goal-directed activities])

Contributing to the overall deterioration is a decline in psychosocial functioning.

Schizophrenia typically first appears in late adolescence or early adulthood. Schizophrenia affects men and women almost equally, though men usu-

Early Warning Signs of Schizophrenia

Deterioration of personal hygiene
Depression
Bizarre behavior
Irrational statements
Sleeping excessively or inability to sleep
Social withdrawal, isolation, and reclusiveness
Shift in basic personality
Unexpected hostility
Deterioration of social relationships
Hyperactivity or inactivity or alternating between the two
Inability to concentrate or to cope with minor problems
Extreme preoccupation with religion or with the occult
Excessive writing without meaning
Indifference
Dropping out of activities or out of life
Decline in academic or athletic interests
Forgetting things
Losing possessions
Extreme reactions to criticisms

British Columbia Schizophrenia Society: Schizophrenia: *Youth's greatest disabler.* British Columbia Schizophrenia Society, ed 6, January 2000, p. 6.

| Box 28-1 | Epidemiology of Schizophrenia

1. One percent of the population suffers from schizophrenia.
2. For 95% of sufferers, the disease lasts a lifetime.
3. Individuals with schizophrenia occupy 25% of inpatient hospital beds.
4. Approximately one third of all homeless Americans suffer from schizophrenia.
5. Of the individuals with schizophrenia, 15% do not respond to traditional antipsychotic medications and 70% are only partial responders.
6. Fifty percent experience serious side effects to medications.
7. Between 20% and 50% of the individuals with schizophrenia attempt suicide, and 10% are successful in killing themselves.
8. Schizophrenic individuals have a 20% shorter life expectancy.

Adapted from News in mental health nursing, *J Psychosoc Nurs* 35(2):6, 1997; American Psychiatric Association: Practice guidelines for the treatment of patients with schizophrenia, *Am J Psychiatry* 154(Suppl 4):1, 1997.

ally have an earlier age of onset by about 4 to 6 years, and new onset schizophrenia after age 50 is almost always seen in women (Seeman, 1995). Studies have shown that approximately 1% of the population will experience schizophrenia during their lifetime. Though the prevalence rate and symptom presentation for schizophrenia are fairly constant worldwide, inner-city residents, those from lower socioeconomic classes, and individuals who experience difficulties *in utero* (e.g., mother with influenza) are more likely to be affected or diagnosed or both (American Psychiatric Association [APA], 2001). Economic costs are in the tens of billions of dollars each year. The cost in human suffering is incalculable. Box 28-1 outlines the statistical realities of schizophrenia.

Morel was the first to name the psychiatric symptoms of schizophrenia. In 1860, while treating an adolescent boy, Morel used the phrase *dementia praecox* (precocious senility) to describe the group of symptoms he observed (Kolb, Brodie, 1982). Kahlbaum (in 1871) and Hecker (in 1874) added to the psychiatric nomenclature with their diagnostic categories catatonia and hebephrenia, respectively (Kaplan, Saddock, 1995). In 1878, Kraepelin added the term *paranoia* and engaged in a rigorous study of what is now called schizophrenia. Kraepelin found

commonalities among these three mental disorders (catatonia, hebephrenia, and paranoia) and, in 1899, grouped them under the diagnostic term that Morel had coined 40 years before, dementia praecox (Kaplan, Saddock). Kraepelin believed that schizophrenia was the result of neuropathologic factors; he envisioned a progressive deteriorating course resulting in disabling mental impairment with little hope of recovery.

It was left to Bleuler in the early 1900s to coin the term schizophrenia in a book subtitled *The Group of Schizophrenias.* Bleuler believed that schizophrenia does not always follow a course of deterioration (thus dementia was inappropriate), nor does it always occur early in life (hence praecox was inappropriate). Bleuler broadened Kraepelin's concept by focusing on symptoms rather than on outcomes (Harding, Zubin, Stauss, 1987). Bleuler identified four primary symptoms that he believed were present in all individuals with schizophrenia. All of these classic symptoms begin with the letter "A," which facilitates memorization (Box 28-2).

These two giants of psychiatric history founded two divergent views of schizophrenia. Kraepelin, in using the diagnostic category of dementia praecox, revealed a conceptual alignment between schizophrenia and disorders such as Alzheimer's disease, which

| Box 28-2 | Bleuler's Four A's

- **Affective disturbance.** Inappropriate, blunted, or flattened affect
- **Autism.** Preoccupation with the self with little concern for external reality
- **Associative looseness.** The stringing together of unrelated topics
- **Ambivalence.** Simultaneous opposite feelings

have a less optimistic prognosis. Bleuler, on the other hand, developed a school of thought that was much broader and more optimistic than that of Kraepelin. Based on Bleuler's wider grouping, pessimism eased, and some clinicians began to see improvements in their patients. Although Kraepelin based his views on biology, Bleuler, influenced by the master analyst Freud and other psychodynamic theorists, sought psychologic explanations for schizophrenia. For most of the twentieth century, Freud's psychoanalytic explanations, and by extension, Bleuler's thinking, dominated the understanding of schizophrenia. However, as the "limitations of talking" cures became more evident, the psychodynamic approach began to lose its grip on mental health professionals.

In recent years, a resurgence of interest in biologic research has resulted in renewed respect for Kraepelin's work. In fact, Kraepelin's term dementia praecox is again used by some clinicians to provoke powerful images of the deteriorative course associated with approximately 10% of the schizophrenic population (Kopelowicz, Bidder 1992).

COURSE OF ILLNESS

Schizophrenia typically first occurs in adolescence or early adulthood, a time during which brain maturation is almost complete. There are three overlapping phases of the disorder. Most patients alternate between acute and stable phases. During periods of stabilization, patients may experience complete remission. Essentially, individuals burdened with schizophrenia experience an acute phase, a stabilization phase, and a stable phase.

- *Acute phase.* The patient experiences severe psychotic symptoms. Although these symptoms may appear abruptly, it is not uncommon to discover a history of social deterioration.
- *Stabilizing phase.* The patient is getting better.
- *Stable phase.* In this phase, the patient may still experience hallucinations and delusions, but

the hallucinations and delusions are not as severe nor as disabling as they were during the acute phase. Other patients may be asymptomatic in regard to psychotic symptoms but find themselves anxious and depressed.

CLINICAL EXAMPLE (STABLE PHASE)
Billy is a 39-year-old man living in a psychiatric residential facility who attends a day-treatment program Monday through Friday. Though Billy experiences hallucinations frequently, most often visual hallucinations, he is indeed stabilized. All staff members agree that Billy is not a danger to himself or others and that the day-treatment program is more appropriate for him than a state hospital would be.

Critical **Thinking Question**
Why do you think Kraepelin was so pessimistic about the patients he saw with dementia praecox?

DSM-IV-TR TERMINOLOGY AND CRITERIA

The DSM-IV-TR criteria for schizophrenia are found in the box on page 314. Since the inception of schizophrenia as a diagnostic entity, attempts have been made to divide it into homogeneous subtypes. Early attempts to identify homogeneous groups resulted in the subtypes catatonic, hebephrenic, paranoid, and simple schizophrenia. This early thinking is still reflected in official diagnostic classifications. The DSM-IV-TR identifies five subtypes of schizophrenia: catatonic, disorganized (similar to the old "hebephrenia"), paranoid, disorganized, undifferentiated (similar to the old "simple"), and residual (see the box titled, "Criteria for Schizophrenia Subtypes" on page 314). The North American Nursing Diagnosis Association (NANDA) nursing diagnoses and the DSM-IV-TR diagnoses related to schizophrenia are listed in the box on page 314.

Although the DSM-IV-TR approach has been carefully crafted, the authors find the subtyping approach based on positive-versus-negative symptoms helpful in the clinical arena because it can be predictive of medication response. The student should realize that most patients are not "either-or," but have a mixture of positive and negative symptoms (Breslin, 1992). Recently, a third category, dis-

DSM-IV-TR Criteria for Schizophrenia

A. Characteristic symptoms (at least two of the following):
   Delusions
   Hallucinations
   Disorganized speech
   Grossly disorganized or catatonic behavior
   Negative symptoms
B. Social-occupational dysfunction: work, interpersonal, and self-care functioning is below the level achieved before onset
C. Duration: continuous signs of the disturbance for at least 6 months
D. Schizoaffective and mood disorders are not present and are not responsible for the signs and symptoms
E. Not caused by substance abuse or a general medical disorder

Adapted from the American Psychiatric Association: *Diagnostic and statistical manual of mental disorders*, ed 4, text revision, Washington, DC, 2000, APA.

DSM-IV-TR and NANDA Diagnoses Related to Schizophrenia and Other Psychoses

DSM-IV*	NANDA†
Schizophrenia	Adjustment, impaired
Paranoid type	Anxiety
Disorganized type	Caregiver role, strain
Catatonic type	Communication, impaired
Undifferentiated type	verbal
Residual type	Coping, compromised family
Schizophreniform	Coping, disabled family
disorder	Coping, ineffective
Schizoaffective disorder	Identity, disturbed personal
Delusional disorder	Role performance, ineffective
Brief psychotic disorder	Self-care, deficit (bathing and
Shared psychotic	hygiene, feeding, toileting)
disorder	Self-esteem, situational low
	Sensory perceptual, disturbed
	(specify)
	Social interaction, impaired
	Social isolation
	Thought processes, disturbed

*American Psychiatric Association: *Diagnostic and statistical manual of mental disorders*, ed 4, text revision, Washington, DC, 2000, APA.
†North American Nursing Diagnosis Association: *NANDA nursing diagnoses: definitions and classifications 2001-2002*, Philadelphia, 2001, NANDA.

DSM-IV-TR Criteria for Schizophrenia Subtypes

PARANOID	A. Preoccupation with one or more delusions or frequent auditory hallucinations (content frequently persecutory and/or grandiose) B. None of the following is prominent: disorganized speech, disorganized behavior, flat or inappropriate affect, catatonic behavior
DISORGANIZED	A. All of the following are prominent: disorganized speech, disorganized behavior, flat or inappropriate affect B. Does not meet criteria of catatonic type
CATATONIC	At least two of the following are present: A. Motoric immobility, waxy flexibility, or stupor B. Excessive motor activity (purposeless) C. Extreme negativism or mutism D. Peculiar movements stereotype of movements, prominent mannerisms, or prominent grimacing E. Echolalia or echopraxia
UNDIFFERENTIATED	Characteristic symptoms (see box at right, criteria A) are present, but criteria for paranoid, catatonic, or disorganized subtypes are not met.
RESIDUAL	A. Characteristic symptoms (see box titled, "Criteria for Schizophrenia," criterion A) are no longer present; criteria are unmet for paranoid, catatonic, or disorganized subtypes B. There is continuing evidence of disturbance, such as the presence of negative symptoms or criteria A symptoms, in an attenuated form (e.g., odd beliefs, unusual perceptual experiences)

Adapted from the American Psychiatric Association: *Diagnostic and statistical manual of mental disorders*, ed 4, TR Washington, DC, 2000, APA.

organized, has been added because careful analysis differentiated it from positive schizophrenia. Disorganized schizophrenia is characterized by disorganized speech, disorganized behavior, and poor attention (APA, 2001).

POSITIVE VERSUS NEGATIVE SCHIZOPHRENIA

Positive, or type I, schizophrenia has a different constellation of symptoms than does negative, or type II, schizophrenia (Box 28-3). Type I is positive in the sense that symptoms are an embellishment of nor-

|Box 28-3 | Positive and Negative Symptoms of Schizophrenia

Symptom Category	Symptoms
Positive (type I)	
Prognosis: better	Abnormal thought form
Precipitating factors: yes	Agitation, tension
Onset: acute	Associational disturbances
Sensorium: dreamlike quality	Bizarre behavior
Intellectual impairment: none	Conceptual disorganization
Pathophysiology: D_2 hyperactivity	Delusions
Pathoanatomy: ventricular brain ratios may be normal	Excitement
Response to typical neuroleptics: fair to good	Feelings of persecution
Effect of levodopa: increases symptoms	Grandiosity
	Hallucinations
	Hostility
	Ideas of reference
	Illusions
	Insomnia
	Suspiciousness
Negative (type II)	
Prognosis: poor	Alogia
Onset: chronic	Anergia
Family history: more so than type I	Anhedonia
Sensorium: clear	Asocial behavior
Intellectual impairment: yes	Attention deficits
Pathophysiology: possibly hypodopaminergic, decreased cerebral blood flow	Avolition
Pathoanatomy: increased ventricular brain ratios, other changes (see text)	Blunted affect
Response to typical neuroleptics: varies	Communication difficulties
Response to atypical neuroleptics: better	Difficulty with abstractions
Effect of levodopa: minimal	Passive social withdrawal
	Poor grooming and hygiene
	Poor rapport
	Poverty of speech

From Harris D, Keltner NL: Medication management. In Worley NK, editor: *Mental health in the community,* St Louis, 1997, Mosby.

mal cognition and perception. The symptoms are "additional." Positive symptoms are believed to be the result of a subcortical dopaminergic process (too much dopamine) affecting cortical areas.

CLINICAL EXAMPLE

John is sitting in the dayroom on the psychiatric unit when his eyes begin to dart back and forth, and he becomes increasingly anxious. You ask, "John, are you hearing something that I cannot hear?" "Can't you hear them?" he replies. "They are going to get me." John's auditory hallucination is a positive symptom because it is an exaggeration of a normal perception (he is "hearing" without an auditory stimulus).

Type II is labeled negative because symptoms are essentially an absence or diminution of that which

should be, that is, lack of affect, lack of energy, and so on. Type II may be a hypodopaminergic process (Ichikawa, Meltzer, 2001) and also caused by cortical structural changes (e.g., cerebral atrophy). Pathoanatomy consistently mentioned in the literature includes decreased cerebral blood flow (CBF), particularly in frontal areas, and increased ventricular brain ratios (VBRs). Decreased frontal blood flow and a hypometabolic state are most pronounced in the dorsolateral prefrontal cortex. Ventricular enlargement can be detected on computed tomography (CT) and magnetic resonance imaging (MRI) film with the naked eye. Other pathoanatomic features observed in some studies that may contribute to negative symptoms include a reduction in brain weight by 5%, a slight decrease in brain length, and neuronal loss in some cortical areas (Roberts, Leigh, Weinberger, 1993).

Philip Wilson has a long history of mental problems and was first diagnosed with schizophrenia in 1963. Mr. Wilson is a patient in the state hospital system. The summary note written by the nursing team leader includes the following observation: "Mr. Wilson is isolative and, for the most part, expressionless. He spends long hours sitting and staring out of the window. Attempts to engage Mr. Wilson in unit activities have not been successful."

An unfortunate side effect of the positive versus negative subtyping approach has been the tendency by a few professionals to be too pessimistic about the prognosis of type II patients. The outcome of negative schizophrenia is not invariably poor (Soni et al, 1992). Kopelowicz and Bidder (1992), who caution nurses and others against such rash and uninformed thinking, divide negative symptoms into primary and secondary. The secondary symptoms are therapeutically accessible, particularly early in the course of the illness. These symptoms arise from some of the consequences of a schizophrenic diagnosis: medications, hospitalizations, loss of social supports, and a socioeconomic decline. If assessed early, secondary negative symptoms can be arrested.

CLINICAL EXAMPLE
Merritt Burgone is a homeless man with a long history of mental illness. He has not seen his family in many years. Although his family was supportive at one time, they simply grew tired of trying to cope with Mr. Burgone. At this point, even modest improvements in his mental health are compromised by his lack of social support.

According to biologic theory, typical antipsychotic drugs (drugs that antagonize primarily dopamine D_2 receptors) are likely to be beneficial for positive symptoms because positive schizophrenia is a hyperdopaminergic process (see Box 28-3). Negative schizophrenia, on the other hand, is thought to be more structurally related and possibly a hypodopaminergic process. Dopamine antagonists (i.e., traditional antipsychotics) have relatively less effect and may actually cause the negative symptoms to worsen. Accordingly, the more florid the psychotic symptoms are (as in positive schizophrenia), the greater the likelihood of a favorable response will be to antipsychotics. As was noted in Chapter 20, atypical antipsychotic drugs

such as clozapine (Clozaril), risperidone (Risperdal), olanzapine (Zyprexa), quetiapine (Seroquel), and ziprasidone (Geodon) benefit negative symptoms, apparently because they affect different dopamine receptors. Furthermore, these drugs also antagonize serotonin receptors, which theoretically liberates dopamine in cortical areas, "correcting" the hypodopaminergic state. Unfortunately, some of these newer drugs are so expensive that some health maintenance organizations (HMOs) and governments are refusing to pay for them. For example, a 30-day supply of Zyprexa costs $350 or more, whereas the same amount of Haldol costs only $2.50 (News, 1997). Box 28-4 provides an overview of the evolution of schizophrenic subtyping.

As is true of all fields, there are special psychiatric terms you must know to communicate effectively with nurses and other professionals. A list of these key terms is provided at the beginning of the chapter.

BEHAVIOR

"My identity began to fragment and seemed to blend with my environment. Rather than just enjoying the wind, for instance, I thought I had merged with it. I had to stare at the sun to appreciate its warmth. Yet gradually I was able to see myself separate from those things. As I neared discharge, I began to feel some stirring of belief in myself. It was not until much later that I made a conscious effort to develop a sense of control, realizing that I had the power to decide what form my life would take and who I would be" (Leete, 1987, p. 486).

People who are treated for mental problems come to the attention of mental health professionals in one of two ways. The first way is when patients seek help. Patients who seek help do so because they have experienced such troubling subjective symptoms that they want professional intervention. Often, professional help is not sought until patients have exhausted self-help aids, friends, and family. The second way in which people come to the attention of the mental health system is by drawing attention to themselves through behavior that bothers, concerns, or frightens other people. These indicators of a mental disorder are apparent to others and are called objective signs. As discussed in the chapter on legal issues, help is sometimes resisted, and the person must be treated on an involuntary basis.

| Box 28-4 | Evolution of Schizophrenic Subtyping

1860	Morel coins the term *dementia praecox*.
1871	Kahlbaum uses the term *catatonia* to describe patients immobilized by psychologic factors.
1874	Hecker uses the term *hebephrenia* to describe patients with silly, bizarre, and regressed behaviors.
1878	Kraepelin adds the term *paranoia* to describe highly suspicious patients. He recognizes commonalities among catatonic, hebephrenic, and paranoid individuals.
1899	Kraepelin groups all three patient categories under the heading *dementia praecox*.
1900s	Bleuler introduces the term *schizophrenia* to describe these mental disorders. He adds the subtype *simple schizophrenia*.
1952	DSM-I: The first attempt to develop a diagnostic manual for nationwide use. DSM-I includes nine subtypes.
1968	DSM-II: Developed in an effort to articulate more efficiently a common diagnostic language. DSM-II has a total of 11 subtypes.
1980	DSM-III: The authors streamline the diagnostic subtypes to five: disorganized, catatonic, paranoid, undifferentiated, and residual.
1982	Andreasen, Crow, and others suggest a new subtyping approach. They categorize schizophrenia, based on symptoms, into positive (type I) and negative (type II).
1987	DSM-III: Revised; same subtypes.
1994	DSM-IV: Same subtypes as DSM-III.
1997	The APA practice guidelines on treating patients with schizophrenia recognize the addition of the subtype "disorganized" to the positive and negative subtyping concept.
2000	DSM-IV-TR is published; same subtypes.

From Harris D, Keltner NL: Medication management. In Worley NK, editor: *Mental health in the community,* St Louis, 1997, Mosby.
DSM, The Diagnostic and Statistical Manual of Mental Disorders.

| Box 28-5 | Objective and Subjective Behavioral Disorders in Schizophrenia

Objective Signs

Alterations in personal relationships
- Decreased attention to appearance and social amenities related to introspection and autism
- Inadequate or inappropriate communication
- Hostility
- Withdrawal

Alterations of activity
- Psychomotor agitation
- Catatonic rigidity
- Echopraxia (repetitive movements)
- Stereotypy (repetitive acts or words)

Subjective Symptoms

Altered perception
- Hallucinations
- Illusions
- Paranoid thinking

Alterations of thought
- Flight of ideas
- Retardation
- Blocking
- Autism
- Ambivalence
- Loose associations
- Delusions
- Poverty of speech
- Ideas of reference
- Mutism

Altered consciousness
- Confusion
- Incoherent speech
- Clouding
- Sense of "going crazy"

Alterations of affect
- Inappropriate, blunted, flattened, or labile affect
- Apathy
- Ambivalence
- Overreaction
- Anhedonia

Subjective and objective categories are not as discrete as they may appear at first. Hallucinations, for example, are subjective phenomena but may easily cause objective signs that get the attention of others (e.g., a person who talks back to an auditory hallucination). Nonetheless, dividing the expressions of schizophrenia into subjective symptoms and objective signs is a rational and convenient approach to understanding this mental disorder.

Six significant "alterations" occur in schizophrenia and can be grouped into objective signs or subjective symptoms (Box 28-5). Alterations in personal relationships and alterations of activity are highly visible to others (objective signs), whereas altered perception, alterations of thought, altered consciousness, and alterations of affect are more subjective in nature.

Objective Signs
Alterations in personal relationships

Patients with schizophrenia often have altered interpersonal relationships. Often, these problems develop over a long period, well before schizophrenia is diagnosed, and become more pronounced as the illness progresses. It is not uncommon to hear that a person was asocial, a loner, or a social "misfit" premorbidly.

Frequently, patients become less concerned with their appearance and may not bathe without persistent prodding. Table manners and other social skills may diminish to the point at which patients are disgusting to others. These behaviors are related to introspection (autism) and extreme self-absorption. Patients are focused on internal processes to the extent that their external social world collapses. Schizophrenia can cause a diminished energy level (anergia), which also complicates social interactions.

Interpersonal communication becomes inadequate and may be inappropriate. Again, internal processes are at work. Hostility, a somewhat common theme, also distances patients from others. Finally, patients with schizophrenia withdraw, further compromising their abilities to engage in meaningful social interactions.

Alterations of activity

Patients with schizophrenia also display alterations of activity. Patients may be too active (psychomotor agitation); that is, they are unable to sit still and continually pace, or they may be inactive or catatonic. These signs respond to antipsychotic drugs but can also be caused by them. The following example illustrates this point.

CLINICAL EXAMPLE
The nurse must be careful in assessing alterations in activity. Restlessness may be caused by akathisia (an extrapyramidal side effect [EPSE] of antipsychotic drugs) or may be a manifestation of schizophrenia. Rigidity, on the other hand, may be a warning sign of neuroleptic malignant syndrome (NMS), not catatonia. Both EPSEs and NMS are side effects of antipsychotic drugs. Hence accurate assessment is critical: though it is appropriate to administer an as-needed (prn) dose of haloperidol for psychomotor agitation or catatonia, it only serves to intensify akathisia and may prove fatal for patients with NMS.

Subjective Symptoms

Subjective symptoms are, by definition, experienced by patients in a personal way. Patients may hide these symptoms from others. For example, if a patient suffers from the delusion that he is a famous person, he may be able to keep it to himself. In fact, some clinicians advise patients who resist psychiatric care to "keep your symptoms to yourself, and no one will ever know." Presumably, there are individuals in society who are not reporting their subjective symptoms to anyone and thus are avoiding psychiatric intervention. For the most part, however, subjective symptoms of schizophrenia spill over into behavior that is noticeable to others. Subjective symptoms can be grouped into the four categories previously mentioned.

Altered perception ·

Altered perception includes hallucinations, illusions, and paranoid thinking. Hallucinations are false sensory perceptions and can be auditory, visual, olfactory, tactile, gustatory, or somatic (strange body sensations). Auditory hallucinations are the most common in schizophrenia and often take the form of accusations ("You slut," "Hey, queer") or commands ("Get away from these people"). Visual hallucinations are not as common in schizophrenia as are auditory hallucinations. The nurse may suspect a toxic process (drugs, fever) if visual hallucinations are present. Hallucinations are probably caused by a hyperdopaminergic state in the limbic areas.

Illusions are misinterpretations of real external stimuli. For example, a tree might be mistaken for a threatening person. Illusions are often associated with physical illness, as well as schizophrenia.

CLINICAL EXAMPLE
Delirium: While lying in bed with a low-grade fever, Gladys, a 68-year-old woman, asked, "Are those cobwebs on the wall?" Her son responded, "No, Mama, those are just shadows from your bedside lamp." Gladys laughed and said, "I guess my mind is going."

CLINICAL EXAMPLE
Schizophrenia: Tim, a patient in a day-treatment program mistakes a tennis shoe on the porch for a rat.

Paranoid thinking is characterized by a persistent interpretation of the actions of others as threatening or demeaning. Paranoid themes can color delusions and hallucinations, as well as the ordinary behavior of others. It is important for the student to differentiate paranoid thinking associated with a paranoid personality disorder from paranoid delusions. Paranoid thinking is less severe than paranoid delusions. Paranoid thinking may be "corrected" with facts, whereas paranoid delusions cannot.

CLINICAL EXAMPLE

Paranoid personality: Bill, a voluntary patient on the adult unit, sought help because of trouble on the job and at home. His ability to get along with people has deteriorated to the point that he has no friends. Bill's wife has started divorce proceedings, and he has sought treatment, hoping that she will change her mind. Over the last few years, Bill has been obsessed with the thought that his wife is cheating on him. He follows her when she leaves the house, sometimes listens to her telephone calls, and has confronted her with accusations of infidelity. Whenever he finds he is mistaken, he is relieved for a while and apologizes for not trusting her; but soon he begins to have the same paranoid thoughts. His paranoid thinking has caused alterations in his personal relationships.

CLINICAL EXAMPLE

Paranoid schizophrenia: Fred is a 28-year-old, unemployed laborer. The police recently brought Fred to the emergency department. Fred had been at the downtown bus station preaching loudly to all who passed. He spoke of a conspiracy of blacks and Jews who plan to take over America. Fred told the emergency room nurse that he feared for his life. He went on to explain that he had proof that the FBI was behind President Kennedy's assassination.

A final example of altered perception is based on the observation that the ability to adapt perceptually (or attend selectively) is altered in patients with schizophrenia.

CLINICAL EXAMPLE

A patient was looking out of a seventh-floor window. The nurse approached to look and noticed activity in the yard below. The nurse assumed that the patient was observing the same activity and commented. The patient, however, was not looking beyond the wire mesh screen in the window. He was unable to filter out what for most people would not be a distraction. The inability to filter out extraneous stimuli (ability to attend selectively) is a perceptual problem for some patients.

Alterations of thought

Alterations of thought are common in schizophrenia and are disturbing and frightening at times. Antipsychotic drugs are often beneficial. Often, insomnia diminishes as these symptoms subside, indicating that insomnia may be a secondary symptom. Common thought disorders include flight of ideas, thought retardation, blocking, autism, ambivalence, loose associations, delusions, poverty of speech, and concrete thinking.

Flight of ideas is a rapid process in which a patient's speech changes abruptly from topic to topic, with the changes usually based on superficial or chance associations, distracting stimuli, or plays on words.

Retardation is a slowing of mental activity. A patient may state, "I just can't think."

Blocking is the interruption of a thought and the inability to recall it. This disorder is very disturbing to patients and, at times, frightening. Blocking may be caused by the intrusion of hallucinations, delusions, or emotional factors. The following is a common example of blocking that might happen to anyone.

CLINICAL EXAMPLE

Joe, a 49-year-old teacher, was in the middle of a lecture when he lost his "train of thought." He could not remember what point he was developing or where to go next. He stalled for time, realizing that he was in a potentially embarrassing situation. Finally, he found his notes and proceeded, a little shaken and distracted but able to continue.

Autism occurs when patients are introspective to the extent that they are distracted from external events. Patients are preoccupied with themselves and may be oblivious to the reality around them, which results in a personalized view of reality.

Ambivalence is a state in which two opposite, strong feelings exist simultaneously. Patients may be both attracted to and repelled by a person, object, or goal. Ambivalence (e.g., love-hate) toward a domineering parent is common. Another common example is the simultaneous need for and fear of people, resulting in immobilization. Schizophrenic patients may be immobilized by their ambivalence regarding a matter as simple as deciding whether to drink orange juice or apple juice for breakfast. In these cases, it is therapeutic for the nurse to make decisions for patients if the patients will allow this. The following clinical example illustrates ambivalence that occurs in some families and is not meant to depict schizophrenic ambivalence.

CLINICAL EXAMPLE

Joyce, a 38-year-old librarian, has ambivalent feelings toward her father. He still tells her what to do, and she has a hard time standing up for herself. Joyce realizes that her periodic need for financial assistance is partially responsible for her predicament. Joyce also finds that she avoids calling her father and, because he calls her excessively to find out what she is doing, she cringes when the telephone rings. Although Joyce is not suffering from schizophrenia, she does experience ambivalence. She loves her father but, in her words, "He is driving me crazy."

Loose association is a pattern of speech in which a person's ideas slip off the track onto another that is completely unrelated or only slightly related. An occasional change of topic without obvious connection does not indicate loose associations.

Delusions are fixed, false beliefs and can take many forms. Delusions are described as fixed beliefs because they cannot be changed by logical persuasion. Delusions are described as false because they are not based in reality. Delusional content often relates to life experiences and can include somatic, grandiose, religious, nihilistic, referential, and paranoid content. An example of each type follows:

- *Somatic delusions.* A patient, after medical tests confirm otherwise, still insists, "I have cancer in my stomach."
- *Grandiose delusions.* A patient states, "I am Napoleon."
- *Religious delusions.* A woman attempts to kill her children because she believes the devil wants her to do so: "The devil told me to kill my children."
- *Nihilistic delusions.* A patient states, "I am dead." In response to saying, "If you are dead, how can you talk?" the patient says, "I don't know, but I'm dead."
- *Delusions of reference.* "The TV is talking about me. The guests on 'Oprah' are making fun of me."
- *Delusions of influence.* "I can control her with my thoughts."
- *Paranoid delusions.* "They all think that I am a homosexual."

Related phenomena sometimes found are the schizophrenic delusions that thoughts can be inserted or withdrawn by others: "Other people can read my mind"; "My thoughts are being broadcast so that everyone can hear."

Poverty of speech is manifested by the inability to formulate and articulate thoughts that are relevant to the discussion at hand. Vocabulary is markedly limited in individuals who experience poverty of speech.

Concrete thinking is the inability to conceptualize the meanings of words and phrases. For example, a concrete response to the proverb "People who live in glass houses should not throw stones" might be construed as "The glass would break." These individuals are likely to misinterpret jokes or smiles. For example, the meanings of "a diamond in the rough" or "cool as a cucumber" may be lost completely on a person exhibiting concrete thinking.

Altered consciousness

Altered consciousness is perhaps the symptom that is most troubling to patients; fortunately, it is also the most responsive to antipsychotic drugs. Manifestations of altered consciousness include confusion, incoherent speech, clouding, and a sense of "going crazy." The last manifestation of altered consciousness, "going crazy", deserves special mention. Many students are surprised when they enter a psychiatric facility to find that patients are not "crazy." In fact, although psychiatric patients are, by definition, struggling with mental disorders, psychiatric units are not wild, bizarre environments. Patients can readily differentiate between the "normal struggle" of dealing with a mental disorder and the feeling of going crazy (loss of control). The student will observe that patients on the psychiatric unit define a fellow patient who has become "wild" or who is loudly talking to himself or herself as crazy. In other words, this behavior is unusual—even on a psychiatric unit. Referring to the discussion of incompetence in Chapter 4, the student can appreciate why the designation of "incompetence" is reserved for only a few individuals.

Alterations of affect

Alterations of affect are varied and include inappropriate, flattened, blunted, or labile affects; apathy; ambivalence; and overreaction. For example, responding to bad news with laughter is an affective response that does not match the circumstances and is inappropriate. If a patient is unable to generate much affect, and the response to the bad news is weakly appropriate, the affect is blunted or dull. The inability to generate any affective response is referred to as flattened affect. Labile affect is a condition in which emotional tone changes quickly. A patient may be telling a happy story, suddenly begin to cry, and then quickly return to a happy disposition.

Apathy, which can be defined as a lack of concern or interest, is the inability to generate a normal response to people, situations, or the environment.

Ambivalence, as discussed earlier, is a condition in which patients are immobilized by the coexistence of opposite feelings. The immobilization can lead to an affective expression that approaches indifference or indecision.

Another alteration of affect is the tendency to overreact to events. An analogy is the small child who must put so much energy into closing a car door that the door slams shut, offending the ears and "nerves" of adults nearby. Because of physical limitations, the child has to push as hard as possible to overcome inertia. Because of emotional limitations, schizophrenic patients overreact to normal events to overcome mental and social inertia; and, like the child, these patients may offend the sensitivities of those nearby.

ETIOLOGY

Many authorities suggest that multiple factors must cause schizophrenia, because no single theory satisfactorily explains the disorder. Explanations can be categorized broadly into biologic or psychologic (psychodynamic) causes. These two categories parallel the "nature versus nurture" debate discussed in Chapter 27. Biologic theories and psychodynamic theories are discussed here, followed by a vulnerability-stress model, an eclectic approach that seems to capture the major forces at work in the genesis and outcomes of schizophrenia.

Biologic Theories

"People don't cause schizophrenia, they merely blame each other for doing so" E. Fuller Torrey (quoted in British Columbia Schizophrenia Society, [BCSS] 2000).

Biologic theorists posit that schizophrenia is caused by anatomic or physiologic abnormalities. Biologic explanations include biochemical, neurostructural, genetic, perinatal risk factors, and other theories. Biologic explanations have driven the development of biologic interventions, such as psychotropic drugs and somatic therapies.

Some clinicians have been reluctant to endorse biologic theories because the exclusive use of biologic approaches, such as psychotropic and somatic therapies, excludes interpersonal factors. The psychotherapeutic management model, however, recognizes the importance of both biologic and interpersonal interventions.

A positive result of biologic theories has been the minimization of the "blaming" that is inherent in other explanations. Just as viewing alcoholism as an illness has helped clinicians, families, and patients to get beyond blaming and on to treatment, biologic theories have facilitated the treatment of schizophrenia. To illustrate, just as diabetic or cardiac patients must learn to cope with illness (e.g., change in life style, threat of death), psychiatric patients must learn to cope with the limitations of their illness.

Biochemical theories

Biochemical theory can be traced to 1952, when Delay and Deniker reported the antipsychotic effects of chlorpromazine. Andreasen and Olsen (1982), Crow (1982), and others have postulated that a biochemical process accounts for the positive symptoms of schizophrenia. The prevailing biochemical explanation is referred to as the dopamine hypothesis. According to this hypothesis, excessive dopaminergic activity in cortical areas causes acute positive (type I) symptoms of schizophrenia (hallucinations, delusions, and thought disorders). Excessive dopamine may be a result of increased dopamine synthesis, increased dopamine release or turnover, or an increase in the number and activity of dopamine receptors (Brown, Mann, 1985). It is also known that drugs that increase dopamine, such as levodopa and the amphetamines, can cause a psychotic state (see the box titled, "Cigarette Smoking and Schizophrenia). This hypothesis is attractive because it is easy to grasp, and because drugs that block dopamine seem to be extremely effective in the treatment of schizophrenia. However, these drugs take days, weeks, or months to establish their clinical effectiveness, whereas the central nervous system (CNS) dopamine receptors are blocked within a few minutes. Therefore it seems that the dopamine hypothesis is too simplistic and that other factors are involved in the effectiveness of antipsychotic drugs.

Cigarette Smoking and Schizophrenia

People with schizophrenia tend to smoke a lot. Although approximately 30% of the general public smokes, studies indicate up to 81% of individuals suffering from schizophrenia do so (Hughes, Hatsukami, Mitchell, 1986). The difference in cigarette use between this population and the general population is significant, yet there are noticeably fewer attempts at smoking cessation. Some researchers argue that to deprive the schizophrenic person of the joys of smoking would be unduly cruel—smoking presumably being one of the few pleasures they have (Dalack, Healy, Meador-Woodruff, 1998).

The question becomes, "Why do people with schizophrenia smoke so much?"

The answer probably lies in the biochemical changes provoked by nicotine. All drugs of abuse, for instance, cause changes in brain dopamine levels. Dopamine axons from the ventral tegmental area are afferents through the reward pathway, including the putative pleasure nucleus, the nucleus accumbens. Nicotine increases the release of dopamine in the nucleus accumbens (Addington, 1998). This action is accomplished because nicotinic receptors synapse on dopamine afferents in the reward pathway, that is, nicotine modulates dopamine release (Dalack et al, 1998). Nicotine also modulates dopamine afferents to the prefrontal cortex (mesocortical tract). When coupled with the supposition that negative symptoms may be related to a hypodopaminergic process, nicotinic stimulation of dopamine in prefrontal areas may produce a therapeutic effect. In other words, the answer to the question, "Why do patients with schizophrenia smoke so much?" is simply this: it makes them feel better.

Selected Structural Brain Imaging Findings in Schizophrenia

1. Cerebral ventricular enlargement
2. Smaller cerebral and cranial size
3. Hypoplasia of the medial (limbic) temporal structures, especially the hippocampus

Nasrallah HA: Neurodevelopmental pathogenesis of schizophrenia, *Psychiatr Clin North Am* 16(2):269, 1993.

and Shaw suggested a role for serotonin in schizophrenia. Serotonin inhibits dopamine synthesis therefore serotonin antagonists potentially increase dopamine levels. This characteristic is one of the neurophysiologic properties that are presumed to cause atypical antipsychotics to be effective (see Chapter 20). These agents are now referred to as serotonin-dopamine antagonists (SDAs) by some clinicians (and by manufacturers).

Reduced levels of glutamate, a product of the Krebs cycle, have been proposed as a factor in schizophrenia (Kim et al, 1980). Both glutamate and glycine contribute to regulate N-methyl-D-aspartate (NMDA) receptors, receptors necessary for cognitive processes. Theories suggest that when NMDA receptors are normalized, schizophrenic symptoms are reduced (Ereshefsky, Lacombe, 1993). Neither treatment with glutamate nor glycine has proven particularly promising.

Neurostructural theories

The neurostructural theorists propose that schizophrenia, particularly negative (type II) schizophrenia, is a result of pathoanatomy. The three specific neurostructural changes mentioned most often are increased VBRs, brain atrophy, and decreased CBF. CT, MRI, positron emission tomography (PET), and single photon emission computed tomography (SPECT) are techniques used to develop images of the brain. CT and MRI provide images of brain structure (e.g., for VBRs and brain atrophy). PET and SPECT provide information on both brain structure and brain activity. Box 28-6 summarizes the most commonly used imaging techniques.

Ventricular brain ratios

The finding that a significant subgroup of individuals with schizophrenia have enlarged ventricles, according to CT scan, was first reported by Johnstone and

The dopamine hypothesis, though limited in explanatory power, continues to have great educational value for the following reasons:

1. Dopaminergic drugs (e.g., levodopa, amphetamines) can cause psychotic symptoms.
2. The degree of clinical improvement is correlated to D2 receptor blockade; at about 70% to 80% of these receptors (Kapur et al, 2000). This characteristic suggests that dopamine is a causative factor.
3. Postmortem studies of individuals with schizophrenia reveal increased numbers of dopamine receptors.

Other proposed neurotransmitter contributors to schizophrenia include serotonin, glutamate, and glycine (Yamada, 2000). As early as 1954, Woolley

|Box 28-6| Commonly Used Brain Imaging Techniques

1. Computed tomography (CT) is the most widely used x-ray method for imaging the living brain and is approximately 100 times more sensitive than conventional radiography. A number of contrast mediums can be used in conjunction with this procedure to enhance the image. The procedure does not cause pain but does expose patients to radiation.
2. Magnetic resonance imaging (MRI) provides clearer and more complete pictures than a CT scan, but it is more expensive to perform. In this procedure, patients are surrounded by a strong magnetic field through which pulses of radio frequency irradiation are projected that realigns hydrogen atoms. The altered radio frequency caused by the realignment is converted into an image by a computer.
3. Positron emission tomography (PET) is the most sophisticated physiologic imaging technique available. PET has a resolution capability of less than 5 mm in the brain. Glucose-containing radioactive atoms are given to the patient, and a computerized image of brain activity is developed. Because glucose is the primary source of body energy, the extent of metabolic activity in specific brain sites can be traced. PET technology is expensive.
4. Single-photon emission computed tomography (SPECT) also uses radioactive atoms that are tagged onto larger molecules. This technology is not as advanced as PET, but it is less expensive.

▌ Key Objectives for Treating Persons with Schizophrenia

- Work with the family.
- Treat depression.
- Minimize stressful interactions.
- Treat substance abuse.
- Avoid lengthy, intense verbal interactions.

colleagues (1976). Individuals with enlarged ventricles have a poor prognosis and exhibit the negative (type II) symptoms (Crow, 1982; Andreasen et al, 1982; Andreasen, 1985; Rabins et al, 1987).

Although ventricular enlargement is not peculiar to schizophrenia, anatomic findings are substantially different than those for neurodegenerative disorders, such as Alzheimer's disease. Ventricular enlargement in schizophrenia is not associated with a neuro-degenerative process (Bogerts, Lieberman, Ashtari, 1993; Casanova et al, 1993; Marsh et al, 1994); that is, one would not necessarily expect to find a gradual increase in ventricular volume over time in a patient with schizophrenia. In the patient with Alzheimer's disease, however, ventricles continue to increase in volume as brain cells die. It must be noted that not all patients with schizophrenia have abnormally enlarged ventricles. About 50% of these patients fall within the range of control or "normal" subjects (Cannon, Marco, 1994). This overlapping

effect has led researchers to study monozygotic twins when one twin suffers from schizophrenia. In documented cases in which the affected twin had ventricles falling within the "normal" range, pathoanatomic deviance can be demonstrated only when contrasted to the ventricles of the unaffected (i.e., nonschizophrenic) twin. Roberts, Leigh, and Weinberger (1993) clearly demonstrate that an otherwise "normal"-appearing ventricle was in actuality enlarged when compared with the "perfect" control—the ventricles of the monozygotic twin.

Brain atrophy

Over 100 years ago, Alzheimer described brain cell loss in schizophrenia. Anatomic pathology in cortical and subcortical areas has been suggested by brain imaging techniques and confirmed by postmortem examinations of individuals with schizophrenia. Limbic, hippocampal, thalamic structures, temporal lobes, the amygdala, and the substantia nigra are specific lobes and nuclei found to have neuropathologic changes.

Cerebral blood flow

Individuals with atrophic changes also have decreased cortical blood flow, particularly in the prefrontal cortex, with a consequent decrease in metabolic activity (BCSS, 2000; Berman et al, 1987; Ingvar, Franzen, 1974). Cognitive demands, such as organizing, planning, learning from experience, problem solving, introspection, and critical judgment, are compromised (Berman et al, 1987). A significant subgroup of schizophrenic patients with negative symptoms has decreased brain activity, as demonstrated by in vivo studies of CBF and glucose metabolism (Berman et al, 1987; Ingvar, Franzen, 1974).

Genetic theories

Individuals with schizophrenia seem to inherit a predisposition to the disorder because schizophrenia runs in families (Staal et al, 2000). The relatives of

|Box 28-7| Genetic Risk for Schizophrenia

Identical twin affected	50%
Fraternal twin affected	15%
Brother or sister affected	10%
One parent affected	15%
Both parents affected	35%
Second-degree relative affected	2%-3%
No affected relative	1%

Adapted from Roberts GW, Leigh PN, Weinberger DR: *Neuropsychiatric disorders,* London, 1993, Mosby Europe.

individuals with schizophrenia have a greater incidence of the disorder than chance alone would allow (Schultz, Andreasen, 1999). The genetic risk for schizophrenia is shown in Box 28-7. Of particular interest to clinicians is the risk associated with having a parent afflicted with schizophrenia. Though the risk reaches 35% if both parents have schizophrenia, this higher incidence alone does not adequately address the debate of nature (genetics) versus nurture (upbringing). For instance, a mentally disordered parent may rear children inadequately to the extent that the children are predisposed to schizophrenia based on the parenting skills, not genetics.

To control the "nurture" variable, researchers have studied twins. Both monozygotic (identical) and dizygotic (fraternal) twins have been studied. Monozygotic twins have consistently reported a higher concordancy rate (meaning both twins do or do not have symptoms of schizophrenia). Concordancy rates are 50% for monozygotic twins. This rate is 50 times greater than is the risk for the general population, and three times higher than is the risk for dizygotic twins.

These findings seem to establish the genetic or nature basis of schizophrenia; however, there are still extraneous variables that cannot be explained. For instance, many monozygotic twins are dressed alike and often are misidentified; their upbringing may be identical, too. Some argue that it is no wonder that monozygotic twins have a high concordancy rate. Unless researchers can control the environment variable, the relative impact of nature and nurture cannot be reported with confidence.

To control for the variable of environment, studies have been conducted of situations in which monozygotic twins have been separated at birth and reared apart. Monozygotic concordancy rates remain significantly higher in these studies.

Critical Thinking Question

Why do people with type I schizophrenia often evolve into type II schizophrenia?

Perinatal risk factors

Multiple nongenetic factors influence the development of schizophrenia (McNeil, Cantor-Graae, Weinberger, 2000; Rapoport, 2000). Some researchers believe that schizophrenia can be linked to the prenatal exposure to influenza, birth during the winter, minor malformations developing during early gestation, and complications of pregnancy particularly during labor and delivery (McNeil, 1995; Andreasen, 1999; Talan 2001). The research about large influenza epidemics is far from conclusive, but there is evidence that individuals with schizophrenia are more likely to have been born in the winter months. Research of cohorts conceived during devastating influenza epidemics reveals a meaningfully higher incidence of schizophrenia in products (i.e., children) of conceptions during this time. Other researchers suggest a high incidence of birth trauma and injury among individuals with schizophrenia. These studies suggest a relationship between schizophrenia and birth problems, particularly when adverse events occur during the second trimester of pregnancy (Roberts, Leigh, Weinberger, 1993).

Other biologic considerations

In addition to the foregoing, a number of neurologic abnormalities, such as poor motor coordination (e.g., balance, hopping, finger-thumb opposition), are found among individuals with schizophrenia. Eye tracking abnormalities are thought to be a distinguishing biologic feature as well.

Psychodynamic Theories of Schizophrenia

Psychodynamic theories of schizophrenia focus on the individual's responses to life events. The common theme of these theories is the internal reaction to life stressors or conflicts. These etiologic explanations include developmental and family theories.

Developmental theories of schizophrenia

During the early part of the twentieth century, two men—Adolph Meyer and Sigmund Freud—held to the significance of developmental psychiatry. These two men believed that the seeds of mental health and illness are sown in childhood, and that to understand the current functioning of individuals, it is important to understand their upbringing or development (Bowlby, 1988). Freud focused on mental processes, on the unconscious forces that influence individuals. The primary difference between the views of the two men was that Freud focused on fantasy, and Meyer focused on real-life events. An extension of their arguments is that events in early life can cause problems that are as severe as schizophrenia. Freudian concepts are still used meaningfully in discussions of schizophrenia. These concepts include poor ego boundaries, fragile ego, ego disintegration, inadequate ego development, superego dominance, regressed or id behavior, love-hate (ambivalent) relationships, and arrested psychosexual development.

Two later developmental theorists whose work more directly explains schizophrenia are Erikson (1968) and Sullivan (1953). Erikson, who theorized an eight-stage model of human development, saw the first step, "trust or mistrust," as crucial to later interpersonal relationships. The child who is deprived of a nurturing, loving environment, who is neglected or rejected, is vulnerable to mental disturbances. Inadequate passage through this stage predisposes the child to mistrust, isolative behaviors, and other asocial behaviors. Therapeutic intervention focuses on the reestablishment of trust through consistent, anxiety-free relationships.

Sullivan, using different terms, expressed essentially the same ideas. The absence of warm, nurturing attention during the early years blocks the expression of these same affective responses in later years. Without this capacity, a person exhibits disordered social interactions, as well as other disturbances. These individuals learn to avoid interpersonal interactions because these interactions are painful.

Family theories of schizophrenia

Family theories of schizophrenia are linked naturally to developmental theories. If early-life experiences are crucial in development, the argument is made that the family—the environment in which most people grow—is significant to the development of mental health or illness. Lack of a loving and nurturing primary caregiver, inconsistent family behaviors, and faulty communication patterns are thought to be responsible for mental problems in later life.

Outdated and harmful theories specifically tailored to the families of schizophrenic individuals were the schizophrenogenic mother theory and the double-bind theory. The word schizophrenogenic literally means to cause schizophrenia. Perhaps this definition has been the greatest single disservice of psychodynamic theories. Essentially, this notion states that the blame for schizophrenia can be placed on the mother. The double-bind theory described family practices in which the child was "damned if he did and damned if he didn't." An example used often was the child who was expected to do well in school but was criticized for taking time away from the family to study. Acocella (2000) captures some of the ideology behind these assertions. "Psychoanalysis took a while to conquer the United States, but once it did, after the Second World War, its dominance was unquestioned, and its arrogance breathtaking. Schizophrenia, autism, and numerous other disorders were blamed on the mother, with no evidence, just utter certainty" (p. 11).

Geiser, Hoche, and King (1988) called the family theories blame theories and described a bias by mental health professionals toward the families of patients with schizophrenia. Families have been viewed as causative agents, saboteurs of treatment, toxic influences, and as patients themselves. Sometimes, families have been treated with hostility and distrust. Because families bear the brunt of preprofessional and postprofessional care of these patients, it is important to work with families without alienating them.

CLINICAL EXAMPLE
Many of us think back to our childhood and remember birthday parties, hide and seek, baseball games, and so forth. Al thinks back to his past and remembers molestation, cruelty, and punishment. Al has been diagnosed with undifferentiated schizophrenia since the age of 20.

Al is the next to youngest of eight children. According to Al, more than one half of these siblings suffer from major mental illness. Al stated, "My mama had schizophrenia for 10 years, then God saved her." When asked about his relationship with his mother now, Al states that she left the rest of the family after "daddy" died. When questioned about his father, Al speaks of the way his father used to beat his mother and the children. Al recalls seeing his father beat one

Continued

brother so severely he thought the boy might die. Al further described a beating he received from his father that left him bleeding. When asked why he thought his father beat him, Al responded, "He got mad a lot. I forgot to get fire wood like he asked me to."

In discussing his illness, Al was asked to describe when he first started hearing voices. He replied, "When I was little, after those boys did that to me. I was out fixing my bicycle and I heard the devil talk to me over and over." Al reported numerous incidents of abuse during his life. At one point during the interview, Al stated his belief that his schizophrenia was God's punishment for what he had done.

Al's first documented psychiatric episode occurred in the early 1980s. In the psychologic evaluation emanating from this experience, the psychiatrist noted the presence of hallucinations and delusions; Al described spaceships, command hallucinations, and stated he had killed Christ. His condition deteriorated further and he was committed to a public hospital. During his hospitalization, Al was diagnosed as having undifferentiated schizophrenia.

Today, Al lives in a residential group home and attends day treatment. He continues to manifest both auditory and visual hallucinations. Though prescribed two atypical antipsychotic drugs, symptom control varies from day to day (From Keltner et al, 2001).

Unfortunately, some families are dysfunctional and contribute to later emotional problems. Muenzenmaier and colleagues (1993) studied chronically mentally ill patients and found that 65% had been sexually or physically abused as children. The exact meaning of these findings in the current climate is not known. Many more people, especially women, are coming forward to reveal an abusive childhood. Mental health professionals believe that child abuse, especially sexual abuse, is widespread and underreported (Jaroff, 1993), but it remains unclear whether such abuse plays a causative role in schizophrenia. A marginally related issue is the fact that some psychiatric and lay articles now include discussions of the false memory of abuse, which serves to illustrate yet another way in which families can be unfairly maligned.

Vulnerability-Stress Model of Schizophrenia

As previously stated, no single etiologic theory adequately answers the questions about the genesis of schizophrenia. The vulnerability-stress model ad-

dresses the variety of forces that cause schizophrenia in some cases, and in other cases, that cause the broader schizophrenia-spectrum problems of schizoaffective disorders and schizophrenia-related personality disorders. This model recognizes that both biologic and psychodynamic predispositions to schizophrenia, when coupled with stressful life events, can precipitate a schizophrenic process. According to this model, people with a predisposition to schizophrenia may (but not always) avoid serious mental disorder if they are protected from the stresses of life. Individuals with a similar vulnerability may succumb to schizophrenia if exposed to stressors. To illustrate the point, a wealthy person might be spared the brunt of some stressors because of wealth, whereas a poor member of society, struggling to meet basic needs, finds confrontation with stressors a daily event. According to this model, the second person is more likely to display symptoms of schizophrenia.

"An enduring and consistent finding has been the strong association between schizophrenia and lower socioeconomic status" (Cohen & Henkin, 1993, p. 178). Individuals with schizophrenia tend to "drift downward" socioeconomically. This unenviable status enhances their vulnerability by exposing them to constant stressors. In an article entitled, "Daily Hassles of Persons with Severe Mental Illness," Segal and Vander Voort (1993) describe some of the daily problems besetting seriously mentally ill persons. Table 28-1 lists some of those daily problems.

| Table 28-1 | Daily Stressors for Seriously Mentally Ill Individuals |

Daily Problem	Percent Reporting this Problem
Rising cost of common goods	48%
Loneliness	45%
Troubling thoughts about the future	42%
Too much time on hands	42%
Crime	40%
Filling out forms	39%
Not enough money for entertainment	39%
Regrets over past decisions	35%
Inability to express self	35%
Fear of rejection	31%
Trouble with reading, writing, and spelling	31%

Adapted from Segal SP, Vander Voort DJ: Daily hassles of persons with severe mental illness, *Hosp Community Psychiatry* 44(3): 276, 1993.

SPECIAL ISSUES RELATED TO SCHIZOPHRENIA

A number of special issues need to be clarified to help the student focus on the breadth of concerns involved in the psychiatric nursing care of patients with schizophrenia.

Families of Schizophrenic Individuals

Families, particularly mothers, have often been blamed for the problems of individuals with schizophrenia. It is no wonder that some families are suspicious of professionals who may view the family as a villain, nor is it any wonder that many of these families have little desire to be "studied."

Although research substantiates the state of turmoil in these families, many clinicians argue that dysfunctional families are not the cause of schizophrenia, but rather, the result of having a family member with this illness. Nevertheless, once a family becomes "destabilized," there is a high probability that the dysfunctional family will have a negative effect on the schizophrenic member.

Families of people with schizophrenia tend to have inappropriate family cohesion, and family members may be emotionally overinvolved, hostile, and critical. These families often demonstrate poor communication patterns. There is a tendency to be unclear, to lack focus, and to participate in incomplete communication. Arguably, many families without a schizophrenic member also have these attributes. What other variables are still at work is not clear. Nonetheless, with education and therapy, families can diminish their negative impact on patients. When working with a family, it is important for the nurse to avoid any message that places blame on the family.

Individuals with schizophrenia, on the other hand, can be a disruptive influence on the family, particularly when they are noncompliant with prescribed medications or when they use mind-altering drugs. Although there is consensus that the family characteristics previously described are present in many families of schizophrenic patients, it should be noted that these families are studied after schizophrenia is identified—years after the family may have been disrupted by the illness. This observation leads to the "chicken or egg" question raised previously: Do disruptive families cause individuals to have schizophrenia, or do individuals with schizophrenia cause families to become disruptive?

Although "blame" may be warranted in some family situations, in most instances, it is not. Blaming the family leads to a sense of alienation between the family and the treatment team. Nurses should remember that families bear the brunt of care outside the hospital. Most discharged psychiatric patients are sent home to live with their families, therefore the family's stake in the patient's care is obvious. As time goes on, these families tend to become more and more isolated and to feel more and more frustrated, helpless, and hopeless, even though they care very much about the patient.

CLINICAL EXAMPLE

Pete is 24 years old. At age 19 he began having symptoms that eventually led to a diagnosis of schizophrenia. Through several hospitalizations and outpatient treatment programs, he continued to live at home with his parents. Pete started having delusions that people were watching him. His paranoid thinking reached such levels that his presence in the home completely disrupted family life. Pete would barricade himself in his room, believe his parents were part of a conspiracy to spy on him, and become physically violent on occasion. Two years earlier, after a fourth hospitalization, Pete's parents informed the treatment team that he was no longer welcome in their home. They verbalized fear of Pete and worried about how he was affecting his younger siblings in the home. Although his parents live within 50 miles of Pete, they seldom visit.

Depression and Suicide in Schizophrenia

Depressive symptoms are frequently a part of the psychopathology of schizophrenia, and studies, on average, suggest 25% or more of schizophrenic patients experience depression (APA, 1997; Keck et al, 2000). These symptoms can occur at any time during the illness, including years after the acute phase and respond to antidepressants (Mason, Gingerich, Siris, 1990; Menzies, 2000; Sands, Harrow, 1999). A related phenomena is the high incidence of suicide (10%) among schizophrenic patients (APA, 1997). Suicide is the leading cause of premature death in schizophrenia. There are three explanations for this high prevalence of depression (APA, 1997):

1. Depression is a natural part of schizophrenia but is masked during the acute phase of the disorder.

2. Depression is a reaction to schizophrenia in the same way that depression is a reaction to a physical illness. Warnes (cited in APA, 1997) refers to this reaction as a "hopeless awareness of their own pathology" (p. 45).
3. The biologic nature of the disorder (schizophrenia is more than a "dopamine" problem) and the drugs used to treat it produce a depressive syndrome.

Cognitive Dysfunction

That patients with schizophrenia suffer cognitive impairment is well established. For instance, memory, attention, and executive function are affected (Andreasen, 1999). Research reveals that cognitive deficits are a better predictor of declining abilities to engage in basic activities of daily living than are positive or negative symptoms (Velligan et al, 1999). Because cognitive ability directly influences so many aspects of successful living, it is important to discuss this aspect of schizophrenia. Traditional antipsychotics do not reduce cognitive symptoms and, in fact, may exacerbate them. For example, EPSEs such as akinesia cause cognitive slowdown. Atypical agents are known to improve performance on some tests of cognitive ability, however significant deficits remain (Velligan et al, 1999; Velligan, Miller, 1999).

Relapse

Both clinical opinion and research studies support the observation that many patients with schizophrenia experience relapse and remission of symptoms throughout their illness. A patient in remission described her relapse as having occurred in stages. She reported the following sequence:

"In the first stage, I feel just a bit estranged from myself.... In the second stage, everything appears a bit clouded.... In the third stage, I believe I am beginning to understand why terrible things are happening to me; others are causing it.... In the fourth stage, I become chaotic and see, hear, and believe all manner of things. I no longer question my beliefs, but act on them" (Lovejoy, 1984, p. 809).

People most likely to suffer relapse include those exposed to significant stressors and those not taking prescribed antipsychotics. Important prophylactic activities of professionals include developing strategies to ensure compliance with medications and manipulating the environment (e.g., moving from a crime-ridden neighborhood, remedial three Rs).

Stress

One of the three "inescapable facts" noted in the opening paragraph is the "...role of stress in onset and relapse." According to the vulnerability-stress model, people with schizophrenia are vulnerable to stress. Common stressors can be categorized as:

1. Biologic (e.g., medical illness)
2. Psychosocial (e.g., loss of a relationship)
3. Sociocultural (e.g., homelessness)
4. Emotional (e.g., persistent criticism)

The therapeutic mandate is to minimize the impact of stress on vulnerable individuals. Two basic strategies are used:

1. Reducing stress and stressor accumulation
2. Developing coping skills

Because of their economic and social status, many individuals face major stressors routinely. Stated another way, some of those most vulnerable to stress have more stress to handle. Helping patients learn to identify and avoid stressful events is an important task for the psychiatric nurse.

Substance Abuse among People with Schizophrenia

Substance abuse is the most common co-morbid psychiatric condition associated with schizophrenia and seems to be increasing. A high percentage of people with schizophrenia abuse alcohol or other drugs or both. Alcohol abuse in these patients is

Family Issues | in Schizophrenia: Support Groups

The National Alliance for the Mentally Ill (NAMI) or an individual state's Alliance for the Mentally Ill (AMI) are groups that help family and friends of the severely mentally ill to understand the illness. NAMI provides support and has become a powerful advocate for the severely mentally ill. This self-help group has influenced mental health legislation, as well as the way society views the severely mentally ill. For more information, families can write:

NAMI
200 N. Glebe Rd, Suite 1015
Arlington, VA 22203-3754
703-524-7600

thought to be 30% or more (Roeber, 1997). Alcohol, marijuana, and cocaine accounted for most of the drugs abused. Unlike the general population, schizophrenic individuals have little chance of using alcohol in a social manner.

Drug abuse has a negative effect on the treatment of these patients and is associated with poor outcomes. It may also account for the overrepresentation of schizophrenic individuals in jail. Alcohol, for example, causes a disinhibition effect, aggressiveness, and poor judgment. These symptoms are already present in patients with severe mental illness. Furthermore, these very symptoms and related lack of social skills hinder patients with schizophrenia from fully benefiting from treatment programs such as Alcoholics Anonymous and Narcotics Anonymous.

Critical Thinking Question

Why do you think the rate of substance abuse is so high among individuals with schizophrenia?

Work

The lack of work, the inability to work, and the lack of a desire to work are all features of schizophrenia. Because work, or what one does for a living, is a major defining characteristic in this society, the fact that many people with schizophrenia do not work adds to their inability to "fit in." According to Lysaker and colleagues (1993), the major problem confronting these individuals is not so much a lack of skill, but an inability to cope socially on the job. Routine behaviors such as joking, inviting someone out, or having insight into the way one is affecting others are the major obstacles to a productive work life for the schizophrenic population.

Psychosis–Induced Polydipsia

Psychosis-induced polydipsia or compulsive water drinking (between 4 and 10 liters per day) occurs in 6% to 20% of patients with psychosis (APA, 1997).

As early as the 1930s, it was recognized that patients with schizophrenia urinate twice as much as do other patients (Shah, Greenberg, 1992). The desire to drink probably occurs because of thirst and osmotic dysregulation and is characterized by a compulsive approach to water ingestion. Patients report a variety of reasons for polydipsia, including cleansing the body, washing away evil spirits, and relief of dry mouth caused by medication (Snider, Boyd, 1991).

The major concern associated with polydipsia is hyponatremia. Hyponatremia causes light-headedness, weakness, lethargy, muscle cramps, nausea and vomiting, confusion, convulsions, and coma. Treatment includes frequent weighings, restricted fluid intake, sodium replacement, and positive reinforcement.

CONTINUUM OF CARE FOR PEOPLE WITH SCHIZOPHRENIA

"Rather than starting to release patients in a few locales and measuring the outcome, officials implemented the policy in cities and counties across the United States virtually simultaneously, based on widespread hope that the new drugs would cure people and the widespread belief in state legislatures that the policy would save taxpayers money" (Torrey, 1997, p. 663).

By "policy," Torrey means deinstitutionalization, and driven by this policy, an array of services, or a continuum of care, has developed. Most clinicians agree that a community setting is good for some patients; the institutional setting may be better for others. The continuum of care for people with schizophrenia includes (APA, 1997):

- Hospitalization for acute symptoms
- Long-term hospitalization for patients (10% to 20%) who are treatment resistant
- Day hospitalization for individuals who are acutely psychotic but not at risk of harming self or others
- Day treatment for patients needing ongoing supportive care as they stabilize
- Supportive housing for individuals who do not or cannot live with their family but who need some level of supervision. Varieties of supportive housing include:
  - Foster care
  - Board and care home
  - Nursing home

Psychotherapeutic Management

Most schizophrenics go on for years struggling alone without anyone to help them become stronger than their symptoms.

Ruocchio, 1989, p. 188

Psychotherapeutic management is aimed at helping patients become stronger than their symptoms. The nursing interventions used in the treatment of patients with schizophrenia are derived from the appropriate development of the nursing care plan.

Psychotherapeutic nurse-patient relationship

"Pharmacotherapy can improve some of the symptoms of schizophrenia but has limited effect on social impairments that characterize the disorder and limit functioning and quality of life" (Huxley et al, 2000, p. 187).

The objective of the psychotherapeutic nurse-patient relationship is to build a therapeutic alliance with patients. A long-term relationship in which trust has developed is probably more significant and therapeutic than is a particular theory of care. It is known that "insight" therapy has limited usefulness with this population, whereas less invasive modalities such as supportive therapy, problem solving, and reality-adaptive social skills training that focuses on behavior and not "meaning" are more helpful. Long-term, trusting relationships yield better compliance to medications and better outcomes on psychological resources.

The objective of this section is to provide basic concepts for working with patients with schizophre-

---

Key Nursing Interventions for Developing the Therapeutic Nurse-Patient Relationship

The following are specific interventions and examples for developing a therapeutic nurse-patient relationship, including examples of appropriate responses. These examples are meant to illustrate some of the common situations described in the text. Obviously, each patient is unique, and that uniqueness might necessitate a variation of the response suggested below.

Intervention	Rationales
Do not argue about delusions.	Arguing tends to reinforce delusions and can make patients angry. Reflect reality, and attempt to distract patients in a matter-of-fact manner. *Patient:* The FBI and the Mafia are both after me. *Nurse:* I know your thoughts seem real to you; however, it does not seem reasonable to me. I also want you to know that you are safe here. Let's go into the dayroom and talk. Proceed to talk about occupational therapy efforts (or a similar topic) that focus on the patient's real world.
Do not reinforce hallucinations.	*Patient:* The voices are calling me terrible names. *Nurse:* I do not hear anything but your voice and mine.
If a patient is acting odd and the nurse suspects he or she is hallucinating, the patient should be asked about it.	*Patient's behavior:* Looks around the room, eyes darting to the corners of the room. *Nurse:* It looks like you might be listening to something. Are you hearing voices?
Help patients identify the stressors that might precipitate hallucinations or delusions.	This effort might lead to identifying and avoiding triggering events. *Patient:* Nurse, I started hearing the voices last night right after I went to bed. *Nurse:* Tell me about your evening last night. There may be a link between something that happened and your hearing voices again.
Focus on real people and real events.	This helps patients stay in touch with reality. *Patient:* I keep hearing the voices. *Nurse:* I understand, but I want to help you focus away from those voices. Let's go to the dayroom and talk. Proceed to bring patients closer to reality by talking about daily life.
Be diligent in attempting to understand patients.	It is therapeutic to help patients communicate what they want to say; however, use good judgment. Pushing too hard to understand can be frustrating for the patient. *Patient:* I could have been bitten. It was never a dog's day. *Nurse:* I am not sure what you are saying, but I want to understand. Are you talking about almost being hurt?
Attempt to balance siding with inappropriate behavior and crushing a fragile ego.	Time and effort help the nurse to learn to negotiate artfully between these potentially negative outcomes. *Patient:* I am going to hit that bastard if he says another word to me. *Nurse:* I know you are upset with him. Let's talk about other ways you can deal with this situation.

nia. General principles for developing a therapeutic nurse-patient relationship are presented. In addition, the box on the previous page lists some of these specific principles with patient comments the student may encounter. Examples of therapeutic responses by the nurse are also listed.

General principles for developing a therapeutic nurse-patient relationship include the following:

- Be calm when talking to patients. *Rationale:* Anxiety is contagious and counterproductive when working with patients who have schizophrenia.
- Accept patients as they are, but do not accept all behaviors. *Rationale:* Everyone wants to be accepted. The focus is on behaviors, which communicates very directly that behaviors can change.
- Keep promises. *Rationale:* Dependability builds trust.
- Be consistent. *Rationale:* Consistency increases trust.
- Be honest. *Rationale:* Honesty increases trust.
- Do not reinforce hallucinations or delusions. *Rationale:* The nurse should simply state his or her perception of reality, voice doubt about the patient's perceptions, and move on to discuss "real" people or events.

Patient and Family Education

Schizophrenia

Illness:

Schizophrenia is a brain disease that disrupts perceptions, thinking, feelings, and behaviors. It can cause distortions of reality, false beliefs, hallucinations, and changes in speech patterns, moods, and behaviors. It disrupts the person's ability to function, socialize, and work.

Medications:

1. Some of the medicines for schizophrenia may cause temporary, but uncomfortable, side effects. Some of these side effects can be lessened with other medications or nondrug interventions or both.
2. As a result of these side effects, the person may not want to take the prescribed medicines. The doctor needs to know this immediately.
3. It is crucial for the person to continue taking the medicines even after the person feels better or the illness symptoms are no longer evident.

Other Issues:

Discuss with the person early symptoms, which may indicate a beginning relapse. Make an agreement with the person about the actions that family, friends, or both will take to get the person appropriate help.

- Orient patients to time, person, and place, if indicated. *Rationale:* Orientation reinforces reality. However, use good judgment. To be continually reminded that you are "disoriented" takes an emotional toll.
- Do not touch patients without warning them. *Rationale:* Patients who are suspicious may perceive a touch as a threat and retaliate.
- Avoid whispering or laughing when patients are unable to hear all of a conversation. *Rationale:* Have you ever wondered whether you were the subject of discussion when around people who whisper or giggle? Suspicious patients will interpret these actions as a personal affront.
- Reinforce positive behaviors. *Rationale:* Appropriate reinforcement can increase positive behaviors.
- Avoid competitive activities with some patients. *Rationale:* Competition is threatening and can lead to decreased self-esteem.
- Do not embarrass patients. *Rationale:* Persons with schizophrenia often avoid contacts because they fear embarrassment. Just calling on some patients during an educational program may cause great discomfort.
- For withdrawn patients, start with one-to-one interactions. *Rationale:* Even in group situations, it is probably most therapeutic for interactions to be a series of nurse-to-patient rather than patient-to-patient interactions. Nurse-to-patient interactions are less threatening to patients and can evolve into a wider circle of social interaction.
- Allow and encourage verbalization of feelings. *Rationale:* Patients are helped if they can say what they think without the nurse becoming defensive.

Psychopharmacology

"The discovery of antipsychotic drugs in 1950 is unrivaled as a breakthrough in the treatment of mental illness. The magnitude of this therapeutic advance in psychiatry has been compared to the discovery of insulin for diabetes, antibiotics for infectious disease, and anticonvulsants for epilepsy" (Lieberman, 1997, p. 1).

The student is encouraged to review Chapter 20, which provides a complete discussion of antipsychotic drugs. Schizophrenic patients need to take psychotropic drugs as prescribed. As many as 46% of psychiatric inpatients and 60% of psychiatric

Key Nursing Interventions to Increase Compliance

- Observe patients for side effects and intervene accordingly. Akathisia is a troubling side effect that patients cannot tolerate.
- When giving tablets or pills, make sure patients do not "cheek" the medications (hide the medication in cheeks or mouth) to spit them out or hoard them for later.

- Teach patients and their families about drugs, including side effects, potential interactions, dosage schedules when discharged, and so on.
- Depot drugs are effective for patients who do not comply with drug therapy.

| Box 28-8 | Review of Major Side Effects of Antipsychotic Drugs

Extrapyramidal side effects from high-potency drugs
  Parkinsonism
  Akathisia
  Dystonias
  Neuroleptic malignant syndrome
Anticholinergic effects from low-potency drugs
  Dry mouth
  Blurred vision
  Constipation
  Urinary hesitation
  Tachycardia
Tardive dyskinesia
Amenorrhea and galactorrhea
Sedation (associated with low-potency drugs)
Orthostatic hypotension (associated with low-potency drugs)

outpatients do not comply with their medication regimens. (See the above box for nursing interventions to help ensure compliance.) A review of major side effects is found in Box 28-8. For a full review of these side effects, the student is referred to Chapter 20. Because of racial and ethnic variation, Asians and Hispanics with schizophrenia may need less antipsychotic medications than Caucasians to achieve the same blood levels (Surgeon General, 1999).

Milieu management

"Thus intensely active, highly staffed units may be disruptively intense for schizophrenic patients, who more often benefit from decreased stimulation and a greater measure of solitude and clear role models" (Simpson, May, 1982, p. 148).

Milieu management is an important dimension of the psychiatric nursing care of schizophrenic patients. With the dramatic introduction of psychotropic drugs in the 1950s, other forms of treatment were abandoned. Now that psychopharmacologists have had free reign for many years, it is clear that drugs alone are not enough. A therapeu-

tic treatment approach is best developed with all three components of psychotherapeutic management in place.

Environmental manipulation for therapeutic gain can occur both at the inpatient and outpatient levels and helps patients function better in the hospital and in the community (Breslin, 1992). General principles that specifically address the environment of schizophrenic patients follow.

For disruptive patients:
- Set limits on disruptive behavior.
- Decrease environmental stimuli. Place escalating patients in a low-stimulus environment, and give prn medication if indicated.
- Frequently observe escalating patients to intervene. Intervention (e.g., medication) before acting out occurs protects patients and others physically and prevents embarrassment for escalating patients.
- Modify the environment to minimize objects that can be used as weapons. Some units use furniture so heavy that it cannot be lifted by most people.
- Be careful in stating what the staff will do if a patient acts out; however, follow through once a violation occurs (e.g., "If you break the window, we will place you in restraints").
- When using restraints, provide for safety by evaluating the patient's status of hydration, nutrition, elimination, and circulation.

For withdrawn patients:
- Arrange nonthreatening activities that involve these patients in "doing something"; for example, a walking tour of a park, leather work, and painting.
- Arrange furniture in a semicircle or around a table, which "forces" patients to sit with someone. Interactions are permitted in this situation but should not be demanded. Sit in silence with patients who are not ready to respond. Some will move the chair away despite the nurse's efforts.
- Help patients to participate in decision making as appropriate (e.g., selecting the menu for the next day's meals).

- Provide patients with opportunities for non-threatening socialization with the nurse on a one-to-one basis.
- Reinforce appropriate grooming and hygiene (assist at first, if needed).
- Provide remotivation and resocialization group experiences. Often, students work with occupational or recreational therapists to provide these services.
- Provide psychosocial rehabilitation, that is, training in community living, social skills, and health care skills. Occupational and recreational therapists often are involved in these activities.

For suspicious patients:
- Be matter-of-fact when interacting with these patients.
- Staff members should not laugh or whisper around patients unless the patients can hear what is being said. The nurse should clarify any misperceptions that patients have.
- Do not touch suspicious patients without warning. Avoid close physical contact.
- Be consistent in activities (time, staff, approach).
- Maintain eye contact.

For patients with impaired communication:
- Be patient and do not pressure patients to make sense.
- Do not place patients in group activities that would frustrate them, damage their self-esteem, or overtax their abilities.
- Provide opportunities for purposeful psychomotor activity (e.g., painting, ceramic work, exercise, gross motor games).

For patients with disordered perceptions:
- Attempt to provide distracting activities.
- Discourage situations in which patients talk to others about their disordered perceptions.
- Monitor television selections. Some programs seem to cause more perceptual problems than do others (e.g., horror movies). If staff members cannot censor programs, they should be available to patients for discussion and clarification following programs.
- Monitor for command hallucinations that may increase the potential for patients to become dangerous.
- Have staff members available in the dayroom so that patients can talk to real people about real people or real events.

For disorganized patients:
- Remove disorganized patients to a less stimulating environment.

Case Study

The police brought Bill, a 25-year-old man, to the hospital. He was in a downtown bus station preaching loudly. He stated in the emergency room that he had spoken to God and that God had told him to save San Francisco. He admitted to hearing both God and Satan arguing and was terrified at times. In talking with his family, staff members discover that Bill was a solid student until about a year ago. He began to struggle in school but continued to pass his course work. He dropped out of school 3 months ago. His family believes his problem started when his girlfriend of 4 years broke off their engagement.

Bill began hearing voices a couple of weeks ago, according to his family, but the family lost contact with him until they were notified of this hospitalization. Bill's family is committed to helping him. On admission to the unit, Bill is oriented to time, place, and person, but states: "God has chosen me to be his special angel. I must save the sinners of San Francisco." Bill then stands up and turns his head rapidly from side to side. When asked why, he says: "God and Satan are arguing about what I should do."

See Bill's nursing care plan on page 334.

- Provide a calm environment; the staff should appear calm.
- Provide safe and relatively simple activities for these patients.
- Provide information boards with schedules, and refer to them often thus patients can begin to use this as an orienting function.
- Help protect each patient's self-esteem by intervening if a patient does something that is embarrassing (e.g., a patient who takes off his or her clothes or becomes overtly sexual).
- Assist with grooming and hygiene.

For patients with altered levels of activity:
Hyperactivity
- Allow patients to stand for a few minutes during group meetings.
- Provide a safe environment and a place where patients can pace without inordinately bothering other patients.
- Encourage participation in activities or games that do not require fine motor skills or intense concentration.

Immobility
- Provide nursing care for catatonic or immobile patients to minimize circulatory problems and loss of muscle tone.
- Provide adequate diet, exercise, and rest.

Care Plan

Name: Bill Wilson _____ **Admission Date:** June 2002 _____

DSM-IV-TR Diagnosis: Schizophrenia: undifferentiated type _____

Assessment	**Areas of strength:** past accomplishments; past good heterosexual interpersonal relationships (IPRs); alert, oriented to time, place, person; acute symptoms respond to medications; family support. **Problems:** religious hallucinations, religious delusions, thought disorder; broken engagement; dropped out of school.
Diagnoses	• Disturbed sensory perception (auditory) related to thought disturbance, as evidenced by hallucinations. • Anxiety related to disturbed perceptions, as evidenced by fear and extraneous movements.

Outcomes		Date met
	Short-term goals:	
	• Patient will voice freedom from hallucinations.	_____
	• Patient will report lack of fear of others.	_____
	• Patient will discuss feelings about loss of girlfriend.	_____
	Long-term goals:	
	• Patient will verbalize need for medication and counseling.	_____
	• Patient will make appointment for outpatient program assessment in mid-July.	_____
	• Patient will return to school in September.	_____

Planning/ Interventions	**Nurse-patient relationship:** Do not reinforce hallucinations and delusions; voice doubt; encourage identification of strengths and accomplishments; encourage expression of feelings about broken engagement; discuss plans for immediate future. **Psychopharmacology:** Zyprexa 10 mg qd. **Milieu management:** Provide distracting activities; monitor television, particularly religious programming and movies with satanic themes; encourage participation in self-esteem group and anger-management group.
Evaluation	Patient responding to Zyprexa.
Referrals	Will see Ms. White, RN, CS, once a week as outpatient. Appointment in 3 weeks with R. Jones for education counseling.

• Maintain bowel and bladder function and intervene before problems arise.

• Observe patients to prevent victimization (physical and verbal) by others.

OTHER PSYCHOTIC DISORDERS

In addition to schizophrenia, several other psychotic disorders are described in the DSM-IV-TR with which the student should be familiar. Interventions for these disorders are directed at prominent symptoms and are the same as the interventions used for those symptoms of patients with schizophrenia.

Schizoaffective Disorder

Schizoaffective disorder is a psychosis characterized by both affective (mood disorder) and schizophrenic (thought disorder) symptoms, with substantial loss of occupational and social functioning. Because this disorder is a hybrid of two disorders thought to have different biochemical origins, schizoaffective disorder is somewhat of a puzzle to many clinicians. Affective disorders cause people to be extremely depressed or elated, and schizophrenia is expressed as positive, negative, or disorganized symptoms. The fact that patients with affective disorders can experience positive and negative symptoms, plus the fact that patients with schizophrenia experience mood changes, partially explains the difficulty in diagnosis (Levinson et al, 1999). Furthermore, patients are not infrequently switched from a diagnosis of schizophrenic to a mood disorder diagnosis or vice versa. The diagnosis of schizoaffective psychosis helps bridge the gap between the affective disorders and schizophrenia and underscores the fluidity of

Case Study

A 40-year-old woman with a history of multiple admissions is admitted to the floor. Emma Rice was found wandering downtown incoherent and disheveled. During the assessment interview, Emma is noted to have a flat affect and is withdrawn. She reports not seeing her family for 5 years and cannot remember when she last held a job. There is no history of hallucinatory or delusional thought content in this recent occurrence. The staff knows Emma and knows that, during past admissions, she has responded to haloperidol. After admission, Emma says, "Let me go. Go on, onward, backward. (pause) Emma hide, died." When asked where she lives, Emma slowly responds, "Over there, somewhere, anywhere, nowhere." Emma's board and care operator knows her well and has indicated that a bed is being held for Emma.

See the next page for Emma's nursing care plan.

human emotion and behavior (Harvard Mental Health Letter, 1996). "The essential feature of schizoaffective disorder is an uninterrupted period of illness during which, at some time, there is a major depressive, manic, or mixed episode concurrent with symptoms that meet Criterion A for schizophrenia" (APA, 2001, p. 319).

In this disorder, schizophrenic symptoms are dominant but are accompanied by major depressive or manic symptoms. Patients with schizoaffective disorder will have experienced delusions or hallucinations in the absence of a prominent mood disturbance, but symptoms of a mood disorder will be present for a significant period. Substance abuse or a general medical condition must be ruled out before this diagnosis can be made. Whether the disorder is bipolar (more common in young adults) or depressive (more common in older adults) should be specified.

This disorder probably occurs more often in women than it does in men and may be partially accounted for by the differences in brain lateralization between men and women (Crow, 1995). Epidemiologic studies indicate the disorder is heritable (Gerson, 1994). The prognosis for schizoaffective disorder is better than that of schizophrenia but significantly less optimistic than the prognosis for mood disorders (APA, 1997).

CLINICAL EXAMPLE

Patty is a 42-year-old white woman referred to the county mental health department by her sister after Patty had attempted suicide by combining a large number of benzodiazepines with a six pack of beer. Patty states that most of her "mental" problems began when she became pregnant at age 18. At the time, she was unmarried and alienated from her parents. Patty raised her young daughter, Billie, alone until she eventually married another man. At age 25, Patty became pregnant again and gave birth to a son. Her husband, an alcoholic, had abused Patty to some extent, but the abusive behavior became more frequent and more severe as Patty entered her early 30s. There had been suspicion that he had sexually abused Billie, but nothing conclusive was documented. Patty and her husband divorced when the young boy was 7 years old. The court awarded the child to the husband. Today, Patty has little contact with her daughter, son, ex-husband, or parents. She frequently has auditory hallucinations telling her to kill herself and has nightmares about killing her son and ex-husband. She attends a day treatment program 5 days a week and lives in a one-bedroom apartment alone. Patty is very sad and always looks at the floor. She is consumed with guilt. She does not initiate conversation with others at the day treatment program. She states that she continues to hear voices and thinks about suicide all of the time.

Delusional Disorder

People with delusional disorder display symptoms similar to those seen in patients with schizophrenia. However, substantial differences exist and necessitate a diagnostic differentiation. The following symptoms differentiate delusional disorders from schizophrenic disorders:

- Delusions have a basis in reality.
- The patients have never met the criteria for schizophrenia.
- The behavior of these patients is relatively normal except in relation to their delusions.
- If mood episodes have occurred concurrently with delusions, their total duration has been relatively brief.
- The symptoms are not the direct result of a substance or a medical condition.

Brief Psychotic Disorder

The category of brief psychotic disorder includes all psychotic disturbances that last less than 1 month and are not related to a mood disorder, a general medical condition, or a substance-induced disorder (First et al, 1994). At least one of the following psychotic disturbances must be present: delusions, hallu-

Care Plan

Name: Emma Rice _____   Admission Date: _____

DSM-IV-TR Diagnosis: Schizophrenia, disorganized type _____

Assessment	**Areas of strength:** Board and care operator knows Emma well and wants her back. Staff knows and understands Emma.
	Problems: Affective flattening, loose associations, withdrawn, chronic course of illness, no family support.
Diagnoses	• Impaired verbal communication related to thought disturbance, as evidenced by impaired articulation and loose association of ideas.
	• Bathing and hygiene self-care deficit related to thought disturbance, as evidenced by inability to maintain appearance at satisfactory level.
	• Social isolation related to lack of trust, as evidenced by absence of supportive significant other.

Outcomes

Short-term goals:	*Date met*
• Patient will talk in coherent manner.	_____
• Patient will carry out ADLs.	_____
• Patient will participate in nonthreatening activities.	_____
Long-term goals:	
• Patient will maintain outpatient program.	_____
• Patient will return to board and care.	_____
• Patient will comply with medication regimen.	_____

Planning/ Interventions	**Nurse–patient relationship:** Be patient; treat as adult; encourage hygiene and appropriate dress; reinforce positive social behaviors; start with one-to-one interactions with nurse, and then encourage independent social behaviors.
	Psychopharmacology: Haldol 5 mg bid PO (concentrate). May need long-acting form on discharge.
	Milieu management: Start patient in occupational therapy by the end of the week; invite patient to sit with staff and other patients; encourage her to make decisions about meals or some other simple tasks; provide resocialization group experience and community living education.
Evaluation	Patient stabilized on medications.
Referrals	Will see Ms. Brown, RN, CS, once a week and will attend outpatient resocialization group five times a week. Board and care operator will monitor drugs and arrange transportation.

cinations, disorganized speech, or grossly disorganized or catatonic behavior. The DSM-IV-TR cautions against applying these standards to people from a culture in which they are exhibiting acceptable behavior.

Schizophreniform Disorder

Schizophreniform disorder displays symptoms that are typical of schizophrenia and last at least 1 month, but no longer than 6 months. Patients' prognoses should be specified as good or poor. Features of a good prognosis include the onset of psychotic symptoms within 4 weeks of the initial change in behavior, confusion at the height of the psychotic episode, absence of a flat affect, and a history of good social and occupational functioning before the occurrence.

Critical Thinking Question

If a first-degree relative of yours suffered from schizophrenia, what behavior might cause you to refuse to live with that person?

Principles of Psychotherapeutic Management

Nurse-Patient Relationship Principles	Psychotropic Drugs	Milieu Management Principles
Focus on behavior not "meaning." Long-term relationship most therapeutic. Accept patient but not all behaviors. Be consistent. Do not reinforce hallucinations and delusions. Avoid whispering or laughing if patient cannot hear all of conversation.	Traditional antipsychotics haloperidol (Haldol) fluphenazine (Prolixin) chlorpromazine (Thorazine) Atypical antipsychotics clozapine (Clozaril) risperidone (Risperdal) olanzapine (Zyprexa)	Modify environment to decrease stimulation and for safety. Staff consistency is crucial. Arrange environment to reduce withdrawn behavior. Monitor television watching. Protect patients' self esteem.

Key Concepts

1. The concept of schizophrenia has evolved over the last 100 years as a result of the contributions of early theorists, such as Kraepelin and Bleuler, and modern theorists, such as Andreasen.
2. The DSM-IV-TR identifies five subtypes of schizophrenia: catatonic, disorganized, paranoid, undifferentiated, and residual.
3. Bleuler contributed what he thought to be the four primary symptoms of schizophrenia: affective disturbances, loose associations, ambivalence, and autism (also known as Bleuler's four As).
4. Andreasen (Andreasen, Olsen, 1982), Crow (1982), and others have conceptualized schizophrenia as having only two subtypes: type I (positive symptoms and usually treatable with traditional antipsychotic drugs) and type II (negative symptoms). More recently, some researchers have added the subtype labeled as disorganized.
5. Objective signs of schizophrenia include alterations in personal relationships and activity.
6. Subjective symptoms of schizophrenia include alterations in perception, thought, consciousness, and affect.
7. Etiologic explanations for schizophrenia are numerous and include both biologic theories (dopamine hypothesis, pathoanatomy, and genetic theories) and psychodynamic theories (developmental theory and family theory).
8. The dopamine hypothesis—the view that schizophrenia is a result of increased bioavailability of dopamine in the brain—is a widely held theory of schizophrenia.
9. Traditional antipsychotic drugs block dopamine receptors and relieve acute symptoms of schizophrenia.
10. Nursing interventions include developing a therapeutic nurse-patient relationship. Several general principles undergird the nurse's interactions with patients who have schizophrenia. These principles include being calm, accepting, dependable, consistent, and honest.
11. In addition to these basic principles, several basic interventions are therapeutic for most patients with schizophrenia. These basic interventions include the following that the nurse should not do: do not reinforce hallucinations and delusions, do not touch patients without warning, do not whisper or laugh when patients cannot hear the conversation, do not compete with patients, and do not embarrass patients; and the following that the nurse should do: provide reality testing, assist with orientation when appropriate, reinforce positive behaviors, and encourage verbalization of feelings.
12. Psychopharmacology is an important part of the nurse's role in caring for patients with schizophrenia. Understanding therapeutic versus toxic dose levels, side effects, interactions, patient teaching issues, use in older adults, and appropriateness of drugs for use during pregnancy are significant nursing activities.
13. Nurses help shape the milieu of patients with schizophrenia. Strategies for working with disruptive, withdrawn, suspicious, and disorganized patients are crucial for developing a therapeutic environment. Special considerations for patients with impaired communication, disordered perceptions, and altered levels of activity are important.
14. Other psychoses listed in the DSM-IV-TR include schizoaffective disorder, delusional disorder, brief psychotic disorder, and schizophreniform disorder.

References

Acocella J: The empty couch, *The New Yorker* 8:11, 2000.

Addington J: Group treatment for smoking cessation among persons with schizophrenia, *Psychiatr Serv* 49(8):925, 1998.

American Psychiatric Association: *Diagnostic and statistical manual of mental disorders, text revision,* ed 4, Washington, DC, 2001, APA.

American Psychiatric Association: Practice guidelines for the treatment of patients with schizophrenia, *Am J Psychiatry* 154(suppl 4):1, 1997.

Andreasen NC: Positive vs. negative schizophrenia: a critical evaluation, *Schizophr Bull* 11:380, 1985.

Andreasen NC: Understanding the causes of schizophrenia, *N Engl J Med* 340(8):645, 1999.

Andreasen NC, Olsen S: Negative vs. positive schizophrenia, *Arch Gen Psychiatry* 39:789, 1982.

Andreasen NC et al: Ventricular enlargement in schizophrenia: relationship to positive and negative symptoms, *Am J Psychiatry* 139:297, 1982.

Becker RE: Depression in schizophrenia, *Hosp Community Psychiatry* 39:1269, 1988.

Berman KF et al: A relationship between anatomical and physiological brain pathology in schizophrenia: lateral cerebral ventricular size predicts cortical blood flow, *Am J Psychiatry* 144:1277, 1987.

Bogerts B et al: Hippocampus-amygdala volume and psychopathology in chronic schizophrenia, *Biol Psychiatry* 33(4):236, 1993.

Bowlby J: Developmental psychiatry comes of age, *Am J Psychiatry* 145:1, 1988.

Breslin NA: Treatment of schizophrenia: current practice and future promise, *Hosp Community Psychiatry* 43(9):877, 1992.

British Columbia Schizophrenia Society: Schizophrenia: youth's greatest disabler, *BCSS* 6(1):11, 2000.

Brown RP, Mann JJ: A clinical perspective on the role of neurotransmitters in mental disorders, *Hosp Community Psychiatry* 36:141, 1985.

Cannon TD, Marco E: Structural brain abnormalities as indicators of vulnerability to schizophrenia, *Schizophr Bull* 20(1):89, 1994.

Casanova MF et al: A topographical study of senile plaques and neurofibrillary tangles in the hippocampi of patients with Alzheimer's disease and cognitively impaired patients with schizophrenia, *Psychiatry Res* 49(1):41, 1993.

Cohen CI: Poverty and the course of schizophrenia: implications for research and policy, *Hosp Community Psychiatry* 44(10):951, 1993.

Cohen E, Henkin I: Prevalence of substance abuse by seriously mentally ill patients in a partial hospital program, *Hosp Community Psychiatry* 44(2):178, 1993.

Crow TJ: Brain changes and negative symptoms in schizophrenia, *Psychopathology* 28(1):18, 1995.

Crow TJ: Two dimensions of pathology in schizophrenia: dopaminergic and nondopaminergic, *Psychopharmacol Bull* 18:22, 1982.

Dalack GW, Healy DJ, Meador-Woodruff JH: Nicotine dependence in schizophrenia: clinical phenomena and laboratory findings, *Am J Psychiatry* 155(11):1490, 1998.

Drake RE, Wallach MA: Moderate drinking among people with severe mental illness, *Hosp Community Psychiatry* 44(5):780, 1993.

Ereshefsky L, Lacombe S: Pharmacological profile of risperidone, *Can J Psychiatry* 38(suppl 3):S80, 1993.

Erikson E: *Childhood and society,* New York, 1968, WW Norton.

First MB et al: Changes in substance-related, schizophrenic, and other primarily adult disorders, *Hosp Community Psychiatry* 45(1):18, 1994.

Geiser R, Hoche L, King J: Respite care for the mentally ill patients and their families, *Hosp Community Psychiatry* 39:291, 1988.

Gerson ES: Genetics of schizoaffective disorders, *Current Approaches to Psychoses* 3:8, 1994.

Harding CM, Zubin J, Stauss JS: Chronicity in schizophrenia: fact, partial fact, or artifact? *Hosp Community Psychiatry* 38:477, 1987.

From Harris D, Keltner NL: Medication management. In Worley NK, editor: *Mental health in the community,* St Louis, 1997, Mosby.

Harvard Mental Health Letter: Schizoaffective disorder, *Harv Ment Health Lett* 10:1, 1996.

Hughes Jr et al: Prevalence of smoking among psychiatric outpatients, *Am J Psychiatry* 143:933, 1986.

Huxley NA, Rendall M, Sederer L: Psychosocial treatments in schizophrenia: a review of the past 20 years, *J Nerv Men Dis* 199(4):187, 2000.

Ichikawa J, Meltzer HY: Relationship between dopaminergic and serotonergic neuronal activity in the frontal cortex and the action of typical and atypical antipsychotic drugs, *Eur Arch Psychiatry Clin Neurosci* 249(suppl 4):IV90, 2001.

Ingvar DH, Franzen G: Abnormalities of cerebral blood flow distribution in patients with chronic schizophrenia, *Acta Psychiatr Scand* 50:425, 1974.

Jaroff L: Lies of the mind, *Time* 142(23):52, 1993.

Johnstone EC et al: Cerebral ventricular size and cognitive impairment in chronic schizophrenia, *Lancet* 2:924, 1976.

Kaplan HI, Saddock BJ: *Comprehensive textbook of psychiatry/IV,* ed 6, Baltimore, 1995, Williams & Wilkins.

Kapur S et al: Relationship between dopamine D2 occupancy, clinical response, and side effects: a double-blind PET study of first episode schizophrenia, *Am J Psychiatry* 157(4): 51, 2000.

Keck PE, Strakowski SM, McElroy SL: The efficacy of atypical antipsychotics in the treatment of depressive symptoms, hostility, and suicidality in patients with schizophrenia, *J Clin Psychiatry* 61(suppl 3):4, 2000.

Keltner NL et al: Nature vs nurture: brothers with schizophrenia, *Perspect Psychiatr Care* 37(3):88, 2001.

Kim JS et al: Low cerebrospinal fluid glutamate in schizophrenia patients and a new hypothesis on schizophrenia, *Neurosci Lett* 20:379, 1980.

Kolb LC, Brodie HKH: *Modern clinical psychiatry,* Philadelphia, 1982, WB Saunders.

Kopelowicz A, Bidder TG: Dementia praecox: inescapable fate or psychiatric oversight? *Hosp Community Psychiatry* 43(9):940, 1992.

Kraepelin E: *Clinical psychiatry: a textbook for students and physicians,* New York, 1902, Macmillan (translated by AR Defendorf).

Lee DT: Help through Recovery, Inc, *Hosp Community Psychiatry* 44(1):83, 1993.

Leete E: The treatment of schizophrenia: a patient's perspective, *Hosp Community Psychiatry* 38:486, 1987.

Levinson DF, Umapathy C, Musthaq M: Treatment of schizoaffective disorder and schizophrenia with mood symptoms, *Am J Psychiatry* 156(8):1138, 1999.

Liberman RP et al: Polydipsia and hyponatremia, *Hosp Community Psychiatry* 44(2):184, 1993 (letter).

Lieberman JA: Atypical antipsychotic drugs: the next generation of therapy, *Decade Brain* 8(3):1, 1997.

Lovejoy M: Recovery from schizophrenia: a personal odyssey, *Hosp Community Psychiatry* 35:809, 1984.

Lysaker P et al: Work capacity in schizophrenia, *Hosp Community Psychiatry* 44(3):278, 1993.

Marsh L et al: Medial temporal lobe structure in schizophrenia: relationship of size to duration of illness, *Schizophr Bull* 11(3):225, 1994.

Mason SE, Gingerich S, Siris SG: Patient's and caregiver's adaptation to improvement in schizophrenia, *Hosp Community Psychiatry* 41:541, 1990.

McGrath J, Emmerson WB: Fortnightly review: treatment of schizophrenia, *BMJ* 319(7216):1045, 1999.

McNeil TF: Perinatal risk factors and schizophrenia: selective review and methodological concerns, *Epidemiol Rev* 17(1):107, 1995.

McNeil TF, Cantor-Graae E, Weinberger DR: Relationship of obstetric complications and differences in size of brain structures in monozygotic twin pairs discordant for schizophrenia, *Am J Psychiatry* 157(2):203, 2000.

Menzies V: Depression in schizophrenia: nursing care as a generalized resistance resource, *Issues Ment Health* 21:605, 2000.

Muenzenmaier K et al: Childhood abuse and neglect among women outpatients with chronic mental illness, *Hosp Community Psychiatry* 44(7):666, 1993.

Nasrallah HA: Neurodevelopmental pathogenesis of schizophrenia, *Psychiatr Clin North Am* 16(2):269, 1993.

News: Schizophrenia drug cut off by a California HMO, *J Psychosoc Nurs* 35(3):8, 1997.

North American Nursing Diagnosis Association: *NANDA nursing diagnoses: definitions and classifications 2001-2002,* Philadelphia, 2001, NANDA.

Rabins P et al: Increased ventricle-to-brain ratio in late-onset schizophrenia, *Am J Psychiatry* 144:1216, 1987.

Rapoport JL: The development of neurodevelopmental psychiatry, *Am J Psychiatry* 157(2):159, 2000.

From Regier DA et al: The de facto U.S. mental and addictive disorders service system: epidemiological catchment area prospective, 1-year prevalence rates of disorders and services, *Arch Gen Psychiatry* 50:85, 1993.

Roberts GW, Leigh PN, Weinberger DR: *Neuropsychiatric disorders,* London, 1993, Mosby Europe.

Roeber CR: Schizophrenics who abuse alcohol: dilemmas of treatment, *Clin Care Rev* 9(2):3, 1997.

Ruocchio PJ: How psychotherapy can help the schizophrenic patient, *Hosp Community Psychiatry* 40:188, 1989.

Sands JR, Harrow M: Depression during the longitudinal course of schizophrenia, *Schizophr Bull* 25(1):157, 1999.

Schultz SK, Andreasen NC: Schizophrenia, *Lancet* 353(9162):1425, 1999.

Seeman MV: Schizophrenia in women and men, *Curr Approaches Psychoses* 4:10, 1995.

Segal SP, Vander Voort DJ: Daily hassles of persons with severe mental illness, *Hosp Community Psychiatry* 44(3):276, 1993.

Shah PJ, Greenberg WM: Polydipsia with hyponatremia in a state hospital population, *Hosp Community Psychiatry* 43(5):509, 1992.

Simpson G, May P: Schizophrenic disorders. In Greist J, Jefferson J, Spitzer R, editors: *Treatment of mental disorders,* New York, 1982, Oxford University.

Snider K, Boyd MA: When they drink too much: nursing interventions for patients with disordered water balance, *J Psychosoc Nurs Ment Health Serv* 29(7):10, 1991.

Soni SD et al: Differences between chronic schizophrenic patients in the hospital and the community, *Hosp Community Psychiatry* 43(12):1233, 1992.

Staal WG et al: Structural brain abnormalities in patients with schizophrenia and their healthy siblings, *Am J Psychiatry* 157(3):416, 2000.

Sullivan HS: *The interpersonal theory of psychiatry,* New York, 1953, WW Norton.

Surgeon General: *Mental health: a report of the Surgeon General,* Washington, DC, 1999, Department of Health and Human Services.

Talan J: Schizophrenia fight leads experts to a retrovirus. *The Brain in the News,* January-May (special issue):1, 2001.

Torrey EF: The release of the mentally ill from institutions: a well-intentioned disaster, *Chron High Educ* 43(240):B4, 1997.

Velligan DI et al: Randomized controlled trial of the use of compensatory strategies to enhance adaptive function in outpatients with schizophrenia, *Am J Psychiatry* 157(8): 1317, 1999.

Velligan DI, Miller AL: Cognitive dysfunction in schizophrenia and its importance to outcome: the place of atypical antipsychotics in treatment, *J Clin Psychiatry* 60(suppl):25, 1999.

Weinberger DR: Implications of normal brain development for the pathogenesis of schizophrenia, *Arch Gen Psychiatry* 44:660, 1987.

Woolley DW, Shaw E: Biochemical and pharmacological suggestion about certain mental disorders, *Proc Natl Acad Sci USA* 40:228, 1954.

Yamada S: *The role of serotonin in schizophrenia.* www.medscape.com/medscape/cno/2000/CINP/Story.cfm?story_id=1497. Accessed 4/19/01.

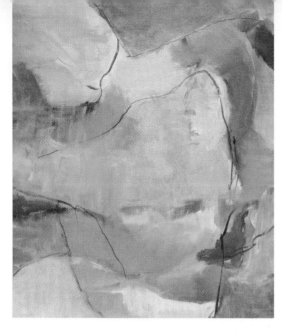

Chapter 29

Depression

Norman L. Keltner, Barbara Jones Warren

Learning Objectives

After reading this chapter, you should be able to:

- Recognize *The Diagnostic and Statistical Manual of Mental Disorders, Fourth Edition, Text Revision* (DSM-IV-TR) criteria and terminology for depressive disorders.
- Compare and contrast major depressive disorder and dysthymic disorder.
- Describe the biological and psychodynamic explanations for depressive disorders.
- Describe effective nursing interventions for depressed patients.
- Recognize warning signs of suicide.
- Describe interventions to prevent suicide.
- Describe the family issues related to this disorder.

Two major types of depressive disorders are recognized by the American Psychiatric Association (APA): major depressive disorder and dysthymic disorder. However, in reality, it might be more accurate to think in terms of many "depressions." The ability to recognize underlying pathologies is growing, and with these advancements come more precise understanding of the variability among depressive disorders. Major depressive disorder and dysthymia are defined as follows:

Major depressive disorder is characterized by one or more major depressive episodes, which is defined as at least 2 weeks of depressed mood or loss of interest accompanied by at least four additional symptoms of depression (APA, 2001). Major depression is a disorder of *severity* and is easily treatable, with 80% able to resume normal activities within a few weeks (National Institute of Mental Health, 2001).

Dysthymic disorder is characterized by at least 2 years of depressed mood for more days than not (i.e., >50%) accompanied by additional depressive symptoms that do not meet the criteria for major depression (APA, 2001). Dysthymia is a disorder of *chronicity*.

Normally, every individual experiences different types and levels of moods or emotional states. Brief periods of highs, lows, and sadness occur for everyone, because mood is a person's state of mind that is exhibited through feelings and emotions (APA, 2001). However, mood is considered "disordered" and may be diagnosed as such when an individual has problems with daily functioning because of the presence of exaggerated feelings and emotions. The DSM-IV-TR defines a mood disorder as one in which the predominant feature is the disturbance in a person's mood (APA, 2001). The DSM-IV-TR

Key Terms

Affect Individual's external response to changing states of moods.

Anhedonia Inability to experience pleasure.

Apathy Lack of feeling, concern, interest, or emotion; inability to be motivated.

Atypical depression Subtype of depression occurring more often among younger individuals and is expressed by "atypical" symptoms; for example, increased appetite, weight gain, hypersomnia.

Bipolar disorder Disturbance in mood in which the symptoms of mania have occurred at least one time; an episode of depression may or may not occur.

Clinical depression Another term for major depressive disorder that defines the disturbance of a person's mood according to DSM-IV-TR criteria.

Cortisol Glucocorticoid hormone formed in the adrenal cortex that participates in carbohydrate and protein metabolism; cortisol hypersecretion occurs in many depressed individuals; excretion of this hormone is not suppressed in a significant number of persons with major depression after an injection of dexamethasone.

Cyclothymia Mood swing that alternates between hypomania and depression.

Dexamethasone suppression test (DST) Diagnostic test for clinical depression that measures the function of the hypothalmic-pituitary-adrenal (HPA) axis.

Dysphoria Disorder of affect characterized by depression, malaise, and anguish.

Dysthymic disorder Disorder resulting in depressed mood with a duration of at least 2 years.

Electroconvulsive therapy (ECT) Form of somatic therapy that uses electrical-induced seizures to relieve person's intractable depressive symptoms.

Euphoria Subjective, exaggerated feeling of well-being characterized by confidence, elation, and assurance.

Hypersomnia Increased and prolonged sleeping.

Hypomania Milder form of mania that is less intense and severe than mania.

Insomnia Inability to sleep or disrupted sleep patterns.

Mania Individual's state of extreme or exaggerated excitement and euphoria that results in accelerated mental and physical activity.

Melancholic depression Subgroup of depression generally occurring in older persons, often misdiagnosed as dementia; more often associated with dexamethasone nonsuppression; depression usually worse in the morning, early morning as awakening occurs, psychomotor retardation or agitation, excessive or inappropriate guilt, and significant anorexia or weight loss are symptoms of melancholia.

Monoamine oxidase inhibitors (MAOIs) Classification of antidepressant drugs that inhibit the action of monoamine oxidase, which results in increased levels of norepinephrine, dopamine, and serotonin.

Mood Individual's internal state of mind that is exhibited through feelings and emotions.

Mood disorder Disorder whose predominant feature is the disturbance or alteration in a person's mood.

Mood disorder as a result of a general medical condition Disorder resulting in a disturbance or alteration of a person's mood that is due to a specific medical and physiologic consequence.

Postpartum depression Subgroup of depression occurring 30 days or less in the postpartum period.

Psychotic depression Subtype of depression in which a person experiences delusions and hallucinations, often misdiagnosed as schizophrenia or schizoaffective disorder.

Seasonal affective disorder Subtype of depression occurring in late autumn or winter and lasting until spring.

Selective serotonin reuptake inhibitors (SSRIs) Classification of antidepressants that inhibit the reuptake of serotonin into the presynaptic neuron and increase serotonin in the brain.

Substance-induced mood disorder Disorder resulting from the disturbance or alteration of a person's mood that is due to the ingestion of a prescribed or nonprescribed drug or medication or exposure to a toxic substance.

Tricyclic antidepressants Drug classification of antidepressants that block the reuptake of norepinephrine and serotonin into the presynaptic neuron.

categorizes mood disorders according to four overarching categories: depressive disorders, bipolar disorders, mood disorder resulting from a general medical condition, and substance-induced mood disorder.

This chapter considers the cause, diagnostic criteria, and treatment of depressive disorders. Chapter 30 addresses these same issues related to bipolar disorders.

- Box 29-1 summarizes criteria for major depressive disorders.
- Appropriate interventions for patients who suffer from these disorders will also be discussed.
- Key terms for understanding mood disorders are listed above.
- DSM-IV-TR and North American Nursing Diagnosis Association (NANDA) diagnoses are listed in the box on page 342.

12-Month Prevalence Rate of Mental Disorders in the United States

Diagnosis	Percentage of Population Over 17 Years of Age	Number of People
Anxiety disorders	12.6	20,034,000
Phobia disorders*	10.9	17,331,333
Mood disorders	9.5	15,143,000
Alcohol disorders	7.4	11,766,000
Major depression[†]	5.0	7,950,000
Drug disorders	3.1	4,929,000
Cognitive impairment	2.7	4,293,000
Obsessive-compulsive disorder	2.1	3,339,000
Antisocial disorder	1.5	2,385,000
Panic disorders*	1.3	2,067,000
Bipolar disorder[†]	1.2	1,908,000
Schizophrenia	1.1	1,749,000
Somatization	0.2	365,000

*Also calculated in anxiety statistics.
[†]Also calculated in mood disorders statistics.
From Regier DA et al: The de facto U.S. mental and addictive disorders service system: epidemiological catchment area prospective, 1-year prevalence rates of disorders and services, *Arch Gen Psychiatry* 50:85, 1993; Surgeon General: *Mental health: a report from the Surgeon General,* 1999, Washington DC, Department of Health and Human Services.

| Box 29-1 | Key Features of Major Depressive Disorders

At least a 2-week period of maladaptive functioning that is a clear change from previous levels of functioning. At least five of the following symptoms must be present during that 2-week period, one of which must be (1) or (2):
1. Depressed mood
2. Inability to experience pleasure or markedly diminished interest in pleasurable activities
3. Appetite disturbance with weight change (change >5% of body weight within 1 month up or down)
4. Sleep disturbance
5. Psychomotor disturbance
6. Fatigue or loss of energy
7. Feelings of worthlessness or excessive or inappropriate guilt
8. Diminished ability to concentrate or indecisiveness
9. Recurrent thoughts of death or suicidal ideations
   The mood disturbance causes marked distress or significant impairment in social or occupational functioning or both.
   No evidence of a physical or substance-induced cause exists for the patient's symptoms or of the presence of another major mental disorder that accounts for the patient's depressive symptoms.

Adapted from the American Psychiatric Association: *Diagnostic and statistical manual of mental disorders,* ed 4, text revision, Washington, DC, 2000, APA.

DSM-IV-TR | DSM-IV-TR and NANDA Diagnoses Related to Depression

DSM-IV*
Dysthymic disorder
Major depressive disorder

NANDA[†]
Anxiety
Communication, impaired verbal
Coping, ineffective
Grieving, anticipatory
Grieving, dysfunctional
Hopelessness
Injury, risk for
Nutrition, less than body requirements, imbalanced
Powerlessness, risk for
Self-care deficit
Self-esteem, chronic low
Sexual dysfunction
Sleep pattern, disturbed
Social isolation
Spiritual distress
Thought processes, disturbed
Violence, risk for self-directed

*Adapted from the American Psychiatric Association: *Diagnostic and statistical manual of mental disorders,* ed 4, text revision, Washington, DC, 2001, APA.
[†]North American Nursing Diagnosis Association: *NANDA nursing diagnoses: definitions and classifications 2002,* Philadelphia, 2001, NANDA.

DEPRESSIVE DISORDERS

Depression is the oldest and most frequently described psychiatric illness (Belcher, Holdcraft, 2001). The existence of depression has been documented since biblical times and has been defined by religious writers, philosophers, and scientists (Mahendra, 1986). Historically, many important individuals have experienced the devastating symptoms of depression, including King Saul, Job, Elijah, Jeremiah, Mary and Abraham Lincoln, and Winston Churchill. More recently, Mrs. Colin Powell, the wife of the nation's Secretary of State, and newscaster Mike Wallace are known to have suffered from this disorder. Of course, normal feelings of sadness are quite appropriate in many situations. In fact, it would be abnormal not to feel sad in certain situations, for example, when a loved one dies or when other losses occur in an individual's life. However, these feelings are typically short lived and do not completely and permanently alter a person's functioning ability.

| Table 29-1 | Demographic Variables Associated with Mood Disorders (15 to 54 Years of Age) |

Demographic Variable	Most Likely to be Depressed	Least Likely to be Depressed
Sex	Women	Men
Age	35-44	15-24
Race	Caucasian, Hispanic	African American
Income	Low income	>$70,000
Education	Less than high school education	High school or more
Geography	Urban	Rural

Adapted from Kessler RC et al: Lifetime and 12-month prevalence of DSM-III-R psychiatric disorders in the United States: results from the national comorbidity survey, *Arch Gen Psychiatry* 51:8, 1994.

The DSM-IV-TR categorizes depressive disorders into major depressive disorder (MDD), dysthymic disorder, and depressive disorder not otherwise specified. Depression can manifest itself as a single or recurrent episode and varies somewhat according to age, race, and gender (APA, 1993; 2001). The connection between MDD and suicide is alarming. A discussion of suicide and depression is presented at the end of the chapter. Demographic factors associated with mood disorders are found in Table 29-1.

Criteria and Symptoms of Major Depressive Disorder

MDD involves psychologic, biologic, and social symptoms that impair a person's functioning ability and social interactions (Box 29-2 lists common and other symptoms of MDD). The DSM-IV-TR describes MDD as a mood disorder characterized by symptoms that persist over a minimal 2-week period. A person must have at least five of the nine criteria, one of which must be a depressed mood or anhedonia. The criteria for MDD are:

1. Depressed mood
2. Anhedonia (or apathy)
3. Significant change in weight
4. Insomnia or hypersomnia
5. Increased or decreased psychomotor activity
6. Fatigue or energy loss
7. Feelings of worthlessness or guilt
8. Diminished concentration or indecisiveness
9. Recurrent death or suicidal thoughts

Nurses can be instrumental in the assessment of depression. A variety of instruments may be used for assessment purposes. One of these, the Geriatric Depression Scale, can be found in Appendix C.

| Box 29-2 | Symptoms of Depression |

Common Symptoms	Other Symptoms
Apathy	Fatigue
Sadness	Thoughts of death
Sleep disturbances	Decreased libido
Hopelessness	Ruminations of inadequacy
Helplessness	Psychomotor agitation
Worthlessness	Verbal beratings of self
Guilt	Spontaneous crying
Anger	Dependency, passiveness

The DSM-IV-TR categorizes MDD into several variants called specifiers. These variants include MDD with atypical features, melancholic features, catatonic features, postpartum onset, psychotic features, and seasonal patterns (i.e., seasonal affective disorder). Overarching symptoms are the same across these subgroups, but variances in expression occur. The DSM-IV-TR description helps define the population, time frame, and symptoms for these subgroups.

Atypical depression is a mood disturbance of depression that generally occurs in younger populations and is more common in women compared with men. This type of depression is expressed by increased appetite or weight gain, hypersomnia, leaden paralysis, and extreme sensitivity to interpersonal rejection. Mood reactivity in which the mood brightens considerably with positive events is another characteristic. Hypersomnia is defined as sleeping 10 hours a day or at least 2 hours more than usual. Leaden paralysis is defined as feeling heavy, leaden, or weighted down in the arms or legs. Feelings of personal rejection tend to be a symptom of long-standing and tend to persist after depressive symptoms subside (APA, 2001)

Melancholic depression is a disturbance of depression occurring most often in older adults and may be misdiagnosed as dementia. This type of depression is characterized by anhedonia and an inability to be cheered up. The mood does not improve even temporarily. At least three of the following depressive symptoms are found in melancholic patients: depression worse in the morning, early morning awakening, psychomotor retardation or agitation, significant anorexia or weight loss, and excessive or inappropriate guilt. This diagnosis is more likely to be associated with dexamethasone nonsuppression (mentioned later) and elevated cortisol levels (also mentioned later) (APA, 2001).

Catatonic features are marked by significant psychomotor alterations, including immobility, excessive motor activity, mutism, echolalia (parrotlike repetition of words), and inappropriate posturing. Though this sign is more often associated with schizophrenia, more cases actually occur in patients with mood disorders (APA, 2001).

Postpartum depression is a mood disturbance that occurs in the first 30 days postpartum. Postpartum "blues" affects approximately 50% to 80% of new mothers (Kennedy, Suttenfeld, 2001). Symptoms include feeling anxious, irritable, or tearful but also having periods of normalcy. Postpartum depression is more serious compared with postpartum blues. Postpartum depression can present with or without psychotic features (far less than 1% are afflicted with psychosis). Over concern or even delusional thoughts about the baby's health are not uncommon features of this disorder. Infanticide is most often associated with command hallucinations to kill the infant or delusions that the infant is possessed by Satan (APA, 2001).

In *psychotic depression,* a person has delusions and hallucinations in conjunction with the mood disturbance. These perceptual problems tend to be mood congruent, that is, delusions of guilt, delusions of deserved punishment, nihilistic delusions (e.g., personal destruction), somatic delusions ("My brain is dying."), and delusions of poverty. Psychotic depression is associated with a poorer prognosis compared with other forms of depression (APA, 2001).

Seasonal affective disorder (SAD) is a depression occurring in conjunction with a seasonal change most often beginning in fall or winter and remitting in spring (in the Northern Hemisphere). As might be expected, the higher the latitude, the more likely SAD will occur. Women are much more likely to be affected by seasonal changes than are men (APA, 2001).

Adult populations

Depression (all types) is one of the most prevalent mental health problems within the United States, with about 18 million people affected at any given time (APA, 2001; Horwath et al, 1994; Kessler et al, 1994; U.S. Department of Health and Human Services [DHHS], 1993a). Depression is predicted to become the leading cause of disability in the future (Venarec, 2000). Women's lifetime risk for depression is 10% to 20% compared with men's lifetime risk of about 5% to 10% (APA, 2001; Nemeroff, 1998). Although depression can occur at any age, the average age of adult onset is in the mid to late 20s. Some individuals will have a single episode of clinical depression, recover, and never become depressed again. However, about 80% will eventually have recurrent episodes. Five to ten percent will experience manic phases in addition to depressive episodes (about 1.2% of Americans) (Nemeroff, 1998). The prevalence rates appear unrelated to ethnicity (though differences in expression occur); however, low-income groups and individuals with a positive family history of depression are at increased risk (up to three times more common).

Children and adolescents

The occurrence of depression in children and adolescents can be even more devastating than it is in adults. Children of parents who incur depression are at greater risk of developing the disorder than are children whose parents are not diagnosed with the disorder (Depression Guideline Panel [DGP], 1993). The onset of childhood depression predisposes a child to develop recurrent adult depression. Nurses need to be able to assess children and their families for possible symptoms of depression and then develop appropriate interventions for them. Certain events may predispose children and adolescents to develop depressive symptoms or MDD, including:

1. Loss of parents through divorce, separation, or death
2. Death of other individuals close to the child, such as siblings, grandparents, other relatives, or friends
3. Death of a pet
4. Move to another neighborhood or town
5. Academic problems or failure
6. Physical illness or injury that might require hospitalization (Hyde, 1993; Kahan, 1993)

Culture, age, and gender

Little data is available regarding depression in people from different ethnic, racial, or cultural groups; yet, it is known that individuals from certain groups may display depressive symptoms differently. Depression may be experienced in somatic terms in some ethnic, racial, or cultural groups. People from Hispanic, Latino, and Mediterranean groups may describe their sadness or guilt in terms of being nervous or having headaches or stomachaches. Individuals from Asian cultures may describe themselves as being out of balance or feeling weak and nervous. Native-

American and Asian-American groups withdraw for meditation and personal growth as part of their culture, thus symptoms of depression may be overlooked, ignored, or denied. Please refer to Chapter 16 for more specific information on expression of emotional states in different ethnic, racial, and cultural groups.

Nurses and other health care providers can misinterpret symptoms of depression in children, adolescents, women, and older adults. For example, depressive symptoms in children and adolescents may mimic normal developmental emotional and physical changes. On the other hand, women's reports of depression may be dismissed as symptoms of conditions expressed in ways similar to depression. The gender disparity for depression is puzzling, and some research has suggested this overrepresentation may well be considered a social disease (Schreiber, 2001). That is, the devaluation of women in North America is a primary contributor to the higher incidence of depression among women. Finally, recognizing symptoms of depression in older adult populations is particularly challenging because many symptoms of depression are similar to those found in dementia, diabetes, and cardiac conditions (DGP, 1993).

Critical Thinking Question

What factors do you think contribute to the high levels of depression in the United States?

DYSTHYMIC DISORDER

Dysthymic disorder is diagnosed when a person has a depressed mood for at least 2 years, for more days than not. The distinction between dysthymia and MDD is subtle, and diagnostic confusion is common. Dysthymic disorder is essentially a disorder of chronicity, whereas severity is the distinguishing factor for MDD. In addition, because a less severe depression might be expected as a patient is recovering from MDD, the DSM-IV-TR criteria reduce the possibility of confusing a gradual recovery from MDD with the less severe dysthymic disorder. The DSM-IV-TR (APA, 2001) criteria for dysthymia include:

A. Depressed mood for most of day, for more days than not

B. Presence of two or more of the following:
   - Poor appetite or overeating
   - Insomnia or hypersomnia
   - Low energy or fatigue
   - Low self-esteem
   - Poor concentration or difficulty making a decision
   - Feelings of hopelessness

BEHAVIOR SYMPTOMATIC OF DEPRESSION

Depression results in both objective and subjective behaviors. Objective signs, such as agitation, can be observed by the nurse. Subjective symptoms, such as hopelessness, are painful but may be hidden by depressed individuals. The differentiation between objective and subjective symptoms in depression is difficult to develop, perhaps more than it is in schizophrenia. Objective signs are typically extensions of a subjective state. The nurse is encouraged to observe for visible signs of depression and to be aware of, assess for, and expect subjective anguish and anger.

CLINICAL EXAMPLE

Mrs. Lewis is a 50-year-old woman who presents with dysphoria, tearfulness, suicidal ideation, loss of energy and sexual interest, and insomnia. Although she feels hopeless about the future and worries that she will never get better, she denies that she is "really" depressed. Mrs. Lewis is an extremely devout woman and believes that someone truly walking with the Lord would not find himself or herself in her situation. Mrs. Lewis believes that she is a burden to her family; she also has fears related to her physical health. Mrs. Lewis also feels guilty for not being able to handle her situation. Her husband, also a religious person, has been dutifully patient through all of this turmoil but is growing tired of her pessimism, crying, and lack of interest in sex. The nurse fears a breakup of this 25-year marriage may occur if Mrs. Lewis does not respond to treatment.

Objective Signs

Depressed patients often demonstrate behavior that is noticeable to others, but these patients may not want to talk to anyone and may seek to be alone. If someone intrudes into the obsessive thinking of their inner world, depressed patients may become irritable and aggressive and actually strike out at the "intruder." Two general areas of objective signs are alterations of activity, including activities of daily living (ADLs), and altered social interactions.

Alterations in activity

Patients may exhibit psychomotor agitation; they may be unable to sit still; and they may pace and engage in hand-wringing. These patients may pull or rub their hair, skin, clothing, or other objects. Tying and retying shoes and buttoning and unbuttoning a shirt or blouse are typical behaviors. Psychomotor retardation is marked by a slowing of speech, increased pauses before answering, soft or monotonous speech, decreased frequency of speech (poverty of speech), and muteness. In addition, a general slowing of body movements occurs. Patients may state they "are tired all the time," even when they are not physically active. For example, a patient may have difficulty getting up from a chair to turn off the television. Even the smallest task may seem unbearable.

ADLs suffer as well. Depressed individuals often defer basic personal hygiene, such as bathing, shaving, putting on clean clothes, or wiping their mouths after eating. However, these latter objective signs are probably a result of more than a lack of energy. Apathy, a lack of feeling, absence of emotion, or an inability to be motivated, plays an important role in these behaviors as well. An extreme extension of these anergic symptoms is seen in cases in which depressed people lie in bed and become incontinent or constipated because of the inability to muster the energy (both physical and psychic energy) to walk to the bathroom.

Depressed people usually experience a change in eating behaviors that results in either weight loss or gain. Sleeping patterns change as well. Depressed individuals may experience insomnia (difficulty falling asleep), middle insomnia (difficulty remaining asleep), or terminal insomnia (early morning awakening). Hypersomnia (increased or prolonged sleeping or both) is an atypical symptom of depression. Depressed people may deny they are depressed yet spend hours by themselves. In this case, the nurse should not confuse a request to "go to my room and lie down" with hypersomnia. Many depressed people want to lie down but do not sleep. There, in the solitude of an empty room, these individuals descend into uninterrupted, self-defeating ruminations.

CLINICAL EXAMPLE
Stan Treback is a 60-year-old Caucasian man who has been successful in business for many years. He recently has become "blue" and does not seem to care about anything. He is cooperative and desires treatment.

Stan's symptoms are decreased energy, anxiety, agitation, insomnia, and a weight loss over the past year of 54 pounds. He has many somatic complaints.

Altered social interactions

Depressed individuals often suffer from poor social skills that are linked directly to other symptoms of depression. Underachievement causes a lack of productivity on the job and at home. The self-absorbing nature of depression causes these individuals to be easily distracted and reduces their interest in people, their ideas, or problems. Depression causes problems with thinking, idea development, and problem solving. In addition, conversations are difficult to maintain, and only with great effort can a depressed person sustain a facial expression of interest and concern. Depressed individuals are also withdrawn and often seek social isolation over social interaction with others. Hobbies and avocations that were once actively pursued become unimportant and may be abandoned or engaged half-heartedly. Finally, the body language of depression (e.g., saddened facial expression, drooping posture) serves as a social barrier.

Subjective Symptoms
Alterations of affect

Alterations of affect are the symptoms primarily associated with depression, which is reasonable because these disturbances dominate the internal world of a depressed person. Anxiety, doom and gloom, fear, self-destructive thoughts, and panic attacks are all products of the depressed mind. Because of this anguish, depressed individuals vacillate between sadness and apathy. When the pain becomes too great, patients shut down and become apathetic. Finally, although most laypeople consider sadness to be the universal symptom of distress, apathy actually comes closer to being continually present in depressed individuals.

The overall affective sense is one of low self-esteem. Guilt may include an overreaction to some current failing or may be associated with an indiscretion in the distant past that cannot be forgiven. Guilt can also take the form of accepting responsibility for occurrences in which the person had little impact or take the form of obsessional preoccupation with "What if I had only...?" The person becomes immobilized with "should haves, could haves." An even more morbid extension of guilt is the psychotic delusion of guilt for calamities that happened continents away.

Anxiety is a companion of depression. Depressed individuals are filled with anxiousness and dread. A ringing telephone holds the potential for catastrophic news. A siren might mean a loved one has been injured; a child at school might not return. Although these terrible things do happen, most go on with life somewhat comforted by the knowledge that they will probably not happen if unusual risks are not taken. However, for many depressed individuals, the ringing telephone causes the same anxious reaction each time.

Worthlessness can range from a feeling of inadequacy to total devaluation. Depressed individuals may scan the environment for clues to their inadequacy and as one person remarked, "I knew I wasn't any good; it just took a while to figure out why."

Alterations of cognition

Alterations of cognition include ambivalence and indecision, inability to concentrate, confusion, loss of interest and motivation, memory problems, pessimism, self-blame, self-depreciation, self-destructive thoughts, thoughts of death and dying, and uncertainty. The inability of depressed individuals to make a decision is particularly difficult for others to understand. Faced with even a simple decision, much vacillation is expressed. Once a decision is made, depressed individuals may be obsessed with "what if" questions. Major decisions can be immobilizing.

Alterations of a physical nature

Alterations of a physical nature are common in the depressed individual. Almost all parts of the body can be affected. Common physiologic disorders include abdominal pain, anorexia, chest pain, constipation, dizziness, fatigue, headache, indigestion, insomnia, menstrual changes, nausea and vomiting, and sexual dysfunction. Additionally, as mentioned in the previous section of this chapter on cultural aspects, some ethnic and racial groups' cultural practices may mimic depressive symptoms, or depression may be expressed somatically.

These subjective symptoms come to the attention of the nurse because of the numerous somatic complaints of depressed individuals. Some people become preoccupied with their bodies to the extent that every twinge, every body change is greeted with great alarm and dread. One recovering depressed patient joked, "I have had a hundred heart attacks." Monitoring of body functions is not uncommon in the general population and is no doubt related to a variety of factors, including perhaps this society's obsession with fitness. However, overinvestment in self-assessment by depressed individual is pathologic, and it is the degree of this thinking that sets those who are depressed apart. Chest pain, an unusual spot on the face or abdomen, and stomach pain all can precipitate a panic attack in some people. Panic attacks occur in 15% to 30% of individuals with MDD (APA, 1993).

Alterations of perception

Some depressed individuals suffer from altered perceptions. Delusions and hallucinations are typically congruent with the depressed mood (e.g., a delusion of persecution because of a moral mistake). Somatic delusions (e.g., "My body is full of cancer.") and nihilistic delusions (e.g., "My brain is dying.") are not uncommon forms of psychotic delusions in depressed individuals. Hallucinations tend to be less elaborate than are those of schizophrenia and tend to focus on personal faults, for example, "You are no good. You don't deserve your family."

ETIOLOGY OF DEPRESSION

Biologic Theories of Depression

The etiology of depression has been biologically attributed to alterations in neurochemical, genetic, endocrine, and circadian rhythm functions. These alterations produce physical and psychologic changes expressed as depression (Warren, 1997).

Neurochemical theories

Research findings suggest that a neurochemical depression results when levels of certain neurotransmitters are altered. The biogenic amines norepinephrine and serotonin are most often mentioned, but dopamine, another biogenic amine, is indicated as well. Figure 29-1 illustrates the proposed roles of the three key monoamines. Furthermore, dysregulation of acetylcholine and gamma-aminobutyric acid (GABA) may contribute to the development of biochemical depression as well. More specifically, when the levels of these neurotransmitters are altered at receptor sites, or when receptor sensitivity changes, a neurochemi-

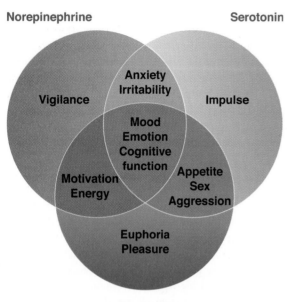

Proposed Roles for the Three Key Monoamine Systems

Norepinephrine   **Serotonin**

Vigilance

Anxiety
Irritability

Impulse

Mood
Emotion
Cognitive
function

Motivation
Energy

Appetite
Sex
Aggression

Euphoria
Pleasure

Dopamine

Figure 29-1 Proposed roles for the three key monoamine systems. (From Healy D, McDonagle T: The enhancement of social functioning as a therapeutic principle in the management of depression, *J Psychopharmacology* 11(Supp): S25-S31, 1997.)

cal depression may result (Keltner, 2000a). The serotonergic receptors originate in the raphe nuclei of the brainstem and are located near the midline for most of the length of the brainstem (Keltner, Hogan, Guy, 2001a). The more rostral neurons (towards the head) project throughout the cortex. Each serotonergic neuron sends over 500,000 terminals to the limbic system and to the cortex (Dubovsky, 1994). Hence serotonin contributes to the regulation of many psychologic functions (Dubovsky, 1994). Norepinephrine or noradrenergic pathways originate in the locus ceruleus and innervate all areas of the cortex, the hypothalamus, and the hippocampus (Keltner et al, 2001). As is the case with serotonin, norepinephrine neurons innervate and contribute to regulation of brain areas with a variety of functions.

It might be appealing to conceptualize depression as a decreased level of serotonin and norepinephrine or to suggest that by increasing the bioavailability of these amines, depression can be successfully treated. However, doing so oversimplifies both the problem and the solution. Other hypotheses include the sensitivity of both presynaptic and postsynaptic receptors and the modulating effects of acetylcholine and GABA on aminergic systems (Keltner, Hogan, Guy, 2001a; Keltner et al, 2001). It is thought, for example, that beta autoreceptors, which normally inhibit the release of norepinephrine, are downregulated by antidepressants, thus disinhibiting norepinephrine release (i.e., increasing synaptic norepinephrine). Too many norepinephrine or serotonin receptors might be thought of as a positive situation. However, excessive (i.e., upregulation of) receptors indicate insufficient levels of these neurotransmitters. This action is an example of the body compensating for decreased monoamine availability (Nemeroff, 1998). Finally, peptides, dietary practices, and nutritional status are being examined for their biochemical roles in the development of depression because food intake affects the development of precursors (i.e., amino acids) for neurotransmitters. In summary, there is much to learn about the biochemistry of depression. (Chapter 21 provides a detailed explanation of antidepressants.)

Genetic theories

Other researchers have contended that depression may be genetically based and that heredity may predispose individuals to develop depression (Kendler et al, 1993; Shuchter, Downs, Zisook, 1996). Several studies have examined the incidence of depression in twins. Findings have indicated that the concordancy rate for MDD ranges from 32% to 67% in twins in which one or both of the biological parents had been diagnosed with MDD (Shuchter, Downs, Zisook, 1996).

Endocrine theories

Endocrine changes, in relationship to depression, have also been investigated. Normally, the hypothalamic-pituitary-adrenal (HPA) axis is a system that mediates the stress response. However, in some depressed people, this system malfunctions and creates cortisol, thyroid, and hormonal abnormalities. Dysregulation of the HPA axis results in hypercortisolemia (in about 40% to 60% of depressed patients), nonsuppression by dexamethasone, and elevated corticotropin-releasing factor (CRF) (Keltner et al, 2001). The hypersecretion of cortisol is the result of an overexpression of the CRF gene (leading to increased CRF synthesis) and an increase in CRF-producing neurons in the hypothalamus. This action, in turn, leads to increased pituitary release of adrenocorticotropic hormone (ACTH) and the subsequent hypersecretion of cortisol by the adrenal glands. Nemeroff (1998) believes early life exposure to overwhelming trauma literally changes the expression of CRF neurons in the hypothalamus. Events such as early loss of parents, inadequate parenting, or childhood sexual and physical abuse create an adult who is overly responsive to stressors and vulnerable to depression. Essentially, a physical change brought about by childhood stressors causes a long-term or even permanent hyperactivity of central corticotropin-releasing hormones, leaving the adult highly vulnerable to stress. Nemeroff calls this phenomenon the "stress–diathesis model of depression."

The dexamethasone suppression test (DST) will fail to suppress cortisol in about 40% of depressed patients; however, this test is not conclusive for depression. This malfunctioning and its results are more pronounced in severely depressed patients (Shuchter, Downs, Zisook, 1996). In addition, the presence of endocrine disease, caused by disease in any component of the HPA axis, has also been associated with the development of depressive symptoms (Maes et al, 1994; Shuchter, Downs, Zisook, 1996). Controversy exists regarding the role of genetics and hormonal explanations of depression in women; some researchers have contended that women have a predisposition to develop depressive symptoms and MDD because of fluctuations in hormones (McGrath et al, 1992). Other researchers have contended that these fluctuations influence the development of MDD through their interaction with neurotransmitters, psychosocial factors, and the stress system (Beeber, 1996; Cockerman, 1992).

Circadian rhythm theories

Individuals experiencing circadian rhythm changes are at increased risk for developing depressive symptoms and MDD. These changes may be caused by medications, nutritional deficiencies, physical or psychologic illnesses, hormonal fluctuations associated with women's reproductive system, or aging (Buysse et al, 1994; Cartwright, Lloyd, 1994; McEnany, 1995a, 1995b; Warren, 1997). Circadian rhythms are responsible for the daily regulation of wake-sleep cycles, arousal and activity patterns, and hormonal secretions associated with these regulatory mechanisms. In depressed individuals, these regulatory mechanisms are altered, which leads to shortened latency in rapid eye movement (REM) and sleep disturbances such as insomnia, frequent waking, and increasingly intensified dreaming (Shuchter, Downs, Zisook, 1996).

Psychologic Theories of Depression

The psychologic explanations for depression flow from psychoanalytic, cognitive, interpersonal, and behavioral perspectives. In addition, related psychosocial-psychodynamic views explain depression from three general themes: adverse early life experiences, intrapsychic conflicts, or reactions to life events or combinations of these (i.e., stressors).

Psychoanalytic theorists have contended that depression occurs as a result of an early life loss (Freud, 1957). Freud viewed depression as the aggressive instinct inappropriately directed at the self, often triggered by the loss of a loved person or object ("object loss"). This loss predisposes the adult to depression when adult losses trigger the "memory" of the childhood loss. By understanding (i.e., gaining insight into) one's thoughts, feelings, and motives, one can heal. It should be noted that many clinicians believe this approach is not in the patient's best interest because it focuses on problems in the past and often creates more issues than it solves.

Cognitive theorists have contended that depression results when a person perceives all stressful situations as being negative (Beck, 1991; Beck et al, 1979). In addition, a depressed person reacts to all situations as if they are stressful and sees himself or herself, others, and daily events in a negative light. This reaction to stress is grounded in early childhood losses (e.g., often the loss of the parent through death, leaving the home, or divorce) and serves as the basis for the way in which the depressed person makes decisions and sees himself or herself in relationship to other persons and occurrences. Cognitive therapy aims at symptom removal by identifying and correcting distorted, negative, moment-by-moment maladaptive thinking and seeks to prevent recurrence by correcting silent assumptions (DGP, 1993; Ford-Martin, 2002). Most clinicians, even those heavily steeped in a biologic framework, believe medications serve the purpose of preparing the mind to work on faulty thinking. Cognitive approaches are ideal when used in conjunction with antidepressants.

Interpersonal theorists believe that when a person has interpersonal difficulties, coping with individuals, life events, and life changes can be inordinately stressful and lead to depression (Klerman, 1989). Role dispute, social isolation, prolonged grief reaction, and role transition are major interpersonal themes. Interpersonal difficulties are viewed as causal, concomitant, or exacerbating in maintaining factors for depression (DGP, 1993).

Behavioral theorists propose that a person develops depression when he or she develops feelings of helplessness and unworthiness and then learns to use these attitudes to evaluate life outcomes (Abramson, Seligman, Teasdale, 1978).

As noted, psychologic or psychodynamic explanations of depression can be categorized under three general themes: debilitating early life experiences, intrapsychic conflicts, or reactions to life events.

Debilitating early-life experiences

According to traditional psychiatric thought, events in early life can lay the foundation for adult depression. The developmental theorists view the early years of life as the foundation of lifelong mental health. Although these theorists use different words to designate life stages, their views of the importance of a solid, nurturing early life environment are similar. Early losses, maternal inconsistency, the giving and withholding of love by the caregiver, and various types of abuse are all explained as causative agents for depression.

Intrapsychic conflict

Intrapsychic conflict refers to the conflicts people have when they have mixed emotions about a behavior, event, or situation. For instance, an individual who has been brought up to refrain from sexual activity, but who also has strong urges to experience sex, has a conflict. To refrain from sexual activity increases sexual frustration; and to engage in sexual activity may cause anxiety, guilt, and fear. People are faced with intrapsychic conflicts all the time. Persistent unsuccessful resolution of these conflicts can lead to depression.

Reactions to life events

Most people view depression as a reaction to life stress. Loss is a major theme: of a loved one, of a job, of self-esteem, and of familiar surroundings. Reacting to loss with grief and sadness is normal; overreacting is abnormal. However, exactly when normal becomes abnormal is unclear. (See box titled "Dysfunctional Grief" below.)

| Dysfunctional Grief

If you live long enough you will experience grief—an intense but normal response to loss—typically the loss of someone very close to you. Typically, we think of grief as a reaction to death, but it can also be a reaction to divorce, relocation to another part of the country, terminal illness (e.g., anticipatory grief), or a natural disaster (Anonymous, 2002; Zeitlin, 2001). As noted, grief is normal. To lose someone close—for example, a mother, father, brother, sister, wife, husband, or child—and not experience grief is abnormal.

Typically, the grief response lasts about 6 months. People experiencing grief report a choking sensation, emptiness, shortness of breath, weakness, and sighing (Anonymous, 2002). They also use the term "waves" to verbalize how these feelings roll over them. After about 6 months, the grieving person begins to return to normal, but waves of grief can continue to occur for some time (Anonymous, 2002).

During my (NLK) teenage years (i.e., the early 60s) I was acquainted with an older woman in my hometown of Manteca, California. She had lost her only boy in World War II, and his photograph was displayed on her piano. Not often but on occasion, she would pick up his photograph and begin to cry. Twenty years later, she still experienced a wave of grief from time to time.

Dysfunctional grief is said to occur when these "symptoms" extend beyond 6 months. Zeitlin (2001) outlines the risk factors for dysfunctional grieving (p. 423):
1. History of psychiatric disorders
2. Ambivalent, overly close, or intense relationship with deceased
3. History of multiple, recent losses
4. Loss of a parent or a significant person during childhood
5. Lack of social support
6. Deaths by suicide, AIDS, murder, or other unexpected means

Differentiating grief and depression is not always simple, but the following guidelines can be useful (Anonymous, 2002, p. 19):

Grief	Depression
Natural response to death	An illness
Self-limited and improves with time	Persistent and can worsen
Responsive to social contacts	Burdened by social contacts
Rarely suicidal	Suicidal ideations common
Typically does not need antidepressants	Responsive to antidepressants

Anonymous: Coping with grief, *Psychiatr Serv* 53(1):19, 2002.
Zeitlin SV: Grief and bereavement, *Primary Care: Clinics in Office Practice* 28(2):415, 2001.

CLINICAL EXAMPLE

Elle Jones is a 45-year-old, well-educated, intelligent Caucasian woman who has been in and out of therapy for a long time (15 to 20 years). Elle grew up in northern Mississippi with two brothers and a very physically and emotionally abusive father. Elle reports that, when she was quite young, her mother left home and did not return for several years. Elle left home at age 17 and was married twice and divorced shortly after each marriage. She has a history of depression, and she attempted suicide 20 years ago. After many turbulent years, she started going to bars in hopes "that I might get killed." She refers to this period as her "death-hunt days." After emotional and financial collapse, Elle has recently returned to her father's home. He continues to control her life in every way. She has commented that her life is so futile that she would rather be dead.

ASSESSMENT OF DEPRESSION

Assessment of depression may be accomplished through both nonbiologic and biologic assessment methods. The DGP (1993) and Shuchter, Downs, and Zisook, (1996) recommend that patients be examined in a "profile" manner for an accurate diagnosis of depression. The profile should address DSM-IV-TR criteria and biologic findings, including:

1. History of onset of symptoms
2. Presence of co-morbid substance, alcohol, and medication use (Box 29-3)
3. Physical examination to rule out possibility of the presence of medical conditions (Box 29-4 provides a list of medical conditions)
4. The presence of nonmood psychiatric disorders
5. Patient resources and social support systems
6. Interpersonal and coping abilities
7. Level of stressors
8. Presence or level of suicidal ideation

Nurses can be instrumental in collecting all of this information because they are often the health care professionals who initially assess patients and develop the database for use in the general diagnostic and nursing processes.

Cultural Issues and Assessing Depression

Instrument selection is based on the nurse's clinical knowledge and experience, as well as on the age and mental capacity of the person being assessed. Unfortunately, only limited measures have been developed and "normed" for use in different ethnic, racial, and cultural groups (Jones, 1996). The lack of measurement specificity for these populations can lead to misdiagnosis or underdiagnosis. Because some researchers contend culturally competent measures

Box 29-3 | Drugs and Toxins that May Induce Depression

Analgesics	Antihypertensives	Antiparkinsonian Agents	Miscellaneous
Pentazocine	Alpha-methyldopa	Amantadine	Baclofen
	Calcium-channel	Levodopa	Choline
Antibiotics	blockers (possibly)		Cimetidine
Aminoglycosides	Clonidine	**Antituberculosis agents**	Disulfiram
Chloramphenicol	Hydralazine (possibly)	Isoniazid	Phenylephrine
Sulfonamides	Propranolol		Physostigmine
	Reserpine	**Cardiovascular agents**	
Anticonvulsants		Digitalis	**Psychotropic and Central Nervous**
Carbamazepine (rare)	**Antiinflammatory Agents**	Disopyramide	**System Agents**
Clonazepam	Corticosteroids	Procainamide	Aliphatic phenothiazines
Phenobarbital	Nonsteroidal antiinflam-		Amphetamines
Phenytoin	matory drugs		Appetite suppressants (fenfluramine,
Primidone			phenmetrazine)
Succinimide			Barbiturates
			Benzodiazepines
			High-potency neuroleptics

Adapted from Ford CV, Folks DG: Psychiatric disorders in geriatric medical/surgical patients. II. Review of clinical experience in consultation, *South Med J* 78(4):397, 1985.

|Box 29–4| Medical Illnesses Commonly Associated with Depression

Central Nervous System Disorders	**Toxic-Metabolic Disturbances and Endocrinopathies—cont'd**
Alzheimer's disease	Parathyroid disorders
Amyotrophic lateral sclerosis	Uremia
Brain tumor	
Cerebrovascular accident (stroke)	**Infections**
Chronic subdural hematoma	Acquired immunodeficiency syndrome
Multiple sclerosis	Encephalitis
Normal-pressure hydrocephalus	Hepatitis
Parkinson's disease	Infectious mononucleosis
Subarachnoid hemorrhage	Influenza
	Syphilis
Collagen Vascular Disease	Tuberculosis
Polymyalgia rheumatica	Viral pneumonia
Rheumatoid arthritis	
Systemic lupus erythematosus	**Neoplastic Disorders**
Temporal arteritis	Carcinoma of head of pancreas
	Chronic myelogenous leukemia
Toxic-Metabolic Disturbances and Endocrinopathies	Lymphoma
Addison's disease	Other malignant disease
Cushing's disease	Small-cell carcinoma of lung
Diabetes mellitus	
Electrolyte disorders	**Other**
Hypoglycemia	Chronic fatigue syndrome
Hypothyroidism	Chronic obstructive pulmonary disease
Metal intoxication	

Adapted from Ford CV, Folks DG: Psychiatric disorders in geriatric medical/surgical patients. II. Review of clinical experience in consultation, *South Med J* 78(4):397, 1985.

predict relevant criteria more accurately than do nonculturally competent measures, this assessment deficiency should be viewed as clinically significant. Routine review of cultural competence issues will facilitate accurate and valid assessment for all patients.

Culture is the internal and external manifestation of an individual, group, or community's beliefs, values, and norms that are used as premises for everyday functioning. Tseng and Streltzer (1997) recommend that clinicians distinguish between normal cultural behavior and psychopathology by using:

1. Cultural competence guidelines or a panel of experts or both (i.e., someone who understands the culture)
2. DSM-IV-TR criteria
3. A functional status measurement
4. The affected person's perception of self and what he or she considers "normal"

Assessment of Depression in Older Adults

Depression among older adults is a major health concern. The prevalence of MDD declines with age (probably <5%), but symptoms of depression

increase (Surgeon General, 1999). Depressive symptoms are relatively common, but because of the overlapping symptoms of physical illness and the depressive side effects of many medications, diagnosis is complex. To acquaint the nurse with potential confounding variables, a list of depression-causing medications and a list of illnesses that share symptoms with depression are presented (see Boxes 29-3 and 29-4, respectively). It should be noted that late life depressions (i.e., first depressive episode occurring in late life) are thought to be more likely associated with brain abnormalities rather than genetic or psychologic factors.

If the depression is related to a treatable medical illness, elimination of the illness often returns the depressed mood to normal. On the other hand, MDD and medical illness can coexist, and, in these cases, treatment needs to be instituted. The nurse should also be aware that some people who are diagnosed with dementia are, in reality, depressed (referred to as pseudodementia). Hence it is important to differentiate between depression and dementia. Again, depression and dementia can occur co-morbidly, in which case, both disorders must be treated. Co-morbid MDD and dementia tend to occur early in the course of Alzheimer's disease (DGP, 1993).

Finally, older adults are at increased risk of suicide. Men are at increased risk over women, with older Caucasian men having the highest risk of suicide in the United States. A discussion of suicide is presented at the end of this chapter.

Nonbiologic Assessment Measures of Depression

Nonbiologic assessments are composed of standardized verbal and pen-and-paper measurement scales. Obtained data can be used in conjunction with the DSM-IV-TR criteria and biologic assessments to give a more accurate diagnosis regarding MDD.

Biological Assessment Measures of Depression

Dexamethasone suppression test

Although not frequently ordered, the DST is a diagnostic test for MDD in adults that measures the function of the HPA axis. Urine and blood samples are collected before the test to determine baseline levels of cortisol. Then, a single injection of the drug dexamethasone is given to the patient. Urine and blood cortisol levels are monitored for 24 hours. A positive result occurs when cortisol levels do not fall (i.e., are not suppressed) or return to 5 µg/dl or above within 24 hours. Forty percent of severely depressed patients fail to suppress cortisol. The DST is not specific for depression because individuals suffering from dementia, alcohol withdrawal, and bulimia do not suppress either urine or blood cortisol levels.

Growth hormone assessment

Growth hormone secretion is often used as a biologic assessment measure in childhood depression. Past research has indicated that some depressed children may have decreased secretion of the growth hormone during the day and increased secretion while asleep. This test is not useful in adolescent and adult populations.

Polysomnographic measurements

Polysomnographic findings (i.e., examination of sleep patterns) are used to assess depression in adult populations. The REM stage usually begins within 70 to 100 minutes of a person falling asleep and increases in length throughout the night. However, in depressed adults, the REM latency phase is shortened, which results in frequent night and early morning wakening. Antidepressants can restore the normal pattern of REM sleep.

Psychotherapeutic Management

The nurse uses the nursing process to develop appropriate nursing interventions and strategies, expected outcomes, and evaluation of the outcomes for depressed patients. The intervention strategy described in this book, psychotherapeutic management, emphasizes the nurse-patient relationship, psychopharmacology, and milieu management. These concepts are discussed in detail in Units 3, 4, and 5, respectively. The case study and care plan presented in this section on depression are geared toward the nursing management of a depressed patient who is residing in a psychiatric hospital environment. However, it is important to realize that the majority of psychiatric patients, in the current managed care environment, are hospitalized for short periods or may not be hospitalized at all. Consequently, nursing management of depressed individuals may occur in medical settings or outpatient clinics. In addition, it is imperative that nurses in any setting be familiar with the DSM-IV-TR criteria of MDD and the information regarding mood disorders presented in this chapter. Finally, it is recommended that the reader refer to Chapter 39 for a detailed explanation of electroconvulsive therapy used in the treatment of depression.

Nurse-patient relationship

The objective of this section is to provide specific principles of therapeutic communication for nurses who work with depressed patients.

1. Depressed individuals suffer from low self-esteem. The most effective approach to bolster self-esteem is to accept patients as they are (negative attitude and all), to help them to focus on the positive (accomplishments, good points), to provide successful experiences with positive feedback, to keep self-help strategies simple, and to help patients avoid embarrassing social blunders (e.g., smelly clothes, unkempt appearance).
2. Development of a meaningful relationship in which depressed individuals are valued as human beings is important to their sense of

personal worth. It is important for the nurse to be honest and to work on developing trust. Doing specific things that are in the best interest of each patient develop the "trusting relationship." For instance, a patient may wish to tell the nurse something of clinical significance but does not want the nurse to share the information with other staff members. The nurse builds trust by telling the patient that significant information will be shared only with staff members who have a need to know. The patient learns to trust the nurse as a professional whose dominant concern is the patient's best interest.

3. The nurse who works effectively with depressed patients must have sincere concern for patients and be empathic. For instance, it is not unusual for a nurse to feel a little sad when working with depressed or suicidal patients. The nurse acknowledges the emotional pain and suffering conveyed by patients and offers to help patients work through the pain. It is important for the nurse to discuss personal feelings with a colleague.

4. It is usually not effective to outline logically why a patient is a worthwhile human being. The nurse does, however, point out even small visible accomplishments and strengths, for example, "I'm glad you combed your hair today." A patient may agree with everything the nurse says but may remain just as depressed. Intellectual understanding does not help severely depressed patients. Cognitive behavior therapists, however, have been successful in helping some depressed individuals learn to "reprogram" negative thoughts, for example, to progress from "I can't do anything right." to "I can learn from my mistakes."

5. Depressed individuals are typically dependent. The nurse may notice that he or she (i.e., the nurse) is taking on responsibility for the depression of patients. The nurse should recognize, but not resent, this tendency in depressed individuals to become dependent. The nurse should reward even small decisions and independent actions.

6. The nurse should not attempt to "embarrass" patients out of being depressed. For example, pointing out less fortunate people in the hope that such an action might bring depressed individuals to their senses provides, at best, short-lived relief based on the misfortune of others.

7. Never reinforce hallucinations, delusions, or irrational beliefs: the nurse cannot agree, and arguing seems to reinforce them. The nurse should state his or her perception of reality, voice doubt about the patient's perceptions, and move on to discuss real people and events.

8. Depressed individuals tend to be angry (Figure 29-2). Sometimes, they surprise even themselves with the hateful or hostile things that they say. It is important for the nurse to learn to handle hostility therapeutically by recognizing the anger, not taking it personally and not retaliating in word, deed, or some passive-aggressive form. Encouraging verbal expressions of anger helps release patients' tension.

9. The nurse can help withdrawn patients emerge from their social isolation by spending time with them (even without speaking) by providing a nonthreatening one-to-one relationship, by practicing assertiveness interactions, and by being accepting.

10. Depressed individuals can have difficulty in making even simple decisions. It is not therapeutic to badger patients into making a deci-

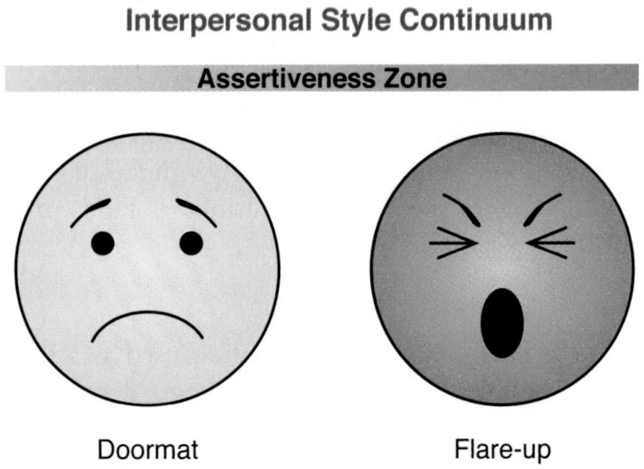

Interpersonal Style Continuum

Assertiveness Zone

Doormat   Flare-up

Figure 29-2 Depressed individuals often adopt an interpersonal style that causes them to be "doormats"—that is, they allow people to walk all over them. Sometimes the doormat personality will explode when they have had "too much." These outbursts are typically followed by even more recrimination and regret. The nurse can help the patients learn to avoid these extremes of interpersonal behavior by teaching them to use assertiveness techniques.

sion; but it is therapeutic to provide decision-making opportunities as patients are able to comply. Initially, the nurse may need to make decisions for patients, for example, "It is time for your bath"; "Here is your apple juice." When possible, the nurse helps guide patients to appropriate decisions by using problem-solving techniques, that is, identifying options, the advantages and disadvantages of each option, and the potential consequences of each decision. (A summary of key nursing interventions is found in the box below.)

Psychopharmacology

To understand the range of information required for effective psychopharmacologic intervention, the student is encouraged to review Chapter 21, which provides a complete discussion of antidepressant and antimanic drugs A brief review of critical parameters of antidepressant drug administration is given in Box 29-5 and in the side effects box on page 356.

Milieu management

Milieu management is an important dimension of the psychiatric nursing care of depressed patients. The student is referred to Unit Five for a complete discussion of milieu management. General principles that specifically address the environment of depressed patients include the following.

For patients with low self-esteem:

- Encourage patients with low self-esteem to participate in activities, including group activities, in which they will be able to experience accomplishment and receive positive feedback. Most people develop a sense of self-worth through mastery or accomplishment. Simply telling patients that they are "OK" is not convincing. Provide successful experiences, however small.
- Provide assertiveness training. Many depressed individuals feel like doormats because of their interactional problems; their communication history is typically a lifetime of being "taken advantage of," punctuated by periodic outbursts

Key Nursing Interventions   for Depressed Patients

The psychiatric nurse should consider the following intervention principles when working with depressed patients.

Intervention	Rationales
Accept patients where they are and focus on their strengths.	Depressed persons have low self-esteem, and this is the best approach to recapturing some sense of value.
Reinforce decision making by patients.	Depressed patients struggle to make even simple decisions. By reinforcing patients' efforts to make simple decisions, the nurse helps patients move toward health.
Never reinforce hallucinations or delusions.	Confronting these psychotic symptoms tends to reinforce them. The best approach is for the nurse to state his or her view of reality and to begin discussing real people and events.
Respond to anger therapeutically.	Depressed persons are typically angry. By understanding that anger is a symptom of depression, the nurse can focus on the issue at hand and help patients to move toward a more acceptable style of interaction.
Spend time with withdrawn patients.	Withdrawn patients are aware of their surroundings. By spending time (frequent but brief contact) with these patients, the nurse communicates patients' worth and, consequently, may be available during a time when patients feel comfortable with initiating dialogue.
Make decisions for patients that they are not ready to make for themselves.	Some patients cannot make a decision. Simply present situations to these patients that do not require decision making (e.g., "It's time to go for a walk").
Involve patients in activities in which they can experience success.	People can feel good about themselves in several ways. One way to develop self-worth is through accomplishment.

|Box 29-5| Important Points for Administering Antidepressant Drugs

- Most antidepressants have a lag time of 2 to 4 weeks before a full clinical effect occurs.
  1. During that time, patients gradually begin to feel better and have more energy.
  2. Suicidal tendencies may be increased because antidepressants increase energy and motivation.
- Monitor patients for "cheeking" or hoarding of drugs. At amounts not much greater than the therapeutic amount, TCAs become toxic.
- Monitor vital signs of patients who take TCAs and monoamine oxidase inhibitors (MAOIs).
  1. TCAs can cause orthostatic hypotension, reflex tachycardia, and arrhythmias.

  2. MAOIs have the potential for triggering a hypertensive crisis.
- Monitor sexual side effects of selective serotonin reuptake inhibitors (SSRIs) because they occur fairly frequently and lead to noncompliance.
- Be aware of the drug-drug and food-drug interactions associated with MAOIs.
- Observe for early signs of toxicity:
  1. TCAs. Drowsiness, tachycardia, mydriasis, hypotension, agitation, vomiting, confusion, fever, restlessness, sweating.
  2. MAOIs. Dizziness, vertigo, fatigue.
  3. SSRIs. Have low probability for causing toxicity.

Side Effects for Antidepressant Drugs

Antidepressants (TCAs, SSRIs)

Dry mouth
Nasal congestion
Urinary hesitancy
Urinary retention
Blurred vision
Constipation
Sedation, ataxia
Confusion
Orthostatic hypotension
Arrhythmias, tachycardia, palpitations
Decreased sweating

MAOIs

Overstimulation such as agitation, hypomania
Blurred vision, hypotension, dry mouth, constipation
Hypertensive crisis related to food-drug or drug-drug interactions

MAOIs, Monoamine oxidase inhibitors; *SSRIs,* selective serotonin reuptake inhibitors; *TCAs,* tricyclic antidepressant.

of anger when they become "fed up." Assertiveness training helps these patients learn to take care of their needs and to express their feelings along the way; thus the extremes of "doormat" and "flare-up" are avoided.

- Help patients avoid embarrassing themselves through socially unacceptable appearance or behavior. Many appearance problems are related directly to depressed individuals' preoccupation, apathy, and decreased energy level. For instance, food stains on clothes, food in one's beard, an unattended runny nose, uncombed hair, urine on trousers, and an unzipped fly may be seen among depressed individuals who "cannot" pay attention to these hygienic concerns. Help patients shower and dress appropriately. Remind patients to go to the bathroom. In some cases, it is better to encourage patients to walk with the nurse (e.g., to the bathroom area or to the shower).

For withdrawn patients:

- Keep contacts with withdrawn patients brief but frequent. Depressed patients often do not want anyone around or, at least, anyone to talk to them. Unfortunately, their wishes are not a good indicator of what should be done. Spending time with patients is constructive; allowing patients to isolate themselves is not. Patients may need to increase physical activity before they are able to verbalize issues.
- Many patients are insistent about going to their rooms to lie down. They may stay there all day if the nurse does not intervene. Locking a patient's room during the day may be required to keep the withdrawn or isolative patient from disappearing for hours at a time. Sitting in silence during an activity is better than ruminating in isolation.

For anorectic patients:

- The nursing staff must take responsibility for ensuring that depressed patients eat. It is irresponsible to set a tray down in front of a depressed person, particularly in his or her room, and then leave. The nurse must encourage patients to eat and may even spoon-feed them if required.

Case Study

Bill W. is a 35-year-old African-American man who has been in and out of mental health facilities for several years. Before his formal entrance into the mental health system, he had had several brushes with the law, primarily related to driving under the influence (DUI) of alcohol. It is thought that Bill was actually self-medicating with alcohol and with other substances long before he was able to admit he had a problem. One year after being diagnosed with major depression, Bill developed hepatitis B through sexual activity. Subsequent to this diagnosis, Bill attempted to kill himself on at least five occasions. During a brief period of his affliction with depression, he developed auditory hallucinations accusing him of being gay. Although this was a relatively brief episode and did not recur, Bill is very troubled by it, believing these hallucinations make him "certifiably crazy." Bill now lives with his widowed father who seems to be very pleased to have Bill "back home again." Bill continues to attend an outpatient program 3 days per week. He verbalizes wanting to go back to work but cannot seem to get moving. A long-standing fear of crowds and people remains. As Bill says, "I'm not out of the woods, but I am a lot better than I was."

Care Plan

Name: Bill W.   Admission Date: February 12, 2002

DSM-IV-TR Diagnosis: Major depression

Assessment

Areas of strength: Bill understands his disease, has a good relationship with his father, is financially stable, is willing to acknowledge his problems and work on them, and is motivated to go back to work.
Problems: Bill verbalizes motivation but seems "stuck"; he enjoys living with his father, but he is too dependent for a 35-year-old man; he continues to be intimidated by crowds and people and has a suicidal history.

Diagnoses

• Risk for self-injury related to depression as evidenced by history of suicide attempts.
• Social isolation related to anxiety, as evidenced by withdrawal from people and uncommunicative behavior.

Outcomes

Short-term goals: *Date met*
• Learn and develop coping skills for dealing with other patients at mental health treatment program.   _____
• Participate in class activities at the mental health center.   _____
• Develop socialization skills.   _____
• Continue to comply with medication regimen.   _____
Long-term goals:
• Seek out information about jobs at his skill level.   _____
• Practice coping skills learned at mental health center in public areas.   _____
• Make steps to return to a more independent lifestyle.   _____

Planning/ Interventions

Nurse-patient relationship: Develop a trusting relationship based on honesty and genuine concern for the patient. Spend time with him, and reinforce his strengths and accomplishments. Help patient develop coping skills, and work with him to obtain job information.
Psychopharmacology: Risperidone 3 mg qd; sertraline 50 mg qd; alprazolam 1 mg tid.
Milieu management: Minimize patient's tendency to isolate himself by encouraging social interaction. As tolerated, draw patient into group situations. Keep environment safe, should patient attempt self-injury.

Evaluation

Patient is doing better but still tends to avoid large groups of people. He is compliant with medications, and no psychotic behavior has been observed or reported.

Referrals

Patient is a candidate for a mental health system sponsored apartment in the near future.

- Allow patients to participate in selecting preferred foods from the menu.
- Promote a proper diet, adequate fluids, and exercise. Provide small, frequent meals. Record intake.
- Constipation is a side effect not only of antidepressants, but also of depression. A diet with adequate fiber content and sufficient fluids is important. Monitoring and recording bowel elimination is also important.
- If patients will eat food brought from home, permit them to do so.

For patients with sleep disturbances:

- Depressed individuals want to sleep, but many suffer from insomnia. The tremendous fatigue is real to these patients because the sleep they manage to get is usually not restful. Patients often wake up looking and feeling exhausted. The nursing staff should record the amount and quality of patients' actual sleep. Patients who lie down during the day are not necessarily sleeping but may be isolating themselves. An accurate understanding of the amount of sleep being obtained helps the nurse formulate an intervention strategy.
- For patients taking a sedating tricyclic antidepressant (TCA), combining the daily dose into a single bedtime dose is known to decrease daytime sedation.

 Family Issues | Living with the Depressed Person

Living with a depressed mother

Living with a depressed person can be very difficult. The person is often irritable, moody, isolative, and pessimistic. Family members may struggle to get along with the person, co-workers may find the person impossible to please, and children may assume responsibility for their depressed parent's mood. Grunebaum and Cohler (1983) found that children of depressed mothers were more vulnerable to emotional problems than children of mothers with schizophrenia. Schizophrenia, they suggested, is exhibited in such a clearly abnormal fashion that children can recognize the parent as mentally disturbed (i.e., this behavior is abnormal, this behavior is normal). This level of insight affords some degree of emotional insulation from the parent's disruptive behavior. Grunebaum and Cohler further reasoned that because the depressed parent is not clearly "abnormal" but rather basically unhappy, moody, sad, and irritable, children are less able to set these boundaries. Hence, living with a depressed parent can trigger emotional insecurity and self-doubt and cause a myriad of intrafamilial communication problems. Two brief clinical examples follow to illustrate the difficulties encountered in families with depressed individuals.

Living with a depressed wife

Joan is a 40-year-old college professor. She has been married for 15 years and has two children, a 13-year-old daughter and an 11-year-old son. Joan admits to a few close friends and to her husband that she is depressed. She has never "officially" sought help for her depression, but her physician has ordered a TCA at bedtime for "sleep." The problems her family faces that are related to her depressed mood are subtle but beginning to take their toll. Joan is never happy nor can she become excited about anything the family does together. She spends much of her time at home either soaking in the bathtub or in her bedroom reading. She seems to have energy for her research at the university, but for little else. She resents her husband for many things; some are real, others are not. She is often critical of her daughter and then feels remorseful. Joan has great difficulty talking with her family. Her husband, also a professional, realizes that something is wrong, but he is losing patience with his wife. He perceives her lack of interest in sex or even talking with him as signs of a failing marriage. What is not clear is whether the failing marriage precipitated Joan's depressed mood (a reactive depression), whether Joan's depressed mood is causing the marriage to fail (an endogenous depression), or whether there is a synergistic combination of the two.

Living with a depressed husband

Tom is a 60-year-old white man who has been hospitalized numerous times over the years for depression. He has not worked for over 12 years. The past 6 years have been punctuated with threats of suicide and suicidal gestures. He talks about suicide often and has taken out a gun at home on several occasions while talking about killing himself. Tom is the father of four children, three boys and a girl, ages 15 to 32 years. Three children still live at home. Judy, his wife of 35 years, does not know what to do. When Tom's "suicide talk" becomes "serious," she either takes him to the hospital or calls the sheriff's office. The hospital staff, sheriff's deputies, children, Judy, and even Tom are tired of these frequent emergencies. Every time Judy leaves the house and returns, she admits to a fear of finding Tom dead. She is angry with Tom, but she keeps her feelings to herself, for fear of precipitating a suicide attempt. The children living at home become very anxious if they do not see their father as soon as they return from school each day. Judy states that she feels like a prisoner in her own home and cannot take it anymore.

- People suffering from insomnia often engage in self-defeating behaviors, such as daytime napping and drinking stimulants (e.g., coffee, colas). Eliminating these behaviors increases the likelihood of nighttime sleep.
- Depressed patients who sleep too much (hypersomnia) should have restricted access to their rooms. The goal of working with patients who cannot sleep or who sleep too much is adequate rest (6 to 8 hours per night). Activities can be substituted for daytime sleeping. Exercise often increases energy levels.

Critical Thinking Questions

Do you think physicians have the right to help terminally ill patients end their lives? Should adults in their right minds be allowed to commit suicide?

SUICIDE AND DEPRESSION

Suicide is a complex phenomenon influenced by a person's cultural beliefs, values, and norms. Suicide may occur in children, adolescent, and adult populations. Nurses need to assess the following:

Suicidal ideation level: suicidal ideation includes a person's thoughts regarding suicide, as well as suicidal gestures and threats.

Suicidal gestures: suicidal gestures are a person's nonlethal self-injury acts, including cutting or burning of skin areas or ingesting small amounts of drugs. Others often see these gestures as "attention-getting" measures and do not consider them serious problems that may lead to a suicide attempt or completion.

Suicidal threats: suicidal threats are a person's verbal statements that may declare their intent to commit suicide. Threats often precede an actual suicidal attempt.

Patient and Family Education

Depression

Illness:

Depression is a life-altering process or state. Depression may be precipitated by overwhelming life stresses including loss (e.g., divorce, death, job), medications, medical illnesses, and specific chemical deficiencies in the brain. These precipitating factors are not mutually exclusive and may interact to produce depression. For example, it is thought that chronic exposure to intense stress can alter brain chemistry. Support for the chemical-deficiency view has increased over the last two decades because medications known to relieve and correct depressive states correct the chemical deficiencies previously noted. Nine cardinal symptoms define depression: depressed mood, apathy, changes in weight, sleep disturbances, movement disturbances, lack of energy, sense of worthlessness, inability to concentrate, and thoughts of death. An individual with a majority of these symptoms (depressed mood or apathy must always be present) should be diagnosed as suffering from depression.

Medications:

1. The most popular antidepressants are the SSRIs. Well-known drugs in this category include Prozac, Zoloft, Paxil, and Celexa. These drugs are effective and have few side effects. However, sexual dysfunction, defined as a loss of interest in sex or the inability to perform sexually, is quite common and disturbing to many patients. This side effect moves some patients to stop taking their SSRI. Fortunately, other medications can be added that may restore sexual vitality, (e.g., Wellbutrin, Viagra).
2. An older group of medication, referred to as TCAs is still commonly prescribed (e.g., Elavil, Pamelor, Norpramin). Although they have a higher rate of side effects than do the SSRIs, the TCAs are as effective and are considerably less expensive. The most common side effects are a drop in blood pressure when standing, dry mouth, constipation, and a racing heart (at times).
3. A number of newer and very promising agents are now available (e.g., Wellbutrin, Effexor, Remeron). All these drugs seem to be effective and cause fewer side effects for most people.

Other issues:

It is easy to be angry with a depressed person—to wonder why that person simply cannot "snap out of it." If a family member feels this way, it may help to compare the situation to someone with diabetes. Individuals with diabetes have a reduced level of insulin. They cannot just snap out of it. A depressed person with changed levels of brain chemicals cannot just snap out of it either. On the other hand, just as the person with diabetes is not powerless, neither is the person who is depressed. For instance, individuals with diabetes who will not adhere to a diabetic diet or take medications as prescribed can make their conditions worse. So, too, the individual with depression may need to avoid certain substances, associations, and situations.

SSRIs, Selective serotonin reuptake inhibitors; *TCAs,* tricyclic antidepressants.

Suicidal attempt: suicidal attempts are the actual implementation of a self-injurious act with the express purpose of ending the person's life.

Suicide is a significant cause of death: it is the ninth leading cause of death in the United States (Pearson, 1998) and is among the three leading causes of death for people aged 15 to 34 years (Mann, 1998). The overall ratio of attempted to complete suicide is approximately 7:1 (USDHHS, 1993b). The annual number of suicides in this country is about 11 per 100,000, or roughly 30,000 individuals (Center for Disease Control and Prevention [CDC], 2000).

The prototypical suicide victim is an unemployed male Caucasian, living alone, who has made a serious suicide attempt in the past. Men are four times as likely as are women, and Caucasians are twice as likely as are African Americans, to complete a suicide attempt successfully (Cugino et al, 1992; News and Notes, 1994). Over 70% of all suicides are committed by Caucasian men (Pearson, 1998).

The overall suicide rate for the general adult population in the United States is high, but it is still considerably lower than it is for people with psychiatric disorders. Psychiatric diagnosis is the most reliable risk factor for suicide. Approximately 90% of all suicides are committed by individuals with a diagnosable mental or substance abuse disorder. It is estimated that, over a period of 10 to 15 years, 10% to 15% of all patients with depression, schizophrenia, or alcoholism will die by suicide. Table 29-2 compares the suicide rates by diagnostic entity of the general population with those for mentally disordered individuals (Clark et al, 1987). Box 29-6 provides a list of other risk factors that have been related empirically to suicide (DHHS, 1993b).

Critical Thinking Question
Why do you think the prevalence of suicide is higher in Caucasians than it is in other races?

The death by suicide of psychiatric patients is of particular importance to the nurse because of opportunities for assessment and intervention. The psychiatric nurse must continually assess for suicide potential among all patients, but especially among schizophrenic, depressed, and alcoholic patients.

Although there are separate suicide rates for schizophrenics, the depressed, and alcoholics, Hendin

Table 29-2 Clinical Risk Factors for Suicide in the United States

Population	Suicides per 100,000
Adult general public	<20
Schizophrenic	140
Depressed	230
Alcoholic	270

Box 29-6 Risk Factors of Completed Suicide

Hopelessness
General medical illness
Severe anhedonia
Male
Caucasian and Native American
Living alone
Prior suicide attempts
Age 60 and older
Unemployed or financial problems

(1986) points out that, when schizophrenic individuals kill themselves, they are typically in a depressed phase, and the act typically is not a product of psychosis. Alcoholics kill themselves usually in response to loss (e.g., divorce, separation, being fired) and when they have been drinking. Hendin makes the point that suicide most often is the result of depression, diagnosed or not.

The major themes of suicidal patients are loss, unbearable psychic pain, helplessness, hopelessness, loneliness, and abandonment ("nobody cares"). These themes complement the common suicidal expressions of a loss of self-esteem, a cry for help, or suicide as a threat (Box 29-7 provides a more complete list of suicidal expressions). Hendin (1986) underscores that suicidal patients view and use death differently than do other people. Suicidal patients tend to use their own death to control others and to maintain control over their own lives. Hence, death is viewed as a means of ensuring control.

Suicide and Older Adults

The suicide rate for the general population is 11 per 100,000 (CDC, 1999). The rate for men over age 65 is 28.8 per 100,000; for white men over age 85, the rate is 65 per 100,000 (CDC, 2000; News and Notes, 1994). This age group has a high attempt-to-completion ratio that is accounted for probably by

| Box 29-7 | Common Expressions of Suicidal Individuals

Cry for help	Admission of inability to handle problem.
Escape	"I can't put up with this mess any longer" (especially with embarrassing or traumatic situations).
Heroic	To gain respect; some cultures view suicide as a manly alternative to failure; occasionally a male patient who is ambivalent about suicide has been taunted into showing he is a real man.
Loss of self-esteem	Failure in an area of great personal investment.
Manipulation	This is a coercive measure. "You had better come back to me or I will kill myself." An attempt to control.
Martyrdom	"Nobody cares about me. Everyone would be better off without me."
Rebirth	Fantasy of getting a new start in life. "Heaven has got to be better than this."
Redemption	An attempt to make up for some wrong; for example, a man responsible for the death of a child might kill himself.
Relief of pain	"I can't stand the pain (emotional or physical) any longer" (especially with terminal illness).
Retaliatory	Suicide is viewed as getting even. "I'll show them."
Reunion	Joining a loved one in heaven. "I can't live without her."

the seriousness of the intent and the lethality of the means (Mellick, Buckwalter, Stolley, 1992). Whereas the general attempt-to-completion ratio is 7:1, in older adults, the ratio is 2:1 (Gomez, Gomez, 1993). Although the upsurge in recent years of suicide among the young has resulted in much media coverage, the suicide rate among older adults is more widespread. Young people may use the suicide gesture as a cry for help; older people may just want to die, and they often do.

Assessment of Suicidal Patients

It is important for the nurse to assess the suicidal potential of psychiatric patients because these patients are at an increased risk of suicide. Most facilities provide the nurse with a format for evalu-ating suicidal lethality. The crucial variables are the plan, the method, and the provision for rescue.

Plan

The more developed the plan is, the greater the risk will be of suicide. People who have carefully developed a suicidal plan are more serious about suicide and present a greater risk compared with those who have no plan. Although impulsive suicide attempts can result in death, they are generally less often lethal because the lack of planning sometimes foils the effort.

Method

Some methods of attempting suicide are more lethal than are others. Accessibility of the means to commit suicide is important as well. Having three bottles of pills on hand is more lethal compared with having to make an appointment with a doctor to ask for a prescription. A crucial factor in determining the lethality of a particular method is the amount of time between initiation of the suicide method and delivery of the lethal impact of that method. For instance, the person using a gun has no opportunity to avoid the bullet once the trigger is pulled. On the other hand, sitting in the garage with the motor running affords some time to choose an alternative to self-destruction, as does taking an overdose of certain drugs. Lethal methods of suicide include the use of guns, jumping from high places, hanging, drowning, carbon monoxide poisoning, and overdose with certain drugs (e.g., barbiturates, alcohol, several central nervous system depressants). Methods that are less likely to be lethal include wrist cutting and overdosing on aspirin or Valium.

Rescue

The person who deliberately attempts to deceive would-be rescuers has an increased lethality potential. For instance, a woman who says she is going to the ocean for the weekend and then drives to the mountains makes it difficult for family and friends to intervene. A person who leaves a note or makes a telephone call before making an attempt is more likely to be rescued.

In summary, the more detailed the plan is, the more lethal and accessible the method is, and the more effort that is exerted to block rescue, the greater the likelihood will be of the suicidal effort being successful. However, impulsive efforts of suicidal individuals with rescuers in sight have proved fatal, particularly when a lethal method (e.g., a gun) has been selected.

Suicide Interventions

Face-to-face

In working face-to-face with suicidal patients, several general guidelines are useful to the nurse.

1. Suspect suicidal ideation in most depressed patients (DHHS, 1993b).
2. Ask patients if they plan to hurt themselves. It is important for the nurse to understand the following:
   a. Talking to patients about their suicidal intentions will not drive them to suicide. Asking patients directly provides useful information and often provides patients with a sense of relief, for example, "Finally, someone hears me."
   b. Many people who have died from suicide did not mean to die; they tragically miscalculated. It can be said accurately that many people who die from suicide do so accidentally. The nurse must take all suicidal threats seriously.
3. If a patient is considering suicide, the nurse should ask about the plan (when and where), method, and how the patient intends to accomplish the suicide. (Is the plan to frustrate rescue attempts?) If the patient wants to use a gun, ask someone at the patient's home to remove the gun. If the patient plans to overdose, ask someone in the home to throw away the pills. Do not offer a weekend pass to this patient. Some clinicians believe that if the method of choice can be blocked, many suicidal patients will not use another method. For example, a woman who might use a drug overdose would not consider jumping off a building.
4. Ask about previous suicide attempts. Ask about the "when" and the "how." How did the patient feel concerning rescue? How was the response to treatment? Previous attempts put individuals at an increased risk.
5. Evaluate patients for depression, recent loss or threat of loss, self-destructive hallucinations, and alcohol or drug use, all of which place individuals at an increased risk for suicide.

6. Once patients are hospitalized, many units protect them by using one of two levels of suicide prevention:
   a. Level 1 is used for patients who are not considered to be at immediate risk of suicide. The nursing staff provides periodic observation (every 10 minutes) and monitors drug taking, eating utensils, shaving gear, and other potentially dangerous devices in the environment. The staff communicates concern and control with this close observation of patients and their environment. Patients are asked to sign a contract with the staff stating that they will not harm themselves during hospitalization and will seek out a staff member should they begin to contemplate self-injurious behavior. Clinicians are divided in their view of the efficacy of "no-suicide" contracts (Valente, 1997).
   b. Level 2 is used for patients who present an immediate and serious threat of suicidal behavior. Level 2 also may be initiated for patients who refuse to sign a "no-suicide" contract. Restraints may be used occasionally, as can neuroleptic drugs. Continuous observation is typically required. This approach is an expensive use of manpower but provides the needed control and human interaction. Patients at serious risk are usually confined to the unit and have restrictions on visitors, where meals are taken, and so on. Harmful objects are removed from the environment.

Over the telephone

Former patients frequently call the psychiatric unit or outpatient clinic in which psychiatric nurses work. Helpful guidelines for nurses who work with suicidal individuals over the telephone are as follows (Green, Wilson, 1988).

1. Express genuine concern and a desire to work with callers. ("Let's see what we can do.") Give callers your full attention.
2. Acknowledge how difficult and painful recent losses must be. ("It's been a tough time for you lately.")
3. Assess lethality, especially if the suicidal attempt has begun.

4. Focus on the healthy side of callers. ("You called for help. That tells me you want help, and that's what we want to do.")
5. Ask about alcohol or drug use. If present, these substances increase the lethality level.
6. Ask callers for their ideas about immediate solutions to the current situation. Assess feasibility, appropriateness, and availability. Suggest alternatives if needed.
7. Obtain each caller's name, telephone number, address, and whereabouts during the call. Ask callers how they want to be addressed. ("Your name is Mr. Robert Smith. What would you like for me to call you?")
8. If other staff members are available, the nurse may need to direct them to notify the police or send an ambulance. Ask for consent to do so, or, at least, inform the caller of the plan.
9. Ask if anyone is with the caller. If someone is present, ask to speak to that person to obtain assistance in planning instructions.
10. If family members can be reached, they should be asked to go to the caller and intervene if it is safe to do so (ask for caller consent).
11. Refer callers to walk-in crisis services or a regular outpatient counselor.
12. If a caller refuses further help, give the telephone number of a crisis center or a suicide-prevention hotline.

Key Concepts

1. Major depression and dysthymia are the most significant depressive disorders.
2. The DSM-IV-TR defines major depression as an episode of depression (apathy, weight changes, sleep changes, psychomotor changes, fatigue, feelings of worthlessness or guilt, decreased cognitive ability, and recurrent thoughts of death) without a history of manic episodes.
3. Dysthymia is characterized by its chronicity.
4. Reacting to a disappointment or loss with sadness, guilt, or "depression" is normal; however, if any of these reactions persist too long, then a diagnosable condition (either dysthymia or major depression) exists.
5. A high correlation exists between depression and suicide.
6. There are several variants of major depression, including atypical depression, melancholic depres-

sion, catatonic depression, postpartum depression, psychotic depression, and seasonal depression.
7. Depression is common in the United States. Women have a lifetime risk of 10% to 20%. Men have a lifetime risk of about 5% to 10%.
8. A number of early life traumas are associated with depression in children.
9. People from different ethnic and cultural groups may experience depression differently.
10. Objective signs of depression include alterations in activity and social interactions.
11. Subjective symptoms of depression include alterations in affect, cognition, physical nature (somatic concern), and perception.
12. Biologic explanations for depression include neurotransmitter, genetic, endocrine, and circadian rhythms dysfunctions. Psychodynamic explanations concern debilitating early life experiences, intrapsychic conflicts, and reaction to life events.
13. Assessment of depression includes consideration of cultural influences, age (older adults are particularly vulnerable), nonbiologic standardized tests, and biologic indices (DST, growth hormone tests, and polysomnography).
14. Psychotherapeutic management includes developing a therapeutic nurse-patient relationship, administering antidepressant drugs when appropriate, and providing a well-managed milieu with particular emphasis on safety.
15. The psychiatric nurse should suspect suicidal ideation in most depressed patients because suicide is a prevalent theme among this population.
16. The prototypical suicide victim is an unemployed, Caucasian man living alone. Over 70% of all suicides are committed by Caucasian men. Elderly men are at particularly high risk.
17. In assessing the lethality of suicide consider the plan, the method, and the prevention of rescue.
18. It is important to ask depressed patients if they are contemplating suicide. Asking this question will not drive the patient to suicide.
19. Psychiatric inpatient units typically have two levels of "suicide contracts." Level 1 usually involves checking on the patient every 10 minutes. Level 2 usually involves continuous direct observation of the patient.
20. Both face-to-face and telephone strategies are important for the nurse to use in working with suicidal patients.

References

Abramson LY, Seligman ME, Teasdale JD: Learned helplessness in humans: critique and reformulation, *J Abnorm Psychol* 87:48, 1978.

American Psychiatric Association: *Diagnostic and statistical manual of mental disorders, text revision,* ed 4, Washington, DC, 2001, The Association.

American Psychiatric Association: Practice guidelines for major depressive disorder in adults, *Am J Psychiatry* (supplement) 150(4):1, 1993.

Beck AT: *Depression: causes and treatment,* Philadelphia, 1991, University Press.

Beck AT et al: *Cognitive therapy of depression,* New York, 1979, Guilford.

Beeber LS: Depression in women. In McBride AB, Austin JS, editors: *Psychiatric mental-health nursing: integrating the behavioral and biological sciences,* Philadelphia, 1996, WB Saunders.

Belcher JVR, Holdcraft C: Web-based information for depression: helpful or hazardous? *J Am Psychiatric Assoc* 7(3):61, 2001.

Bourdan KH et al: Estimating the prevalence of mental disorders in US adults from the Epidemiological Catchment Area Survey, *Public Health Rep* 107(6):663, 1992.

Buysse DJ et al: Do ECG sleep studies predict reoccurrence in depressive patients treated with psychotherapy? *Depression* 2:105, 1994.

Cartwright RD, Lloyd SR: Early REM sleep: a compensatory change in depression, *Psychiatry Res* 51:245, 1994.

Centers for Disease Control and Prevention: *Suicide and suicidal behavior: fact book for year 2000.* www.CDCgov/ncipc/pub-res/FactBook/Suicide/HTM accessed 5/3/02.

Clark DC et al: A field test of Motto's risk estimator for suicide, *Am J Psychiatry* 144:923, 1987.

Cockerman WC: *Sociology of mental disorder,* ed 3, Englewood Cliffs, NJ, 1992, Prentice-Hall.

Cugino A et al: Searching for a pattern: repeat suicide attempts, *J Psychosoc Nurs Ment Health Serv* 30(3):2326, 1992.

Depression Guideline Panel: *Depression in primary care. Detection and diagnosis,* vol 1, DHHS Pub No 93-0550, Washington, DC, 1993, US Government Printing Office.

Dubovsky SL: Beyond the serotonin reuptake inhibitors: rationales for the development of new serotonergic agents, *J Clin Psychiatry* 55(suppl 2):34, 1994.

Ford CV, Folks DG: Psychiatric disorders in geriatric medical/surgical patients. II. Review of clinical experience in consultation, *South Med J* 78(4):397, 1985.

Freud S: *Mourning and melancholia,* standard ed, vol 14, London, 1957, Hogarth Press.

Gomez GE, Gomez EA: Depression in the elderly, *J Psychosoc Nurs Ment Health Serv* 31(5):28, 1993.

Green LW, Wilson CR: Guidelines for nonprofessionals who receive suicidal phone calls, *Hosp Community Psychiatry* 39:310, 1988.

Grunebaum H, Cohler B: Children of parents hospitalized for mental illness. I. Attentional and interactional studies. In Frank M, editor: *Children of exceptional parents,* New York, 1983, Haworth.

Hendin H: Suicide: a review of new directions in research, *Hosp Community Psychiatry* 37:148, 1986.

Hirschfeld RMA, Russell JM: A synopsis of the assessment and treatment of suicidal patients, *Decade of the Brain* 8(4):7, 1998.

Horwath EM et al: What are the public implications of subclinical depressive symptoms? *Psychiatr Q* 65(4):323, 1994.

Jones RL editor: *Handbook of tests and measurements for black populations,* vols 1, 2, Hampton, Va, 1996, Cobb & Henry.

Kahan BB: Not just another stage, *Insight* 14(2):7, 1993.

Keltner NL: Mechanisms of antidepressant action: in brief, *Pers Psychiatric Care* 36(2):69, 2000b.

Keltner NL: Neuroreceptor function and psychopharmacologic response, *Issues in Ment Health Nurs* 21:31, 2000a.

Keltner NL et al: Adrenergic, cholinergic, GABAergic, and glutaminergic receptor function in the CNS, *Pers Psychiatric Care* 37(4):140, 2001.

Keltner NL et al: *Psychobiological foundations of psychiatric care,* St Louis, 1998, Mosby.

Keltner NL, Hogan B, Guy DM: Dopaminergic and serotonergic receptor function in the CNS, *Pers Psychiatric Care* 37(2):65, 2001a.

Kendler KS et al: The lifetime history of major depression, *Arch Gen Psychiatry* 50:863, 1993.

Kennedy R, Suttenfeld K: Postpartum depression, *Medscape Ment Health* 6(4):1, 2001.

Kessler RC et al: Lifetime and 12-month prevalence of DSM-III-R psychiatric disorders in the United States: results from the national comorbidity survey, *Arch Gen Psychiatry* 51:8, 1994.

Killeen MR, Bongarten CF: Caring for depressed children and adolescents. In McBride AB, Austin JS, editors: *Psychiatric mental-health nursing: integrating the behavioral and biological sciences,* Philadelphia, 1996, WB Saunders.

Klerman GL: Overview of affective disorders. In Kaplan HI, Freedman AM, Sadock BJ, editors: *Comprehensive textbook of psychiatry III,* vol 2, Baltimore, 1980, Williams & Wilkins.

Klerman GL: The interpersonal model. In Mann JJ, editor: *Models of depressive disorders,* New York, 1989, Plenum Press.

Maes M et al: A further investigation of basal HPT axis function in unipolar depression: effects of diagnosis, hospitalization, and dexamethasone administration, *Psychiatry Res* 51:185, 1994.

Mahendra B: *Depression: the disorder and its associations,* Boston, 1986, MTP Press Limited.

Mann JJ: Brain biology influences the risk for suicide. The decade of the brain, Arlington, Va, *NAMI* 8(4):3, 1998.

McEnany GW: *Neuropsychiatric disorders: dementia versus depression versus drug intoxication.* Invited paper presented at Contemporary Forums Tenth Anniversary Conference on Psychiatric Nursing, Boston, May 1995a.

McEnany GW: *Restless nights: understanding and treating sleep disturbances.* Invited paper presented at Contemporary Forums Tenth Anniversary Conference on Psychiatric Nursing, Boston, May 1995b.

McGrath E et al: *Women and depression: risk factors and treatment issues,* Washington, DC, 1992, American Psychological Association.

Mellick E, Buckwalter KC, Stolley JM: Suicide among elderly white men: development of a profile, *J Psychosoc Nurs Ment Health Serv* 30(2):29, 1992.

Metcalfe M: The personality of depressive patients. In Coppen A, Walk A, editors: *The psychology of depression: contemporary therapy and research,* New York, 1974, John Wiley & Sons.

National Institute of Mental Health: *Depression information.* [Online] Available at: www.nimh.nih.golv/publicat/depression-menu.cfm. Accessed October 11, 2001.

Nemeroff CB: The neurobiology of depression, *Sci Amer* 278(6):42, 1998.

News and Notes: Cost of depression estimated at nearly $44 billion: time lost from work accounts for largest share, *Hosp Community Psychiatry* 45(1):85, 1994.

Pearson J: Suicide in the United States, the decade of the brain, Arlington, VA. *NAMI* (8)4:1, 1998.

Regier DA et al: The de facto US mental and addictive disorders service system: epidemiologic catchment area prospective 1-year prevalence rates of disorders and services, *Arch Gen Psychiatry* 50:85, 1993.

Schreiber R: Wandering in the dark: women's experiences with depression, *Health Care Women Intl* 22:85, 2001.

Shuchter SR, Downs N, Zisook S: *Biologically informed psychotherapy for depression,* New York, 1996, Guilford Press.

Surgeon General: *Mental health: a report of the Surgeon General.* Depart-ment of Health and Human Services, Washington, DC, 1999.

Tseng W, Streltzer J: *Culture and psychopathology: a guide to clinical assessment,* New York, 1997, Brunner/Mazel, Inc.

US Department of Health and Human Services: Depression in primary care: detection, diagnosis, and treatment, *J Psychosoc Nurs Ment Health Serv* 31(6):19, 1993a.

US Department of Health and Human Services: *Depression in primary care, treatment of major depression,* vol 2, Washington, DC, 1993b, USDHHS.

Valente SM: Preventing suicide among elderly people, *Am J Nurse Pract* 1(4):15, 1997.

Venarec E: Depression in the workforce. Part I, *Business Health* 4:48, 2000.

Warren BJ: Depression, stressful life events, social support, and self-esteem in middle class African American women, *Arch Psychiatr Nurs* 11(3):107, 1997.

Weiss KJ, Valdiserri EV, Dubin WR: Understanding depression in schizophrenia, *Hosp Community Psychiatry* 40:849, 1989.

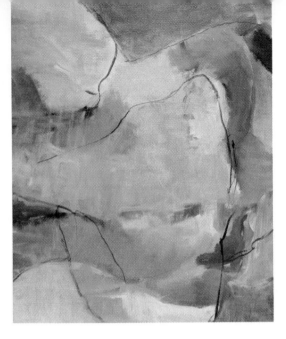

Chapter 30

Bipolar Disorders

Norman L. Keltner

Learning Objectives

After reading this chapter, you should be able to:

- Recognize the DSM-IV-TR criteria and terminology for bipolar disorder.
- Describe the objective and subjective symptoms of bipolar disorder.
- Explain the biologic and psychodynamic hypotheses for bipolar disorder.

- Describe the psychotherapeutic management issues related to bipolar disorder.
- Formulate a nursing care plan for bipolar disorder using the psychotherapeutic management model.

Bipolar disorder is a recurrent mood disorder in which one or more episodes of mania or mixed episodes of mania and depression occur (Surgeon General, 1999). Bipolar disorders are classified in *The Diagnostic and Statistical Manual of Mental Disorders-Fourth Edition-Text Revision* (DSM-IV-TR) as bipolar I, bipolar II, cyclothymic disorder, and bipolar disorder not otherwise specified (NOS) (American Psychiatric Association [APA], 2000).

GENERAL DESCRIPTION OF BIPOLAR DISORDER

Bipolar disorders are those in which individuals experience the extremes of mood polarity. Individuals may feel very euphoric or very depressed (Box 30-1). Bipolar disorder can be traced from earliest recorded history to the present day. Thousands of years ago, the Greeks recognized the vacillation

between extremes of elation and depression. Other people have also observed and recorded wide mood swings for the historic record. Although the term bipolar disorder is the accepted diagnostic terminology, many professionals, and much professional literature, still use the terms manic-depressive or bipolar affective disorder. Accordingly, the terms are used somewhat interchangeably in this chapter.

Epidemiologic research indicates that approximately 2 million women and men experience bipolar disorder yearly (or about 1.2% of the adult population; see table titled "12-Month Prevalence Rate of Mental Disorders in the United States"). Approximately 1.6% of the population will have this mental disorder at some point during their lifetime (APA, 2000; Kessler et al, 1994). Onset tends to be in the early 20s, and for 90% of these individuals, symptoms will be recurrent. Bipolar I disorders

Key Terms

Affect Individual's external response to changing states of mood.

Bipolar disorder Disturbance in mood in which the symptoms of mania have occurred at least one time. An episode of depression may or may not occur.

Cyclothymia Mood swing that alternates between hypomania and depression (but not major depression).

Euphoria Subjective, exaggerated feeling of well being characterized by confidence, elation, and assurance.

Hypomania Milder form of mania that is less intense and severe than mania.

Insomnia Inability to sleep or disrupted sleep patterns.

Labile affect Unstable or readily changeable affect.

Mania Individual's state of extreme or exaggerated excitement and euphoria that results in accelerated mental and physical activity.

Mood Individual's internal state of mind that is exhibited through feelings and emotions.

Mood disorder Disorder in which the predominant feature is the disturbance or alteration in a person's mood.

Mood disorder caused by a general medical condition Disorder resulting in a disturbance or alteration of a person's mood that is the result of a specific medical or physiologic consequence.

Substance-induced mood disorder Disorder resulting from the disturbance or alteration of a person's mood that is a result of the ingestion of a prescribed or nonprescribed drug or medication or exposure to a toxic substance.

---

appear to be equally common among men and women but with evidence of a difference in order of expression. In men, the first episode is more likely to be a manic episode, but for both women and men, depression is more likely to be experienced first (APA, 2002). There are no reports of differential incidence based on ethnic or racial groupings; however, findings suggest bipolar disorder may occur more commonly in higher socioeconomic groups (Simmons-Alling, 1996). Conversely, some ethnic groups and younger individuals are often misdiagnosed as suffering from schizophrenia when a diagnosis of bipolar disorder would be more appropriate. Because schizophrenia is a more stigmatizing illness compared with bipolar disorder, occurrences such as these are unfortunate and potentially hurtful. As with depressive disorders, many individuals with bipolar disorder do not seek treatment. Sadly, about 10% to 15% of individuals with bipolar I and bipolar II disorders will end their own lives (APA, 2002).

DSM-IV-TR TERMINOLOGY AND CRITERIA

The DSM-IV-TR defines several variations under the category of bipolar disorders, as previously noted. To understand the DSM-IV-TR diagnostic categories, the student must be able to distinguish the basic syndromes presented, such as the manic episode and the hypomanic episode.

12-Month Prevalence Rate of Mental Disorders in the United States

Diagnosis	Percentage of Population Over 17 Years of Age	Number of People
Anxiety disorders	12.6	20,034,000
Phobia disorders*	10.9	17,331,333
Mood disorders	9.5	15,143,000
Alcohol disorders	7.4	11,766,000
Major depression[†]	5.0	7,950,000
Drug disorders	3.1	4,929,000
Cognitive impairment	2.7	4,293,000
Obsessive-compulsive disorder	2.1	3,339,000
Antisocial disorder	1.5	2,385,000
Panic disorders*	1.3	2,067,000
Bipolar disorder[†]	1.2	1,908,000
Schizophrenia	1.1	1,749,000
Somatization	0.2	365,000

*Also calculated in anxiety statistics.
[†]Also calculated in mood disorders statistics.
From Regier DA et al: The de facto U.S. mental and addictive disorders service system: epidemiological catchment area prospective, 1-year prevalence rates of disorders and services, *Arch Gen Psychiatry* 50:85, 1993; Surgeon General: *Mental health: a report from the Surgeon General,* 1999, Washington, DC, Department of Health and Human Services.

Critical Thinking Question

Can a person fall within the bipolar spectrum but not meet the DSM-IV-TR criteria for bipolar disorder?

| Box 30-1 | Symptoms Occurring during Manic and Depressive Episodes

Manic episode	Other symptoms	Depressive episode—cont'd
Elevated mood	Labile mood	Diminished interest in activities;
Grandiosity, inflated self-esteem	Delusions	inappropriate or excessive guilt
Irritability	Hallucinations	Decrease in speech
Anger	Depressed mood	Fatigue
Insomnia	Low self-esteem	Decreased interest in sex
Anorexia		High rate of suicide
Flight of ideas, racing thoughts	**Depressive episode**	
Distractibility	Withdrawal	**Other symptoms**
Hyperactivity	Passivity	Memory loss
Involvement in pleasurable activities	Insomnia, daytime sleepiness	Abnormal thoughts about death
Loud, rapid speech; talkative	Anorexia	Weight loss
High energy	Sluggish thinking	
Increased interest in sex	Difficulty concentrating, distractibility	
High rate of suicide	Inertia	

DSM-IV-TR and NANDA Diagnoses Related to Mood Disorders

DSM-IV-TR*

Bipolar I disorder
Bipolar II disorder
Cyclothymic disorder
Dysthymic disorder
Major depressive disorder

NANDA†

Anxiety
Communication, impaired verbal
Coping, ineffective individual
Grieving, anticipatory
Grieving, dysfunctional
Hopelessness
Injury, risk for
Nutrition, less than body requirements, imbalanced
Powerlessness
Self-care deficit
Sexual dysfunction
Sleep pattern disturbed
Social isolation
Thought processes, disturbed
Violence, risk for self-directed

*Adapted from the American Psychiatric Association: *Diagnostic and statistical manual of mental disorders,* ed 4, text revision, Washington, DC, 2000, APA.
†North American Nursing Diagnosis Association: *NANDA nursing diagnoses: definitions and classifications 2001-2002,* Philadelphia, 2001, NANDA.

Manic Episodes

Manic episodes are characterized by an elevated, expansive, or irritable mood and are fundamental to the diagnosis of bipolar I disorder. To meet diagnostic criteria, the symptoms must persist for at least 1 week (or shorter if hospitalization is required). Symptoms are listed in Box 30-1. Manic episodes usually begin suddenly, escalate rapidly, and last from a few days to several months. Judgment is impaired, social blunders occur, and involvement with alcohol and drugs is common (often as an attempt at self-medication). Onset usually occurs in the early 20s. Individuals experiencing a manic episode have an inflated view of their importance, sometimes reaching grandiosity. ("I'm so important that the President needs my advice on international affairs.") The impairment is sufficiently serious that functioning deteriorates at home, work, school, or in social contexts. Other symptoms include a decreased need for sleep, talkativeness, flight of ideas, and distractibility. The mind races and seems to go faster and faster. Individuals experiencing a manic episode may engage in risky behavior, such as sexual relationships that are not in keeping with their normal conduct. People may speculate on a risky business venture because they "understand" the big picture of business. People have lost everything in these periods of manic thinking. Excess is common: spending sprees, sexual indiscretions, loud clothing, and excessive make-up are often seen in individuals in a manic state. Hospitalization is fre-

DSM-IV-TR	Criteria for Bipolar Disorders

I. Manic episode:
   A. A distinct period of abnormal and persistent elevated, expansive, or irritable mood that lasts at least 1 week (or less if hospitalization is required).
   B. At least three of the following symptoms must occur during the episode (or four if the patient is only irritable).
      1. Inflated self-esteem or grandiosity
      2. Decreased need for sleep
      3. Very talkative
      4. Flight of ideas or subjective feeling that thoughts are racing
      5. Distractibility
      6. Increase in goal-directed activity (social, occupational, educational, or sexual) or psychomotor agitation
      7. Excessive involvement in pleasurable activities that have a high potential for personal problems (e.g., sexual promiscuity, spending sprees, bad business investments)
   C. Mood disturbance severe enough to cause problems socially, interpersonally, or at work, or the person has to be hospitalized to prevent harm to self or others
   D. Not due to a substance

II. Hypomanic episode: The person experiencing a hypomanic episode meets most of the criteria for manic episode, with two major exceptions: the symptoms must be present "only" 4 days and the person must manifest an unequivocal change in functioning that is observable by others. A hypomanic episode is not severe enough to result in significant impairment or to require hospitalization.

III. Bipolar disorders:
   A. Bipolar episodes are divided into bipolar I and bipolar II. There are six categories of bipolar I. In bipolar I, the patient must have a history of a manic episode.
   B. Bipolar II: The patient has experienced major depression and a hypomanic episode (but not a manic episode)

IV. Cyclothymic disorder: For a period of 2 years, the patient has had numerous periods of hypomanic symptoms and numerous periods of a depressed mood. The patient is never symptom-free for more than 2 months at a time. The patient has never experienced major depression.

Adapted from the American Psychiatric Association: *Diagnostic and statistical manual of mental disorders,* ed 4, text revision, Washington, DC, 2000, APA.

quently required to prevent harm to the person or to others. Manic episodes can also be part of organic mental disorders, a general medical condition (Box 30-2), another psychotic process, or may be substance induced.

Fieve (1975), in his highly respected book, *Moodswings,* points out that many creative people in this society ride the energy from their manic state to success. Fieve points out that successful producer Joshua Logan (the musical, "South Pacific") and astronaut Buzz Aldrin (first moon landing) used the tremendous energy from their elevated moods to accomplish great things. Unfortunately, for patients suffering from a manic episode, the climb up the emotional ladder does not stop with elation, and excessive energy moves into psychotic thinking and unacceptable behavior. In addition, an equally extreme depression can follow these highs. Both Logan and Aldrin required professional help to restore their moods to normal. The following clinical example outlines the success and then the failure of a successful businessman.

Box 30-2	General Medical Conditions that Cause Mania

Anoxia
Hyperthyroidism
Hemodialysis
Lyme disease
Hypercalcemia
Acquired immunodeficiency syndrome
Stroke
Brain tumor
Multiple Sclerosis
Normal pressure hydrocephalus
Medications
Other neurologic disorders

From Keltner NL, Folks DG: *Psychotropic drugs,* ed 3, St Louis, 2001, Mosby.

CLINICAL EXAMPLE

Bill Smith is a 46-year-old former chief executive officer of a computer software company. Mr. Smith built the company from scratch into a multimillion-dollar-a-year endeavor. In fact, it was Mr. Smith's second time to develop a profitable business from the ground up. In the

Continued

late 80s while in his early 30s, Mr. Smith left a nationally recognized computer company and went into business on his own. Within 3 years, his company was remarkably profitable with what seemed as unlimited potential. Four years later, the business was bankrupt. He started the second business in 1998 and experienced even more success with it. Eventually, the new business became insolvent as well. The reason both businesses failed is directly linked to Mr. Smith's bipolar disorder. Although he credits the energy and goal-directed drive associated with the illness for helping him achieve great success, grandiose (e.g., unwarranted expansion, excessive spending) and unrealistic (e.g., he believed the government could not function without his computer applications) thinking eventually drove his business into the ground. As he puts it, "I also lost two business, two wives, and three children because of this illness." Both episodes of bipolar disorder required hospitalization.

Mr. Smith has never really "recovered" from the financial and personal setbacks of his last "nervous breakdown." He now lives in a county-operated apartment complex with other people who suffer from persistent mental disorder. Mr. Smith has a limited income and, though significantly improved, continues to display mood lability and other residual symptoms. Mr. Smith volunteers at a community mental health center and acknowledges that he most likely will never be a "wheeler-dealer" again. He is able to laugh about the good old days when he would drive into a Cadillac dealership and buy two cars, one for himself and one for his girlfriend of the moment.

Hypomanic Episodes

The hypomanic episode is similar to the manic episode but denotes a less severe level of impairment. Both bipolar II disorder and cyclothymia diagnoses require evidence of a hypomanic episode. Because the level of severity is somewhat subjective, the DSM-IV-TR attempts to differentiate hypomanic from manic episodes with more objective criteria. For a hypomanic episode to be diagnosed, the length of the episode must be at least 4 days in duration, but not severe enough to warrant hospitalization. Additionally, the episode is not severe enough to cause major problems at home, work, school, or in the social milieu, but is observable by others and

is distinct from the person's typical behavior. The episode is characterized by an abnormal period of persistent elevated, expansive, or irritable mood. Furthermore, the individual must experience at least three of the following symptoms:

- Increased self-esteem or grandiosity
- Decreased need for sleep
- Flight of ideas or subjective sense that thoughts are racing
- Distractibility
- Increase in goal-directed activity (typically social, occupational, educational, or sexual) or motor agitation
- Excessive involvement in pleasurable activities that have a high potential for painful consequences

At times, it may be difficult to distinguish severe hypomania from mania (Keltner et al, 1998).

BIPOLAR DISORDERS

The DSM-IV-TR bipolar diagnoses are based on an understanding of manic episodes, hypomanic episodes, and major depression. As noted, the DSM-IV-TR divides bipolar diagnoses into bipolar I, bipolar II, cyclothymic disorders, and bipolar disorder NOS. There are six variants of bipolar I disorder, one type of bipolar II disorder, and one type of cyclothymic disorder. Bipolar disorder NOS will not be discussed.

Bipolar I disorder. Bipolar I disorder is the most significant of these disorders. In bipolar I, the patients experience swings between manic episodes (defined earlier) and major depression (defined in Chapter 29). Figure 30-1 visually depicts the subtle differences in the bipolar disorders. The bipolar I diagnosis can be based on a single manic episode subtype or on several subtypes. The subtypes are:

- Bipolar I disorder, single manic episode
- Bipolar I disorder, most recent event a manic episode
- Bipolar I disorder, most recent event a hypomanic episode
- Bipolar I disorder, most recent episode mixed (both manic and depressive symptoms)
- Bipolar I disorder, most recent episode depressed
- Bipolar I disorder, most recent episode unspecified

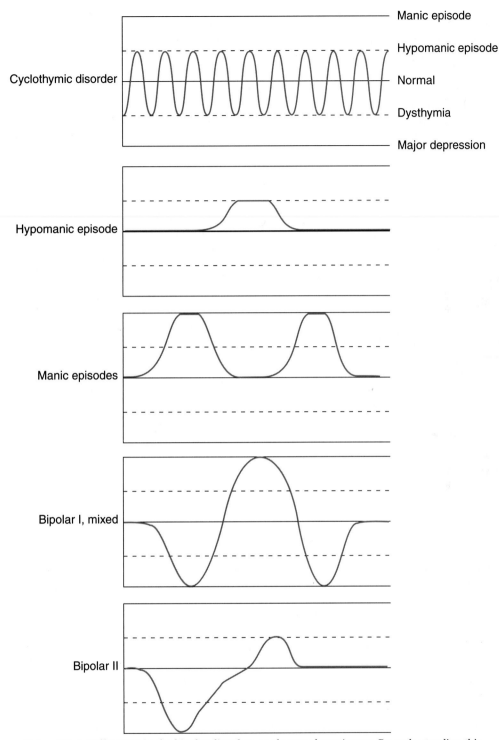

Figure 30-1 Differences in the bipolar disorders on the mood continuum. By understanding this figure, the student will be able to conceptualize the differences among these bipolar disorders.

Perhaps an additional word is warranted for the bipolar I: *mixed subtype*. This disorder is characterized by both manic and depressive symptoms. A designation of "rapid cycling" is given if four or more episodes of mania and depression have occurred in 1 year (Kuyler, 1988; APA, 2000).

Bipolar II disorder. Bipolar II disorder is similar to bipolar I disorder, with the major exception being that the person has never experienced a manic episode but "only" a hypomanic episode. In this disorder, the person has experienced major depression but has experienced a hypomanic episode, rather than a full manic episode on the other side of the mood continuum (APA, 2002). There may be a higher incidence of this disorder among women. The lifetime risk for bipolar II disorder is about 0.5%. Over the course of a few years, 5% to 15% of these individuals go on to develop a full manic episode (APA, 2000).

> ### *Critical* Thinking Question
>
> What do you think of the following statement? "There are many people in American society who could be diagnosed as hypomanic. Many high-level, 'workaholic' executives are hypomanic and just don't know it."

Cyclothymic disorder. Cyclothymic disorder is defined as a swing between a hypomanic episode and depressive symptoms. The swings in either direction are not quite severe enough to warrant the ultimate diagnoses of manic episode and major depression. Using a pendulum as a metaphor, the person experiencing cyclothymic disorder swings from one side to the other but never quite reaches the extremes of the arc. The person is elated and expansive but does not meet the criteria for manic episode. Cyclothymic disorder is characterized by symptoms that have occurred for at least 2 years without symptom remission for more than 2 months. The person experiences numerous hypomanic episodes and numerous dysthymic-level episodes. Cyclothymic disorder is equally distributed between men and women with a lifetime risk below 1%.

Behavior

Objective behavior

The person experiencing a manic episode appears enthusiastic and euphoric. Other people around the person recognize these behaviors as excessive. Objec-

---

> **CLINICAL EXAMPLE**
>
> Sue Miller is a 45-year-old Jewish woman who is admitted for bipolar disorder. Police were called to the Greyhound bus station where they found Ms. Miller annoying customers. She claimed to be a Messianic Jew and was preaching to anyone that would politely listen. She resisted the officers and repeatedly stated that she was the "woman at the well" and had married Christ. On arriving on the unit, it was noted that Ms. Miller had excessive bright red lipstick on, dramatically enhanced eyebrows, and turquoise eye shadow. The rest of her clothing appeared unattended to, and she was dirty and smelly. Ms. Miller is known to the hospital staff and, after her initial physical assessment, was prescribed and received lithium. This particular drug had been quite effective in the past.

tive behaviors include disturbances of speech; disturbances of the individual's social, interpersonal, and occupational relationships; and disturbances of activity and appearance. Accordingly, violent behavior, divorce, spouse and child abuse, job loss, and academic failure are relatively common features of this illness.

Disturbed speech patterns

- Rapid speech
- Loud speech
- Pressured speech
- Easily distracted

Manic patients may speak loudly in a rapid-fire fashion; they monopolize the dialogue and deflect attempts by others to contribute. Conversations are filled with jokes and puns. Sarcastic and biting remarks are not uncommon. In fact, even though mental health professionals are aware of this tendency, the ability of manic patients to find a "weak spot" often frustrates, embarrasses, and angers mental health professionals. The tendency to complain often and loudly is also present. Manic patients have the ability to engage staff members in debate and place them on the defensive. Speech is often dramatic, and it is not uncommon for manic individuals to burst into song. Speech is often pressured (a compulsion or strong need to talk).

These patients also are quite easily distracted. For example, while in the middle of an apparently meaningful discussion, a patient may be distracted by a bird flying outside the window and change the topic of the conversation to flying. This phenomenon, in which patients jump from topic to topic, is referred to as flight of ideas.

Altered social, interpersonal, and occupational relationships

- Failed relationships
- Job loss and job failure
- Overbearing behavior
- Increased sex drive
- Alienation of family

It is not surprising that manic patients irritate others with their fault-finding, anger, and blaming. This disorder destroys relationships. In a classic article entitled, "Playing the Manic Game," Janowsky, Leff, and Epstein (1970) identify five tendencies of manic patients.

1. Manipulation of the self-esteem of others. Patients use coercive techniques to increase or decrease another's self-esteem. It is easy to fall prey to the manipulation of praise. ("No one here really understands me but you.") It is just as easy to feel the ego-deflating wrath when plans are thwarted. Some insightful nurses have disclosed the feeling of "having been played like a yo-yo."
2. Ability to find vulnerability in others. Manic patients can exploit weakness in others or create conflicts among staff members.
3. Ability to shift responsibility. Through the technique mentioned earlier, patients somehow shift personal responsibility (e.g., not arriving at breakfast on time) to someone else. Nurses are particularly vulnerable in this area because they are trained to take responsibility for many concerns of their patients.
4. Limit testing. Manic patients keep pushing the limits established by the treatment setting. If a limit is relaxed, these patients will push it even more.
5. Alienation of family. Manic patients drive away their families with their behavior (Dore, Romans, 2001). The cyclic nature of the disorder, at first, inspires hope in the family. After numerous "cycles," families often sink into a demoralized state. Divorce and child and spousal abuse are not uncommon occurrences during severe manic episodes.

Janowsky, Leff, and Epstein (1970) noted the tendencies that cause manic-depressive patients to have difficulty socially, interpersonally, and occupationally. The same behaviors that drive away family also drive away friends, lovers, bosses, co-workers, ministers, and nonpsychiatric health care providers. Several trends have been noted among individuals with bipolar disorder:

1. Failed relationships are commonplace for those who do not receive adequate treatment.
2. Most report difficulties maintaining long-term friendships.
3. Job loss and job change are common occurrences.
4. A need to engage people, even strangers, in conversation characterizes bipolar disorder. Although at first, behavior such as this engages others, soon the overbearing and intrusive nature of the conversation alienates and even frightens people.
5. Mood lability can cause these individuals "to fall in and out of love" rapidly with all the associated pains to themselves and others.

Obviously, the effects of bipolar illness permeate all types of relationships. The expansive mood overflows into excesses as well. The otherwise faithful spouse may become sexually promiscuous; the otherwise thrifty homemaker may go on a shopping or spending spree; and the conservative investor may make a dangerously speculative investment. Divorce rates are two to three times higher than among comparable couples (APA, 2002).

Alterations in activity and appearance

Manic patients are often hyperactive and agitated. Overt manifestations, such as pacing, flamboyant gestures, colorful dress, singing, and excessive use of make-up, are relatively common. Patients also may dress sloppily and omit personal grooming; they may not need sleep, or perhaps need only a few hours per night. Some patients have gone for days without sleep, and, at one time, reports of manic patients dropping from exhaustion were not uncommon. Many manic patients suffer from poor nutrition because they quit eating; they simply do not have the patience, the ability to sit still long enough, or the desire to eat.

Subjective behavior

Alterations of affect

Manic patients experience euphoria and a high regard for the self. The inflated self-image can reach levels of grandiosity. Subjectively, the person going through a manic episode experiences an elevated mood, a feeling of joy, and greatness. A certain sense of invincibility leads to the social, interpersonal, and occupational problems already discussed.

Another significant symptom is a labile or quickly changing affect. Rapid mood swings are exhibited as changing from elation to irritability or from happiness to anger. For example, a 64-year-old woman was laughing and talking about her personal acquaintance with the president. "You know, my husband's name was George." She abruptly began to cry. "He is dead, you know." She quickly returned to the topic of her importance, becoming very excited, with an elevated mood.

Alterations of perception

Delusions and hallucinations occur, and their content is typically consistent with mood. For example, if a patient is grandiose about his importance to the government, a mood-congruent delusion might include paranoid thinking related to being pursued by enemy forces.

Etiology

Psychodynamic theories

At one time, most psychiatric professionals believed that bipolar illness, or manic-depressive illness, was caused by psychologic difficulties. Developmental theorists have hypothesized that faulty family dynamics during early life are responsible for manic behaviors in later life. According to this view, the mother (or primary caregiver) enjoys being the "giver of life" and resents autonomy. As the child grows independent, the mother becomes unhappy; to please the mother, the child becomes more dependent; that is, to gain affection, the child at an early age learns to deny his or her own natural tendencies. The unnatural tension between dependence and independence, and the inherent ambivalence in this family environment, can be a causative factor in bipolar illness, according to this view. Others have suggested that the polar events (e.g., approval or disapproval) of childhood are significant for some people to the extent that an adult emotional counterpart to the emotional roller coaster is caused, for example, receiving approval (elation) and disapproval (depression). Although some of the psychodynamic explanations seem more credible than others, many professionals believe that family dynamics play an important role in the genesis of manic-depressive illness.

Another psychodynamic hypothesis explains manic episodes as defense against or massive denial of depression. According to this view, manic-depressive individuals go through life appearing to be independent and excessive to others (too pushy, too talkative, and too manipulative) only to be eventually blocked by someone who no longer tolerates being pushed, talked to, or manipulated. When this event happens, the manic individual (who is actually overdependent) may become psychotic.

Neurotransmitter and structural hypotheses

Although some professionals still hold to the importance of psychologic influences, most are aware of the role of biology. Just as depression seems to be caused by neurotransmitter deficiency, manic episodes also seem to be related to excessive levels of norepinephrine and dopamine or an imbalance between cholinergic and noradrenergic systems. Goodwin and Jamison (1990) believe serotonin is deficient in bipolar disorder, just as it is in depression. Biologic findings also suggest lesions are more common in this population in areas of the brain such as the right hemisphere or bilateral subcortical and periventricular gray matter. Knowing what to make of these structural findings is difficult, but the neurotransmitter hypotheses are consistent with putative mechanisms of some antimanic drugs.

Genetic considerations

It seems clear that genetics has a role in bipolar disorder (APA, 2002). Monozygotic (identical) twins have a very high concordancy rate, whereas dizygotic (fraternal) twins have a higher rate than normal siblings and other close relatives. Siblings and close relatives have a higher incidence of manic-depressive illness than the general population, and cyclothymic characteristics are common among family members of bipolar patients. The following risks have been established for developing bipolar disorder (Craddock, Jones, 1999):

1. First degree relative 5% to 10% chance
2. Unrelated person, about 0.5% to 1.5% chance
3. Identical twin with bipolar disorder, about a 40% to 70% chance

Significant issues arise surrounding family planning counseling for women with bipolar illness, including the heritability of the disease, the stress of parenthood, and the effect an ill parent has on a child. Furthermore, teratogenicity of lithium, carbamazepine, and valproic acid is a concern when treating a pregnant woman who has bipolar disorder.

Consequently, pregnant women with bipolar disorder should be prescribed these drugs only when the risk of not doing so is greater than the risk of fetal insult. Because of these teratogenic effects, olanzapine (Zyprexa) is more likely to be prescribed to a pregnant woman.

Co-Morbidity

Abuse of alcohol and other substances is more common among individuals with bipolar disorder than it is in any other DSM-IV-TR Axis I diagnosis (Suppes, Denehy, Gibbons, 2000). Of people diagnosed with bipolar disorder, 60% abuse drugs according to the landmark National Institute of Mental Health Epidemiologic Catchment Area study (Regier et al, 1993). Additionally, individuals known to abuse drugs are five to eight times more likely to suffer from bipolar disorder than the general public (Kessler et al, 1997; Regier et al, 1993a). Some clinicians believe most first-time diagnoses of bipolar disorder occur in the emergency department related to consequences of alcohol or other substance abuse. Strakowski and DelBello (2000) forward four hypotheses to account for high rates of substance abuse among bipolar patients.

1. Substance abuse occurs as a symptom of bipolar disorder.
2. Substance abuse is an attempt by bipolar patients to self-medicate.
3. Substance abuse causes bipolar disorders.
4. Substance use and bipolar disorders share a common risk factor.

The use and abuse of alcohol and other substances cause several problems for the bipolar patient: relapse rates increase, response to lithium decreases, remission is delayed, poor treatment compliance occurs, and poor treatment outcomes are common (Suppes, Denehy, Gibbons, 2000).

Psychotherapeutic Management

Nurse-patient relationship

The box titled "Key Nursing Interventions" lists specific interventions to be used with patients who experience manic episodes.

- *Matter-of-fact tone.* A matter-of-fact tone minimizes the need for the patient to respond defensively and avoids power struggles. By providing emotional support and responding to patients in a matter-of-fact manner, the nurse conveys both control of the situation and empathy.
- *Clear, concise directions and comments.* Working with hyperactive patients who are highly talkative, easily distracted, experience flight of ideas, and who have poor judgment and a labile affect is difficult. When the nurse is confronted with talkative patients, it is not unusual for the nurse to attempt to use familiar skills. For example, most people learn not to interrupt another person until a pause. The pause may never come with manic patients. To be effective, the nurse may need to raise his or her hand and say, "Wait just a minute. I do not want to be rude, but I would like to say something." As a patient starts improving, the nurse may be able to work out a nonverbal signal to indicate when the patient needs to stop and let someone else speak.

Key Nursing Interventions for a Manic Episode

Patients too Busy to Eat

The nurse should use the following interventions to maintain patient's body weight:
1. Provide patients with foods that can be eaten on the run (sometimes referred to as finger foods) because some patients cannot sit long enough to eat.
2. Provide high-protein, high-calorie snacks for patients. A vitamin supplement may be indicated.
3. Weigh patients regularly (sometimes weighing daily is needed).

Patients Who Cannot Sleep

Manic patients experience insomnia. The nurse can help patients to maximize the opportunity for sleep by doing the following:
1. Provide a quiet place to sleep.
2. Structure patient's days so that there are fewer stimulating activities toward bedtime.
3. Do not allow caffeinated drinks before bedtime.
4. Assess the amount of rest patients are receiving. Manic patients are not capable of judging the need for rest, and exhaustion and death have resulted from lack of rest.

Although manic patients are talkative, there is a tendency for the talk to be superficial. When talking to hyperactive patients, the nurse should keep remarks brief and simple. Many patients literally cannot tolerate a lengthy discussion of any subject.

- *Limit setting.* When the nurse is leading a group, a talkative patient can be disruptive because of these tendencies:
  - Manipulation of the self-esteem of others
  - Ability to find vulnerability of others
  - Ability to shift responsibility to others
  - Limit testing

These patients have the ability to damage the self-esteem of other patients, to ridicule the nurse, to blame others, to pick fights, to create problems between patients, and to manipulate others. The nurse needs to protect vulnerable patients and to keep them from being drawn into the anger that manic patients feel. When the nurse is able to remain calm instead of becoming angry, it helps manic patients and the other patients in the group. This calmness should be based on an understanding of psychopathology; otherwise, it may be simply an unhealthy defense by the nurse. ("You cannot bother me; you are not important enough.") The nurse absolutely does not want to convey that she is engaged in an adult version of the childish behavior of plugging the ears and saying, "I can't hear you." It is also important to avoid arguing with patients about unit rules and limits. Do not debate these issues with patients. Simply state the unit policy and move on. Debating and arguing reinforces the tendencies mentioned earlier.

Patient and Family Education

Bipolar Disorder

Illness:

Bipolar disorder is a brain disorder that disrupts mood. The patient may experience extreme moods—bouncing from depression to euphoria (or mania) or may primarily exhibit symptoms of mania. A little over 1% of the adult population suffers from bipolar disorder. Manic episodes are characterized by an elevated mood, irritability, inflated self-esteem, decreased need for sleep, talkativeness, distractibility, and excessive involvement in pleasurable activities. The disorder is typically diagnosed first in the early 20s and occurs about equally between men and women. Because of the pursuit of pleasurable activities, many bipolar patients overspend, become sexually involved in situations they would normally avoid, and invest in unwise business dealings. Both dress and language can become loud and excessive. Involvement with drugs and alcohol is fairly common.

Medications:

Lithium has been the mainstay of treatment for patients with bipolar disorders. It is a naturally occurring element and is located on the periodic table in the same column as sodium and potassium. Lithium is so similar to sodium that the nervous system confuses it for sodium. However, because lithium reacts more slowly than sodium, it can be given to slow the nervous system down. Lithium works but causes some fairly predictable side effects (e.g., fine tremor, thirst, frequent urination). Although lithium is effective for most patients, it can also cause problems because the difference is slight between a therapeutic dose and a harmful dose (or toxic dose). Because of this concern, patients diagnosed with bipolar disorder must have their blood examined frequently for its lithium content. After chronic and stable use of lithium, blood draws become less frequent.

Antiepileptic drugs are also used to treat bipolar disorder. A number of these agents are used, but the most commonly prescribed are Depakene (or Depakote) and carbamazepine (Tegretol is the most familiar trade name for this product). These drugs have a wider margin of safety than lithium, but they can also produce some significant and serious side effects.

Zyprexa, an antipsychotic agent, is a different category of drug used to treat bipolar disorder. The FDA has recently approved its use in the treatment of bipolar disorder. Zyprexa is effective but has been known to cause substantial weight gain.

Other issues:

Patients with bipolar disorder can be very difficult to live with. Their self-importance, nonstop behavior, talkativeness, style of dress, and irritability can overwhelm a family member. On the other hand, these individuals can be remarkably creative and productive. It is important when living or dealing with individuals with this diagnosis to be matter-of-fact, clear, and concise in communication, to set limits, and to redirect critical negativism into healthier activities. Although difficult at times, it is important to avoid personalizing negative, sarcastic, and rude comments that these individuals might direct toward you.

- *Reinforcement of reality.* Manic patients also experience disturbances in perception. The intervention strategies outlined for other patients with disturbed perceptions are recommended for manic patients as well.
- *Provide a homogeneous group if possible.* Working with a group of inpatients with exclusively bipolar disorder may be beneficial because patients feel "understood." In addition, topics can be focused into an area of relevance for this group of patients. Although this homogeneity may not always be possible or even desirable, the psychiatric nurse may wish to explore this approach for working with bipolar patients.
- *Respond to legitimate complaints.* Although many frivolous complaints arise, the nurse must respond to legitimate complaints to defuse irritability and develop trust.
- *Redirect patients into more "healthy" activity.* The bipolar patient's distractibility serves as an intervention tool when the patient engages in nonproductive behavior.

Psychopharmacology

The efficacy of lithium in the treatment of bipolar disorder has been recognized for years. Traditionally, lithium has been the most prescribed drug for manic patients. At one time, 80% to 90% of patients responded to lithium; but now only about 50% seem to respond (Surgeon General, 1999). The starting dose is usually 600 mg three times daily. The typical maintenance dose is 900 to 1200 mg a day (Keltner, Folks, 2001). Maintenance blood levels are 0.6 to 1.2 mEq/L. There are several alternatives to lithium; two are anticonvulsants and one is an atypical antipsychotic. The anticonvulsants are valproic acid (Depakote, Depakene) and carbamazepine (Tegretol). Valproic acid seems to be the more effective of the two and is particularly beneficial in cases of rapid cycling. Newer anticonvulsants such as gabapentin (Neurontin), lamotrigine (Lamictal), and topiramate (Topamax) are also used on occasion. Olanzapine, an atypical antipsychotic, has recently been approved for treatment of acute manic episodes. Overall, these agents have a treatment success rate of about 80%. A full discussion of these drugs is found in Chapter 22.

Milieu management

Milieu management is an important dimension of the nursing care of manic patients because they test the unit perhaps more than any other group of patients.

1. Safety. It is important for the nurse to prevent manic patients from hurting themselves or others. Manic patients can become angry when things do not go their way. This pathologic irritability leads to arguments, fights, self-injury (e.g., hitting the wall, not paying attention to the environment), and hurting others. It is reassuring to patients to realize that the staff will not let them harm themselves or others.
2. Consistency among staff. Because manic patients tend to create conflict, to pick on vulnerable individuals (patients and staff), to blame others, to test limits, and to shift responsibility to others, the nurse must carefully develop a plan of care. Nursing and other staff members should meet often to defuse conflict and clarify communication. All staff members should be aware of intervention strategies and agree to abide consistently by team decisions.

Side Effects and Nursing Interventions | for Lithium

Side Effects	Interventions
Confusion, restlessness, sleeplessness	Withhold lithium
Gastrointestinal symptoms	Give lithium with meals
Nausea	Give lithium with meals
Thirst	Instruct patients to drink 10 to 12 glasses of water each day
Diarrhea	Observe patient closely for depletion of electrolytes, which can cause increased serum lithium levels
Weight gain	Weigh patient weekly; patient may need to be placed on structured diet

Case Study

Mr. Casey Tubbs, a 44-year-old electrician, was admitted to the unit with the diagnosis of bipolar I disorder, manic type. The police arrested him after he started a fight with three Hispanic men in a bar. He had been drinking heavily. He was hyperactive, distractible, irritable, talkative, and demanding upon admission. He demonstrated flight of ideas and was verbally hostile concerning a Hispanic co-worker, whom he accused of sleeping with his wife. Mr. Tubbs has vowed to get even. He made several comments about Hispanics in general while looking at Mr. Azteca, a Hispanic nurse.

This is Mr. Tubbs' third hospitalization. The first occurred 12 years ago when he contracted a *Candida* infection after having sexual intercourse with his wife. The second hospitalization occurred in 1998. No precipitating event was recorded; nor does Mr. Tubbs recollect anything unusual about the second admission.

Mr. Tubbs has responded well to lithium in the past, and during his last hospitalization, he was also given olanzapine because of his agitation. Between hospitalizations, Mr. Tubbs has functioned well and is considered a good worker. His boss appreciates his perfectionistic tendencies. Mrs. Tubbs states that Mr. Tubbs has not slept in 3 days and has not stopped to eat for some time (the actual length of time is not clear). She reports a good marriage until Mr. Tubbs stopped taking his lithium, which he says he will no longer take. She wants him to "get better and come home." The head nurse decides to streamline the admission process because of Mr. Tubbs' agitated state. He is taken to a quiet area and given peanut butter crackers and milk.

Inexperienced staff members must guard against falling prey to esteem-building statements that tend to split the staff, for example, "You're the only one who understands."

3. Reduce environmental stimuli. Because manic patients are hyperactive, talkative, irritable, and angry, it is important to decrease environmental stimuli. Patients are distractible and respond to all sorts of environmental cues; it is therefore important to modify the environment as much as possible. Helpful environmental modifications include private (if possible), quiet rooms; limited activities with others and scheduled rest periods; gross motor activities (e.g., walking, sweeping, aerobics) to discharge some of the need to be active; and a public room free from a television or stereo.

4. Do not escalate patients. Manic patients can become hostile and aggressive. It is important for the staff to deal with this aggressiveness in a calm, confident manner. For patients who are escalating, an antipsychotic drug, such as haloperidol, can be administered to prevent physical aggressiveness, and potential weapons (e.g., chairs, pool cues) can be removed. Limits and the consequences of violating these limits should be reviewed. Do not include limits that are not significant. It is counter therapeutic to defend a poor policy, and it is also counter therapeutic to allow patients to debate a unit issue. It is therapeutic to follow through with appropriate action should a patient violate a unit norm.

5. Reinforce appropriate hygiene and dress. Bipolar patients often forget hygiene behaviors, thus appearing disheveled and unclean at times. Simple reminders to shower, brush teeth, and wear clean clothes can correct some problems. The nurse should also monitor for flamboyant and suggestive dress that might ultimately embarrass the patient.

6. Nutrition and sleep issues. Both inadequate nutrition and inadequate sleep patterns plague bipolar patients. (See the "Key Nursing Interventions" box for appropriate nursing interventions.)

Critical Thinking Question

Can a person fall within the bipolar spectrum but not meet the DSM-IV-TR criteria for bipolar disorder?

Key Concepts

1. Bipolar disorders (e.g., bipolar disorder, hypomania, cyclothymia, bipolar disorder NOS) occur in about 1.2% of adult population in any given 12-month period. About 1.6% of Americans will be affected by this disorder in their lifetime.

2. Manic episodes are characterized by a distinct period (1 week at least or less if hospitalized) during which there is an abnormal and persistent elevated, expansive, or irritable mood. These symptoms tend to occur suddenly and escalate rapidly, lasting from a few days to several months. At least three other symptoms are required (see Box 30-1).

Care Plan

Name: <u>Casey Tubbs</u>   Admission Date: _____

DSM-IV-TR Diagnosis: <u>Bipolar I disorder, most recent episode manic</u>

Assessment	**Areas of strength:** Patient's marriage is solid between hospitalizations. Patient's boss likes him and is eager for him to return to work. Good adjustment between hospitalizations. He has responded well to lithium in the past.
	Problems: Patient is threatening and irritating others. Patient has legal problems from bar fight. Patient is threatening to get even with his wife's alleged lover. Patient has not complied with medication regimen recently and states that he will not take lithium.

Diagnoses
- Violence, high risk for, related to manic dyscontrol and delusions, as evidenced by irritability and verbal hostility.
- Fatigue related to insomnia, as evidenced by lack of sleep for 3 days.
- Nutrition, altered: less than body requirements related to anorexia and hyperactivity, as evidenced by lack of interest in food.

Outcomes

Short-term goals: *Date met*
- Patient will not hurt anyone while in hospital.   _____
- Patient will comply with medication regimen.   _____
- Patient will become less agitated.   _____
- Patient will comply with unit norms and limits.   _____

Long-term goals:
- Patient will remain free of manic episodes.   _____
- Patient will continue to take lithium on outpatient basis.   _____
- Patient will resolve legal problems.   _____
- Patient will join manic-depressive support group.   _____

Planning/
Interventions

Nurse-patient relationship: Talk to patient in matter-of-fact tone, and clearly indicate that aggressive behaviors are not acceptable. Set firm, clear limits. Do not engage in debates over unit policy or limits. Keep comments brief and simple. Do not respond to sarcastic remarks with anger. Reinforce good behavior and confront (carefully) unacceptable behavior.

Psychopharmacology: Lithium carbonate, 600 mg tid, PO (concentrate); olanzapine 15 mg HS.

Milieu management: Provide quiet room and decrease stimuli. Do not include in-group activities for a few days. Provide opportunities for rest and monitor sleep. Provide finger foods and weigh daily. Set limits.

Evaluation

Mr. Tubbs is less agitated and is taking lithium on schedule. Patient is beginning to talk less about his wife's alleged infidelity. Has not lost weight. Patient continues to test limits.

Referrals

Schedule outpatient appointment and give patient and wife telephone number for manic-depressive support group.

---

3. Hypomanic episodes are characterized by the set of symptoms that occur in manic episodes, except the symptoms are not as severe; occur over a 4-day period; do not cause significant social, occupational, or interpersonal problems; and do not require hospitalization.

4. Bipolar I disorder is described as a swing in mood from a manic episode to major depression.

5. Bipolar II disorder is described as a swing in mood from a hypomanic episode to major depression.

6. Cyclothymic disorder is described as a swing in mood from a hypomanic episode to depressive

symptoms (but not as severe as those with major depression).

7. Objective signs of bipolar illness include altered speech patterns; altered social, interpersonal, and occupational relationships; and altered activity and appearance.

8. Subjective symptoms of bipolar illness include alterations in affect and perception.

9. Psychodynamic theories of bipolar illness include theories about family dynamics and psychoanalytic explanations that view manic behavior as a defense against overwhelming feelings of depression.

10. Biologic explanations of bipolar disorder include excessive levels of neurotransmitters (norepinephrine, serotonin, and dopamine) and genetics (up to 80% concordancy rates among identical twins in some studies).

11. Lithium is the drug of choice for the treatment of bipolar disorders; however, valproates (e.g., Depakene, Depakote) are also used extensively. Olanzapine (Zyprexa) is the most recently approved agent for bipolar disorder. Carbamazepine (Tegretol) is also used.

References

American Psychiatric Association: *Diagnostic and statistical manual of mental disorders,* ed 4, Revised Text, Washington, DC, 2000, APA.

American Psychiatric Association; Practice guidelines for the treatment of patients with bipolar disorder, *Am J Psychiatry* 159(4 suppl):16-36, 2002.

Craddock N, Jones I: Genetics of bipolar disorder, *J Med Genet* 36(8):585, 1999.

Dore G, Romans SE: Impact of bipolar affective disorder on family and partners, *J Affect Disord* 67(1-3):147, 2001.

Fieve RR: *Moodswings,* New York, 1975, Bantam.

Goodwin FK, Jamison KR: *Manic-depressive illness,* New York, 1990, Oxford University Press.

Janowsky DS, Leff M, Epstein RS: Playing the manic game, *Arch Gen Psychiatry* 22:252, 1970.

Keltner NL et al: *Psychobiological foundations of psychiatric care,* St Louis, 1998, Mosby.

Keltner NL, Folks DG: *Psychotropic drugs,* ed 3, St Louis, 2001, Mosby.

Kessler RC et al: Lifetime and 12-month prevalence of DSM-III-R psychiatric disorders in the United States: results from the national comorbidity survey, *Arch Gen Psychiatry* 51:8, 1994.

Kessler RC et al: Lifetime co-occurrence of DSM-III-R alcohol abuse and dependence with other psychiatric disorders in the National Comorbidity Survey, *Arch Gen Psychiatry* 4:231, 1997.

Kuyler PL: Rapid cycling bipolar I illness in three closely related individuals, *Am J Psychiatry* 145:114, 1988.

Regier DA et al: Comorbidity of mental disorders with alcohol and other drug abuse: Results from the Epidemiologic Catchment Area (ECA) Study, *JAMA* 264:2511, 1993a.

Regier DA et al: The de facto US mental and addictive disorders service system: epidemiologic catchment area prospective 1-year prevalence rates of disorders and services, *Arch Gen Psychiatry* 50:85, 1993b.

Simmons-Alling S: Bipolar mood disorders. In McBride AB, Austin JS, editors: *Psychiatric mental-health nursing: integrating the behavioral and biological sciences,* Philadelphia, 1996, WB Saunders.

Strakowski SM, DelBello SP: The co-occurrence of bipolar and substance use disorders, *Clin Psych Rev* 20(2):191, 2000.

Suppes T, Denehy EB, Gibbons EW: The longitudinal course of bipolar disorder, *J Clin Psychiatry* 61(suppl 9):23, 2000.

Surgeon General: *Mental health: a report from the Surgeon General,* Washington, DC, 1999, U.S. Department of Health and Human Services.

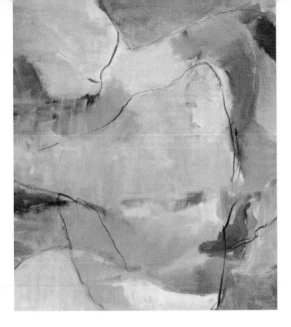

Chapter 31

Anxiety-Related, Somatoform, and Dissociative Disorders

Carol E. Bostrom; Lee H. Schwecke

Learning Objectives

After reading this chapter, you should be able to:

- Recognize the special terms related to anxiety disorders, somatoform disorders, and dissociative disorders.
- Describe *The Diagnostic and Statistical Manual of Mental Disorders-Fourth Edition-Text Revision* (DSM-IV-TR) criteria for these disorders.
- Describe objective and subjective symptoms of these disorders.

- Develop nursing care plans for individuals with these disorders.
- Evaluate the effectiveness of nursing interventions for individuals with these disorders.
- Recognize issues related to the care of individuals with these disorders.
- Describe the family issues related to these disorders.

The disorders discussed in this chapter are classified in the DSM-IV-TR as anxiety-related disorders, somatoform disorders, and dissociative disorders. Interventions for each disorder are included. First, to understand anxiety-related disorders, it is crucial to understand *what* anxiety is, *where* it comes from, *why* it is difficult to manage, and *how* individuals normally cope with it. (See Chapter 12 for a conceptualization of the dynamics of anxiety-related disorders.) To understand these dynamics and to provide effective treatment, it is important to understand the concepts of *primary gain* and *secondary gain*. Primary gain refers to the individual's desire to relieve anxiety to feel better and more secure. Secondary gain refers to the attention or support the individual derives from others because of illness. For example, "If I am sick, I cannot leave home to go grocery shopping, so I will call my husband at work and tell him to stop at the grocery store on his way home to buy the needed items." The assistance from the husband is a secondary gain.

Sometimes the attention or the benefit of the secondary gain becomes more important than reducing the anxiety. This phenomenon immeasurably complicates the treatment of these patients.

GENERALIZED ANXIETY DISORDER

In generalized anxiety disorder (GAD), the symptoms of anxiety are directly felt and expressed. GAD is the most common anxiety disorder and is frequently seen with depression and other anxiety disorders that increase impairment in functioning (Ballenger et al, 2001). The anxiety or worry is chronic and excessive and may concern everyday events,

Key Terms

Primary gain Relief or expression of anxiety through symptoms of disorder.

Secondary gain Support received from others while one is ill.

Flashbacks Cognitive, emotional, and physical reexperiencing of traumatic events.

Derealization Feelings of unreality.

Depersonalization Feeling detached from oneself.

Dissociation Removal from conscious awareness of painful feelings, memories, thoughts, or aspects of identity.

DSM-IV-TR Criteria for Generalized Anxiety Disorder

1. Excessive worry and anxiety
2. Difficulty in controlling the worry
3. Anxiety and worry are evident in three or more of the following:
   - Restlessness
   - Fatigue
   - Irritability
   - Decreased ability to concentrate
   - Muscle tension
   - Disturbed sleep

Adapted from the American Psychiatric Association: *Diagnostic and statistical manual of mental disorders,* ed 4, text revision, Washington, DC, 2000, APA.

12-Month Prevalence Rate of Mental Disorders in the United States

Diagnosis	Percentage of Population Over 17 Years of Age	Number of People
Anxiety disorders	12.6	20,034,000
Phobia disorders*	10.9	17,331,333
Mood disorders	9.5	15,143,000
Alcohol disorders	7.4	11,766,000
Major depression†	5.0	7,950,000
Drug disorders	3.1	4,929,000
Cognitive impairment	2.7	4,293,000
Obsessive-compulsive disorder	2.1	3,339,000
Antisocial disorder	1.5	2,385,000
Panic disorders*	1.3	2,067,000
Bipolar disorder†	1.2	1,908,000
Schizophrenia	1.1	1,749,000
Somatization	0.2	365,000

*Also calculated in anxiety statistics.
†Also calculated in mood disorders statistics.
From Regier DA et al: The de facto U.S. mental and addictive disorders service system: epidemiological catchment area prospective, 1-year prevalence rates of disorders and services, *Arch Gen Psychiatry* 50:85, 1993; Surgeon General: *Mental health: a report from the Surgeon General,* 1999, Washington, DC, Department of Health and Human Services.

such as work or school. These individuals have great difficulty in controlling the anxiety, and worrying becomes a habitual way of coping. The anxiety causes significant distress and impairment in interpersonal, social, or occupational functioning. Because of the sense of helplessness that results from the anxiety, these patients can also experience feelings of depression. Frequently, patients have used alcohol or other drugs to the point of dependence in an attempt to feel better. The following box lists the DSM-IV-TR criteria for GAD.

When anxiety is caused by or related to a medical condition, the diagnosis of *anxiety disorder caused by a general medical condition* is used. Presumably, successful treatment of the medical illness will result in a reduced level of anxiety.

Etiology

Recent twin studies suggest a genetic link to the development of GAD (American Psychiatric Association [APA], 2000). In patients with GAD, there may be an abnormal response to stress with neurochemical abnormalities in the gamma-aminobutyric acid (GABA-)-benzodiazepine, norepinephrine, and serotonin systems (Nutt, 2001). Some evidence exists that in GAD and panic disorder, patients may have alterations in a number of benzodiazepine receptors. Further research is needed to clearly explain the neurobiologic mechanisms involved in GAD.

Psychotherapeutic Management

Nurse-patient relationship

The first step in the nurse-patient relationship is for the nurse to assist patients in reducing their level of anxiety. Anxiety must be reduced before problem solving can occur. The nurse's ultimate goal is to assist patients with developing adaptive coping responses.

Initially, patients need support and reassurance from the nurse. The nurse promotes trust through acceptance of patients' positive and negative feelings and acknowledgment of their discomfort. Conveying empathy tells patients that the nurse is concerned and understanding and does not minimize the level of distress. For example, the nurse might say, "This must be uncomfortable and painful for

DSM-IV and NANDA Diagnoses Related to Anxiety-Related Disorders

DSM-IV*	NANDA†
Anxiety disorders	Adjustment, Impaired
Generalized anxiety disorder	Anxiety
Panic disorder with or without agoraphobia	Body image, Disturbed
Agoraphobia without panic disorder	Breathing pattern, Ineffective
Specific phobia	Communication, Impaired verbal
Social phobia	Coping, Ineffective
Obsessive-compulsive disorder	Coping, Ineffective community
Acute stress disorder (ASD)	Fear
Posttraumatic stress disorder (PTSD)	Injury, Risk for
Anxiety disorder due to a general medical condition	Pain, Chronic
	Posttrauma syndrome, Risk for
Somatoform disorders	Powerlessness
Somatization disorder	Role performance, Ineffective
Pain disorder	Self-esteem, Chronic low
Hypochondriasis	Self-esteem, Situational low
Conversion disorder	Self-esteem, Risk for situational low
	Sensory perception, Disturbed
	Sleep pattern, Disturbed
Dissociative disorders	Social interaction, Impaired
Dissociative amnesia	Social isolation
Dissociative fugue	Spiritual distress
Depersonalization disorder	Thought processes, Disturbed
Dissociative identity disorder (Multiple personality disorder)	Violence, Risk for self-directed or Risk for other-directed

*From the American Psychiatric Association: *Diagnostic and statistical manual of mental disorders,* ed 4, text revision, Washington, DC, 2000, APA.
†From the North American Nursing Diagnosis Association: *NANDA nursing diagnoses: definitions and classifications 2000,* Philadelphia, 1997, NANDA.

you." To help patients manage and reduce their level of anxiety, the nurse should use the interventions found in the boxes titled "Key Nursing Interventions to Reduce Anxiety" and "Key Nursing Interventions in Problem Solving" on page 384.

After the anxiety level is reduced to a more manageable and comfortable level, the nurse should begin to assist patients in examining their coping behaviors. Through the use of problem-solving methods, adaptive coping skills can increase.

The process of helping patients learn to use adaptive coping behaviors requires patience and the awareness that individuals learn and change at their own pace. The nurse must also be aware of his or her own verbal and nonverbal behavior when working with these patients, because anxiety is contagious. The nurse should manage his or her own stress and anxiety so that the work between the nurse and the patient is not compromised. The nurse educates the patient about the illness, including the effects of anxiety on the patient's life and also on the members of the family.

Psychopharmacology

Antidepressants, such as serotonin reuptake inhibitors, serotonin-norepinephrine reuptake inhibitors, and nonsedating tricyclic antidepressants are most appropriate for treating GAD because of the presence of co-morbid disorders such as depression (Ballenger et al, 2001). Because GAD is a chronic disorder, antidepressants are better than benzodiazepines because of the possibility of dependency and tolerance with long-term use of benzodiazepines (Davidson, 2001). Sometimes, benzodiazepines are used on a short-term basis when a quick-acting medication is needed.

Milieu management

The patient with GAD can benefit from a variety of milieu activities. Recreational activities help reduce tension and anxiety. The use of relaxation exercises and tapes and meditations helps decrease bodily tension and promotes relaxation and comfort.

Groups that focus on stress management, problem solving, self-esteem, assertiveness, and goal setting are helpful with stress. Cognitive-behavioral therapy has

Key Nursing Interventions   to Reduce Anxiety

1. Provide a calm and quiet environment. *Rationale:* to identify and reduce stimulation, which includes exposure to situations and interactions with other patients that might provoke anxiety.
2. Ask patients to identify what and how they feel. *Rationale:* to help patients increase their recognition of what is happening to them.
3. Encourage patients to describe and discuss their feelings with you. *Rationale:* to help patients increase their awareness of the connection between feelings and behaviors.
4. Help patients identify possible causes of their feelings. *Rationale:* to assist patients in connecting their feelings with earlier experiences.

5. Listen carefully for patients' expressions of helplessness and hopelessness. *Rationale:* to assess for self-harm; patients might be suicidal because they want to escape their pain and do not think that they will ever feel better.
6. Ask patients whether they feel suicidal or have a plan to hurt themselves. *Rationale:* same as above and to initiate suicide precautions, if necessary.
7. Plan and involve patients in activities such as going for walks or playing recreational games. *Rationale:* to help patients release nervous energy and to discourage preoccupation with the self.

Key Nursing Interventions   for Problem Solving

1. Discuss with patients their present and previous coping mechanisms. *Rationale:* to reinforce effective adaptive behaviors.
2. Discuss with patients the meaning of problems and conflicts. *Rationale:* to help patients appraise stressors, explore their personal values, and define the scope and seriousness of their problems.
3. Use supportive confrontation and teaching. *Rationale:* to increase patients' insight into the negative effects of their maladaptive and dysfunctional coping behaviors.
4. Assist patients with exploring alternative solutions and behaviors. *Rationale:* to increase adaptive coping mechanisms.

5. Encourage patients to test new adaptive coping behaviors through role-playing or implementation. *Rationale:* to provide an opportunity for patients to practice new behaviors.
6. Teach patients relaxation exercises. *Rationale:* to reduce the level of anxiety. These techniques help patients manage or control anxiety on their own.
7. Promote the use of hobbies and recreational activities. *Rationale:* to help patients deal with routine feelings of stress and anxiety.

---

been found to be helpful in reducing symptoms and improving coping (Falsetti, Davis, 2001). Therapeutic touch and acupressure may be useful in reducing anxiety (La Torre, 2001). Depending on the issues and concerns of each patient, a variety of groups can be beneficial.

PANIC DISORDER

Patients with panic disorder experience recurrent panic attacks and are worried about having more attacks. A panic attack develops suddenly, is accompanied by intense fear or discomfort, and peaks within 10 minutes. In addition to somatic symptoms, patients who experience panic attacks fear they are losing control over themselves, "going crazy," having a heart attack, or dying. Panic attacks can occur during sleep, resulting in exhaustion. (See box listing the DSM-IV-TR criteria for panic disorder.)

DSM-IV-TR Criteria for Panic Disorder
1. Recurrent, unexpected panic attacks
2. Panic attacks are followed by a month or more of worry about having additional attacks, worry about the results of the attacks, and behavior changes related to the attacks
3. Panic disorder can be accompanied by agoraphobia

Adapted from the American Psychiatric Association: *Diagnostic and statistical manual of mental disorders*, ed 4, text revision, Washington, DC, 2000, APA.

According to the DSM-IV-TR, panic attacks are (1) unexpected, occur "out of the blue," or occur spontaneously or (2) are situationally bound, meaning that they occur in anticipation of or on exposure to a trigger situation. Panic attacks that occur in response to a situation or trigger are related to social and specific phobias. Some panic attacks occur later after exposure to a cue or situation.

Panic disorder can result in agoraphobia because patients fear having a panic attack in a place where embarrassment might occur, where help might not be available, or where escape is impossible. Patients who have panic disorder with agoraphobia restrict their activities outside of the home or require another person to be with them when outside the home. Thus these patients become agoraphobic as a result of the fear of having an attack outside the home.

Etiology

Panic disorder may be genetically transmitted. Genetic factors, coupled with environmental factors, may be associated with vulnerability to this disorder, while brain and biochemical factors may account for its development. Abnormalities in the brain's benzodiazepine receptors are implicated in the origin of anxiety disorders. In patients with panic disorder, panic attacks can be induced with caffeine, carbon dioxide, and sodium lactate. Some patients experience anxiety sensitivity because they interpret symptoms of anxiety as signs of impending catastrophe (Grinspoon, 2001). Patients are less likely to panic when informed about the symptoms they will experience. This tendency suggests a psychologic as well as a biologic component to panic disorder.

Psychotherapeutic Management

Nurse-patient relationship

The therapeutic relationship between the nurse and patients with panic disorder is centered on the same issues and interventions discussed for patients with GAD. Interventions specific to patients experiencing a panic attack are described in the box below. The rationale for the interventions is to help patients get through the panic attack safely with as little discomfort as possible. With the nurse's assistance, patients' anxiety can be reduced to more manageable levels.

The nurse educates patients about panic disorder to reassure them that they are not losing their minds or dying during an attack. Patients experience relief when given information about the disorder and about medications that can block symptoms. The nurse should help patients realize that attacks are time limited and that symptoms will abate. Cognitive restructuring helps the patient reinterpret and reappraise beliefs regarding the danger of an event or bodily sensations.

Psychopharmacology

Antidepressants are most commonly used in long-term treatment of panic symptoms. Benzodiazepines such as clonazepam (Klonopin) and lorazepam (Ativan) are used for an immediate effect until the antidepressants start working. The selective serotonin reuptake inhibitors (SSRIs) are mostly used because of the relatively few side effects.

Patients with panic disorder may resist drug therapy because it may mean a loss of control at a time when they are struggling to maintain control over themselves and their symptoms. Some patients fear medications and their side effects. A good, simple explanation of the disorder and its biologic components can often convince patients that medication is helpful and not a sign of "weakness."

The nurse must differentiate symptoms of increased anxiety levels from medication side effects. Anxiety symptoms increase when pertinent issues are addressed or stressors are present. When symptoms of anxiety remain constant, or decrease immediately before the next dose of medication, the symptoms are probably related to the medication. Anxiety-reduction strategies (e.g., relaxation exercises) may help patients manage anxiety.

Key Nursing Interventions   for Panic Attack

1. Stay with the patient who is having a panic attack and acknowledge the patient's discomfort.
2. Maintain a calm style and demeanor.
3. Speak in short, simple sentences, and give one direction at a time in a calm tone of voice.
4. If the patient is hyperventilating, provide a brown paper bag and focus on breathing with the patient.
5. Allow patients to pace or cry, which enables the release of tension and energy.
6. Communicate to patients that you are in control and will not let anything happen to them.
7. Move or direct patients to a quieter, less stimulating environment. Do not touch these patients; touching can increase feelings of panic.
8. Ask patients to express their perceptions or fears about what is happening to them.
   Rationale: to help patients reduce anxiety to a more manageable and comfortable level.

Case Study

Sandra Johnson, a 41-year-old white woman, is admitted to the psychiatric unit of a general hospital. She is accompanied by her husband and is coming from the emergency department. Her symptoms in the emergency department were shortness of breath, hyperventilation, palpitations, chest pain, and fear of dying. She stated that these symptoms occurred unexpectedly while she was cooking dinner. She thought she was having a heart attack.

These attacks had happened three times before. The first attack occurred 2 months ago, after which she went to her family physician, who performed an electrocardiogram, a stress test, and conducted a complete physical examination. All results were negative for any physiologic causation of the symptoms. After the second attack, Mrs. Johnson stated that she took 2 weeks off from work because she was worried about having another "attack." She had been employed for 5 years as a secretary for a small insurance agency. Just before she was about to return to work, she experienced another attack. After this third attack, she decided not to return to work and to quit her job. She was unable to leave the house to go grocery shopping, to drive the children to activities, or to

go out socially with her friends. Her husband, who is 42 years old, stated that he and their three daughters, aged 15, 12, and 9 years, were very concerned about her and had been helping her with daily tasks.

After her husband leaves, Mrs. Johnson begins to cry and states that she is letting her family down. They have tried to help her and she cannot do anything at home; she cannot work or even leave the house because she is so afraid of being unable to control the possibility of another attack. She does not understand what is happening to her and wants medication to help her feel better.

On the third day of her hospitalization, Mrs. Johnson tells the nurse that she is upset because her husband has not visited her since her admission. As she continues to talk about her husband, she starts to cry and states that she is afraid of losing him. She reports that 2 or 3 months ago, she noticed a change in her husband. He was less affectionate and was spending more time away from home. Suddenly he had more business trips. She is afraid he is having an affair. She says, "What am I going to do if he leaves? I can't support myself and my children alone. I don't even have a job. I can't go out of the house. I've lost contact with my friends."

Care Plan

Name: <u>Sandra Johnson</u>   Admission Date: _____

DSM-IV-TR Diagnosis: <u>Panic disorder with agoraphobia</u>

Assessment	**Areas of strength:** Managing her role as mother, homemaker, and secretary; was socially active with her friends; is in relatively good health.
	Problems: Fear of dying related to fear of heart attack; unable to leave home; fear of losing her husband; feelings of inadequacy.
Diagnoses	• Anxiety: panic related to life stress, as evidenced by somatic symptoms and fear of dying.
	• Self-esteem disturbance related to feelings of helplessness, as evidenced by inability to function.
	• Fear related to avoidance, as evidenced by inability to leave home.

Outcomes

Short-term goals: *Date met*

• Patient will discuss fears, her sense of inadequacy and helplessness, and anger.   _____

• Identify relationship between anxiety and physiological responses.   _____

• Develop strategies for reducing anxiety, such as relaxation techniques.   _____

• Use problem-solving techniques for life stresses.   _____

Long-term goals:

• Patient will meet with husband and social worker to discuss marital issues.   _____

• Schedule appointment with outpatient therapist for systematic
   desensitization or self-exposure training.   _____

• Identify schedule for attending an agoraphobia support group.   _____

Care Plan—cont'd

Name: <u>Sandra Johnson</u>   Admission Date: _____

DSM-IV-TR Diagnosis: <u>Panic disorder with agoraphobia</u>

Planning/ Interventions	**Nurse-patient relationship:** Empathy and supportive-suppressive techniques to keep anxiety at a minimum; encourage ventilation of feelings and issues; help patient to identify relationships among stress, anxiety, and physiological responses; assist with adaptive coping strategies. **Psychopharmacology:** Ativan 1 mg q 4 hr prn; Prozac 20 mg q AM. **Milieu management:** Decrease stimuli and provide quiet, calm atmosphere; monitor anxiety level to prevent escalation; encourage recreational and diversional activities; use quiet room if necessary; later encourage problem-solving assertiveness, communication, problem-centered, self-esteem, and stress management groups.
Evaluation	Patient reports being less anxious for the past 2 days. Met with husband and social worker.
Referrals	Outpatient appointments for cognitive therapy and self-exposure training.

Milieu management

As a patient's anxiety decreases from the panic level to other levels of anxiety, gross motor activities, such as walking, jogging, basketball, volleyball, or the use of a stationary bicycle, are appropriate to help decrease tension and anxiety. Other milieu interventions are located in the section about GAD.

OBSESSIVE-COMPULSIVE DISORDER

According to the DSM-IV-TR, obsessions are recurrent and persistent thoughts, ideas, impulses, or images that are experienced as intrusive and senseless. (See box on "Criteria for Obsessive-Compulsive Disorders.") Individuals with obsessive-compulsive disorder (OCD) recognize that the thoughts are products of their own minds; they know that the thoughts are trivial, ridiculous, or aggressive but cannot stop, forget, or control them. The thoughts are distressful and anxiety provoking. An example of an aggressive obsession is a woman experiencing an obsession to kill her child. An example of a silly obsession is the rhyme "Sticks and stones may break my bones, but words will never hurt me."

Compulsions can be defined as repetitive behaviors that are performed in a particular manner in response to an obsession. The compulsions are performed to prevent discomfort and to bind or neutralize anxiety. Individuals with OCD experience anxiety if they try to resist the obsessions or the compulsions. Some examples of compulsions are repetitive hand washing, checking the locks on doors, counting, and

---

DSM-IV-TR — Criteria for Obsessive-Compulsive Disorders

A. Obsessions
   1. Intrusive, inappropriate, recurrent, and persistent thoughts, impulses, or images that are distressful or produce anxiety
   2. Unsuccessful attempts to ignore or neutralize thoughts or impulses by other thoughts or actions
   3. Recognition that obsessions are produced by own thoughts
   4. Not simply excessive worry about real-life problems
B. Compulsions
   1. Repetitive behaviors, such as hand washing, or mental acts, such as counting, are performed in response to an obsession
   2. Excessive behaviors or mental acts are used to reduce distress or prevent dreaded events
C. Recognition that obsessions or compulsions are unreasonable or excessive
D. Obsessions or compulsions cause distress, are time-consuming, and interfere with usual daily functioning

Adapted from the American Psychiatric Association: *Diagnostic and statistical manual of mental disorders,* ed 4, text revision, Washington, DC, 2000, APA.

---

touching. These individuals know or recognize that their actions are absurd, but they are compelled to perform the rituals to avoid an extreme increase in tension and anxiety. These individuals have a great need to control themselves, others, and their environment. Some individuals with OCD find it difficult to express emotions and to be introspective. Depression is a feature associated with this disorder because of its impact on self-esteem and self-worth.

An important feature to remember about OCD is that the obsessions or compulsions are severe to the extent that they significantly interfere with the patient's normal routine and are time consuming to the extent that they interfere with occupational and social functioning. The obsessions and compulsions also interfere with these patients' interpersonal relationships because they do not have time to relate to others—they are too busy thinking or doing. People who experience *magical thinking* believe that thinking *equals* doing.

CLINICAL EXAMPLE

John is watching a football game on television. As his favorite player prepares to attempt a field goal, John experiences severe anxiety because he thinks the player will miss the field goal. John is afraid that his thinking will cause the player to miss.

Thinking processes in individuals with OCD may also be rigid, and these individuals may be task oriented. Relaxation is difficult. Patients with OCD are extremely overcontrolled and have a strong sense of right and wrong.

In this society, value is placed on performing well in school and at work. Being responsible and perfectionistic is often rewarded by the boss or by family members. Thus, at times, anyone may be "compulsive." Generally, however, people do not allow their compulsiveness to rule their lives; they are able to maintain a balance between work and play, between role expectations and performance. There is a difference between having characteristics or traits and having an illness. Occasional brooding, rumination, or steadfastness to a task is not usually considered ridiculous or excessively bothersome. These thoughts and feelings do not rule most people's lives.

Critical Thinking Question

A patient with OCD washes her hands after each time she touches anything. Her skin is cracked and bleeding. She states to the nurse, "I can't get my hands free of germs." What would you say and do when this patient approaches the sink to wash her hands?

Etiology

Current views concerning the origin of OCD point to genetic transmission. OCD may run in families (Grinspoon, 1998). Biologic findings in OCD identify increased brain activity in the frontal lobe and basal ganglia (Glod, Cawley, 1997). Serotonin dysregulation is involved in the formation of OCD. This action may account for the effectiveness of clomipramine (Anafranil) and the SSRIs.

Psychotherapeutic Management

Nurse-patient relationship

Basic nursing interventions for hospitalized patients with OCD are listed in the box below.

Therapeutic work involves the nurse increasing patients' abilities to verbalize feelings, solve problems, and make decisions concerning stressors and problems. The nurse focuses on teaching and helping patients develop adaptive coping behaviors to deal with anxiety. Patients need to learn to substitute

---

Key Nursing Interventions   for Obsessive-Compulsive Disorder

1. Ensure that basic needs of food, rest, and grooming are met. *Rationale:* patients are too busy to attend to these tasks. Reminders and specific directions are usually necessary.
2. Provide patients with time to perform rituals. *Rationale:* patients need to keep anxiety in check. Later, work to decrease the rituals by setting limits, but never take away a ritual, or panic may ensue.
3. Explain expectations, routines, and changes. *Rationale:* to prevent an increase or escalation of anxiety.
4. Be empathic toward patients and aware of their need to perform rituals. *Rationale:* to convey acceptance and understanding.

5. Assist patients with connecting behaviors and feelings. *Rationale:* to promote the ability to identify and understand feelings.
6. Structure simple activities, games, or tasks for patients. *Rationale:* to help patients focus on alternatives to their thoughts and actions.
7. Reinforce and recognize, positive nonritualistic behaviors. *Rationale:* to increase patients' self-esteem and self-worth.

positive, anxiety-reducing behavior for obsessions and rituals. A variety of positive behaviors can include physical exercise, such as walking or using a stationary bicycle. Positive coping behaviors are slowly introduced into each patient's schedule, allowing time for rituals, as well as normal activities. The nurse supports patients and positively reinforces nonritualistic behavior. Hobbies and social activities are introduced slowly as patients are able to handle them.

Psychopharmacology

The antidepressant clomipramine (Anafranil) and the SSRIs, such as fluoxetine (Prozac), sertraline (Zoloft), fluvoxamine (Luvox), paroxetine (Paxil), are effective in treating OCD. Patients tolerate the SSRIs better than they do clomipramine (Anafranil) because of a better side effect profile. The treatment of patients with OCD with SSRIs is unique in that a selective efficacy exists. Other antidepressants are ineffective, a longer therapeutic lag occurs, and higher doses are often required than in treating patients with other disorders (Hollander et al, 2001).

Milieu management

A variety of milieu activities and groups are beneficial to patients. Of particular importance are stress-management groups, relaxation exercises, recreational or social skills groups, cognitive therapy groups, problem-solving groups, and communication or assertiveness training groups. Care is always based on the individual needs of patients.

Behavior therapies are effective for patients with OCD and can be performed on an outpatient basis. These approaches are encouraged to slowly contact feared stimuli and then to limit the rituals or the number of repetitions. Exposure treatment is explained in Chapter 38 on behavior therapy. A form of cognitive therapy such as thought stopping can be used. When an intrusive thought occurs, the patient says "stop" and snaps a rubber band on the wrist or substitutes an adaptive behavior, such as deep breathing, for the ritual. A 7-week group exposure and response prevention therapy was also found to be effective (Himle et al, 2001).

PHOBIC DISORDERS

Phobic disorders are intense, irrational fear responses to an external object, activity, or situation. Anxiety is experienced if the person comes into contact with the dreaded object or situation. Similar to all anxiety disorders, a phobia is a response to experienced anxiety and is characterized by a persistent fear of *specific* places or things, as opposed to GAD, in which the anxiety is free-floating; thus anxiety is displaced or externalized to a source outside the body.

Phobias persist even though phobic individuals recognize that they are irrational. People can control the intensity of anxiety simply by avoiding the object or situation they fear.

In the DSM-IV-TR, phobias are categorized into three types:

1. Agoraphobia without history of panic disorder: a fear of being in public or open spaces, places, or situations in which escape might be difficult or help might not be available, for example, if the person should faint.
2. Social phobia: fear of being humiliated, scrutinized, or embarrassed in public, for example, choking while eating in front of others or stumbling while dancing in view of others.
3. Specific phobia: fear of a specific object or situation that is not either of the above. Examples are a fear of animals, flying, or heights.

Exposure to the stimulus results in an anxiety response. It is common to have some fears or phobias about certain objects or situations. Some people are afraid of public speaking, while some may be afraid of elevators or heights. However, these fears do not ruin most people's lives to the extent that they can never leave home. Most people are still able to function and fulfill role expectations, responsibilities, and relationships. Phobic symptoms become phobic disorders when they cause severe distress and impair functioning.

Etiology

Research has led to theories that specific individual factors, environment, family environment, and genetic factors underlie phobic disorders. Types of phobias develop based on the influence of environment and genetic predisposition.

Psychotherapeutic Management

Nurse-patient relationship

Patients with phobic disorders are usually treated on an outpatient basis. If the phobia incapacitates a patient to a severe extent, as in panic disorder with agoraphobia, the patient may be hospitalized. Another example in which hospitalization is indicated is the person who has a phobia about germs and may not eat or drink. Some interventions useful for individuals experiencing phobic disorders are the following:

1. Accept patients and their fears with a noncritical attitude.
2. Provide and involve patients with activities that do not increase anxiety but will increase involvement rather than avoidance.
3. Help patients with physical safety and comfort needs.
4. Help patients recognize that their behavior is a method of coping with anxiety.

Psychopharmacology

Behavior therapies are the most successful treatments of phobic patients, and drugs traditionally have no effect on avoidant behaviors. Medication that reduces or blocks panic attacks or reduces depression is used if those features are present.

Milieu management

Assertiveness-training and goal-setting groups are beneficial. Social skills groups and other milieu activities help patients redevelop social skills and decrease avoidance.

Behavior therapy, such as systematic desensitization, flooding, exposure, and self-exposure treatments, is most therapeutic for phobic patients. Self-exposure treatment is being used more often to avoid frequent therapy sessions (see Chapter 38).

ACUTE STRESS DISORDER AND POSTTRAUMATIC STRESS DISORDER

Acute stress disorder (ASD) and posttraumatic stress disorder (PTSD) are somewhat different from the other anxiety disorders. ASD and PTSD are disorders that can develop after exposure to a clearly identifiable traumatic event that threatens the self, others, resources, and/or a sense of control or hope and that overwhelms the individual's usual coping strategies. Some of the traumatic stressors that may precipitate the development of ASD and PTSD are community violence, war, terrorist attack, being a hostage or prisoner of war, torture, natural and man-made disasters, bombings, fatalities in fires or accidents, catastrophic illness, gross injury to self or others, childhood sexual abuse, chronic abuse, rape, assault, and sudden or major personal losses (Everly, Flannery, Mitchell, 2000; Kaplan, Iancu, Bodner, 2001).

Anyone experiencing events such as these would be distressed, with intense fear, horror, and a sense of helplessness. (The box on the following page lists the DSM-IV-TR criteria for ASD and PTSD). To an extent, the type and degree of the initial and later reactions to trauma depend on the individual's pre-existing characteristics and conditions, usual coping style and defense mechanisms, personal and social resources, previous exposure to trauma, and the meaning of the event to the individual.

The diagnosis of ASD is made when an individual has dissociative symptoms *during or immediately after* the distressing event: amnesia, depersonalization, derealization, decreased awareness of surroundings, numbing, detachment, or lack of emotional response. The diagnosis of PTSD is not made because of any initial reactions at the time of the trauma but is based on the characteristic symptoms that occur *1 month or more after* the trauma. It is common for PTSD to be unrecognized for years, sometimes even 10 to 20 years, which is a result, in part, of the major characteristic of both ASD and PTSD:"numbing of responsiveness" to or reduced involvement with the external world. There is a persistent attempt to avoid situations, activities, and, sometimes, people who evoke memories of the trauma. These efforts include trying to avoid thoughts and feelings related to the event.

Denial, repression, and suppression are common in both disorders. A constricted or blunted affect, or a limitation in the range of feelings, may occur, such as being unable to show affection. Patients may feel detached or estranged from family and friends. An inability to trust and to love may lead to withdrawal. Interest in activities, even those unrelated to the traumatic event, is often lost. The individual's perceptions about the future may also change—a kind of hopelessness, for example, hopelessness about having a family or a career.

A second major characteristic of ASD and PTSD is reexperiencing the traumatic event in some way, which may occur as intrusive, unwanted memories; upsetting dreams or nightmares; illusions; or suddenly feeling as if the event were reoccurring (flashbacks). With PTSD, there may be hallucinations related to the traumatic event. It is not known precisely why these unpleasant, frightening experiences begin to break through the denial, repression, or suppression. The triggers for the reexperiencing episodes may have obvious connections to the trauma or may not resemble the original situation at all. In the latter case,

DSM-IV-TR Criteria for Acute Stress Disorder and Posttraumatic Stress Disorder	

Acute Stress Disorder
1. Exposure to a traumatic event involving threat of death/injury to self or others, or actual injury to self or others
2. Responses of horror, helplessness, or fear
3. Dissociative symptoms during or immediately after the event:
  • Absence of emotions, numbing, detachment
  • Decreased awareness of surroundings (in a "daze")
  • Derealization or depersonalization
  • Amnesia
4. Reexperiencing or reliving the traumatic event: distressing thoughts, dreams, flashbacks, illusions
5. Avoidance of stimuli related to trauma: feelings, thoughts, people, conversations, places, and activities. Distress when exposed to reminders of the event
6. Increased arousal or anxiety: sleep disturbance, hypervigilance, startle response, irritability, restlessness, decreased concentration
7. Impairment or distress in functioning: occupational, social, or other important areas
8. Onset: within 4 weeks after the event
9. Duration: 2 days to 4 weeks
	Posttraumatic Stress Disorder
	1. Same criteria as ASD
	2. Some criteria as ASD (in children, may be seen as agitated or disorganized behavior)
	3. Numbing of responsiveness
	  • Restricted affect, such as not being able to love or detachment
	  • Sense of "foreshortened future" (lack of expectations about the future)
	  • Inability to recall aspects of the event
	4. Same criteria as ASD plus
	  • Hallucinations (in children may be seen as repetitive play with reenacting aspects of trauma or frightening dreams with no particular theme)
	5. Same criteria as ASD, plus
	  • Decreased participation and interest in activities
	  • Estrangement and detachment from others
	6. Same criteria as ASD plus
	  • Outbursts of anger
	7. Same criteria as ASD
	8. Onset:
	  • Acute: within 6 months after the event
	  • Delayed: 6 months or more after the event
	9. Duration:
	  • Acute: 1 to 3 months
	  • Chronic: 3 months or more

Adapted from the American Psychiatric Association: *Diagnostic and statistical disorders*, ed 4, text revision, Washington, DC, 2000, APA.

patients may try to avoid all activities and people in an effort to prevent reexperiencing the flashback.

CLINICAL EXAMPLE

Three days after a tornado had destroyed her home and seriously injured her son, Joan Marin was found wandering around the hospital in which her son was a patient. She was not injured but complained of nightmares and irritability. She said she could not bear to see her son because he "just wanted to talk about what happened—things I can't remember." Joan had not been to work since the tornado. She was taken to the crisis unit and diagnosed with ASD.

Other criteria of ASD and PTSD include increased arousal, anxiety, restlessness, irritability, disturbances in sleep, and impairment in memory or concentration. Especially with PTSD, there may be occasional outbursts of anger or rage and "survivor guilt," that is, guilt about surviving or the actions taken to survive (Kaplan, Iancu, Bodner, 2001). For example, disaster or terrorist victims and combat soldiers may feel they survived because of cowardly acts; rape victims may feel guilty for not resisting their attacker.

Another consequence of ASD and PTSD can be psychologic and physiologic symptoms that develop during exposure to situations resembling the original trauma, such as anxiety or panic attacks or psychophysiologic illnesses (e.g., gastrointestinal disorders, headache). Differentiating ASD and PTSD from other disorders is sometimes difficult.

Individuals experiencing posttraumatic symptoms may develop problems with grief, depression, suicidal ideations and attempts, impulsive self-destructive behaviors, anxiety-related disorders, and substance abuse (Foa, Keane, Friedman, 2000; McMillan, North, Smith, 2000). Patients may appear avoidant, schizoid, schizophrenic, paranoid, or even manic. These symptoms complicate treatment, especially if the ASD and PTSD are ignored and only the other diagnoses are treated.

Preexisting psychiatric disorders, including personality disorders, can increase the risk of developing ASD and PTSD after a traumatic event (Tucker et al, 2000). A history of previous traumas, including childhood abuse, rape, and abuse by a partner, leads to an increased risk for PTSD after later traumas. On the other hand, events later in life may trigger previously unrecognized PTSD. For example, some World War II and Korean veterans had not shown PTSD symptoms until after experiencing retirement, losses, and other processes associated with aging (Snell, Padin-Rivera, 1997). Activation and reactivation of PTSD symptoms has also been reported in veterans following the Persian Gulf War and in people who survived the Oklahoma City bombing (Moyers, 1996), as well as some who witnessed the World Trade Centers and Pentagon tragedies.

There may be difficulties such as arrests, unemployment, homelessness, abusiveness, divorce, and paranoia toward authority figures or other persons whom patients perceive as directly and indirectly responsible for not helping with the original traumatic situation (Amaya-Jackson et al, 1999; Beckham, Moore, Reynolds, 2000). Mistrust, isolation, abandonment fears, workaholism, focusing on the needs of others, feelings of inadequacy, anger toward God, unresolved grief, and fear of losing control of emotions are common (Bille, 1993).

The family members, friends, and co-workers of individuals with ASD or PTSD may develop problems as well, as "secondary victims" (see box below on Family Issues). In some cases, these individuals experience the same trauma (e.g., accident, fire, disaster) and develop symptoms themselves. The family may or may not be able to help in the treatment of their family member with ASD or PTSD. The whole family or selected members may need treatment.

After a community disaster or a tragedy affecting the nation, many people may experience acute stress or posttraumatic symptoms and initially find it difficult to get support from others. When the danger is over, small groups of victims may gather for mutual support and assistance. Fear, concern, uncertainty, frustration, anger, grief, and humor are all to be expected. Disaster personnel often encourage and facilitate debriefing in groups, including groups of emergency personnel. With the World Trade Centers and Pentagon tragedies, the firefighters, emergency medical technicians, and police were not only rescuers, but they were also victims.

Neurochemical Basis of Acute Stress Disorder and Posttraumatic Stress Disorder

It is proposed that fear conditioning, a failure of extinction (of the fear-anxiety response), and behavioral sensitization may be important in the development of ASD and PTSD symptomatology following exposure to a traumatic event (Charney et al, 1993; van der Kolk, 1997). It has been shown that *fear conditioning* to auditory and visual stimuli can last for years and produce relatively indelible emotional and visceral memories. If *extinction* of fear responses does not occur, the responses continue even when the traumatic event is absent (Beckham, Moore, Reynolds, 2000). Normally, associations leading to the conditioned response would be "erased," or new associations would "mask" the response-producing associations over time. Conditioned fear responses, after being dormant for years, can be reactivated by trauma-associated stimuli.

Family Issues | Acute Stress Disorder and Posttraumatic Stress Disorder

Family members, friends, and colleagues of patients with acute stress disorder (ASD) or posttraumatic stress disorder (PTSD) need to be assessed along with patients. Issues to be addressed include the following:

1. Assess whether any or all members of the family or others have been exposed to the same trauma as the patient and, if so, if family members may be experiencing symptoms of ASD or PTSD as well.
2. Assess whether any or all of the family members or others are having reactions to the behaviors of the member with ASD or PTSD.
3. Teach family members and others about the causes, symptoms, and treatment of ASD and PTSD.
4. Educate family members and others about ways to help the patient(s) with ASD or PTSD.
5. Referring family members and others to a support group for families of ASD or PTSD survivors or a related group, if available.
6. Referring members for couple or family counseling if needed.

Sensitization is the increased magnitude of response to one stimulus, but especially to repeated traumatic stimuli. This behavioral sensitivity produces increased arousal *(hyperarousal)* and stress sensitivity that can endure for a long time (Beckham, Moore, Reynolds, 2000). *Cross-sensitization* can occur such that there is overreaction to other, even minor, stimuli that resemble the original traumatic stimulus (Beckham, Moore, Reynolds, 2000; Charney et al, 1993; Friedman, 1997; van der Kolk, 1997).

Avoidance (behavioral), numbing (emotional), autonomic hyperarousal (somatic), and reexperiencing of the trauma (cognitive, emotional, somatic, and behavioral) are characteristic symptoms of ASD and PTSD. Avoidance and numbing (in response to fear conditioning and behavioral sensitization) are likely to be related to increased endogenous opiate release (Friedman, 1997), producing emotional blunting, physical analgesia, and depersonalization. Autonomic hyperarousal (also in response to fear conditioning and behavioral sensitization) is related to increased noradrenergic and dopaminergic system activity and decreased serotonergic activity, causing fear, anxiety, and "fight or flight" readiness. Reexperiencing the trauma (in response to fear conditioning and failure of extinction) is related to activation of the amygdala, locus ceruleus, thalamus, and hippocampus, which enhances encoding of traumatic memories, and sensory and cognitive memory retrieval (Charney et al, 1993; Friedman, 1997; van der Kolk, 1997). Prolonged stress eventually results in downregulation of the corticotropin-releasing factor (CRF) and adrenergic receptors and decreased adrenocorticotropin-releasing hormone (ACTH) release, so that the fear-anxiety response may become blunted and desensitization induced (Friedman, 1997; van der Kolk, 1997).

Hyperarousal may cause memories to be dissociated, repressed, or stored as bodily sensations that are not available at a conscious level. Fragments of these memories may appear later as physiologic reactions, nightmares, flashbacks, and emotional reenactments of the trauma (van der Kolk, 1997). ASD and PTSD patients typically have more psychophysiologic symptoms, sleep disturbances, and altered immune function than individuals who do not have ASD and PTSD (van der Kolk, 1997).

The incidence of alcohol, opiate, and benzodiazepine abuse in individuals with posttraumatic symptoms may be related to attempts to reduce the symptoms that result from increased noradrenergic and dopaminergic activity. Conversely, "addiction" to trauma (compulsively exposing oneself to traumatic events) may be explained, in part, by the recurrent increase in endogenous opiates. Individuals with posttraumatic symptoms also have an exaggerated response to amphetamines and cocaine because of their preexisting hyperarousal. After taking these drugs, individuals with posttraumatic symptoms are more vulnerable to paranoia and psychosis (Bremner et al, 1996).

Critical Thinking Questions

Ron Jenkins's workplace was severely damaged by an explosion. He was found staring at the cars in the parking lot and repeating that he had to find his car and wife. He was unable to give his address or say where his wife would be at that time of day. He refused to be treated for cuts and bruises until he could find his wife. What interventions would you use at the scene? What referrals and recommendations would you make to prevent ASD and PTSD?

Psychotherapeutic Management

The most effective approach with ASD and PTSD is to prevent or minimize the symptoms. Principles of Critical Incident Stress Management (CISM) are often applied to natural and manmade disaster situations (including the World Trade Centers and Pentagon attacks) in which the development of posttraumatic symptoms in some victims is likely. This model provides a wide range of services for primary and secondary victims, including "seven core integrated elements: (1) precrisis preparation (including individuals and organizations who will assist in CISM); (2) large-scale demobilization procedures for use after mass disasters; (3) individual acute crisis counseling; (4) brief small-group discussions called defusings, designed to assist in acute symptom reduction; (5) longer small-group discussions, called critical incident stress debriefing (CISD), designed to assist in achieving a sense of psychological closure post crisis and/or facilitate the referral process; (6) family crisis intervention techniques; and (7) follow-up procedures and/or referral for psychological assessment or treatment." (Everly, Flannery, Mitchell, 2000, p. 24). The National Organization of Victims Assistance (NOVA Model) and the American Red Cross have developed similar models.

The element of CISM related to crisis counseling is similar to the crisis intervention strategies described in Chapter 12, but places more emphasis on mobilizing community resources to assist in crisis management (Everly, Flannery, Mitchell, 2000). Group psychologic debriefing technologies (usually implemented in 2 to 7 days after the traumatic event) "seek to restore reasonable mastery, the support network of caring attachments, and victims' sense of meaning in life, as well as to stabilize the situation and provide symptomatic relief" (Everly, Flannery, Mitchell, 2000, p. 26). This group work is an organized and structured approach, beginning with a discussion of the goals, rules, and roles of the leaders (who are often both mental health workers and trained peers of the victims). Then, there is a cognitive-oriented discussion of the facts of the incident, beginning with thoughts group members experienced when arriving on the scene. The discussion then moves to an emotional phase that allows for the expression of the full range of feelings. The final stage of the group focuses on discussing any symptoms of ASD or PTSD, which are being experienced, teaching coping strategies to use with any further stress reactions, and ways to prepare for return to work. Ideally, the goal for group debriefing is psychologic closure related to the critical event and a return to a precrisis (or an even more functional) level of adaptation. After the group debriefing, the leaders also debrief among themselves about what they heard and felt while listening to the traumatic experiences being discussed and about the effectiveness of the group debriefing (Everly, Flannery, Mitchell, 2000). With large-scale disasters, such as the World Trade Centers, closure is much more difficult because of the extended length of time required for location and identification of victims and for the final cleanup of the debris.

The treatment of patients who do develop ASD or PTSD must be individualized according to age or developmental level or both (Adams et al, 1999; Tierney, 2000), the predominant symptoms, and the associated problems, such as disorganized behaviors, depression, suicidal ideation, or substance abuse. (See Chapter 36 for working with dually diagnosed patients and Chapter 41 on Survivors of Violence for specific traumas, such as workplace violence, cults, ritual abuse, rape, partner abuse, and childhood sexual abuse, as well as the stages of recovery from trauma.) The goals of treatment are progressive,

intensive review of the traumatic experiences and then integration of the feelings and memories, often from the least to the most painful. This approach involves moving from a victim status to a survivor status, from "I can't go on because of this" to "I have learned from it and can go on with my life." As with any crisis, there is a potential for growth and the development of improved coping skills, appreciation of the value of life, and enhanced relationships.

Nurse-patient relationship

The first priority in the relationship with patients experiencing ASD or PTSD is the development of trust. Because these patients have a tendency to be withdrawn, to feel alienated, and to be suspicious of others, developing trust may be difficult. Seeking help or accepting it when offered is also sometimes difficult for patients. When a patient is aware of the current influence of the trauma, there is often a tendency for him or her to believe that "No one can understand what I've been through unless they have been through it too." Therefore the nurse needs to be nonjudgmental, honest, empathic, and supportive. The nurse can convey the message, "I haven't been through what you have, but the more you tell me, the better I will understand what you have been through and are experiencing." It is important to acknowledge any unfairness or injustices that were part of the trauma.

These patients also need to hear that they are not "crazy" but that they are having typical reactions to a serious trauma. Teaching about the dynamics of ASD or PTSD is often appropriate (Creamer, 2000). Depending on the nature of the trauma, the nurse must be prepared to hear "horror stories" about hideous injuries, unpredicted behaviors, and gross destruction. If the nurse cannot tolerate the stories of atrocities, patients are not free to process all of the losses and changes that have occurred in their lives as a result of the trauma. Nurses may need help themselves to avoid vicarious victimization (secondary PTSD) or burnout when working with trauma victims in setting such as emergency departments, burn units, neonatal intensive care units, accidents, or disaster scenes (Hospital Focus, 2000; Lyttle, 2001; Badger, 2001).

It may take time for patients to recognize the relationship between current problems and the original traumatic event. When patients are not initially aware of the connection between the original trauma and current feelings and problems, the nurse should gently clarify these connections as they emerge.

Patients need to evaluate their past behaviors according to the original context of the situation, not by current values and standards (Figley, 2000). For example, a rape victim who did not resist her knife-wielding attacker needs to judge her behavior in the context of the life-or-death situation, not by an acquaintance's comment that she "must have asked for it." Another example is the Vietnam veteran who must evaluate his experience of killing a woman who was holding a grenade within the context of war, not by society's current view of that war as immoral. Developing a new perspective on the original trauma, which involves clarifying facts, feelings, and values, is not always easy for patients.

Specific techniques are sometimes used to help patients with ASD and PTSD: systematic desensitization described in the Behavior Therapy chapter (Creamer, 2000); cognitive-behavioral therapy described in Chapter 3; and eye movement desensitization and reprocessing (EMDR) (Barron, Curtis, Grainger, 1998; Creamer, 2000).

Patients need significant help in safely verbalizing feelings, particularly anger, that have often been ignored or repressed. This circumstance is especially true if there have been destructive outbursts or patients are trying desperately to remain in control. Writing in a journal is often helpful. Expressive therapy (psychodrama, art, music, and poetry) can facilitate externalizing painful emotions that are difficult to verbalize (Clark, 1997; Hines-Martin, Ising, 1993).

As patients struggle through the sometimes lengthy process of reexperiencing, reintegrating, and processing memories of and feelings about trauma experiences, patients need empathy and reassurance that they will be safe and not overwhelmed with anxiety (Figley, 2000). It is also important to take "time-outs" to focus on emergent problems and potential solutions. These problems, such as finances, housing, divorce, and their associated feelings, can be as stressful as the original event.

Patients need to be involved in problem solving, decision-making, and taking specific actions toward overcoming these stresses. Patients' adaptive coping skills and use of relaxation strategies need to be encouraged, whereas dysfunctional ones, especially avoidance of responsibility for one's actions and the abuse of alcohol and drugs, are discouraged. For patients plagued by intrusive thoughts, it may be helpful to have them imagine the word "stop" or to snap a rubber band on their wrist to interrupt these thoughts (Clark, 1997).

Patients also need to establish or reestablish relationships that provide support and assistance. Couple or family education and counseling may be recommended if appropriate. Hospitalization of ASD and PTSD patients is normally necessary only if they are suicidal, homicidal, self-mutilating, or unable to function in daily activities. The following box titled, "Key Nursing Interventions for Acute Stress Disorder and Posttraumatic Stress Disorder" lists additional nursing interventions to use with ASD and PTSD.

Key Nursing Interventions for Acute Stress Disorder and Posttraumatic Stress Disorder

1. Be nonjudgmental and honest; offer empathy and support; acknowledge any unfairness or injustices related to the trauma. *Rationale:* building trust may be difficult for patients.
2. Assure patients that their feelings and behaviors are typical reactions to serious trauma. *Rationale:* patients often believe that they are "going crazy."
3. Help patients recognize the connections between the trauma experience and their current feelings, behaviors, and problems. *Rationale:* patients often are unaware of these connections.
4. Help patients evaluate past behaviors in the context of the trauma, not in the context of current values and standards. *Rationale:* patients often have guilt about past behaviors and are judgmental of themselves.

5. Encourage safe verbalization of feelings, especially anger. *Rationale:* feelings are or have been repressed or suppressed.
6. Encourage adaptive coping strategies, exercise, relaxation techniques, and sleep-promoting strategies. *Rationale:* patients may have been using maladaptive or dysfunctional coping to avoid dealing with feelings and issues.
7. Facilitate progressive review of the trauma and its consequences. *Rationale:* review helps patients integrate feelings and memories and begin the grieving process.
8. Encourage patients to establish or reestablish relationships. *Rationale:* relationships (needed for assistance and support) may have been affected by patients' suspiciousness or fear of asking for help.

Case Study

Billy Craig was 19 years old when he spent a year in heavy combat in Vietnam. Although he was upset when his buddies were killed, he was secretly relieved when his wounds got him sent home. He studied forestry and became a ranger in a national forest. He was considered a loner and showed no interest in marriage. He never talked about his experiences in Vietnam with anyone.

During the television coverage of the World Trade Centers and Pentagon tragedies, Billy began to have nightmares and flashbacks about killing the enemy and about a friend who was dismembered. Billy became angry more frequently and startled easily. After a month of not seeing him, other rangers found Billy in his cabin, very depressed, and surrounded by old guns and grenades. He kept repeating that he should have died in Nam too. He admitted that he was intending to shoot himself. With effort, the rangers convinced him to come with them to the mental health center, where he was admitted and diagnosed with delayed posttraumatic stress disorder and major depression.

Psychopharmacology

Medications for patients experiencing ASD or PTSD are used generally for short-term therapy during the acute crisis or for intensive counseling periods to prevent or reverse neurochemical fear conditioning and sensitization. The choice of medications depends on the primary symptoms.

Benzodiazepines, such as clonazepam, may be prescribed to reduce levels of conditioned fear and anxiety symptoms. These medications also may help patients with sleep disturbances and nightmares. Of course, there is a risk of dependence, especially with patients who are already abusing alcohol or drugs. Other benzodiazepines, such as lorazepam, are usually prescribed on an as-needed (prn) basis for short periods rather than on a fixed schedule.

Clonidine and *propranolol* may produce responses similar to those of the benzodiazepines. Propranolol can help to diminish the peripheral autonomic response associated with fear.

Valproic acid or *carbamazepine* are sometimes given to patients who are experiencing explosive outbursts and intense feelings of being out of control. These drugs can help decrease hyperarousal, startle response, and nightmares.

SSRIs (paroxetine and sertraline) may reverse continued emergency responses and decrease repetitive behaviors, images, and somatic states.

Tricyclic antidepressants (TCAs) are used if depression, anhedonia, and sleep disturbances are primary problems. TCAs, especially amitriptyline, are usually given in one dose at bedtime. Trazodone may be used instead of the TCAs.

Antipsychotics are used if patients also have psychotic thinking. These drugs may be used for hyperarousal in acute crisis periods. Low doses of risperidone can help decrease flashbacks and nightmares (Charney et al, 1993; Davidson, 1997; Famularo, 1997; Friedman et al, 2000).

Milieu management

Patients experiencing ASD or PTSD can benefit from many inpatient or outpatient milieu activities. Social activities can help to rebuild social skills that have been damaged by suspiciousness and withdrawal. Recreational and exercise programs can help reduce tension and promote relaxation. Groups that may be useful are those that focus on self-esteem, decision-making, assertiveness, stress-management, and relaxation techniques. Victims of a variety of traumas may benefit from group meetings that focus on the similarities in their reactions and feelings, such as mistrust, helplessness, fear, guilt, numbing, detachment, nightmares, and flashbacks.

Community resources

A particularly useful therapeutic aid for patients experiencing ASD and PTSD is group therapy or self-help groups with others who have experienced the same or a similar trauma. A community may have a veterans outreach center for Vietnam veterans and their spouses, as well as groups for victims of rape, incest, or torture and their family members. A community may hold meetings for victims after a community disaster or national tragedy. There also may be a victim's assistance program for crime victims.

Care Plan

Name: Billy Craig   Admission Date: _____

DSM-IV-TR Diagnosis: Axis I—Posttraumatic stress disorder; major depression

Assessment	**Areas of strength:** Intelligent, enjoys his work, has supportive co-workers.
	Problems: Suicidal ideation, flashbacks of and anger about Vietnam; disturbed sleep; lives in an isolated area.
Diagnoses	• Potential for self-directed and other-directed violence related to suicidal ideation and anger, as evidenced by suicidal behavior and statements.
	• Sleep pattern disturbance related to nightmares, as evidenced by interrupted sleep, increasing irritability.
	• Posttrauma response related to war experiences, as evidenced by reexperience of traumatic events in flashbacks and nightmares.

Outcomes	*Short-term goals:*	*Date met*
	• Patient will state that he is no longer suicidal and will appropriately verbalize feelings of anger and sadness.	_____
	• Patient will describe his experiences in Vietnam.	_____
	Long-term goals:	
	• Patient will schedule outpatient appointments at the veteran's outreach center and at the mental health center.	_____

Planning/ Interventions	**Nurse-patient relationship:** Assess and monitor suicidal ideations. Assist patient with identification and verbalization of feelings, especially anger. Assist patient in describing Vietnam experiences.
	Psychopharmacology: Paroxetine (Paxil) 20 mg 8 AM; risperidone (Risperdal) 1 mg bid; lorazepam (Ativan) 1 mg q4hr prn.
	Milieu management: Groups focusing on stress and anger management, relaxation techniques, social skills, and self-esteem.
Evaluation	Patient verbalizes that he is no longer suicidal. Patient is beginning to verbalize his anger and sadness about Vietnam and the loss of his buddies.
Referrals	His appointment at the veteran's center is January 12; his appointment at the mental health center is on January 25.

ADJUSTMENT DISORDERS

This separate group of adjustment disorders is *not* part of the anxiety disorders category but is included here because of its contrasts with ASD and PTSD. The diagnosis of adjustment disorder may be made when symptoms develop within 3 months after an identifiable life event, and the reaction is not severe enough to fit the criteria of ASD or PTSD. Common events or circumstances that may precipitate an adjustment disorder are divorce, moving, marriage, retirement, illness or disability, financial problems, or difficulties in child rearing.

The symptoms of maladaptive reactions to a stressful event or circumstances are not defined as specifically as those for ASD and PTSD, but they are still considered more severe than a "normal" stress response or grief reaction. The acute reaction interferes with functioning but lasts no longer than 6 months *after* the stressor and its consequences have ended. Chronic symptoms may persist more than 6 months if the consequences of the stressor are more enduring, such as a chronic illness or difficulties resulting from a divorce.

The diagnosis of adjustment disorder is based on subcategories according to the predominant feature of the patient's maladaptive stress reaction. The major feature may be a mood disturbance of *anxiety* or *depression,* or it may be a disturbance with *mixed anxiety and depressed mood.* There may be a *disturbance of conduct:* violation of societal norms or the rights of others. There is a subcategory of *mixed disturbance of emotions and conduct.*

The psychotherapeutic interventions for patients with adjustment disorders are generally similar to those used for patients experiencing ASD and PTSD. The major goals are to recognize the relationship between the stressful situation and current problems and to review and reintegrate feelings and memories of the original situation.

SOMATOFORM DISORDERS

The major characteristic of somatoform disorders is that patients have physical symptoms for which there is *no known organic cause or physiologic mechanism.* Evidence is present or a presumption exists that the physical symptoms are connected to psychologic factors or conflicts. These patients are not in control of their symptoms, which are unconscious and involuntary. Patients express conflicts through bodily symptoms and complaints using the defense of somatization.

Patients with these disorders repeatedly seek medical diagnosis and treatment, even though they have been told that there is no known physiologic or organic evidence to explain or fully explain their symptoms or disability.

Traditional views concerning somatoform disorders consider repression, denial, and displacement as defense mechanisms used in these disorders. Repression occurs in reference to feelings, conflicts, and unacceptable impulses. Denial of psychologic problems is present even though these patients have been told that there is no physiologic cause or basis for their symptoms. Displacement occurs when the anxiety is transformed into bodily symptoms.

Current research suggests that genetic, developmental-learning, personality, and sociocultural factors can predispose, precipitate, and maintain somatoform disorders. Emotional and social stress can precipitate these disorders. Individuals with somatoform disorders often appear to be needy and dependent on others.

The somatoform disorders discussed here are somatization disorder, pain disorder, hypochondriasis, and conversion disorder. (See box titled, "DSM-IV-TR Criteria for Somatoform Disorders.")

SOMATIZATION DISORDER

According to the DSM-IV-TR, the main characteristic of somatization disorder is that these individuals

---

DSM-IV-TR   Criteria for Somatoform Disorders
Somatization disorder. Many physical complaints over several years, resulting in treatment being sought or impairment in functioning. It is characterized by 4 pain, 2 gastrointestinal, 1 sexual, and 1 pseudo-neurological symptom.   **Pain disorder.** Pain in one or more areas of the body that is severe enough to seek treatment; causes impairment in functioning or significant distress   **Conversion disorder.** One or more symptoms or deficits affecting voluntary motor or sensory function that suggest a neurologic or general medical condition   **Hypochondriasis.** Preoccupation with fear of having, or the idea that one has, a serious disease, includes misinterpretation of bodily symptoms; preoccupation persists despite medical evaluation and reassurance

Adapted from the American Psychiatric Association: *Diagnostic and statistical manual of mental disorders,* ed 4, text revision, Washington, DC, 2000, APA.

---

verbalize recurrent, frequent, and multiple somatic complaints for several years without physiologic cause. This type of disorder usually begins before the age of 30 years. These patients see many physicians through the years and may even have exploratory and unnecessary surgical procedures. Impairment in social and occupational functioning may be present.

PAIN DISORDER

The chief complaint in pain disorder is severe pain in one or more anatomic sites that causes significant distress or impairment in functioning (APA, 2000). The location or complaint of the pain does not change, unlike the complaints voiced in somatization disorder. Psychologic factors play a role in the development and maintenance of pain disorder. No organic basis for this disorder exists.

There may be underlying psychologic factors related to pain disorder that patients may not recognize consciously. For example, feelings connected with the loss of a job or status may occur before the development of pain disorder. This type of pain disorder is classified as *pain disorder associated with psychologic factors.* In some cases, the pain may allow patients to avoid something that they do not want to do; for example, a woman's chest pain may prevent her from going to work.

Sometimes, there is a physiologic disorder, but the amount of pain or impairment is greatly exaggerated or out of proportion. For example, a patient who has experienced a mild myocardial infarction (MI) is now convinced that he or she can no longer engage in recreational activities such as bicycling or swimming, resulting perhaps from feelings of inadequacy or fear of suffering another MI. This pain disorder would be classified as *pain disorder associated with both psychologic factors and a general medical condition.*

Patients with pain disorder are often "doctor shoppers" and may use analgesics excessively without experiencing any relief from their pain. These patients are often anxious about their symptoms and depressed about ever getting better.

HYPOCHONDRIASIS

Hypochondriacs are worried about having, or believe that they have, a serious disease based on the misinterpretation of bodily signs and sensations (APA, 2000). Medical evaluation and reassurance does not help dispel the fear. These patients displace anxiety onto their bodies and misinterpret bodily symptoms. Hypochondriacs "check" for reassurance from physicians or friends in ways that are similar to the compulsive behavior of patients with OCD. Hypochondriacs are afraid that they have a disease, whereas patients with OCD fear getting an illness and constantly check for germs. Similar to patients with OCD, hypochondriacs constantly check for reassurance about their illness.

CONVERSION DISORDER

The major characteristic of conversion disorder is a

CLINICAL EXAMPLE

Roberta is worried about having an ulcer. She experiences acid ingestion on occasion after dinner. The uncomfortable feeling in her stomach causes her to fear that her stomach acid will burn a hole in the stomach lining. After each episode, Roberta visits her doctor for a physical examination. Based on the negative results from examinations and tests, the doctor has repeatedly told her that she does not have an ulcer.

---

deficit or alteration in voluntary motor or sensory function that suggests a neurologic or medical condition (APA, 2000). Psychologic factors, conflicts, or stressors are associated with or precede the development of this disorder. The most common conversion symptoms suggest neurologic disease such as paralysis, blindness, or seizures. As mentioned earlier,

primary gain refers to the alleviation of anxiety that the disorder provides because conflict is kept out of conscious awareness. Secondary gain is the gratification received as a result of the way people in these patients' environment respond to their illness.

Another characteristic of this disorder is that the symptom often is determined by the situation that produced it. For example, a soldier suddenly develops paralysis of his hand. As a result, he can no longer engage in combat because he cannot pull the trigger on his gun. The symptom is related to the conflict. This soldier can discuss combat, but he cannot connect his feelings about fighting to the development of his paralysis.

This patient also may have an attitude of *la belle indifference,* meaning that he expresses little concern or anxiety about his distressing disorder. This lack of concern occurs because his symptom binds his anxiety so that it is not behaviorally expressed. It may seem as though patients with conversion disorder minimize their illness.

Psychotherapeutic Management

Nurse-patient relationship

The focus of the nurse-patient relationship is to improve patients' overall levels of functioning by building adaptive coping behaviors. Patients with somatoform disorders are often unable to identify and express their feelings, needs, and conflicts. Teaching them ways to verbalize feelings appropriately helps eliminate or diminish the need for physical symptoms.

Patients need time to understand their need for physical symptoms. Awareness and insight develop slowly as they begin to verbalize their needs. For some patients, this awareness and insight take longer to develop.

The physician or psychiatrist orders tests and laboratory workups to thoroughly assess patients physically for the presence of any physiologic or organic disease or causation (if this has not been done before admission). The absence of any relevant medical findings strongly suggests that somatization is present.

The nursing interventions used for patients with somatoform disorders are described in the box on page 400.

Psychopharmacology

Because patients with somatoform disorders may be using too much medication and taking a variety of

Key Nursing Interventions for Somatoform Disorders

1. Use a matter-of-fact, caring approach when providing care for physical symptoms. *Rationale:* to decrease secondary gains and to decrease focusing on physical symptoms.
2. Ask patients how they are feeling and ask them to describe their feelings. *Rationale:* to increase the use of verbalization about feelings (especially negative ones), needs, and anxiety rather than about somatization.
3. Assist patients with developing more appropriate ways to verbalize feelings and needs. *Rationale:* to increase adaptive coping through assertiveness.
4. Use positive reinforcement and set limits by withdrawing attention from patients when they focus on physical complaints or make unreasonable demands. *Rationale:* to increase noncomplaining behavior.
5. Be consistent with patients, and have all requests directed to the primary nurse providing care. *Rationale:* to decrease attention-seeking or manipulative behaviors.
6. Use diversion by including patients in milieu activities and recreational games. *Rationale:* to decrease rumination about physical complaints.
7. Do not push awareness of or insight into conflicts or problems. *Rationale:* to prevent an increase in anxiety and the need for physical symptoms.

Case Study

William Robinson, a 62-year-old white man, was admitted to the psychiatric inpatient unit on June 15 at 10 AM. He walked onto the unit limping and supported by his wife, Harriet. He stated that he was experiencing horrible pain in his left leg and foot. Anger and irritability were evident in his voice.

Mr. Robinson's pain started suddenly about 7 months ago. Since that time, he has seen numerous physicians to obtain treatment and relief from his pain. The last physician told him that his pain was due to stress, and it was recommended that he be hospitalized to obtain treatment from a physician who was trained to manage stress-related disorders. The patient stated that he hoped this physician would know what to do; that none of the others did.

Mrs. Robinson brought her husband's medications to the hospital. The nurse found that a number of analgesics had been prescribed, along with sleeping medication. Mr. Robinson said that he took what he wanted, when he wanted it, and that it was better than not taking anything at all.

The next day, after visiting her husband, Mrs. Robinson told the nurse that Mr. Robinson needed a lot of help with everything. In fact, she had been so physically tired that she had called their only daughter, Sheila, for assistance. Sheila lives 400 miles away, and they had not seen her for 3 years. Their daughter was so concerned about her parents that she had come to help for 2 weeks last month.

As the conversation continued, Mrs. Robinson told the nurse that her husband had been in good health, except for an occasional cold, until about 8 months ago, when he suddenly started to complain about awful pain in his leg and foot. He had never in all his years working for a cabinet manufacturer experienced anything like this before. Mrs. Robinson did not know why all of this pain was happening now, especially since her husband had retired 9 months earlier. He had been forced to retire early, because the company he worked for had not been doing well and all employees aged 60 and over were forced to retire. She stated that her husband had never said too much about it, and she thought that now they would have time to travel and take fishing trips, which her husband had always enjoyed. They had taken many fishing trips as a family while their daughter was growing up and had enjoyed them immensely. Periodically, her husband went fishing with some friends. Since the onset of her husband's pain, however, they had not done anything socially, together or with friends.

From the time he was admitted to the hospital, Mr. Robinson refused to do anything but sit in a lounge chair in the community room. He needed much assistance from staff members to walk to the dining room and to the restroom. At times, his food was brought to him in the community room because he refused to walk to the dining room.

Interactions with the nurse centered on his pain and on requests for pain medication. He described his pain in detail and would talk of little else.

Mr. Robinson was getting Darvon for pain, and an antidepressant as ordered by his physician.

Care Plan

Name: <u>William Robinson</u>   Admission Date: _____

DSM-IV-TR Diagnosis: <u>Pain disorder</u>

Assessment	**Areas of strength.** Enjoyed fishing and traveling; had been in good health; wife is very supportive; had worked for many years. **Problems.** Experiencing pain in his left leg and foot; social functioning has declined; focus with staff is about his pain; secondary gains maintain his sick role.
Diagnoses	• Ineffective coping related to anger, as evidenced by complaints of physical pain. • Chronic pain, related to low self-esteem, as evidenced by inability to verbalize feelings. • Severe anxiety, related to dependency, as evidenced by inability to care for self.

Outcomes

Short-term goals: *Date met*
• Patient will verbalize feelings and needs.   _____
• Patient will verbalize underlying anger as a result of early retirement.   _____
• Patient will verbalize awareness about connecting conflict with physical   _____
  symptoms.
• Patient will develop adaptive coping behaviors.   _____
Long-term goals:
• Patient will assume responsibility for self-care and independent functioning. _____
• Patient will schedule appointments for joint counseling with his wife.   _____
• Patient will identify plans to volunteer in his community.   _____
• Patient will plan leisure activities.   _____

Planning/ Interventions	**Nurse-patient relationship.** Convey interest and support, focus on assisting the patient to verbalize feelings and needs related to anxiety, self-esteem, and anger, give positive feedback when the patient focuses on issues other than pain; set limits on need for attention and medication. **Psychopharmacology.** Decrease the use of analgesics. Paxil 20 mg q AM. **Milieu management.** Encourage participation in assertiveness and communication groups, as well as problem-solving, discharge-planning, and social skills groups, diversional occupational therapy and recreational activities.
Evaluation	Patient's focus on pain is decreasing and is able to assume self-care activities with little assistance.
Referrals	Appointments for outpatient group therapy and counseling with wife.

---

drugs, medication for pain should be used temporarily and sparingly. SSRIs are helpful for treating anxiety and depression.

Milieu management

For patients with conversion disorder, hypnosis may be used to help identify the source of the conflict. Psychologic testing and relaxation exercises also may be helpful. Relaxation exercises and behavior modification may help patients with other somatoform disorders. Assertiveness, decision-making, goal-setting, stress-management, and social skills groups often benefit these patients.

Outpatient therapy is also necessary for most patients. Because patients with somatoform disorders are usually overusers of medical care, some hospitals and clinics provide psychotherapy groups as part of the medical care. These groups focus on underlying psychosocial needs, not on physical needs. The success of this type of treatment approach can result in decreasing hospital costs, while providing more appropriate patient care. The hope is that the efficacy of these groups will be recognized and thus used in more hospitals to provide optimal and appropriate patient care.

DISSOCIATIVE DISORDERS

Dissociation, which is the removal from conscious awareness of painful feelings, memories, thoughts, or aspects of identity, is an unconscious defense mechanism that protects an individual from the emotional pain of experiences or conflicts that have been repressed. This "splitting off" helps these individuals endure and survive intense emotion or physical pain or both.

Dissociation occurs in extreme stress or trauma, such as war or abuse in childhood and adulthood. Everyone uses dissociation at times. For example, a person may be engrossed in a book or a movie that they do not hear anything or anyone around them. This instance is not pathologic. Everyone forgets things or daydreams. However, this circumstance does not indicate an illness. Abnormal dissociative states are the dissociative disorders when identity, memory, or consciousness are disturbed or altered. Dissociative disorders in the DSM-IV-TR are dissociative amnesia, dissociative fugue, depersonalization, and dissociative identity disorder (multiple personality disorder) The box titled, "Criteria for Dissociative Disorders" summarizes the main characteristics of dissociative disorders.

DSM-IV-TR Criteria for Dissociative Disorders

Dissociative amnesia. Loss of memory of important personal events that were traumatic or stressful in nature

Dissociative fugue. Sudden, unexpected travel away from home or work with a loss of memory about the past; confusion about identity or assumption of partial or completely new identity is present

Depersonalization. Experiences of feeling detached from, or an outside observer of, one's body or mental processes; reality testing is intact

Dissociative identity disorder. Presence of two or more identities or personalities that take control of the person's behavior; loss of memory for important personal information

Adapted from the American Psychiatric Association: *Diagnostic and statistical manual of mental disorders,* ed 4, text revision, Washington, DC, 2000, APA.

DISSOCIATIVE AMNESIA

Amnesia is the loss of memory or the inability to recall important personal information. Recent amnesia can occur immediately after a traumatic event, such as a car accident. Localized amnesia occurs when the individual cannot remember what occurred during a specific period of time (e.g., not being able to remember what happened for hours after a car accident). The ability to recall some events during a specific period is called selective amnesia (APA, 2000). It is important to remember that patients are sometimes found by the police; these patients wander aimlessly and are confused and disoriented. These individuals may be taken to a hospital and may be frightened and perplexed. The precipitant is usually something that causes severe psychosocial stress, such as the threat of physical injury or death.

The DSM-IV-TR describes dissociative amnesia as one or more episodes of the inability to recall important personal information that is beyond ordinary forgetfulness. The information is usually stressful or traumatic in nature. The amnesia does not occur only during the course of dissociative identity disorder, nor is it the result of a substance (drug or medication) or a medical condition, such as head trauma (APA, 2000).

DISSOCIATIVE FUGUE

The major feature of dissociative fugue is sudden, unexpected travel away from home or locale with the assumption of a new identity (partial or complete) or a confusion about one's identity. The travel and behavior appear normal to casual observers, thus the person does not seem to be wandering in a confused state.

Fugue states last from a few hours to several days. These episodes are usually accompanied by amnesia; consequently, patients do not remember what happened during the fugue state. Sometimes, depression is also present.

Dissociative fugues usually follow severe psychosocial stress, such as marital quarrels, personal rejections, military conflict, or natural disaster. The fugue state then allows escape or flight from an intolerable event or situation.

DEPERSONALIZATION

According to the DSM-IV-TR, depersonalization is included in this group of disorders because the sense of one's reality is changed, but the person is oriented to time, place, and person. In depersonalization, individuals feel detached from parts of their body or from mental processes. Depersonalization involves an altered sense of self such that individuals feel unreal or strange or feel that danger is not happening to them but to someone else. Therefore as a response to overwhelming stress, these individuals are protected from overwhelming anxiety. Depersonalization can also involve feeling like a robot or feeling as though one is in a dream. Depersonalization is often accompanied by symptoms of derealization in which individuals feel that the outside world is changed or unreal. For example, buildings may appear to be leaning, or everything may seem gray and dull.

A diagnosis of depersonalization is made only when the prevalence or intensity of the disorder causes marked distress, interferes with daily functioning, and occurs in the absence of other disorders. An imaging study of depersonalization disorder suggests abnormalities on limited cortical areas (Simeon et al, 2000). Little research has been done on this disorder to date.

DISSOCIATIVE IDENTITY DISORDER

The major feature of dissociative identity disorder is the existence of two or more identities or personalities that take control of the person's behavior (APA, 2000). The person, or "host," is unaware of the other personalities, but the other personalities may be aware of each other in varying degrees.

Traditional views of this disorder consider dissociation to be a defense against extreme anxiety that is aroused in highly painful and emotionally traumatic situations, such as physical, emotional, and sexual abuse. The "splitting off" of these painful events allows the person to survive the trauma but leaves an impaired personality with disconnected parts or "alters." The alter personalities contain feelings and behaviors associated with the trauma.

Each personality is quite different from the others and from the original personality. Each personality has its own name, behavior traits, memories, emotional characteristics, and social relations. The primary identity may carry the person's name and be depressed, dependent, and guilty, while alternate personalities may be hostile, controlling, and self-destructive (APA, 2000).

A shy, quiet woman may have alternate personalities that are promiscuous or flamboyant, childlike, and aggressive. A woman may awaken one morning and find the living room of her apartment littered with toys or strewn with empty alcohol bottles and leftover food. She does not remember what happened because she has amnesia for the span of time when another personality has taken over or "come out."

Sometimes, a switch to another personality is preceded by a headache, or individuals may cover their face and eyes with their hands. For example, the patient or original personality may state that he or she hears voices talking to one another in his or her head. This instance may be misdiagnosed as auditory hallucinations, and the disorder misdiagnosed as schizophrenia.

These patients are admitted to inpatient psychiatric units when they are suicidal, meaning that an alter personality is trying to harm or kill one of the other personalities for revelations, or when mutilation or uncontrollable impulses to harm the self are present. Severe anxiety or depression related to the coming out of upsetting alters may also be a reason for admission. Sometimes, the safe structure of a hospital setting provides emotional security when working with difficult or overwhelming material.

Some patients experience numerous hospitalizations with different diagnoses before they are finally and accurately diagnosed with dissociative identity disorder. The array of symptoms these patients present may be one reason for inaccurate diagnoses. Another reason may be that patients do not recognize their symptoms or know what they mean. Patients may think that they are "going crazy" or "losing their minds" because they do not understand what their symptoms mean or represent. Thus these individuals might delay seeking treatment until their disorder severely interrupts their functioning in life. Others around them, such as family members, may not understand what is occurring, may not know how to help, or may want to keep the disorder a secret, especially if the perpetrator of abuse is among them.

Psychotherapeutic Management

Nurse-patient relationship

The nurse's relationship with individuals experiencing amnesia and fugue includes interventions to establish trust and support. Patients have physiologic and neurologic workups to rule out organic causations. The nurse assists with gathering data regarding feelings, conflicts, or situations that patients experienced before the amnesia or fugue state. Patients also may have sessions under hypnosis to gather data about forgotten material. The nurse should slowly help patients deal with anxiety and conflicts in their lives.

Patients with depersonalization disorder are not usually found in an inpatient setting unless they have become suicidal, extremely anxious, or depressed. Nurses may work with these patients in outpatient settings.

The treatment goal of dissociative identity disorder, ultimately, is to integrate the personalities or memories, if possible, thus they can survive or coexist in the original personality. Therapy, combined with hypnosis, assists in this process.

The nurse works with patients to establish trust because the relationships of these patients with authority figures may have been inconsistent, rigid, and unpredictable. A contract should be initiated for patients' safety and to reduce self-harm and violence. An alter may be homicidal because of revelations concerning abuse. Self-mutilation and suicidal behaviors also may be present when overwhelming anxiety or depression occurs. The nurse must also be alert to "splitting" by staff members regarding patients' diagnoses. The staff may divide into groups of believers and nonbelievers regarding the validity of patients' diagnoses. Education about diagnoses, management of feelings, especially anger and rage, and consistency of approach assist the staff with developing a caring, supportive environment for patients so that trust increases and a predictable positive learning environment ensues.

Psychopharmacology

The symptoms of the dissociative identity disorder are not alleviated by medication. Patients' response to medication may be partial, and alters' response to medication may be different and inconsistent. If symptoms of anxiety, and depression are present in these patients, medication may alleviate them.

Milieu management

The nurse assumes an important role in the care of patients who are hospitalized in an inpatient psychiatric unit because of suicidal or uncontrollable attempts to harm themselves. Provisions for a safe environment and a trusting relationship are basic to helping these patients, who usually have not had trusting relationships with anyone. Assisting with therapy sessions, providing emotional security, acceptance, support, and helping patients cope with daily living are all involved in nursing care.

For patients with dissociative identity disorder, ongoing process-oriented groups may be nontherapeutic when patients reveal too much and overwhelm the group or regress. Individual therapy should be in progress and may have been initiated before hospitalization. Task-oriented groups are beneficial. Occupational therapy and art therapy provide patients with a means of nonverbal expression to reveal material that cannot be verbally accessed. Attendance at milieu meetings decreases isolation from the community. Patients should attend activities that they and their alters can cooperate and participate in appropriately.

Before discharge, a safety plan and "no-harm" contract may be necessary, as well as initiating or continuing a system of support for the patient. Self-help support groups provide outpatients the opportunity to learn social skills and problem solving to develop a sense of empowerment and control.

Critical Thinking Question

A patient with dissociative identity disorder is admitted to the inpatient unit because of self-mutilating behavior. Before admission, the patient has stated to a friend, "I'll kill you and kill myself." The patient refuses to sign a "no-harm" contract. What type of initial care plan would you design, including types of precautions?

| Key Concepts

1. The issues of primary and secondary gains are important to patients because primary gain relieves discomfort, while secondary gain may encourage patients to maintain their sick role.
2. Patients' anxiety must be reduced to a mild or moderate level before the nurse can work with them on problem solving and adaptive coping.

3. In the category of anxiety disorders, symptoms of anxiety are directly felt or expressed.
4. With somatoform disorders, anxiety is expressed through physical symptoms.
5. In dissociative disorders, anxiety is "split off" (or removed) from conscious awareness, which helps patients survive extreme emotional pain.
6. Uncovering and linking feelings with conflicts and managing feelings are important aspects of recovery and nursing care plans.

References

Adams SM et al: Mental health response: nursing interventions across the lifespan, *J Psychosoc Nurs* 37(11):11, 1999.

Amaya-Jackson L et al: Functional impairment and utilization of services associated with posttraumatic stress in the community, *J Trauma Stress* 12(4):709, 1999.

American Psychiatric Association: *Diagnostic and statistical manual of mental disorders*, ed 4, text revision, Washington, DC, 2000, APA.

Badger JM: Understanding secondary traumatic stress, *AJN* 101(7):26, 2001.

Ballenger JC et al: Consensus statement on generalized anxiety disorder from the international consensus group on depression and anxiety, *J Clin Psychiatry* 62(suppl 13):47, 2001.

Barron J, Curtis MA, Grainger RD: Eye movement desensitization and reprocessing, *J Am Psychiatr Nurs Assoc* 4(5):140, 1998.

Beckham JC, Moore SD, Reynolds V: Interpersonal hostility and violence in Vietnam combat veterans with chronic posttraumatic stress disorder, *Aggression and Violent Behavior* 5(5):451, 2000.

Bille DA: Road to recovery, posttraumatic stress disorder: the hidden victim, *J Psychosoc Nurs Ment Heath Serv* 31(9):19, 1993.

Bremner JD et al: Vietnam vet's PTSD experience, *J Psychosoc Nurs Ment Health Serv* 34(6):48, 1996.

Charney DS et al: Psychobiologic mechanisms of posttraumatic stress disorder, *Arch Gen Psychiatry* 50(4):294, 1993.

Clark C: Posttraumatic stress disorder, *Am J Nurs* 97(8):27, 1997.

Creamer M: Posttraumatic stress disorder following violence and aggression, *Aggression and Violent Behavior* 5(5):431, 2000.

Davidson JR: Pharmacotherapy of generalized anxiety disorder, *J Clin Psychiatry* 62(suppl 11):46, 2001.

Davidson JRT: Biological therapies for posttraumatic stress disorder: an overview, *J Clin Psychiatry* 58(9):29, 1997.

Everly GS, Flannery RB, Mitchell JT: Critical incident stress management (CISM): a review of the literature, *Aggression and Violent Behavior* 5(1):23, 2000.

Falsetti SA, Davis J: The nonpharmacologic treatment of generalized anxiety disorder, *Psychiatr Clin North Am* 24(1):99, 2001.

Famularo R: What are the symptoms, causes, and treatments of childhood posttraumatic stress disorder? *Harv Ment Health Lett* 13(7):8, 1997.

Figley CR: Families coping with trauma, clinical update: posttraumatic stress disorder, *Am Assoc Marriage Family Ther* 2(5):1, 2000.

Foa EB, Keane TM, Friedman MJ: Guidelines for treatment of PTSD, *J Trauma Stress* 13(4):539, 2000.

Friedman MJ: Posttraumatic stress disorder, *J Clin Psychiatry* 58(9):33, 1997.

Glod C, Cawley D: Psychobiology perspectives: the neurobiology of obsessive-compulsive disorders, *J Am Psychiatr Nurs Assoc* 3(4):120, 1997.

Grinspoon L, editor: Obsessive compulsive disorder. Part II, *Harv Ment Health Lett* 15(5):4, 1998.

Grinspoon L, editor: Panic disorder, *Harv Ment Health Lett* 17(9):1, 2001.

Himle JA et al: Group behavioral therapy of obsessive-compulsive disorder: seven vs. twelve-week outcomes, *Depress Anxiety* 13:161, 2001.

Hines-Martin VP, Ising M: Use of art therapy with post-traumatic stress disordered veteran clients, *J Psychosoc Nurs Ment Health Serv* 31(9):29, 1993.

Hollander E et al: Pharmacotherapy for obsessive-compulsive disorder, *Psychiatr Clin North Am* 23(3):643, 2001.

Hospital Focus: Avoiding secondary trauma in the emergency department, *RN* 63(12):24, 2000.

Kaplan Z, Iancu I, Bodner E: A review of psychological debriefing after extreme stress, *Psychiatr Serv* 52(6):824. 2001.

La Torre MA: Therapeutic approaches to anxiety-a holistic view, *Perspect Psychiatr Care* 37(1):28, 2001.

Lyttle V: Why ED nurses have *that* attitude, *RN* 64(9):49, 2001.

McMillen JC, North CS, Smith EM: What parts of PTSD are normal: intrusion, avoidance, or arousal? *J Trauma Stress* 13(1):57, 2000.

Moyers F: Oklahoma City bombing: exacerbation of symptoms in veterans with PTSD, *Arch Psychiatr Nurs* 10(1):55, 1996.

Nutt DJ: Neurobiological mechanisms in generalized anxiety disorder, *J Clin Psychiatry* 62(suppl 11):22, 2001.

Simeon D et al: Feeling unreal: a PET study of depersonalization disorder, *Am J Psychiatry* 157:1782, 2000.

Snell FI, Padin-Rivera E: Group treatment for older veterans with post-traumatic stress disorder, *J Psychosoc Nurs Ment Health Serv* 35(2):10, 1997.

Tierney JA: Post-traumatic stress disorder in children: controversies and unresolved issues, *J Am Psychiatr Nurs Assoc* 13(4):147, 2000.

Tucker P et al: Predictors of post traumatic stress symptoms in Oklahoma City: exposure, social support, peri-traumatic responses, *J Behav Health Serv Res* 27(4):401 2000.

van der Kolk BA: The psychobiology of post traumatic stress disorder, *J Clin Psychiatry* 58(9):16,1997.

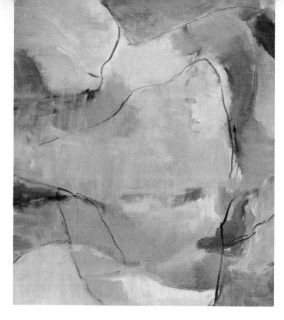

Chapter **32**

Cognitive Disorders

Judith A. Wilson; Catherine S. Childers

Learning Objectives

After reading this chapter, you should be able to:

- Describe the biologic and functional changes associated with the dementias (including Alzheimer's disease and vascular dementia).
- Describe the etiologic aspects and behaviors associated with delirium.
- Be able to use *The Diagnostic and Statistical Manual of Mental Disorders,* fourth edition, text revision

(DSM-IV-TR) to understand the diagnostic criteria used for cognitive disorders.
- Differentiate dementia from delirium.
- Discuss appropriate pharmaceutical interventions with patients with dementia.
- Develop a care plan for a patient with dementia.
- Develop effective caregiver interventions.
- Discuss family issues related to cognitive disorders.

INTRODUCTION

Cognitive disorders comprise a variety of assaults on the human brain. Cognition revolves around learning and memory. Loss of these fundamental abilities is a common thread in all cognitive disorders. In some disorders these losses may be temporary. However, for most disorders, loss of memory is the harbinger of things to come. This chapter describes the most common cognitive disorders that the nurse may confront.

Other changes in cognition commonly take place. Disorientation, decreased concentration, the loss of abstract thinking, and language disturbances may be present. Delusions, hallucinations, and misidentification may frighten the patients. These individuals might not be able to perform routine activities because they have forgotten how to do them in spite of intact motor skills.

Cognitive disorders are divided into reversible and irreversible types. These disorders can span a few hours to many years and may or may not be imminently life threatening. To cloud the diagnostic picture, patients may have more than one cognitive disorder or a coexisting psychiatric illness. Depression and anxiety are common in these patients.

Patients who exhibit a marked change of mental status often have a cognitive disorder. The DSM-IV-TR (American Psychiatric Association [APA], 2000) provides diagnostic criteria for all of these disorders. The DSM-IV-TR criteria for both delirium and dementia are included in boxes in this chapter. Table 32-1 compares and contrasts dementia and delirium. Key terms are included, and the student should also consult the glossary in the back of this text. The 12-month prevalence rate of mental disorders in the United States is also included.

|Table 32-1 | Dementia and Delirium: Contrast and Comparison

Characteristics	Delirium	Dementia
Onset	Occurs quickly, obvious	Slow, unnoticeable at first
Course	Acute: rapid development, hours to days usually but can last for months	Chronic: slow development over months and years with a progressive deterioration spanning 3-10 years until death
Causes	Usually the result of other physical reasons (e.g., illness, post surgical, toxins)	Usually the primary disorder, but may be related to other illnesses (e.g., AIDS)
Memory	Short-term memory is impaired; when it is assessed during an interim lucid or clear moment	Short-term memory is lost initially; long-term memory fails slowly
Level of consciousness	Fluctuating level of consciousness; alert at times; sleep is erratic; no pattern	No change; sleep patterns are usually consistent; day-night reversal is common
Thought content	Matches level of consciousness	Normal at first; later may be difficult to assess because of confusion or expressive or receptive aphasia and poverty of content
Thought process	Logical alternating with illogical, depending on the level of consciousness	Logical at first, then loss of abstraction (e.g., understanding a joke); concrete thinking occurs as the disease progresses
Speech	Slurred speech	Normal speech
Perceptual differences	Hallucinations—*visual:* seeing animals or unusual colors, also picking at the air is a sign; *tactile:* feeling bugs on or under the skin Delusions—grandiose, paranoid	Misidentification: (calling one relative another's name, for example, calling a daughter "mama"); hallucinations may occur in the later stage, usually not at first Delusions: pathologic jealousy, interfering with belongings and property
Mood	Anxiety and fear	Wide range of feelings
Affect	Appears bewildered, frightened	Appearance matches feeling

From Wilson J, Helton B: *PSYCHed: continuing education and consultation, dementia and delirium module,* Birmingham, Ala, 2001. Unpublished.

| 12-Month Prevalence Rate of Mental Disorders in the United States

Diagnosis	Percentage of Population over 17 Years of Age	Number of People
Anxiety disorders	12.6	20,034,000
Phobia disorders*	10.9	17,331,333
Mood disorders	9.5	15,143,000
Alcohol disorders	7.4	11,766,000
Major depression†	5.0	7,950,000
Drug disorders	3.1	4,929,000
Cognitive impairment	2.7	4,293,000
Obsessive-compulsive disorder	2.1	3,339,000
Antisocial disorder	1.5	2,385,000
Panic disorders*	1.3	2,067,000
Bipolar disorder†	1.2	1,908,000
Schizophrenia	1.1	1,749,000
Somatization	0.2	365,000

*Also calculated in anxiety statistics.
†Also calculated in mood disorders statistics.
From Regier DA et al: The de facto U.S. mental and addictive disorders service system: epidemiologic catchment area prospective, 1-year prevalence rates of disorders and services, *Arch Gen Psychiatry* 50:85, 1993; Surgeon General: Mental Health: A Report from the Surgeon General. DHHS, 1999, Washington, DC.

Pertinent DSM-IV-TR diagnoses and 2001 North American Nursing Diagnosis Association (NANDA) diagnoses, which facilitate care planning, are listed in the box on page 409.

In dementia research, dozens of diagnostic tools are available from pen-and-pencil examinations to sophisticated neuroimaging studies. The Geriatric Depression Scale can be found in Appendix C. Genetic studies have isolated chromosomes and genes that are related to certain diseases. Since 1993, four different medications for Alzheimer's disease have reached the market. However, no other medications have been approved for any other cognitive disorders.

OVERVIEW OF NONDEMENTIA COGNITIVE DISORDERS

Mild Cognitive Impairment

Mild cognitive impairment (MCI) is a regression in cognition that is not a result of normal aging. Petersen (2000) refers to mild cognitive impairment as the transitional zone between normal aging and very probable early Alzheimer's disease. Currently, no

DSM-IV-TR diagnosis exists for MCI. Forgetfulness is the hallmark behavior. Nonmemory areas of function are not impaired enough to lead to a dementia diagnosis. Jack and colleagues (1999) found that, in the patient with MCI, premorbid hippocampal atrophy was predictive of subsequent conversion to Alzheimer's disease. Ten to fifteen percent of patients with MCI converted to Alzheimer's disease in 5 years or less, according to Petersen (2000). Other reports have had even higher percentages. The *National Institute of Aging [NIA] 2000 Progress Report on Alzheimer's Disease* states that 40% of all patients with MCI develop Alzheimer's disease in 3 years. Morris et al, (2001) also concluded that patients with MCI are generally in the early stage of Alzheimer's disease.

No medications are specifically indicated for MCI, but several clinical trials are underway. Antioxidants such as vitamins C and E, estrogen, ibuprofen, and some of medications that the U.S. Food and Drug Administration (FDA) has approved for Alzheimer's disease are currently being tested. Although no treatments are available, the patient with MCI should consider staying active, exercising at the appropriate level, eating a well-balanced diet, curbing alcohol consumption, and stopping tobacco usage. Challenging the brain with mental exercises such as comparing and contrasting things, playing board games, putting together puzzles, and solving word games may enhance cognitive functioning.

Key Terms

Alzheimer's disease More correctly referred to as dementia of the Alzheimer type (DAT). DAT is the most common type of dementia. The characteristic symptoms are amnesia, aphasia, apraxia, and agnosia (the four As).

Cognitive disorder A disorder that affects consciousness, memory, and other cognitive processes.

Dementia A cognitive disorder that causes pronounced memory and cognitive disturbances. Typically, dementias are gradual in onset and progressive in course.

Delirium A disorder with alterations in consciousness and changes in cognition that are usually caused by a general medical condition or are substance induced. Typically, deliria develop over a short period of time and are treatable.

Vascular dementia (formerly multiinfarct dementia) Dementia resulting from interruption of blood to the brain, which causes anoxia, ischemia, and subsequent infarction.

CLINICAL EXAMPLE OF A PATIENT WITH MILD COGNITIVE IMPAIRMENT

Mr. Hawkins, a 67-year-old retired accountant, had trouble balancing his checkbook. He had forgotten to enter the amounts in the ledger. Mr. Hawkins was aware that he was forgetful and started asking his wife to help him. He did not have any other noticeable change in behavior. However, 3 years later he was diagnosed with Alzheimer's disease.

Delirium

The word *delirium* literally means "out of one's furrow," which refers to the dramatic behavioral changes the person might experience. The hallmark sign of delirium is its acute onset. This sign is key because the disorder rapidly develops in most cases. Other signs include a fluctuating level of consciousness, slurred speech, nonsensical thoughts, and day-night sleep reversal. The delirious patient may have visual hallucinations, for example, seeing multicolored rats or tactile hallucinations during which the patient may feel bugs under the skin. The patient may pick at the air as if trying to do some routine task, such as opening a prescription bottle. The patient may be able to follow a conversation for a short period followed by an acute bout of confusion. Emotions are on edge, and the patient may startle easily. The nurse should intervene quickly when delirium is suspected. Assessment and treatment of any underlying physical problem or illness should be addressed because delirium can be life threatening. In one retrospective study, Tasman (1997) found that 28% of patients with untreated delirium died within 3 months. One half of those patients died within 1 year.

DSM-IV-TR   Criteria for Delirium

Delirium is characterized by:
1. Disturbances of consciousness (i.e., reduced clarity of awareness of the environment) with reduced ability to focus, sustain, or shift attention.
2. Changes in cognition (e.g., memory deficit, disorientation, language disturbance, perceptual disturbance).
3. Developments over a short period of time (usually hours to days) and with a tendency to fluctuate during the course of the day.

Adapted from the American Psychiatric Association: *Diagnostic and statistical manual of mental disorders*, ed 4, text revision, Washington, DC, 2000, APA.

Delirium is the most common complication of the hospitalized older adult patient (Inouye, 2000). "ICU psychosis" is another name for hospital-based delirium. Acute changes in the patient's mental status may serve as a sign that a serious underlying medical illness exists (Inouye et al, 1999). Delirium is associated with numerous physical illnesses, especially pneumonia, myocardial infarction, and urinary tract infection. Toxic response to medications occurs with prescribed and over-the-counter (OTC) medications (e.g., anticholinergic, antihistaminic medications). Diphenhydramine is a common ingredient in OTC sedatives, allergy medicines, and cough syrups. Using one or more of these preparations increases the likelihood of developing delirium. Taking amitriptyline, a tricyclic antidepressant, and hydroxyzine, a medication used for anxiety and itching, places the older adult patient at risk as well. Benztropine and trihexyphenidyl, medications for extrapyramidal effects, may also lead to delirium. Mood stabilizers such as

Diagnoses Related to Cognitive Disorders

DSM–IV–TR*

Delirium types
Alcohol
- Induced persisting amnestic disorder
- Intoxication delirium
- Withdrawal delirium
Amphetamine (or amphetamine-like)
- Intoxication delirium
Delirium
- Cannabis intoxication
- Cocaine intoxication
- Inhalant intoxication
- Opioid intoxication
- Phencyclidine (or phencyclidine-like) intoxication delirium
- Sedative, hypnotic, or anxiolytic intoxication delirium
Delirium due to multiple etiologies
Sedative, hypnotic, or anxiolytic withdrawal delirium
Delirium due to [indicate the general medical condition]
Delirium NOS (not otherwise specified)

Dementia Types

Dementia
- Substance-induced persisting
- Dementia due to multiple etilogies
Dementia due to Creutzfeldt-Jakob disease
Dementia due to head trauma
Dementia due to HIV (human immuno-deficiency virus)
Dementia due to Huntington's disease
Dementia due to Parkinson's disease
Dementia due to Pick's disease

Dementia due to [indicate other general medical condition]
Dementia NOS
Dementia of the Alzheimer's type
- With early onset
- With late onset
Vascular Dementia

Other Disorders

Amnestic disorder NOS
Amnestic disorder due to [indicate the general medical condition]
Cognitive disorder
Other (or unknown) substance-induced persisting amnestic disorder
Sedative-, hypnotic-, or anxiolytic per-sisting amnestic disorder

NANDA**

Anxiety
Anxiety, Death
Caregiver role strain, Risk for
Comfort, Impaired
Communication, Impaired verbal
Confusion,
   Acute
   Chronic
Coping,
   Ineffective
   Ineffective community
   Compromised family
   Disabled family
   Readiness for enhanced family
Denial, Ineffective
Diversional activity, Deficient

Family processes,
   Alcoholism, dysfunctional
   Interrupted
Fear
Grieving,
   Anticipatory
   Dysfunctional
Hopelessness
Knowledge, Deficit
Loneliness, Risk for
Memory, Impaired
Noncompliance
Powerlessness, Risk for
Self care deficit,
   Bathing/Hygiene
   Feeding
   Toileting
Self-esteem,
   Chronic low
   Situational low
Sensory perception, disturbed
Sleep pattern, disturbed
Social interaction, impaired
Social isolation
Spiritual distress, Risk for
Suicide, Risk for
Therapeutic regimen management,
   Effective
   Ineffective
   Ineffective community
   Ineffective family
Thought processes, disturbed
Violence,
   Risk for other-directed
   Risk for self-directed
Wandering

*From the American Psychiatric Association: *Diagnostic and statistical manual of mental disorders*, ed 4, text revision, Washington, DC, 2000, APA.
**From the North American Nursing Diagnosis Association: *NANDA-Approved nursing diagnoses: definitions and classifications 2001*, Philadelphia, 2001, NANDA.

lithium and divalproex sodium (or valproic acid) in older adults may become toxic at lower serum levels than the laboratory reference range. Malnourishment, dehydration, constipation, and impactions increase the possibility of developing delirium. The nurse, during the initial medication assessment, should ask the patient or family member about prescription *and* OTC medications. The nurse should also ask about cough syrup, dietary supplements, sleeping pills, and pain medications in particular.

Dementia is the most consistent risk factor for delirium. Of the patients who have delirium, 30% to 50% have dementia. If the cause of the delirium is the result of a physical illness, treatment should be started to stabilize the patient. Alcohol and drug withdrawal require strict protocols to reduce the likelihood of its occurrence.

If at all possible, delirium prevention is the best medical option. Epling and Taylor (1999) identify six risk factors: cognitive impairment, hearing impairment, sleep deprivation, immobility, visual impairment, and dehydration. These researchers also developed protocols that addressed each risk factor. Of their subjects who used these protocols, 87% did not develop delirium.

CLINICAL EXAMPLE OF A PATIENT WITH DELIRIUM
Ms. Helton, a 64-year-old woman, was found crawling around her bedroom. She thought her husband was plotting to kill her. She found his pistol, took it, and was waiting to shoot him when her daughter found her. At that time, she was taking three different OTC preparations that contained diphenhydramine: a sedative, a cough syrup, and a pill for allergies. Discontinuation of the diphenhydramine resulted in a return to the patient's premorbid level of cognitive function.

Pseudodementia

Pseudodementia is a type of cognitive disorder that is most often linked to an underlying functional psychiatric illness, such as depression (Tasman, 1997). These patients are often depressed to the extent that they seem demented. They are also typically withdrawn and apathetic. Patients with pseudodementia may be anxious and agitated. A common answer when responding to a question is, "I don't know" or other vacant responses. In contrast, the patient with dementia usually tries to answer questions.

The patient with pseudodementia usually responds favorably to treatment. The nurse can provide support, therapeutic activities, and structure. Medications can be given that target symptoms such as anxiety and depression. Once the clinical symptoms start resolving, the patient usually becomes more functional. However, many clinicians now agree with Reifler (2000) that pseudodementia is really predementia, which explains why some patients continue to decline.

CLINICAL EXAMPLE OF A PATIENT WITH PSEUDODEMENTIA
Mr. Howell, a 75-year-old man, refused to answer any assessment questions. He said, "I don't know" repeatedly throughout the interview. His wife tried to answer the questions for him. He had stopped taking the antidepressant prescribed for him 2 months before; he could not remember why. Mr. Howell also stopped playing dominoes with his friends. After he stabilized on the antidepressant medication, Mr. Howell resumed all of his usual activities. Two years later, he was diagnosed with Alzheimer's disease.

DEMENTIA

The word *dementia,* from Latin, literally means "out of one's mind." Dementia is a type of illness that has a progressive deteriorating course that ultimately affects cognition, perception, language, behavior, and motor abilities. Over 70 types of dementia have been identified, of which Alzheimer's disease is the most prevalent (Geldmacher, 1997).

A dementia can be either reversible or irreversible. Unfortunately, most dementing illnesses are irreversible, and those that can be reversed may not be completely reversible. Normal pressure hydrocephalus (NPH) and vitamin B_{12} deficiency are two of the dementias that are potentially reversible. Dementias related to endocrine dysfunction, other metabolic disturbances, and neoplasms may show some improvement after treatment (Perkin, 1998).

REVERSIBLE DEMENTIAS

Normal Pressure Hydrocephalus

NPH usually presents with this classic triad of symptoms: urinary incontinence, apraxic gait, and dementia. These patients have enlarged ventricles seen on

---

DSM-IV-TR Criteria for Dementia

A. The development of multiple cognitive deficits manifested by both
   1. Memory impairment (impaired ability to learn new information or to recall previously learned information).
   2. One (or more) of the following cognitive disturbances:
      a. Aphasia (language disturbance)
      b. Apraxia (impaired ability to carry out motor functions despite intact motor function)
      c. Agnosia (failure to recognize or identify objects despite intact sensory function)
      d. Disturbance of executive functioning (e.g., planning, organizing, sequencing, abstracting)
B. The cognitive deficits in criteria A1 and A2 each cause significant impairment in social or occupational functioning and represent a significant decline from a previous level of functioning.
C. The course is characterized by a gradual onset and continuing cognitive decline.

Note: The above are the common criteria for diagnosing a dementia. Delirium must be ruled out before a dementia can be diagnosed. A dementia related to a general medical condition must first rule out Alzheimer's disease and vascular dementia.

Adapted from the American Psychiatric Association: *Diagnostic and statistical manual of mental disorders,* ed 4, text revision, Washington, DC, 2000, APA.

---

either computed tomography (CT) or magnetic resonance imaging (MRI) scan of the brain (Tulberg et al, 1998). The cause of NPH is impaired return of cerebral spinal fluid to the spinal column from the brain. The cerebral spinal fluid has normal pressure or is slightly elevated when monitored. Urinary urgency or frequency, common signs of a urinary tract infection, may instead be a precursor to incontinence. Gait apraxia may be described as magnetic or as if the patient were walking over a sticky floor.

Impairment in activities of daily living is a common presenting problem. Another common early sign is a dulling of personality with lack of motivation (Perkin, 1998). Judgment and insight may be lacking. Memory loss is the last of three symptoms to appear. If untreated, these symptoms will progress until the patient is bed bound (Moore, Jefferson, 1996).

If caught early, NPH may be reversed. Unfortunately, the patient, family, and clinicians often ignore the initial symptoms. Treatment requires neuro-

surgery. A ventricular shunt is placed in one of the lateral ventricles in the brain, which then leads to the peritoneum (VP shunt). A small pump is implanted just under the scalp behind the ear. The caregiver activates the pump for the prescribed number of times and frequency each day. The surgery has a 50% success rate (Perkin, 1998). If NPH has progressed and is no longer reversible, the shunting procedure may not arrest further decline.

CLINICAL EXAMPLE OF A PATIENT WITH NORMAL PRESSURE HYDROCEPHALUS

Mrs. Burkhalter, a 66-year-old woman, was admitted for evaluation. Her husband said that she had been diagnosed with Alzheimer's disease. She was bed bound, incontinent of urine, and in a fetal position. Mrs. Burkhalter was unable to walk or talk. An MRI scan of her brain was suggestive of NPH. After surgical placement of a VP shunt, the patient was able to have meaningful conversation. She was able to ambulate with assistance. Although the illness was not completely reversed, the patient regained significant function.

Vitamin B_{12} Deficiency

Although vitamin B_{12} deficiency is common in older adults; the dementing disorder related to this deficiency is not. If anything interferes with the absorption of vitamin B_{12} in the stomach, malabsorption may occur. Pernicious anemia is the most prevalent cause of this deficiency.

Dementia related to vitamin B_{12} deficiency is rare. When the deficiency proceeds to this level, demyelinization occurs, leading to axon loss in the brain and in the spinal cord. Paresthesias start in the lower extremities, followed by upper extremity involvement. Behavioral and mood changes occur. On MRI of the brain, lesions may be found in the optic nerve and cerebral white matter. Perkin (1998) and Moore and Jefferson (1996) call this type of vitamin B_{12} deficiency encephalomyelopathy.

Vitamin B_{12} replacement should be started immediately and should be continued throughout the patient's lifetime. Changes take several months to appear. Because vitamin B_{12} supplementation treats the deficiency, the goal is to prevent dementia from developing. The nurse should educate the patient and family of the importance of routine health assessments.

CLINICAL EXAMPLE OF A PATIENT WITH VITAMIN B$_{12}$ DEFICIENCY

Mrs. Washington, an 84-year-old woman, was admitted for cognitive evaluation after the adult protective custody agency found her living in squalor. She was malnourished and dehydrated with a low vitamin B$_{12}$ level. The patient had forgotten to eat. She was also unstable because of weakness in her upper and lower extremities. Vitamin B$_{12}$ replacement therapy was started and continued in the nursing home after discharge.

IRREVERSIBLE DEMENTIAS

Presently, no cure is available for any of the following dementing disorders, but medications have been developed with FDA indications for Alzheimer's disease. Medications for vascular dementia are in clinical trials. The course of the irreversible dementias may be slowed and it may plateau, but cognitive decline is inevitable. Through education and support, the nurse can play a pivotal role in assisting both the patient and the family with this devastating diagnosis. Additionally, the nurse can inform patients and family members of the local and national resources available.

Each illness is different in origin and clinical manifestation, yet they also share some common behaviors. Effective interventions are featured in this chapter, as well as important issues that patients and their families face.

Alzheimer's disease is by far the most prevalent dementia, representing 50% of all demented patients. Individuals with vascular dementia comprise approximately 20%. Another 25% of patients with dementia have both Alzheimer's disease and vascular dementia. The remaining dementias account for the rest (Gruetzner, 2001). This small percentage of dementias include frontal lobe dementias (e.g., Pick's disease), dementia related to Parkinson's disease, diffuse Lewy body disease, dementia related to acquired immune deficiency syndrome (AIDS), Huntington's disease, dementia related to alcoholism, and Creutzfeldt-Jakob disease. Creutzfeldt-Jakob disease, although rare, sparks interest because of its connection with "mad cow" disease (Tasman, 2000).

Alzheimer's Disease

Alzheimer's disease is the most prevalent dementia. Alois Alzheimer, a German neurologist, first diag-

nosed a patient with this disease in 1907. Yet, the disease did not attract much attention for many years. Biddle and van Sickel in a 1948 psychiatric nursing text, included only three sentences about Alzheimer's disease. None of the other dementias were mentioned. Interest in this disease has had a resurgence in the last 20 years (Rosen et al, 2000). Now that Alzheimer's disease has been studied extensively, it is known that the course from onset to death of a patient with Alzheimer's disease may exceed 10 years. The patient with the illness the shortest time will generally have the most precipitous drop in cognition and function. The patient with a 10-year course usually has a more gradual and subtle decline.

Alzheimer's disease, as well as the other types of dementia, is diagnosed after all other disorders have been ruled out. Pseudodementia, mild cognitive impairment, delirium, and other psychiatric illnesses are considered before a dementia diagnosis is made. As previously stated, a patient may have more than one illness, which makes assessment and treatment that much more difficult.

Age is the most significant risk factor for Alzheimer's disease (Gruetzner, 2001). A history of head injury, lower levels of education, and being female are also risk factors (Plassman et al, 2000). Longevity and smaller head size were reasons given for the increased number of women having Alzheimer's disease. However, Snowdon (2001) asserts that gender alone does not explain this difference.

The three stages of Alzheimer's disease are mild, moderate, and severe. Each stage has characteristics that typify them, but symptoms may occur outside their expected stage.

Table 32-2 provides information related to the stages of Alzheimer's disease. When nurses and caregivers understand the different stages, they can then plan appropriate interventions.

What causes Alzheimer's disease?

Theories abound regarding the cause of Alzheimer's disease. The cholinergic hypothesis is perhaps the most recognized and accepted theory. Simply stated, the level of the neurotransmitter acetylcholine is reduced in the brain. Acetylcholine is the primary neurochemical that affects an individual's ability to acquire new information, make simple and complex decisions, and retain memories. The nucleus basalis of Meynert in the basal forebrain is the major site of

|Table 32-2| Stages of Alzheimer's Disease

Stage	Duration	Changes
Mild (MMSE* score = 20-30)	2-3 years	Decreased short-term memory. Word- and name-finding difficulties Decision-making, concentration, reasoning, and judgment problems Difficulty performing usual activities Denial Getting lost Repetitive questioning
Moderate (MMSE score = 10-19)	3-4 years	Apraxia, agnosia, aphasia with poor comprehension, disorientation, blunting of affect, misidentification, sleep disturbance, delusional, needs assistance with activities of daily living Redirectable, extreme emotional lability, self-absorption, supervision with meals, wandering, urinary incontinence, requires supervision
Severe (MMSE score = 0-9)	5-10 years or more	Gait disturbance, unable to feed self, double incontinence, bowel impaction, bed bound, difficulty swallowing, fetal position; requires 24-hour supervision or close observation or both

Adapted from Folstein M et al: Mini-mental state: a practical method for grading the cognitive status of patients for the clinician, *J Psychiatr Res* 12:189, 1975; Wilson J, Helton B: *PSYCHed: continuing education and consultation, dementia module,* Birmingham, Ala, 2001. Unpublished; Snowdon D: *Aging with grace,* New York, 2001, Bantam Books.
*MMSE, Mini-mental state examination.

cholinergic cell bodies. Axons communicate from this area to the hippocampus, amygdala, and neocortex. Deficiency in acetylcholine reduces the messages between these areas (Cummings et al, 1998; Stahl, 2000).

Oxidative stress plays a major part in this destructive process. Free radicals are produced that become killer proteins in these cholinergic-producing neurons (Stahl, 2000). Tau protein is altered and forms twisted ropelike bundles within the cell, resulting in neurofibrillary tangles. These distorted tubules are then unable to transport molecules through the cell that keep it alive. Consequently, less acetylcholine is available.

Other possible causes of Alzheimer's disease involve beta amyloid plaque deposits. The patient with Alzheimer's disease is thought to have an abnormality in deoxyribonucleic acid (DNA) that provides the basis of amyloid precursor protein (APP). When the Alzheimer's disease process starts, an inevitable cascade of events follows. The APP is cut by one of the secretases (enzymes). After this cut, the fragment becomes beta amyloid that forms the core of the amyloid plaques (Gruetzner, 2001; Stahl, 2000). Cell death results from an over abundance of this plaque formation, which clumps on the exterior of the cell.

It is unknown if plaques or neurofibrillary tangles play a more critical role in the development of Alzheimer's disease. In fact, researchers are uncertain if these tangles and plaques are the cause or the result of the disease (Stahl, 2000). Researchers usually identify themselves as being on one side of the "plaque versus tangle" debate or the other (Garber, 2001).

Genetics plays a part in Alzheimer's disease development. Genes on chromosomes 1, 14, 19, and 21 have been linked to Alzheimer's disease. Additionally, the protein apolipoprotein E4 (Apo-E4) has been linked to the development of amyloid plaque (Cummings et al, 1998). The more amyloid plaque deposited in the brain, the greater the impairment is thought to be. Inheriting the Apo-E4 allele from one or both parents increases the likelihood that the person will develop Alzheimer's disease. In contrast, however, a person who does not inherit the gene for Apo-E4 may also develop the disease (Snowdon, 2001; NIA, 2000).

The Alzheimer's brain is also shrinking, weighing about two thirds the weight of the normal brain. This atrophy begins in the temporal and parietal regions and progresses throughout the entire brain (Snowdon, 2001). Smaller gyri and corresponding larger sulci are atrophic changes (Figure 32-1, *A-E,* and Figures 32-2 through 32-4). Atrophy is also occurring in the subcortical areas, which is most apparent in the lateral ventricles. The more the brain shrinks, the larger the ventricles become.

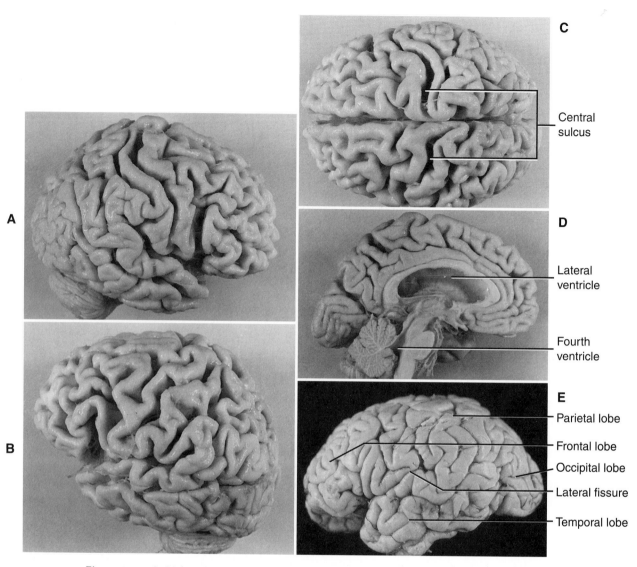

Figure 32-1 A, Right side of the brain of a patient with Alzheimer's disease. Narrow gyri and larger sulci are demonstrated. B, Left side of the same brain demonstrates even narrower gyri and larger sulci. C, Superior view. Central sulcus is very wide. D, Midsaggital view of the left hemisphere. The greatly enlarged lateral and fourth ventricles are demonstrated. E, Normal brain. (Photographs A to D by Berto Tarin, Western University of Health Science; E courtesy Dr. Richard E. Powers, University of Alabama at Birmingham Brain Resource Program [UAB-BRP].)

Environmental issues related to Alzheimer's disease

Research on exposure to excessive aluminum from using aluminum cookware has not been conclusive. Dental amalgams do not cause Alzheimer's disease either (NIA, 2000; Snowdon, 2001). No viral agent that transmits Alzheimer's disease has been identified (Gruetzner, 2001).

Nontraditional findings

The traditional roots of Alzheimer's disease development have been discussed. The cause of Alzheimer's disease is not without controversy. The Nun Study, a longitudinal research study that has explored topics related to normal aging and Alzheimer's disease, has generated new questions. David Snowdon of the Sanders-Brown Center on

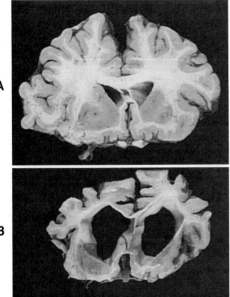

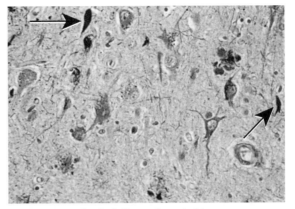

Figure 32-3 The dark flame-shaped objects are neurofibrillary "tangles" or dead neurons *(arrows)*. Tangles are twisted fibrils inside the neuron that disrupt cellular processes and eventually kill the cell. (Courtesy Dr. Richard E. Powers, UAB-BRP.)

Figure 32-2 A, Brain is normal. The sulci and gyri are not atrophied. B, Brain shows the effects of Alzheimer's disease. Widened sulci and narrowed gyri are demonstrated. In addition, the lateral ventricles are increased in size because of the decrease in brain mass associated with Alzheimer's disease. (Courtesy Dr. Richard E. Powers, UAB-BRP.)

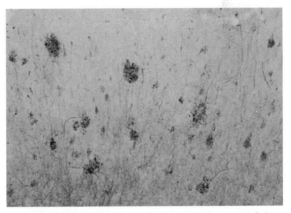

Figure 32-4 The darker objects are plaques, one of the two microscopic findings in Alzheimer's disease (the other are the tangles seen in Figure 32-3). Since plaques can be found in about 50% of older individuals over age 70, it is the quantity of plaques in relation to the person's age that is significant. (Courtesy Dr. Richard E. Powers, UAB-BRP.)

Aging at the University of Kentucky began the study in the mid-1980s. In the order of School Sisters of Notre Dame, 678 nuns volunteered to undergo annual assessments and at death to donate their brains for autopsy. This study has been widely covered in both the professional and lay press (Snowdon, 2001).

The Nun Study has had two unexpected findings. One sister who had lived to be over 100 showed no signs of cognitive decline, although her brain autopsy showed an abundance of both plaque and tangle formations. Another nun who died in her 70s had profound dementia yet had few tangles and plaques. The Nun Study researchers are exploring reasons for these unusual findings. The following background issues have been isolated in the nuns having the highest cognitive ability: advanced education, use of complex language, and a positive attitude. The way these variables relate to cognitive preservation is under investigation (Snowdon, 2001).

Classic behaviors of Alzheimer's disease

Memory loss is the most noticeable initial problem. Impairment of short-term memory occurs first. The patient and family may think this loss is a minor problem because the long-term memory remains intact at first. Word-finding difficulty is the easiest problem for the nurse to assess. The patient often describes an object rather than naming it. "The thing you tell time with" for a watch is a typical response. Impaired concentration often follows memory problems and word-finding difficulty. Trouble understanding a conversation, comprehending the plot in a book, or following a television program frequently occurs. Withdrawing from previous routine and pleasurable activities because of a lack of interest and a lack of initiative contributes to further cognitive decline. Box 32-1 outlines what is referred to as the four "A"s of Alzheimer's disease.

| Box 32-1 | Four "A"s of Alzheimer's Disease* and Adaptive Actions

Agnosia. Impaired ability to recognize or identify familiar objects and people in the absence of a visual or hearing impairment.
- Assess and adapt for visual impairment.
- Do not expect patient to remember you; introduce yourself.
- Cover mirrors or pictures if they cause distress.
- Name objects and demonstrate their use.
- Keep area free of ingestible hazards (toiletries, cleaning chemicals, checkers, buttons, unmonitored medicine).

Aphasia. Language disturbance are exhibited in both expressing and understanding spoken words. Expressive aphasia is inability to express thoughts in words; receptive aphasia is the inability to understand what is said.
- Assess and adapt for hearing loss.
- Observe and use gestures, tone, and facial expressions.
- Provide help with word finding.
- Restate your understanding of behaviors, word fragments.
- Acknowledge feelings expressed verbally and nonverbally.
- Use simple words and phrases; be concise and organized.
- Allow time for response.
- Listen carefully and encourage with nonverbal praise.
- Use pictures, symbols, and signs.

Amnesia. Inability to learn new information or to recall previously learned information.
- Do not expect patient to remember you; introduce yourself.
- Do not test the patient's memory unnecessarily.
- Operate in the here and now.
- Provide orientation cues.
- Remember *you* must adapt when the patient cannot change.
- Compensate for patient's lost judgment or reasoning.

Apraxia. Inability to carry out motor activities despite intact motor function.
- Assess and adapt for motor weakness, swallowing difficulties.
- Simplify tasks; give step-by-step instructions and time for response.
- Initiate motion for patient with gentle guidance or touch.

*May also be present in other cognitive disorders.

One of the unusual problems associated with Alzheimer's disease is *misinterpreting the environment.* Visual hallucinations are the most common types of hallucinations seen in Alzheimer's disease. The Charles Bonnet syndrome refers to a specialized type of visual hallucinations. Many patients *see* images of deceased relatives, little people, animals, or strangers in the house (Pliskin, 1996). Auditory hallucinations are less common but do occur. The *voices* or *sounds* typically go along with the visual hallucinations, for example, the perceived deceased relative is *speaking* to the patient. Olfactory, tactile, and gustatory hallucinations are the least common types of hallucinations.

Delusions are common. Paranoia about spouses having extramarital affairs, stealing money, rearranging things in the home, and somatic preoccupations are frequent observations the nurse makes. Whether any of these accusations have any basis in reality must be assessed.

Calling a family member or friend by another person's name is known as *misidentification.* Family members are often devastated when the patient cannot remember their names. The nurse can educate the family about misidentification and dispel any ideas that it may be a humorous attempt by the patient.

The sundown syndrome is the phrase that describes the period, usually in the afternoon and early evening, during which a patient becomes more agitated and less redirectable. This phenomenon is also called *sundowning.* Researchers have yet to find the cause of this behavioral change. The behavior is further confusing to families because the patient may have "good" and "bad" days.

Loss of the ability to care for oneself is particularly difficult for all parties. Over time, the patient forgets how to take care of all personal care needs. Bowel and bladder incontinence are two of the most unmanageable behaviors and often result in nursing home placement.

CLINICAL EXAMPLE OF A PATIENT WITH ALZHEIMER'S DISEASE

Mrs. Jefferson, a 62-year-old woman, has had difficulty recalling the names of people in her church. She described the choir as "those people who sing at church." At home, she placed her purse in the oven. Each one of these occurrences is not diagnostic of Alzheimer's disease. However, the cluster of these signs should make the nurse consider this diagnosis.

Critical Thinking Question

When assessing patients and their families with cognitive disorders, what skills of the nurse are the most essential?

Vascular Dementia

The second most prevalent dementia is vascular dementia. Before the DSM-IV (APA, 1994), vascular dementia was known as multiinfarct dementia. The diagnosis of vascular dementia is made when the brain has multiple vascular lesions in the cortex and subcortical areas (APA, 2000). These affected areas are sometimes called "small strokes."

Memory loss is the most common presenting complaint. Unlike Alzheimer's disease, the patient with vascular dementia usually maintains the ability to speak without word-finding difficulty. The cognitive changes that occur with vascular dementia are directly related to the location of the lesions. In contrast, the patient with Alzheimer's disease has a more global pattern of deterioration. The time the patient remains at a particular level may be months and years, or vascular changes may occur over a shorter period. If the cognitive levels are plotted on a graph, the decline usually assumes a stair-step pattern of deterioration. Although the predictability is impossible, a further decline is likely because the original risk factors are usually still present.

The major risk factors for vascular dementia are hypertension, diabetes mellitus, previous stroke, cardiac arrhythmias, coronary artery disease, tobacco usage, and alcohol and substance abuse. Aspirin, antiplatelet medications, and endarterectomy are symptomatic treatments for this disease (Folstein, 1997).

CLINICAL EXAMPLE OF A PATIENT WITH VASCULAR DEMENTIA

Mr. Babb, a 76-year-old man, is hospitalized for depression. During the initial interview he had difficulty understanding why he was admitted. He did not know the day, date, month, or year; however, he was able to do serial calculations. One week before admission, he had an automobile accident because he pulled out into traffic without looking.

Frontotemporal Lobe Dementia

Frontotemporal lobe dementia (FLD) is a type of dementia caused by atrophy of the frontal and ante-rior temporal lobes of the brain. This atrophy may be symmetric or asymmetric. Pick's disease is a subtype of FLD. This type of dementia features Pick's cells and Pick's bodies in the brain. Pick's cells are "swollen, ballooned neurons that display central chromatolysis. The Pick body is a well-defined argentophilic inclusion found within the neuronal cytoplasm" (Moore, Jefferson, 1996). Chromosomes 3 and 17 have genetic material that shows familial linkage to Pick's disease. This disease is usually diagnosed when patients are in their 60s, and the patient may live from 2 to 15 years (Rosen et al, 2000).

The area of the brain affected is responsible for executive functioning. These behaviors include judgment, decision making, impulse control, and social norms (Litvan et al, 1997). Behavioral changes are the first signs that something is wrong. Disinhibition is the most shocking. Disrobing in public, extreme impatience, or openly masturbating typifies FLD behaviors. Difficulties with abstraction, reasoning, and planning occur as well. Apraxia, agnosia, and visual-spatial abilities—common signs seen in Alzheimer's disease—are not usually found because of the preservation of the parietal region of the brain. Later in the illness, speech disturbance, memory problems, and gait disturbance occur in a sharp progressive decline (Tasman, 1997).

CLINICAL EXAMPLE OF A PATIENT WITH FRONTOTEMPORAL LOBE DEMENTIA (PICK'S DISEASE)

Ms. Brewer, a 66-year-old woman, was found nude in the foyer of her assisted-living facility. She had taken her clothes off three times in a week. Before this occurrence, she had been quite modest. A few days later, she cursed the housekeeper. Ms. Brewer was diagnosed with Pick's disease based on her behavior, her relatively good memory, and neuroimaging that showed both frontal and anterior temporal lobe atrophy.

Dementia Related to Parkinson's Disease

Parkinson's disease is a complex neurologic disorder that affects the extrapyramidal system. All diseases that affect this system have associated aberrant movements. Parkinson's disease is usually diagnosed when patients are in their 50s or 60s, although patients in their 30s, such as the actor Michael J. Fox, have developed the disease. The substantia nigra has approximately a 50% reduction in neurons. The remaining cells contain Lewy bodies, which are eosinophilic intracellular structures (Knopman, 2001). Acetylcholine reduction is also a possibility as are neurofibrillary tangles and senile plaques (Moore, Jefferson, 1996). Dementia occurs in 15% to 20% of patients with Parkinson's disease (PD) (Geldmacher, 1997). Parkinsonian behaviors include muscular rigidity, masklike facies, and stooped posture. Shuffling gait, pill rolling (rubbing the thumb up and down across the tips of the fingers), and drooling are also signs associated with PD (Knopman, 2001). Poor postural reflexes may also be present, which makes these patients prone to falls. Tremor may or may not be present. Freezing refers to the rigid posture that alternates with more fluid movements. Many patients with PD also have depression that is related to neurologic changes and the grieving process that occurs as these patients become less functional.

Patients with PD may develop cogwheel rigidity with or without tremor (Young, 1999). One way to assess cogwheel rigidity begins with asking the patient to extend his or her arm. Next, the patient should be asked to flex his or her arm slowly. At the same time, the nurse tries to extend the patient's arm with one hand. The nurse's other hand should hold the elbow of the extending and flexing arm. Cogwheel rigidity, if present, feels like a ratcheting motion in the patient's elbow.

Fifteen years is the usual course of PD (Moore, Jefferson, 1996), making the decline more gradual than most other dementias. Many pharmaceutical agents used are dopamine enhancers (dopaminergics), but these medications are only for movement enhancement (Keltner, Folks, 2001).

CLINICAL EXAMPLE OF A PATIENT WITH PARKINSON'S DISEASE

Mr. McGreevy, a 72-year-old man, has had PD for 7 years. He has a blunted affect, excessive drooling, and a shuffling gait. Mr. McGreevy has intermittent freezing when he cannot move. He can no longer remember where he is.

Diffuse Lewy Body Disease

Diffuse Lewy body disease (DLBD) is the form of dementia that has both cognitive impairment with extrapyramidal signs. In addition to Lewy bodies, these patients also have senile plaques; both cause neuronal dysfunction or death. Lewy bodies are found in the frontal and temporal cortex primarily but can also occur in the subcortical areas (Gomez-Tortosa, 1998).

To a lesser extent, Lewy bodies are found in hippocampus and the substantia nigra. The hippocampus is an area of high acetylcholine concentration. The substantia nigra is the area of the brain that is most affected in PD. These patients have many parkinsonian signs (see the previous section). DLBD can occur as a sole dementia or can be combined with Alzheimer's disease. This combination is called a Lewy body variant of Alzheimer's disease.

Differentiating DLBD from Alzheimer's disease is difficult. Many signs are the same. However, 80% of patients with DLBD have severe visual hallucinations, a tendency to fall, and fluctuation in alertness early in the disease (Gomez-Tortosa, 1998; Lopez et al, 2000). These patients are also highly sensitive to neuroleptic medications, even at small doses. DLBD follows a downward course that is much more precipitous than Alzheimer's disease. After the mild stage, the extrapyramidal signs separate the two diseases. The course of diffuse Lewy body disease is usually 5 to 8 years (Gomez-Tortosa, 1998).

CLINICAL EXAMPLE OF A PATIENT WITH DIFFUSE LEWY BODY DISEASE

Mr. Hall, a 68-year-old man, started having vivid visual hallucinations. He had fallen twice as a result of his gait disturbance. Mr. Hall has both short- and long-term memory loss after taking a small dose of an anitpsychotic mediation. He also became agitated after taking a small dose of an antipsychotic medication.

Creutzfeldt-Jakob Disease

Until "mad cow" disease became headline news, little information appeared in the media about Creutzfeldt-Jakob disease (CJD). Now, a variant of CJD has been identified. This disease is known as v-CJD and is the human form of "mad cow" disease. These patients contract this variant after ingesting meat infected with bovine spongiform encephalopathy. Subacute spongiform encephalopathy is a feature of both "mad cow" disease and CJD.

On microscopic examination, these cells appear like sponges. The cells are stripped of their intracellular material. The infecting agent is the prion, a protein particle, which is unlike either a bacterium or virus. CJD is 1 of at least 12 prion-related diseases, all of which are transmittable from one person to another. A genetic component also exists, but this accounts for 10% or less of patients with CJD. Of the individuals who develop this disease, 85% have no known risk factors (National Institute of Neurological Disorders and Stroke [NINDS], 2001). CJD is potentially transferable between people when blood and body fluids are present (Moore, Jefferson, 1996; Perkin, 1998). Health care workers who are involved in surgery or autopsy are vulnerable.

Dementia is inevitable and occurs early in the disease (NINDS, 2001). Initially, personality changes, seizures, and myoclonic movements occur. Impairment of vision and even blindness is not unusual. The course is rapid; on average most patients die within 6 months to a year (Perkin, 1998). Only 10% live past a year (NINDS, 2001). The nurse should focus on anticipatory grief for the family and the patient if he or she is cognitively able.

CLINICAL EXAMPLE OF A PATIENT WITH CREUTZFELDT-JAKOB DISEASE

Mrs. Henderson, a 65-year-old woman, became openly hostile to her husband while they were dining out. She had never had outbursts such as this one. In 2 months, her vision was affected, and 3 months later, she was blind. Mrs. Henderson also developed myoclonic jerks that were not controlled with medication. Based on the change in personality, visual impairment, and movement disorder, she was diagnosed with CJD. She died 9 months later.

AIDS Dementia Complex

AIDS dementia complex (ADC) occurs in approximately 20% to 30% of patients with AIDS (Brew, 1999). ADC is a subcortical dementia that presents with motor disturbance initially. Cognitive and behavioral changes occur later. Development of dementia takes several years. However, once ADC occurs, the patient rarely lives over a year. A theory about ADC development is that the human immunodeficiency virus (HIV) crosses the blood-brain barrier. White matter changes, cerebral atrophy, and infiltration of macrophages also occur in patients with ADC (Perkin, 1998). See Chapter 44 for a complete review of psychiatric disorders associated with HIV infection.

Mania is often the first sign of the ADC. Other behaviors may include forgetfulness, ataxia, speaking difficulties, and problems concentrating (Brew, 1999).

AIDS can occur in all age groups. Presence of the behavioral and cognitive changes in the younger patient should alert the nurse to consider ruling out this disease.

CLINICAL EXAMPLE OF A PATIENT WITH AIDS DEMENTIA COMPLEX

Mrs. Browning, a 46-year-old woman, has had AIDS for 8 years. Her family reported that she had been raped 10 years ago. Now, Mrs. Browning is agitated, does not eat, and does not sleep well. In the last 6 months, Mrs. Browning's memory began to fail. She died 11 months after she was diagnosed with ADC.

Dementia Associated with Alcoholism

This dementia usually occurs decades after the person starts drinking alcohol. Similar to many other dementias, personality changes typically precede memory disturbance. The decline is similar to the course of Alzheimer's disease.

Thiamine deficiency is the main cause of alcohol-related changes. Additionally, the toxic effects of years of drinking alcohol finally take their toll in multiple end-stage organ damage including the brain. Wernicke's encephalopathy results in motor problems related to alcohol abuse. Most often, the patient develops motor impairments such as ataxia and nystagmus. Korsakoff's syndrome is often associated with Wernicke's encephalopathy. Patients with Korsakoff's syndrome confabulate as they attempt to answer questions (Moore, Jefferson, 1996). This delay is an attempt to cover their severe short-term memory loss. Superficially, these patients seem to know what they are saying. Unless the facts are known, these patients make statements that will seem truthful to the nurse.

The brain of a patient with Wernicke-Korsakoff syndrome has several changes. The affected areas of the brain are the medial thalamus and hypothalamus, some of the mid-brain gray matter, and the periventricular pons and medulla (Brust, 1998). Other researchers have found that some of the brain structures (e.g., hippocampus, mammillary bodies), may have reduced volume, whereas the third ventricle is increased in volume (Visser et al, 1999).

With abstinence, improvement of cognitive function is possible. However, if the dementia is diagnosed, these patients may have an inability to process new information, hindering their rehabilitation and participation in support groups such as Alcoholics Anonymous (AA).

CLINICAL EXAMPLE OF PATIENT WITH DEMENTIA RELATED TO ALCOHOLISM

Mr. Kelly, a 75-year-old man, was admitted to a general hospital for chest pain. Three days later, he was transferred to a geriatric psychiatry unit with altered mental status. Mr. Kelly was unable to speak rationally; he made gestures in the air as if he were having visual hallucinations. His spouse said that he did not have a "drinking problem," but he did drink wine each evening. After 3 days of unexpected abstinence, Mr. Kelly was experiencing delirium related to alcohol withdrawal and was placed on an alcohol withdrawal protocol.

Two years later, the patient returned to the hospital with short-term memory loss. He said that he was in Hawaii when asked where he had been before admission. His wife confirmed that Mr. Kelly had not gone to Hawaii. He was confabulating. He had developed Korsakoff's syndrome.

Huntington's Disease

All of the dementing illnesses have a sorrowful course. Perhaps none is more tragic than is Huntington's disease (HD). This illness is particularly devastating because it is transmitted only through the autosomal dominant gene that either parent may provide. As such, HD does not skip generations. This illness is not usually diagnosed until the patients are in their 30s and 40s, but it can develop before or after these ages (Snowdon, 2001). By the time patients are diagnosed with HD, they may have children and even grandchildren. The child has a 50% chance of inheriting the gene and thus the disease. Personality changes are usually the first signs to appear. A mild-tempered person may develop mood swings or start drinking alcohol. Most of the time, the movement disorder occurs after the personality changes. These movements, known as choreiform movements, begin with facial twitches or involuntary limb movement and progress to myoclonus (jerking movements) of all extremities (Moore, Jefferson, 1996). These movements place the patient at risk for falling out of a chair or bed.

Chromosome 4 is the point at which the gene associated with HD is located (Snowdon, 2001). Genetic testing involves a simple laboratory serum test. A positive test result means the patient will develop HD. Testing poses an ethical dilemma. For example, should individuals at risk be tested before having children, should they decide not to have children, or should they proceed and take the chance that a child will not have HD? The nurse should be supportive when these issues are raised.

The dementia may develop before or after the choreiform movements begin. Short-term memory is affected first, followed by long-term memory loss. The course is unpredictable because the illness may occur over a short period, or it may last decades.

CLINICAL EXAMPLE OF PATIENT WITH DEMENTIA RELATED TO HUNTINGTON'S DISEASE

Mrs. Thompson, a 57-year-old woman with HD, was admitted to the psychiatric unit for unmanageable behavior. She had severe myoclonus to the extent that she almost fell out of her wheelchair. She could no longer feed herself and was incontinent of bowel and bladder. She did not know where she was. Based on the previous diagnosis of HD and this recent onset memory loss, Mrs. Thompson was diagnosed with dementia.

Other Dementias

The most prevalent dementias have been described. Dozens of other types of dementia have been identified. Some dementias are caused by diseases, for example neurosyphilis, systemic lupus erythematosus, and Wilson's disease. Other dementias may be related to metabolic imbalances, such as hypothyroidism and hypocalcemia. Another class of dementias is related to head injuries, toxic effects of medications, heavy metals, or carbon monoxide poisoning (Perkin, 1998).

FAMILY CONSIDERATIONS

Family-focused interventions affect quality of life for patients with cognitive impairments. Families devote 3 to 8 hours of care daily for at least two thirds of all dementia patients (Farlow, 1999; Hendryx-Bedalov, 2000). Replacing family caregivers with paid home care staff would cost $45 to $94 billion per year

(Administration on Aging [AoA], 2001). Caring for a patient with Alzheimer's disease at home has been described as the toughest job in the world. Stress, exhaustion, inadequate self-care, and social isolation are commonly cited. Family caregivers, often spouses, suffer depression at three times the rate of others in their own age group and endure more health problems as well (AoA, 2001). Assisting families to manage the burden of care can delay long-term care placement and prevent other negative sequelae.

The prevalence of abuse in older adults is estimated at 4% to 10% (Wolf, 2001). Cognitively impaired patients are at risk of abuse by family and professional caregivers in all settings. Abusers may think demented victims of verbal or physical attacks, neglect, or exploitation may not comprehend or remember what is happening (Hogstel, Curry, 1999). Precipitating factors may include the stress of providing care and previous patterns of coping. Nurses should be familiar with the potential for abuse, its signs, and actions required by law when abuse is identified.

Families confront many difficult decisions from the time a cognitive disorder is diagnosed to its endpoint, usually death. Physicians and families are reluctant to inform dementia patients of their diagnosis and prognosis. Some patients may choose not to know the underlying cause of their deficits (Marzansi, 2000). Withholding information can be based on the best intentions. Anxiety, depression, psychotic reactions, and even suicides have been reported by individual learning of their irreversible disorder. On the other hand, patients who are informed early in the disease can participate in important decisions. Planning for changes in living arrangements and the end of driving, fiercely defended staples of independence, allows the patient a degree of control and sometimes makes the transition easier. Patient input into financial, legal, and end-of-life care decisions can reduce caregivers' burden. Nurses can assist with the grief process, a response to the anticipated and actual losses experienced by patients and family members. In the early phases, patients may mourn the loss of cognitive and physical abilities; however, with disease progression, they may no longer recognize deficits. Family members, however, watch their loved one's life disappear. When the diagnosis has a strong genetic link, such as HD, children face the implications for their own future as well.

Daily care is a significant challenge for caregivers. Nurses can help by assessing needs, educating about specific disorders and care management, and facilitating caregiver's access to other sources of information and support. The government has instituted multiple initiatives to support family caregivers. The Family and Medical Leave Act was signed into law in 1993. The enactment of the Older Americans Act Amendment of 2000 supported the development of the national Family Caregiver Support Program by the AoA, which focuses on information to caregivers, counseling, respite care, and limited supplemental services. The Area Agency of Aging and numerous support organizations for Alzheimer's disease and other cognitive disorders provide a variety of services, including support groups and links to experts. Information about adult day care, community centers, home health agencies, and other sources of respite may be beneficial. *The 36-Hour Day* is an excellent source of information (Mace, Rabins, 1991). The "Family Issues" box on page 422 provides important excerpts from this book.

Psychotherapeutic Management

Nurse-patient relationship

Because of the tremendous variation in presentation and progressions of cognitive disorders, nursing care must be highly individualized. The highest priority for a patient with delirium is given to life-sustaining interventions. The focus of care for a patient with dementia is on maintaining optimal function. Meeting basic physiologic and safety needs is essential for patients who are unable to do so independently. Tailored plans of care begin with the identification of unique patient characteristics, such as concurrent medical and psychiatric conditions, cultural and religious values and beliefs, past interests and preferences, and social supports. These characteristics are then integrated into more generic plans of care for manifestations of specific cognitive disorders (Hall, 1999). Patients profit when clinicians work as partners with family caregivers, share information, and work toward mutual goals. An understanding of the pathophysiologic aspects of cognitive disorders and the patient as a unique individual with both abilities and deficits are basic to planning and providing effective interventions.

Family Issues | Strategies for Coping with Alzheimer's Disease and Dementia

Be informed. The more you know about the nature of dementing illnesses, the more effective you will be in devising strategies to manage behavior problems.

Share your concerns with the patient. When a person is mildly impaired, he or she can take part in managing his or her problems. Together you may be able to devise memory aids that will help the patient remain independent.

Try to solve your most frustrating problems one at a time. Day-to-day problems often seem to be the most insurmountable. Getting the person to take his or her bath or getting a meal prepared, eaten, and cleaned up can become daily ordeals. If you are at the end of your rope, single out one thing that you can change to make life easier and work on that.

Get enough rest. One of the dilemmas families often face is that the caregiver may not get enough rest, which can make the caregiver less patient and less able to tolerate irritating behaviors.

Use your common sense and imagination. Adaptation is the key to success. If a thing cannot be done one way, ask yourself if it must be done at all. For example, if a person can eat successfully with his fingers but cannot use a fork and spoon

appropriately, do not fight the problem. Serve as many finger foods as possible.

Maintain a sense of humor. The sick person is still a person. He or she needs and enjoys a good laugh too. Sharing your experiences with other families will help you.

Try to establish an environment that allows as much freedom as possible but also offers the structure that confused people need. Establish a regular, predictable, simple routine for meals, medication, exercising, bedtime, and other activities.

Remember to talk to the confused person. Speak calmly and gently. Avoid talking about the person in front of him or her, and remind others to avoid this also.

Have an identification (ID) necklace or bracelet made for the confused person. This is one of the single most important things you can do. Many confused people get lost or wander away, and an ID can save you hours of frantic worry.

Keep the impaired person active but not upset. Activity helps maintain physical well being and may help prevent other illnesses and infections. Being active helps the ill person continue to believe that he or she is involved in the family and that his or her life has meaning.

From Mace NL, Rabins PV, editors: *The 36-hour day,* Baltimore, 1991, Johns Hopkins University Press.

| Box 32-2 | Communication Strategies

Sending
- Attract and sustain attention
- Position at or below eye level
- Minimize distractions
- Consider vision and hearing limitations
- Use short, clear, and direct sentences
- Attend to expression, tone, pace, and volume
- Match verbal and nonverbal messages
- Allow time for processing and response

Receiving
- Listen respectfully
- Use verbal and nonverbal messages to encourage effective communication
- Assist with word finding
- Search for meaning in nonverbal behaviors
- Restate perceived message received
- Respond to content and feelings conveyed

Effective communication, one of the most valuable therapeutic tools, is also one of the biggest challenges for caregivers of the cognitively impaired. Communication is complicated by the expressive and receptive problems common in these disorders (Hendryx-Bedalov, 2000). Patients whose ability to communicate thoughts and feelings verbally is compromised because of memory loss, aphasia, or dysarthria communicate in other ways. The challenge for caregivers is to seek the patient's perspective to find meaning in verbal and nonverbal communication within the environmental context (Curry et al, 2000; Acton et al, 1999). This text's chapter on communication provides more detail about this concept. Box 32-2 offers strategies to facilitate communication. Problematic behaviors such as aggression are best viewed as messages to be interpreted and managed rather than symptoms to be treated. Validation of the caregiver's understanding of messages may come only from the responses to interventions. Patients may understand more than they can express. Patronizing terms, sarcasm, false reassurance, and negative remarks should be avoided in all circumstances. Falsehoods and harsh confrontations of delusional content are not therapeutic. (To a patient looking for her mother, "Your mother will be here to see you in a while" or "Your mother is dead.")

Through the careful use of verbal and nonverbal messages, caregivers with an understanding of the patient's losses and retained abilities can assist patients with receptive aphasia in understanding messages. The value of a smile, positive phrases, and a pleasant unhurried tone cannot be overstated. Gentle touch and affection are generally positively received if in keeping with the patient's past preferences. It is important to remember that, in cognitive disorders, the ears or eyes are not necessarily impaired; the brain's ability to interpret is lost. Talking louder will not help the patient with receptive aphasia understand. Treat all patients with respect and unconditional regard. Address patients by their preferred name, which might be the title and last name; however, with cognitive decline, some patients recognize only childhood nicknames. Dressing patients in their own clothes and assisting or insuring appropriate grooming enhances self-esteem in the patient and is an acknowledgment of individuality. Memory books containing pictures familiar to the patient may be comforting and facilitate reminiscence. Participation in life review is valuable for patients and caregivers, whose increased knowledge about their patients aids the development of a therapeutic relationship.

Psychopharmacology

Aging produces numerous physiologic changes that alter the absorption, distribution, metabolism, and excretion of drugs. Older adult patients with cognitive disorders are likely to have coexisting physical disorders for which they are taking other prescription or OTC medications. Problems associated with many expected side effects are amplified in older adults. These factors and the effects of cost and dosing schedules on compliance are factors in drug selection and administration.

Antipsychotics

Antipsychotic medications or neuroleptics are often effective in treating psychotic symptoms, as well as disturbed and unsafe behaviors associated with dementia. Nonpsychotic symptoms such as agitation, aggression, uncooperativeness, and hostility usually show improvement, but antipsychotics are less effective on wandering, apathy, and hypersexuality (Tariot, 1999). The avoidance of side effects typically influences selection of an antipsychotic. Newer atypical antipsychotics such as clozapine (Clozaril), olanzapine (Zyprexa), risperidone (Risperdal), and queti-

apine (Seroquel) are gaining favor over older drugs in this class because of their favorable side effect profiles and efficacy (Maixner et al, 1999). The low-potency agents such as chlorpromazine (Thorazine) cause sedative, anticholinergic, and antiadrenergic effects to which the older adults are particularly sensitive. On the other hand, high-potency agents such as haloperidol (Haldol) cause the neurologic extrapyramidal effects to which people with neurodegenerative processes are highly sensitive as well.

Anticonvulsants

Anticonvulsants are being prescribed for agitation with increasing frequency (Tariot, 1999). Valproic acid (Depakene), its sustained release derivative divalproex sodium (Depakote Sprinkles), and carbamazepine (Tegretol) have psychotropic properties similar to lithium when used in patients with mania but have a more favorable side effect profile.

Antidepressants

Antidepressants are used to treat depression-related symptoms associated with cognitive disorders. The selective serotonin reuptake inhibitors (SSRIs) are favored over older drugs in this classification for treatment of depression and depression-related symptoms in older adults. Fluoxetine (Prozac), paroxetine (Paxil), sertraline (Zoloft), and citalopram (Celexa) are effective, have a generally favorable side effect profile, and are not lethal in overdose (Compton et al, 2001). Additionally, bupropion (Wellbutrin), mirtazapine (Remeron), and venlafaxine (Effexor) have been effective. The last three drugs have multiple actions at the neurotransmitter level. Tricyclic antidepressants (TCAs) have anticholinergic, antiadrenergic, and antihistaminic properties. Because cognition is compromised when acetylcholine is blocked, antidepressants with significant anticholinergic properties are best avoided. A TCA-induced delirium resulting from anticholinergic effects is relatively common among older adult patients receiving these drugs. Patients with diagnosed cognitive impairments are at even greater risk. Monoamine oxidase inhibitors (MAOIs) are rarely used in older adults because of dietary restrictions, potentially serious side effects, and lethality in overdose (Compton et al, 2001).

Antianxiety agents

Benzodiazepines continue to be prescribed for agitation, anxiety, and insomnia despite that in cognitively impaired patients, their use may exacerbate confusion and produce paradoxical agitation. The common side effects of sedation and ataxia lead to an increased risk of falls (Wang et al, 2001). Tolerance and withdrawal are also issues connected to long-term use of benzodiazepines. Lorazepam (Ativan) and oxazepam (Serax) are the generally favored drugs in this class because they are less likely to accumulate with repeated dosing (Tariot, 1999). The nonbenzodiazepine buspirone (BuSpar) has considerably fewer side effects than benzodiazepines and is not subject to restrictions of the Omnibus Budget Reconciliation Act (OBRA) of 1987.

Treatment of Alzheimer's disease

The first four medications with FDA approval for Alzheimer's disease are acetylcholinesterase inhibitors. Tacrine (Cognex), donepezil (Aricept), rivastigmine (Exelon), and galantamine (Reminyl) have been released since 1993. However, although tacrine is still available, it is not widely used because of potential liver disease (Raskind, Perskind, 2001).

Antioxidants have been found to promote healthy neurons. Free radicals, oxygen fragments that are produced in the dying neuron, start a chain reaction that ends with nerve cell destruction. Vitamin C and vitamin E plus the nonsteroidal antiinflammatory drugs such as ibuprofen, have some neuroprotective effects (NIA 2000).

The discovery of a specific secretase, which is a type of enzyme related to plaque formation, has garnered additional interest (Garber, 2001). An Alzheimer's disease vaccine had reached the Phase IIA clinical trial level when the FDA stopped it. Several subjects had developed brain inflammation. At publication, no medication has FDA approval for augmentation with another; however, the use of two acetylcholinesterase inhibitors was in trials (NIA, 2000).

Alternative therapies

Because of their exposure in the popular press and potential cost savings over prescription drugs, a number of patients with cognitive disorders may choose to take agents such as ginkgo biloba and St. John's wort for depression or memory loss. Formulation and additives are not consistent or controlled. Few formal trials of effectiveness have been done. Use of these should be assessed because they can be the source of symptoms and cause significant drug interactions.

Milieu management

Patients with cognitive disorders require a milieu designed to maximize functional capability, which requires attention to potential hazards and a balance between overstimulation and understimulation. Good judgment based on an understanding of patients' perceptual, cognitive, and physical deficits should guide the nurse. Patients need a warm, caring atmosphere that will facilitate their development of a trusting interpersonal relationship with the caregivers. Emphasis has been placed in long-term care on making facilities more "homelike" by encouraging personal belongings and pictures, along with the use of warm colors, textures, plants, birds, and aquariums. Although these modifications are not always possible, caregivers in all setting should attempt to create a patient-focused environment. Careful attention should be focused on lighting, floor coverings, and the elimination of hazards that increase the risk of falls. Potentially harmful items, such as chemicals, sharp objects, and electrical devices along with small or toxic items that might be placed in the mouth or swallowed, should be available only with supervision. Sturdy furniture, chosen to promote independent mobility, is best grouped for socialization. To provide a positive treatment area, the nurse must be aware of milieu related issues: stress, safety, wandering, agitating, and passivity.

Stress

Stress has been shown to be a cause of anxious behavior in patients with cognitive impairments. If the level of stress continues or increases, dysfunctional behavior and catastrophic reactions may follow. Hall (1988) lists five types of stressors that produce dysfunctional behavior in this population. Any combination of these stressors will cause the cognitively impaired person to perform at a lower level of functioning than would occur as a result of the cognitive disability alone. In other words, to help cognitively impaired patients perform at their highest potential, the nurse needs to structure the environment to minimize these stressors. A discussion of these stressors and examples of milieu management follows:

1. Fatigue
2. Change of environment, routine, or caregiver
3. Overwhelming or competing stimuli
4. Demands that exceed capacity to function
5. Physical stressors

Patient and Family Education

Alzheimer's Disease

Illness:

Alzheimer's disease and other cognitive disorders have profound effects on the individual and family. As a group, these disorders are most often referred to as dementias (de = loss; mentia—mind). Individuals affected by dementia struggle with then lose their ability to remember. Since memory is the cornerstone of intellectual life, learning, concentration, and orientation to surroundings soon begin to crumble as well. An alliteration has been developed that captures the losses of Alzheimer's disease: amnesia (loss of memory), aphasia (loss of the ability to understand or speak the spoken word), apraxia (loss of the ability to use familiar objects such as a door knob), and agnosia (loss of the ability to recognize once familiar objects). With Alzheimer's disease the brain actually changes. There is a loss of brain tissue—the brain actually shrinks in most if not all patients. Although brain cells (or neurons) do not regenerate, some of the functions caused by these losses can be treated. For example, it is known that a consequence of brain loss is a reduction in the amount of a brain chemical called *acetylcholine*. Acetylcholine is important for many cognitive or thinking processes.

Medications:

1. The most important group of medications now used in the treatment of Alzheimer's disease are those that increase the level of the chemical acetylcholine. Donepezil (Aricept) and rivastigmine (Exelon) are examples of these drugs. These medications prevent the metabolic breakdown of acetylcholine. They are referred to as acetylcholinesterase or cholinesterase inhibitors; in other words, they inhibit the enzymes that breakdown acetylcholine, thus actually increasing the net amount of acetylcholine available to the brain. These drugs seem to work best in the mild-to-moderate stages of Alzheimer's disease.
2. A number of drugs are used to treat agitation and other behavioral disturbances associated with Alzheimer's disease. Benzodiazepines, mood stabilizers, and antidepressant medications are often used to treat patients with behavioral disturbances.
3. Other drugs have been used with some success in treating cognitive decline. Vitamin E, estrogens, antiinflammatory drugs, and ginkgo biloba have some support as treatments for Alzheimer's disease.

Other issues:

Perhaps the most difficult job is having the primary (if not sole) responsibility for the care of an individual with Alzheimer's disease. Beyond the hard work, constant vigilance, and exhausting schedule, the patient may not understand the caregiver's actions or even recognize the caregiver's face (i.e., agnosia). If a significantly impaired individual is to be cared for at home, it is critical that the caretaking duties be shared. To leave an older spouse as sole caretaker for an individual with Alzheimer's disease is unfair and creates a health risk for the "healthy" partner. Local support groups can be an excellent resource for gaining ideas on managing everyday issues and for emotional support. At minimum, the extended family should assume caretaking responsibilities while the primary caregiver attends such meetings.

Fatigue

Fatigue may be the result of activity, co-morbidities, and a disrupted sleep-wake pattern. Sleep disturbances are common in patients with dementia. Sleep deprivation may cause excessive fatigue, decreased motivation, increased use of pharmaceuticals, and disruptive behaviors (Beck, Vogelpohl, 1999). Practices that promote improved sleep include restricting daytime napping, eliminating caffeine, and limiting fluids near bedtime. A warm bath within 2 hours of bedtime may also be helpful (Friedman et al, 2000). A daily routine, interspersing activities with short rest periods in the morning and afternoon should be planned. These quiet times should be in comfortable chairs, such as recliners, to avoid confusing the patient with nighttime cues.

Change of environment, routine, or caregiver

Change of any sort can be stressful for patients because of their altered ability to plan, initiate, and carry through voluntary activities. Memory loss can cause patients to feel lost in the familiar environment of their own home. When relocated, patients often exhibit distress. Moving the patient from home to home to accommodate multiple caregivers can yield catastrophic results. Routine schedules may provide orientation cues and be a source of comfort. Flexibility in the schedules is necessary; however, because rushing or forcing patients to complete a task can cause stress. Consistent caregivers are important for dependent patients. Those who know the patient best are more able to understand the patient, anticipate typical responses, and identify changes. Even though patients might not remember the name (or recognize the face) of their caregivers, they respond more positively to those who are comfortably familiar with tasks and maintain a set routine.

Overwhelming or competing stimuli

Making sense of internal stimuli, such as hallucinations and external stimuli, is difficult for patients with cognitive disorders. Patients may react strongly or misperceive sounds that staff members easily ignore, such as the public address system. Unable to differentiate a violent television scene from reality, patients might respond to a violent news report as they would to a real crime taking place in front of them. Competing stimuli can cause profound problems in even the simplest task. For example, serving foods that mix consistencies such as a crunchy cereal with milk can cause choking when the patient is unable to determine whether to chew the solid or simply swallow the liquid. Eliminating high noise levels, crowds of people, multiple activities, and conflicting stimuli, will minimize anxious behaviors.

Demands that exceed capacity to function

Just as students experience frustration and stress when, despite their best efforts, they are unable to perform to an instructor's expectations; cognitively impaired patients can be devastated by demands that exceed their functional capacity. Some families and staff members think that frequent testing of patient's memory and orientation is important. However, being asked questions they cannot answer—especially when corrected and told they are wrong—can be frustrating. Reality orientation is essential for patients with delirium and generally helpful for patients with mild cognitive impairments. When memory loss is severe and the patient cannot retain new information, however, reality orientation may be a stressor. Simple tasks can be overwhelming. Activities as simple as oral care require a great deal of recall and motor skill. Caregivers can foster independence by limiting choices, breaking tasks into small steps, providing step-by-step instructions with demonstration or gestures, allowing time for the patient to understand and respond, and praising results. Activities planned that are based on the patient's abilities promotes optimal function without overreaching ability (Wells et al, 2000)

Physical stressors

Physical stressors are anything that causes physiologic changes, such as pain, illness, chemicals, and extremes in temperature. Physical changes associated with normal aging, co-morbid medical conditions, and dependency place patients at risk for multiple physical stressors. Patients with dementia are at risk for under identification of pain, yet the prevalence of painful musculoskeletal disorders is high in older adults (Miller et al, 2000; Wynne et al, 2000). Research indicates that many patients with profound cognitive impairments are unable to use words to describe pain or participate in pain assessment using scaled instruments (Wynne et al, 2000). Administration of mild analgesic medications for patients with painful conditions may be preferred to giving the medication on an as-needed (prn) basis. Secondary effects of dementia, which cause the majority of deaths for patients with cognitive disorders, are infection, immobility, malnutrition, and dehydration. Adhering to the principles of basic nursing care for geriatric patients can increase comfort and reduce the incidence of delirium.

Safety

Maintaining the patient's personal safety is a caregiver's foremost responsibility. An understanding of the losses associated with cognitive disorders and physical co-morbidities can serve as a basis for modifications to the environment and care regime. The false assumption that physical and chemical restraints contribute to safety has led to overuse in older adults. Evidence demonstrates that restraints and overmedication contribute to increased numbers and severity of falls, confusion, and a host of other serious problems, even death. Following OBRA 1987, which outlined the patient's right to be free from any physical or chemical restraints imposed for purpose of discipline or convenience and not required to treat medical symptoms, emphasis was placed on finding other ways to manage behaviors and preserve safety. Still, the use of physical restraints and antipsychotic drugs remains prevalent (Middleton et al, 1999). The Health Care Financing Administration (HCFA, now known as Centers for Medicare and Medicaid Services) has mandated an examination of side rails used as an unnecessary restraint, as well as issuing stringent guidelines for other restraints in acute care (Capezuti et al, 1999). Caregiver education on the risks of restraints and unnecessary medication coupled with alternate interventions is effective in increasing patient safety without unnecessary restrictions.

Behavioral manifestations of needs

Patient behaviors may stem from milieu issues and contribute to its disruption. A useful approach is re-

case study

Blaire Holt, a thin 72-year-old woman, was brought from her home to the emergency department accompanied only by ambulance personnel. Her speech was garbled and nonsensical, and she was unable to provide information. She was unable to focus and was picking the air. Her clothing was stylish but mismatched and smelled of urine. Her hair was dirty and unkempt. She was admitted with a diagnosis of altered mental status. After 2 days of treatment for dehydration and a urinary tract infection, she was transferred from the medical unit to a geriatric psychiatry unit. She displayed multiple cognitive deficits. She could not perform activities of daily living (ADLs) without assistance and often got lost in the unit. Her communication was limited to social pleasantries.

An extensive evaluation resulted in a diagnosis of dementia, Alzheimer's type, and community resources were used to acquire information about Mrs. Holt. Her son's telephone number was in her purse. Living in a distant state and estranged for many years, he was able to provide the name of the family attorney and said friends could probably be located through the country club close to Mrs. Holt's home. Former friends said that since her husband's death 4 years earlier, Mrs. Holt had become less active. She stopped playing bridge because it bored her, stopped visiting friends because she hated to drive, quit golf after repeatedly accusing others of cheating, and, over time, stopped returning phone calls. Her accusations and her increasingly slovenly dress and manners caused friends to distance themselves. Wait staff members at the club said that for the past 6 months, Mrs. Holt had eaten lunch alone every day. The last time she had been in, she left angrily when someone else was sitting at her "regular" table. She did not come to the club for 2 weeks until a groundskeeper said he saw her trying to get into the building at 6:00 AM saying she wanted lunch. Club management said her bill had not been paid for 3 months. The attorney reported that although Mrs. Holt's finances were in disarray and her utilities had been shut off for 2 months, she had more than adequate funds for whatever care she needed. The son refused to be involved with his mother's care.

Care Plan

Name: <u>Blaire Holt</u>   Admission Date: _____

DSM-IV-TR Diagnosis: <u>Dementia, Alzheimer's type</u>

Assessment	**Areas of strength:** Adequate financial resources for necessary care. **Problems:** Severe confusion, recent and remote memory loss, agnosia, impaired judgment, inadequate social supports.
Diagnoses	• Self-care deficit (bathing and hygiene, feeding, toileting) related to cognitive impairment as evidenced by agnosia, confusion, and inability to perform any ADLs without prompting. • Impaired social interaction, related to communication barriers and altered thought processes as evidenced by observed discomfort in different social settings. • Nutrition, less than body requirements as evidenced by Ideal body weight.

Outcomes	*Short-term goals:*	*Date met*
	• Patient will remain safe and free of injury.	_____
	• Patient's needs for social interaction will be met.	_____
	Long-term goals:	
	• Patient will remain active and as independent as possible.	_____
	• Appropriate placement will be found.	_____

Planning	**Nurse-patient relationship:** Provide a set routine for care Spend time with patient, especially at mealtime, use pictures. **Psychopharmacology:** Monitor effects of antioxidants and acetylcholinesterase inhibitors; prepare information literature to accompany patient to long-term care (LTC) facility. **Milieu management:** Monitor and provide safe care in all ADLs, work with attorney to get appropriate clothing purchased or from home; monitor legal guardianship issues.
Evaluation	Patient remains safe and secure; monitor for weight gain; maintain patient care until room in LTC special Alzheimer's unit is available.
Referrals	Contact Department of Human Services/Adult Protection Division.

maining "actively calm": giving the patient the time the illness needs and using the time to observe, interpret, and plan actions from the patient's point of view (Skog et al, 2000). Although patients who have lost the ability to plan and organize do not have the ability to plot stubborn or angry attacks, unfortunately, some caregivers personalize behavioral symptoms. The first question in assessment should be, "Whose problem is it?" In many cases, patient behaviors may be troublesome to the caregiver but not for the patient. In these cases, caregivers may choose to reframe their perception, channel the patient's activity in another way, or elect not to act. Often, creative strategies borne from a search for the patient's perspective may reduce the need for pharmacologic intervention, enhance quality of life for the patient, and provide rich satisfaction to caregivers.

Wandering

Research has linked wandering to multiple deficits common in patients with cognitive deficits (Algase, 1999a; Algase, 1999b). For example, patients exhibiting memory deficits may walk looking for a specific location, or they may start purposefully then forget their destination. Although wandering is different from pacing, patients with difficulty in shifting visuospatial attention may start walking and lack the ability to stop unless interrupted. Environmental adaptations should be planned to minimize risk and promote patient independence. Walking paths that do not dead-end but do have strategically placed seats for rest can reduce frustration and exhaustion. The use of directional signs, pictures, and universally recognized symbols to both guide and stop patients might be helpful. A common solution for many patients is to place them within visual range of frequent destinations, such as the bathroom. Diverting or redirecting to other activities can sometimes interrupt wandering. Camouflaging exits with patterns or simple doorknob covers plus exit alarms can prevent unauthorized exit. The patient, in the event of separation from caregivers, should wear some form of identification. Nurses should teach families about alert systems formulated for the cognitively impaired and recommend that a recent photograph be maintained for identification.

Agitation

Agitation is a term used to encompass a spectrum of verbal and nonverbal behaviors, ranging from nonaggressive irritability, negativity, resistance, and restlessness to verbal or physical aggression. These behaviors may be the result of unmet needs, an inability to inhibit behavior because of structural brain damage, or an accentuation of the patient's premorbid pattern of dealing with stress (Kolanowski, 1999). Agitation occurs during the course of dementia in about one half of all cases, aggression in approximately one quarter of cases (Tariot, 1999).

Personal care, which involves touch, close intimate contact, and high demands on patients, is a frequently identified precipitating factor (Wells et al, 2000). Disruptive vocalizations (e.g., screaming, cursing, crying for help) are among the most frequent, persistent, and annoying behaviors of patients with dementia (Beck, Vogelpohl, 1999). Aggressive behaviors, including physical assault and verbal attacks, can cause adverse effects on caregivers, especially when the behaviors are perceived as deliberate. Specific interventions should be planned after a careful assessment of the nature, frequency, and intensity of the behavior. This information can help identify aggravating factors, thus triggers can be eliminated or at least minimized. Nursing research to identify other effective interventions such as slow-stroke massage or white noise is ongoing (Rowe, Alfred, 1999; Beck, Vogelpohl, 1999).

Passivity

Caregivers often overlook passive behaviors or fail to regard them as problematic (Colling, 1999). Apathy, lack of energy, and lack of purpose significantly interfere with the quality of life and require intervention. Caregivers who take over and provide total care without patient involvement may be motivated by the desire to spare the patient from stressful decisions and laborious effort or to satisfy their own need to get tasks completed quickly. This practice and the unnecessary use of indwelling catheters, restraints, and sedating medications, however, increase confusion and decrease function (Cutillo-Schmitter et al, 1996). Every effort should be made to engage the patient in self-care, interaction, and recreational activities planned for the patient's functional ability.

> ### *Critical* Thinking Question
> Decisions regarding the need for placement in a long-term care facility depend on the degree to which the patient's needs can be met in the home. What is the first priority for consideration when moving to a long-term care or another type of facility?

Key Concepts

1. Cognitive disturbances include amnesia, aphasia, agnosia, apraxia, alterations in abstract thinking, judgment, and perception.

2. Delirium is acute and imminently life threatening. If diagnosed and treated promptly, delirium is generally reversible.

3. Many forms of dementia have been identified. Some dementias are chronic, progressive, and irreversible; others may be reversed with appropriate and early intervention.

4. MCI may be a precursor to Alzheimer's disease.

5. Alzheimer's disease, which is the most prevalent of the dementias, is chronic and irreversible. The cholinergic hypothesis is the most accepted cause of Alzheimer's disease. Acetylcholinesterase inhibitors can slow, but not stop, progressive deterioration.

6. Symptoms of all dementing illnesses are caused from damage to the brain. Each illness causes unique structural damage, thus each illness has characteristic symptoms that aid diagnosis and guide the choice of nursing interventions. Although some symptoms are shared in all forms of dementia, onset and severity may differ.

7. Vascular dementia is caused by small strokes. The course is a step-wise progression with plateaus between cerebral events. Risk factors for stroke should be eliminated or reduced.

8. PD is a degenerative motor disorder related to the loss of dopamine-generating cells in the substantia nigra. Dementia and depression often coexist.

9. HD is a rare hereditary disorder involving deterioration of both motor and cognitive functions.

10. Family members care for most patients with dementia. Outcomes are improved when professional and family members work together. Caregivers are at risk for developing physical illnesses and psychiatric disorders, such as anxiety and depression.

11. Nursing care must be planned to meet the basic safety and physiologic needs of patients. Priority nursing interventions for patients with delirium are those that maintain life and return patients to their premorbid state. Nursing care for patients with dementia is focused on maintaining an optimal level of functioning.

12. Patients with cognitive disorders require a caring, structured milieu that minimizes stress and provides for safety.

13. Disruptive behaviors are not deliberate; they are symptoms of the illness and may signal unmet needs.

References

Acton G et al: Communicating with individuals with dementia: the impaired person's perspective, *J Gerontol Nurs* 25(2):6, 1999.

Administration on Aging (AoA): *Family Caregiving Fact Sheet*, May 2001.

http:www.aoa.dhhs.gov/may2001/factsheets/family-caregiving.html Retrieved June 5, 2001.

Algase D: Wandering in dementia, *Ann Rev Nurs Res* 17:185, 1999a.

Algase D: Wandering: a dementia-compromised behavior, *J Gerontol Nurs* 25(9):51, 1999b.

Alzheimer's Association: *"Alzheimer's vaccine" trials are stopped.* http://www.alz.org/whatsnew/alzvacstop.htm. Retrieved May 15, 2002.

American Psychiatric Association: *Diagnostic and statistical manual of mental disorders,* ed 4, text revision, Washington, DC, 2000, APA.

American Psychiatric Association: *Diagnostic and statistical manual of mental disorders,* ed 4, Washington, DC, 1994, APA.

Beck C, Vogelpohl T: Problematic vocalization, *J Gerontol Nurs* 25(9):17, 1999.

Biddle W, van Sickel M: *Introduction to psychiatry,* ed 2, Philadelphia, 1948, WB Saunders.

Brew J: Central nervous system infections: AIDS dementia complex, *Neurol Clin* 17(4):861, 1999.

Brust J: Neurologic emergencies-acute neurologic complications of drug and alcohol abuse, *Neurol Clin* 16(2):503, 1998.

Capezuti E et al: Individualized interventions to prevent bed-related falls and reduce siderail use, *J Gerontol Nurs* 25(11):6, 1999.

Colling K: Passive behaviors in dementia: clinical adaptation of the need driven dementia compromised behavior model, *J Gerontol Nurs* 25(90):27, 1999.

Compton M et al: The evaluation and treatment of depression in primary care, *Clin Cornerstone* 3(3):10, 2001.

Cummings J et al.: Alzheimer's disease: etiologies, pathophysiology, cognitive reserve, and treatment opportunities, *Neurology* 51(suppl 1):S2, 1998.

Curry L et al: Individualized care: perceptions of certified nurse's aides, *J Gerontol Nurs* 26(7):45, 2000.

Cutillo-Schmitter T et al: Formulating treatment partnerships with patients and their families, *J Gerontol Nurs* 22(6):23, 1996.

Epling J, Taylor H: Preventing delirium in hospitalized older patients, *J Fam Pract* 48(6):417, 1999.

Farlow M: *Therapeutic advances for Alzheimer's disease and other dementias,* 1999. http://www.medscape.com/medscape/N...ate/ 1999/to03/public/toc.tu03.html. Retrieved June 19, 2001.

Folstein M: Differential diagnosis of dementia-the clinical process, *Psychiatr Clin North Am,* 20(1):45, 1997.

Folstein M et al: Mini-mental state: a practical method for grading the cognitive status of patients for the clinician, *J Psychiatr Res* 12:189, 1975.

Friedman L et al: An actigraphic comparison of sleep restriction and sleep hygiene treatments for insomnia in older adults, *J Geriatr Psychiatry Neurol* 13(1):17, 2000.

Garber K: An end to Alzheimer's? *MIT Magazine Innovat Technol Rev* 70, 2001.

Geldmacher D: Differential diagnosis of Alzheimer's disease, *Neurology* 48(5):PS002, 1997.

Gomez-Tortosa E: Dementia with Lewy bodies, *J Am Geriatr Soc* 46(11):1449, 1998.

Gruetzner H: *Alzheimer's: a caregiver's guide and sourcebook,* New York, 2001, John Wiley and Sons.

Hall G: Alterations in thought process, *J Gerontol Nurs* 14(30):38, 1988.

Hall G: When traditional care falls short—caring for people with atypical presentations of cortical dementia, *J Gerontol Nurs* 25(2):22, 1999.

Hendryx-Bedalov P: Alzheimer's Dementia: coping with communication decline, *J Gerontol Nurs* 26(8):25, 2000.

Hogstel M, Curry L: Elder abuse revisited, *J Gerontol Nurs* 27(1):10, 1999.

Inouye S: Delirium and other mental status problems in the older patient. In Goldman L, editor: *Cecil textbook of medicine,* ed 21, Baltimore, 2000, WB Saunders.

Inouye S et al: A multicomponent intervention to prevent delirium in hospitalized older patients, *N Engl J Med* 340(9):669, 1999.

Jack C et al: Prediction of AD with MRI-based hippocampal volume in mild cognitive impairment, *Neurology* 52(7):1397, 1999.

Keltner N, Folks D: *Psychotropic drugs,* ed 3, St Louis, 2001, Mosby.

Knopman D: An overview of common and non-Alzheimer dementias, *Clin Geriatr Med* 17(2):281, 2001.

Kolanowski A: An overview of the need-driven dementia-compromised behavior model, *J Gerontol Nurs* 25(9):7, 1999.

Litvan I et al: What are the obstacles for an accurate clinical diagnosis of Pick's disease, *Neurology* 49(1):62, 1997.

Lopez OL et al: Severity of cognitive impairment and the clinical diagnosis of AD with Lewy bodies, *Neurology* 54(9):1780, 2000.

Mace N, Rabins P: *The 36-hour day,* Baltimore, 1991, Johns Hopkins University Press.

Maixner S et al: The efficacy, safety and tolerability of antipsychotics in the elderly, *J Clin Psychiatry* 60(suppl 8):29, 1999.

Marzanzi M: Would you like to know the truth what is wrong with you? On telling the truth to patients with dementia, *J Med Ethics* 26(2):108, 2000.

Middleton H et al: Physical and pharmacologic restraints in long-term care facilities, *J Gerontol Nurs* 25(7):26, 1999.

Miller L et al: Comfort and pain relief in dementia: awakening a new beneficence, *J Gerontol Nurs* 26(9):32, 2000.

Moore P, Jefferson J: *Handbook of medical psychiatry,* St Louis, 1996, Mosby.

Morris J et al: Mild cognitive impairment represents early-stage Alzheimer's disease, *Arch Neurol* 58(3):397, 2001.

National Institute of Aging (NIA): *2000 progress report on Alzheimer's disease,* Bethesda, MD, 2000, NIA.

National Institute of Neurological Disorders and Stroke (NINDS): *Creutzfeldt-Jakob disease fact sheet,* Bethesda, MD, 2001, NINDS.

North American Nursing Diagnosis Association: *NANDA-Approved nursing diagnoses: definitions and classifications 2001,* Philadelphia, 2001, NANDA.

Perkin G: *Mosby's color atlas and text of neurology,* London, 1998, Times Mirror International Publishers.

Petersen R: Aging, mild cognitive impairment and Alzheimer's disease, *Neurol Clin* 18(4):789, 2000.

Plassman B et al: Documented head injury in early adulthood and risk of Alzheimer's disease and other dementias, *Neurology* 55(8):1158, 2000.

Pliskin N et al: Charles Bonnet syndrome: an early marker for dementia, *J Am Geriatr Soc* 44(9):1055, 1996.

Raskind M, Perskind E: Alzheimer's disease and related disorders, *Med Clin North Am* 85(3):803, 2001.

Regier D et al: The de facto US mental and additive disorders service system: epidemiologic catchment area prospective 1-year prevalence rates of disorders and services, *Arch Gen Psychiatry* 50:85, 1993.

Reifler B: A case of mistaken identity: pseudodementia is really predementia, *J Am Geriatr Soc* 48(5):593, 2000.

Rosen H et al: Frontotemporal dementia, *Neurol Clin* 18(4):979, 2000.

Rowe M, Alfred D: The effectiveness of slow-stroke massage in diffusing agitated behaviors in individuals with Alzheimer's disease, *J Gerontol Nurs* 25(6):22, 1999.

Skog M et al: The patient as "teacher": learning in the care of patients with dementia, *Nurse Education Today* 20(4):288, 2000.

Snowdon D: *Aging with grace: what the nun study teaches us about leading longer, healthier, and more meaningful lives,* New York, 2001, Bantam Books.

Stahl S: *Essential psychopharmacology: neuroscientific basis and practical applications,* Cambridge, UK, 2000, Cambridge University Press.

Tariot P: Treatment of agitation in dementia, *J Clin Psychiatry* 60(suppl):11, 1999.

Tasman A et al: *Psychiatry,* ed 1, Baltimore, 1997, WB Saunders.

Tasman A et al: *Psychiatry: behavioral science and clinical essentials. Dementia, delirium, and other cognitive disorders,* Baltimore, 2000, WB Saunders.

Tulberg M et al: CSF neurofilament and glial fibrillary acidic protein in normal pressure hydrocephalus, *Neurology* 50(4):1122, 1998.

Visser P et al: Brain correlates of memory dysfunction in alcoholic Korsakoff's syndrome, *J Neurol Neurosurg Psychiatry* 67(6):774, 1999.

Wang P et al: Hazardous benzodiazepine regimens in the elderly: effects of half-life, dosage and duration on risk of hip fracture, *Am J Psychiatry* 158(6):892, 2001.

Wells D et al: Effects of an abilities-focused program of morning care on residents who have dementia and on caregivers, *J Am Geriatr Soc* 48(4):442, 2000.

Wilson J, Helton B: *PSYCHed: continuing education and consultation, dementia module,* Birmingham, Ala, 2001. Unpublished.

Wolf R: *The nature and scope of elder abuse,* 2001. http://www. asaging. org/generations/gen-24-2/intro.html. Retrieved 5/15/02.

Wynne C et al: Comparison of pain assessment instruments in cognitively intact and cognitively impaired nursing home residents, *Geriatric Nursing* 21(1):20, 2000.

Young R: Update on Parkinson's disease, *Am Family Physician* 59(8): 2155, 1999.

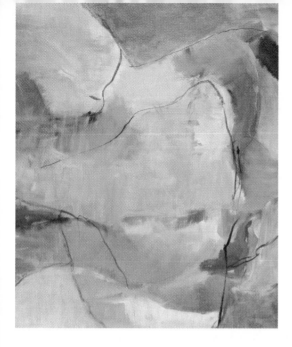

Chapter 33

Personality Disorders

Carol E. Bostrom

Learning Objectives

After reading this chapter, you should be able to:

- Recognize characteristics of each personality disorder.
- Describe behaviors of individuals with personality disorders.
- Describe nursing interventions for patients with personality disorders.
- Recognize issues related to the care of patients with personality disorders.

This chapter focuses on patients with personality disorders hospitalized in the inpatient psychiatric setting or treated in outpatient programs. Except for the patient with a borderline disorder, these patients are not usually hospitalized because of their personality disorders but because of other mental disorders diagnosed on axis I. The interventions focus primarily on the nurse-patient relationship unique to each personality disorder; however, this chapter does not repeat the general nurse-patient interventions described in Chapter 10. Neither milieu issues nor psychopharmacologic factors will be addressed for each disorder because milieu and pharmacologic interventions are not appropriate for all disorders. Medication may be given if the patient has an axis I diagnosis or a symp- tom severe enough to interfere with functioning, such as severe anxiety or depression.

All individuals have personality traits and characteristics that make them unique and interesting human beings. Traits are exhibited in the way individuals think about themselves and others and in the way they behave. When traits are inflexible and dysfunctional, individuals generally have problems in functioning and experience subjective distress. Patients with personality disorders suffer lifelong, inflexible, and dysfunctional patterns of relating and behaving. These dysfunctional patterns and behaviors usually cause distress to others. However, individuals with personality disorders may not find their behaviors distressing to themselves; they become distressed because of other people's reactions or behaviors toward them. This reaction affects these individuals by causing immense emotional pain and discomfort. The nurse conveys acceptance of the individual and empathy for emotional pain regardless of the patient's behavior. Patients with personality disorders have more psychiatric inpatient, outpatient, and pharmacologic treatment than do patients with major depressive disorder (Bender et al, 2001). Difficulty in managing complicated symptoms and significant impairment in functioning have resulted in increased contact with the mental health system and use of services. Patients do not seek treatment to change their personality but want help for depression, anxiety, alcoholism, and for dif-

12-Month Prevalence Rate of Mental Disorders in the United States

Diagnosis	Percentage of Population Over 17 Years of Age	Number of People
Anxiety disorders	12.6	20,034,000
Phobia disorders*	10.9	17,331,333
Mood disorders	9.5	15,143,000
Alcohol disorders	7.4	11,766,000
Major depression[†]	5.0	7,950,000
Drug disorders	3.1	4,929,000
Cognitive impairment	2.7	4,293,000
Obsessive-compulsive disorder	2.1	3,339,000
Antisocial disorders	1.5	2,385,000
Panic disorders*	1.3	2,067,000
Bipolar disorders[†]	1.2	1,908,000
Schizophrenia	1.1	1,749,000
Somatization	0.2	365,000

*Also calculated in anxiety statistics.
[†]Also calculated in mood disorders statistics.
From Regier DA et al: The de facto U.S. mental and addictive disorders service system: epidemiologic catchment area prospective, 1-year prevalence rates of disorders and services, *Arch Gen Psychiatry* 50:85, 1993; Surgeon General: Mental health: a report from the Surgeon General, *DHHS,* 1999, Washington, DC.

ficulties in work and personal relationships (Grinspoon, 2000).

Personality disorders are listed on axis II. Axis II can also be used to designate developmental disorders, personality traits, or habitual use of particular defense mechanisms. For example, compulsive traits are not the same as obsessive-compulsive personality disorder, which, in turn, is not the same as obsessive-compulsive disorder. Many high-functioning people have compulsive traits, whereas only a few have compulsive personality disorders. Patients benefit from the fact that some nurses may have compulsive traits, for example, rechecking labels, dressings, and drainage tubes.

Criteria for a personality disorder include experiences and behaviors that are very different from that which is usually expected in an individual's culture. The individual must have disturbances in two of the following areas: cognition, affect, interpersonal functioning, and impulse control. *The Diagnostic and Statistical Manual of Mental Disorders,* fourth edition, text revision (DSM-IV-TR) box titled "Criteria for a Personality Disorder" presents general criteria for a personality disorder.

DSM-IV-TR Criteria for a Personality Disorder

Disturbances in two or more of the following must be present:
A. Cognition (thinking about self, people, and events)
B. Affectivity, (range, intensity, lability, and appropriateness of emotional response)
C. Interpersonal functioning
D. Impulse control

Adapted from the American Psychiatric Association: *Diagnostic and statistical manual of mental disorders,* ed 4, text revision, Washington, DC, 2000, APA.

GENERAL ETIOLOGY: CONTEMPORARY VIEWS

Between 10 and 15 years ago, the causes of personality disorders were thought to be psychologic in origin based on reactions to childhood experiences and the reaction of the interpersonal and family environment to the experiences. Child development, family, and environment were key to developing personality disorders.

With the explosion of biologic research within the past 10 to 15 years, a different approach to the study of biologic dimensions underlying the development of personality disorders is emerging. Disturbances in cognition, impulsivity and aggression, affective lability, and chronic anxiety in patients with personality disorders are being studied across many personality disorders rather than for a specific personality disorder. This approach will add biologic data or another dimension to psychodynamic theory to increase our understanding of the psychopathology of these disorders (Silk, 2000).

Biologic factors alone are not totally responsible for the occurrence of these disorders. Twin studies indicate that specific traits, rather than disorders, are inherited.

The social environment coupled with psychologic vulnerability strongly influences the individual. The effects of societal changes, a stressful environment, and negative childhood experiences, along with biologic factors, are important in the genesis of personality disorders.

PERSONALITY DISORDER CLUSTERS

According to the DSM-IV-TR, the personality disorders are grouped into three clusters based on descriptive features. Cluster A includes the schizoid,

DSM-IV-TR and NANDA Diagnoses Related to Personality Disorders

DSM-IV-TR*	NANDA†
Cluster A—Odd, Eccentric Behaviors	Anxiety
Paranoid personality disorder	Communication, Impaired verbal
Schizoid personality disorder	Coping, Defensive
Schizotypal personality disorder	Coping, Ineffective
	Family processes, Interrupted
Cluster B—Dramatic, Emotional, Erratic Behaviors	Hopelessness
Antisocial personality disorder	Powerlessness
Borderline personality disorder	Self-esteem, Chronic low or Situational low or
Histrionic personality disorder	Risk situational low
Narcissistic personality disorder	Self-mutilation, Risk for
	Social isolation
Cluster C—Anxious, Fearful Behaviors	Violence, Risk for self-directed or Risk for other-directed
Avoidant personality disorder	
Dependent personality disorder	
Obsessive-compulsive disorder	

*From the American Psychiatric Association: *The diagnostic and statistical manual of mental disorders,* ed 4, text revision, Washington, DC, 2000, APA.
†From the North American Nursing Diagnosis Association: *NANDA nursing diagnoses: definitions and classifications 1997-1998,* Philadelphia, 1997, NANDA.

Key Terms

Dissociation Separation of mental or behavioral processes from the rest of the person's consciousness or identity.
Idealization Viewing others as perfect, exalting others.
Devaluation Criticism of others, which defends against own feelings of inadequacy.
Splitting Inability to integrate good and bad aspects of self and others; viewing self and others as all good or all bad.
Projective identification Blames others to justify own expression of feelings.

schizotypal, and paranoid disorders characterized by odd or eccentric behaviors. Cluster B includes the narcissistic, histrionic, antisocial, and borderline disorders characterized by dramatic, emotional, or erratic behaviors. Cluster C includes the dependent, avoidant, and obsessive-compulsive disorders characterized by anxious or fearful behaviors (American Psychiatric Association [APA], 2000).

When a person exhibits features of more than one specific personality disorder or does not meet the full criteria for any one disorder, the classification of "personality disorder not otherwise specified" is used. DSM-IV-TR diagnoses and potential North American Nursing Diagnosis Association (NANDA) nursing diagnoses for personality disorders are listed in the above box.

CLUSTER A: ODD-ECCENTRIC

PARANOID PERSONALITY DISORDER

Suspiciousness and mistrust of people characterize the person with a paranoid personality disorder. These individuals interpret the actions of others as personal threats, which results in an increase in anxiety and the need to scan the environment. They are hypersensitive to other people's motives but externalize their own feelings by projecting their own desires and traits to others. They feel vulnerable because they think others treat them unfairly. Individuals with paranoid personality disorders are unable to laugh at themselves and are often humorless and serious. Speech is logical and goal directed, although the basis of arguments are false because of their suspiciousness. Other symptoms include prejudice and sometimes ideas of reference. These individuals have a blunted affect, so they may appear to be cold, but they are capable of close relationships with a select few. However, they may be suspicious of people close to them. For example, these individuals may unjustifiably believe their spouse is having an affair. The DSM-IV-TR box on the following page, "Criteria for Paranoid Personality Disorder," presents the diagnostic criteria for this disorder.

Unlike paranoid schizophrenia, people with paranoid personality disorders do not have fixed delu-

A. Suspicious of others
B. Doubt trustworthiness or loyalty of friends and others
C. Fear of confiding in others
D. Suspicious, without justification, of spouse's or sexual partner's fidelity
E. Interpret remarks as demeaning or threatening
F. Hold grudges toward others
G. Become angry and threatening when they perceive they are attacked by others

Adapted from the American Psychiatric Association: *Diagnostic and statistical manual of mental disorders,* ed 4, text revision, Washington, DC, 2000, APA.

A. Lacks desire for close relationships or friends
B. Chooses solitary activities
C. Little interest in sexual experiences
D. Avoids activities
E. Appears cold and detached
F. Lacks close friends
G. Appears indifferent to praise or criticism

Adapted from the American Psychiatric Association: *Diagnostic and statistical manual of mental disorders,* ed 4, text revision, Washington, DC, 2000, APA.

sions or hallucinations. Transient psychotic symptoms may be precipitated by extreme stress. People with paranoid personality disorders are hospitalized when their behavior is out of control in response to a threat perceived as overwhelming or immediate. Because they are quick to respond with anger or rage if they feel severely threatened, these individuals may be brought to the hospital because of their loss of control and potential for violence.

Unique Etiology

Some evidence suggests that the paranoid personality disorder tends to occur in biologic relatives of identified schizophrenic patients and is diagnosed more often in men than it is in women (APA, 2000).

CLINICAL EXAMPLE
James Sneed is admitted to the hospital accompanied by a female friend. Mr. Sneed states, "My neighbor is taking my land. He built a fence on my property instead of his." The female friend states that James had barricaded himself in his house and was surrounded by his collection of shotguns and was threatening to "blow away" his neighbor.

SCHIZOID PERSONALITY DISORDER

People with schizoid personalities do not want to be involved in interpersonal or social relationships. These individuals rarely have close friends and appear uncomfortable interacting with others; they may be thought of as hermits because of their shyness and introversion; they respond with short answers to questions and do not initiate spontaneous conversation; they can function at work successfully, especially if little verbal interaction is required; and although they are reality oriented, fantasy and daydreaming

may be more gratifying compared with real persons and situations. The above DSM-IV-TR box titled, "Criteria for Schizoid Personality Disorder" presents additional characteristics.

If a person with schizoid personality disorder is hospitalized, the nurse-patient relationship will focus initially on building trust, followed by the identification and appropriate verbal expression of feelings. At first, the patient may be able to participate only on the fringe of unit activities because of discomfort and anxiety. Slowly involving the patient in milieu and group activities may help increase social skills.

SCHIZOTYPAL PERSONALITY DISORDER

Individuals with schizotypal personality disorder appear similar to patients with schizophrenia with the major exception being that psychotic episodes are infrequent and less severe. These patients have problems in thinking, perceiving, and communicating. Their outward appearance may be eccentric and their behavior odd; they are sensitive to the behaviors of others, especially rejection and anger, and feel they are different and do not "fit in." Fantasies about imaginary relationships may be substituted for real relationships. The DSM-IV-TR diagnostic criteria for this disorder are listed in the box titled, "Criteria for Schizotypal Personality Disorder" on the following page.

Schizotypal personality disorders are more common in the biologic relatives of schizophrenics (APA, 2000). Genetic studies indicate that patients with this disorder show disturbances (behaviors) similar to those found in people with schizophrenia.

When a person with schizotypal personality disorder is hospitalized, interventions offering support, kindness, and gentle suggestions will help the patient

DSM-IV-TR — Criteria for Schizotypal Personality Disorder

A. Ideas of reference
B. Magical thinking or odd beliefs
C. Unusual perceptual experiences, including bodily illusions
D. Odd thinking and vague, stereotypical, overelaborate speech
E. Suspicious
F. Blunted or inappropriate affect
G. Odd or eccentric appearance or behavior
H. Few close relationships
I. Excessive social anxiety

Adapted from the American Psychiatric Association: *Diagnostic and statistical manual of mental disorders*, ed 4, text revision, Washington, DC, 2000, APA.

DSM-IV-TR — Criteria for Antisocial Personality Disorder

A. Deceitfulness as seen in lying or conning others
B. Engages in illegal activities
C. Aggressive behavior
D. Lack of guilt or remorse
E. Irresponsible in work and with finances
F. Impulsiveness
G. Reckless disregard of safety for self or others

Adapted from the American Psychiatric Association: *Diagnostic and statistical manual of mental disorders*, ed 4, text revision, Washington, DC, 2000, APA.

become involved in activities with others. It is essential for the nurse to help the patient improve interpersonal relationships, social skills, and appropriate behaviors. Social situations are uncomfortable and cause discomfort and anxiety because of the reactions of others to the patient's appearance and behavior. These patients can benefit from socializing experiences if the interactions are carefully orchestrated. Vocational counseling and assistance with job placement increase the patient's opportunity for success. Low doses of antipsychotic drugs may decrease the severity of symptoms exhibited in the transient psychotic state in relation to thinking, perception, and anxiety.

Psychotherapeutic Management

Nurse-patient relationship

The most important psychotherapeutic task centers on dealing with trust issues. A professional demeanor coupled with honesty and nonintrusiveness will assist in developing some trust. Clear, simple explanations and requests will reduce the patient's feelings of being threatened or controlled. These patients do not tolerate group therapies that expect or involve confrontation or much emotional involvement.

CLUSTER B: DRAMATIC-ERRATIC

ANTISOCIAL PERSONALITY DISORDER

The main feature of antisocial personality disorder is a pattern of disregard for the rights of others, which is usually demonstrated by repeated violation of the law. Before age 15, these behaviors are diagnosed as conduct disorder. Affected individuals engage in unlawful behavior as evidenced by driving while intoxicated and engaging in spouse or child abuse. They are also promiscuous and have no guilt about hurting others. Lying, cheating, and stealing are common. Their criminal behavior places them within the court and prison system more than it does the mental health system. Not all criminals, however, have antisocial personality disorders.

The diagnosis of the antisocial personality disorder is based on history of disordered life functioning rather than on mental status. These individuals may experience distress and anxiety because of others' hostility toward them, but they see the problem as being within others and not themselves. People with an antisocial personality disorder may appear to be charming and intellectual; they are smooth talkers and deny and rationalize their behavior. Expected anxiety over their predicament is absent. Guilt, sorrow for offenses, or loyalty is nonexistent, as if they do not have a conscience. These individuals do not behave as responsible, mature, and independent adults. The DSM-IV-TR diagnostic criteria for this disorder are listed in the above box titled, "Criteria for Antisocial Personality Disorder."

Critical Thinking Question

A patient with antisocial personality disorder is verbally threatening to the staff when limits are set on his manipulative behaviors. How would the nurse manage the patient's threatening behavior?

Unique Etiology

Both genetics and the environment are known to influence the development of antisocial personality disorder. Parents establish an environment in which the parent-child relationship is unstable, resulting in delinquency in their children. Genetic studies of twin or adoptive siblings and family history data provide significant evidence that suggests a genetic predisposition to this disorder. In other words, children inherit traits that may lead to the development of an antisocial personality disorder. Substance abuse and dependency problems are highly correlated with the antisocial personality disorder (Grinspoon, 2000a).

A common biologic finding seen in individuals with antisocial personality disorder is a weak response to stress in the autonomic nervous system evidenced by a low heart rate and a lack of increase in level of anxiety. They are insensitive to the emotional connotations of language, which may explain their inability to learn from reward and punishment. Brain scans of individuals with antisocial personality disorder show lower than average activity in the frontal lobes, which govern judgment and decision making (Grinspoon, 2000b).

Psychotherapeutic Management

Nurse-patient relationship

Long-term treatment is necessary for any type of lasting changes to occur. With short-term hospitalization, the nurse can initiate the therapeutic process by setting firm limits. These patients try to manipulate staff and bend rules for their wants and needs. The nurse must be steadfast and consistent in confronting behaviors and enforcing rules and policies. Consequences of behavior, both for the unit and for the patient's life, are also a point of focus. Helping the patient to be aware of consequences is a concrete way to assist the patient in realizing what the results of behaviors are or will be. Pointing out the effects that the patient's behaviors have on others is also part of the therapeutic process. The patient must begin to understand the way others feel and react to his or her behaviors and the reasons they react the way they do. The nurse avoids moralizing and assists the patient in identifying and verbalizing feelings that may reflect anxiety and depression. Group membership can help the patient feel accepted as a person, even if the patient's behaviors are not acceptable. Groups of other individuals with this same diagnosis can be effective in confronting inappropriate and manipulative behavior because these individuals are "experts" in spotting smooth talking, rationalizing, and lying. These groups can be effective in helping the antiso-

cial patient. In summary, the keys to working with the antisocial patient are consistency by the nursing staff and accountability by the patient.

BORDERLINE PERSONALITY DISORDER

Of all personality disorders, the borderline personality disorder (BPD) is the most commonly treated. However, because the full range of symptoms and behaviors is not typically demonstrated during one short-term inpatient hospitalization, it is often difficult to fully appreciate the complexity of these individuals' mental disorder. These patients usually require hospitalization when they are in a crisis or exhibit self-mutilating or suicidal behaviors.

The patient with a BPD has problems with identity, self-image, relationships, thinking, mood, and impulsive behaviors (Livesly, 2000). Identity problems are apparent in the patient who is uncertain about his or her self-image, career goals, personal values, and sexual orientation. Interpersonal relationship problems exist in choosing unhealthy relationships and in short-term intimate relationships. The patient alternates between overidealization and devaluation of individuals. For example, the patient with BPD "falls in love" with the perfect person and, shortly thereafter, can find no redeeming qualities in the formerly idealized person. The person with BPD cannot appreciate the "mixed-bag" of qualities most people have.

Manipulation and dependency commonly occur. This patient has great difficulty in being alone and therefore seeks intense but brief relationships. Mood disturbances are exhibited in symptoms of depression, intense anger, and labile mood. Projective identification is used to protect the self. Patients displace their angry feelings onto others to justify their own feelings. Blaming others helps the patient deal with feelings even though it is dysfunctional and inappropriate. Intense emotional pain contributes to mood shifts, which range from euphoria to crying to acting-out behaviors, such as displays of temper and physical fights, self-mutilation, and suicidal behaviors. Impulsiveness is exhibited in the use of substances and anorexia-bulimia. Other relatively common impulsive activities include overspending, promiscuity, compulsive overeating, and unhealthy risk taking and decision making. DSM-IV-TR criteria for this disorder are listed in the box titled, "Criteria for Borderline Personality Disorder" on the following page.

DSM-IV-TR | Criteria for Borderline Personality Disorder

A. Frantic avoidance of abandonment; real or imagined
B. Unstable and intense interpersonal relationships
C. Identity disturbances
D. Impulsivity
E. Affective instability
F. Recurrent suicidal behavior or self-mutilating behavior
G. Rapid mood shifts
H. Chronic feelings of emptiness
I. Problems with anger
J. Transient dissociative and paranoid symptoms

Adapted from the American Psychiatric Association: *Diagnostic and statistical manual of mental disorders*, ed 4, text revision, Washington, DC, 2000, APA.

Research findings indicate that as many as 75% of individuals with BPD are women and victims of childhood sexual abuse (APA, 2000). This finding is significant because it suggests the possible dynamics of BPD behaviors, which, in turn, determine nursing interventions. The dissociation used by a child sex abuse victim may result in "splitting," which is found in the BPD. The defense mechanism of splitting is defined as the inability to view both self and others as having both good and bad qualities. Therefore self and others are viewed as either all good or all bad. Splitting helps the individual avoid the pain and feelings associated with past abuse and current situations involving threats of rejection or abandonment. The complexity of behaviors associated with BPD can include severe symptoms of posttraumatic stress disorder and dissociative disorder. See Chapter 41 on victims of violent behavior and Chapter 31 on anxiety-related disorders for related discussions.

On admission to an inpatient psychiatric unit, the person with a BPD may exhibit a need for attention and affection by contradictory behaviors of manipulation, dependency, or acting out. Frustration on the part of the staff may be seen as rejection. This perception by the patient can lead to increased anger and withdrawal. Shifts between depression, anxiety, euphoria, and anger are seen in the patient's labile mood. Under stress, the patient regresses to immature behaviors and is unable to cope with conflict. The patient vacillates between clinging and disengaged behaviors, as demonstrated by desiring the staff to solve all problems or by the patient viewing the inpatient treatment as unnecessary and meaningless. When progress seems to be occurring, the patient with a BPD may suddenly exhibit opposite behaviors, and it may seem as if the staff will need to start over.

Patients with BPD use self-mutilation for the purpose of self-punishment, tension reduction, improvement in mood, and distraction from intolerable affects (Stanley et al, 2001). After self-mutilating behaviors such as cutting and burning, the patient feels better and relieved.

Patients who mutilate themselves are at a serious risk for suicide. Their feelings of hopelessness, despair, and depression contribute to their suicidality, and their self-mutilation should never be interpreted as manipulation or as attention-seeking behavior. Patients with BPD are at risk for suicide because of their depression, aggression, underestimation of the lethality of their behavior, and longer and more frequent occurrence of suicidal thoughts. These patients are often unaware of the likelihood of death and misperceive the lethality of their attempts. The lethality of individuals who self-mutilate and attempt suicide is as serious as those who do not self-mutilate and attempt suicide (Stanley et al, 2001). Self-mutilation and suicide attempts should never be minimized or ignored.

Unique Etiology

The development of the borderline personality disorder may be the result of a combination of temperament, childhood experiences, and neurologic and biochemical dysfunction (Zanarini, 2000). Biologic, environmental, and stress-related factors contribute to the complexity of the disorder. Biologic studies indicate neurotransmitter dysregulation of the serotonin system as seen in affective disturbances and impulsive behaviors. Abnormalities of cholinergic and adrenergic systems predispose individuals to dysphoria, emotional lability, and hyperreactivity related to environmental stimuli (Gurvits, Koenigsberg, Siever, 2000). Increased norepinephrine leads to increased reactivity to the environment, which may contribute to affective instability.

Environmental factors include a traumatic home environment, such as emotional discord in the family; neglect of the child's feelings and needs; or verbal, emotional, physical, and sexual abuse.

Stress-related events may trigger the individual's vulnerable temperament and create misery and frustration. The individual is reminded of earlier stress or trauma, which results in the development of the borderline symptoms and condition (Grinspoon, 2000).

Psychotherapeutic Management

Nurse-patient relationship

The use of empathy by the nurse is important in establishing a relationship with the patient diagnosed with BPD. The nurse acknowledges the reality of the patient's pain, offers support, and empowers and works with the patient to understand, control, and change dysfunctional behaviors. The patient is ultimately in control of his or her own behaviors even when the behaviors seem out of control (Smith, Ruiz-Sancho, Gunderson, 2001). With the nurse's assistance, the patient can identify and verbalize feelings, control negative behaviors, and slowly begin to replace them with more appropriate actions.

The patient is usually in a crisis situation when hospitalized because of suicidal ideation or behavior, self-mutilation, acute personality disorganization, or inability to function. The nurse provides a safe environment to decrease self-harm and contain impulses and then works with the patient to find alternatives to express anger and rage. Alternatives may include ventilation and discussion of feelings, punching pillows, and the use of foam bats. For self-harm behaviors to diminish, the nurse helps the patient identify feelings and verbally express them nonaggressively, which enables the patient to understand that his or her actions are habitual responses to handling emotions. Recognizing behavioral and emotional cues can help the patient decrease impulsive and self-harm behaviors. The nurse then discusses with the patient safe, alternative methods to handle feelings. The use of a behavioral contract to decrease self-mutilation in inpatient and outpatient settings provides the patient with clear expectations of behavior.

Patients can be helped with understanding themselves and their feelings by writing in a notebook on a daily basis. In sharing the journal with the nurse, the patient gains an understanding of self and a sense of autonomy and responsibility. This technique can be useful for many patients with BPD.

Patients with BPD who are victims of abuse need to talk about their trauma in a safe environment. The nurse should acknowledge their pain and convey empathy and the appropriateness of their feelings. When patients understand that current behaviors are linked to past trauma, they can learn to recognize and then work toward changing dysfunctional actions toward self and others. See Chapter 41 on victims of violent behavior for more detailed interventions.

The patient with BPD is often manipulative. Consistency, limit setting, and supportive confrontation are necessary interventions to provide clear expectations regarding patient behaviors. These patients are adept at sidestepping rules, avoiding consequences, and pitting staff members against each other, all for the sake of getting what they want. Enforcing unit rules, providing clear structure, and placing the responsibility for appropriate behaviors on the patient, though vigorously resisted, will benefit the person with a BPD. The need to help the patient develop realistic short-term goals must be part of the treatment plan if the patient's responsibility for self is to increase.

The psychiatric nurse is in a perfect position to help the patient with BPD with the daily give-and-take issues of life that create the many problems for this patient. The nurse should work with the patient on appropriate verbal expression of feelings and assertiveness, even though the nurse's ability to be empathetic, nonjudgmental, and therapeutic is sometimes severely tested by the patient's behaviors. The nurse may feel frustrated and ineffective as a caregiver because of the patient's behaviors and defenses. Hence offering superficial solutions to problems, pointing out rules, and interacting superficially may be less frustrating and "safer." However, understanding and working with the patient therapeutically can result in a positive experience for the nurse and be of lasting import to the patient.

Psychopharmacology

Psychopharmacology is used for specific symptoms for the patient with BPD. The symptoms are divided into three domains: cognitive-perceptual symptoms, affective or emotional dysregulation, and impulsive-behavioral dyscontrol (Lively, 2000; Soloff, 2000). Medications are only part of the treatment plan and will not solve all of the patient's problems. Cognitive-perceptual symptoms may include transitory hallucinations, suspiciousness, paranoid thinking, and delusions. Transient psychot-

Case Study

Sherry Morgan, a 27-year-old woman, is brought to the psychiatric inpatient unit from the emergency department. Both wrists were bandaged after suturing. She is complaining of nausea and heartburn. She vacillates between being angry and crying. Sherry states, "I know I am bad. I should not have done it. I do not want to die, but I am tired of the hassles." She has brought with her three suitcases filled with her belongings. During the admission interview, the nurse finds that Sherry has had three previous admissions to this inpatient unit during the past 8 years. Sherry states that she refuses to return to work because her boss accuses her of bothering the other employees instead of doing her own work. She states that her boss is falsely accusing her of using alcohol and drugs and does not accept her reasons for being absent from work. On the morning of admission, she called her outpatient therapist, whom she had not seen in a year and a half; he agreed to see her at 3:00 PM. When she called the therapist back at noon and found he was at lunch, she used her scissors to cut her wrists. "I used to think he understood me, but now I know he doesn't care." Her parents are on vacation out of state, and her only close friend is busy going through a divorce. She had taken some of her mother's Valium, but it did not calm her down. She has averaged only 3 to 4 hours of sleep each night for the past 5 days and has been unable to eat regular meals. Her attempts to clean her parents' house were not completed. She could not even finish watering her mother's plants. A male acquaintance of 2 weeks was no longer calling her, so she was frequenting several bars and inviting men home. She never heard from these men again, even though she thought that their relationships were sexually satisfying.

Sherry completed 2 years of college and is dressed attractively. She enjoys reading romance novels and has brought five of her favorite books.

Care Plan

Name: Sherry Morgan _____   Admission Date: _____

DSM-IV-TR Diagnosis: Axis I—Major Depression; Axis II—Borderline Personality Disorder _____

Assessment **Areas of strength:** Well-groomed, neat and clean, intelligent, enjoys reading.
Problems: Self-mutilating behavior, absence of support system, loss of job, decreased sleeping and eating, irresponsible and impulsive sexual behavior.

Diagnoses • High risk for self-mutilation related to absence of support systems as evidenced by cutting wrists.
• Defensive coping related to low self-esteem as evidenced by angry and labile emotions.

Outcomes *Short-term goals:*   *Date met*
• Patient will eliminate self-mutilating behavior and appropriately verbalize   _____
  feelings of anger and sadness.
Long-term goals:
• Patient will schedule outpatient appointment and meeting with boss   _____
  regarding job problems.

Planning/ Interventions **Nurse-patient relationship:** Monitor and set limits on acting-out behaviors. Assist patient with identification and verbalization of feelings. Discuss fears about accepting responsibility for self and decision-making. Discuss behaviors interfering with job performance.
Psychopharmacology: Prozac 20 mg q AM, Desyrel 50 mg q hs.
Milieu management: Groups focusing on self-esteem, stress and anger management, assertiveness training, social skills, problem-solving skills, discharge planning.

Evaluation Patient has not engaged in self-mutilating behavior. Patient is beginning to verbalize feelings of anger and sadness.

Referrals Appointment weekly after discharge with therapist at outpatient mental health clinic.

ic states resulting from overwhelming stress are treated with low-dose typical and atypical antipsychotics for 3 to 12 weeks to decrease symptoms.

Affective or emotional dysregulation may include depression, labile mood, anger, anxiety, hostility, and mistrust. Selective serotonin reuptake inhibitors (SSRIs) are used to reduce anger, anxiety, chronic emptiness, and temper outbursts. Clonazepam may be useful for anxiety management if needed (Soloff, 2000). Lithium, valproic acid, and carbamazepine can be used for rapid mood swings.

Impulsive-behavioral dyscontrol symptoms may include suicidal threats and attempts, assaultiveness, impulse-aggression, and binge behaviors involving alcohol, drugs, or sex. SSRIs are used to decrease impulsive behaviors.

Milieu management

Interventions mentioned in the nurse-patient relationship discussion regarding firm limits, consistency, and clear structure are basic to the milieu for the BPD patient. The patient's manipulation of other patients must be confronted because the BPD patient can mobilize others against the staff. Consistent communication among staff members is essential to minimize the patient's attempts to divide the staff.

Group sessions that include cognitive-behavioral techniques, assertiveness training, problem solving, stress management, anger management, and victimization are some of the therapeutic activities that are important for these patients in both inpatient and outpatient settings.

Referral to self-help groups that are applicable for alcohol and drug problems, eating disorders, and victimization is also important. Vocational counseling and training are important to foster autonomous and independent functioning. Residential treatment may need to be considered particularly for patients with chronic self-destructive behavior.

> ### *Critical* Thinking Question
>
> Staff members on the unit are frustrated and angry with a patient who is attempting to split members on the various shifts against each other. They are even beginning to be angry with each other for the inconsistencies occurring with this patient's care. What strategies should the head nurse employ to help the staff and ultimately the treatment of the patient?

NARCISSISTIC PERSONALITY DISORDER

The patient with a narcissistic personality disorder displays grandiosity about his or her importance and achievements. This grandiosity is unlike the delusions of grandeur found in schizophrenia or bipolar disorders. The grandiosity of the narcissistic personality disorder is based somewhat in reality but is distorted, embellished, or convoluted to meet the patient's needs of self-importance. For example, the male patient may say that he was a star football player in high school and that he could have played for the Indianapolis Colts; he does not tell the nurse that he barely made the second-string football team in high school.

The narcissistic patient overvalues himself or herself, needs to be admired, is arrogant, and seems indifferent to the criticism of others. Those around this person are often viewed as superior or inferior. For example, the patient views the nurse who is understanding and supportive as competent or superior, whereas the nurse who questions or confronts is viewed as incompetent or inferior.

The patient may appear nonchalant or indifferent to criticism while hiding feelings of anger, rage, or emptiness. Relationships with others seem shallow but may be meaningful if the patient's self-esteem is positively enhanced. The patient cannot empathize with others, and the feelings of others are not understood or considered. These individuals use others selfishly to meet their own needs but do not reciprocate. This type of patient has a sense of entitlement and expects special treatment. The patient uses rationalization to blame others, makes excuses, and provides alibis for self-centered behaviors. See the box below for DSM-IV-TR criteria box titled, "Criteria for Narcissistic Personality Disorder."

> **CLINICAL EXAMPLE**
> The patient has been admitted to the unit and insists on a private room with a telephone and television because he needs to keep up with the reports on the financial news network.

Unique Etiology

Studies of biologic and genetic factors in the narcissistic personality disorder have not been conducted. Some theorists believe that the self-centered person is arrested at an early developmental stage because the parents fail to mirror that which is appropriate or inappropriate back to the child (Gunderson, 1988). Consequently, the child develops without any feedback about his or her behaviors.

DSM-IV-TR Criteria for Narcissistic Personality Disorder

A. Grandiose self-importance
B. Fantasies of unlimited power, success, or brilliance
C. Believes he or she is special or unique
D. Needs to be admired
E. Sense of entitlement (i.e., deserves to be favored or given special treatment)
F. Takes advantage of others for own benefit
G. Lacks empathy
H. Envious of others or others are envious of him or her
I. Arrogant or naughty

Adapted from the American Psychiatric Association: *Diagnostic and statistical manual of mental disorders*, ed 4, text revision, Washington, DC, 2000, APA.

Psychotherapeutic Management

Nurse-patient relationship

If this patient is hospitalized, the nurse must deal with decreasing the constant recitation of self-importance and grandiosity. The nurse must mirror what the patient sounds like, especially if contradictions exist, and help the patient focus on the identification and verbal expression of feelings. Supportive confrontation is used to point out discrepancies between that which the patient says and that which actually exists to increase responsibility for self. Limit setting and consistency in approach are used to decrease manipulation and entitlement behaviors. Realistic short-term goals focused on the here-and-now are important to decrease the patient's use of fantasy and rationalization and to increase responsibility for self. The patient needs to be taught that no one is perfect and that everyone has worth even if he or she makes mistakes and has imperfections.

HISTRIONIC PERSONALITY DISORDER

The patient with the histrionic personality disorder dramatizes all events and draws attention to self. This patient is extroverted and thrives on being the center of attention. Behavior is silly, colorful, frivolous, and seductive. Speech is vague, descriptive, superficial, and overembellished but lacking in detail, insight, and depth. The patient seems to be in a hurry and restless. Temper tantrums and outbursts of anger are seen, as well as overreaction to minor events. This patient may use somatic complaints to avoid responsibility and support dependency. Dissociation is a common defense to avoid feelings. Therefore this patient cannot deal with his or her true feelings. The patient views relationships with others as special or possessing greater intimacy than is real. Recently met individuals are thought of as being dear friends. The DSM-IV-TR box on the following page titled, "Criteria for Histrionic Personality Disorder" presents additional criteria.

The causes of histrionic personality disorder are unknown but are probably a result of many factors. In the early mother-child relationship, the mother negates the child's inner feelings. The child then turns to his or her father for nurturance, and the father responds to the child's dramatic emotional behaviors (Gunderson, 1988).

DSM-IV-TR — Criteria for Histrionic Personality Disorder

A. Needs to be center of attention
B. Displays sexually seductive or provocative behaviors
C. Shallow, rapidly shifting emotions
D. Uses physical appearance to draw attention
E. Uses speech to impress others but is lacking in depth
F. Dramatic expression of emotion
G. Easily influenced by others
H. Exaggerates degree of intimacy with others

Adapted from the American Psychiatric Association: *Diagnostic and statistical manual of mental disorders*, ed 4, text revision, Washington, DC, 2000, APA.

DSM-IV-TR — Criteria for Dependent Personality Disorder

A. Unable to make daily decisions without much advice and reassurance
B. Needs others to be responsible for important areas of life
C. Seldom disagrees with others because of fear of loss of support or approval
D. Problem with initiating projects or doing things on own because of little self-confidence
E. Performs unpleasant tasks to obtain support from others
F. Anxious or helpless when alone because of fear of being unable to care for self
G. Urgently seeks another relationship for support and care after a close relationship ends
H. Preoccupied with fear of being alone to care for self

Adapted from the American Psychiatric Association: *Diagnostic and statistical manual of mental disorders*, ed 4, text revision, Washington, DC, 2000, APA.

Positive reinforcement in the form of attention, recognition, or praise is given for unselfish or other-centered behaviors. Because the patient needs much reassurance and feels helpless, the nurse must provide support to facilitate independent problem solving and daily functioning. Because the patient is unaware of and does not deal with feelings, the nurse must help clarify the patient's true feelings and help the patient learn the appropriate way to express them. Working with this type of patient can be frustrating for the nurse because the patient needs time to internalize the meaning of that which the nurse is trying to accomplish.

CLUSTER C: ANXIOUS-FEARFUL

DEPENDENT PERSONALITY DISORDER

The main characteristic of the dependent personality disorder is a "pervasive and excessive need to be taken care of that leads to submissive and clinging behaviors and fears of separation" (APA, 2000, p. 721). Dependent individuals want others to make everyday decisions for them, for example, type of clothes to wear and type of job to seek. They need direction and reassurance. These individuals feel inferior and cling to others excessively because they are afraid they will be left alone. Avoiding responsibility and expressing helplessness, the patient maintains the need to rely on others. They perceive themselves as being unable to function without the help of others.

Dependent individuals also expect that if they perform good deeds for others, they will be rewarded by someone doing something for them. An intimate relationship with a spouse who is abusive, unfaithful, or an alcoholic is tolerated so as not to disturb the sense of attachment. Passivity and concealing of sex-

ual feelings and anger are a means of avoiding conflict. DSM-IV-TR criteria are listed in the box titled, "Criteria for Dependent Personality Disorder."

CLINICAL EXAMPLE
The patient has been telling the nurse about her alcoholic, abusive husband. She has been married to him for 16 years. She expresses sadness and frustration about her marriage but states, "How could I leave him? What would I do? Who will take care of me? I could never live alone."

Biochemical and genetic factors have not been correlated with dependent personality disorders. Psychosocial theories consider culture to be the basis of the development of this disorder. Certain cultures dictate that women should maintain a dependent role. Parents or society may believe that the child should not exhibit certain autonomous behaviors, and the child, in turn, may believe disapproval or loss of attachment are consequences of these behaviors. Individuals with dependent personality disorder assume a passive role regarding self but do so for others to foster attachment.

Psychotherapeutic Management

Nurse-patient relationship

The nurse slowly works on decision making with the patient to increase responsibility for self in day-to-day living. The patient needs assistance with managing anxiety because it will increase as the

DSM-IV-TR	Criteria for Avoidant Personality Disorder

A. Avoids occupations involving interpersonal contact because of fears of disapproval or rejection
B. Uninvolved with others unless certain of being liked
C. Fears intimate relationships due to fear of shame or ridicule
D. Preoccupied with being criticized or rejected in social situations
E. Inhibited and feels inadequate in new interpersonal situations
F. Believes self to be socially inept, unappealing, or inferior to others
G. Very reluctant to take risks or engage in new activities due to possibility of being embarrassed

Adapted from the American Psychiatric Association: *Diagnostic and statistical manual of mental disorders,* ed 4, text revision, Washington, DC, 2000, APA.

DSM-IV-TR	Criteria for Obsessive-Compulsive Personality Disorder

A. Preoccupied with details, rules, lists, organization
B. Perfectionism that interferes with task completion
C. Too busy working to have friends or leisure activities
D. Overconscientious and inflexible
E. Unable to discard worthless or worn-out objects
F. Others must do things his or her way in work- or task-related activity
G. Reluctant to spend and hoards money
H. Rigid and stubborn

Adapted from the American Psychiatric Association: *Diagnostic and statistical manual of mental disorders,* ed 4, text revision, Washington, DC, 2000, APA.

patient assumes more responsibility for self. Assertiveness is an important area of the nurse's teaching, which enables the patient to clearly state his or her feelings, needs, and desires. Verbalization of feelings and ways to cope with them are essential.

AVOIDANT PERSONALITY DISORDER

Patients with the avoidant personality disorder are timid, socially uncomfortable, withdrawn, and they feel inadequate and hypersensitive to criticism. Although they are fearful and shy, patients with the avoidant personality disorder desire relationships and challenges. To keep their anxiety at a minimal level, these individuals avoid situations in which they might be disappointed or rejected. When interacting with someone, this person sounds uncertain and lacks self-confidence. This person is afraid to ask questions or speak up in public, withdraws from social support, and conveys helplessness. The above DSM-IV-TR box titled, "Criteria for Avoidant Personality Disorder" presents criteria for this disorder.

Few biologic, genetic, and psychologic studies have been conducted. Shyness is common in childhood, but increased shyness and avoidant behavior during adolescence may lead to this disorder. The nurse helps the patient gradually confront his or her fears. Discussing the patient's feelings and fears before and after doing something that he or she is afraid to do is an essential part of the relationship. The nurse supports and directs the patient in accomplishing small goals. Helping patient to be assertive and to develop social skills is necessary. The nurse includes the patient in interac-

tions with others and then progresses to small groups as the patient is able to tolerate them. Because of the patient's anxiety, relaxation techniques are taught to enable the person to be successful in interactions. The nurse will give positive feedback to the patient for any real success or will attempt to engage in interactions with others to promote self-esteem.

Obsessive-Compulsive Personality Disorder

Individuals with obsessive-compulsive personality disorder are perfectionistic and inflexible. These patients are overly strict and often set standards for themselves that are too high, thus their work is never good enough. They are preoccupied with rules, trivial details, and procedures. They find it difficult to express warmth or tender emotions. There is little give-and-take in their interactions with others, and they are rigid, controlling, and cold. The patient is serious about all of his or her activities, thus having fun or experiencing pleasure is difficult. Because the person is afraid of making mistakes, he or she can be indecisive or will put off decisions until all the facts are accumulated. The person's affect is constricted, and he or she may speak in a monotone. The above DSM-IV-TR box titled, "Criteria for Obsessive-Compulsive Personality Disorder" presents the criteria for this disorder.

Early parent-child relationships around issues of autonomy, control, and authority may predispose a person to this disorder. Recent genetic studies indicate that this malady and the more severe obsessive-compulsive disorder may be inherited.

The nurse needs to support the patient in exploring his or her feelings and in attempting new experiences and situations. The nurse helps the patient with decision making and encourages follow-through behavior. At times, a need exists to confront the patient's procrastination and intellectualization. The nurse teaches the patient the importance of leisure activities and exploring interests in this area. Because the patient lacks awareness of the way he or she affects others, the patient needs to look at and understand other's view of him or her. Teaching the patient that he or she is human and that it is all right to make mistakes helps decrease irrational beliefs about the necessity to be perfect.

Key Concepts

1. Personality traits are enduring approaches to the world expressed in the way the person thinks and feels and that which the person does.
2. When personality traits become rigid, dysfunctional, and cause distress in self and others, they may be diagnosed as a personality disorder. Personal discomfort arises primarily from others' reactions to or behaviors toward that person.
3. The odd-eccentric cluster of personality disorders includes the following:
   a. Paranoid, characterized by suspiciousness and mistrust
   b. Schizoid, characterized by hermitlike lifestyle, aloneness
   c. Schizotypal, characterized by symptoms similar to but less severe than those of schizophrenia
4. The dramatic-erratic cluster includes the following:
   a. Antisocial, characterized by disregard of others' rights without guilt
   b. Borderline, characterized by problems with self-identity, interpersonal relationships, mood shifts, and self-destructiveness
   c. Narcissistic, characterized by overevaluation of self, arrogance, and indifference to the criticism of others
   d. Histrionic, characterized by dramatic behaviors, attention seeking, and superficiality

5. The anxious-fearful cluster includes the following:
   a. Dependent, characterized by submissiveness, helplessness, fear of responsibility, and reliance on others for decision making
   b. Avoidant, characterized by timidity, social withdrawal behavior, and hypersensitivity to criticism
   c. Obsessive-compulsive, characterized by indecisiveness, perfectionism, inflexibility, and difficulty expressing feelings
6. Nursing interventions for individuals with personality disorders help the patient focus on specific behaviors distressing to self or others or both and awareness of dysfunctional and self-defeating patterns.

References

American Psychiatric Association: *Diagnostic and statistical manual of mental disorders,* ed 4, text revision, Washington, DC, 2000, APA.

Bender DS: Treatment utilization by patients with personality disorders, *Am J Psychiatry* 158(2):295, 2001.

Grinspoon L, editor: Antisocial personality—part I, *Harv Ment Health Lett* 17(7):1, 2000a.

Grinspoon L, editor: Antisocial personality—part II, *Harv Ment Health Lett* 17(7):1, 2000b.

Grinspoon L, editor: Personality disorders—part II, *Harv Ment Health Lett* 16(10):1, 2000.

Gunderson JG: Personality disorders. In Nicholi A, editor: *The new Harvard guide to psychiatry,* Cambridge, Mass, 1988, The Belknap Press.

Gurvits IG, Koenigsberg HW, Siever LJ: Neurotransmitter dysfunction in patients with borderline personality disorder, *Psychiatr Clin North Am* 23(1):27, 2000.

Lively WJ: A practical approach to the treatment of patients with borderline personality disorder, *Psychiatr Clin North Am* 23(1):211, 2000.

Silk KR: Overview of biologic factors, *Psychiatr Clin North Am,* 23(1):61, 2000.

Smith GW, Ruiz-Sancho AR, Gunderson JG: An intensive outpatient program for patients with borderline personality disorder, *Psychiatr Serv* 52(4):532, 2001.

Soloff PH: Psychopharmacology of borderline personality disorder, *Psychiatr Clin North Am* 23(1):169, 2000.

Stanley B et al: Are suicide attempters who self-mutilate a unique population? *Am J Psychiatry* 158(3):427, 2001.

Zanarini MC: Childhood experiences associated with the development of borderline personality disorder, *Psychiatr Clin North Am* 23(1):89, 2000.

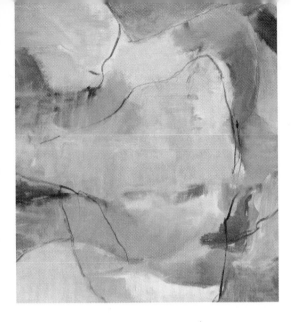

Chapter 34

Sexual Disorders

Carol E. Bostrom

Learning Objectives

After reading this chapter, you should be able to:

- Recognize the importance of the nurse's role in assessing patients' sexual concerns and problems.
- Describe the categories of sexual dysfunctions, sexual disorders, and gender identity.
- Identify the issues related to the care of patients with sexual disorders.
- Demonstrate an understanding of the need for referral for in-depth assessment and treatment of patients with sexual disorders.

This chapter presents an overview of sexual disorders and sexual dysfunctions. Normal sexuality and sexual preference issues, such as homosexuality, are not included.

Individuals engage in a wide range of sexual activities, resulting in a wide range of sexual responses. Sexual activity may focus on objects or people; it is unacceptable legally when it involves a nonconsenting individual, a child, or the use of objects in a way that might interfere with healthy relationships. Sexual activity is unacceptable morally when it violates the norms, standards, and values of the culture. Sexual activity should be evaluated according to its effects on the individual and others, such as the level of functioning, self-esteem, and relationships with others.

Considering coercion versus consent between sexual partners is important. An individual's rights and needs should never be violated. Power and control issues affect the definition of consent and the degree of coercion. For example, some clinicians believe that a sexual relationship between a powerful political figure and a young female office worker, though apparently consensual, is actually coercive at its core.

DSM-IV-TR CRITERIA AND TERMINOLOGY

The Diagnostic and Statistical Manual of Mental Disorders, fourth edition, text revision, (DSM-IV-TR), American Psychiatric Association [APA], 2000) categorizes sexual disorders according to sexual dysfunctions, the paraphilias, and gender identity disorders. Sexual dysfunctions are characterized by the inhibition of sexual appetite or psychophysiologic changes that compromise the sexual response cycle. Paraphilias are characterized by intense sexual urges focused on (1) nonhuman objects, (2) the suffering or humiliation of oneself or one's partner, or (3) children or other nonconsenting individuals. Gender identity disorders are characterized by a discomfort with one's biologic sex or the desire to have the characteristics of the other sex.

Diagnoses Related to Sexual Disorders

DSM-IV*

Sexual dysfunction disorders
Paraphilias
Gender identity disorders

NANDA†

Altered family process
Altered sexuality patterns
Anxiety
Ineffective coping
Knowledge deficit
Potential for violence: self-directed or other
Sexual dysfunction
Social isolation

*From the American Psychiatric Association: *Diagnostic and statistical manual of mental disorders,* ed 4, text revision, Washington, DC, 2000, APA.
†From the North American Nursing Diagnosis Association: *NANDA nursing diagnoses: definitions and classifications,* 1999-2000, Philadelphia, PA, 2000, NANDA.

SEXUAL DYSFUNCTIONS

As part of the admission interview, the nurse assesses each patient for potential or actual problems with sexual functioning. Box 34-1 lists initial questions the nurse may use to assess the patient's feelings and concerns about sexuality. Potential or actual problems can occur as a result of emotional or physiologic factors or both. Medications and chemicals can also alter sexual desire and functioning. A more thorough assessment or evaluation is necessary for appropriate referral and treatment. Treatment is individualized according to the cause or combination of causes. For example, the individual who becomes impotent because of a medical illness or a medication side effect may also have diminished self-esteem and self-confidence that compounds the problem. Therefore treatment would focus on both the physiologic aspects and emotional needs of the individual.

The phases of human sexual activity have been called the sexual response cycle. There are four phases: the desire phase, the excitement phase, the orgasm phase, and the resolution phase. Sexual dysfunctions are grouped into disorders that compromise one of these phases. Sexual desire disorders effectively stop the sexual response cycle from beginning. Sexual arousal disorders sidetrack the sexual response cycle at the excitement phase. Orgasm disorders arrest the progression of the cycle

Box 34-1 | Initial Nursing Assessment of Sexual Concerns

Describe any difficulties you have experienced with sexual performance or satisfaction.
What are your feelings and concerns about sexuality?
How satisfied are you with your sexual relationship?
What kind of changes would you like to make in your sexual relationship?
What kind of negative sexual experiences have you had?

in the orgasm phase. Finally, sexual pain disorders can abort the sexual response cycle at any phase.

Sexual Desire Disorders

Individuals with these disorders have little or no sexual desire for or have an aversion to sexual contact.

Sexual Arousal Disorders

Individuals with these disorders cannot maintain the physiologic requirements for sexual intercourse. Women cannot maintain the lubrication-swelling response of sexual excitement, and men cannot maintain an erection.

Orgasm Disorders

Individuals with these disorders cannot complete the sexual response cycle because of the inability to achieve an orgasm. In premature ejaculation, a man reaches orgasm with minimal sexual stimulation, frustrating both himself and his partner.

Sexual Pain Disorders

Individuals with these disorders suffer genital pain (dyspareunia) before, during, or after sexual intercourse. Vaginismus—involuntary spasm of the outer third of the vagina—interferes with sexual intercourse.

PARAPHILIA

Paraphilia is a condition in which the sexual instinct is expressed in ways that are socially prohibited or unacceptable or are biologically undesirable (APA, 2000).

Critical Thinking Question

A patient with insulin-dependent diabetes states, "After I leave the hospital, I'm going to use only half of the prescribed insulin because I heard insulin might affect my sexual performance." What are your interventions with this patient?

Individuals with paraphilia may seek inpatient treatment because of a distinct axis I diagnosis that does not reflect a sexual disorder. The nurse on an inpatient unit may encounter individuals admitted with major depression and suicidal ideation who may be trying to avoid criminal prosecution or to obtain a minimized sentencing by seeking psychiatric treatment. Others may be admitted to inpatient or outpatient care because of Axis I disorders and not their paraphilia. Mood disorders, anxiety disorders, and substance disorders may be the reason for seeking treatment. Individuals with paraphilias do not consider their sexual activities or interests a disorder and do not seek psychiatric treatment for them. Dementia may be associated with the onset of paraphilias, and some professionals are considering paraphilias to be part of the obsessive-compulsive spectrum (Lehne et al, 2001). Therefore the nurse intervenes with behaviors reflective of the axis I diagnosis rather than specifically addressing the paraphilia.

Treatment for pedophilia, exhibitionism, and voyeurism generally occurs on an outpatient basis. Information about paraphiliacs comes from individuals who have been arrested and incarcerated, and from their victims. Outpatient treatment programs and programs for incarcerated individuals also provide information about assessment and treatment.

Paraphiliacs may be men or women, and paraphiliac activity may be limited to a period of stress rather than following a chronic or repetitive pattern. Generally, chronic paraphiliacs have a large number of victims. Little new research has been conducted between 1999 and 2000 about treatment or evaluation of paraphilias. There is a lack of funding in this area and is usually dealt with as a legal rather than a legal or medical issue in this society. The DSM-IV-TR box titled, "Criteria for Paraphiliacs" presents the criteria for the various paraphilias.

Pedophilia

Pedophilia involves recurrent intense sexual urges and sexually arousing fantasies involving sexual activity with children. The individual acts on the urges or is distressed by them (APA, 2000). By definition, the victim of pedophilia must be younger than 13 years of age and the pedophile 16 years or older and at least 5 years older than the victim. Pedophilic behavior can be expressed for opposite-sex children, same-sex children, or both. Pedophilia also can be limited to incest. Fondling and oral sex

---

DSM-IV-TR   Criteria for Paraphiliacs

The following paraphiliac activities last over a period of 6 months and cause distress or impairment in social, occupational, or other important areas of functioning.

Exhibitionism
- Recurrent, intense sexually arousing fantasies, sexual urges, or behaviors involving exposing one's genitals to unsuspecting strangers.

Fetishism
- Recurrent, intense sexually arousing fantasies, sexual urges, or behaviors using nonliving objects.

Frotteurism
- Recurrent, intense sexually arousing fantasies, sexual urges, or behaviors involving touching and rubbing against a nonconsenting person.

Pedophilia
- Recurrent, intense sexually arousing fantasies, sexual urges, or behaviors that involve sexual activity with a child or children generally 13 years of age or younger.
- The person is at least 16 years of age and at least 5 years older than the child or children involved.

Sexual masochism
- Recurrent, intense sexually arousing fantasies, sexual fantasies, urges, or behaviors involving the act of being humiliated, beaten, restrained, or otherwise made to suffer.

Sexual sadism
- Recurrent, intense sexually arousing fantasies, urges, or behaviors involving acts in which the psychological or physical suffering of the victim is sexually exciting to the person.

Voyeurism
- Act of observing an unsuspecting person who is naked, in the process of disrobing, or engaging in sexual activity.

Adapted from the American Psychiatric Association: *Diagnostic and statistical manual of mental disorders*, ed 4, text revision, Washington, DC, 2000, APA.

---

are typical pedophilic behaviors. Vaginal and anal penetration are usually found in incest.

Much controversy exists regarding the personality profiles of sex offenders against minors. Accurately stating the personality characteristics that are present in all sex offenders is impossible. Some of the characteristics reported are shyness, sensitivity, and isolation in social situations; low self-esteem; dependency; depression; low self-confidence; and use of alcohol and drugs. These individuals often have many paraphilias and histories of being abused and neglected. Witnessing violence in the family is associated with increased risk of abusing others (Wood et al, 1999). To compensate for feelings of powerlessness, the pedophile may need to feel power over the victim through control and domination. Some sex offenders are nonaggressive; others use aggression in the form of trickery or bribery. The threat of violence may be used to encourage the victim's silence. The use of physical violence may indicate that the offender is a child rapist. The pedophile may seek an occupation that provides easy access to children. Typical occupations are teaching school, working in a day care setting, coaching, or scout leadership. The presence of Axis I and Axis II disorders in this population is high and if untreated plays a role in treatment failure and recidivism of sexual offenders (Raymond et al, 1999).

Treatment includes a combination of group therapy, behavioral methods, and antiandrogen medication to lower sexual desires. Specialized groups may include victim empathy development, psychoeducation about the illness and medication, coping and social skills training, and relapse prevention (Replique, 1999).

Incest

Incest is pedophilia with child and adolescent relatives and involves relationships by blood, marriage (step-parents), or live-in partners. Incest is traumatic to children because they are victimized by someone they depend on and trust and are unable to escape their victimization.

The characteristics of the perpetrator of incest are as varied as those of the pedophile. Families in which incest occurs may be generally disorganized and exhibit disturbed relationships. Although sex is always involved between the perpetrator and the victim, the perpetrator turns to the child for gratification, intimacy, emotional fulfillment, power, and control. Unlike pedophiles, perpetrators of incest do not typically select occupations for access to potential victims because their victims are easily accessible. Treatment is offered to victims and spouses. Some family studies indicate that victims and spouses do not hate the abuser and do not want others to condemn them (Scheela, 1999).

Critical Thinking Question

A patient with pedophilia attends a self-esteem group on the inpatient unit. Three members of the group are victims of childhood sexual abuse. What would you discuss with the patient regarding the way he might benefit from the group without upsetting the other members?

Exhibitionism

The primary characteristic of exhibitionism is sexual pleasure derived from exposing one's genitals to an unsuspecting stranger. The stereotypical offender is a young man in a raincoat who "flashes" women while walking down the street. No other sexual activity is attempted. The exhibitionist is stimulated by the effect of shocking his victims.

Fetishism

The primary characteristic of fetishism is the sexual pleasure derived from inanimate objects. Common fetish objects are bras, underpants, stockings, and shoes. Less common fetish objects include urine-soaked and feces-smeared items. The individual with fetishism often masturbates while holding or rubbing these items.

Frotteurism

The primary characteristic of frotteurism is sexual pleasure derived from touching or rubbing one's genitals against a nonconsenting individual's thighs or buttocks. The individual with frotteurism may also attempt to fondle the person's breasts or genitals. Frotteurism usually occurs in a crowded place in which escape into the crowd is possible.

Sexual Masochism

The primary characteristic of sexual masochism is the sexual pleasure derived from being humiliated, beaten, or otherwise made to suffer. Some sexually masochistic individuals enjoy being urinated or defecated on and may pay prostitutes to do so. Hypoxyphilia is the act of enhancing sexual arousal by strangulation or other oxygen-depleting activities. Apparently, sexual response is heightened by these activities. People have died in their search for enhanced orgasms.

Sexual Sadism

The primary characteristic of sexual sadism is sexual pleasure derived from inflicting psychologic or physical suffering on another. Partners can be consenting or masochistic. Sadistic behaviors include spanking, whipping, pinching, beating, burning, and restraining. Some sadistic individuals derive great pleasure from torturing or even killing their victims and may be sadistic rapists. The so-called snuff films, found in the underground of the pornography world, apparently show the actual rape, torture, and murder of women and children for the convenient viewing of sadistic individuals.

Voyeurism

The primary characteristic of voyeurism is sexual pleasure derived from observing unsuspecting people who are naked or undressing or who are engaged in sexual activity. The voyeur is commonly referred to as a "peeping Tom." The voyeur may masturbate during peeping or after returning home.

GENDER IDENTITY DISORDER

Gender identity disorder in adults involves discomfort with one's sex or the gender role of that sex. In adults, this disorder can include the desire to live as the other sex or can involve feelings and reactions of the other sex (APA, 2000). The following DSM-IV-TR box presents the criteria for gender identity disorder. Another characteristic is a preoccupation with getting rid of primary and secondary sexual characteristics. These individuals believe that they were born as the wrong sex, and they desire hormones and surgery to become the opposite sex.

Sexual reassignment surgery is not undertaken immediately on request. The individual must be thoroughly assessed for the presence of other psychiatric disorders that may involve problems with gender identity. The individual desiring sexual reassignment is generally in psychotherapy for 6 to 12 months. Some gender identity programs require a

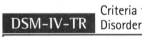

Criteria for Gender Identity Disorder

A. A strong and persistent cross-gender identification
  1. In children:
     a. Stated desire or insistence that he or she is the other sex
     b. In boys, dressing in female attire; in girls, wearing only masculine clothing
     c. Make-believe play or fantasies of being the other sex
     d. Desire to participate in games and pastimes of other sex
     e. Prefers playmates of other sex
  2. In adolescents and adults:
     a. Stated desire to be the other sex
     b. Frequently passes as the other sex
     c. Desires to be treated as the other sex
     d. Conviction that he or she has typical feelings and reactions of other sex
B. Feelings of discomfort with own sex or inappropriateness in gender role of own sex

Adapted from the American Psychiatric Association: *Diagnostic and statistical manual of mental disorders*, ed 4, text revision, Washington, DC, 2000, APA.

written second opinion from another physician or psychologist before proceeding with surgical reassignment. Hormonal treatment and living and relationship changes are slowly made over months while the individual is in therapy. During this time, the individual's attitudes toward sexual reassignment may change and sexual reassignment surgery is not chosen. People who do choose surgery can be helped to live more comfortable and productive lives.

Psychotherapeutic Management

Nurse-patient relationship

The nurse must have an accepting, empathic, and nonjudgmental attitude if patients are to be comfortable enough to disclose problems with sexuality. This trust comes about only after the nurse has reconciled and accepted his or her own feelings related to sexuality. Patients may interpret the nurse's discomfort with sexual issues and sexuality as disapproval of them and of their sexual issues and concerns. A private area in which to discuss fears or concerns about sexuality and victimization helps patients disclose and discuss their feelings. The nurse discusses options for dealing with sexual issues and problems. Clarification and education may be needed about sexual functioning, effective communication, and healthy relationships. The nurse may also need to intervene to discuss self-esteem issues, anxiety, guilt, and empathy for victims.

Helping patients who are perpetrators deal with physical and emotional dimensions is necessary. Physical dimensions may include anorexia, insomnia, and weight loss. Emotional dimensions may include guilt, helplessness, shame, and relief about getting caught. Setting limits on the extent to which the patient discloses in a group setting, especially if other group members may be victims of sexual assault, must be discussed.

The nurse is involved in the planning of patients' care regarding the specific issues and problems that are addressed during an inpatient stay versus that which is addressed in outpatient treatment. The nurse also collaborates with social workers and chaplains, if patients choose, about feelings and religious views. The nurse is legally obligated to report suspected and actual sexual abuse of children to police or appropriate agencies. All states have mandatory child abuse reporting statutes. The nurse discusses possible referrals with patients and family members and refers patients to sex therapists if necessary. Referrals to outpatient treatment programs or therapy groups for specific disorders may be necessary. Individual, group, and family treatment for incest and support groups for perpetrators and victims may be appropriate.

Critical Thinking Question

What issues about sexual disorders would you discuss in an education session for staff?

Psychopharmacology

Patients with axis I diagnoses are prescribed psychotherapeutic medication for their specific disorders. The nurse assesses all medications for side effects that affect sexual performance or dysfunction. The use of pharmacologic agents for the treatment of sexual disorders is controversial, and effectiveness is variable. Men with paraphilias can be treated with agents to lower testosterone levels, thereby reducing their sex drive. Antiandrogen therapy with oral and parenteral preparations has been shown to reduce recidivism rates in male sexual aggressors (Lehne, Thomas, Berlin, 2000). The use of selective serotonin reuptake inhibitors (SSRIs), including fluoxetine (Prozac) and sertraline (Zoloft), are being used for paraphiliac and related disorders with unproven effectiveness.

Milieu management

Patients with sexual disorders and dysfunctions benefit from groups dealing with self-esteem, assertiveness, anger management, social and relationship skills, sex education, and stress management. Referrals may be indicated as mentioned previously. Self-help groups such as Sex Addicts Anonymous can benefit those with paraphilias. A multidimensional treatment plan using a combination of education and cognitive-behavioral and family intervention needs to be used to reduce recidivism for sexual offenders. Longitudinal research studies will eventually help determine treatment factors that are effective in reducing recidivism rates.

Case Study

Bill Wood, 62 years old, has been admitted to the inpatient unit. His wife died 2 years earlier; he has one daughter and three grandchildren. Bill is presently employed but has few friends or hobbies. He visits his daughter and grandchildren approximately once a month. He does not date and does not have any female companions. For the past year, he has noticed an increase in sexual fantasies concerning children. He did not act on the fantasies until a week ago when he was babysitting for his youngest grandchild, 8-year-old Stephanie. He admits to fondling Stephanie's breasts but denies other sexual contact with her. Bill states to the nurse, "I never thought I could be capable of such a horrible thing. I deserve to die. I even thought of killing myself."

▌Care Plan

Name: <u>Bill Wood</u> _____   Admission Date: _____

DSM-IV-TR Diagnosis: <u>Major depression and pedophilia</u> _____

Assessment	**Areas of strength:** Employed, visits daughter and grandchildren, remorse for contact with child, first offense. **Problems:** Death of wife, few friends, disturbing sexual fantasies, suicidal ideation.
Diagnoses	• Potential for self-directed violence related to guilt, as evidenced by suicidal ideation. • Sexual dysfunction related to lack of significant other, as evidenced by fondling child. • Social isolation related to lack of social support, as evidenced by loneliness.
Outcomes	*Short-term goals:* • Patient will state he no longer has thoughts of suicide. • Patient will discuss sexual concerns and needs, and methods to satisfy these needs.

Date met

_____

_____

Care Plan—cont'd

Name: <u>Bill Wood</u>   Admission Date: _____

DSM-IV-TR Diagnosis: <u>Major depression and pedophilia</u>

Outcomes	*Long-term goals:*	*Date met*
	• Patient will contact support groups and senior, citizen organizations.	_____
	• Patient will schedule outpatient appointment, for further assessment of sexual disorder.	_____

Planning/
Interventions

Nurse–patient relationship: Instruct patient to approach staff when suicidal thoughts occur. Discuss feelings of guilt, remorse, anger, loneliness, and low self-esteem. Discuss the patient's beliefs and values about sexuality with him. Discuss and help the patient to identify sexual concerns, needs, and methods to satisfy needs.

Psychopharmacology: Prozac 20 mg q AM.

Milieu management: Groups focusing on self-esteem, stress and anger management, assertiveness training, social skills, and discharge planning.

Evaluation   Patient reports he is no longer suicidal.

Referrals   He will attend senior citizen activities at his church with a friend. Appointment scheduled at a sexual disorders clinic.

Key Concepts

1. Sexual dysfunctions may occur as the result of psychologic, physiologic, and pharmacologic factors.
2. Paraphilias involve sexual activity with objects, children, and consenting or nonconsenting adults.
3. Efforts to achieve sexual pleasure do not give individuals the right to violate the rights of others through coercion and control.
4. Gender identity disorder in adults involves persistent discomfort with one's biologic sex.
5. The nurse's role in the treatment of sexual disorders is primarily one of referral.

References

American Psychiatric Association: *Diagnostic and statistical manual of mental disorders,*ed 4, text revision, Washington, DC, 2000, APA.

Lehne G, Thomas K, Berlin F: Treatment of sexual paraphilias: a review of the 1999-2000 literature, *Curr Opin Psychiatry* 13(6):569, 2000.

Raymond NC et al: Psychiatric comorbidity in pedophilic sex offenders, *Am J Psychiatry* 156(5):786, 1999.

Replique RJ: Assessment & treatment of persons with pedophilia, *J Psychosoc Nurs Ment Health Serv* 37(5):19, 1999.

Scheela RA: A nurse's experiences, working with sex offenders, *J Psychosoc Nurs Ment Health Serv* 37(9):25, 1999.

Wood RM et al: Sexual offenders in custody for control, care and treatment, *Curr Opin Psychiatry* 12:659, 1999.

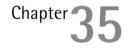

Chapter 35

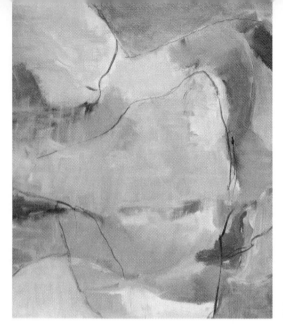

Substance-Related Disorders

Norman L. Keltner, Gordon I.G. Pugh, Beverly K. Hogan*

Learning Objectives

After reading this chapter, you should be able to:
- Recognize the personal and societal toll of the abuse of alcohol and other drugs.
- Recognize *The Diagnostic and Statistical Manual of Mental Disorders-Fourth Edition-Text Revision* (DSM-IV-TR) criteria and terminology for substance-related disorders.
- Recognize and describe objective and subjective symptoms of substance dependence and abuse.
- Describe physiologic, emotional, and interpersonal theoretical explanations for the development of substance-related disorders.

- Develop a nursing care plan for patients with substance-related disorders.
- Evaluate the relative effectiveness of nursing interventions for patients with substance-related disorders.
- Understand the contributions of nonmedical interventions in recovery from substance-related disorders.
- Understand the impact of substance-related disorders on the family.

INTRODUCTION TO SUBSTANCE-RELATED DISORDERS

Drug abuse statistics vary from time to time and from culture to culture. Because of the enormity of these numbers, most people find it difficult to grasp the extent of societal and individual suffering produced by substance abuse and dependence. As Joseph Stalin noted, "A single death is a tragedy; a million deaths is a statistic." Collectively, the statistics of substance-related disorders produce many costs, but even one person's pain is tragic. The vignettes of real patients

---

*This chapter is a revision of the text originally written by MaryLou Scavnicky-Mylant and revised by Virginia M. Spaulding.

you will meet in these pages represent the individuals who make up these "statistics." The effects of their drug and alcohol abuse ripple through our society, touching everyone to some degree.

Human beings have used mood-altering substances at least since the beginning of recorded history. Whether using Far Eastern opium, South American cocaine, North American peyote, French wine, or modern pharmaceuticals, human beings consistently find ways to alter their mood. Use of mind-altering substances can lead to diverse complications and problems. Often, however, these mind-altering effects provide therapeutic benefit (e.g., pain relief, decreased anxiety), clouding the distinction

Key Terms

Abstinence syndrome Physical signs and symptoms that occur when the addictive substance is reduced or withheld; also referred to as withdrawal.

Abuse Excessive use of a substance that differs from societal norms.

Blackouts A period of time in which the drinker functions socially but for which there is no memory.

Cirrhosis Disease of the liver typically caused by abuse of alcohol.

Co-dependency Stress-related preoccupation with an addicted person's life, leading to extreme dependence on that person.

Dependence A state in which a drug abuser must take a usual or increasing dose of a drug to prevent the onset of abstinence symptoms or withdrawal. The patient feels normal only when the drug is "on board."

Metabolic tolerance (pharmacokinetic tolerance) Occurs when the body is more efficient at metabolizing the substance.

Pharmacodynamic tolerance Occurs when higher blood levels are required to produce a given effect.

Tolerance The need for increasing amounts of a substance to achieve the same effects.

Withdrawal Physical signs and symptoms that occur when the addictive substance is reduced or withheld; also referred to as an abstinence syndrome.

|Table 35-1| The Numbers Game

Substance	Number Who Used in Past Month
Heroin	200,000
Amphetamines	800,000
Cocaine/crack	1,500,000
Marijuana	10,000,000
Alcohol	11,000,000 (abusers)
Nicotine	61,000,000
Caffeine	130,000,000

Adapted from Nash JM: Addicted: why do people get hooked? *Time*, p 68, May 5, 1997.

between therapeutic and abusive use. This chapter concentrates on maladaptive uses of alcohol and other drugs, both legal and illegal, commonly referred to as "drug abuse." Table 35-1 outlines the extent of drug use in a given month.

As a nurse, you will see patients suffering from the consequences of substance abuse as part of your work. You probably know people personally who suffer from substance-related disorders and who have experienced problems associated with substance abuse; you may suspect that other people suffer from it as well. Your ability to recognize the possibility and to suggest appropriate referrals or interventions may save a home, a family, or a life. Furthermore, as a nurse, friends and acquaintances may turn to you first when they realize that their use has become problematic. Hence we hope you take the time to study this information carefully and diligently. The road to recovery begins with the initial assessment.

| 12-Month Prevalence Rate of Mental Disorders in the United States

Diagnosis	Percentage of Population Over 17 Years of Age	Number of People
Anxiety disorders	12.6	20,034,000
Phobia disorders*	10.9	17,331,333
Mood disorders	9.5	15,143,000
Alcohol disorders	7.4	11,766,000
Major depression†	5.0	7,950,000
Drug disorders	3.1	4,929,000
Cognitive impairment	2.7	4,293,000
Obsessive-compulsive disorders	2.1	3,339,000
Antisocial disorders	1.5	2,385,000
Panic disorders*	1.3	2,067,000
Bipolar disorders†	1.2	1,908,000
Schizophrenia	1.1	1,749,000
Somatization	0.2	365,000

*Also calculated in anxiety statistics.
†Also calculated in mood disorders statistics.
From Regier DA et al: The de facto U.S. mental and addictive disorders service system: epidemiologic catchment area prospective, 1-year prevalence rates of disorders and services, *Arch Gen Psychiatry* 50:85, 1993; Surgeon General; Mental Health: A Report from the Surgeon General. DHHS, 1999, Washington DC.

CLINICAL EXAMPLE
Robert had an average childhood and made good grades in school. He grew up in a home with both parents and with other siblings. His parents were active in the community. In high school, he was particularly talented in sports and was popular among his peers. Robert was, and is, an immensely likable fellow. He

Continued

began drinking beer when he was 15 years of age with his baseball teammates. After graduation from high school with honors, he went to college on a baseball scholarship. In college, he was known to smoke some marijuana, but "never let it get in the way" of his sports or his studies. He was good at hiding his drug use. It would never have occurred to him that he "had a problem," not even later when his self-destruction was blatantly apparent to everyone else in his life except himself. Robert has since learned, however, that he suffers from addiction and has learned how to manage his condition.

At first, he stayed out a little too late one night before a big game, and he had a bad game or two because of his slightly decreased performance. Eventually, he was introduced to cocaine, discovered intravenous (IV) use ("mainlining"), lost his promising sports career, was divorced by his wife, stole from people, lied to his family, tried to kill himself, and spent time in prison. While he was incarcerated, he realized how self-destructive his drug use had become, and he vowed to do whatever it would take to become and remain drug free. He reasoned that he had been willing to do a great many things in his search for dope, so he ought to be willing to exert the same amount of energy in his search to break free from its grip on his life. Robert had been hospitalized for detoxification in the past but "wasn't ready." When he attended a small treatment group at the county jail, however, he was ready to listen and learn.

Today, Robert is in his early 30s, has earned his bachelor's degree, has a good job, makes a good salary, is no longer on parole, plays ball with a local community league, is married to a wonderfully supportive spouse, and—most importantly—remains drug free. Robert's life did not get back together overnight, however. Undoing most of the damage that his drug use caused took several years. Some of the damage he caused can never be repaired, but he is far better off now than he was before he recognized the extent of the problems caused by his drug use.

Assessment Strategies for Chemical Dependency

As a component of every assessment, the nurse should inquire about the amount and type of alcohol and other drugs (AOD) used by the patient or the family. The nurse should always ask about the amount of prescription medication the patient actually takes (not simply the amount prescribed because many people abuse prescription medications as well). The nurse should also question the patient about medical problems associated with AOD use by the patient or family members. Furthermore, because many substance abusers tend to minimize their level of AOD use (as well as the consequences of their use), many facilities routinely use blood or urine drug screens to obtain objective information (Schiller et al, 2000). The importance of this objective data lies in its prevention of AOD minimization. Probably 40% to 60% of AOD users underreport use during their initial interview. Many addicted patients will not readily reveal in an initial interview more than what the nurse can already discover by other means. For instance, someone referred to treatment because alcohol use has led to problems with the legal system often does not admit to cocaine or marijuana use until objective testing reveals it. Even then, some patients deny use of the substance detected (Longo et al, 2000). Signs and symptoms raising the index of suspicion of a substance-related disorder may include the following:

- Absenteeism, especially after off days
- Frequent accidents or injuries
- Drowsiness
- Slurred speech
- Inattention to appearance
- Increasing isolation
- Frequent "secretive" disappearances
- Tremors
- Flushed face
- Watery or reddened eyes
- "Spaciness"
- Odor of alcohol on the breath or strong mouthwash or breath mint smell
- High number of physical complaints
- Disappearing prescriptions (raiding the medicine cabinet)

Although signs and symptoms suggestive of a substance-related disorder can represent other problems, considering the presumptive signs along with other subjective and objective data may point to substance abuse as the culprit.

Denial occurs when the dependent person does not recognize the destructive nature of AOD use, though blatantly obvious to others. Denial prevents the individual from linking the problems in his or her

| Table 35-2 | Period of Time After Ingestion that Drugs Can Be Detected in the Urine |

Drug	Detection Period
Opioids	
Heroin	2-4 days
Morphine	2-4 days
Meperidine (Demerol)	2-4 days
Methadone	2-4 days
Fentanyl	Can be < 1 hour
Depressants	
Barbiturates	12 hours to 3 weeks
Benzodiazepines	Up to 1 week
Stimulants	
Amphetamines	2-4 days
Cocaine	2-4 days
Hallucinogens	
Marijuana	3 days to < 1 month
PCP	1 day to 1 month

Adapted from Sullivan E, Bissell L, William E: *Chemical dependency in nursing*, Redwood City, Calif, 1998, Addison-Wesley.

| Box 35-1 | Defense Mechanisms at Work: Denial |

An intoxicated 60-year-old Madison, Wisconsin, woman, who was dressed as a clown on her way to entertain children at a birthday party, tried to kill her 83-year-old mother-in-law over a beer. "I've had 40 years of hell because of you," she is reported to have told the victim. When asked about her long-standing alcohol problem, she indicated that she has no "problem," except for the mother-in-law.

Adapted from "Whatdyaknow," Wisconsin Public Radio, June 4, 1994. The story is from *USA Today*, p 10A, June 3, 1994. (Chris Bannon, the producer of "Whatdyaknow," is available at Bannon@VILAS.uwex.edu or [608] 262-3970.)

life causally with AOD use. This inability to see self-destructive behavior and attitudes, or to link life problems with AOD use, defines substance dependence.

Urinalysis often provides the most objective measure of recent drug use (Table 35-2). Blood levels can also detect recent use and trigger treatment protocols. Hair toxicology effectively determines long-term patterns of use but costs more than other methods of detection. Hair samples of Henri Paul, the driver of the car in which Diana, Princess of Wales, died in 1997 underwent testing in an attempt to find objective evidence about his actual long-term AOD use (Sancton, 1997). Hair toxicology kits available on the retail market enable parents to test the hair of children they suspect of drug abuse. Blonde hair does not seem to accumulate certain drugs such as cocaine as effectively as does darker hair (Muha, 1997).

Interview Approaches

Because underreporting can lead to misdiagnosis, it is important for the nurse to approach the patient in a manner that encourages forthrightness. The nurse should be matter-of-fact and nonjudgmental while eliciting information that might carry with it some feelings of shame. Most nurses are not prepared for the defensiveness that the person with substance-related problems displays, but some genuine concern for the patient can help overcome this barrier. Furthermore, because drugs and alcohol have personally affected many nurses, it is important for them to be aware of their own feelings and avoid projecting any negative attitudes onto the patient.

Gathering accurate information during the interview claims high priority. As a nurse, you may find it difficult to elicit accurate clinical information from the woman in Box 35-1. Phrases such as "problem with drinking" or "difficulties with drug use" might be more palatable compared with the labels "addict" or "alcoholic," but these, too, may not elicit the accurate information the nurse seeks. It may also be helpful initially to focus more on legally or culturally accepted substances such as caffeine and nicotine. The patient's consumption should be evaluated in more detail if the initial assessment data identify the patient as being more at risk for substance-related problems. The authors suggest using the terms "problems because of drinking" or "using more than intended" as more accurate and diagnostic, less threatening, and more likely to link patients' AOD use with the problems in their lives. This factor is important both in effective care planning and in providing the patient with good internal motivation.

Various assessment guides are available to the nurse, including both subjective interviews and objective assessment instruments. Early diagnosis of substance-related disorders is often missed because of misdiagnosing or underdiagnosing related to misunderstandings about AOD disorders or inadequate training or both. Selected instruments are covered later in this chapter.

Substance abuse is widespread in North America and demands the attention of psychiatric nurses, both as a singular phenomenon and as a variable in other psychiatric disorders. For example, estimates indicate that one third to one half of all patients undergoing psychiatric treatment abuse alcohol or drugs or both (Ananth et al, 1989; Carey, 1989; Surgeon General, 1999). Co-morbidity or a dual diagnosis is such an important issue that a separate chapter addresses the subject (Chapter 36). Additionally, patients admitted to hospitals because of health problems directly related to alcohol abuse occupy an estimated 25% to 40% of U.S. hospital beds (Wegscheider, 1981).

The use and abuse of alcohol and drugs among the general population is one of the most significant social issues of our time. Because of the significance of the problem, this chapter addresses the general issues surrounding substance abuse. To treat the substance-abusing person's condition effectively, the nurse must understand three areas important to effective intervention:

1. The DSM-IV-TR criteria used to assess substance-related disorders
2. The nature of the substance being abused
3. The treatment of patients with substance-related disorders

Drugs of abuse fall into several classes: alcohol, barbiturates and other central nervous system (CNS) depressants, opioids, stimulants, and hallucinogens (Table 35-3). More detailed descriptions of these drugs are found in Appendix F.

DSM-IV-TR CRITERIA

The DSM-IV-TR specifies criteria for classifications of substance dependence, substance abuse, substance intoxication, and substance withdrawal. Dependence is often marked by physiologic need for the substance, usually in increasing amounts, to gain the same effect; a persistent desire to cut down, which is met with little success; and continued substance use even though physical, social, and emotional processes are compromised. Regardless of the substance, behavior patterns that meet these criteria indicate a problem. The term *dependence* has generally replaced the term addiction for describing compulsive drug use because it more precisely defines the condition. Heroin addiction and alcoholism are therefore correctly referred to as drug dependencies.

In 1987 the American Medical Association declared all drug dependencies to be diseases. When chemical dependencies are viewed as diseases, their treatment and understanding are facilitated. This view also reduces the guilt and blame traditionally associated with chemical dependency. Although not all psychiatrists and psychiatric nurses embrace the disease concept of drug dependence, there are convincing arguments for accepting it (www.ama.assn.org/ama/pub/article/3342-3627. Accessed 6/4/02).

Some professionals use a working definition of chemical dependency that is less rigid compared with the criteria outlined in the DSM-IV-TR (see box on page 458). These researchers define use of substances as a problem when the effects of such use interfere with and disrupt family, work, or social relationships. If these areas of a person's life are being adversely affected, then the person is viewed as having a problem and as being in need of treatment. Still other professionals simply define dependence as a state in which "the person feels normal only when the drug is on board."

ALCOHOL ABUSE

Alcohol abuse is the primary drug problem in North America and is addressed separately because of the enormity of the problem it poses. The cost to the United States in terms of health problems, lost work hours, family disruption and disintegration, and criminal activity (Box 35-2) is estimated at more than $100 billion annually. An estimated 7.4% of the adult population in America exhibits symptoms of alcoholism, and along with cardiovascular disease and cancer, it ranks as one of the leading causes of death and disability in the United States. Alcoholics have a premature death rate 2 to 4 times higher than nonalcoholics. Approximately 100,000 deaths each year are directly related to alcohol. Cirrhosis, other medical problems, homicides (50% alcohol related), and suicides (25% alcohol related) are directly linked to alcohol use (see Box 35-2). Furthermore, accidental deaths such as those from motor vehicle accidents (50% alcohol related), fires and burns (47% alcohol related), drownings (34% alcohol related), and falls (28% alcohol related) are examples of the different ways alcohol use is lethal (Cherpitel, 1992). In motor vehicle accidents in which pedestrians are killed, 40% of the pedestrians are under the influence of alcohol (Feldman, 1994).

Table 35-3 | Drug Information

Class	Examples or Other Names	Withdrawal Syndrome	Withdrawal Treatment	Psychiatric Symptoms During Chronic Use	Overdose Fatal?	Unassisted Withdrawal Fatal?	Overdose Symptoms
CNS depressants	Benzodiazepines Barbiturates Other depressants	Tremors, sweats seizures, anxiety, irritability, hallu-cinations, death*	Long-acting benzodiazepine, Vistaril	Mood disorder, depression, psychosis, dementia	Yes*	Yes*	Shallow respirations, clammy skin, dilated pupils, weak and rapid pulse, coma, death
Opioids	Demerol, heroin, morphine, opium, codeine	Lacrimation, runny nose, diaphoresis, chills, muscle aches, n/v, diarrhea, leg spasm, goose bumps	Clonidine, supportive medications	Psychosis, mood disorder	Yes	No	Respiratory depression, pulmonary edema, pinpoint pupils, seizures, coma, death
Cannabinoids	Marijuana, hash	Craving, irritability		Psychosis, paranoia	No	No	Hallucinations, paranoia, insomnia, hyperactive
Cocaine	Crack, coke, snow	Anhedonia, craving, irritability, fatigue, mood disorder, anxiety	Dopamine agonists, catecholamine precursors	Psychosis	Yes	No	Delirium, psychosis, violence, tachycardia, hypertension, coma, hyperreflexia, myocardial infarction
Methamphet-amine	Oral: speed, meth Smokable: ice, crystal, crank	Dysphoria, fatigue, insomnia	Supportive	Psychosis, mood disorder, anxiety disorder	Yes	No	Delirium, psychosis, violence, tachycardia, hypertension, coma, hyperreflexia, myocardial infarction
Inhalants	Gasoline, freon, paint, and others	Mouth ulcers, gastrointestinal s problems, anorexia, confusion, headache	Supportive	Psychosis, panic, memory loss	Yes	No	Seizures, coma
Hallucinogens	LSD, psilocybin, PC	None specific	Supportive	Psychosis, panic	No	No	Seizures, panic, depression

CNS, Central nervous system; n/v, Nausea and vomiting; LSD, lysergic acid diethylamide; PCP, phencyclidine.
*For barbiturates.

DSM-IV-TR Criteria for Substance-Related Disorders

Substance Dependence

A. A maladaptive pattern of substance use as manifested by three or more of the following:
   1. Tolerance
   2. Withdrawal
   3. A need for more of the substance than was intended
   4. Inability to stop using even when wanting to do so
   5. A great deal of time is spent in acquiring the substance or in recovering from its effects
   6. Substance use causes social, occupational, or recreational problems
   7. Continued substance use despite knowledge that the substance is causing physical or psychological problems

Substance Abuse

A. A maladaptive pattern of substance use leading to clinically significant impairment or distress as manifested by one or more of the following:
   1. Failure to fulfill major role obligations at work, school, or home
   2. Recurrent substance use in hazardous situations

   3. Recurrent substance-related legal problems
   4. Continued substance use despite problems
B. Has never met the criteria for substance dependence for this class of substance

Substance Intoxication

A. The development of a substance-specific syndrome due to a recent ingestion of a substance
B. Clinically significant maladaptive behavioral or psychological changes due to the effect of the substance on the central nervous system
C. Not due to a general medical condition and not better accounted for by another mental disorder

Substance Withdrawal

A. The development of a substance-specific syndrome due to the cessation of or reduction in the intake of a substance
B. The substance-specific syndrome causes clinically significant distress or impairment
C. Not due to a general medical condition and not better accounted for by another mental disorder

Adapted from the American Psychiatric Association: *Diagnostic and statistical manual of mental disorders, text revision,* ed 4, Washington, DC, 2000, APA.

|Box 35-2| Alcohol and Crime

The statistics are striking. Approximately 60% of convicted homicide offenders drank just before committing the offense. Sixty percent of prison inmates drank heavily just before committing the violent crime for which they were incarcerated. The relationship between poverty and homicide is stronger in neighborhoods with higher rates of alcohol consumption than in those with average or below-average rates. Numerous studies report a strong association between sexual violence and alcohol, finding that "anywhere between 30% and 90% of convicted rapists are drunk at the time of the offense." Juveniles, especially young men, who drink to the point of drunkenness are more likely than those who do not drink to get into fights, get arrested, commit violent crimes, and recidivate later in life. Alcohol-dependent male factory workers are more than three times as likely to physically abuse their wives than are otherwise comparable, non–alcohol-dependent counterparts. The high incidence of drinking among convicted criminals does not necessarily prove that drinking stimulates crime; it may be nearer to being evidence that criminals who drink are more likely to get caught and convicted than those who do not. However, it is important not to discount or deny the probable, and in some cases patently obvious, connection between alcohol abuse and crime.

From Dilulio JJ Jr: Broken bottles: alcohol, disorder, and crime, *Brookings Review* (The Brookings Institution), p 14, Spring 1996.

Etiologic Theories
Psychodynamic theories

A number of psychologic theories have attempted to explain the ways people become substance dependent. People who are alcohol dependent have often been viewed as individuals who easily succumb to the escape that alcohol provides. Psychoanalytic theory describes people with alcohol dependency as having strong oral tendencies related to unresolved needs for early attachments (Frosch, 1985). Drinking alcohol is thought to be an attempt to satisfy those unconscious oral needs. More recent theories have described people likely to become alcohol dependent as more phobic and inferior feeling compared with social drinkers. Over time, the search for an "alcoholic personality" has given way to a multivariate model that incorporates the biopsychosocial components of addiction. Current researchers believe that many of the stereotypical characteristics found among alcohol-dependent people (e.g., dependency, low self-esteem, passivity, introversion) are the result of and not the cause of substance dependence. Psychodynamically oriented treatment tends to emphasize behavioral management techniques and rejects the disease model of substance dependence.

Biologic theories

Heredity as an etiologic factor has been studied for many years and continues to provide insight into understanding the genesis of alcoholism. Genetic predisposition is considered to be the single most significant piece of information in identifying alcoholism. Researchers have known for a quarter of a century that children of alcoholic parents, even if raised in an alcohol-free environment, are more likely to become alcoholics than are the children of nonalcoholic parents (Goodwin et al, 1973). Although studies indicate different degrees of effect, hereditary explanations, at the very least, provide a good basis for understanding a person's vulnerability to alcohol dependency. However, predisposition means neither fatalism nor determinism. Even patients who are genetically predisposed to certain types of cancer, for example, can take steps to minimize their risk. Recognizing their familial predisposition to alcoholism or addiction, individuals can avoid use of alcohol and drugs.

Pharmacokinetics of Alcohol

Absorption

Alcohol is absorbed partially from the stomach but mostly from the small intestine. If a person with an empty stomach ingests alcohol, it is in the bloodstream within 20 minutes. The form of alcohol consumed affects the rate of absorption. Alcohol in beer and wine is absorbed more slowly compared with alcohol in liquor. This characteristic may be a result, in part, to dilution; beer contains 4% ethanol; wine, 12% ethanol; and whiskey, 40% to 50% ethanol. However, dilution of the alcohol in its beverage medium cannot completely account for slower absorption. Food also slows alcohol absorption.

Distribution

Ethanol is distributed equally in all body tissue according to water content. Larger individuals (who have greater amounts of body water) can therefore ingest more alcohol than can smaller people, who have less body water. Alcohol affects the cerebrum and cerebellum before it affects the spinal cord and the vital centers because the former areas contain more water.

Metabolism

Although the rate of absorption largely determines how quickly a person will become intoxicated, a person's metabolic rate largely determines how long

alcohol will affect the body. The healthy body can metabolize 15 ml of alcohol an hour or roughly the alcohol content a shot of whiskey, can of beer, or glass of wine. In individuals who drink alcohol frequently over a number of years, hepatic drug-metabolizing levels are increased to hasten alcohol metabolism (pharmacokinetic tolerance). Hot coffee, "sweating it out," and other home remedies do not increase alcohol metabolism, nor do they speed the "sobering up" process. Attempts by scientists to develop a pill to prevent or decrease intoxication have been unsuccessful. In late-stage alcoholism, tolerance decreases as the abused liver finally can no longer adequately metabolize the alcohol.

The chemical name for alcohol is ethanol (CH_3CH_2OH). Alcohol is primarily metabolized in the liver. The oxidation process can be described chemically as follows:

- Alcohol= ethanol (CH_3CH_2OH)
- **Enzyme = alcohol dehydrogenase**
- Products = acetaldehyde (CH_3CHO) and hydrogen (H_2)
- **Enzyme = aldehyde dehydrogenase**
- Product = acetic acid (CH_3COOH)

At each step of the metabolizing process, an enzyme breaks down the chemical. Alcohol dehydrogenase breaks down CH_3CH_2OH to CH_3CHO and H_2. The H_2 molecule causes the liver to bypass normal energy sources (the H_2 from fat) and to use the H_2 from CH_3CH_2OH. Fat accumulates (since it is not being used as a primary energy source) and leads to fatty liver, hyperlipemia, hepatitis, and, ultimately, cirrhosis. CH_3CHO is toxic to the body; it compromises normal cell function in the liver. If the metabolism of CH_3CHO is impaired, it accumulates in the liver, causing cell death and necrosis. CH_3CHO also interferes with vitamin activation. Aldehyde dehydrogenase breaks down CH_3CHO to CH_3COOH, which is an innocuous substance. When enzymatic action on CH_3CHO is blocked by the aldehyde dehydrogenase blocker disulfiram (Antabuse), CH_3CHO accumulates, causing severe sickness.

Research confirms an age-old suspicion that women become intoxicated more easily than do men, even when studies are controlled for size differences. Frezza and colleagues (1990) discovered that the gastrointestinal tissue of women and of alcohol-dependent men contains little alcohol dehydrogenase. The alcohol dehydrogenase in the gastrointestinal tissue of men who are not dependent on alcohol oxidizes a significant amount of CH_3CH_2OH in the gut before it enters the bloodstream. The inability of women's bodies to make this "first-pass metabolism" accounts for their enhanced vulnerability to alcohol.

Blood alcohol levels

Blood alcohol levels accurately indicate the amount of ethanol to which the brain is exposed. Behavioral and physiologic effects are predictable for most drinkers. For example, at 0.05% blood alcohol levels, most individuals are predictably feeling good and experience disinhibition (i.e., they may do and say things they would typically just "think or think about doing"). The box below outlines the typical responses for a given blood alcohol level.

Tolerance to Alcohol

Tolerance to alcohol is probably related to elevated hepatic enzyme levels and to cellular adaptation (pharmacodynamic tolerance). At the point at which the normal drinker might be noticeably drunk after 10 to 12 drinks, the long-term drinker with pharmacodynamic tolerance might seem unaffected by drinking the same amount. However, tolerance to the respiratory depressing effects of alcohol does not develop appreciably. Blood levels just slightly higher than those required to get a "buzz on" have killed long time, pharmacodynamically tolerant drinkers.

Physiologic Effects

People generally begin consuming alcohol because it causes a reaction they desire. Disinhibition, impaired judgment, and fuzzy thinking are initial responses to alcohol ingestion. These signs represent cerebrum intoxication. In many situations, this men-

Clinical Effects of Alcohol

Blood alcohol level (%)	Physiologic effect
0.05	Euphoria, decreased inhibitions
0.10-0.15	Labile mood, talkative, impaired judgment
0.15-0.20	Decreased motor skills, slurred speech, double vision
0.25	Altered perceptions
0.30	Altered equilibrium
0.35	Apathy, inertia
0.40	Stupor, coma
0.40-0.50	Severe respiratory depression, death

Adapted from Lehne RA: *Pharmacology for nursing care*, ed 4, Philadelphia, 2001, WB Saunders.

tal relaxation is pleasant. Alcohol also depresses psychomotor activity. Alcohol has been described as a "social lubricant" because it relaxes self-imposed barriers that inhibit sociability. Anxiety and tension are relieved, usually for a couple of hours after a drink is taken. Eventually, at least for the alcoholic, drinking becomes defensive; that is, the alcoholic often drinks to avoid the effects of many years of drinking. For instance, once the anxiety-reducing effect wears off, more tension and anxiety are produced, thus the drinker must consume more alcohol to regain the "anxiety-free" state. Many alcohol-dependent people, even after drinking all they "can hold," are not able to quell the rebound psychomotor upheaval caused by years of alcohol-related CNS irritation. The presenting complaint of many of those who seek treatment for alcohol dependence is "nervousness" or "depression."

Central nervous system effects

The adverse effects of alcohol can be categorized as central or peripheral. CNS effects are related to sedation and toxicity. As the vital centers become affected, a slowed, stuporous-to-unconscious mental state develops. Large amounts of alcohol can cause sleep, coma, deep anesthesia, and death. Other common symptoms of intoxication include slurred speech, short retention span, loud talk, and memory deficits. Blackout is a period in which the drinker functions socially but for which the drinker has no memory.

Historically, the brain damage that is associated with alcoholism was thought to be caused by alcohol-related nutritional deficiencies. Alcohol-dependent people tend to eat poorly, and no doubt this behavior leads to pathologic change. It is now known, however, that brain damage occurs with drinking, even when a nutritious diet is maintained. In fact, all alcohol-dependent drinkers will have some brain cell loss.

Increased psychomotor activity as a consequence of alcohol is called the alcohol-withdrawal syndrome. Sedation is the predominant effect of alcohol, but as sedation wears off, psychomotor activity increases. This state is referred to as a rebound phenomenon. As the CNS becomes more irritated, the normal drinker feels sick and irritable (a hangover) but lives through it, perhaps vowing "never again." The heavy drinker and the alcoholic have to drink again to "resedate" the psychomotor system. Eventually, the alcohol-dependent person has to drink larger amounts to feel somewhat "normal." Some drinkers reach the point at which they cannot drink enough alcohol, and CNS irritability is not "sedatable." Then, alcoholic tremors, sweating, palpitations, and agitation occur. Although these symptoms usually occur when alcohol ingestion has stopped (Table 35-4), in some cases, they occur while the alcohol-dependent person is drinking.

Alcoholic hallucinosis, a state of auditory hallucinations, is a phenomenon that alcohol-dependent people can sometimes experience. The brain begins to "invent" sensory input. Alcoholic hallucinosis usually begins 48 hours or so after drinking has stopped. Usually within the context of a clear sensorium, frightening voices or sounds are heard.

The ultimate level of CNS irritability is delirium tremens (DTs). In DTs, the body not only invents sensory input, but also has extreme motor agitation. Hallucinations become visual (e.g., the proverbial pink elephants), and the sufferer is tremulous and terrified. Tonic-clonic seizures (grand mal) can occur.

Wernicke-Korsakoff syndrome is a mental disorder characterized by amnesia, clouding of consciousness, confabulation (falsification of memory) and memory loss, and peripheral neuropathy. This disorder results from the poor nutrition of the alcoholic (specifically, inadequate amounts of thiamine

and niacin in the diet) and from the neurotoxic nature of alcohol.

Peripheral nervous system effects

Peripheral effects are varied and cause great suffering. For a complete discussion of these various processes, the reader is directed to a medical-surgical textbook. Cirrhosis and peripheral neuritis are the physical health problems most commonly associated with alcohol. As the alcohol-dependent person's liver functions become impaired, he or she is less able to "tolerate" alcohol. The person who once boasted of drinking exploits becomes drunk after only a few beers. Physical consequences of cirrhosis include obstructed blood flow (which leads to portal hypertension, ascites, and finally esophageal varices), decreased liver cell function, low serum albumin levels, high ammonia and high bilirubin serum levels, and clotting problems. Peripheral neuritis causes numbness and subsequent injury in the legs, as well as changes in gait.

Alcohol is also an irritant; it burns the mouth and throat and prompts the stomach to secrete more hydrochloric acid. Gastric ulcers are caused and then worsened by alcohol. Alcoholics can experience ulcers, gastritis, bleeding, and hemorrhage in the

|Table 35-4| Courses of Withdrawal from Addictive Drugs

Drugs	Length of Acute Detoxification	Common Detoxification Agents	Withdrawal Signs and Symptoms
CNS depressants			
Alcohol	3-5 days	Librium, Serax, Valium, Vistaril, alcohol	Anxiety, sweats, tremors, flushed face irritability, sleeplessness, confusion, seizures, delirium
Valium	Slow drug taper, up to 2 wks	Librium, Valium	
Phenobarbital	Slow drug taper, 2-4 wks	Librium, phenobarbital	
Opioids			
Heroin	3-5 days	Methadone or other tapering opioid or nonopioid withdrawal regimens	Yawning, dilated pupils, gooseflesh, vomiting, diarrhea, runny nose and eyes, sleeplessness, anxiety, irritability, elevated blood pressure and pulse, craving for narcotics
Morphine	3-5 days		
Demerol	3-5 days		
Methadone	2 weeks		
Stimulants			
Amphetamines	3-5 days	Drug intervention usually not required	General fatigue, apathy, depression, drowsiness, irritability, paranoia
Cocaine	3-5 days		
Hallucinogen			
Marijuana	2-3 days (metabolites remain in the body up to 2 wks)	Drug intervention usually not required	Few signs of withdrawal, craving for marijuana, general anxiety and restlessness

From Mueller LA, Ketcham K: *Recovering: how to get and stay sober*, New York, 1987, Bantam Books.

stomach. Ulcers can eventually perforate, creating a life-threatening situation.

The pancreas is affected by alcohol in many direct and indirect ways. Pancreatitis and diabetes are not uncommon consequences of alcoholism. A malabsorption syndrome is caused by irritation of the intestinal lining. This condition seems to affect B vitamins generally and to lead to a deficiency of vitamin B$_1$ (thiamine) in particular. Thiamine deficiency contributes to peripheral neuritis. Alcohol also has a direct effect on muscle tissue, a condition known as alcoholic myopathy. Other organs affected by alcohol include the eyes (loss of peripheral and night vision), the heart (hypertension, enlarged left ventricle), and reproductive organs. As a depressant, alcohol can cause impotence. Furthermore, prolonged drinking shrinks the testicles and decreases testosterone. Sexual potency is further compromised by a failing liver that is unable to detoxify female hormones, thus increasing the level of these hormones and adding to the male's sexual decline. As many men have experienced, alcohol can increase the interest in sex but can decrease the performance of sex.

CLINICAL EXAMPLE

Anthony is a 36-year-old suffering from alcohol abuse with physiologic dependence. As alcohol predominates, a primary diagnosis of polysubstance dependence is not appropriate. He has a long history of presentations at the emergency room for suicidal ideations. Alcohol and other drugs are always found in his system. He presents at a local treatment facility saying, "I just can't keep it up any more. I've been drinking for 23 years and my life is falling apart. Everyone I know hates me. I can't keep a job. No one trusts me. I have to have some help." First, Anthony needed detoxification. He then went through a 28-day treatment program. He attends Alcoholics Anonymous (AA) five times each week and has a sponsor, someone in whom he can confide and from whom he can "learn to live life on life's terms." He also attends an after-care treatment group three times per week to focus on dealing with his shame. After 108 days of sobriety, Anthony began to think that he was cured and no longer needed his sobriety support system. He drank again. Just before he was pulled over for driving under the influence, he managed to throw away the cocaine he had just bought. Five months later, the conse-

quences of his past lifestyle are catching up with him. He is considered a habitual offender and has been offered 20 years in prison by the district attorney. The AA program teaches responsibility for one's actions and surrender of self-will to one's higher power. After getting the alcohol out of his system and reconnecting with AA, Anthony is now, rather than trying to run from his obligations, prepared to go to prison, if necessary. "I did it. I don't want to go to prison, but if that's what God has in mind for me because of my foolish decisions, then so be it. Maybe there's somebody out there who needs to hear my story. I can share my experience, strength, and hope, and let them know that God is a way-maker." These attitudes of surrender of self-will to one's "higher power" are characteristic of 12-step programs and are considered essential to recovery.

Nursing Issues

Overdose

People die from overdoses of alcohol because it depresses the CNS. Vital centers become anesthetized, compromising breathing and heart rate, leading to a comatose state or death. Gastrointestinal bleeding or hemorrhage can occur. As a vasodilator, alcohol also leads to heat loss; many people have succumbed to hypothermia in colder climates. People consistently underestimate the potency of alcohol, and deaths have occurred simply because individuals have consumed too much. Almost every year, newspapers report the death of a college student by alcohol poisoning. Although alcohol alone can kill, most overdose-related deaths are the result of combining alcohol with other CNS depressants.

Disulfiram: A drug that makes drinking painful

Disulfiram (Antabuse) inhibits the breakdown of CH_3CHO by the enzyme aldehyde dehydrogenase. Because CH_3CHO is toxic to the body, the person who drinks alcohol while taking disulfiram will become ill (as evidenced by sweating, flushing of the neck and face, tachycardia, hypotension, throbbing headache, nausea and vomiting, palpitations, dyspnea, tremor, weakness, or any combination). Disulfiram and alcohol can also cause arrhythmias, myocardial infarction, cardiac failure, seizures, coma, and death. The unpleasant response to alcohol is intended to help reinforce the alcoholic's efforts to stop drinking alcohol. Basically, the patient taking disulfiram has to make only one decision a day about drinking: once the pill is taken, the patient dare not drink. Disulfiram is usually started with a single 500-mg dose at bedtime. After 1 or 2 weeks, the dose is reduced to a maintenance dose of 250 mg per day. Anecdotal accounts note that some alcoholics will experience an ostensibly spontaneous relapse episode that coincides with their "forgetting" to take disulfiram for a couple of weeks before their return to alcohol use. Disulfiram is most effective in patients with significant internal motivation for long-term change.

Naltrexone hydrochloride: A drug that decreases the pleasure of drinking

Naltrexone hydrochloride (ReVia) is an opioid-receptor antagonist, formerly used to treat narcotic dependence, now approved for the treatment of alcohol dependence. Naltrexone increases abstinence and reduces alcohol craving when used as a part of a comprehensive treatment plan (Sinclair, 2001). Naltrexone interferes with opioid functioning, which probably compromises the pleasurable effects of alcohol. Naltrexone has been known to cause liver toxicity if taken at higher than recommended levels and is contraindicated for patients who have abused narcotics within 7 to 10 days because it will precipitate opioid withdrawal (FDA Consumer, 1995). Typically, patients receive 500 mg per day.

Interactions

Alcohol taken with other CNS depressants causes profound CNS depression, often leading to death. For instance, diazepam, which is not lethal when taken alone, has led to death when combined with alcohol. Alcohol should be avoided when a person is taking barbiturates, antipsychotic drugs, antidepressants, benzodiazepines, and other sedatives. Chloral hydrate and lorazepam (Ativan) have been associated with intentional sedating of unsuspecting persons in bars. A chloral hydrate and alcohol combination (the legendary "knockout drops") was used years ago to "recruit" men for ship duty or for robbery. An updated version with Ativan, replacing chloral hydrate, has been used by young women to rob men who thought they were going out for a good time.

Use by Older Adults

Alcoholism in older adults can be roughly divided into two groups:

1. Lifelong users
2. Late-onset users responding to stress

Lifelong users tend to have increased physical, cognitive, and emotional problems associated with their drinking. Late-onset alcoholics include individuals who, as they grow older, tend to cope with the many and persistent losses of later life by drinking. These individuals, if not effectively treated, can deteriorate rapidly. On the other hand, late-onset alcoholics have a robust response when treated.

Alcohol use in older adults is underreported, frequently unrecognized, and rarely treated (Box 35-3). As the population of older adults has grown, so have the substance-related problems many of these people bring with them. People with impaired liver function do not metabolize alcohol efficiently and can therefore tolerate little of the drug alcohol. Decreased liver function is a product of aging, and, consequently, many older individuals cannot drink much alcohol without becoming inebriated, confused, and sedated. The nurse should be particularly watchful for combinations of alcohol with other CNS depressants among patients in this age group.

Fetal Alcohol Syndrome

Pregnant women who drink alcohol run the risk of seriously harming their unborn child. Fetal alcohol syndrome (FAS) is the result of alcohol's inhibiting

| Box 35-3 | Older Alcoholics

Older alcoholics are divided into two groups. About two thirds are "early-onset" drinkers who have abused alcohol much of their lives and have survived into an unhealthy, unhappy old age. The "late-onset" group—about one third of all drinkers over age 60—is unlike the general alcoholic population. This group has an excellent chance for recovery.

"They are not as impaired physically, emotionally, or cognitively as the early-onset drinkers... With abstinence, proper diet, and time, recovery can be complete" (Robertson, 1992).

Heavy drinking in the late-onset group is usually triggered by traumatic loss. The deterioration is rapid, only a 1- to 2-year progression, compared with alcoholics who have been drinking for 20 to 40 years.

From Robertson N: The intimate enemy: will that friendly drink betray you? *Modern Maturity* 35(1):28, 1992.

fetal development during the first trimester. FAS is the third most commonly recognized cause of mental retardation and the only one that is preventable. Characteristic signs of FAS include microcephaly and an associated severe mental retardation. The risk of FAS is directly related to the amount of alcohol the mother drinks during pregnancy.

Withdrawal and Detoxification

Withdrawal from alcohol can be painful, scary, and even lethal (see Table 35-4). As the person abstains from alcohol, he or she begins to reap the consequences of CNS irritation caused by alcohol: tremulousness, nervousness, anxiety, anorexia, nausea and vomiting, insomnia and other sleep disturbances, rapid pulse, high blood pressure, profuse perspiration, diarrhea, fever, unsteady gait, difficulty concentrating, exaggerated startle reflex, and a craving for alcohol or other drugs. As the withdrawal symptoms become increasingly pronounced, hallucinations can occur. The body is undergoing alcohol withdrawal and needs detoxification.

The level of supervision depends on the severity of alcoholism. Mild dependence can be handled on an outpatient basis. Even more heavily dependent cases of alcoholism have been managed "cold turkey" without medical supervision. In years past, it was not uncommon for former alcoholics to take turns sitting with an individual going through the misery of withdrawal from alcohol. Having gone through this same process, these recovering alcoholics were both sensitive when needed and firm when needed; they understood the pain but knew it was usually survivable; and they knew that individuals had died from withdrawal occasionally when medical assistance was not used.

Because of the misery and risk of death associated with unattended withdrawal, most cases today have medical supervision of some sort. Drugs that have a cross-dependence with alcohol, that is, other CNS depressants, can be used to avoid diminished symptoms of withdrawal. The most commonly used medications are the benzodiazepines, specifically chlordiazepoxide (Librium), lorazepam (Ativan), and diazepam (Valium). These agents minimize symptoms of withdrawal, prevent DTs, and decrease the risk of seizures.

CENTRAL NERVOUS SYSTEM DEPRESSANTS

Barbiturates

Barbiturates depress the CNS. Barbiturates were first used medicinally as sedatives in the last half of the nineteenth century. It was not until 1950 that researchers were able to confirm their ability to produce physical dependence. CNS depressants decrease the awareness of and response to sensory stimuli. Antipsychotic drugs and antianxiety agents, which also depress the CNS, are discussed elsewhere.

Barbiturates are used to relieve anxiety or to produce sleep. Examples of common barbiturates are secobarbital (Seconal), pentobarbital (Nembutal), amobarbital (Amytal), and phenobarbital

Case Study

E.F., a 28-year-old Caucasian man, was brought to treatment by his wife after his third driving-under-the-influence offense in which he ran off the road and into a neighbor's mailbox. He has a history of alcohol and drug use since age 14. Although neither of his parents drank, he had a grandfather who died from cirrhosis of the liver and bleeding esophageal varices.

E.F. has been in counseling twice before in an effort to salvage his previous marriage. After the breakup of the marriage, he lost his business and became extremely depressed. However, when E.F. drank, he became belligerent and, at one point, threatened his ex-wife and child, forcing her to file for sole custody of their son. During this period, he also began gambling in an effort to make quick money.

E.F. says that he is willing to enter treatment at this time so that he does not lose his wife and because he fears the men to whom he owes gambling debts. He knows that he will be safe in the hospital until he can figure out what to do. He does not believe that he has a problem with alcohol, drugs, or gambling and attributes his misfortunes to the ill will of others. He denies suicidal ideation at this time. Blood level alcohol on admission was 0.02%.

E.F.'s current lifestyle involves hunting and doing things with his wife and two step-children, Ann, 4, and Steve, 6. He misses his 2-year-old son, who lives with his ex-wife.

(Luminal). Barbiturates are also used in the migraine medications Fiorinal and Fioricet. Slang names for these barbiturates include yellow jackets, reds, blues, Amy's, and rainbows. These drugs have a narrow therapeutic index, the lethal dose being only slightly higher than the therapeutic dose. The long-term effects of barbiturate intoxication can be severe because of hypoxia secondary to shallow or absent respirations during intoxication and overdose. Most people recover if treatment is begun early. These drugs produce both physical and psychologic dependence. Barbiturates are classified according to their duration of action: ultrashort (30 minutes to 3 hours), short (3 to 4 hours), intermediate (6 to 8 hours), and long (10 to 12 hours). Barbiturates with short to intermediate duration have the highest abuse potential. Barbiturates in this category include amobarbital, pentobarbital, and secobarbital.

Barbiturates, usually taken orally, are metabolized by the liver and excreted by the kidneys. When barbiturates are combined with alcohol, dangerous levels of CNS depression can occur.

Physiologic Effects

Barbiturates cause CNS depression, primarily by increasing gamma-aminobutyric acid (GABA) activity. GABA stimulation decreases awareness of external stimuli, shortens the attention span, and decreases intellectual ability. Barbiturates are used to treat insomnia, to soften withdrawal from heroin, and as anticonvulsants. Drug abusers take barbiturates to maintain a state of relatively anxiety-free living. These drugs are also taken to counteract the effects of amphetamines, "to come down," or in place of heroin when it is not available. The acutely intoxicated person will have an unsteady gait, slurred speech, and sustained nystagmus. Chronic users can have mental

▌Care Plan

Name: <u>E.F.</u>   Admission Date: _____

DSM-IV-TR Diagnosis: <u>Alcohol dependence (or alcoholism)</u> _____

Assessment	**Areas of strength:** Has no medical problems and denies suicidal ideation. Has also been in counseling twice and enjoys hunting and doing things with his family. **Problems:** Has a genetic history of chemical dependency and long-time use of alcohol and drugs. Denies that alcohol is a problem in his life despite family and occupational problems.
Diagnoses	• Ineffective individual coping related to alcohol abuse as evidenced by legal and financial problems. • Ineffective family coping: disabled related to alcohol abuse as evidenced by potential marriage separation and financial difficulties.

Outcomes	*Short-term goals:* *Date met*
	• Patient will state that his marital and occupational problems are due to _____
	  drinking.
	Long-term goals:
	• Patient will remain chemical free on monthly testing, which will be _____
	  assessed through urine testing by his probation officer.

Planning/ Interventions	**Nurse-patient relationship:** Recognize initial need to use denial; discuss the natural consequences of his drinking and the need for total abstinence; educate regarding the diagnosis of alcoholism, offering hope for long-term recovery; encourage attendance at AA meetings. **Psychopharmacology:** No caffeine or sugar; multivitamin daily. **Milieu management:** Family treatment; encourage ADLs.
Evaluation	According to probation officer, E.F. is sober after 1 month.
Referrals	Refer to AA and make appointment with substance abuse counselor.

How Abused Drugs Work in Brief

Abused Substance	Mechanism of Action
Barbiturates	Increase the effect of GABA
Opioids	Mimic endogenous neurotransmitters by stimulating opioid receptors; increase the release of dopamine in the nucleus accumbens
Cocaine	Decreases the reuptake of dopamine
Amphetamines	Increase the release of norepinephrine; enhance dopamine release; block the reuptake of dopamine; methamphetamine blocks the breakdown of dopamine
Ecstacy	Increases the release of serotonin; increases the release of dopamine
Marijuana	Stimulates dopamine pathways in the nucleus accumbens
LSD	Binds tightly to $5HT_2$ receptors, causing a more pronounced effect

symptoms that include confusion, irritability, and insomnia. People who regularly use barbiturates develop a tolerance to the psychologic effects but not to respiratory depression effects. Hence the user must consume more and more barbiturate to achieve a pleasurable effect but eventually increases the dose to the point of depressing respirations.

Nursing Issues

Overdose

The toxic dose of barbiturates varies, but in general, an oral dose of 1 g results in serious poisoning, and doses of 2 to 10 g can be fatal. Acute overdose is characterized by CNS and respiratory depression. Coma and death are possible. Treatment is supportive.

Interactions

Barbiturates interact with many other drugs, but the most significant are those that increase CNS depression. Other CNS depressants such as alcohol, sedatives, tranquilizers, and antihistamines can cause serious CNS depression.

Use by older adults

Barbiturates frequently cause excitement in older adults. Older adults are also more prone to confusion caused by barbiturates.

Use during pregnancy

Barbiturates can cause fetal abnormalities. These drugs cross the placental barrier, and fetal serum levels approach maternal blood levels. Infants born to mothers who take barbiturates during the last trimester of pregnancy can experience withdrawal symptoms.

Withdrawal and Detoxification

Symptoms of withdrawal from barbiturates are severe and can cause death. Symptoms usually begin 8 to 12 hours after the last dose. Because barbiturates subdue the CNS, a rebound effect can occur when a person stops taking them. Minor withdrawal symptoms include anxiety, muscle twitching, tremor, progressive weakness, dizziness, distorted visual perception, nausea and vomiting, insomnia, and orthostatic hypotension. More serious withdrawal symptoms include convulsions and delirium. Untreated, withdrawal symptoms may not decline in intensity for about a week (Lehne, 2001). Detoxification requires a cautious and gradual reduction of these drugs. One approach is to reduce the patient's regular dose by 10% each day.

Benzodiazepines

Benzodiazepines have many legitimate uses and are thoroughly reviewed in Chapter 23. One benzodiazepine, flunitrazepam or Rohypnol (also known as roofies, rophies, roche, roaches, and ruffies) is known primarily for its abuse potential (Taylor, Donoghue, 2001). Because of both its sedative and its amnesic effects, Rohypnol has been used for date rape. Until relatively recently, Rohypnol was manufactured as a colorless, odorless, and tasteless substance when mixed with liquids. Sexual predators were able to easily slip it into the beverage of an unsuspecting woman and then perform date rape. Again, the amnesia associated with this drug interfered with prosecution of the perpetrator. Although Rohypnol is not sold in the United States, an active smuggling operation makes it available on the black market.

Gamma Hydroxybutyrate

Gamma hydroxybutyrate (GHB) (also known as G, liquid X, liquid Ecstasy, Georgia homeboy), is a CNS depressant and is popular among youth as a club drug (Allen, 2001; Taylor, Donoghue, 2001). GHB is taken orally, injected, or snorted. Sexual predators use GHB to incapacitate their victims and render them incapable of remembering the assault. GHB is manufactured from products available in health food stores and has been used as a performance-enhancing drug for athletic competition (Allen, 2001). Interestingly, millions of men and women currently use a number of potential drugs, sold as athletic supplements, despite known deleterious effects (Kanayama et al, 2001). GHB, usually when used with alcohol, has been linked to over 60 deaths (Whitten, 2001).

INHALANTS

Inhalants are inhaled and are common because they are cheap, readily available, and typically legal. Examples of inhalants include airplane glue, gasoline, rubber cement, polyvinylchloride cement, hair sprays, air fresheners, spot remover, polish remover, paint remover, and lighter fluid. Inhaled substances can be broken down into three basic groups: hydrocarbon solvents (gasoline and glues), aerosol propellants (propellants in spray cans), and anesthetics and gases (chloroform, nitrous oxide [laughing gas]). Inhalants usually depress the CNS and increase hilarity; they can also cause excitability. Inhalants are also particularly dangerous because the amount inhaled cannot be controlled. Deaths from asphyxiation, suffocation & choking (e.g., on vomit) have been reported. Inhalants cross the blood-brain barrier quickly. Common side effects include mouth ulcers, gastrointestinal problems, anorexia, confusion, headache, and ataxia. Because of their accessibility, children are at a special risk of coming into contact with substances in this category. Some inhalants are highly lipid soluble to the extent that they become sequestered in fatty tissues, thus having a prolonged effect. Brain damage has been reported with inhalants, including frontal lobe, cerebellar, and hippocampal damage, leading to diminished problem solving, ataxic gait, and memory dysfunction respectively. Inhalatants can be breathed in by sniffing fumes from a container, by "bagging" (inhaling fumes from a paper bag), and by "huffing" (inhaling fumes from an inhalant-soaked rag stuffed in the mouth).

OPIOIDS (NARCOTICS)

Opioids include opium, morphine, codeine, heroin, hydromorphone (Dilaudid), meperidine (Demerol), methadone (Dolophine), and oxycodone (Oxycontin). Opioids are widely abused. Until the "cocaine crisis," the general public viewed heroin as the most significant drug of abuse. Although heroin abuse has been relegated to a lower status for some time, it is again becoming the focus of attention because drug users find it less expensive compared with cocaine and less devastating. Using cocaine and heroin together ("speed-balling") has grown in popularity. Opioids can be swallowed, smoked, snorted, injected into soft tissue ("skin popping"), and "mainlined" (IV).

Parenteral use of heroin, for example, involves (1) "cooking" the substance in a spoon or bottle cap, (2) filtering it with a cotton ball, (3) "sterilizing" a needle with a match, and (4) injecting the drug into a vein. Initially, veins in the antecubital space are used, but as vein membranes break down and sclerose (form "tracks"), they "get used up," and other veins are selected for injection. The needle is frequently passed from one user to another. Infections, including acquired immunodeficiency syndrome (AIDS), have been relatively common. Because of AIDS and hepatitis, snorting is increasing in popularity as a route of administration. However, sharing of straws also poses a risk resulting from trauma of the highly vascular mucous membranes in the nasal passages (Gorski, 1996).

CLINICAL EXAMPLE

Sam Jones is a 32-year-old maintenance man. He has a history of drinking and using marijuana since junior high. He began showing a strong preference for opioids after a visit to the dentist to have a tooth extracted. Since that visit, Sam has had several other teeth extracted and has been to the emergency room several times for various situations requiring treatment for one type of intense pain or another. Sam has lost several jobs because of suspected stealing. Actually, he was only trying to get people's prescriptions they weren't using anyway and "would never steal from people." Sam recently started injecting drugs and became obviously impaired fairly quickly. When he was found wandering around the apartment complex with slurred speech and confused thinking, his boss fired him. He left angrily and had a motorcycle accident in which he almost lost his life. He was taken to the trauma unit of the medical center where he began to exhibit narcotic withdrawal the following day. Sam's injuries were severe to the extent that he was "sobered" into agreeing to be evaluated for treatment in the substance abuse treatment program of the medical center. Sam has a long way to go to successfully recover, but exposing him to treatment will at least help him learn more about another way of life, even if he is not ready to fully participate in recovery right now.

Physiologic Effects

Opioids relieve pain by increasing the pain threshold and by reducing anxiety and fear. These drugs accomplish this task by stimulating opioid receptor sites in the brain. The naturally occurring neurotransmitters, the endorphins, among other responses, mediate pain and regulate mood by activating opioid receptors (Lowinson et al, 1992). The opioids are endorphin agonists. Drug abusers are attracted by the drug's effect on mood (a feeling of euphoria). Drug abusers frequently refer to the euphoric mood created by morphine and heroin as "better than sex." In fact, intravenous (IV) heroin delivers a "rush" (less than 1 minute) that is described as similar to a sexual orgasm. In addition to the euphoria, an overall CNS depression occurs. Drowsiness or "nodding" and sleep are common effects.

Heroin has a higher abuse potential compared with morphine and other opioids because it more readily passes the blood-brain barrier. Once heroin enters the brain, its chemical structure is changed to that of morphine thus it becomes "trapped" in the brain, causing a more sustained high. CNS effects of opioids include respiratory depression related to decreased sensitivity to carbon dioxide stimulation by the medullary center for respiration. Respiratory depression is the primary cause of death when opioid-caused death occurs. Peripheral nervous system (PNS) effects include constipation; decreased gastric, biliary, and pancreatic secretions; urinary retention; hypotension; and reduced pupil size. Pinpoint pupils are a sign of opioid overdose. Another opioid, meperidine, is typically the drug of choice for physicians and nurses. Readily available in the health care setting, this drug produces less pupil constriction (hard to detect), is effective if taken orally, and causes less constipation than do other opioids (Lehne, 2001).

Nursing Issues
Overdose

At therapeutic doses prescribed and administered by professionals, morphine and meperidine are helpful and safe analgesics. However, drug abusers who buy on the streets cannot be sure of the amount of opioid they are taking. Street purchases are not standardized, and users occasionally obtain "purer" drug than they anticipated. Inadvertent overdose may thus occur. The primary effect of overdose is respiratory

depression. A respiratory rate below 12 breaths per minute is cause for concern. A recognizable symptom pattern for overdose is documented:

- The person becomes stuporous and then sleeps.
- The skin is wet and warm.
- Next, a coma develops, accompanied by respiratory depression and hypoxia.
- The skin becomes cold and clammy.
- The pupils dilate.
- Death quickly follows at this point.

Provision of adequate airway and assisted ventilation, if needed, are treatment priorities. A narcotic antagonist is administered to reverse the effects of opioids.

Narcotic antagonists: antidote to opioids

The opioids are the only class of commonly abused drugs that have a specific antidote. Naloxone (Narcan), a narcotic antagonist, is the intervention of choice if opioid overdose is suspected. Naloxone blocks the neuroreceptors affected by opioids, thus the patient responds in a few minutes to an IV injection of naloxone. Respiration improves, and the patient consciously responds. However, because most opioids have a longer lasting effect than naloxone has, it is often necessary to repeat the antagonist to maintain adequate respiration. The nurse who administers naloxone must carefully observe the patient to determine whether additional antagonist will be needed. If the dose of the antagonist is proportionately greater than that of the opioids in the system, it is possible to precipitate a state of narcotic withdrawal.

CLINICAL EXAMPLE
A hospice team member told the following story. The patient was a 70-year-old man suffering from prostate cancer with painful bone metastases. A nursing concern is maintaining a balance between the need for pain management and the risk of respiratory suppression. The patient built up tolerance to his pain medication. His family members were afraid that he was becoming an "addict," thus they decided to reduce his medication intake without consulting the physician. Cutting in half and administering a time-release pain pill (a synthetic morphine that lost its "time release" characteristic when broken), they quickly noticed that Dad was not very responsive. He was taken to the hospital, and Narcan was administered. Because it blocks the opioid

receptor sites, there was no effective pain relief for this patient. The man was in extreme physical pain, because his family was afraid of the legitimate medical uses of pain medication. Additionally, lack of knowledge about the way in which time-release medications work led to an erratic and fatal dose being administered.

Interactions

The effects of opioids are increased when they are combined with other CNS depressants. Because the use of multiple drugs is common among drug abusers, the potential for deadly combinations is real. If it is known that heroin was taken and that naloxone does not reverse CNS depression, it can be safely assumed that other depressants (e.g., barbiturates) were taken also. In cases such as these, supportive nursing care is indicated.

Use by older adults

Some older patients may have chronic medical conditions associated with chronic pain for which long-term narcotic pain medication has been used. Older adults are particularly at risk for decreased pulmonary ventilation associated with opioids.

Use during pregnancy

Women who abuse opioids give birth to babies who suffer withdrawal symptoms. These drugs can cross the placental barrier and produce respiratory depression in neonates.

Withdrawal and detoxification

The unassisted withdrawal from alcohol or barbiturates can be fatal, but the unassisted withdrawal from opioids is rarely fatal, though often painful. The term "kicking the habit" comes from the leg spasms associated with the withdrawal from opioids. Withdrawal symptoms are related to the degree of dependence and the abruptness of the discontinuance. Maximal intensity is reached within 36 to 72 hours and subsides in about a week. Withdrawal symptoms include yawning, rhinorrhea, sweating, chills, piloerection (goose bumps), tremor, restlessness, irritability, leg spasm, bone pain, diarrhea, and vomiting.

Clonidine has been used successfully for withdrawal by relieving some of the autonomic symptoms (e.g., vomiting and diarrhea). Clonidine does not reduce craving, however. Buprenorphine (Buprenex) and

naloxone (Narcan) have been found helpful in the detoxification of these individuals (Mathias, 2001). Treatment is primarily symptomatic and supportive.

Specific Drugs

Other opioids include hydromorphone (Dilaudid), a more potent derivative of morphine; levorphanol (Levo-Dromoran), a drug with an action that is identical to that of morphine but is used for less severe pain; meperidine (Demerol), a synthetic narcotic analgesic; pentazocine (Talwin), which has weaker analgesic effects and is less addicting compared with other narcotic drugs and is not supposed to cause euphoria; and several other related drugs. Fentanyl (Sublimaze), an anesthetic, is similar to but 100 times stronger compared with morphine and 50 times stronger compared with heroin. Many deaths have been attributed to fentanyl analogues (Lowinson et al, 1992). These drugs are typically "marketed" as purer heroin.

Methadone

Methadone (Dolophine), although an opioid similar to morphine, is used specifically to prevent withdrawal symptoms; it is also used as an analgesic in conditions associated with severe pain, such as cancer. Methadone is given orally and is poorly metabolized in the liver. Accordingly, methadone has a much longer half-life (15 to 30 hours) than does morphine (~2 hours). Because of the long half-life, once-a-day dosing is effective and conducive to outpatient care. When used to aid in lessening physiologic dependence on opioids, methadone is of great benefit. A longer acting related drug, levo-alpha-acetylmethadol (LAAM) (Orlaam) can be administered three times a week instead of every day. This dosing schedule may be preferable for some individuals.

Heroin

Heroin, which was originally a trade name developed by the Bayer Company in 1898 (Lowinson et al, 1992), was derived from morphine to be a cure for morphine addiction but proved to be more addictive by comparison.

Codeine

Codeine is used primarily as a cough suppressant; its abuse preceded the general drug abuse of the middle to late 1960s because it was easily available in over-the-counter cough syrups. Ease of access was eliminated at about the same time that drug abuse became recognized as an emerging national problem. Codeine is still a drug of choice for many substance abusers today.

Oxycodone

Oxycodone (OxyContin), an effective painkiller, has received much attention in the media the last several years. OxyContin is a time-released form of oxycodone. Oxycodone has been available in other medications such as Percocet, Percodan, and Tylox for some time. By crushing OxyContin, then swallowing, snorting, or injecting the powder, substance abusers have found another way to achieve a high. Unfortunately, the widespread media coverage of these individuals has made clinicians reluctant to prescribe OxyContin for people suffering from severe pain.

STIMULANTS

Use of stimulants containing caffeine such as soda pop, coffee, and tea is widespread. Many people feel sluggish if they do not start their day with a cup of coffee. Other, more powerful stimulants, such as amphetamines, cocaine, and so on, cause immeasurable harm to society in the United States.

Cocaine

Coca plants grow high in the Andes mountains, and the Incas chewed coca leaves long before the Spanish explorers arrived. It should be noted that this plant is not cocoa, from which we get chocolate, but coca. Cocaine is still in legitimate use today in some parts of Andean South America. Used as a mild tea, cocaine can help bring relief for altitude sickness. Cocaine is a fine, white, odorless powder with a bitter taste that was introduced to Western medicine as an anesthetic in 1858. Sigmund Freud was known to use cocaine and believed it to be a remedy for morphine addiction. Freud reported on the effects of cocaine in his book, *Cocaine Papers*. Cocaine was once used in some cola drinks (e.g., Coca-Cola), and advertisements extolled the ability of cola, as well as of other "brain tonics," to "refresh." After the Pure Food and Drug Act was passed in 1906, cocaine was eliminated from these beverages. Cocaine (cocaine hydrochloride) and its offspring, crack (freebase cocaine), have caused a major drug problem today. The list of famous and not-so-

famous people struck down in their youth by this stimulant is lengthy. The problems associated with cocaine extend to every level of society.

Physiologic effects

Cocaine and its derivatives are addicting stimulants. Cocaine's exhilarating effect is related to its ability to block dopamine reuptake (Castaneda et al, 2000), particularly in the nucleus accumbens pleasure center in the brain (see Chapter 5). Although physical dependence is less severe than it is with opioid abuse, psychologic dependence is intense. Abusers become tongue-tied when attempting to describe the sensations of this drug. Euphoria, increased mental alertness, increased strength, anorexia, and increased sexual stimulation are desired effects of these drugs. Increased motor activity, tachycardia (up to 200 bpm), and high blood pressure are PNS effects. CNS effects include deep respirations (from medulla stimulation), euphoria, increased mental alertness, dilated pupils, anorexia, and increased strength. The cocaine user can be loquacious and stimulated sexually (libido is increased, ejaculation retarded). This latter characteristic undoubtedly adds to the drug's overall appeal. Intense paranoia is common. This paranoia, in combination with other factors such as decreased inhibitions, explains, at least in part, the reason that many drug deals "go bad" and result in someone being murdered.

Less common reactions are specific hallucinations and delusions. Cocaine users report "bugs" crawling beneath the skin (formication) and foul smells. Nasal septum perforation has been associated with snorting cocaine and is the result of extreme vasoconstriction, which impedes blood supply to this area and thus causes nasal necrosis. Death from cocaine is linked to metabolic and respiratory acidosis and hyperthermia associated with prolonged seizures. Tachyarrhythmias and coronary artery spasm have also led to death.

Tolerance to CNS and PNS effects develops quickly because neuronal norepinephrine stores are depleted, causing a need to increase drug amounts to create the desired effect. Tolerance develops to otherwise lethal amounts. Children born to mothers using cocaine are more likely to score lower on tests that measure alertness, attention, and intelligence than do children of mothers who do not use cocaine (Zickler, 1999).

Case Study

J.R. is a 25-year-old unemployed carpenter who lives with his aunt. One night, he began tearing the house apart, then locked himself in the bathroom yelling that he was going to kill himself. His aunt called the police, who delivered J.R. to the emergency room of the local hospital. The emergency room examiner noted that J.R. was suicidal and having auditory hallucinations, delusions of persecution, disorganized thinking, anorexia, insomnia, anxiety, and agitation. He had been threatening the police and continued to be extremely agitated and threatening the emergency room personnel. Following some history from the aunt, the diagnosis of cocaine intoxication was made.

J.R.'s aunt stated that she had been concerned about possible drug use for the last couple of years but had never pursued the issue with J.R. He was often belligerent and was fired from his job until he was able to get "cleaned up." She had noticed things missing around the house but never questioned J.R. about this.

The emergency room physician decided to keep J.R. in the emergency room until his thinking cleared and to monitor him for tachycardia, cardiac arrhythmia, and seizure activity. The physician ordered 5 mg of diazepam (Valium) to be given IV for 2 to 3 minutes every 10 to 15 minutes if needed for seizures and propranolol (Inderal) IV (0.1 to 0.15 mg/kg at a rate of 0.5 to 0.75 mg every 1 to 2 minutes) should the patient experience cardiac arrhythmias. J.R. was transferred to the psychiatric unit following 4 hours of observation in which there was no seizure activity or cardiac abnormalities.

On arrival at the unit, J.R. was noticeably irritable, agitated, anxious, and complained of a headache. His responses to questions indicated continuing difficulty in concentration and some disorganized thinking. The care plan on the following page was developed.

Routes of cocaine use

Cocaine passes the blood-brain barrier quickly, causing an instantaneous high. When administered IV (mainlining), cocaine is rapidly metabolized by the liver, thus the "rush," though exhilarating, does not last long. Cocaine exerts both CNS and PNS effects because of its ability to block norepinephrine and dopamine reuptake into presynaptic neurons; it depletes these neurotransmitters. Cocaine can also be swallowed (but is poorly absorbed this way) and snorted. Snorting, in which cocaine is absorbed through the nasal mucosa, was the preferred route of administration especially glamorized in the 1980s. With the discovery of smoking an adulterant-free cocaine crystalline base, freebasing became popular and paved the way for the advent of "crack" or "rock" cocaine.

Crack

Crack is a less expensive way of using cocaine compared with snorting or mainlining, primarily because it is sold and marketed in smaller packages, most commonly as $10 or $20 rocks. Crack is purported to be the most addictive drug on the streets today. Crack is produced in a relatively uncomplicated procedure (mixed with baking soda and water, heated, and hardened) and then smoked; it is reported to produce an instantaneous high and almost as instantaneous a "crash." An intense desire to smoke again is produced. It is thought that the faster a drug's effect builds and then diminishes, the more addictive it is, thus explaining the reason that crack is considered the most addictive drug (Wright, 1999).

Crack is cheap on a per-dose basis, but the user wants more immediately, thus it is not an inexpensive drug to use. Crack is also easy to find. When the user's money is gone, however, the crash often gives way to cocaine-induced depression. This depression is sometimes severe to the extent that users attempt suicide.

CLINICAL EXAMPLE

Gladys is a 32-year-old woman who suffers from cocaine dependence and was referred to outpatient treatment through the legal system because of a possession charge. After her second group therapy session, she requests an individual session with her counselor. There, she reveals that 1 month earlier, other "customers" at the local crack house that she has frequented had raped her. Gladys is frightened and embarrassed; her urge to escape the emotional pain she feels by using is strengthened by her traumatic experience at the crack house. Although Gladys says that she has a supportive family, she is further ashamed and terrified because she

Continued on page 473

Care Plan

Name: J.R._____   Admission Date: _____

DSM-IV-TR Diagnosis: Substance intoxication and dependence_____

Assessment	**Areas of strength:** Young (25 years old); lives with aunt who wants him to return once he begins to feel better; previous employer would hire him if he gets "clean."
	Problems: Suicidal ideation, hallucinations (auditory), delusions that someone wants to kill him, thinking disorganized (has difficulty completing thoughts), anorexia, insomnia, anxious (has exaggerated startle reflex), agitated.
Diagnoses	• Potential for self-directed violence related to substance abuse or CNS agitation as evidenced by history of suicide attempt.
	• Alterations in perception related to substance abuse or CNS agitation as evidenced by suicidal ideation, disorganized thinking, and hallucinations and delusions.
	• Alteration in nutrition: less than body requirements related to anorexic effect of cocaine as evidenced by loss of weight.

Outcomes

Short-term goals: *Date met*
• Patient will not experience physical injury during hospitalization.   _____
• Patient will not experience symptoms of cocaine withdrawal.   _____
• Patient will sleep 6 to 8 hours per night.   _____
• Patient will admit that cocaine is a problem in his life.   _____
Long-term goals:
• Patient will maintain optimal levels of nutrition and maintain at least
  90% of normal weight.   _____
• Patient will attend outpatient Cocaine Anonymous meetings.   _____
• Patient will practice abstinence from psychoactive drugs.   _____
• Patient will verbalize and show some evidence of developing
  non-drug-using friends.   _____

Planning/
Interventions

Nurse-patient relationship: Develop a contract with patient to report to nurse if suicidal thoughts occur. Establish trusting relationship with patient. Provide reality-based conversation. Accept patient. Set limits on behavior; confront the patient with inconsistencies; and do not allow patient to manipulate. All staff must be consistent. Allow patient to verbalize anxiety and fear. Teach patient the effects of drugs on his body. Encourage independence in self-care, and reinforce examples of self-denial and delayed gratification.

Psychopharmacology: Desipramine 50 mg bid for cocaine withdrawal for 2 weeks. Haldol 5 mg po q4h prn agitation; Cogentin 2 mg po with first dose of Haldol on the days it is given. Tylenol tabs 2 q4h prn headache.

Milieu management: Provide patient with a quiet room to decrease stimulation and agitation. Provide safe environment, including frequent observation by staff, monitoring of smoking, assessing vital signs prn. Monitor the environment for dangerous objects such as glass, razors, and belts. Provide foods the patient likes to increase interest in food. Provide group setting for patient to explore the issues of substance abuse with other patients and to help the patient get past the notion that no one understands his problems. Orient to surroundings.

Evaluation

Patient has not experienced significant cocaine withdrawal; appetite is returning. Beginning to sleep better (4 to 6 hours). Patient has not attempted self-injury and denies suicidal intent.

Referrals

Outpatient treatment for after care, including Cocaine Anonymous meetings and random urine screens for increased accountability.

thinks that she is pregnant. In her helplessness, Gladys experiences some suicidal ideation and talks about aborting the pregnancy. After she is calm, Gladys agrees to consult with her physician. After she does not return to treatment, no one answers the telephone, and there is no response to letters sent, Gladys is lost to contact. Six months later, Gladys calls her counselor to say that she laid aside her shame and talked with her pastor, her mother, and her 12-year-old daughter. She reports that all is going well, although the baby was stillborn. She has not used since that time.

Critical Thinking Question

The older generation of former cocaine abusers seems to be turning to heroin as they have grown older. Can you think of a reason why this might be so?

Amphetamines and Related Drugs

Amphetamines, which were developed in 1887, have medicinal uses, such as short-term treatment of obesity, attention-deficit disorders in childhood, and narcolepsy. Amphetamines and some variants referred to as "speed," "meth," "ice," or "crank," are widely abused. Examples of amphetamines include dextroamphetamine (Dexedrine), amphetamine (a 50-50 combination of D-amphetamine and L-amphetamine), methamphetamine (Desoxyn), and an amphetamine mixture (Adderall). Related drugs include methylphenidate (Ritalin), a drug used in the treatment of attention deficit disorder, and 3-4-methylenedioxymethamphetamine or Ecstasy.

Metabolism

Amphetamines are taken orally, are well absorbed from the gastrointestinal tract, are excreted basically unchanged by the kidney, and continue to have an effect until cleared. Therapeutic parenteral administration is illegal in the United States, but many speed users self-administer amphetamines IV.

Physiologic effects

Amphetamines are indirect-acting sympathomimetics that cause the release of norepinephrine from nerve endings. Amphetamines also block norepinephrine reuptake in presynaptic nerve endings. Similar to cocaine, amphetamines also have a pro-

found effect on the pleasure pathway by enhancing dopamine, sometimes referred to as the pleasure neurotransmitter. Amphetamines block dopamine reuptake but also stimulate excess release of dopamine and retard its enzymatic breakdown. This affect on dopamine and the dopamine system probably accounts for amphetamines' "addicting" effects. CNS effects include wakefulness, alertness, heightened concentration, energy, improved mood to euphoria, insomnia (sometimes desired, sometimes not), and amnesia. The most common side effects of amphetamine use are restlessness, dizziness, agitation, and insomnia. PNS effects are palpitations, tachycardia, and hypertension. Respirations also increase because, similar to cocaine, the amphetamines stimulate the medulla. A psychiatric side effect of amphetamine use is amphetamine-induced psychosis. In the emergency room, this psychotic presentation can be almost indistinguishable from paranoid schizophrenia.

Methamphetamine

Methamphetamine (referred to as speed, meth, chalk, crystal, crank, or ice) produces a longer high than does cocaine and is typically less expensive by comparison. Methamphetamine is frequently used as an adulterant of cocaine; it can be snorted, swallowed, injected, or smoked (as in the ice, crank, or crystal versions). Methamphetamine causes an intense feeling of pleasure, which is followed by an equally intense "crash" as the drug wears off. Users become paranoid and may hallucinate. Long-term use of methamphetamine can cause damage to dopaminergic systems and other brain areas (Zickler, 2000). As Mathias (2000, p. 10) has noted, "Speed does kill."

Ecstasy

Ecstasy or 3-4-methylenedioxymethamphetamine (MDMA) (also known as XTC, E, X, rolls, or Adam) was synthesized in the early 1900s and was briefly used sometime later as an adjunct to psychotherapy. The chemical structure of Ecstasy is closely related to methylenedioxymethamphetamine (MDA) and methamphetamine. Ecstasy is the most popular club drug (Allen, 2001), promoted as enhancing closeness to others, affection, and communication abilities. At higher doses, an amphetamine-like stimulation occurs, including euphoria, heightened sexuality, diminished self-consciousness, and disinhibition.

Ecstasy also produces a psychedelic effect as well. Unpleasant amphetamine-type side effects also occur, such as tachycardia, increase in blood pressure, anorexia, dry mouth, and teeth grinding (creatively ameliorated by candy pacifiers) (Taylor, Donoghue, 2001). Ecstasy results in memory impairment and appears to have profound impact on the serotonin system (Mathias, 1999). Ecstasy has made headlines related to its use at "raves." Raves are all-night dances in which drugs are used to enhance dancing and other activities. Hyperthermia, dehydration, rhabdomyolysis, renal failure, and deaths have been reported. Ecstasy is taken orally, and its effects last up to 6 hours (Taylor, Donoghue, 2001). Some research now indicates an Ecstacy-related loss of serotonin-producing neurons (Hess, DeBoer, 2002). Although the long-term consequences of altered serotonin neurons are not known, decline in memory and mood are likely.

Nursing Issues
Overdose

Cocaine and amphetamine "overdose" has resulted in a number of deaths, resulting primarily from cardiac arrhythmias and respiratory collapse (Wray, 2000). Smoked cocaine adds to the problem because large amounts reach the system quickly. Toxic levels of amphetamines cause tachycardia, severe hypertension, cardiac ischemia, cerebral hemorrhage, seizures, and coma. Treatment includes induction of vomiting, acidification of the urine, and forced diuresis. In patients with amphetamine psychosis related to toxic levels of these drugs, chlorpromazine or haloperidol given intramuscularly will antagonize the amphetamine effect.

Interactions

The effects of cocaine and amphetamines are augmented when they are combined with other CNS stimulants. Many over-the-counter products such as hay fever medications and decongestants contain stimulants. Urinary alkalinizing agents such as sodium bicarbonate decrease the elimination of amphetamines, whereas urinary acidifying agents increase the elimination of amphetamines.

Use during pregnancy

Amphetamines should be used during pregnancy only if clearly needed, because harm to the fetus has been demonstrated. Cocaine-addicted mothers give birth to addicted babies with multiple problems, withdrawal and physical problems of the neonate being only the beginning of a lifetime of resulting effects. About 400,000 infants born each year in the United States are exposed to cocaine in the womb (Clinical News, 1998). As "crack babies" have reached school age, impaired neurologic development of the exposed fetus has become apparent and is associated with an explosion of children with behavior and learning problems in special education programs.

Withdrawal and detoxification

Although cocaine and amphetamines are highly addictive, physical withdrawal is relatively mild. Psychologic withdrawal is severe, however, because the drugs are highly pleasurable and because of depletion of monoamines known to be associated with depression. For individuals withdrawing from amphetamines under medical supervision, the withdrawal process is gradual and safe. "Cold turkey" withdrawal without medical supervision causes agitation, irritability, and severe depression, frequently with suicidal ideation. As a rule of thumb, the "low" of withdrawal will be inversely proportional to the "high" experienced. Withdrawal from cocaine causes intense craving for the drug. A number of approaches are used, all of which aim to restore depleted neurotransmitters. Amino acid catecholamine precursors such as tyrosine and phenylalanine, tricyclic antidepressants, and the dopamine agonist bromocriptine are three approaches used to increase the availability of neurotransmitters.

HALLUCINOGENS

Hallucinogens, also referred to as psychotomimetics or psychedelics, cause hallucinations. Hallucinogens are divided into two basic groups: natural and synthetic. Natural hallucinogenic substances include mescaline (peyote [from cactus]), psilocybin (psilocin [from mushrooms]), and marijuana (*Cannabis sativa*). Synthetic or semisynthetic substances include lysergic acid diethylamide (LSD) and phencyclidine (PCP). In general, hallucinogens can heighten awareness of reality or can cause a terrifying psychosis-like reaction. Users report distortions in body image and a sense of depersonalization. Particularly frightening is a loss of the sense of reality. Hallucinations depicting grotesque creatures, such as a "dog with a snake for a tongue," can be extremely frightening. Emotional consequences of these effects are panic, anxiety, confusion, and paranoid reactions. Some individuals have experienced frank psychotic reactions after minimal use. In the jargon of the hallucinogens, this experience is a "bad trip." The drugs discussed here do not represent an exhaustive accounting of hallucinogens. Consult Appendix F for a more definitive review of these agents.

Mescaline

Mescaline (peyote) is derived from cactus plants found in America. Native Americans harvested peyote "buttons" from cacti and used them in their religious ceremonies. This religious practice was protected by law as part of their worship until 1990, when the U.S. Supreme Court ruled that states can prohibit its use. Mescaline is taken orally; its site of action is probably the norepinephrine synapses; and its effects last up to 12 hours.

Physiologic effects

With mescaline, colors are vivid, music is beautiful, and sounds become intense. When users close their eyes, colors and images can be seen. A distorted sense of space and time occurs. A young person who drove his car after taking peyote stated that it seemed to take an eternity to reach a stop sign no more than 50 feet away. The experience is directly related to preingestion expectations. "Good" experiences include hilarity and joy. The user may feel especially insightful. The answers to questions such as those involving the "meaning of life" may seem clear. These insights can easily add to a sense of an almost "religious" experience. If the conversation were recorded and replayed later, however, the users would not be as impressed with their having encountered what they believed to be ultimate truth (this is also true of marijuana). "Bad" trips are the side effects of concern. Although peyote is less potent than is LSD, it still can cause panic, paranoid thinking, and anxiety if the trip is too intense. Dependence does not occur in the strict sense, yet users enjoy the experience and seek to repeat it. Pupil dilation and tremors sometimes occur.

Psilocybin, Psilocin

Psilocybin is derived from mushrooms *(Psilocybe mexicana)* and converted to psilocin in the stomach.

The effects last up to 8 hours. Hallucinations and time, space, and perceptual alterations are experienced and are the basis of some Native American groups continued use in religious and other sacred ceremonies (to facilitate integration of body, mind, and spirit). Psilocybin dilates the pupils and increases heart rate, blood pressure, and body temperature. Tingling of the skin and involuntary movements can occur. Similar to other hallucinogens, a sense of unreality can occur. An inability to concentrate may add to feelings of anxiety and lead to panic and paranoia. Hallucinations and illusions may occur. Although no deaths from psilocybin toxicity have been reported, deaths related to perceptual distortions have occurred.

Marijuana

Cultivation of marijuana (also known as pot, weed, grass) has taken place for over 5000 years. Marijuana is the drug most widely used illegally in the United States. Marijuana and other related drugs (hashish and tetrahydrocannabinol) come from an Indian hemp plant. Marijuana is difficult to categorize. Placement with the hallucinogens seems appropriate, but other categorizations can be defended as well. Marijuana varies significantly in strength dependent on climate and soil conditions in which it is grown.

Metabolism

The active ingredient in marijuana is delta-9-tetrahydrocannabinol (THC). THC, which is changed to metabolites in the body and is stored in fatty tissues, remains in the body for up to 6 weeks after it is smoked and can be detected in blood and urine from 3 days to about 4 weeks, depending on level of use. The effects of smoked marijuana last between 2 and 4 hours. If marijuana is ingested, effects may last up to 12 hours.

Physiologic effects

Marijuana produces a sense of well being, is relaxing, and alters perceptions. Euphoria results and is the cause of drug-seeking behaviors. Increased hunger ("the munchies") is an effect that makes marijuana useful for anorexic individuals (e.g., patients with cancer who are undergoing chemotherapy). Marijuana's antiemetic properties make it useful for treating nausea and vomiting associated with chemotherapy.

Marijuana Makes People Inattentive and Stupid

Fanning the Flames about the Medical Use of Marijuana Produces More Heat than Light

Former "Drug Czar" Dr. William J. Bennett tells the following story: He was invited to Alaska, where personal possession of marijuana was legal, and was asked "to weigh in on behalf of a new initiative seeking to recriminalize possession of marijuana. Not surprisingly, the percentage of high school students using dope in Alaska was much higher than in the rest of the nation." He continues, "When I accepted the invitation, the prolegalization forces went into action. The 'pothead lobby,' as I called it, distributed fliers in Anchorage and Fairbanks saying 'Confront the Drug Bizarre.' But when I arrived, there was very little opposition.... It later became apparent why. When the 'pothead lobby' passed out fliers announcing my visit, they had put the wrong date on them. I had been saying for a long time that marijuana makes people inattentive and stupid. I rested my case."

Proponents say it is "natural." Critics point out that lead, radiation, and hemlock are also natural. Three primary medical benefits are noted: (1) it eases the extreme nausea associated with many treatments, such as with chemotherapy; critics point out that wine is commonly prescribed for this purpose; (2) it reduces intraocular pressure associated with glaucoma; critics point out that the synthetic form of the drug has the same benefits; and (3) pain management (e.g., with migraine headaches) is purported to be superior to more established medications; critics point out that alternatives are available that do not run the risk associated with smoking marijuana (the preferred route of administration for most of these patients), including the inhalation of smoke and fungal spores, tar ("resin"), and other negative side effects.

Bennett WJ: *The de-valuing of America: the fight for our culture and our children,* New York, 1992, Summit Books.

Balance and stability are impaired for up to 8 hours after marijuana use. Short-term memory, decision making, and concentration are also impaired. Dry mouth, sore throat, increased heart rate, dilated pupils, conjunctival irritation (i.e., red eyes), and keener sight and hearing are physical responses to marijuana. Marijuana has also been thought to be amotivational, but not all research supports this thinking.

Other effects associated with the use of marijuana include harmful pulmonary effects (bronchitis), weakening of heart contractions, immunosuppression, and reduction of serum testosterone and sperm count. Anxiety, impaired judgment, paranoia, and panic are not uncommon reactions to marijuana. Memory is also impaired related to occupation of THC receptors on the hippocampus. These experiences may culminate in some health-compromising behavior. Flashbacks, more commonly associated with LSD, have also been reported. A flashback is a spontaneous reliving of feelings experienced during a "high."

Critical Thinking Question

If you believe that marijuana is benign, would you want your neurosurgeon to "take the edge off" by taking a few tokes just before surgery to remove your mother's brain tumor? Yes or no? Explain and justify your answer.

Lysergic Acid Diethylamide

Lysergic acid diethylamide (LSD), which stimulates the nervous system by binding tightly to serotonin receptors (i.e., $5HT_2$), is taken orally, and the effects are experienced for up to 12 hours. LSD causes a phenomenon known as synesthesia. Synesthesia is the blending of senses (e.g., smelling a color or tasting a sound). Expectations and environment govern the "quality" of the LSD "trip." LSD causes an increase in blood pressure, tachycardia, trembling, and dilated pupils. CNS effects include a sense of unreality, perceptual alterations and distortions, and impaired judgment. Another problem with LSD is flashbacks. Flashbacks are scary and can heighten a sense of "going crazy." Bad trips from LSD cause anxiety, paranoia, and acute panic. Some users have suffered psychotic "breaks" from LSD and have never fully recovered. A number of individuals have killed themselves while under the influence of LSD (Box 35-4).

Phencyclidine and Ketamine

Phencyclidine (PCP, angel dust, hog), a synthetic drug, has been traditionally used in veterinary medicine as an anesthetic. Many emergency room nurses are familiar with this drug because PCP-intoxicated individuals are often brought to the emergency room. The unpredictable outbursts of violent behavior of PCP patients are legendary; they literally change from coma to violent behavior and back.

|Box 35-4| Research Gone Wrong!

The 40-year-old remains of a scientist who fell to his death after he was given LSD in a CIA experiment were found in good condition when they were exhumed.... A government commission investigating the CIA indicated that the agency had experimented with LSD and other hallucinogens in the early 1950s and that a number of experiments were conducted on unwitting federal employees, including [the] civilian biochemist involved in biological warfare research.... Forensic experts plan to analyze hair, brain tissue, fingernails and bones...for toxins and drugs, including LSD and other hallucinogens.

From the Associated Press: Body of man in 1953 LSD test exhumed, *Los Angeles Times*, p A-4, June 5, 1994.

Caution must be exercised when providing care to these patients because of their unpredictable behavior. PCP is taken orally, IV, is smoked, and snorted. Effects last for 6 to 8 hours.

The PCP user experiences a high. Euphoria and a peaceful, easy feeling can occur and are sought after. Perceptual distortions are common. Undesired effects of PCP can be serious. Blood pressure and heart rate are elevated. Other PNS effects include ataxia, salivation, and vomiting. A catatonic-type of muscular rigidity alternating with violent outbursts is particularly frightening to bystanders. Psychologic symptoms include hostile, bizarre behavior, a blank stare, and agitation.

Ketamine (K, Special K) is a general anesthetic used for minor surgery. It causes a dissociative effect. Bad experiences with ketamine are called a K-hole. Because of its amnesic properties, ketamine has also been implicated in date rapes.

CLINICAL EXAMPLE
Mary Sky is an 18-year-old high school student who has recently become involved with peers who use various hallucinogenic drugs to help them with their spiritual quests. Mary attended a ceremony last night during which she had LSD for the first time. Initially, she experienced anxiety as the sky became a brilliant blue and particular stars seemed to shine brightly as if they were directly in front of her. Mary soon began smiling a lot and realized the depth of "this process called life" and how we are all "a part of the stars." This heightened experience continued throughout the evening. By the next day, all that remained was memory of bliss

and insights, but Mary's actual state of consciousness had returned to usual with all her previously standing inner conflicts.

Nursing Issues
Overdose

High doses of mescaline are not generally toxic. Deaths, however, have occurred. Psilocybin overdose has not been associated with any deaths, and usually a calm environment is all that is needed to assist withdrawal. LSD- and PCP-related deaths are not uncommon. Deaths can be caused by overdose but are more likely to be associated with perceptual disorientation and unresponsiveness to environmental stimuli. Confusion and acute panic can result from an overdose of marijuana, LSD, and other hallucinogens. Diazepam (Valium) can be administered for psilocybin, LSD, and mescaline overdoses and is known to terminate panic attacks caused by these drugs (Hollister et al, 1993). PCP presents greater problems. Diazepam may be given for seizures and agitation and haloperidol (Haldol) for psychotic behavior. Acidifying the urine to a pH of 5.5 accelerates its excretion. Urine screening is the best means of identifying abused substances.

Interactions

Mescaline, psilocybin, and LSD can enhance the effects of sympathomimetics. Marijuana should not be used with alcohol, because marijuana masks the nausea and vomiting associated with excessive alcohol consumption. Respiratory depression, coma, and death can occur.

Use during pregnancy

A number of birth defects have been associated with these drugs. Obviously, hallucinogenic drugs should not be taken during pregnancy.

Withdrawal and detoxification

Hallucinogens do not produce physical dependence, thus no withdrawal symptoms exist. Symptoms of withdrawal from marijuana can include extreme irritability, insomnia, restlessness, and hyperactivity. One of the biggest concerns for the nurse is development of an approach for dealing with the intoxicated person. Basically, the nurse should provide a calm, reassuring environment.

SUBSTANCE-RELATED DISORDERS

FAMILY ISSUES

Although the substance-dependent person is the designated patient, all family members are affected. The family is usually in need of treatment as well. Family members of addicts and alcoholics are referred to as "co-dependent," reflecting the process of participating in behaviors that maintain the addiction or allow it to continue without holding the addict or alcoholic accountable for his or her actions. These behaviors become ingrained to the extent they are difficult to alter when the addict or alcoholic stops using. If the family also gets in "recovery" via Co-dependency Treatment or self-help groups such as AA, Narcotics Anonymous, or Co-dependency Anonymous, they often find many underlying issues of their own that contributed to their selection of a mate with an alcohol or drug problem. For instance, many spouses are children of alcoholics or other dysfunctional family systems in which they, out of necessity for survival, had to take on caretaking responsibilities within the family, setting them up to repeat these behaviors in adult relationships. Dealing with these past traumas and learning ways to let others be responsible for themselves is an important aspect of family recovery.

In some cases, the family has been affected to the extent that the family member may alternate between rescuing (or enabling) the abuser and blaming the abuser. Examples of rescuing include the following: (1) making excuses for the abuser, (2) lying for the abuser, and (3) doing things that the person with a substance-related problem should have done. Oddly enough, living with a recovering addict or alcoholic can sometimes be more difficult than it was when he or she was actively using (see Bill Waters' clinical example). Most units for substance-related disorders have a number of classic stories in which, after abstinence was achieved, the addict or alcoholic was "encouraged" to start using again, or the spouse separated from the addict or alcoholic. Once drug and alcohol free, the person with substance-related problems begins to participate in family functions that have been taken over by other family members. Family roles are difficult to give up, even when they were initially adopted out of necessity. It is sometimes difficult for families and friends to hold the addict or alcoholic accountable; however, on hearing that their loved one is in jail, the family reasons that it is better

than hearing the dreaded words from the police, "Your loved one is dead." The clinical example about Bill represents a situation in which a family resists role changes. Sometimes the family gets well, but the addicted person does not. Conversely, sometimes the addicted person gets well and the family does not.

Children of Alcoholics

Several classic roles have been delineated within alcoholic or substance-abusing homes (Wegscheider, 1981; Wegscheider-Cruse, 2000). As the balance in family responsibilities shifts in response to the irresponsible behavior of the alcoholic or addict, children in particular adopt certain roles in an effort to maintain homeostasis. As children of alcoholics grow, they tend to recreate the same dynamics in their relationships to which they became accustomed as children, thus ensuring reenactment of trauma. For example, the hero role is the child in the alcoholic or addicted family that excels at everything in spite of all the turmoil at home. Table 35-5 describes these roles.

CLINICAL EXAMPLE

Bill Waters was a 48-year-old house painter. He was an alcoholic, and although he was not as productive as he had been in years past, he still made a good living until recently. In the last 6 months, his alcoholism began to have more and more of an effect on his work. He lost one important job because he was unable to meet the deadlines he had established. His home life had been dysfunctional for years. Weekends were only a blur because he drank beer continuously and watched television. His wife Wanda made sure the bills were paid and took care of all the children's needs. Bill never interfered but would occasionally spend money on alcohol before Wanda was able to pay a bill. In recent years, however, Wanda had caught on to all of Bill's tricks, and he rarely had an opportunity to spend household money. When Bill was too hung over to go to work, Wanda called and made up the excuses. Wanda covered for Bill at church and in other situations in which his heavy drinking would be an embarrassment. Wanda alternated between protecting Bill and blaming him for their problems. Her life now revolved around Bill and his problems. After Bill lost an important painting contract, Wanda insisted on treatment. Bill attended a 6-week inpatient treatment program. On his return, Bill was ready to reestablish himself as the husband and father, but Wanda was not ready to trust him. In essence, what had happened, and what happens in many families such as these, is that Wanda

|Table 35-5| Family Roles and Characteristics in Alcoholic Families

Family Role	Characteristics	Example
Caretaker	Tends to everyone's needs in the family; makes sure the family looks normal to the outside	Marjorie gets up at 4:30 in the morning so she can make the kids lunches, clean up her teenager's room, pay the bills, and clean up the mess her husband made when he ran over the flower bed coming in drunk a few hours earlier. She has to be efficient because she has agreed to do all the carpooling during the month and has to lead the parent's meeting at 7:00 this morning.
Hero	Responsible, wants to be the best; may be the teacher's pet; excels in academics, athletics, or some other area	Jenny gets up early so she can practice for the school play. She hopes to get a scholarship to study drama in Europe. She is an A student and has time for many extracurricular activities including drama, debate, and the school newspaper. She was recently elected class president.
Scapegoat	Gets in trouble, breaks rules, defies authority; shifts focus away from the alcoholic or addict	Jimmy is late to school again and was caught smoking in the bathroom. He has been suspended twice this year and is barely passing most of his classes. He slammed the door and ran from the building when the principal was about to call his father.
Mascot	Class clown; diffuses stress; distracts people from problems with humor and foolishness	Mary has lots of friends and loves to be the life of the party. Anytime anyone is down and out, they can always count on Mary for a good laugh. Last night when Mary's dad came home drunk, her mom was really upset and Mary had her laughing before it was over with. Mary keeps everyone in the family guessing what she might say or do next.
Lost Child	Disappears from the activity of the family; does not ever make waves; stays to self, blends in with the "woodwork"	Jane is very quiet and unobtrusive. She sits in the back of the class and rarely speaks. She will answer if called, but otherwise, no one really notices she is there. At home, Jane stays in her room, watches television, and reads and plays alone. She never has friends over and never asks for anything. Jane figures it is best just to try to keep things as calm as possible.

These roles were identified by Sharon Wegscheider Cruse in her books on Adult Children of Alcoholics.

had to take over responsibilities of making decisions, and she was not willing to give them up without long-term proof of Bill's sobriety and responsibility. He had promised to stay sober many times before and failed. Bill, on the other hand, had a clear head for a change and wanted to be the "man of the house" again. Although neither Bill nor Wanda was able to articulate the new problems with which they were struggling, they did recognize emotions they were unable to control. Bill and Wanda soon divorced. A marriage that was able to withstand alcoholism was not able to withstand recovery.

Treating the Chemically Dependent Person

The most common goal of treatment for the chemically dependent person is abstinence from alcohol or drugs. It is thought that the person who is dependent on one substance can easily become dependent on another. The term cross-dependence describes this condition. Professionals working with chemically dependent individuals realize their patients' vulnerability and usually refrain from thinking of anyone as being "cured." Conversely, professionals tend to view treatment as an ongoing, lifelong process in which the person abstaining from formerly abused substances is "recovering." The term recovering indicates a current and dynamic process but also indicates the ever-present possibility of "slipping."

DIAGNOSTIC TOOLS FOR CHEMICAL DEPENDENCY

Many tools exist for the evaluation of chemical dependency. Criteria set forth in the DSM-IV-TR are among the most helpful in diagnosing a person with chemical dependence (see box on page 480). Early diagnosis can mean a better treatment prognosis. Misdiagnosis can lead to unsuspected withdrawal or drug interactions or both. Ultimately, an accurate diagnosis may mean the difference between life and death. It is most important that the nurse look for behavioral and physical clues when making diagnostic evaluations with the treatment team.

DSM-IV-TR and NANDA   Diagnoses Related to Chemical Dependency

DSM-IV-TR*

Alcohol dependence
Alcohol abuse
Alcohol intoxication
Alcohol intoxication delirium
Alcohol withdrawal
Amphetamine (or related substance) dependence
Amphetamine (or related substance) abuse
Amphetamine (or related substance) intoxication
Amphetamine (or related substance) withdrawal
Caffeine intoxication
Cannabis dependence
Cannabis abuse
Cannabis intoxication
Cocaine dependence
Cocaine abuse
Cocaine intoxication
Cocaine withdrawal
Hallucinogen dependence
Hallucinogen abuse
Hallucinogen intoxication
Hallucinogen persisting perception disorder
Inhalant dependence
Inhalant abuse
Inhalant intoxication
Nicotine dependence
Nicotine withdrawal
Opioid dependence
Opioid abuse
Opioid intoxication
Opioid withdrawal
Phencyclidine (or related substance) dependence
Phencyclidine (or related substance) abuse
Phencyclidine (or related substance) intoxication
Sedative, hypnotic, or anxiolytic dependence
Sedative, hypnotic, or anxiolytic abuse
Sedative, hypnotic, or anxiolytic intoxication
Sedative, hypnotic, or anxiolytic withdrawal
Polysubstance dependence
Other (or unknown) substance dependence
Other (or unknown) substance abuse
Other (or unknown) substance intoxication
Other (or unknown) substance withdrawal

NANDA†

Anxiety
Communication, Impaired verbal
Coping, Ineffective
Family processes, Alcoholism, Dysfunctional
Fear
Grieving, Dysfunctional
Growth and development, Delayed
Hopelessness
Infection, Risk for
Injury, Risk for
Knowledge, Deficient
Noncompliance
Nutrition, Less than body requirement, Imbalanced
Nutrition, More than body requirement, Imbalanced
Nutrition, More than body requirement, Risk for imbalanced
Pain, Acute
Pain, Chronic
Parenting, Impaired
Powerlessness
Self-care deficit
Self-esteem, Chronic low
Self-esteem, Situational low
Self-esteem, Risk for situational low
Sensory perception, Disturbed
Sexual dysfunction
Sleep pattern, Disturbed
Social isolation
Spiritual distress
Thought processes, Disturbed
Violence, Risk for other-directed
Violence, Risk for self-directed

*From the American Psychiatric Association: *Diagnostic and statistical manual of mental disorders,* ed 4, text revision, Washington, DC, 2000, APA.
†From North American Nursing Diagnosis Association: *NANDA nursing diagnoses: definitions and classifications 2000-2001,* Philadelphia, 2000, NANDA.

Tools for Alcoholism

Several screening questionnaires have been developed to assist the health care professional in diagnosing alcohol dependency. Among the easiest are the Michigan Alcoholism Screening Test (MAST) and the CAGE questionnaire. Many other tools are available. The purpose of these tools is to provide an objective assessment for identifying alcoholism or addiction. The health care professional must further assess the potential for a problem of alcoholism or addiction in any patient who answers affirmatively to questions about alcohol or drug use.

Michigan Alcoholism Screening Test

The MAST is a good screening tool that can help the unconvinced patient gain insight into at least the possibility of a problem if questions are answered honestly. This test can also aid the clinician in diagnostic assessment and can be easily modified to identify other drug problems.

The CAGE questionnaire

The CAGE questionnaire is another valid instrument. Even easier to administer and possibly perceived as less accusatory compared with the MAST, the following four questions comprise this tool:

1. Have you ever felt you should **C**ut down on your drinking?
2. Have people **A**nnoyed you by criticizing your drinking?
3. Have you ever felt bad or **G**uilty about your drinking?
4. Have you ever had an **E**ye-opener in the morning to steady your nerves or get rid of a hangover?

Two positive responses are suggestive of alcoholism, and three or four positive responses are diagnostic (Whitfield, Davis, Barker, 1986).

Diagnosing Drug Abuse

Alcohol abuse and drug abuse have many similarities; however, there are several significant differences: alcohol is typically legal, whereas many drugs of abuse are illegal (or, if legal, taken out of accordance with the law); stages of drug abuse tend to advance more rapidly as compared with alcohol; and drugs can produce their desired effect almost instantly. See the box of appropriate NANDA diagnoses on page 480.

The problem with most screening tests, particularly for drug abusers, has been their susceptibility to faking and denial on the part of the patient.

Psychotherapeutic Management

Alcoholism is highly treatable. Success of treatment for abuse of other chemical substances varies, but recovery is possible with all chemical dependencies. The success of treatment, however, depends first on the patient's motivation (Box 35-5) and then on the clinician's skill in interpreting data and implementing treatment strategies. The importance of understanding the role of each of the three psychotherapeutic management interventions is crucial. In working with these individuals, the nurse must realize that milieu management has the potential to be more important for this group of patients than it has for other types of patients. With these ideas in mind, it is important to note that two dominant but divergent general philosophies determine the treatment most professionals will provide. In their broadest sense, the two umbrella treatment philosophies are (1) the behavioral model and (2) the disease model.

| Box 35-5 | Motivation

Whether external coercion is a positive influence on treatment outcome is a matter of disagreement. Participants who voluntarily seek treatment are more compliant with their therapists than are those coerced into treatment. Participants who are coerced into treatment may be compliant only while the coercive influence is present and may be compliant only with behaviors specified by the coercive agent. (One example would be the client who does not drive after drinking, but insists on continuing alcohol use, which has proven to contribute to problems in other areas of life.) Data are contradictory about whether coerced and voluntary participants have different treatment outcomes.... [One measure] found that external motivation was related to a positive treatment outcome only when internal motivation was also present....

Internal sources of motivation [included] spouse/family (28.5%), increasing problems with alcohol, wants to stop but can't (17.1%), and mental health affected by drinking (15.9%). Of the 19 participants with external sources of motivation, 18 (90%) were coerced by their spouses to seek treatment.

Steinberg ML, et al: Sources of motivation in a couple's outpatient alcoholism treatment program, *Am J Drug Alcohol Abuse* 23(2): 191, May 1997.

The behavioral model defines addiction as a habit that interferes with work, home, school, health, and relationships; a habit that the addicted individual believes he or she cannot change (Peele, Brodskey, 1991). Adherents of this model point to research that seems to indicate that two brief counseling sessions with a problem drinker's physician can lead to sustained, significantly reduced alcohol consumption (Manissa Communication Group, 1997). One approach of the behavioral model is "moderation management," that is, learning to drink in moderation.

The disease model points to physiologic effects and explanations. The goal of treatment is total abstinence. Obviously, when something as significant as alcohol in an alcoholic's life is removed, something must take its place. This something can be counseling groups facilitated by nurses or other professionals or 12-step programs directed by successfully recovering individuals.

The two camps vehemently disagree on treatment approaches but do agree that substance dependence frequently shows itself in self-destructive behavior. Most professionals are legitimately concerned about this self-destruction and want to be a part of relieving the negative results of AOD use among this population. The authors see validity with both perspectives and believe that a proper approach lies somewhere between the philosophic poles. Although a person's initial exposure to AOD use seems to be influenced by both genetic and environmental factors, it also seems that, once ingested, the substance reinforces continued use by its actions on neurons (Roberts, Koob, 1997).

Nurse-patient relationship

Because most addicted people are experiencing a problem in many areas of their lives at the time they seek treatment, understanding positive motivators will help in establishing new goals and directions for the patient's life. The patient's ability to function at work, at home, in society, and in his or her many roles has been compromised by alcohol and drugs. Stated another way, no one (or hardly anyone) comes to treatment because life is going well. The converse is almost always true; the boss is going to fire him or her, the spouse is going to leave, or the judge is sending the person to jail. Treatment for chemically dependent people is usually initiated out of a crisis. To the degree treatment can help the patient replace ineffective behaviors with new coping skills, the patient has a better chance of getting and staying sober. Coping skills worthy of nursing effort include work skills and habits, job search skills, homemaking, parenting, financial management, family communication, family role responsibilities, and exploration of leisure activities (Stoffel, 1994).

Establishing a trusting therapeutic relationship with the patient in which the rules for treatment are consistently applied is the benchmark for working with chemically dependent individuals. Genuineness is the single most important quality of this relationship. Expressing empathy and providing a safe environment that minimizes anxiety are also important, especially in the early stages of treatment while the patient is going through the painful withdrawal process. Engendering feelings of hope for the future is also necessary as the patient begins to establish new life goals. Nurses working with chemically dependent patients must become skilled at confronting denial and managing manipulation.

Group treatment

Because denial is the most predominant defense of the alcoholic, treating it appropriately is important. A group therapy setting seems to provide the best avenue for treatment because groups are especially effective in breaking down the denial process through confrontation, as well as support of group members who share a common struggle. Confrontation includes telling a patient that which is observed through supportive but reflective listening techniques, irrespective of the strength of a patient's denial.

Here are two fairly common examples of confrontation:

1. "You say you have not been drinking (or using drugs), but I can smell alcohol on your breath (or cocaine was detected in your urine sample)."
2. "I hear you saying that you are in treatment because you believe you need help; so help me understand how you see your need, given your absence from treatment all week without a medical excuse."

What seems to be most effective is when the peers of the patient provide appropriate confrontation, as when Lloyd reported to the group that he had not used alcohol in the last 3 months.

Lloyd's peer, Christy, had used the group well for support earlier that session to process her own recent relapse episode. Christy was able to confront Lloyd directly about his lying, because she had happened to see him at the same club herself the previous weekend!

Personal responsibility

It is important to help the patient learn to foster personal responsibility for recovery. The nurse must cultivate an awareness that responsibility for change lies within the patient himself or herself. Furthermore, while expressing support and concern for the patient in recovery, the nurse must not shield the patient from the negative consequences of the patient's own addictive behavior.

Conscience development

Paradoxically, one of the most effective means for placing responsibility with the patient is in a group that fosters responsibility for another patient in the group. Essentially, patients in these groups are directly told that they have done a poor job of guiding their own lives to the extent that this level of personal responsibility is incomprehensible. However, perhaps they would be able to guide and be responsible for someone else. This idea is novel and intriguing to most patients until a crisis moment occurs. For example, the program has a rule that no one can drink alcohol on pass. Joe is responsible for Bill. Bill drinks over the weekend, and Joe is punished. Punishment can range from a loss of coffee privileges to dismissal from the treatment program. Joe, who has perhaps lied, stolen, and connived for years to pursue his dependency, is speechless at the "unfairness" of the decision. Bill, on the other hand, though feeling some sense of relief at first because he escapes "his punishment," soon begins to feel the anger of other group members for causing the "innocent" Joe to be punished. Bill, who may have perpetrated all kinds of dastardly things in his life with little remorse (a limited internal conscience), begins to have all sorts of feelings because the group is his conscience now (external). Groups such as these are effective, particularly when occupational or legal consequences are dependent on program completion.

Patient and Family Education

Substance-Related Disorders
Illness:

First, there is divided opinion as to whether substance-related disorders should be described as an illness or disease. To name something a disease implies that symptoms of the disease are beyond the control of the individual. Some professionals find this appealing because it allows the patient and his significant others to move beyond blaming and name-calling and on to a focus on treatment. Other professionals disagree. To classify absenteeism, job loss, frequent accidents and injuries to self and others, inattention to appearance, lying, and sneaking around as symptoms of a disease suggests enabling behavior, according to these individuals. Whatever your view, the reality of substance abuse is all around. It devastates lives, wrecks homes, kills innocent bystanders, and stifles society and culture. Whatever is said in these pages is too much—people simply become addicted to substances in order to blur their reality. Whatever is said in these pages is never enough—whatever is said can never capture the enormity, complexity, and gravity of substance-related disorders.

Medications:

A number of drugs are used in the treatment of substance-related disorders. A brief description of those agents follows:

Antabuse—interferes with the metabolic breakdown of alcohol, thus making an individual deathly sick if they should drink while taking this drug.

ReVia—reduces the craving for alcohol.

Benzodiazepines (e.g., Valium, Ativan)—diminish the symptoms of withdrawal from alcohol.

Narcan—used for opioid (e.g., heroin, morphine) overdose.

Methadone—used as a substitute for heroin, thus helping ease the person off heroin.

LAAM—same function as methadone.

Other issues:

All members of the family are affected by substance abuse. Hence, the family is typically in need of treatment. Families often fluctuate between enabling (e.g., making excuses, lying for, doing things for) and blaming the abuser. An interesting point, verified over and over, is the reality that some families are better at coping with a substance abusing family member than with dealing with a "recovered" family member. Awareness of this issue and attempting to think through these dynamics may serve as a preventative mechanism in some homes.

Lifestyle issues

The nurse must teach the patient the effects of chemical abuse on the body and provide for the physical and special nutritional needs of the patient. Exercise is crucial to increase mental and physical vitality as are relaxation, avoidance of stress, and rest. A balanced diet and vitamin and mineral supplements are also essential parts of treatment and recovery. Patients recovering from alcohol or drugs must learn to detach from old "playmates" and "playgrounds" that were representative of their drug use.

Psychopharmacology

Treatment for chemical dependency using medication is becoming increasingly important as knowledge about brain biochemistry increases. Major categories of chemical dependency and pharmacologic approaches to these dependencies are briefly addressed.

Medications used to treat alcohol dependence

Long-acting benzodiazepines (BZs) such as chlordiazepoxide (Librium), diazepam (Valium), and lorazepam (Ativan) are useful for treatment of alcohol withdrawal. The principle behind this treatment is the rapid substitution of the benzodiazepine for the alcohol to suppress withdrawal symptoms. BZs bind to the GABA-benzodiazepine receptor sites, thus the effectiveness of BZs makes sense. The next step is a gradual tapering of BZs over several days. Some clinicians prefer barbiturates for alcohol withdrawal, but respiratory depression and safety concerns dissuade most prescribers.

All patients being treated for alcoholism should be given thiamine. Thiamine specifically prevents the development of Wernicke's encephalopathy and its characteristic ataxia, nystagmus, and mental status changes. Disulfiram (Antabuse), an inhibitor of the enzyme aldehyde dehydrogenase, is effective in preventing drinking because of the severe symptoms it causes when combined with alcohol. Naltrexone (ReVia) functions as an opioid-receptor antagonist that is used to reduce alcohol craving.

Medications used to treat opioid dependence

Drugs used to treat opioid dependence can be divided into those for opioid overdose and those for long-term treatment. Naloxone (Narcan) (see previous discussion) blocks the neuroreceptors affected by opioids. In case of an opioid overdose, naloxone can be given to reverse the opioid-induced CNS depression. Although improvement occurs rapidly in the patient who has taken an overdose, because of naloxone's short half-life, its effect is short lived, and the patient may return to the pre-naloxone state. Maintenance treatment of opioid dependence is accomplished with methadone (Dolophine). Methadone is an opioid with a much longer half-life compared with the prototype opioid morphine and can be given in once-per-day doses. Methadone relieves the "drug hunger" associated with opioid abuse. Typically, no more than 40 mg per day is prescribed. An alternative to methadone is LAAM, a long-acting methadone cogener with a half-life of 96 hours. LAAM can be given on an every-other-day schedule.

Recent evidence suggests buprenorphine, a mild narcotic that is used as a pain killer, can be as effective as is LAAM or methadone in heroin treatment (News & Notes, 2000; Thomas, 2001).

Medications used to treat stimulant dependence

Many medications have been used to treat stimulant dependency. Dopaminergic drugs such as amantadine (Symmetrel) and bromocriptine (Parlodel), anticonvulsants such as carbamazepine (Tegretol), tricyclic antidepressants such as desipramine (Norpramin), and amino acid catecholamine precursors such as tyrosine and phenylalanine have been associated with successful treatment of stimulant dependency (Keltner, Folks, 2001).

Medications used to treat hallucinogen dependence

Diazepam has been found to be effective in terminating episodes of panic, violence, and paranoid ideations induced by LSD and other hallucinogens (Hollister et al, 1993). Initial doses ranged from 10 mg to 50 mg.

Milieu management

The six dimensions of milieu management are all important when shaping the milieu of the chemically dependent inpatient. Some of these dimensions are significant for the patient who receives outpatient care as well. Safety issues such as a drug-free environment are critical. Nurses and others must be vigilant to protect the environment from individuals who would bring drugs into the milieu. Psychiatric units are not necessarily drug-free places. Multiple avenues exist for illicit contraband. Other safety issues such as suicide prevention, thwarting inappropriate sexual behavior, and so forth continue to be the responsibility of nursing staff. Structural considerations such as an active, meaningful schedule provide for less downtime. Box 35-6 outlines a typical structured day for an inpatient setting. People who abuse alcohol, for instance, often structure their day around planning to drink alcohol, drinking alcohol, and being under the influence of alcohol (Stoffel, 1994). Structure then attempts to replace the old structure with a new, therapeutic structure. Effective unit structure maximizes that which the milieu has to offer the patient. Norms of nonviolent behavior, openness, feedback, and the prohibition of nonprescribed drugs are critical to an effective treatment program. As previously noted, confrontation is a useful technique for working with chemically dependent individuals. Many patients will have never truly been held accountable; they certainly will rarely have experienced an environment in which direct and sometimes painful comments are expected to be absorbed and digested. Comments such as these are necessary to penetrate the strong denial and defensiveness of the addict or alcoholic. Strong norms

reinforce the expectation of a reasoned, nonviolent response to such comments.

Limit setting is perhaps the most important and most challenged (i.e., by patients) milieu management technique the nurse will use. Limit setting can be characterized as providing an environment that protects the patient from the self and from other patients. Therefore the nurse needs to recognize the symptoms of a still actively addicted mind (i.e., substance seeking, stubbornness, belligerence, mood swings, and violent and aggressive behavior) and then set limits on these behaviors. Urine drug screens are also a dimension of limit setting because these tests reinforce the no-drug policy (see Table 35-2). If drugs are found, the patient must be confronted and held accountable.

Balance and environmental modification also play significant roles in the well-managed milieu for the chemically dependent patient. Balance is especially important, for example, when using the technique of confrontation. Although confrontation is important and therapeutic, in the hands of some less skilled staff and some patients, it can become little more than a heavy-handed counterpart to the abuse patients may have experienced years ago. The proper technique requires sensitivity to confront without crushing or totally alienating the patient. Skillful confrontation combines knowledge, empathy, and concern, with accurate timing of the confrontation.

ALCOHOLICS AND NARCOTICS ANONYMOUS

Many programs exist for the treatment of chemical dependency. The fact that these various programs exist gives testimony to the complexity and seriousness of chemical dependencies in North America.

The best-known intervention programs are AA and Narcotics Anonymous (NA). These programs use a self-help, support group model made up of fellow users in various stages of "recovery" (Box 35-7). Philosophically, AA and NA view psychosocial problems as stemming from substance abuse and generally reject the idea that an underlying psychopathology is responsible for substance use. AA has established the 12 suggested steps (Box 35-8), which start with a person's admitting personal powerlessness over alcohol and end with the person's being available, night or day, to another alcoholic in need. The popular bumper sticker slogan "Easy does

Box 35-6 Sample Treatment Schedule

Monday-Friday		Saturday and Sunday
7:00 AM	Breakfast	Breakfast
8:00 AM	Morning meditation and spirituality	Community meeting
9:00 AM	Community meeting	Goal setting
11:00 AM	Lecture recovery concepts	Free time
12:00 PM	Lunch	Lunch
1:00 PM	Group therapy	12-step study
3:00 PM	Goal setting, review of 12-step concepts, journaling	
5:00 PM	Recreation and leisure education	Recreation
6:00 PM	Dinner	Dinner
7:00 PM	Family recovery	Visiting hours
8:00 PM	12-step meeting	12-step meeting

This is a sample treatment schedule reflecting typical concepts focused on in most addiction recovery programs. Each program varies but generally includes these basic concepts.

|Box 35-7| AA Works!

The research builds a convincing argument that AA in combination with professional treatment is the most effective form of help. The difference is observable from the very start. Between 50% and 60% of the alcoholics attending only AA will drop out within the first 90 days. The dropout rate is cut in half for patients referred to AA as a part of their professional treatment. AA members who are also active in counseling and therapy relapse less frequently and achieve more comfort and peace of mind in sobriety than do those who attend only AA.

AA has no position for or against professional therapy, but many AA members have benefited from using both. For instance, Bill Wilson, one of the founders of AA, participated in psychiatric treatment for depression after he became sober.

From Gorski TT: *Understanding the twelve steps,* New York, 1992, Simon & Schuster.

|Box 35-8| Twelve Steps of Alcoholics Anonymous

1. We admitted we were powerless over alcohol—that our lives had become unmanageable.
2. Came to believe that a power greater than ourselves could restore us to sanity.
3. Made a decision to turn our will and our lives over to the care of God as we understood Him.
4. Made a searching and fearless moral inventory of ourselves.
5. Admitted to God, to ourselves, and to another human being the exact nature of our wrongs.
6. Were entirely ready to have God remove all these defects of character.
7. Humbly asked Him to remove our shortcomings.
8. Made a list of all persons we had harmed and became willing to make amends to them all.
9. Made direct amends to such people whenever possible, except when to do so would injure them or others.
10. Continued to take personal inventory, and when we were wrong, we promptly admitted it.
11. Sought through prayer and meditation to improve our conscious contact with God as we understood Him, praying only for knowledge of His will and the power to carry that out.
12. Having had a spiritual awakening as the result of these steps, we tried to carry His message to alcoholics, and to practice these principles in all our affairs.

The Twelve Steps are reprinted with permission of Alcoholics Anonymous World Services, Inc. Permission to reprint this material does not mean that AA has reviewed or approved the contents of this publication. AA is a program of recovery from alcoholism only–use of the Twelve Steps in connection with programs and activities that are patterned after AA, but that address other problems, does not imply otherwise.

it" reflects a philosophy of taking life one day at a time and avoiding a frenetic lifestyle. AA and NA subscribe to the belief that only total abstinence can free the chemically dependent person from the bondage of alcohol and drugs, because, they maintain, "A drug is a drug is a drug," meaning that if one is addicted to one substance, one is by definition addicted (at least potentially) to all. AA's relationship with physicians and mental health professionals has become increasingly cooperative over the last few years.

Although AA in particular has a program that has helped many people, it does not appeal to everyone. Reasons vary, but some professionals believe that the spiritual nature of AA is a deterrent to some individuals' seeking help. Specifically, the concept of a higher power, the expectation that one "tell one's story" publicly, and the notion of making a "searching and fearless moral inventory" and then making amends when needed is incongruent with some people's belief systems. AA continues to be an important treatment alternative for thousands of individuals suffering from alcoholism. Other programs, developed by more traditionally oriented mental health professionals, may view underlying problems, such as depression or bipolar illness, as the cause of substance abuse. The goal of this therapy is to treat the underlying problem. Proponents of this approach believe that successful treatment of the underlying problem facilitates resolution of the chemical dependency. These programs may use a group format or individual therapy format (Box 35-9).

Critical Thinking Question

The founders of AA were clear that the recovery process was a spiritual journey. However, we now live in a day in which most people are reluctant to speak of spiritual things for fear of offending others or of imposing their views on others. Do you think that, in our efforts not to "offend" people, we have deemphasized an important part of psychiatric nursing?

SPECIAL NOTE ABOUT PRESCRIPTION DRUG ABUSE

The traditional stereotype of the addict or alcoholic is the "skid row" individual. One forgets or is shocked to find professionals, especially health care professionals, using drugs. A fairly common form of

| Box 35-9 | Maybe AA Does Not Work

At least four studies...have found no differences between groups of alcoholics assigned to Alcoholics Anonymous and no treatment at all.... Consistently negative findings have also come from controlled studies of insight-oriented psychotherapies, antipsychotic drugs, confrontational counseling, most forms of aversion therapy, educational lectures, group therapy, psychedelics, and hospitalization. One sample of something that seems to work is BRIEF INTERVENTION. According to William Miller, "Studies show conclusively that very brief treatment, if designed properly, is highly successful against even moderately severe addictions."

The article continues, "We found this one out the hard way," he recalls. In 1976, in one of his studies of controlled drinking, Miller separated his subjects into two groups. The treatment group got a variety of treatments, including counseling and disulfiram (Antabuse). The control group was given only a brief self-help manual and told to go home, read it, and do their best.

"To our amazement, people in the control group did just as well as the treatment group. We thought we had really messed up the study so we repeated it twice again and got the same results.

"Then we went looking for what was really happening. We gave one group the manual and another group no manual. The manual turned out to be the variable that was the potent treatment. But why? We knew it wasn't the effect of our initial interview with the subjects, or some difference in the patient groups.

"The key was that we had inadvertently motivated the control group and in spite of our expectations, the addicts changed and moderated their drinking. Simply giving them the manual, saying to them that, we believed, they could help themselves, could handle it, you can do this was enough."

Since then, Miller and other therapists have refined and modified "motivational interviewing" and brief-intervention therapy. More than 30 studies in 14 countries have affirmed the value of its key components, dubbed FRAMES: **F**eedback—specific and tailored to the individual, not general; **R**esponsibility—it's up to you, your choice, you are not the helpless victim of a disease; **A**dvice—firm and clear recommendations; **M**enu—there are different ways to work this out; **E**mpathy—the best therapists have this and are neither pushy nor confrontational, but supportive and warm; and **S**elf-efficacy—you can do it; empowerment.

Rodgers JE: Addiction: a whole new view, *Psychology Today* 27(5):77,1994.

drug abuse is addiction to prescription medications, such as pain medications or anxiolytics. People who are addicted to prescriptions have a particularly difficult denial through which to break.

Prescriptions, being legally obtained, are justified as legitimate by the prescription addict. The skills acquired by the prescription addict in maintaining an increasing supply of their drug of choice are accompanied by significant rationalization and sophisticated denial. Because their drugs are acquired legally, prescription drug addicts have a difficult time seeing their use the same as does a "street" addict. Awareness and concern about the problem of prescription drug abuse has risen considerably over the last decade (Meadows, 2001;Vastag, 2001).

SPECIAL NOTE ABOUT ADDICTED HEALTH CARE PROFESSIONALS

The incidence of addiction and alcoholism among health care professionals is a particularly difficult addiction in that there is a violation of the professional's relationship to the patient. Health care professionals who take drugs from patients are particularly scorned (Bachman, 2001). Many states have adopted nonpunitive monitoring programs that allow the nurse an opportunity to work under strict guidelines while actively participating in recovery.

CLINICAL EXAMPLE

Terry is a 39-year-old opioid-dependent registered nurse whose presentation in treatment is precipitated by the state nursing board. Nursing was Terry's life, and her identity centered on being a nurse. Reporting that it was not uncommon to "share medication" with patients, Terry told of how easy it was at first to document giving the maximum "as needed" pain medications in a patient's chart but not always giving them to the actual patient. "I never let one of my patients be in pain, though," Terry reported.

Terry's supervisor did not suspect a problem until medication became unaccounted for. Terry thought that all areas had been covered but was eventually caught, not because of stupidity, but from the kind of impaired judgment that results from drug use.

Terry's nursing license was put on probationary status. Most facilities were unwilling to hire a nurse on probation; the limitations placed by the board were strict. Terry cannot work the night shift and cannot hold the keys to the medication storage; she must also

Continued

submit to random drug testing. Without a job, Terry cannot begin to fulfill the conditions of the probation.

Terry was hired as a nurse at a health care facility and has 6 months remaining until another hearing date can be set.

EVALUATION, RELAPSE, AND FOLLOW-UP CARE

Evaluation

Because abstinence is the overarching goal of most treatments, and because so many people in treatment are referred by the criminal justice system, accurate information is often difficult to acquire. Another complicating factor is deciding exactly which criteria are significant. Unfortunately, there are more questions than answers. Is self-reported abstinence after 6 months, or 1 year, or 5 years best? Is self-report believable? Should police records be consulted for AOD-related arrests? Outcome evaluations for substance dependence are often among the most confusing of statistics.

Relapse

Not only must the chemically dependent person recover from the dependency or addiction, but also the potential for relapse and readmission to treatment must be addressed. This task can best be accomplished by helping the person see the danger signs of relapse. Rawson, Obert, and McCann (1990) outline five warning signs of relapse.

1. Being around other users
2. Severe craving
3. Stopping attendance at AA or NA
4. Not expressing feelings
5. A major emotional crisis

Follow-Up Care

Follow-up care is essential for preventing relapse. Patients and nurses need to be aware that recovery has only begun when an inpatient or outpatient program is completed. The few months immediately following completion of a treatment program can be dangerous for the chemically dependent person. Relapse is most common during this period. The nurse should confirm that arrangements for aftercare, outpatient counseling, and self-help support group meetings are made before discharge.

Critical Thinking Question

Is the "Drug War" worth fighting? Justify your answer.

Key Concepts

1. Chemical dependency is a major physical and mental health problem in North America, and most nurses, whether they want to or not, will take care of chemically dependent people.
2. Drugs of abuse can be categorized into basic groups: alcohol, CNS depressants (e.g., barbiturates), opioids (e.g., morphine, heroin), stimulants (e.g., amphetamines, cocaine, crack, crank), and hallucinogens (e.g., mescaline, marijuana, LSD, PCP).
3. The DSM-IV-TR distinguishes between substance dependence and substance abuse, with substance dependence indicating more severe problems with a substance.
4. Alcohol is the leading drug problem in North America; it exacts a high price economically from this society and is responsible for great suffering and death.
5. Alcohol causes disinhibition and impaired judgment, and it is relaxing when first used. The primary concern with respect to alcohol overdose is severe and often fatal CNS depression. Withdrawal causes tremors, nausea, vomiting, tachycardia, diaphoresis, seizures, anxiety, and depression. Withdrawal can be fatal.
6. Other CNS depressants include barbiturates (downers, reds, blues, and rainbows), benzodiazepines such as Librium (green and whites), antipsychotic drugs, methaqualone (ludes), and inhalants (gasoline and cement for model airplanes).
7. Depressants cause euphoria, disinhibition, and drowsiness. The primary effect of overdose is respiratory depression. Withdrawal from CNS depressants can be life threatening.
8. Opioids (narcotics) come from the juice of the opium poppy, with opium being the natural product and morphine, codeine, and the semisynthetic heroin being easily derived from the poppy juice. Synthetic preparations such as meperidine (Demerol), pentazocine (Talwin), propoxyphene (Darvon), and methadone (Dolophine) have been developed in the vain search for a pain reliever with no addicting qualities.

9. Opioids are taken IV, orally, intramuscularly, and subcutaneously (skin popping). Overdose can be fatal, with respiratory depression being the most serious side effect. Withdrawal, though miserable (influenza-like symptoms), is not particularly life threatening.

10. Naloxone (Narcan) is an opioid-receptor blocker and is given in emergency rooms to treat opioid overdose. Naloxone causes an opioid-abstinence syndrome.

11. Stimulants include amphetamines and cocaine. Stimulants cause elation, grandiose thinking, talkativeness, and other less pleasant effects. The primary concerns in the event of overdose are agitation, tachycardia, cardiac arrhythmias, and convulsions. Withdrawal from stimulants, though miserable, is not particularly serious.

12. Hallucinogens include mescaline, marijuana, LSD, and PCP. Hallucinogens cause illusions, hallucinations, diminished ability to perceive time and distance, anxiety, and paranoid thinking. The primary effects of hallucinogenic overdose are intense "trips," psychotic reactions, and panic. Withdrawal from hallucinogens can cause anxiety, fear, and panic. However, physical withdrawal has not been found to be particularly serious.

13. Although several treatment approaches are effective, the therapeutic goal for most approaches is abstinence from the substance, although the patient might still be seeking a way to engage in "controlled use." (If the patient were able to do that, he or she probably would not qualify as "dependent" in the first place.)

14. Nursing interventions include group work, education, confrontation, tough love (simply not allowing oneself to be a participant in the patient's self-destruction), providing for physical and nutritional needs, and helping the patient become involved in AA and NA.

References

Allen LN: Drugs of abuse. In Keltner NL, Folks DG, editors: *Psychotropic drugs,* ed 3, St Louis, 2001, Mosby.

American Medical Association: Alcoholism and other drug dependencies are treatable diseases. www.ama-assn.org/ama/pub/article/3342-3627. Accessed 6/4/02.

American Psychiatric Association: *Diagnostic and statistical manual of mental disorders,* ed 4, text revision, Washington, DC, 2000, APA.

Ananth J et al: Missed diagnosis of substance abuse in psychiatric patients, *Hosp Community Psychiatry* 40:297, 1989.

Anton RF: Pharmacologic approaches to the management of alcoholism, *J Clin Psychiatry* 62(suppl 20):11, 2001.

Associated Press: Body of man in 1983 test exhumed, *Los Angeles Times,* p A-4, June 5, 1994.

Bachman J: One nurse's story of addiction and recovery, *Colorado Nurse* 101(1):11, 2001.

Bennett WJ: *The de-valuing of America: the fight for our culture and our children,* New York, 1992, Summit Books.

Carey KB: Emerging treatment guidelines for mentally ill chemical abusers, *Hosp Community Psychiatry* 40:341, 1989.

Castaneda R et al: Long-acting stimulants for the treatment of attention-deficit disorder in cocaine-dependent adults, *Psychiatr Serv* 51(2):169, 2000.

Chang PH, Steinberg MB: Alcohol withdrawal, *Med Clin North Am* 85(5):1191, 2001.

Cherpitel LJ: The epidemiology of alcohol-related trauma, *Alcohol Health Res World* 16(3):191, 1992.

Clinical News: Cocaine exposure in utero, *Am J Nurs* 98(6):9, 1998.

FDA Consumer: Drug approved to treat alcoholism, *FDA Consumer* 29(3):2, 1995.

Feldman M: "Whatdyaknow," Wisconsin Public Radio, June 4, 1994.

First MB et al: Changes in substance-related, schizophrenic, and other primarily adult disorders, *Hosp Community Psychiatry* 45(1):18, 1994.

Frezza M et al: High blood alcohol levels in women, *N Engl J Med* 322(2):95, 1990.

Frosch WA: An analytic overview of addictions. In Milkman HB, Shaffer HJ, editors: *The addictions,* Lexington, Mass, 1985, Lexington Books.

Gold M, Tabrah H: Update on the ecstasy epidemic, *J Addictions Nurs* 12(3/4):133, 2000.

Goodwin DW et al: Alcohol problems in adoptees raised apart from alcoholic biological parents, *Arch Gen Psychiatry* 28:238, 1973.

Gorski TT: Alcoholism: disease or addiction? *Professional Counselor,* p 15, Oct 1996. http://www2.cdc.gov/ncidod/aip/HepC/HepC.asp

Gorski TT: *Understanding the twelve steps,* New York, 1992, Simon & Schuster.

Hess D, DeBoer S: Ecstacy, *AJN* 102(4):45, 2002.

Hollister L et al: Clinical uses of benzodiazepines, *J Clin Psychopharmacol* 13(6):1S, 1993.

Kanayama G et al: Over-the-counter drug use in gymnasiums: an underrecognized substance abuse problem? *Psychother Psychosom* 70(3):137, 2001.

Keltner NL, Folks DG: *Psychotropic drugs,* St Louis, 2001, Mosby.

Kines M: The risks of caring too much, *Can Nurs* 95(8):27, 1999.

Lehne RA: *Pharmacology for nursing care,* ed 4, Philadelphia, 2001, WB Saunders.

Longo LP et al: Addiction: part II. Identification and management of the drug-seeking patient, *Am Fam Physician* 61(8):2401, 2000.

Lowinson JH et al: *Substance abuse: a comprehensive textbook,* ed 3, Baltimore, 2001, Williams & Wilkins.

Manissa Communication Group: Extract from kudzu vine curbs alcohol desire, *Addiction Lett* 9(12):4, 1993.

Manissa Communication Group: US trial confirms value of physician advice to reduce drinking, *Brown Univ Addiction Theory Appl* 16(8):4, 1997.

Mathias R: "Ecstasy" damages the brain and impairs memory in humans, *NIDA Notes* 14(4):10, 1999.

Mathias R: Methamphetamine brain damage in mice more extensive than previously thought, *NIDA Notes* 15(4):1, 2000.

Mathias R: NIDA clinical trials network begins first multisite tests of new science-based drug abuse treatment, *NIDA Notes* 15(6):10, 2001.

Meadows M: Prescription drug use and abuse, *FDA Consumer* 35(5):18, 2001.

Mueller LA, Ketcham K: *Recovering: how to get and stay sober,* New York, 1987, Bantam Books.

Muha L: Home drug tests: what concerned parents must know, *Good Housekeeping,* p 137, July 1997.

Nash JM: Addicted: why do people get hooked? *Time,* p 68, May 5, 1997.

News and Notes: New law permits office based heroin treatment, *Psychiatr Serv* 51(12):1583, 2000.

North American Nursing Diagnosis Association: *NANDA nursing diagnoses: definitions and classifications 2000-2001,* Philadelphia, 2000, NANDA.

Ohlms D: *Marijuana in the '90s,* 1993, Gary Whitaker Corp (videotape).

Peele S, Brodsky A, Arnold M: *The truth about addiction and recovery,* New York, 1991, Simon and Schuster.

Rawson R, Obert J, McCann M: *The neurobehavioral treatment manual,* Beverly Hills, Calif, 1990, Matrix Institute on Addictions. Quoted in Corrie D, editor: *CWASAINT trainee notebook,* Atlanta, 1993, Child Welfare Institute.

Regier DA et al: The de facto U.S. mental and addictive disorders service system: epidemiologic catchment area prospective, 1-year prevalence rates of disorders and services, *Arch Gen Psychiatry* 50:85, 1993.

Roberts A, Koob GF: The neurobiology of addiction, *Alcohol Health Res World* 21(2):101, 1997.

Robertson N: The intimate enemy: will that friendly drink betray you? *Modern Maturity* 35(1):28, 1992.

Rodgers JE: Addiction: a whole new view, *Psychology Today* 27(5):77, 1994.

Sancton T: The dossier on Diana's crash, *Time,* p 50, Oct 13, 1997.

Schiller MJ et al: Utility of routine drug screening in a psychiatric emergency setting, *Psychiatr Serv* 51(4):474, 2000.

Sinclair JD: Evidence about the use of naltrexone and for different ways of using it in the treatment of alcoholism, *Alcohol Alcohol* 36(1):2, 2001.

Steinberg ML et al: Sources of motivation in a couple's outpatient alcoholism treatment program, *Am J Drug Alcohol Abuse* 23(2): 191, 1997.

Stoffel VC: Occupational therapists roles in treating substance abuse, *Hosp Community Psychiatry* 45(1):21, 1994.

Surgeon General, Mental Health: *A Report from the Surgeon General,* Washington DC, 1999. Department of Health and Human Services.

Sullivan E, Bissell L, William E: *Chemical dependency in nursing,* Redwood City, Calif, 1998, Addison-Wesley.

Taylor B, Donoghue J: Club drugs—it's effects on our youth, *Alabama Nurse* 28(2):20, 2001.

Thomas J: Buprenorphine proves effective, expands options for treatment of heroin addiction, *NIDA Notes* 16(2):8, 2001.

Vastag B: Mixed message on prescription drug abuse, *JAMA* 285(17):2183, 2001.

Wegscheider S: *Another chance,* Palo Alto, 1981, Science and Behavior Books, Inc. http://www.samhsa.gov/statistics/statistics.html

Wegscheider-Cruse S: *Another chance: hope and health for the alcoholic,* Palo Alto, Calif, 2000, Family Science and Behavior Books.

Whitfield C, Davis J, Barker L: Alcoholism. In Barker LR, Burton JR, Zieve PD, editors: *Principles of ambulatory medicine,* Baltimore, 1986, Williams & Wilkins.

Whitten L: Conference highlights increasing GHB abuse, *NIDA Notes* 16(2):10, 2001.

Wray J: Psychophysiological aspects of methamphetamine abuse, *J Addictions Nurs* 12(3/4):143, 2000.

Wright K: A shot of sanity, *Discover* 9:47, 1999.

Zickler P: Brain imaging studies show long-term damage from methamphetamine abuse, *NIDA Notes* 15(3):11, 2000.

Zickler P: NIDA studies clarify developmental effects of prenatal cocaine exposure, *NIDA Notes* 14(3):5, 1999.

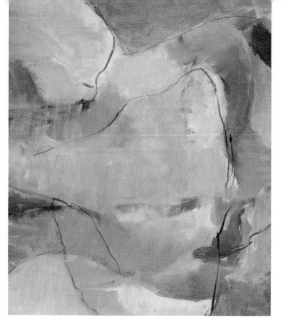

Chapter 36

Dual Diagnosis

Carol E. Bostrom

Learning Objectives

After reading this chapter, you should be able to:
- Define the term dual diagnosis.
- Describe major perspectives related to the etiologies for dual diagnosis.
- Understand issues related to treatment of dual-diagnosis patients.

Traditional psychiatric treatment has divided patients into distinct categories based on the thinking that one type of illness or disorder is primary or more urgent than another. Historically, patients were categorized as having either a mental illness or a substance-abuse or dependency problem. The mental illness or the substance problem was treated without recognition that another diagnosis was appropriate or that there were important issues underlying the substance abuse.

Based on 20 years of research and development, services for patients with mental illness and substance problems have emerged (Drake et al, 2001). The complexity of patients' problems and diagnoses with multiple impairments requires comprehensive therapeutic approaches and individual case management, as well as programming for groups of patients with common needs. Part of this effort is to reduce frequent hospitalization, or the "revolving-door syndrome." Patients with psychiatric illnesses and sub-stance problems have poor treatment outcomes with high rates of relapse, resulting in high costs in multiple settings.

This chapter discusses issues related to patients with dual diagnoses rather than focusing on specific interventions for this population of patients. Three issues in this area will be addressed: the concept of dual diagnosis, etiology, and treatment.

DUAL DIAGNOSIS DEFINED

Dual diagnosis usually refers to the presence of at least one psychiatric disorder in addition to a substance-abuse or dependency problem. The psychiatric disorder may be a mental illness, or a personality disorder. For example, a patient with the diagnoses of major depression and dependent personality disorder is not considered a dual-diagnosis patient. An example of a patient with a dual diagnosis is an individual with chronic schizophrenia and alcohol abuse. Another example is a patient with heroin dependency and antisocial personality disorder. Box 36-1 provides examples of dual-diagnosis combinations. Considering the number of axis I and axis II diagnoses, a multitude of combinations is possible. Therefore patients with dual diagnoses are a heterogeneous group. Research studies indicate that about 50% of patients with severe mental illness are affected by substance problems (Drake et al, 2001). Co-occurrence is common and should be expected (Minkoff, 2001).

Box 36-1 Examples of Dual Diagnoses

Axis I	Schizophrenia
	Alcohol abuse
Axis I	Cocaine abuse
Axis II	Antisocial personality disorder
Axis I	Major depression
	Anxiolytic dependency
Axis I	Major depression
	Marijuana abuse
Axis II	Borderline personality disorder

ETIOLOGY

The origins for diagnoses are discussed in the chapters specific to the disorders. One of the issues that mental health professionals traditionally deal with is which comes first—the mental illness or the substance problem. Because of this dilemma, the treatment of patients has been affected and has followed specific patterns. From the perspective that the mental illness occurred first, many reasons might account for the development of a substance problem. As is true for mental illnesses, heredity and biologic factors may predispose an individual to problems with substances. Some people may be predisposed to develop both a mental illness and a substance-abuse problem.

From the perspective that the substance abuse precedes mental illness, it follows that brain chemistry can be altered, that is, neurotransmitter imbalance or depletion. Chemicals can induce acute and chronic psychiatric problems. Substance-induced psychosis, schizophrenia, depression, and mania can occur in vulnerable individuals. Substance abuse can also lead to feelings of guilt, depression, and altered self-esteem. Repeated stimulant use can alter the dopamine system, and alcohol dependence can increase the positive symptoms of schizophrenia (Addington, Addington, 2001; Littrell, Littrell, 1999).

Many patients with mental illnesses use substances to feel calmer and as a coping strategy when stressed (Gomez et al, 2000). Others use substances to "numb" feelings that are too painful to deal with (Kasten, 1999). For patients experiencing psychotic symptoms, self-medicating with alcohol or drugs can help them feel better, less anxious, and can decrease the intensity of hallucinations temporarily but results in a worsening of symptoms after the effects of the alcohol or drug wears off. Furthermore, using substances does not result in bothersome and uncomfortable side effects when com-

pared with antipsychotics. Patients can also experience some degree of social acceptance when they drink alcohol or use drugs. With the decision to use a substance, the feeling of autonomy or power results in a temporary increase in self-esteem. Problems or issues are avoided, and patients feel better and temporarily in control of themselves.

Individuals with schizophrenia reported using alcohol, cannabis, and cocaine to decrease depression, decrease anxiety, and to decrease side effects of antipsychotic medication (Addington, Addington 2001). Individuals with depression sometimes used stimulants to boost their energy to be able to work or care for their families. The majority of patients who used substances found only temporary relief followed by an exacerbation of symptoms (Kasten, 1999).

Substance-abuse issues are often present in the population of individuals with personality disorders, particularly those with antisocial and borderline personality disorders (Cacciola et al, 2001). Some traits or behaviors of substance abusers are the same as those with personality disorders. Regardless of which disorder or problem came first, the existence of a substance problem, a mental illness, or a personality disorder, complicates diagnosis and treatment, prolongs rehabilitation, increases the incidence of relapse, and is associated with violence, incarceration, homelessness, and human immunodeficiency virus (HIV) and hepatitis (Drake et al, 2001). The complexity of these patients' problems requires a holistic, multifaceted approach.

TREATMENT ISSUES

Traditional models of treatment have focused on one issue at a time or on the most acute problem first. One model assumed that when mental illness was stabilized, substance use would subside. Another idea suggested stabilization of the mental illness would enhance patient participation and benefit from substance-abuse treatment. Some clinicians believed detoxification from chemical substances had to occur before other treatment was possible. All of these assumptions were valid for some patients, some of the time. For example, the severely psychotic patient needs antipsychotic medication before being able to participate in treatment groups. However, many problems exist with these models of treatment. For example, treatment was disrupted when patients had to be transferred from one unit or facility to another. Separate agencies or facilities with different treatment responsibilities did not coordinate and were unable to provide the multiple modalities needed in treatment for patients with dual diagnoses. Continuity of care was difficult to maintain, resulting in gaps in treatment. Consequently, follow-up care was sporadic, and care of patients was not managed effectively or adequately.

Another problem area arises from traditional differences between mental health and substance-abuse programs and staff philosophies. A substance-abuse program may discourage the use of all psychotropic medications, while the psychiatric unit may strongly encourage medication compliance. Confrontational groups on substance-abuse units differ greatly from support groups found in psychiatric units. For example, patients with religious delusions, preoccupations, and distortions find it difficult to participate and work in the 12-step recovery program in Alcoholics Anonymous and similar groups.

In the past, education and training for many staff members focused on the type of unit in which they would be working. As a result, staff members were often unprepared to treat patients with other problems. The lack of understanding of dual-diagnosis patients resulted in the staff having unrealistic expectations of what patients might accomplish during a specific time frame. Within the last 20 years, programs integrating treatment for mental illness and substance use have been increasing. Research is showing that integrated treatment programs have positive results—for example, remission of substance use and improvement in mental health (Drake et al, 2001).

Problems Affecting Program Development

Given the heterogeneity of dual-diagnosis patients, many issues have to be considered regarding program development. In working with these patients, the difficulty lies not so much with individual counseling, but with group programming. Treatment programs must identify which issues pertain to the majority of patients and can be managed in large groups and which issues should be addressed in smaller groups. Unique or highly personal issues are more appropriately handled on a one-to-one basis. For example, education about the disease concept of alcoholism or nutrition may be applicable to an entire group of patients. Education about the side effects of specific antidepressants may be appropriate for a select group of patients. A patient may want to discuss his or her feelings about acquired immuno-deficiency syndrome (AIDS) on a one-to-one basis before talking in a group. On a given day, changes in a patient's mental status may affect his or her ability to participate in a large group. Therefore staff members need to be flexible in assigning patients to specific groups.

Patients with dual diagnoses also need flexibility regarding the length of treatment rather than being assigned a fixed number of treatment days, sessions, or appointments. A program that is open-ended, occurs in stages, and provides support and empowerment may be necessary for patient compliance with treatment. For some patients, abstinence from a substance should be a goal of treatment and not a prerequisite. For example, a patient with chronic schizophrenia may be able to quit smoking marijuana with the nurse's help in developing assertiveness skills. For a patient with antisocial personality disorder, abstinence from alcohol may be required before treatment begins.

The staff needs to be aware of and prepared for dealing with issues and conflicts inherent in this population. In groups and in the milieu setting, patients with personality disorders may try to manipulate more regressed members. Depending on the substances abused, conflict may arise around degrees of addiction and drugs of choice ("Cocaine is worse than alcohol"; "My addiction is worse than yours"). Because most of these patients experience difficulties in concentration and memory, education groups must be structured with concrete concepts, simplified material, and repetition of material. Handouts and homework assignments may be helpful to practice and apply key treatment concepts.

Often, some patients in this group are perpetrators of violence, and others are victims. As a result, victims may find it difficult to participate in or even attend a group with perpetrators. Another problem exists with program funding. Finances are needed for a system of care with standards for treatment for the diverse populations in managed care systems. Some states are providing care for dual diagnosis patients (Minkoff, 2001). Hopefully, additional data will become available on this issue. In dealing with dual-diagnosed patients, it is evident that there are more issues and questions than answers. Continued work and development of models and strategies are necessary for these patients. The hope is that patients will ultimately benefit from more appropriate programming.

What benefits might a patient receive from dual-diagnosis treatment?

Psychotherapeutic Management

Effective treatment for patients with dual diagnoses must be multifaceted and multidisciplinary. Box 36-2 summarizes treatment components. Individual case management for social, medical, and emotional needs requires professional staff members to integrate their knowledge on addictions and mental illness. Education in both areas of mental illness and addictions, communication, cooperation, and collaboration among professional staff responsible for assessing, diagnosing, and treating patients are required.

Nurse-patient relationship

In working with dual-diagnosis patients, the nurse must use interventions specific to patients' individual needs, mental illness, and substance problem. The nurse deals with all of these areas simultaneously.

Trust between the nurse and patient develops if the patient believes that the nurse is knowledgeable, skilled, nonjudgmental, and empathic. Trust is especially important with the short length of inpatient hospitalization and outpatient areas along the continuum of care.

The nurse needs to ask patients about how substances affect their psychiatric symptoms, moods, and medication effects to assist patients with identifying the short- and long-term effects of using substances. The nurse needs to ask patients about physical or sexual abuse and refer for appropriate treatment (Kasten, 1999).

Monitoring patients for symptoms of withdrawal is ongoing. (Specific interventions for the relevant

| **Box 36-2** | Treatment Components for Patients with Dual Diagnosis |

Case management	Vocational counseling
Individual therapy	Referrals to community
Group therapy	resources
Skills training	Self-help groups
Education groups	Housing

mental illness and chemical dependency are found in other chapters.) The nurse is involved in teaching patients about the effects of alcohol and drugs on the mind and body. Patients need education about their mental illness and help with recognizing the signs of relapse regarding their specific mental illness and substance problem. Strategies for relapse prevention are based on each patient's individual needs.

A young male patient with schizophrenia abuses alcohol. How do the behaviors of these individual illnesses complicate treatment?

Psychopharmacology

Medication is specifically prescribed for patients according to their mental illness. Compliance with prescribed medication is supported by the nurse. Assistance with interferences to medication compliance are addressed, such as lack of money or transportation to purchase medications. The nurse teaches patients about side-effect management and about potential problems resulting from using alcohol or other substances with medication. (Refer to chapters on psychopharmacology for specific information.) Caution is used in prescribing anxiolytics, which cause dependence (e.g., benzodiazepines).

Case Study

Barbara Abel is a 28-year-old patient who was transferred from CCU because of imipramine (Tofranil) overdose and alcohol withdrawal. She is weak, shaky, and needs assistance with ambulation. Her diagnoses are major depression and alcohol abuse. Barbara states to the nurse, "I only wanted to sleep, have some peace, and forget my problems. I was so tired and couldn't eat or get out of bed. Ending it all would be better. I'd be happy again and like myself."

Barbara and her husband divorced 3 months ago because "he didn't understand that I needed to have a few drinks to sleep and forget my problems." She is an RN and was employed as a unit manager. She recently lost her job as a result of absenteeism. Barbara moved in with a friend who works as an accountant. Her friend occasionally uses cocaine to "stay on top of things" at work. Two of Barbara's coworkers encouraged her to seek treatment, but she was too tired to make an appointment with her psychiatrist.

Care Plan

Name: Barbara Abel _____   Admission Date: _____

DSM-IV-TR Diagnosis: Alcohol abuse _____

Assessment

Areas of strength: RN who has nursing and leadership skills. Has basic knowledge about her illnesses because of her education. Was medication-compliant before overdose. Two co-workers are supportive of her.

Problems: Suicide attempt with overdose, alcohol abuse, insomnia, anorexia, recently divorced, no place to stay, unemployed, drug-using friend.

Diagnoses

- At risk for violence: self-directed related to depressed mood as evidenced by suicide attempt.
- Low self-esteem related to divorce and job loss as evidenced by statement of not liking self.
- At risk for injury related to Tofranil overdose and alcohol withdrawal as evidenced by weakness and shakiness.
- Altered nutrition: less than body requirements related to depressed mood as evidenced by anorexia.
- Sleep-pattern disturbance related to stress as evidenced by insomnia.

Outcomes

Short-term goals: *Date met*
- Patient will verbalize plans for the future.   _____
- Patient will sleep 6 to 8 hours per night.   _____
- Patient will eat three balanced meals per day.   _____
- Patient will recognize and describe problems associated with drinking alcohol and depression.   _____
- Patient will make plans to live with a friend who does not use drugs or at halfway house.   _____

Long-term goals:
- Patient will practice abstinence from alcohol.   _____
- Patient will attend self-help groups like Double Trouble or Alcoholics Anonymous.   _____
- Patient will attend outpatient treatment.   _____
- Patient will be medication compliant.   _____
- Patient will live at halfway house or with a friend who does not abuse drugs.   _____
- Patient will participate in impaired nurse program through the state nurses' association.   _____

Planning/ Interventions

Nurse-patient relationship: Contract with patient to report to nurse if suicidal thoughts occur. Convey empathy and encourage verbalization of feelings. Reinforce strengths and accomplishments. Teach patient personal signs of relapse and relapse prevention for depression and alcohol abuse. Offer nutritious snacks. Assist patient with ambulation and ADLs when necessary and encourage independence when patient is able to perform own ADLs.

Psychopharmacology: Sertraline (Zoloft) 50 mg q AM; multivitamin 1 qd.

Milieu management: Invite and encourage patient to attend groups on assertiveness, stress management, alcohol, mental illness, medication education, and relapse prevention.

Evaluation

Patient denies suicidal ideation. She is expressing interest in employment and making alternative living arrangement. She is sleeping 6 hours per night and is eating three balanced meals per day. The patient is able to identify some positive characteristics of self and past accomplishments.

Referrals

Patient to attend weekly Double Trouble meetings and appointments for dual diagnosis treatment at a mental health clinic.

Milieu management

Enforcing the rules of the unit or program and setting limits provide structure and clear expectations for patients. Rules and limits help decrease manipulation and conflict among patients on the unit and within group sessions. Treatment groups focus on education about substances, mental illness, and medication. Stress-management, assertiveness, and community living skills are also a focus of treatment. The staff must be flexible in assigning patients to groups because of possible changes in mental status resulting from withdrawal from substances or exacerbation of mental illness symptoms. Supportive, gentle confrontation techniques are more effective than intense confrontation.

Attendance at self-help group meetings such as Alcoholics Anonymous, Narcotics Anonymous, and Double Trouble (for dual-diagnosis patients) begins while patients are on the inpatient unit, if possible. Referral to and involvement with outpatient programs, self-help groups, halfway houses, and vocational counseling is completed before discharge. Sometimes self-help groups are not attended until later in outpatient treatment, when the patient feels more motivated to attend. Continuity of treatment is necessary to prevent relapse and decrease recidivism.

CONTINUUM OF CARE

Dual-Diagnosis Treatment

An outpatient integrated treatment model has led to decreased use of inpatient services, a reduction or elimination of substance use, and improvement in other areas of life (Drake et al, 2001). Treatment that occurs in stages, is open-ended, empowers individuals, and extends beyond weeks or months can be beneficial for individuals with dual diagnoses. The following four-stage model conceptualized by Mueser and Kavanagh (2001) combines mental-health and substance-abuse treatment.

- *Engagement stage.* Establish trust and a working alliance with the patient to enable the patient to express fears and concerns about changing behaviors.
- *Persuasion stage.* At this point, the patient may still be abusing substances, but the nurse works to convince the patient that misuse is an important problem to motivate the patient to begin working on it. Emphasis is on past attempts to control use rather than on failure to address the problem.
- *Active treatment stage.* Treatment shifts to reduce substance use or maintain abstinence. Cognitive-behavioral counseling is used to address high-risk situations, along with attention to self-help groups and social skills training.
- *Relapse prevention stage.* When the patient has achieved substance control for at least 6 months, the goal is to guard against relapse. The focus with the patient is on social relationships, work, and housing. Working with the family to educate and support is a necessary part of treatment.

Key Concepts

1. Dual diagnosis can be defined as the co-morbid presence of a substance disorder and a mental illness or personality disorder.
2. The population of dual-diagnosis patients is heterogeneous.
3. Many issues must be addressed in treating dual-diagnosis patients because of their diverse abilities and needs.
4. Patients with dual diagnoses can benefit from treatment that integrates substance-use and mental-health services.
5. Dual-diagnosis treatment is based on the patient's needs according to stages.

References

Addington J, Addington D: Impact of an early psychosis program on substance use, *Psychiatr Rehabil J* 25(1):60, 2001.

Cacciola JS et al: Psychiatric comorbidity in patients with substance use disorders: do not forget axis I disorders, *Psychiatr Ann* 31(5): 321, 2001.

Drake R et al: Implementing dual diagnosis services for clients with severe mental illness, *Psychiatr Serv* 52(4):469, 2001.

Gomez MB et al: A description of precipitants of drug use among dually diagnosed patients with chronic mental illness, *Community Ment Health J* 36(4):351, 2000.

Kasten BP: Self-medication with alcohol and drugs by persons with severe mental illness, *J Am Psychiatr Nurses Assoc* 5(3):80, 1999.

Littrell KH, Littrell SH: Schizophrenia and comorbid substance abuse, *J Am Psychiatr Nurses Assoc* 5(2): S18, 1999.

Minkoff K: Developing standards of care for individuals with co-occurring psychiatric and substance use disorders, *Psychiatr Serv* 52(5):597, 2001.

Mueser KT, Kavanagh D: *Treating comorbidity of alcohol problems and psychiatric disorder, international handbook of alcohol dependence and problems,* New York, 2001, John Wiley & Sons.

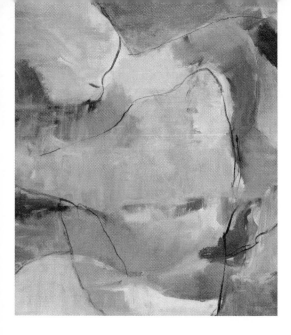

Chapter 37

Eating Disorders

Sandra Wood
Revised from a chapter by Linda K. Hinkle

Learning Objectives

After reading this chapter, you should be able to:

- Recognize the criteria and terminology used in *The Diagnostic and Statistical Manual of Mental Disorders, Text Revision* (DSM-IV-TR) for eating disorders.
- Recognize and describe objective and subjective symptoms of eating disorders.
- Describe current etiologic explanations for eating disorders.

- Describe treatment issues for professionals who deal with eating-disordered patients.
- Develop nursing care plans for patients with eating disorders.
- Evaluate the effectiveness of nursing interventions for patients with eating disorders.

American culture has become preoccupied with food, eating, weight, and fitness. Often, men and women structure their daily schedules around health-club and exercise programs in pursuit of increased attractiveness. Books on diets, nutrition, and fitness are being sold in greater numbers than ever before. All the while, media reports indicate more people are overweight, and there is a greater percentage of Americans, both adult and children, who qualify as obese than ever before (White, 2000). Restaurant portions have increased in size, while computer graphics enable advertisers to make already slender models look even thinner or more enhanced in areas such as the breasts. This practice provides an inaccurate image of the true size and shape of models. Therefore young women and, sometimes, men chase an unrealistic ideal. Life-threatening eating disorders can be the result. In this chapter, clinical examples, case studies, and nursing care plans focus on patients with the specific eating disorders of anorexia nervosa and bulimia nervosa. Although some professionals also consider obesity an eating disorder, discussing it is beyond the scope of this chapter.

ANOREXIA NERVOSA

DSM–IV–TR Criteria

The DSM-IV-TR (American Psychiatric Association, 2000) diagnostic criteria for anorexia nervosa are found in the box on page 498. Some studies suggest that anorexia nervosa is not necessarily a distortion of body image, but rather, a "weight phobia" (Pumariega et al, 1993). Anorectic patients generally do not lose their appetites. If they are hungry, patients with anorexia suppress their appetite in an effort to remain

Key Terms

Amenorrhea Absence of menstruation.

Anorexia nervosa Disorder characterized by restrictive eating resulting in emaciation, amenorrhea, disturbance in body image, and an intense fear of becoming obese.

Binge Eating an unusually large amount of food in a relatively short period.

Binge-eating disorder Disorder in which bingeing occurs without purging. Victims are generally overweight since they do not purge.

Bulimia nervosa Disorder characterized by binge eating, compensatory behavior, and overconcern with body shape and weight.

Emaciated Made excessively thin by the lack of nutrition.

Lanugo Fine, soft hair covering almost all parts of the body; developed for warmth in the absence of body fat.

Obesity Abnormal increase in the proportion of fat cells, mainly in the viscera and subcutaneous tissues of the body.

Purge Attempt to compensate for calories consumed via self-induced vomiting or abuse of laxatives, diuretics, or enemas.

DSM-IV-TR — Diagnostic Criteria for Anorexia Nervosa

A. Refusal to maintain body weight at or above a minimum normal weight for age and height

B. Intense fear of gaining weight or becoming fat, although underweight

C. Disturbance in the way in which one's body weight or shape is experienced, overvaluing of shape or weight, or denial of seriousness of low weight or weight loss

D. In women and female adolescents, the absence of at least three consecutive menstrual cycles

Restricting type: During an episode of anorexia nervosa, individuals do *not* engage in recurrent episodes of binge eating or purging

Binge-eating or purging type: During an episode of anorexia nervosa, individuals engage in recurrent episodes of binge eating or purging

Adapted from the American Psychiatric Association: *Diagnostic and statistical manual of mental disorders,* ed 4, text revision, Washington, DC, 2000, APA.

thin or get thinner. Weight or shape may be the most important influence on the person's sense of worth. They may deny that they are dangerously thin, or they may acknowledge their underweight status but then deny that their condition is problematic.

Menstruation may cease early in the illness, before significant weight loss has taken place, or menstruation may continue but be irregular and spotty. If menarche has not been reached, menstruation may not begin. One theory for the cause of amenorrhea suggests that lack of nourishment significantly slows pituitary functioning, fundamental to the menstrual cycle. Women must maintain a body mass index (BMI) of 18 or more to support menstruation (Muscari, 2002). Levels below this amount can result in amenorrhea, with accompanying reduction of hormone levels and blunting of some secondary sexual characteristics. In anorectic men, low sex drive and low testosterone may be the equivalent of amenorrhea in female patients (Walsh, Garner, 1997).

Anorexia is less common than bulimia, affecting up to 3.7% of women during their lifetime (Finelli, 2001). Women account for approximately 90% of the reported cases of anorexia nervosa, though anorexia in men appears to be increasing, as noted later in this chapter (Cohane, Pope, 2001). Onset varies from preadolescence to early adulthood with peaks at early adolescence (12 to 13 years of age) and later at 17 years of age. These ages correspond with transitional times in young people's lives (Potts, 1995). Initial morbidity and relapse from adolescent episodes is beginning to be seen in adulthood, as well as in adolescence. From 6% to 20% of anorectic patients die as a result of their illness (Grothaus, 1998), which is a rate greater than most other psychiatric disorders.

Behavior

The onset of anorexia is often insidious because the typical adolescent female victim usually portrays an image of being compliant and not causing problems for anyone. Because dieting and fad foods are common themes in adolescence and young adulthood, usually no one notices a change until the young woman has lost a significant amount of weight. A common premorbid personality profile is that of a perfectionistic and introverted girl with self-esteem and peer relationship problems, but victims can also be popular, accomplished, and active in school activities (Beumont, 1995).

Objective signs

The most observable behavior of anorexia nervosa is deliberate weight loss. Patients have such a need to control their weight that their eating behaviors change significantly. Patients with anorexia nervosa are in two groups: the dieters and the vomiters-purgers. The dieters are more often young women in the normal or slightly above normal weight range for height and build before the eating disorder begins. This group views losing weight as more probable if they simply eat less and avoid social situations in which they are expected to eat. Therefore they isolate themselves socially. Other members of this group increasingly isolate themselves from friends and family, often withdrawing to their rooms. It is not uncommon for these young women to be competitive, compulsive, and obsessive about their activities. They may participate in rigid exercise programs to help reduce their weight (Walsh, Garner, 1997).

CLINICAL EXAMPLE
Kristin, age 15, was in the normal weight range when she joined the school volleyball team with her friends. The first time they donned their uniforms, one of Kristin's friends called her "piano legs." Kristin was horrified and began to diet. In addition, she asked her parents to join the local health club so she could exercise to "keep in shape" for the team. Her entire day revolved around participation on the team to the extent that she forfeited all other social opportunities. She did not arrive home until after 9:00 PM on many occasions because she went to the health club to exercise after a volleyball game or after practice. Kristin lost 21 pounds before anyone noticed.

Compared with dieters, vomiters and purgers are more often overweight before the eating disorder begins, and their weight tends to fluctuate (Coners, Remschmidt, Hebebrand, 1999). These young women are more prone to dangerous methods of weight reduction, such as induction of vomiting or excessive use of laxatives or diuretics. These anorectic patients commonly deny concerns about weight and typically eat normally in social situations. After the meal, these individuals retreat to the nearest bathroom and purge themselves of the consumed food. Dental problems frequently occur in these patients because the acidic vomitus decays the enamel on their teeth. This group also may be susceptible to times when they binge eat, or uncontrollably eat large amounts of food, if unsuccessful in maintaining the severe dietary restriction they impose on themselves.

CLINICAL EXAMPLE
Tina was always a "chubby" child. When she was 23 years old, she lost considerable weight by dieting. Shortly thereafter, she began seriously dating and was married. Tina was thrilled with her new look and worked hard to maintain her weight loss, consistently keeping her weight slightly under the ideal for her height. After 2 years of marriage, Tina became pregnant. The thought of gaining weight during her pregnancy upset Tina greatly, and she vowed to herself never to let herself become "chubby" again. Before long, Tina's doctor noticed that she was not gaining weight at her monthly prenatal checkups and asked what she was eating. When she did a food log for the office nurse, her anorectic behavior was revealed.

Because the intake of nutrients is so low in anorectic patients, their bodies try to adjust by using less energy. Consequently, other physiologic processes are affected. Hypotension, bradycardia, and hypothermia are commonly reported. In addition, the skin is often dry, and lanugo may appear. Many patients have delayed gastric emptying, causing them to feel full much longer than do others. Thus these patients do not have the normal desire to eat as often as others. Therefore the belief they can "get by" on one small meal a day is common. Slower abdominal peristalsis combined with decreased intake leads to constipation. Dehydration is also common and can lead to irreversible renal damage. Pitting edema occurs in some anorectic patients, most often after attempts to gain weight by eating more food. Noticing the swelling, the young woman immediately stops trying to increase her weight and may even use diuretics to counteract edema, further complicating the problem. Many anorectic patients become hyperactive and are unable to relax. Insomnia is not uncommon; they often take early morning walks to "burn off" calories. In addition, osteopenia or osteoporosis may develop as a consequence of prolonged amenorrhea (Muscari, 2002). This bone mass loss may be irreversible if the anorexia goes on long enough. Moreover, studies have found ventricular dilatation, decreases in thickness of the left ventricular wall, alterations in the size of the cardiac chambers, and myocardial oxygen uptake that can lead to life-threatening cardiac arrhythmias (Mitchell, Pomeroy, Adson, 1997).

Because of starvation, anorectic patients become preoccupied with food and eating (Beumont, 1995). This preoccupation involves all aspects of life. Patients are often found reading multiple materials on food and dieting and attempting to control family meals because they believe they are the resident nutrition authorities in their households. Patients may engage in bizarre behavior regarding food and eating, such as hoarding food, preparing elaborate meals for others and not eating food they prepare. Going through elaborate rituals before and during eating may become a compulsion.

Subjective symptoms

An outstanding feature of anorexia nervosa is the conscious fear these patients have of losing control over the amount of food eaten, resulting in becoming fat. Patients are concerned about feeling obese, losing weight, or preventing weight gain. Some patients even say they would rather be dead than fat. This fear motivates them to begin dieting. The fear may be triggered by one event that seemed trivial to others, or one or more traumatic events for the patient. These patients may feel abandoned or inadequate, which can precipitate an overall feeling of helplessness (Grinspoon, 1997a). They try to combat feeling helpless by taking control of what they can control (i.e., their weight, the amount of food they eat). Most of the patient's energy becomes invested in this effort.

Besides problems with eating behavior and weight concern, anorectic persons have other psychologic symptoms known to be consequences of semistarvation. These patients exhibit depression, irritability, social withdrawal, lessened sex drive, and obsessional symptoms, those also seen in a research study of starvation. Garner (1998) speculates that the anorectic's bizarre behavior may be the result of the starvation. Fortunately, these symptoms often diminish with weight gain.

Etiology

The psychiatrist Hilde Bruch (1973) believed anorexia was caused by a number of specific disturbances. Today, most experts agree eating disorders causation is multifactorial with significant variance among individuals. Suggested contributing factors include biologic, sociocultural, family, cognitive, behavioral, and psychodynamic factors.

Biologic factors

Earlier in this century, physiologic disturbances were postulated as causative in anorexia. Currently, researchers believe the physiologic abnormalities found in anorectic patients are mostly a result of semistarvation and purging behavior rather than the cause of disordered eating (Fairburn, 1995a). An exception may be increased serotonin levels. Studies have found that, even after long-term weight restoration and recovery, anorectics have increased cerebrospinal fluid (CSF) levels of 5-hydroxyindoleacetic acid (5-HIAA), the major metabolite of serotonin. Serotonin activity is known to have inhibitory effects on a number of areas and may lead to food restriction caused by inhibited appetite, as well as to the rigid, inhibited, anxious, and obsessional behaviors seen in anorectics (Kaye, 1995).

In addition, researchers have found premorbid obesity is a risk factor for anorexia, although this may be a general risk factor for dieting rather than for anorexia in particular. Additionally, approximately 47% of anorectics have severe gastrointestinal problems in their early feeding history, suggesting that early feeding problems may contribute to the development of the disorder (Cooper Z, 1995).

Sociocultural factors

Feminist theorists highlight the role of Western philosophical, political, and cultural history in the development of eating disorders. The increased incidence of eating disorders in this century is recognized as corresponding to an increasingly and unrealistically thin beauty ideal for women (Brumberg, 1997; Rand, Wright, 2000). In addition, the American culture has advanced the notion that body weight is a matter of personal choice and that shape can be changed at will. The advent of computer imaging has resulted in the "enhancement" of photos on the Internet by those responding to the current societal standard of beauty. Thus the images of healthy-looking models can be altered to appear thinner or more "well endowed" in the breasts than they actually are. These images encourage dieting, which, it is widely agreed, is a major predisposing factor to both anorexia nervosa and bulimia nervosa (White, 2000).

Another factor is the relational orientation of women, which creates a vulnerability to the opinions of others, particularly during adolescence (Striegel-Moore, 1995). The American culture stresses the importance of physical attractiveness in obtaining approval, and, because of the thin beauty ideal, girls believe the way to get approval is to try to be thinner. Lack of approval is interpreted as related to a less than ideal body size that causes girls to begin dieting.

Family factors

Several studies of monozygotic (identical) and dizygotic (fraternal) twins suggest a genetic component to the causation of anorexia (Grinspoon, 1997a). Family environment may also play a role. Emotional restraint, enmeshed relationships, rigid organization in the family, tight control of child behavior by parents, and avoidance of conflict are other etiologic factors (Grinspoon, 1997a; Vandereycken, 1995). Odd eating habits and strong concerns about appearance and weight within other family members, especially mothers and sisters, have also been described. However, the extent to which the observed family problems of anorectics are consequences of the disorder rather than causal factors cannot be determined.

Cognitive and behavioral factors

Behavioral theorists hold that anorectic behavior develops and is maintained as a function of environmental contingencies. Rejecting food and losing weight, for example, may be positively reinforced by attention from others. Behavioral treatments such as assertiveness training and cognitive restructuring are widely used and are thought to be beneficial for the anorectic. Treatment may also involve use of reinforcement contingent on weight gain and changed eating behaviors (Grothaus, 1998).

Psychodynamic factors

Modern psychoanalytic theorists have stressed the role of sexuality in anorexia nervosa. In addition, some clinicians have suggested that eating disorders may be related to an early history of sexual abuse. However, research finds the rate of sexual abuse history in individuals with eating disorders is similar to that found in the general psychiatric population. Sexual abuse may therefore predispose one to psychiatric disorders in general, rather than eating disorders in particular (Palmer, 1995).

In addition, some researchers have suggested that anorexia involves a regression to a prepubertal state, so that the adolescent does not mature physically or emotionally. Regression is reinforced when the anorectic adolescent's dependency needs are met. The conscious fear of becoming fat is thought to be the symbolic expression of becoming bigger, or growing up, supposedly the real, unconscious fear of the anorectic. Other psychoanalytic theorists suggest the drive for thinness may be an attempt to reduce the control of an overcontrolling maternal figure (Johnson, 1995).

Another theory describes anorexia nervosa as an obsession with weight stemming from a fear of being out of control. In response to this fear, patients use reaction formation to organize their lives with a set of rules and regulations for everything they do. They experience a tremendous amount of anxiety if one of their rules is broken and attempt to regain control by tightening the rules and punishing themselves for their "failure."

Conclusion

Agreement among experts exists that the etiology of anorexia nervosa is multifactorial. Biologic, sociocultural, family, cognitive, behavioral, and psychodynamic factors all may contribute to the disease. However, factors leading to dieting may differ from factors leading to onset of actual eating-disordered behavior (Cooper Z, 1995). In addition, factors contributing to the maintenance of anorexia may also be different than those leading to its development. Today, most research focuses on factors contributing to the onset of dieting (White, 2000). Greater emphases on factors contributing to the development and maintenance of eating-disordered behavior may yield a better understanding of this disorder and more effective prevention of the disease. Research on adult-onset eating disorders may also prove fruitful.

Critical Thinking Question

Some theorists contend adolescent eating disorders are an expression of ambivalence toward becoming an adult. Explain how this thought might have some validity.

Psychotherapeutic Management

Psychotherapeutic management is geared toward the following three major objectives: (1) increasing self-esteem so that patients do not need the artificial perfection they believe thinness provides; (2) increasing weight to at least 90% of the average body weight for the patient's height and age; and (3) helping patients reestablish appropriate eating behavior.

When patients are in the starvation phase of the illness and malnutrition has become a serious medical problem, treatment usually occurs in a medical environment in which appropriate supplies and equipment, such as intravenous and feeding-tube apparatuses, are readily available for feeding the patient if she will not do so herself. When the medical crisis is resolved, patients are transferred to a psychiatric unit or are seen on an outpatient basis in which effective psychotherapeutic intervention can occur.

Nurses may encounter anorectic patients either on an inpatient basis in a medical or psychiatric unit or on an outpatient basis in a physician's office, clinic, or school. In any setting, a multidisciplinary treatment approach is crucial. Members of the treatment team should include a physician, a nurse, a dietitian, and a psychotherapist specializing in the treatment of eating disorders. These patients need thorough medical and psychiatric assessment, medical monitoring, nutritional education and counseling, and psychotherapy. Assessment should include differential diagnosis of other psychiatric conditions, including affective disorders, personality disorders, schizophrenia, anxiety disorders such as obsessive-compulsive disorders, and substance abuse or dependence. Physical conditions that should be ruled out include thyroid conditions, bowel disease or other gastrointestinal conditions, pancreatitis, cancer, or the effects of medications. If eating behaviors are caused by one of these conditions, effective treatment will consist of different treatments than if the eating behaviors are the result of an eating disorder. Patients with diabetes may also develop eating disorders, thus increasing their risk of serious medical complications of diabetes in the future and the risk of ketoacidosis in the present (Poirier-Solomon, 2001).

Working with anorectic patients presents a challenge to the psychotherapeutic team as patients continue the struggle to maintain control. When the treatment team requires weight gain, patients perceive themselves as losing control, which triggers the unconscious feeling of helplessness. Consciously, patients once again experience the fear of becoming fat. This fear underlies the need to gain more control, restarting the vicious cycle. Key nursing interventions for patients with eating disorders are listed in the box below.

Nurse-patient relationship

Because most anorectic patients are in treatment under duress, the challenge for the nurse is to develop a therapeutic alliance. Patients believe the nurse is there simply to make them gain weight, so the nurse is perceived as an enemy, not an ally. Principles of therapeutic interaction that facilitate the nurse-patient relationship include the following:

- Convey warmth and sincerity. Patients need to believe the nurse genuinely cares about and understands their effort to overcome their ambivalence about being in treatment. Increas-

Key Nursing Interventions for Patients with Eating Disorders

- Monitor daily caloric intake and electrolyte status—patients should not gain too much weight too quickly.
- Observe patients for signs of purging or other compensation for food consumed.
- Monitor activity level, and encourage appropriate levels of activity for patient.
- Weigh daily while in hospital, but encourage patient to diminish focus on weight after refeeding.
- Plan for dietitian to meet with patients to (a) provide accurate information on nutrition, (b) discuss a realistic and healthy diet, and (c) assist the nurses in monitoring the nutritional intake of the patient (particularly crucial to patients who are diabetic or pregnant).
- Encourage use of therapies or support groups to attain healthy weight and prevent relapse.
- Promote patient decision making concerning things besides food.
- Promote positive self-concept and perceptions of body, as well as interactions with others.

ing the patients' self-esteem is a primary objective in recovery.

- Listen empathically. Although patients are likely to deny that weight is a problem, they do admit to feeling extremely lonely and tired of compulsively striving to meet unreachable goals.
- Be honest. Patients enter treatment distrustful of everyone. Honesty is essential to a trusting relationship.
- Set appropriate behavioral limits. Because of control needs, patients may attempt to manipulate the nurse. A clear contract must be established between the nurse and patient to establish trust and to minimize power struggles.
- Assist patients in identifying their positive qualities. Because self-esteem is low, patients need to see concrete evidence of redeeming and positive qualities in themselves.
- Collaborate with patients. To elicit cooperation, engage patients in the planning process, which should foster trust and a sense of control that will diminish the need to maintain control through anorexia.
- Teach patients about their disorder. The information received about anorexia should decrease denial of problems and help patients understand the disease's effects on their bodies and minds.
- Determine the patients' ability to view weighing. Often, anorectics need to be weighed with their backs to the scale. The overall therapeutic goal is to help patients reduce their focus on body weight.
- Initiate a behavior modification program that rewards weight gain with meaningful privileges. Although the idea of gaining weight is stressful to patients, it is crucial to recovery. As soon as a safe weight is attained, allow patients more control of their own progress and program as long as they do not "backslide".
- Model and teach appropriate social skills. Acquiring social skills, particularly expressing emotion assertively, is crucial for patients with anorexia.
- Help patients identify and express bodily sensations and feelings. Typically, anorectic patients have little bodily awareness, other than a distorted perception of their size.
- Identify non–weight-related interests of the patient. If reactivated, these interests can reduce anxiety as patients invest their energies in areas not related to eating.

Tips for Professionals from Persons Recovering from Eating Disorders*

Be wary of rigidly applying DSM-IV-TR criteria in the detection of eating disorders.

- Some patients never binge or purge but control weight with exercise and restriction of intake.
- Some patients do not stop menstruating, though there may be changes in their cycles.
- Depression, anxiety, neglect, and domestic violence may predispose patients to eating disorders or be seen comorbidly with them. If only these disorders are treated without treating the eating disorder, efforts will likely fail.
- Patients' concentration on exactness and perfection may lead them to deny their illness by rationalizing that if they do not exhibit *all* the criteria of the disorder, they do not have the disorder.
- Patients may recognize that their body image is distorted but may be unable to stop their destructive behavior.
- Not all eating-disordered patients have rituals about eating. They may simply avoid being in situations in which they have to eat in front of others.

When educating adolescents about eating disorders, avoid using films or other graphic materials that might teach the teens more ways to "beat the system" regarding eating and maintaining healthy weight.

Dishonesty (lying to self and others) is a hallmark of patients with eating disorders. Honesty toward self and others is the key to recovery and to relapse prevention.

Watch for the onset of eating disorders at times of major life transition with increased pressure on an individual to "fit in" or "adjust." These times include the move to middle school from elementary school, the move to high school from junior high or middle school, and graduation from high school with the move to college or a job.

Patients with eating disorders believe calories are everywhere and go to great lengths to avoid them, including not smelling food or licking stamps for fear calories will be absorbed.

Media images of very thin models and celebrities may be viewed by very young girls as an ideal to be achieved, but most patients use media images of thinness to justify their behavior after becoming eating disordered.

*The author wishes to acknowledge the generous sharing of a local chapter of the Anorexia and Associated Disorders Association of Indianapolis support group who offered ideas from their experience and gave information to help professionals deal with individuals such as themselves. Their input enriched this chapter.

Psychopharmacology

Presently, no psychopharmacologic agent is approved specifically for anorexia nervosa. Management with medication of anxiety, depression, somatic disturbances, or other co-morbid conditions is appropriate and may assist in treatment of the patient's anorexia. Small amounts of anxiolytics may help patients with eating, if given just before meals. Prokinetic agents may assist digestion in patients who experience delayed gastric emptying (Garfinkel, Walsh, 1997). Gastric enzymes to promote digestion may be particularly useful in initial refeeding of anorectic patients.

Milieu management

- Provide a tour of the setting to prepare the patient for inpatient or outpatient treatment so fears will be reduced (Fichter, 1995).
- Provide a warm, nurturing atmosphere. It is important for patients to feel support to reduce anxiety and increase self-esteem.

- Closely observe patients. Avoidance behaviors need to be identified to plan appropriate interventions. Common behaviors include hiding food in a paper napkin to be discarded later, leaving bread crusts on the plate and discarding the rest, discarding food into plants or out of the window, spilling food while eating so it cannot be determined how much the patient really ate, and holding food in the mouth to be discarded when the patient brushes his or her teeth. Respond to these behaviors with nonjudgmental confrontation, conveying understanding of fears of weight gain and other related issues. Neither pity nor punishment will be helpful.
- Encourage the patient to approach a team member if he or she feels the need to purge. Expression of feelings reduces anxiety and helps patients discover other alternatives to vomiting.

Case Study

Sarah, a 17-year-old girl, was brought to the hospital by her parents and her outpatient therapist, whom she had been seeing weekly for 1 month. Sarah and the therapist had a contract of a 2-pound weight gain every week. Sarah, however, had continued to lose weight. On admission, she was 5 feet 5 inches tall and weighed 86 pounds. Sarah was strongly opposed to her hospitalization and denied that she had a problem.

Sarah is the youngest of three daughters, ages 27, 24, and 17, a late addition to her middle-class family. Sarah's parents admitted that she had been steadily losing weight for the last 6 months. At first, Sarah's parents believed that she was "just dieting" as teenagers frequently do; but when they began to see her ribs and vertebrae through her nightgown, they became gravely concerned.

Sarah was recently named recipient of a scholarship to go to college. She has been active in school activities and was well liked by her teachers because of her hard work. Although she appeared to have many friends, Sarah claimed she only had one real friend.

Sarah said her obsession with weight began approximately 6 months ago when the family went to visit the oldest daughter, whom Sarah had always idolized. One afternoon, the three sisters went berry picking, and the oldest told Sarah, "Don't eat all the berries, or you'll grow into a real chub!" Sarah interpreted this to mean that her sister thought she was fat. She became obsessed with food, suddenly deciding to become a vegetarian. She took over the role of planning menus and educating

the family on proper nutrition. When the mother attempted to intervene, Sarah would scream that she knew what she was doing and was tired of being treated like a baby. If the mother attempted further control over Sarah's eating behavior, she refused to eat at all. The situation in the home deteriorated until there was little communication between the family members and Sarah. The family watched helplessly as she engaged in irrational rituals and lost a large amount of weight. At the point that she began to look very thin, they persuaded Sarah to seek help; however, she continued to lose weight during outpatient therapy.

Sarah is a likable young lady. Many of the other adolescents in the hospital were attracted to her and wanted to be her friend. However, the patients noticed Sarah's odd eating habits, such as mixing cornflakes in vanilla pudding and pouring cranberry juice over cereals. Sarah always dressed in baggy overalls and wore oversized sweaters. When other patients asked Sarah if she felt cold, she quietly told them that she did not want them to stare at her fat body, a comment that tended to "put off" her peers.

During break times, Sarah was found writing morbid poetry, which contained subtle suicidal messages. She preferred to be alone and became irritable and rude when asked to participate in group therapy sessions. Sarah tried to be as compliant as she thought others wanted her to be; however, the lack of control she experienced in the hospital made this difficult and added to her anxiety and discomfort.

- Involve the patient's family in treatment, when appropriate. If the family denies the problem or is not supportive of treatment, the family may need to be excluded from the treatment team. If parents, particularly of minors, provide emotional support, treatment efforts have a greater chance of success. Families need to understand the disorder and how to deal with it to help patients recover. Family therapy of anorectic adolescents is a crucial treatment component.

- Respond with consistency. The behavioral program or treatment regimen implemented must be adhered to, at all times, by the entire staff. Otherwise, patients quickly discover areas to manipulate.
- Involve the dietitian in the treatment plan. Proper nutrition can be taught while providing patients with an opportunity to select menus. Increase caloric intake gradually to increase patient cooperation in the weight gain program.

▌Care Plan

Name: <u>Sarah Hopkins</u>   Admission Date: _____

DSM-IV-TR Diagnosis: <u>Anorexia nervosa</u>

Assessment	**Areas of strength:** intelligence; past achievements; likableness; past healthy interpersonal relationships; good personal hygiene; some insight into reasons for hospitalization; family support. **Problems:** low weight, disturbed body image, low self-esteem, depression, lack of accurate knowledge regarding nutrition, manipulativeness.
Diagnoses	• Alteration in nutrition: less than body requirements, related to not eating enough nutrients, as evidenced by continued weight loss and inappropriate eating habits. • Disturbance in body image, related to feeling fat when actually underweight, as evidenced by inappropriate dress and comments about how fat she is. • Disturbance in self-esteem, related to feeling as if she is not a "good girl," as evidenced by suicidal messages in poetry and by social withdrawal. • Knowledge deficit in proper nutrition, related to eating an imbalanced diet, as evidenced by odd eating habits and refusal to eat certain foods.

Outcomes

Short-term goals: *Date met*
- Patient will gain 1 pound per week.   _____
- Patient will identify two positive qualities about herself.   _____
- Patient will discuss feelings of losing control.   _____

Long-term goals:
- Patient will gain at least 20 pounds within 6 months.   _____
- Patient will verbalize knowledge of illness and proper nutrition. _____
- Patient will identify at least three alternative coping mechanisms to use when feeling out of control.   _____
- Patient will verbalize increased comfort in relating to peers.   _____

Planning/ Interventions	**Nurse-patient relationship:** Establish a contract to meet at least 3 times a week to discuss feelings; express concern for the patient; encourage verbalization of feelings about depression and/or lack of control; encourage patient to identify positive qualities about herself. **Milieu management:** Encourage patient to attend meals and sit with peers; encourage participation in group therapy to discuss feelings with peers; encourage patient to share positive qualities of herself with peers; maintain consistency of unit rules and make certain patient is adhering to them.
Evaluation	Patient gained 2 pounds in the first 10 days of hospitalization; attended all unit activities; attended individual therapy with Ms. Mills, R.N.
Referrals	Patient has been given information about an eating disorder support group in her community and a person to contact regarding the group.

- Encourage patient attendance at group therapy sessions. Providing an opportunity for patients to participate in a group with peers helps them see that they are not alone in having difficulty expressing feelings and dealing with developmental issues. Nurse-led support groups encourage patients to share issues, feelings, and fears (Owen, Fullerton, 1995).
- Recommend psychotherapeutic groups and individual psychotherapy with a qualified therapist. These sessions may be particularly beneficial following significant weight gain (Fichter, 1995). Before weight restoration, the patient may have difficulty benefiting from psychotherapy because of impaired cognitive processing (Garner, 1998).
- Facilitate patient's transition to outpatient treatment providers after hospitalization. Anorectic patients may relapse or even die because of lack of appropriate outpatient follow-up (Fichter, 1995). A comprehensive continuum of care provides the best option for relapse prevention in view of the chronic nature of the disease (Cummings et al, 2001).

Critical Thinking Question

A 17-year-old girl remarks to you that she feels fat and repulsive. You do not observe that the patient is overweight. How do you begin to assess if the patient is suffering from an eating disorder?

BULIMIA NERVOSA

DSM-IV-TR Criteria

The DSM-IV-TR box presents the diagnostic criteria for bulimia nervosa. The North American Nursing Diagnosis Association (NANDA) diagnoses that are appropriate for eating disorders are listed in the following box.

The DSM-IV-TR reports bulimia nervosa usually begins in adolescence or early adult life, primarily in women. The prevalence of bulimia among adolescents and young adult women is thought to be approximately 1% in the general population and 4% among young adult women (Grinspoon, 1997a). The usual course of the disorder is chronic and intermittent over a period of many years. Most commonly, the binge periods alternate with periods of restrictive eating.

DSM-IV-TR	Diagnostic Criteria for Bulimia Nervosa

A. Recurrent episodes of binge eating in a short time period with intake much greater than average
B. A feeling of lack of control over eating behaviors during the eating binges
C. Recurrent inappropriate compensatory behavior in order to prevent weight gain, such as self-induced vomiting, use of laxatives or diuretics, strict dieting or fasting, vigorous exercise, or taking diet pills
D. Binge eating and inappropriate compensatory behaviors both occur, on average, at least twice a week for 3 months
E. Self-evaluation is unduly influenced by body shape and weight
   Purging type: Regularly engages in self-induced vomiting or the use of laxatives, diuretics, or enemas
   Nonpurging type: Regularly uses strict diet, fasting, or vigorous exercise, but does not regularly engage in purging

Adapted from the American Psychiatric Association: *Diagnostic and statistical manual of mental disorders,* ed 4, text revision, Washington, DC, 2000, APA.

Behavior

The word bulimia literally means to have an insatiable appetite. The term is often used to describe massive overeating and is used interchangeably with binge eating or bingeing. Other names, such as bulimorexia, have also been associated with binge and vomiting behaviors (Russell, 1997).

Until recently, bulimia nervosa was considered to be a part of anorexia nervosa because almost one half of patients diagnosed with anorexia were observed to have binge-eating episodes. Bulimia nervosa is now accepted as a separate disorder. The true prevalence of bulimia nervosa is unknown because many patients hide their eating-disordered behaviors (Orbanic, 2001). Only individuals who seek medical attention (usually for gastrointestinal or menstrual disturbances) or psychiatric help are actually identified.

The onset of the illness is usually between the ages of 15 and 24 years. The disease may develop after anorexia nervosa but almost always occurs following a period of dieting (Beumont, 1995). The dieting predisposes the individual to binge eating, and purging develops as a means of compensating for calories ingested during the binge and attempting to prevent weight gain. The individual continues restrictive eating during the disorder, which precipitates binge eating and then purging, thus perpetuating the cycle.

DSM-IV and NANDA Diagnoses Related to Eating Disorders

DSM-IV*

Anorexia nervosa
Bulimia nervosa
Eating Disorder NOS/Binge eating disorder

NANDA†

Anxiety
Body image, Disturbed
Coping, Compromised family
Coping, Disabled family
Coping, Ineffective individual
Denial, Ineffective
Fluid volume, Risk for deficient
Fluid volume, Risk for imbalanced
Nutrition, less than body requirements, Imbalanced
Nutrition, more than body requirements, Imbalanced
Powerlessness
Self-esteem, Chronic low
Social isolation

*From the American Psychiatric Association: *Diagnostic and statistical manual of mental disorders*, ed 4, text revision, Washington, DC, 2000, APA.
†From the North American Nursing Diagnosis Association: *NANDA nursing diagnoses: definitions and classifications*, 2000, Philadelphia, NANDA.

CLINICAL EXAMPLE

Mary, age 28, was a young professional with an active social life. Although she was approximately 15 pounds overweight, Mary used her sense of humor to hide any serious concern she had about her appearance. However, Mary worried that her weight might deny her a highly prized job she wanted. Before applying for the job at a prestigious banking firm, Mary began dieting and ate less food than did her friends at lunch. When she arrived home, however, Mary found herself hungry and secretly raided her refrigerator, making several sandwiches before dinner. Despite feeling guilty over her uncontrolled "snacking," Mary ate dinner with her roommate. After dinner, feeling uncomfortably full, Mary retreated to the bathroom and vomited until she felt empty. She vowed to try harder to diet the next day, only to have a similar experience.

It is important to distinguish overeating from binge eating. To meet DSM-IV-TR diagnostic criteria for a binge episode, the eating behavior must qualify as an "objective bulimic episode." That is, the person consumes an unusually large amount of food in a relatively short period (e.g., less than 2 hours). The amount of food eaten is considered by others to be atypically large for the particular situation. Additionally, there is a feeling of lack of control over eating during the binge (Orbanic, 2001).

Objective signs

Most bulimic patients are secretive about their behavior. A variety of foods may be eaten during a binge, but the most common is high-calorie, high-carbohydrate food easily ingested in a short period. Some bulimics visit several different fast-food restaurants or grocery stores during a binge so that no one knows how much they are eating at once. Some patients with bulimia have been caught shoplifting food. Most binges occur in the evening or at night. The amount of calories consumed during a binge varies, but it may be as much as 30 times the recommended daily allowance (Beumont, 1995). There is a tendency to eat rapidly during the binge.

Patients report that their bulimic episodes usually end when they begin to induce vomiting, are physically exhausted, suffer from painful abdominal distension, are interrupted by others, or have simply run out of food. After a binge, patients promise themselves to adhere to a strict diet and vow never to binge again. Many bulimics resume their usual schedules as if they had never been interrupted. The frequency of binges varies greatly, depending on the patient. Some patients report having several episodes a day; others report losing control two or three times a week (Orbanic, 2001).

Medical complications in bulimic patients depend on the form and frequency of purging and can include previously described mechanical irritation and dilatation of the stomach resulting from binge eating. Fluid and electrolyte abnormalities may result from self-induced vomiting or abuse of laxatives or diuretics and may include dehydration, hyponatremia, hypochloremia, hypokalemia, and metabolic alkalosis and acidosis. Self-induced vomiting and laxative abuse can cause mechanical irritation and injuries to the gastrointestinal tract. Abuse of laxatives, diuretics, and diet pills can result in addiction. Laxatives can lead to reflex constipation, and both laxatives and diuretics are associated with rebound edema.

Use of ipecac syrup to induce vomiting is particularly dangerous; it can be toxic and cause fatal cardiomyopathy. Bulimics often have menstrual irregularities or enlarged salivary glands, particularly the parotid glands. Erosion of the dental enamel from chronic vomiting often occurs. Russell's sign, callousing of the knuckles of the fingers used to induce vomiting, is also common. Pancreatitis also has been reported in bulimics (Muscari, 2002).

Subjective symptoms

Although most bulimic patients have a normal body weight, they are gravely concerned about their body shape and weight. Loss of control over eating causes them great distress, and similar to anorectic patients, they express a fear of becoming fat.

Moods vary considerably among bulimic patients. Some bulimics have reported feeling weak and constrained before a binge, followed by either continued anxiety or relief from tension during the binge (Palmer, 1995). Patients report feeling anxious, lonely, bored, or having an uncontrollable craving for food before the binge. The anxiety present before the binge is replaced with guilt after the binge. If the anxiety is not relieved after the binge, patients feel angry and agitated; many become depressed. Because depression is common in bulimic patients, it is discussed in a separate section in this chapter. Substance abuse and anxiety disorders also occur at a higher than normal rate among bulimics.

Most bulimic patients induce vomiting to allay the fear of becoming fat. Many patients begin to self-induce vomiting by sticking their fingers, a toothbrush, or an eating utensil down their throats, a dangerous practice, because patients have swallowed objects used to induce vomiting. Over time, vomiting becomes easier and may require only slight abdominal pressure or no physical manipulation at the end of the binge (Mendell, Logemann, 2001). Some bulimics eat a "marker" food at the beginning of the binge and then vomit until this food comes back up. This practice is ill-conceived because food is quickly mixed in the stomach. Furthermore, although bulimics believe self-induced vomiting rids them of all binge calories, researchers have determined that only a partial amount of calories consumed can be regurgitated. Additionally, abuse of laxatives or diuretics primarily causes fluid loss rather than a reduction in absorbed calories (Orbanic, 2001).

Other compensatory behavior may include the neglect of insulin requirements in patients with diabetes mellitus, misuse of saunas, excessive use of enemas or suppositories, chewing and spitting out food without swallowing, rumination (chewing,

swallowing, regurgitating, and then chewing and swallowing again), and breast-feeding babies for a long time (Garner, 1998).

Etiology

Similar to anorexia, the cause of bulimia nervosa is thought to be multifactorial, with biologic, sociocultural, family, cognitive, behavioral, and psychodynamic contributing factors. Many of the factors thought to precipitate anorexia are also thought to be involved in the cause of bulimia. The focus of this discussion therefore will be on the proposed causes of bulimia that are different than those postulated for anorexia.

Biologic factors

Brain chemistry has been increasingly implicated in studies relating to the cause of eating disorders, with several neuroendocrine and neurotransmitter abnormalities demonstrated in dieters and those demonstrating symptoms of eating disorders. Biologic and genetic factors have also been implicated in the cause of bulimia and anorexia. Most researchers believe that illness symptoms are related to the physiologic state of the victims and will remit when weight is restored. However, serotonin activity appears to be an exception. Serotonin activity continues to be abnormal for some eating-disordered patients even after weight restoration (White, 2000). It has been proposed that, as in depression, there is generally lowered serotonin activity in the brains of bulimics (Pirke, 1995). Binge eating is then seen as a form of self-medication to raise the levels of serotonin. This theory correlates with use of selective serotonin reuptake inhibitor (SSRI) antidepressants, particularly fluoxetine (Prozac) in the treatment of bulimia.

Sociocultural factors

These factors are thought to be the same as those for anorexia nervosa (stated earlier in this chapter).

Family factors

As with anorexia nervosa, a heritable component for bulimia has been proposed. Twin studies have found a higher concordance rate for bulimia in monozygotic than that in dizygotic twins (Strober, 1995). In addition, mood disorders and substance-use disorders are found at a high rate in the families of bulimics (Strober, 1995), which may be a result of both biologic and environmental factors.

From self-report studies, bulimics tend to view their families as having a great deal of conflict and as disorganized, lacking in nurturance, and noncohesive (Vandereycken, 1995). Observations of family interactions yield similar data. In addition, observers often view bulimics as resentfully submissive to parents who are hostile and who neglect them (Vandereycken, 1995). Bulimics tend to remember their early childhood as involving a lack of care by both parents, but particularly mothers. Fathers are seen as being overprotective and controlling, without care and concern for the patient (Vandereycken, 1995).

Cognitive and behavioral factors

Christopher Fairburn and his colleagues (1993) have pioneered work on cognitive-behavioral theory for the maintenance of bulimia nervosa after its onset. According to this theory, bulimia nervosa is maintained by cycles of low self-esteem, extreme concerns about body shape and weight, strict dieting, binge eating, and compensatory behavior, which interact and affect each other. Thus bulimia is maintained by the behaviors of dieting, bingeing, and purging, which, in turn, are both affected by and contribute to distorted and negative cognitions about the self and the body. This theory has led to the development of the highly successful cognitive-behavioral therapy for bulimia nervosa that targets both eating-disordered behaviors and cognitions (O'Dea, Abraham, 2000; Sloan, 1999).

Psychodynamic factors

According to Tobin (1993), the psychodynamic understanding of bulimia nervosa depends on the underlying personality structure of the individual. Emphasis is placed on the role of the unconscious in the formation of symptoms.

Some psychodynamic theorists have placed particular emphasis on ambivalent feelings of self-esteem in bulimics. The binge-eating and purging behavior is thought to express the ambivalence patients feel toward themselves. On one hand, patients believe they are worthy of the nurturing they lack, and, because food is a symbolic form of nurturing, they binge. On the other hand, patients feel unworthy of nurturing, so they purge. Bingeing and purging can also be seen as the patient's attempt to numb themselves from the pain in their lives resulting from abuse, neglect, trauma, and strong feelings (Orbanic, 2001).

Bulimia and Depression

Some theorists have postulated several reasons that bulimia nervosa is a variant of a mood disorder. First, there is a high rate of mood disorders, particularly depression, among bulimics (Cooper PJ, 1995). Next, there is a high rate of mood disorders in the families of bulimics. Last, as discussed earlier, treatment with an antidepressant medication has been shown to be helpful in reducing bulimic symptoms.

The relationship between bulimia and depression may be that one causes the other, or there may be independent contributing factors to both. Experts are doubtful that depression causes bulimia because depression most often develops after the onset of the eating disorder, and depression in bulimia nervosa differs from major depressive disorder (Cooper PJ, 1995). It has also been suggested that low serotonin or low self-esteem (or both) may contribute to both disorders (Cooper Z, 1995). Studies of the families of depressive patients have failed to show an unusually high incidence of eating disorders, which argues against a common pathogenesis (Cooper PJ, 1995). Most experts believe depression is secondary to erratic eating habits and feelings of lack of control (Garner, 1998).

Psychotherapeutic Management

As in the treatment of anorexia nervosa, medical stabilization of the bulimic patient is the initial treatment goal. After medical stabilization, psychotherapy is the treatment of choice. Cognitive-behavioral therapy has the greatest research support, although limited evidence exists suggesting interpersonal psychotherapy may have similar long-term effectiveness (Fairburn, 1995b; McGown, Whitbread, 1996). Pharmacotherapy is used as an adjunct to psychotherapy when indicated (Walsh, 1995).

Similar to the treatment of anorexia, nurses may encounter bulimics in an inpatient setting or as outpatients seen for medical monitoring in a physician's office or clinic. Overall, bulimics are less likely than are anorectics to be inpatients. A multidisciplinary approach, involving physicians, nurses, dietitians, and psychotherapists, is recommended with bulimics. See Tips for Professionals From Persons Recovering From Eating Disorders on page 503.

Nurse-patient relationship

Bulimic patients differ from anorectic patients in the sense that bulimics usually want help. They enter therapy of their own volition, are eager to please, and so behave in a manner that will lead therapists to like them. In trying to please, bulimic patients have a tendency to become manipulative and may tell lies and half-truths regarding their problem. The desire to be helped is the greatest strength of these patients. Specific therapeutic communication techniques helpful for these patients include the following.

- Create an atmosphere of trust. Bulimic patients have a difficult time with trust. The nurse must be honest at all times and follow through with what is said.
- Encourage patients to approach staff if feeling the urge to purge.
- Help patients identify feelings associated with the binge-purge behavior. Once the feelings are identified, patients can begin to explore alternative ways of coping with them.
- Accept patients as worthwhile human beings. Bulimic patients are often ashamed of their behavior and are embarrassed to discuss it. When patients realize there are no negative repercussions, they are more comfortable discussing problems.
- Encourage patients to discuss positive qualities about themselves to improve self-esteem.
- Teach patients about bulimia nervosa. Knowledge can affect behavior and sense of control.
- Encourage patients to explore their interpersonal relationships. Many bulimics complain of loneliness. Patients need to be encouraged to examine their interpersonal problems so they may be resolved and they can seek hobbies and activities that enable them to forge new friendships.
- Encourage patients to participate in individual therapy, particularly with a therapist who is familiar with cognitive-behavioral therapy for bulimia nervosa.
- Encourage patients to participate in ongoing group therapy or group support to maintain any gains made and to prevent relapse.

Psychopharmacology

Recent studies have shown that certain antidepressants, such as imipramine (Tofranil), desipramine (Norpramin), fluoxetine (Prozac), and trazodone (Desyrel), significantly reduce the frequency of binge eating (McGowan, Whitbread, 1996). These drugs have been shown to have a positive effect on associated mood disturbances and preoccupation with shape and weight (Walsh, 1995).

Interestingly, antidepressants appear to be equally effective in both depressed and nondepressed patients with bulimia nervosa. These results suggest that the mechanism of the drug action may not be "antidepressant," but rather, direct central effects on neurotransmitter systems, particularly serotonin and norepinephrine. It should be noted, however, that although antidepressants have beneficial effects in the short term, this improvement does not appear to be maintained long term (Grothaus, 1998). Furthermore, the amount of improvement with cognitive-behavior therapy appears to be greater than that obtained with antidepressants (Fairburn, 1995b). Generally, psychotherapy is recommended before a trial of an antidepressant (Walsh, 1995). Antidepressants are considered when the patient has failed to respond adequately to psychotherapy alone or when there is co-morbidity with severe clinical depression.

Milieu management

Although bulimic patients are typically seen on an outpatient basis, they should be hospitalized in the following circumstances:

- To treat a psychiatric or medical crisis, such as suicidal feelings or serious fluid-electrolyte imbalance
- To provide order to an otherwise chaotic life
- To allow patients to examine their living situations
- To provide treatment to patients who live in an area far away from other services

Fairburn (1995b) has recommended a "stepped care" approach to treatment, wherein patients first participate in a simple treatment, such as guided self-help or a psychoeducational group. Individuals who do not respond are then referred for cognitive-behavior therapy. Patients who do not adequately improve from therapy are then referred for a more intensive form of treatment, such as interpersonal psychotherapy, partial or full hospitalization, and possibly, antidepressant medication.

Some principles for management of the bulimic patient include the following:

- Encourage patients to adhere to planned schedules for meals and snacks. Regularization of eating prevents the precipitation of binge eating that results from dieting or restrictive eating practices. Encourage all patients to follow the advice of dietitians regarding normalization of eating.
- Encourage patients to attend eating-disorder group therapy sessions. This avenue not only provides support to patients, but also facilitates their experiencing and resolving the problems they have with relating to others.
- Encourage family therapy. Communication within families needs to be improved to strengthen these relationships and prevent relapse.
- Encourage participation in art, recreation, and other types of therapy. These modalities teach patients alternative ways to express their feelings and provide activities to do other than focusing on food and dieting.

EATING DISORDERS IN MALES

The incidence of eating disorders among males is currently about 10% of the eating-disorder population, with speculation that this figure may increase (Ricciardelli, Williams, Kiernan, 1999). Although diagnosis, etiology, and treatment of males and females with eating disorders are similar, there appears to be some differences with respect to assessment in males. For example, males are more likely to be involved in athletics and to have a history of obesity before the onset of symptoms of an eating disorder. Males also tend to feel less guilt than females about episodes of bingeing and purging. Dieting or bingeing is more often related to a desire to build a lean body for participation in sports or to compete at a lower weight class in wrestling (Ricciardelli, Williams, Kiernan, 1999).

Although controversial, some research has shown that male patients with eating disorders exhibit a high frequency of concerns about gender or sexual identity, homosexual orientation, and asexuality (Meyer, Blisset, Oldfield, 2001). It should be noted, however, that although approximately 21% of eating-disordered males have a homosexual orientation, this is still a minority of cases.

Treatment for males with eating disorders is similar to that of females. From a psychotherapeutic management standpoint, the following three areas need particular focus with males:

1. Body image and the excessive attention that adolescent boys often place on attaining a masculine physique
2. Healthier dietary habits to promote health, fitness, and muscle mass
3. The ability to express feelings, especially if the patient has an underlying sexual identity concern

Although most adolescents with eating disorders have difficulty expressing their feelings, boys seem to have more difficulty than do girls. A therapeutic nurse-patient relationship can be especially instrumental in the recovery of these young men.

BINGE-EATING DISORDER

The DSM-IV-TR lists binge-eating disorder (BED) as a condition that has not met diagnostic criteria for inclusion in the DSM-IV-TR manual, but may warrant further research and study. BEDs share many criteria of bulimia nervosa (lack of control over intake, patient distress, and guilt over bingeing) but without the regular compensation for excess intake through purging, laxatives, fasting, or overexercise. As a consequence, individuals with BED tend to be overweight to a moderate or greater degree and their weight tends to fluctuate more compared with those with anorexia or bulimia. As with bulimia, the onset of this disorder tends to be later than anorexia, generally beginning in late adolescence to early adulthood. Research has shown that this disorder occurs in approximately 20% of individuals seeking help for weight control (Fairburn, Walsh, 1995). These patients are diagnosed Eating Disorder Not Otherwise Specified (NOS) with the notation that the patient's symptoms meet the research criteria for BED. Other examples of NOS disorders include the patient who meets all criteria for anorexia nervosa except amenorrhea or who has a regular pattern of vomiting for weight control after normal eating. These individuals may not be underweight or demonstrate binge eating and so are not identified as having an eating disorder. Clinicians should recognize the importance of early detection and treatment before the NOS illness becomes more severe.

Web Resources

- These sites represent a small sampling of available resources for professionals, patients, and families. Nurses should evaluate the appropriateness of web resources as with all other resources before giving them to patients and families.
- There is a disturbing trend developing on the Internet known as "pro anorexia" web sites or chat rooms that proclaim anorexia as a lifestyle choice rather than a life-threatening illness. Legitimate hosts such as *Yahoo* have ceased hosting these sites and groups, but some may still exist and be passed on from patient to patient.

Eating Disorders Referral and Information Center (EDRIC)
http://www.edreferral.com

Sponsored and maintained by the International Eating Disorders Referral Organization, a nonprofit organization. The web site contains much information and many links to other resources, as well as referrals to caregivers experienced in treating eating disorders.

Anorexia and Related Disorders, Inc. (ANRED)
http://www.anred.com

Sponsored and maintained by a group of mental health professionals (including a nurse) with many years experience treating eating-disordered patients. This group is nonprofit, provides links to other resources, and exists mainly as an educational resource. The web site cautions patients that direct professional care is needed to overcome their illness.

National Association of Anorexia and Associated Disorders (ANAD)
http://www.anad.org

Sponsored and maintained by the association, ANAD the oldest national nonprofit organization devoted to helping eating-disordered patients and their families through providing networking, support groups, and advocacy for patients and their families.

Eating Disorders Awareness and Prevention, Inc. (EDAP)
http://www.edap.org or 1-800-931-2237

Sponsored and maintained by a national nonprofit organization dedicated to eliminating eating disorders and body dissatisfaction, the web site focuses on awareness, prevention, and advocacy regarding eating disorders and sponsors a yearly media-awareness campaign.

Something Fishy Web Site on Eating Disorders
http://www.something-fishy.org/edaso.html

This site serves as a clearinghouse for eating-disorder resources and information.

Key Concepts

1. Anorexia nervosa is characterized by a refusal to maintain body weight at or above a minimally normal weight for age and height, an intense fear of becoming fat, a distorted body image, and amenorrhea.
2. Anorectic dieters may begin their illness in a normal weight range but then isolate themselves socially from others, become competitive concerning weight loss, and exercise excessively.
3. Bulimia is characterized by episodes of binge eating, a feeling of a lack of control of eating, use of compensatory behavior, and an overconcern with body shape and weight. Depression commonly coexists with bulimia.
4. Anorectic and bulimic patients suffer a variety of physiologic problems that can cause death. Personality and emotional changes are also evident in these patients.
5. The cause of eating disorders is thought to be multifactoral, including biologic, sociocultural, familial, cognitive, behavioral, and psychodynamic factors.
6. Cognitive-behavioral therapy has the most research support in the treatment of bulimia nervosa.
7. The incidence of eating disorders in males is increasing, with speculation that this trend will continue.
8. Nursing interventions with eating disordered patients require caring, supportive relationships; limit setting; a behavior-modification program; and a consistent milieu. Family involvement, individual psychotherapy, and group therapy are also essential. Hospitalization with a structured milieu and antidepressant medications may be needed if weight drops below that which is appropriate for the patient's height or if medical complications of patient's condition are present.

References

American Psychiatric Association: *Diagnostic and statistical manual of mental disorders,* ed 4, text revision, Washington, DC, 2000, APA.

Beumont PJV: The clinical presentation of anorexia and bulimia nervosa. In Brownell KD, Fairburn CG, editors: *Eating disorders and obesity,* New York, 1995, Guilford Press.

Bruch H: *Eating disorders,* New York, 1973, Basic Books.

Brumberg JJ: *The body project: an intimate history of American girls,* New York, 1997, Random House.

Cohane GH, Pope HG: Body image in boys: a review of the literature, *Int J Eat Disord* 29(4):373, 2001.

Coners H, Remschmidt H, Hebebrand J: The relationship between premorbid body weight, weight loss, and weight at referral in adolescent patients with anorexia nervosa, *Int J Eat Disord* 26(2):171, 1999.

Cooper PJ: Eating disorders and their relationship to mood and anxiety disorders. In Brownell KD, Fairburn CG, editors: *Eating disorders and obesity,* New York, 1995, Guilford Press.

Cooper Z: The development and maintenance of eating disorders. In Brownell KD, Fairburn CG, editors: *Eating disorders and obesity,* New York, 1995, Guilford Press.

Cummings MM et al: Developing and implementing a comprehensive program for children and adolescents with eating disorders, *J Child Adolesc Psychiatr Nurs* 14(4):167, 2001.

Fairburn CG: Physiology of anorexia nervosa. In Brownell KD, Fairburn CG, editors: *Eating disorders and obesity,* New York, 1995a, Guilford Press.

Fairburn CG: Short-term psychological treatments for bulimia nervosa. In Brownell KD, Fairburn CG, editors: *Eating disorders and obesity,* New York, 1995b, Guilford Press.

Fairburn CG, Marcus MD, Wilson GT: Cognitive-behavioral therapy for binge eating and bulimia nervosa: a comprehensive treatment manual. In Fairburn CG, Wilson GT, editors: *Binge eating: nature, assessment, and treatment,* New York, 1993, Guilford Press.

Fairburn CG, Walsh BT: Atypical eating disorders. In Brownell KD, Fairburn CG, editors: *Eating disorders and obesity,* New York, 1995, Guilford Press.

Fichter MM: Inpatient treatment of anorexia nervosa. In Brownell KD, Fairburn CG, editors: *Eating disorders and obesity,* New York, 1995, Guilford Press.

Finelli L: Revisiting the identity issue in anorexia, *J Psychosoc Nurs* 39(8):23, 2001.

Garfinkel P, Walsh T: Drug therapies. In Garner DM, Garfinkel PJV, editors: *Handbook of treatment for eating disorders,* ed 2, New York, 1997, Guilford Press.

Garner DM: The effects of starvation on behavior: implications for dieting and eating disorders, *Healthy Weight Journal* Sept/Oct:68, 1998.

Grinspoon L: Eating disorders: part I, *Harvard Mental Health Letter* 14(4):I, 1997a.

Grinspoon L: Eating disorders: part II, *Harvard Mental Health Letter* 14(5):II, 1997b.

Grothaus K: Eating disorders and adolescents: an overview of a maladaptive behavior, *J Child Adolesc Psychiatr Nurs* 11(3):146, 1998.

Johnson C: Psychodynamic treatment of bulimia nervosa. In Brownell KD, Fairburn CG, editors: *Eating disorders and obesity,* New York, 1995, Guilford Press.

Kaye WH: Neurotransmitters and anorexia nervosa. In Brownell KD, Fairburn CG, editors: *Eating disorders and obesity,* New York, 1995, Guilford Press.

McGown A, Whitbread J: Out of control! The most effective way to help the binge-eating patient, *J Psychosoc Nurs Ment Health Serv* 34(1):30, 1996.

Melrose C: Facilitating a multidisciplinary parent support and education group guided by Allen's developmental health nursing model, *J Psychosoc Nurs* 38(9):19, 2000.

Mendell DA, Logemann JA: Bulimia and swallowing: cause for concern, *Int J Eat Disord* 30(3):252. 2001.

Meyer C, Blisset J, Oldfield C: Sexual orientation and eating psychopathology: the role of masculinity and femininity, *Int J Eat Disord* 29(3):314, 2001.

Mitchell JE, Pomeroy C, Adson DE: Managing medical complications. In Garner DM, Garfinkel PJV, editors: *Handbook of treatment for eating disorders,* ed 2, New York, 1997, Guilford Press.

Muscari M: Effective management of adolescents with anorexia and bulimia, *J Psychosoc Nurs* 40(2):23, 2002.

O'Dea JA, Abraham S: Improving the body image, eating attitudes and behaviors of young male and female adolescents: a new educational approach that focuses on self-esteem, *Int J Eat Disord* 28(1):43, 2000.

Orbanic S: Understanding bulimia, *Am J Nurs* 101(3):35, 2001.

Owen SV, Fullerton ML: A discussion group in a behaviorally oriented inpatient eating disorder program, *J Psychosoc Nurs Ment Health Serv* 33(11):35, 1995.

Palmer RL: Sexual abuse and eating disorders. In Brownell KD, Fairburn CG, editors: *Eating disorders and obesity,* New York, 1995, Guilford Press.

Pirke KM: Physiology of bulimia nervosa. In Brownell KD, Fairburn CG, editors: *Eating disorders and obesity,* New York, 1995, Guilford Press.

Poirier-Solomon L: Eating disorders and diabetes, *Diabetes Forecast* 11:43, 2001.

Potts NW: Eating disorders. In Johnson BS, editor: *Child, adolescent and family psychiatric nursing,* Philadelphia, 1995, JB Lippincott.

Pumariega AJ et al: Clinical correlates of body-size distortion, *Percept Mot Skills* 76:1311, 1993.

Rand CSW, Wright BA: Continuity and change in the evaluation of ideal and acceptable body sizes across a wide age span, *Int J Eat Disord* 28(1):90, 2000.

Ricciardelli LA, Williams J, Kiernan MJ: Bulimic symptoms in adolescent girls and boys, *Int J Eat Disord* 26(2):217, 1999.

Russell GFM: The history of bulimia nervosa. In Garner DM, Garfinkel PJV, editors: *Handbook of treatment for eating disorders,* ed 2, New York, 1997, Guilford Press.

Sloan G: Anorexia nervosa: a cognitive-behavioral approach, *Nursing Standard* 13(19):43, 1999.

Striegel-Moore RH: A feminist perspective on the etiology of eating disorders. In Brownell KD, Fairburn CG, editors: *Eating disorders and obesity,* New York, 1995, Guilford Press.

Strober M: Family-genetic perspectives on anorexia nervosa and bulimia nervosa. In Brownell KD, Fairburn CG, editors: *Eating disorders and obesity,* New York, 1995, Guilford Press.

Tobin DL: Psychodynamic psychotherapy and binge eating. In Fairburn CG, Wilson GT, editors: *Binge eating: nature, assessment, and treatment,* New York, 1993, Guilford Press.

Vandereycken W: The families of patients with an eating disorder. In Brownell KD, Fairburn CG, editors: *Eating disorders and obesity,* New York, 1995, Guilford Press.

Walsh BT: Pharmacotherapy of eating disorders. In Brownell KD, Fairburn CG, editors. *Eating disorders and obesity,* New York, 1995, Guilford Press.

Walsh BT, Garner DM: Diagnostic issues. In Garner DM, Garfinkel PE, editors: *Handbook of treatment for eating disorders,* New York, 1997, Guilford Press.

White JH: The prevention of eating disorders: a review of the research on risk factors with implications for practice, *J Child Adolesc Nurs* 13(2):76, 2000.

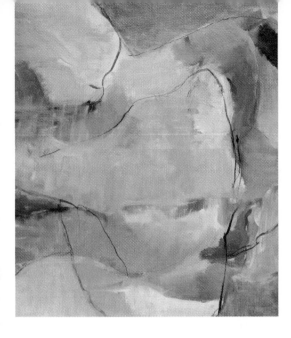

Chapter 38

Behavior Therapies

Lee H. Schwecke*

Lee H. Schwecke*

Learning Objectives

After reading this chapter, you should be able to:
- Identify three techniques for increasing a behavior.
- Describe two schedules of reinforcement.
- Identify three techniques for decreasing a behavior.
- Understand the principles of a token economy.
- Discuss two techniques for helping patients deal with disturbing stimuli.
- Explain the nursing process using behavioral modification principles.

Behavior therapy is a distinctive approach to influencing interactions among individuals and between individuals and their environment. The principles used in behavior therapy were derived from research in conditioned reflex and operant conditioning. Applications of behavior therapy principles are common and effective in psychiatric nursing, especially in helping patients deal with anxiety and change their behaviors. Behavior therapy is typically combined with cognitive therapy and psychotropic medications (Hogarty, 2000).

CLASSICAL CONDITIONING

The origin of classical conditioning is credited to Pavlov (1927) and his research on stimulus and

*Revised from a chapter by Sue Main.

response in laboratory animals. Pavlov was involved in studying reflexes and the various aspects of the secretion of gastric juices in dogs when he discovered that the dogs began salivating before they were presented with food.

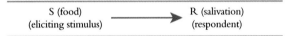

S (food)   →   R (salivation)
(eliciting stimulus)   (respondent)

Pavlov then simultaneously presented food and the sound of a metronome. After several repetitions, the metronome alone was found to elicit the secretion of saliva. *Respondent conditioning* is the process of pairing a neutral stimulus with an eliciting stimulus thus, ultimately, the neutral stimulus alone elicits the response.

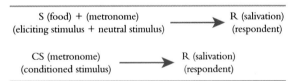

S (food) + (metronome) → R (salivation)
(eliciting stimulus + neutral stimulus) (respondent)

CS (metronome) → R (salivation)
(conditioned stimulus) (respondent)

In an experiment with a young child (Albert) and a white rat (a neutral stimulus), Watson and Rayner (1920) paired the presence of the rat with a loud noise that had been observed to elicit a fear response in Albert. After the noise and the rat were presented simultaneously seven times, the rat alone elicited the fear response in Albert. The fear response was also elicited by stimuli with characteristics similar to

515

those of the rat (rabbit, dog, fur). This process, in which a fear response is elicited by stimuli with similar characteristics, is called *generalization.*

OPERANT CONDITIONING

The basis of the operant learning theory was derived from numerous controlled experiments with animals and was reported originally by B. F. Skinner (1938, 1953, 1956). Attention is directed to the events that immediately precede and follow a person's specific behavior. Theoretical inner causes of behavior, such as psychologic, neurologic, or conceptual states, are not denied; however, they are not viewed as relevant to the analysis of behavior.

A response is any movement or observable behavior. The operant response (the behavior being analyzed) can be described and measured (frequency, duration, magnitude). A stimulus is an event that immediately precedes or follows a behavior. Three types of stimuli include the following:

1. A discriminative stimulus is an event, immediately preceding a behavior, that predicts or indicates that a response will be followed by reinforcement. Discriminative stimuli may be observed, heard, felt, tasted or smelled. Examples include pain, subtle verbal or facial expressions, a tone of voice, posture, dress, or a specific person or situation.
2. A neutral stimulus is an event that is not associated with reinforcement or that which has no effect on changing the probability of behavior.
3. A reinforcing stimulus is an event, following a behavior, that strengthens the behavior and increases the probability of the behavior occurring (e.g., hugs, smiles, attention, an opportunity to play, a paycheck, a chicken dinner).

Primary reinforcers are events of biologic importance (e.g., food, water, sexual contact, coat on a cold day, bed for sleeping). Secondary or generalized reinforcers are events that have been paired repeatedly with a primary reinforcer (e.g., money, tickets, diplomas, attention of others).

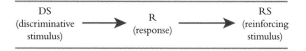

For example, a patient in a hospital room wants the nurse's attention. The patient presses a button labeled "nurse" on the paging apparatus. The voice of the nurse ("This is Mrs. White. May I help you?") is heard.

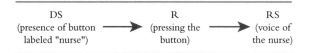

Other buttons labeled "fire," "emergency," or "TV" are neutral stimuli. When a voice responds immediately and consistently following the pressing of the button, learning occurs. If the nurse's voice does not immediately follow pushing the button, extinction occurs. The button-pushing behavior predictably decreases (after a brief period of an increase) and emotional behavior may occur (e.g., yelling loudly for the nurse). If the patient receives a painful electrical shock when pushing the button and the response is suppressed, punishment has occurred. The patient may then exhibit an aggressive response (e.g., throwing the paging apparatus against the wall).

APPLICATION OF BEHAVIOR THERAPY IN PSYCHIATRIC NURSING PRACTICE

Behavior therapy is used with children, adolescents, groups, couples, and families. Behavior modification has been used in inpatient and outpatient settings and in skills-training programs. The use of behavior therapy with specific problematic behaviors has been reported in the treatment of anxiety, sexual disorders, posttraumatic stress disorder (PTSD), and addictions. Additionally, behavioral principles form the basis of self-control treatment programs, such as those used for changes in behaviors (e.g., eating, exercise, assertive communication).

Behavior Modification: Helping Patients Change Behavior

When patients' problem behaviors are reinforced or maintained by consequences of the behavior, operant conditioning, commonly called behavior modification, is the model used. Functional analysis involves a behavioral and reinforcement history. Contingencies that can be controlled by the therapist, patients, or families are altered to create a change in the problematic behaviors.

Increasing the probability that a behavior will recur

Conditioning

Conditioning is the strengthening of a response by reinforcement. Positive reinforcement follows a behavior with a reinforcing stimulus that increases the probability that the behavior will recur. For example, asking for help in an assertive way occurs more frequently when followed by attention and suggestions (reinforcement) in a communication-skills group (specific discriminative stimulus). Negative reinforcement is the process of removing a stimulus from a situation immediately after a behavior occurs, which increases the probability of the behavior occurring. For example, when a person steps into an uncomfortably hot shower and turns the dial to reduce the water temperature, the behavior (turning the dial) is reinforced. The stimulus (uncomfortably hot water) is removed.

The timing of reinforcement is important. Superstitious behavior is a term used for behavior that has been reinforced by accident. Athletes provide common examples of superstitious behaviors when they display peculiar mannerisms such as tapping a shoe with the bat before stepping up to home plate or tapping their fingers on the strings of a tennis racket before receiving a serve. When reinforcers are presented according to a time schedule (rather than being contingent on a particular response), any behavior immediately preceding the reinforcer is strengthened.

Premack principle

When a person is observed often enjoying a particular activity, the opportunity to engage in that activity can be used as a reinforcer for other behaviors that occur less frequently (Premack, 1962). For example, the opportunity to watch television might be used as a reinforcer for cleaning the living area.

Shaping

Shaping is a process of reinforcing successive approximations of responses to increase the probability of a behavior. For example, to increase the probability of a patient saying "no" in an assertive way, each time the patient makes a response that approximates the target response (or gets closer to the target response), reinforcement is presented until that response occurs at a high frequency. Then, reinforcement is withheld until the next response more closely approximates the target behavior and so on until the target behavior is performed. The selective reinforcement of each behavior that more closely approximates the target response is called differential reinforcement.

Schedules of reinforcement

Schedules are the planned sequences for the presentation of reinforcing stimuli.

Continuous reinforcement

Continuous reinforcement is the presentation of reinforcing stimuli following each occurrence of the selected response. Continuous reinforcement is used primarily during the initial phases of conditioning or shaping a behavior and results in a high rate of behavior, such as when a professional provides reinforcement each time a patient uses appropriate comments during a role-play of conflict-management skills.

Intermittent reinforcement

Intermittent reinforcement is the presentation of the reinforcer following the target response according to a selected number of responses (ratio schedule). An example would be after every fifth target response or according to a selected time period (interval schedule) of 5 minutes after every target response. Schedules may vary as well.

Intermittent schedules of reinforcement result in behavior that is more resistant to extinction than behavior that has been reinforced on a continuous schedule. The comparison of inserting coins into vending machines with inserting coins into slot machines illustrates the difference. Normally, inserting coins into a vending machine is reinforced (with food) every time the behavior occurs. When the reinforcer stops (when no food is delivered), the act of inserting coins into that particular machine stops rather quickly. Inserting coins into a slot machine, however, is reinforced with tokens or money on an intermittent schedule, not each time. The act of inserting coins into a slot machine continues for a considerable time, even though reinforcers are not presented.

Decreasing the probability that a behavior will recur

Differential reinforcement of other behavior

Differential reinforcement is a technique used to decrease the frequency of a behavior. When the goal of treatment is to decrease a behavior, another behavior, incompatible with the target behavior, can be reinforced. Target behavior, if emitted, is not reinforced. To decrease the soft speaking of a patient in a group, attention of the group is available only when the patient speaks in a normal, audible voice. The soft speaking voice, incompatible with a normal voice, is ignored.

Extinction

Extinction is the gradual decrease in the rate of responses when reinforcement is no longer available. The rate of responses may increase for a short time, then begin to decrease gradually. Emotional responses characteristically occur during extinction. A familiar example is the behavior that occurs when the button to start an elevator is pushed. When the elevator door fails to close, repeated and sometimes rapid button-pushing behavior occurs for a short period, then stops. Banging or pulling on the elevator door (an emotional response) may occur during this time. Social extinction involves the withdrawal of attention, such as when a patient acts inappropriately.

Negative consequence

Negative consequence is the presentation of an event immediately following a response that decreases the probability of that response recurring, for example, putting a child in his or her room immediately after seeing him or her playing in the street. Another example is having a patient apologize to other patients and mop the floor after throwing food. Negative consequence results in the immediate suppression of the particular response. For inpatients, a common form of this technique is to withdraw privileges or withhold passes as a consequence of acting-out behaviors. Negative consequence may result in emotional behavior or aggressive responses and is used when other techniques are not effective in decreasing the frequency of a particular response or in combination with other procedures.

Time out

Time out is a negative-consequence technique in which the person is removed from a setting in which ongoing reinforcers are available. When a patient is exhibiting aggressive behavior that is followed by social reinforcement from other patients, the patient may be moved to another room in which no social reinforcement is available.

Response cost

Response cost, another negative-consequence technique, is the removal of a reinforcer that is contingent on a specific behavior. Secondary reinforcers, such as points or tokens that were presented for desired behaviors, are removed for inappropriate behaviors. In outpatient settings, the response-cost technique might involve having patients pay a sum of money at the beginning of therapy and returning small amounts contingent on the patient's exhibition of a specific, desired behavior. The money is withheld when inappropriate behavior, such as noncompliance with the treatment contract, is exhibited.

Skills training

When behavioral responses are not appropriate for a person's age and life situation, new behaviors are acquired through the use of social-skills training and problem-solving procedures (Hogarty, 2000). Positive reinforcement and shaping are the basis for these programs; modeling and imitation are also used. Nurses often make individual assessments of the social skills of patients and form small groups to conduct training of skills that are appropriate for the patients but have not been seen in the hospital situation. An example is assertiveness training in which assertiveness is defined, described, and compared with passive and aggressive responses. Assertive responses are modeled. The patients then practice these responses and use them in role-play and homework assignments (Mishra, Gatchel, Gardea, 2000). Reinforcement is given when assertiveness is appropriately demonstrated.

Contingency contracting

Contingency contracting is the arrangement of conditions that enables patients to participate in setting target behaviors and selecting reinforcers. The therapist and the patients jointly specify what, how, when, and where behavioral change will occur. Criteria for the delivery of reinforcement are defined. The type, amount, and schedule of reinforcement are specified. For example, a contract specifies that, if the patient approaches the nurse to ask for his or her medications at the scheduled time, he or she can go for a walk with the nurse after dinner.

Self-control

The direct management of behavioral contingencies by a therapist is usually impractical for adult patients in an outpatient treatment setting. A more frequently used approach is the development of a self-control program with contingency contracting in which patients do the assessment, change their behaviors, provide their own reinforcement, and evaluate the results. This approach can be used with "thought stopping" when patients have "automatic" negative thoughts. Patients are taught to say to themselves, "stop," and to substitute a positive thought (Lyon, 2001). This technique has been adapted for patients with computer addictions as well (Orzack, 1999).

Token economy

Token economy is the term used to describe the use of operant principles in the management of behavior with groups of patients in inpatient or outpatient partial hospital programs (Ayllon, Azrin, 1968).

Tokens (tangible conditioned reinforcers) are presented to patients contingent on specific target behaviors. A simple example is presented in Figure 38-1. Tokens can be exchanged for positive reinforcers, such as privileges and favorite foods.

Critical Thinking Question

Jennifer O'Conner inflicts superficial cuts on her wrists when she receives negative consequences for seductive behavior with male patients. Positive reinforcement for opposing behaviors, social extinction, and "time out" have not been successful. What behavioral approaches would you plan instead?

Critical Thinking Questions

One of the patients in your problem-solving group is silent most of the time. Using contingency contracting principles, describe the gradual progression of desired behaviors you would like for the patient to exhibit and the types and schedules of reinforcements you would use.

Respondent Conditioning: Helping Patients Cope with Disturbing Stimuli

When patients' problem behaviors are related to particular stimuli situations, such as those related to pain, phobias, and PTSD, respondent conditioning is the model used. Treatment may involve making changes in stimuli situations or in control of problematic behaviors.

	S	M	T	W	T	F	S
Get up on time	X	X	X				
Make bed		X					
Complete ADLs	X	X	X				
Go to group on time	X	X	X				
Participate in group			X				
Do own laundry	X						

Figure 38-1 Expected outcomes for patient.

Reciprocal inhibition

The process of strengthening alternative responses to fear or anxiety associated with a stimulus is called reciprocal inhibition or counterconditioning (Yates, 1970). Relaxation techniques, for instance, can be taught to highly anxious patients or those in pain. A person cannot be relaxed and anxious simultaneously. Techniques often taught are positive, affirming self-talk; yoga; deep breathing; meditation; progressive muscle relaxation; and positive or pleasant imagery (Mishra, Gatchel, Gardea, 2000; Nakao et al, 2001). For example, the patient is instructed to tense and relax specific muscle groups, in a sequence, until relaxation is achieved. Several sessions of practice are usually carried out with the therapist, audiotape prompts, written instructions, or any combination of these.

Systematic desensitization

Originally developed by Wolpe (1958) for the treatment of anxiety, systematic desensitization is the planned progressive exposure to stimuli that elicit fear or anxiety while the fear response is suppressed with relaxation techniques. Hierarchies of the fear-eliciting stimuli are constructed through a detailed assessment. For example, a patient with a fear of being in open and crowded places that limits appropriate shopping behavior may report a hierarchy of fear-eliciting situations as follows: standing in the doorway of the house; standing outside several feet from the house, then two blocks away, then several blocks away, being in a small, empty store; being in an empty department store; being in an empty shopping center; being in a small, crowded store, a crowded department store, then a crowded shopping center. The stimulus least likely to evoke fear or anxiety is introduced initially, followed by gradual exposure to more fearful stimuli.

In traditional desensitization procedures and other prolonged exposure models, presentation or imaging of the fearful stimuli is done while an incompatible response, such as relaxation, is used to inhibit the fear or anxiety. A biofeedback program may also be used to reach and maintain a state of relaxation or pain control (Mishra, Gatchel, Gardea, 2000).

Other respondent conditioning techniques

In live (in vivo) exposure, patients actually place themselves, systematically, in the least to the most fearful situations. Usually, patients conduct this self-exposure while using incompatible competing responses to fear, such as relaxation. In using these techniques, the therapist carefully assists patients to experience a gradual decrease of the fear or anxiety response in the presence of the eliciting stimulus. Flooding or implosion is a process in which patients imagine or place themselves in the fearful situation; that is, they immerse themselves in the feared stimuli. For example, an individual with a fear of elevators would stand in an elevator until his or her anxiety subsides.

Critical Thinking Question

What phobias, besides the ones mentioned in this text, might systematic desensitization be successful in overcoming?

BEHAVIORAL INTERVENTION WITH THE NURSING PROCESS

The behavioral nursing process consists of the following: (1) an assessment of behavior and related contingencies; (2) a behavioral nursing diagnosis; (3) outcome identification and planning and implementing an intervention program; and (4) an evaluation of the results of the intervention (Box 38-1). Occasions for conducting this process occur in day-to-day interactions with patients. These interactions focus on providing a well-structured therapeutic milieu, assisting patients with here-and-now living problems, and helping them learn behavioral patterns related to emotional health.

Guidelines for Behavioral Nursing Intervention

The following example illustrates the use of a behavioral approach for skills training in a group of patients with chronic psychiatric disorders who

---

| Box 38-1 | Behavioral Nursing Intervention

Baseline Observations (Assessment)
1. Determine appropriate behavior present.
2. Identify inappropriate behavior present.
3. Determine absent age-appropriate behaviors.
   Assessment of these behavioral categories includes:
   a. Frequency or duration of each response or both
   b. Description of the stimulus conditions that precede responses and follow the behavior
   c. Validation of potential reinforcers

Problem Specification (Behavioral Nursing Diagnosis)
1. Select the response to be changed.
2. Define the response so that everyone can recognize it.
3. Gather baseline data (frequency, duration of behavior, discriminative and reinforcing stimuli).

Formulation of Treatment Plan (Outcome Identification)
1. State the specific response to be changed.
2. State how the response is to be changed (include the present status and the target status of the response):
   a. Increase the rate of the response.
   b. Decrease the rate of the response.
   c. Teach a new response.
3. Identify the discriminative and reinforcing stimuli available for use.
4. Select and write the intervention plan in detail (with rationales).

Intervention
1. Implement the treatment plan as written.
2. Provide reinforcers for the individuals implementing the plan.

Evaluation
1. State the outcome of the intervention.
2. Determine whether the response changed as planned.
3. Specify what additional changes are required.
4. State techniques for maintaining the desirable change.

---

were hospitalized in a facility that used a modified token-economy system.

Baseline observation and assessment

As part of the treatment program, each patient carried a behavioral rating card that listed specific expected behaviors (self-care activities, management of personal items and living area, attendance at prescribed treatment events). When the patients demonstrated these behaviors, a staff member rated the behavior and initialed the card. At the end of each week, each patient's ratings on the behavior cards were tallied, and reinforcement was presented contingent on the score for the week. Examples of the reinforcements were opportunities to engage in the purchase of items at the gift shop and participation in recreation activities. The skills-training groups consisted of four to six patients who met daily. The sessions began with a brief orientation period and an introduction of specific skills relevant to that session. Next, there was a demonstration and role-play using the skills, followed by discussion and homework suggestions.

Problem specification

Skills included assertiveness (patients asking for a staff talk), communication (starting and continuing a conversation in appropriate ways), reporting improvements to staff, making a plan for specific methods of self-care, and contracting with staff about treatment events or outcomes.

Treatment plan

Specific techniques that the nurse used were positive reinforcement (social reinforcement by the nurse or initialing the rating card) contingent on appropriate behavior, modeling and imitation, contingency contracting, homework, self-control, and extinction (withholding of reinforcement) following undesired behaviors.

Evaluation

Each group member's progress was evaluated with the use of a recording form that listed target behaviors. Seven patients showed consistent increases in target behaviors over the period of the group session. One patient demonstrated a relatively high rate of target behaviors during the initial group session and continued this rate. Demonstration of target behaviors by two of the patients was variable and consistently low throughout the sessions. For these two patients, the group-intervention program was not effective in changing target behaviors during the period that they were involved in the group.

Key Concepts

1. Classical conditioning is based on the involuntary stimulus-response reaction. After repeated pairing of eliciting and neutral stimuli, the neutral stimulus alone obtains the expected response.

2. Operant conditioning focuses on the external variables that precede and follow the response to learn which ones control behaviors. Reinforcers are particularly important.

3. Behavior therapy begins with a functional analysis of behavior and environmental contingencies as the basis for developing a treatment program.

4. Behavior modification programs can be used for a variety of problematic behaviors in a variety of settings.

5. Increasing the probability of a desired behavior can occur with conditioning, reinforcement, or shaping.

6. Decreasing the probability of an undesirable behavior can occur with reinforcement of an incompatible behavior, extinction, and negative consequence.

7. New behaviors may be acquired in skills training through the use of modeling and imitation techniques, as well as through reinforcement and shaping.

8. Self-control and token-economy programs are varieties of reinforcement approaches.

9. Respondent conditioning is useful in altering an unpleasant response to a specific stimulus. Reciprocal inhibition, systematic desensitization, in vivo exposure, and flooding are varieties of this approach.

10. Behavioral nursing interventions involve baseline observations, analysis of behaviors, problem specification, formulation of treatment plans, intervention, and evaluation.

References

Ayllon T, Azrin N: *The token economy,* New York, 1968, Appleton-Century-Crofts.

Hogarty GE: Cognitive rehabilitation of schizophrenia, *Harv Ment Health Lett* 17(2):4, 2000.

Lyon, BL: Strategies to enhance positive situational focusing skills, *Reflections on Nursing Leadership,* 3rd qtr, 2001.

Mishra KD, Gatchel RJ, Gardea MA: The relative efficacy of three cognitive-behavioral treatment approaches to temporomandibular disorders, *J Behav Med* 23(3):293, 2000.

Nakao M et al: Somatization and symptom reduction through a behavioral medicine intervention in a mind/body medicine clinic, *Behav Med* (26):169, 2001.

Orzack, MH: Computer addiction: is it real or virtual? *Harv Ment Health Lett* 15(7):8, 1999.

Pavlov IP: *Conditioned reflexes,* London, 1927, Oxford University (Translated by GV Anrep).

Premack K: Reversibility of the reinforcement relation, *Science* 136:255, 1962.

Skinner BF: *The behavior of organisms,* New York, 1938, Appleton-Century-Crofts.

Skinner BF: *Science and human behavior,* New York, 1953, Free Press.

Skinner BF: A case history in scientific method, *Am Psychol* 11:211, 1956.

Watson JB, Rayner R: Conditioned emotional reactions, *J Exp Psychol* 3:1, 1920.

Wolpe J: *Psychotherapy by reciprocal inhibition,* Stanford, Conn, 1958, Stanford University.

Yates AJ: *Behavior therapy,* New York, 1970, Wiley.

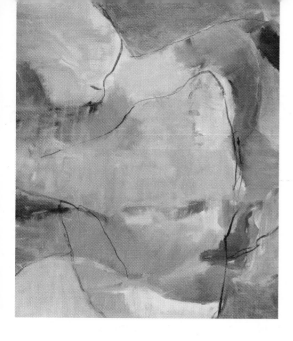

Chapter 39

Somatic Therapies

Norman L. Keltner

Learning Objectives

After reading this chapter, you should be able to:

- Compare modern electroconvulsive therapy (ECT) with "traditional" ECT depicted in some movies.
- Name and understand the purpose of the drugs used in conjunction with ECT.
- Identify three indications for ECT.
- Describe the nurse's role in caring for patients before and after ECT.
- Describe and discuss the ethical, legal, social, and biologic concerns related to psychosurgery.

Electroshock has undergone fundamental changes since its introduction 65 years ago. It is no longer the bone-breaking, memory-modifying, fearsome treatment featured in films. Anesthesia, controlled oxygenation, and muscle relaxation make the procedure so safe that the risks are less than those which accompany the use of psychotropic drugs. Indeed, for the elderly, the systemically ill, and pregnant women, electroshock is a safer treatment for mental illnesses than any alternative.

(Max Fink, *Electroshock*, 1999, p. ix)

Somatic therapies are treatment approaches that use physiologic or physical interventions to effect behavioral change. The most common form of somatic therapy is ECT, which will be dis-

cussed at length. A brief historical mention of insulin-coma therapy and initial convulsive therapies found in Box 39-1 outlines early efforts in somatic therapy. A brief review of psychosurgery, a highly controversial and rarely used therapy, follows the ECT discussion. Psychosurgery's inclusion traces its relevance to historical, ethical, and legal issues profoundly affecting psychiatric care. A brief discussion of other somatic therapies such as transcranial magnetic stimulation and phototherapy concludes the chapter.

ECT and psychosurgery emerged as treatment forms in the 1930s. The roots of ECT lie in the misconception of early twentieth-century psychiatrists that epilepsy and schizophrenia were incompatible (Abrams, 1997; Coffey, Weiner, 1990). Advocates of ECT and psychosurgery envisioned and promised dramatic relief from the curse of mental illness. Over time, inappropriate use and disappointing results, coupled with the development of psychotropic drugs and a growing general distrust of psychiatric hospitals, created a climate of hostility toward these therapies and their practitioners. In the 1960s and early 1970s the use of both therapies came to a virtual standstill. In the last 15 years or so, however, ECT has emerged once again as a useful treatment alternative when more traditional approaches fail. Psychosurgery, on the other hand, remains a treatment of last resort and is infrequent-

| Box 39-1 | Early somatic therapies

Insulin-coma therapy—1933

Insulin-coma therapy was introduced in 1933 by the Viennese physician Manfred Sakel after he accidentally discovered that giving too much insulin to a psychotic diabetic patient produced a reduction in the patient's symptoms. Insulin "shock" therapy gained a wide following for some time in hopes of alleviating the debilitating symptoms of psychosis (Colaizzi, 1996; Dorman, 1995).

First convulsive therapies—1934

Ladislas Meduna, a Hungarian, was the originator of convulsive therapy. In 1934 Meduna introduced camphor oil-induced and then Metrazol-induced convulsion therapy based on his pathologic observation that the glial cells of patients with schizophrenia were different than those of individuals with epilepsy. Meduna erroneously concluded that schizophrenia and epilepsy were mutually exclusive disorders (Abrams, 1997). Fink (1999, p. 88) chronicles one of Meduna's first patients, a 33-year-old man who had been psychotic, mute, and withdrawn for 4 years.

"Two days after the fifth (camphor-oil) injection, on February 10 in the morning, for the first time in four years, he got out of his bed, began to talk, requested breakfast, dressed himself without help, was interested in everything around him, and asked about his disease and how long he had been in the hospital. When the patient was told he had been in the hospital for 4 years he did not believe it!"

---

ly performed. With rigid treatment criteria and careful pretreatment evaluation, many psychiatric patients respond to these somatic therapies.

ELECTROCONVULSIVE THERAPY

Ugo Cerletti and Luciano Bini (Cerletti's assistant), two Italian psychiatrists, introduced ECT in 1938. The first patient suffered from schizophrenia and, after 11 treatments, experienced a full recovery. The first ECT treatment in the United States occurred in 1940.

ECT was once commonly referred to as electroshock therapy (EST) or simply shock therapy. Both terms are considered pejorative today.

During ECT, an electric current is passed through the brain, causing a seizure. Historically, this seizure resulted in a full grand mal convulsion accompanied by the various complications of these convulsions, that is, muscle soreness, fractures, dislocations, sprains, and tongue lacerations. These seizures and the resulting grotesque facial grimaces that occur have been dramatically captured on film and graphically detailed in literature. In films and novels, ECT has been portrayed as a devious tool used by psychiatrists and psychiatric nurses, who are themselves demented. The late Ken Kesey's book, *One Flew over the Cuckoo's Nest* and the 1975 movie of the same name created a firestorm of hostility against the use of ECT. In his book, Kesey portrayed ECT as an agent used to maintain control over sane but highly individualistic patients. This public attack on ECT, linked with reports of inappropriate use, virtually stopped the use of ECT in this country. Inappropriate use of ECT included administering ECT for almost all conditions and, from the accounts of former patients, using it as punishment for noncompliant behavior.

ECT was used most often during the early 1950s (Swartz, 1993a), when it was given to almost every patient who did not respond to other treatment forms. In large state hospitals, ECT was given on Mondays, Wednesdays, and Fridays to as many as 20 or more patients on a psychiatric ward, often without written consent. One patient after another, some under their own power, others literally manhandled and restrained, would take their place on the bed to be given ECT. Nursing staff would hold the patient in place (to decrease fractures, dislocations), insert the mouth guard (to prevent tongue bites), put paste on the electrodes, and hold the electrodes in place on each side of the head (usually the temple area). A nurse would then hold the chin and jaw in proper alignment, and the physician in the background would push a button to deliver the shock. A full grand mal seizure would occur—a tonic seizure followed by a significantly longer clonic seizure. After convulsion activity terminated, the patient was turned on his or her side and tied in place (to prevent aspiration) while a staff member or "helper patient" stayed at the bedside until consciousness returned. The ECT team then moved on to the next patient.

This unforgettable scene, depicted in novels and films and reported by former patients, contributed to a growing public fear of ECT. The use of ECT was all but abandoned in the 1980s.

Despite the negative views, however, ECT remains a viable treatment approach because many mental health professionals know it to be an effective treatment. Unfortunately, in the process of waiting to evaluate the efficacy of other treatments, many patients have suffered needlessly. Many clinicians now argue that ECT should be considered as a treatment choice earlier in the treatment process. About 100,000 patients per year receive ECT treatments in the United States (Smith, 2001).

Modern ECT

During ECT, an electric current is passed through the brain for 0.2 to 8.0 seconds, causing a seizure (Fink, 1999). Induction of a seizure is necessary for a therapeutic outcome (Krystal et al, 2000). The seizure resulting from ECT must be of sufficient quality to produce the best effect. Seizures are timed and subdivided into motor convulsions (at least 20 seconds required), increased heart rate (for 30 to 50 seconds), and a "brain" seizure as monitored by an electroencephalogram (EEG) (for 30 to 150 seconds) (Fink, 1999). The patient is given an oximeter-monitored anesthetic to ensure optimal oxygenation. The events leading up to, during, and after treatment, including nursing responsibilities, follow.

Preparation for ECT

- The patient must have a pretreatment evaluation, including physical examination, laboratory work (blood count, blood chemistries, urinalysis), and baseline memory abilities.
- A consent form must be signed. Because ECT is often given as a treatment of last resort, some patients are profoundly depressed to the extent that, by the time ECT is ordered, a truly "informed consent" is almost a contradiction in terms. In these cases, family members and facility legal staff should be involved.
- The routine use of benzodiazepines or barbiturates for nighttime sedation should be eliminated because of their ability to raise the seizure threshold (i.e., make it more difficult to stimulate a seizure).
- A trained electrotherapist and an anesthesiologist should be available.

Nursing responsibilities before ECT

- The patient should not be given anything by mouth for approximately 6 to 8 hours before ECT, except for cardiac, antihypertensive, and a few other medications.

| Box 39–2 | Drugs Used for Electroconvulsive Therapy

Atropine

Class: Prototypical anticholinergic

Actions: Atropine is used before ECT for several reasons:
1. Inhibition of salivation and respiratory tract secretions to minimize aspiration
2. Decreases the potential for cardiovascular depression resulting from ECT, succinylcholine, methohexital, or any combination

Pharmacokinetics:
   Onset: Orally, 30 minutes; intramuscularly, 15 minutes; intravenously, 1 minute
   Metabolism: Liver; half-life 2 to 3 hours
Dose: 0.4 to 0.6 mg
Side effects: Typical anticholinergic effects

Succinylcholine (Anectine)

Class: Ultrashort-acting neuromuscular blocker

Actions: Prevents the musculoskeletal complications from induced convulsions

Pharmacokinetics:
   Onset: 30 to 60 seconds; duration of action, 5 minutes
Dose: 0.6 mg/kg intravenously
Side effects: Prolonged apnea, respiratory depression, fasciculations

Methohexital (Brevital)

Class: Ultrashort-acting barbiturate

Actions: Induces a light coma preceding delivery of ECT

Pharmacokinetics:
   Onset: 10 to 15 seconds; duration of action 5 to 7 minutes
   Metabolism: Liver, half-life 4 hours
Dose: 1.5 mg/kg (typically 50 to 120 mg)
Side effects: Respiratory depression, hypotension, myocardial depression, decreased cardiac output

---

- Atropine (or glycopyrrolate [Robinul]) should be given as ordered. Atropine can be given 1 hour before treatment or intravenously immediately preceding treatment (Box 39-2). Atropine reduces secretions and subsequent risk of aspiration and counteracts the ECT-induced vagal stimulation.
- The patient should be asked to urinate before the treatment (seizure-induced incontinence is common).
- The patient's hairpins, contact lens, hearing aids, and dentures should be removed.
- Vital signs should be taken.
- The nurse should be positive about the treatment and attempt to reduce the patient's anxiety.

Procedures during ECT

- An intravenous line is inserted.
- Electrodes are attached to the proper place on the head. Electrodes are typically held in place with a rubber strap.
- The bite-block is inserted.
- Methohexital (Brevital) or another short-acting barbiturate is given intravenously. The barbiturate causes immediate anesthesia, preempting the anxiety associated with waiting for the "jolt to hit" and the anxiety caused by succinylcholine (see next).
- Succinylcholine (Anectine) is a neuromuscular-blocking agent and is given intravenously. Succinylcholine causes paralysis but not sedation (it does not cross the blood-brain barrier), thereby leaving the patient conscious but unable to breathe.
- Succinylcholine prevents the external manifestations of a grand mal seizure, thus minimizing fractures, dislocations, but it does not affect the "brain seizure."
- The anesthesiologist mechanically ventilates the patient with 100% oxygen immediately before the treatment.
- The electrical impulse is typically given for 0.2 to 8.0 seconds.
- The seizure should last a certain length of time of therapeutic value (see previous point). If the seizure lasts less than this amount of time, the physician must decide whether to stimulate another seizure. Seizure duration greater than 180 seconds is associated with less favorable outcomes and can be terminated with diazepam or other benzodiazepines.
- Monitoring devices include those for heart rate and rhythm, blood pressure, and electroencephalography.
- Ventilation and monitoring continue until the patient recovers.

Nursing responsibilities after ECT

- The nurse or anesthesiologist mechanically ventilates the patient with 100% oxygen until the patient can breathe unassisted.
- The nurse monitors for respiratory problems.
- ECT causes confusion and disorientation, thus it is important to help with reorientation (time, place, person) as the patient emerges from this groggy state.
- Because approximately 5% to 10% of these patients "awake" agitated, the nurse may need to administer a benzodiazepine as needed (Fitzsimons, 1995).

- Observation is necessary until the patient is oriented and steady, particularly when the patient first attempts to stand.
- All aspects of the treatment should be carefully documented for the patient's record.

An EEG recording monitors seizure activity. Blood pressure, oxygen saturation, and heart rate are also monitored. Oxygen is administered immediately before and then after the treatment because of interruption of breathing caused by the succinylcholine and the electrically induced seizure.

Critical Thinking Questions

ECT has been considered a political issue. Do you think that opponents of ECT tend to be more on the left or the right of the political spectrum?

ECT is more effective than are antidepressants in the treatment of severe depression. Nonetheless, there is reluctance to use ECT. If you or a member of your family were severely depressed, which of these two treatment forms would you want? Carefully consider the stigma of ECT, as well as the effects of anesthesia and memory loss.

How ECT Works

It is not clear how ECT works or why it is so effective, although over 100 theories have been advanced to explain it (Sackiem, 1993). Three of these theories seem most promising (Fink, 1999; Kellner, McCall, 1997; Roberts, Leigh, Weinberger, 1993).

1. ECT alters the endocrine system in ways that promote an antidepressant effect. Hormonal imbalance is common among patients with mental disorders, and ECT appears to stabilize hypothalamic-pituitary-adrenal function.
2. ECT causes changes in monoamine neurotransmitter systems similar to those caused by antidepressant drugs.
3. ECT raises the seizure threshold, which, in turn, causes an antidepressant effect. Promoters of this view believe depression results from abnormal brain activity.

Number of Treatments

Typically, patients are given ECT two to three times a week up to a total of 6 to 12 treatments (or until the patient improves or is obviously not going to improve). Patients often experience relief after two or three treatments, but occasionally up to 20 will be needed. If improvement is not observed after 12 or so treatments, then continuing ECT will not typically be helpful. Although ECT is usually effective, relapse occurs frequently. Many patients require continuation or maintenance ECT treatments to function at their best (see later discussion for expansion of this topic).

Indications for ECT

Although ECT was originally developed for schizophrenia, its primary indication soon shifted to patients who were severely depressed, particularly those manifesting delusions and psychomotor retardation (Potter, Rudorfer, 1993) (Box 39-3). Severely depressed patients account for about 85% to 90% of all patients receiving ECT. These patients respond better and more rapidly to ECT than they do to antidepressants (Bowden, 1985; Coffey, Weiner, 1990). Potter and Rudorfer (1993) suggest a hierarchy of who should receive ECT:

1. Patients who require a rapid response (e.g., suicidal or catatonic patients)
2. Patients who cannot tolerate or be exposed to pharmacotherapy (e.g., pregnant women)
3. Patients who are depressed but have not responded to multiple and adequate trials of medication

Disorders, depressive symptoms, and conditions that respond to ECT are found in Table 39-1. Box 39-4 lists conditions that do not respond to ECT.

|Box 39-3| Indications for Electroconvulsive Therapy

- *Major depression:* ECT is appropriate treatment when associated with:
  1. Nonresponse to an adequate trial of antidepressants
  2. High suicide potential
  3. Dehydration
  4. Depressive stupor
  5. Catatonia
  6. Delusions
- Prophylaxis of recurrent major depression (i.e., maintenance ECT)
- Severe mania not controlled by medications
- Postpartum psychosis after nonresponse to antidepressants
- Schizophrenia (catatonic type) when nonresponsive to medications
- Movement disorders refractory to treatment (e.g., Parkinson's disease, neuroleptic malignant syndrome, tardive dyskinesia)

Adapted from Bezchlibnyk-Butler KZ, Jeffries JJ: *Clinical handbook of psychotropic drugs,* Seattle, 1997, Hogrefe & Huber Publishers.

CLINICAL EXAMPLE

Penny Jones is a 48-year-old woman who worked for the postal service until 3 weeks ago. She was admitted to an acute psychiatric facility accompanied by her daughter, who indicated that her mother had lost 30 pounds during the last 4 months. The daughter further described her mother as having a poor appetite, being isolative, awakening early in the morning with the inability to fall back to sleep, and verbalizing thoughts with suicidal overtones. The daughter stated that her mother's actions scare her.

Ms. Jones states that life is intolerable, and she does not want to live anymore without "Jerry." The daughter explains that Jerry was the patient's husband, who died 5 months ago.

Ms. Jones sought psychiatric help immediately and was prescribed sertraline 25 mg per day for 1 week, then 50 mg qd. She improved slightly but has relapsed into a deeper depression and has lately begun to verbalize suicidal thoughts. Based on her poor response to

Continued

|Table 39-1| Disorders, Depressive Symptoms, and Conditions that Respond to Electroconvulsive Therapy

Disorders	Depressive Symptoms	Conditions
Severe depression	Anhedonia	Tardive dystonia
Treatment-refractory depression	Anorexia	Tardive dyskinesia
	Delusions	Akathisia
	Insomnia	Parkinsonian symptoms
Catatonia	Muteness	
Mania	Psychomotor retardation	Neuroleptic malignant syndrome
Some types of schizophrenia	Suicidal ideations	

From Swartz CM: Seizure benefit: grand mal or grand bene? *Neurol Clin* 11(1):151, 1993b.

|Box 39-4| Conditions that Do Not Respond to Electroconvulsive Therapy

Anxiety disorders
Behavioral disorders
Mild depressions
Personality disorders
Phobic disorders
Somatoform disorders

antidepressants and her suicidal thoughts, a course of six ECT treatments was prescribed. Ms. Jones tolerated the procedures well. Her suicidal ideations ceased, she began interacting with others spontaneously, and regained her appetite. She was discharged during the third week of her hospitalization.

Contraindications for ECT

Coffey and Weiner (1990) state that no absolute contraindications exist for ECT. Ziring (1993) suggests that ECT should be viewed similarly to many lifesaving surgeries; that is, although there may be conditions that place an ECT recipient at risk, the risk may be warranted if the patient's condition is serious (e.g., severe depression, active suicidal ideations). Most clinicians believe the conditions listed in Box 39-5 create some level of risk for a patient who receives ECT.

Advantages of ECT

Historically, ECT has been viewed as providing the fastest relief for depression (Roose, Nobler, 2001).

ECT is a safe procedure; only a few ECT-related deaths have been reported (Sackeim et al, 1993). ECT has about the same risk as that associated with

Box 39-5 | Conditions Resulting in Increased Risk for Patients Receiving Electroconvulsive Therapy

Very high risk:
Recent myocardial infarction
Recent cerebrovascular accident
Intracranial mass

High risk:
Angina pectoris
Congestive heart failure
Extremely loose teeth (aspiration)
Severe pulmonary disease
Severe osteoporosis
Major bone fractures
Glaucoma
Retinal detachment
Thrombophlebitis
Pregnancy
Use of monoamine oxidase inhibitors (severe hypertension)
Use of clozapine (seizures, delirium)

Adapted from Ziring B: Issues in the perioperative care of the patient with psychiatric illness, *Med Clin North Am* 77(2):443, 1993; Bezchlibnyk-Butler KZ, Jeffries JJ: *Clinical handbook of psychotropic drugs,* Seattle, 1997, Hogrefe & Huber Publishers.

general anesthesia, 1 death per 50,000 patients (Gitlin et al, 1993), and is safer compared with tricyclic antidepressants (i.e., less cardiotoxic effects, cannot be used to attempt suicide). Furthermore, ECT is not only safe, but it is also more effective than antidepressants for certain groups of patients. Potter and Rudorfer (1993) state that up to 90% of severely depressed patients respond to ECT. Finally, ECT can be used safely and effectively in older patients, even those regarded as the "old-old" (> 85 years), and in adolescents (Cohen et al, 2000; Tomac, Rummans, Pileggi, 1997).

In addition, because it works faster, ECT may be more economical compared with other treatments. ECT can be given on an outpatient basis in some situations, resulting in additional savings and a greater convenience for the patient (Irvin, 1997).

Disadvantages of ECT

The major disadvantage of ECT is that treatment provides only temporary relief; it does not provide a permanent cure. Certainly, many patients are able to remain free of depression for long periods, and others may never need treatment again. However, some patients receiving ECT may need another series of treatments within a few months. Some psychiatrists order maintenance or continuation ECT (once per month or so for 6 to 12 months or longer); however, there is still much to learn about the benefits of this approach. Studies suggest continued periodic treatments of ECT plus an antidepressant significantly reduces relapse rates (Gagne et al, 2000).

Memory impairment, both retrograde (memory before treatment) and anterograde (memory and the ability to learn new things after treatment), has been frequently cited as a side effect of ECT. Events closest in time to ECT are most frequently affected. Although it is true that memory is impaired for events both before and after each treatment and that confusion occurs immediately after each treatment, there does not seem to be any substantial loss of mental function for most patients once the treatment series is completed. Furthermore, because depression can cause memory loss as well, it is not always clear whether memory impairment is related to ECT or to depression. Unilateral placement of the electrodes, that is, both electrodes placed on the nondominant side of the head (for right-handed individuals, this would be the right side), minimizes treatment impact on memory and learning but may not be as effective (Bailine et al, 2000). Bifrontal placement (placed a few inches apart on the front of the head) also causes fewer problems with memory and learning (Abrams, 1997; Bailine et al, 2000).

Physiologic effects of ECT include cardiac effects such as hypertension, arrhythmias, alterations of cardiac output, and changes in cerebrovascular dynamics. Hemodynamic changes, in combination with increased muscle tone, have been postulated to result in a generalized increase in oxygen consumption. Increases in myocardial oxygen consumption may result in ischemia (Ziring, 1993). Other problems that have been reported include hyponatremia (Greer, Stewart, 1993) and migraine headache (Weinstein, 1993). ECT does not cause brain damage (Abrams, 1997).

OTHER SOMATIC THERAPIES

On November 12, 1935, Almeida Lima, a Portuguese neurosurgeon under the direction of neurologist Egas Moniz, drilled two holes on the frontal aspect of the skull of a mental patient 3 cm anterior to each ear. Into these holes, in the fiber-rich region known as the centrum ovale, 0.2 cc of absolute alcohol was injected. This operation, later called the prefrontal leukotomy, ushered in a new era in the treatment of mental disorders—treatment marked by the procedure known as psychosurgery." (Dorman, 1995, p. 54)

Psychosurgery

This brief introduction to psychosurgery provides the student with an important historical occurrence in psychiatric care. To appreciate today's advances in psychiatric care and patient advocacy, one must understand issues and debates that shaped today's mental health environment.

It is difficult to find an area of psychiatry surrounded by more controversy than psychosurgery. Psychosurgery destroys brain tissue for the purpose of relieving intractable mental disorders not amenable to other therapies. A review of the literature suggests that medical scientists have strongly held views on both the efficacy and ethics of this procedure. Obviously, clinicians should eliminate all other options before using this drastic approach.

Dorman (1995) suggests this radical treatment was adopted because of the convergence of four existing conditions in psychiatric care:

1. The persistent appalling conditions in state hospitals

2. The rivalry between neurology and psychiatry
3. The use of other radical treatments (e.g., ECT)
4. New theories regarding frontal lobe brain function

Historic overview

Gottlieb Burckhardt, director of an insane asylum in Prefargier, Switzerland, first reported on psychosurgery in 1891. Burckhardt operated on six patients: one died and one developed epilepsy. Burckhardt intended to calm highly excitable patients, but the procedure was vigorously opposed by his medical colleagues to the extent that he discontinued this activity (National Commission for the Protection of Human Subjects of Biomedical and Behavioral Sciences [NCPHSBBS], 1977). In 1910, Ludwig Puusepp (NCPHSBBS, 1977), a Russian neurosurgeon, performed psychosurgery on three manic-depressive patients. The results were unsatisfactory, and he did not perform the procedure again or publish his findings for 25 years (Lichterman, 1993; Valenstein, 1980).

The man considered the modern-day pioneer in psychosurgery was Egas Moniz, a Portuguese neurologist. In 1935 Moniz, with the assistance of Lima, performed a series of psychosurgical operations on 20 severely ill institutionalized patients. These researchers reported that 14 members of this cohort showed improvement (Cosgrove, Rauch, 1995) and coined the term psychosurgery. In 1949, Moniz received the Nobel Prize in medicine and physiology for his work.

The Americans, Freeman and Watts, performed the first lobotomy in the United States on September 14, 1936:

"In their development of Dr. Moniz' methods, Drs. Freeman and Watts drilled a small hole in the temple on each side of the patient's head where two skull bones meet. Surgeon Watts then inserted a dull knife into the brain, made a fan-shaped incision upward through the prefrontal lobe, then downward a few minutes later. He then repeated the incisions on the other side of the brain. No brain tissues were removed" (Freeman, Watts, 1942, p. 48). (In two operations, they cut cerebral arteries. Both patients died.)

Walter Freeman, a neurologist, and his neurosurgeon colleague, James Watts, were impressed with the work of Moniz. Although a neurologist, Freeman treated many psychiatric patients and sought treatment approaches that were more efficient compared with standard treatment modalities. Psychosurgery was the procedure he was looking for. Before his retirement, Freeman (1971) performed over 3500 psychosurgeries. Furthermore, Freeman toured the country, stopping at the large state mental institutions to demonstrate his technique. In Freeman's wake, local practitioners began performing psychosurgery. Colaizzi (1996) paints a vivid picture of Freeman's visit to a hospital in 1950.

Freeman's reputation is sullied somewhat by what appears to be high-handed or pejorative language. Dorman (1995) has retrieved some of Freeman's remarks that detract from his work:

> Some patients come to operation at the end of a long and exasperating series of medical treatments, hospital treatments, shock treatments, including endocrines and vitamins mixed with their physiotherapy and psychotherapy. They are still desperate, and will go to any length to get rid of their distress. Other patients can't be dragged into the hospital and have to be held down on a bed in a hotel room until sufficient shock treatment can be given to render them manageable. We like both types. (p. 60)

Freeman also recorded a conversation with a 24-year-old laborer who was awake during the surgery (p. 58).

Freeman: Are you scared?
Patient: Yeh.
(2 minutes later)
Freeman: How do you feel?
Patient: I don't feel anything, but they're cutting me now.
Freeman: You wanted it?
Patient: Yes, but I didn't think you'd do it awake. Oh, gee whiz, I'm dying. Oh, doctor. Please stop. Oh, God. I'm goin' again. Oh, oh, oh. Ow, *(chisel on skull)*, oh, this is awful. Ow, *(grabs Freeman's hand and sinks nails into it)*. Oh, God, I'm goin', please stop.
(After cuts have been made)
Freeman: What's happened to your fear?
Patient: Gone.
Freeman: Why were you afraid?
Patient: I don't know.
Freeman: Feel okay?
Patient: Yes. I feel pretty good right now.

Moreover, in response to critics of his surgical technique, he referred to concerns about sterile procedure as "all that germ crap" (p. 61).

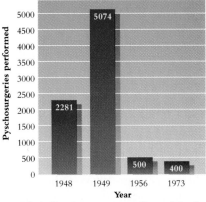

Figure 39-1 Psychosurgery performed in the years before and after the discovery and introduction of antipsychotic drugs. (From Valenstein ES: *The psychosurgery debate,* San Francisco, 1980, WH Freeman.)

Psychosurgical intervention was widely used in the 1940s and 1950s, but a sharp decline occurred after the introduction of psychotropic drugs to state hospitals in the early to mid-1950s (Figure 39-1). As previously mentioned, psychosurgery suffered some of the same public rejection as did ECT. Again, the popular novel *One Flew over the Cuckoo's Nest* depicted the defiant hero as the victim of a treacherous state hospital staff. The patient's defiance eventually resulted in the ultimate punishment—a lobotomy—and he emerged from the lobotomy room a "vegetable," his defiant character finally conquered. This depiction of psychosurgery helped shape public opinion about this procedure. The majority of professionals soon abandoned psychosurgery treatment.

Ethical concerns

As might be expected, many concerns have been voiced regarding the ethics of psychosurgery. To destroy brain tissue constitutes an extreme and irreversible tactic. Without room for error, most clinicians believe psychosurgery should be abandoned. More vocal critics see psychosurgery as a barbaric technique that is out of step with modern thinking. Some opponents suggest that a powerful tool such as psychosurgery should never be used because of the inherent potential for misuse. Most mental health professionals find these arguments against the use of psychosurgery compelling.

Indications for psychosurgery

Only patients with severe, chronic, disabling, and treatment-refractory psychiatric disorders should be considered for psychosurgery (Cosgrove, Rauch, 1995). Psychosurgery is helpful for the following mental disorders if or when traditional treatments have failed (Flor-Henry, 1975; Rappaport, 1992; Reese, 1988; Tueber, 1977; Valenstein, 1980):

- Depression and anxiety
- Depression-related pain
- Obsessive-compulsive disorders
- Aggression

Modern psychosurgery

Psychosurgery has changed considerably in the last 70 years. Four procedures are currently used. Each procedure has different indications, techniques, results, and complications. The review of these specific surgical interventions is beyond the scope of this text.

Phototherapy

Phototherapy exposes patients to intense light a few hours per day. The rationale for this treatment comes from several studies plus anecdotal reports indicating that environmental factors play a role in mood disorders. Seasonal affective disorder (SAD), for instance, results from decreased exposure to sunlight and typically occurs in and around the winter season. Phototherapy applied to SAD sufferers relieves symptoms of depression. Apparently, both morning and midday phototherapy administration provides relief from depression, thus permitting therapy to occur at work or home. The precise mechanism of action of the way exposure to intense light produces an antidepressant effect remains unclear. Other conditions thought to respond to light therapy include bulimia, sleep-maintenance insomnia, and nonseasonal depression. Because phototherapy produces few if any significant adverse effects, the risk-benefit ratio favors its use.

Transcranial Magnetic Stimulation

Transcranial magnetic stimulation (TMS) produces a magnetic field over the brain, influencing brain activity. Apparently, TMS increases the release of neurotransmitters, thus ameliorating depressive symptoms and potentially other disorders. Because

TMS does not require anesthesia, it is an attractive alternative to ECT should conclusive evidence of its efficacy be demonstrated. Adverse effects include seizures in previously seizure-free individuals, headache, and transient hearing loss. Patients with metal implanted in their bodies (e.g., plates), pacemakers, heart disease, or increased intracranial pressure should be carefully evaluated before receiving TMS.

Critical Thinking Question

What are some of the potential abuses of psychosurgery in a society in which physicians are held in high esteem?

Key Concepts

1. Somatic therapies are treatment approaches that use physiologic or physical interventions to effect behavioral change.
2. The most common form of somatic therapy is ECT.
3. During ECT, an electric current is passed through the brain, causing a grand mal seizure.
4. Modern ECT uses anesthesia and muscle relaxants to prevent convulsive jerks that once caused broken bones; oxygen is given to guard against brain damage.
5. ECT is indicated for the treatment of severe depression, depression that is unresponsive to other treatments, mania, catatonia, and some types of schizophrenia.
6. Psychosurgery, a controversial brain surgery, is performed to provide relief from mental disorders that have been resistant to other treatment forms.
7. Critics of psychosurgery have raised many ethical concerns, including its efficacy and the possibility of worsening patients' conditions.
8. Refinements in modern psychosurgery that target precise and limited brain anatomy have made the procedure safer than it was in the past.
9. Some individuals suffer depressive symptoms in response to decrease sunlight availability (i.e., during winter months). Phototherapy, the exposure to intense artificial light, reduces these symptoms.
10. TMS of the brain reduces symptoms of depression, perhaps by increasing levels of neurotransmitters.

References

Abrams R: *Electroconvulsive therapy,* New York, 1997, Oxford University Press.

Bailine SH et al: Comparison of bifrontal and bitemporal ECT for major depression, *Am J Psychiatry* 157(1):121, 2000.

Bezchlibnyk-Butler KZ, Jeffries JJ: *Clinical handbook of psychotropic drugs,* Seattle, 1997, Hogrefe & Huber Publishers.

Bowden CL: Current treatment of depression, *Hosp Community Psychiatry* 36:1192, 1985.

Coffey CE, Weiner RD: Electroconvulsive therapy: an update, *Hosp Community Psychiatry* 41:515, 1990.

Cohen D et al: Absence of cognitive impairment at long-term follow-up in adolescents treated with ECT for severe mood disorder, *Am J Psychiatry* 157(3):460, 2000.

Colaizzi J: Transorbital lobotomy at Eastern State Hospital (1951-1954), *J Psychosoc Nurs Ment Health Serv* 34(12):16, 1996.

Cosgrove CR, Rauch SL: Psychosurgery, *Nurs Clin North Am* 6(1):167, 1995.

Dorman J: The history of psychosurgery, *Tex Med* 91(7):54, 1995.

Fink M: New technology in convulsive therapy: a challenge to training, *Am J Psychiatry* 144:1195, 1987.

Fink M: *Electroshock,* New York, 1999, Oxford University Press.

Fitzsimons L: Electroconvulsive therapy: what nurses need to know, *J Psychosoc Nurs Ment Health Serv* 33(12):14, 1995.

Flor-Henry P: Psychiatric surgery 1936-1973: evolution and current perspectives, *Can Psychiatr Assoc J* 20:157, 1975.

Freeman W: Frontal lobotomy in early schizophrenia: long-term follow-up in 415 cases, *Br J Psychiatry* 119: 621, 1971.

Freeman W, Watts JW: *Time,* p 48, Nov 30, 1942.

Gagne GG et al: Efficacy of continuation ECT and antidepressant drugs compared to long-term antidepressants alone in depressed patients, *Am J Psychiatry* 157(12):1960, 2000.

Gitlin MC et al: Splenic rupture after electroconvulsive therapy, *Anesth Analg* 76:1363, 1993.

Greer R, Stewart R: Hyponatremia and ECT, *Am J Psychiatry* 150(8):1272, 1993.

Irvin SM: Treatment of depression with outpatient electroconvulsive therapy, *AORN J* 65(3):573, 1997.

Kellner C, McCall W: Novel electrode placements: time to reassess, *J ECT* 15(2):115, 1999.

Krystal AD et al: ECT stimulus intensity: are present ECT devices too limited? *Am J Psychiatry* 157(6):963, 2000.

Lichterman L: On the history of psychosurgery in Russia, *Acta Neurochir* 125(1-4):1, 1993.

National Commission for the Protection of Human Subjects of Biomedical and Behavioral Sciences: *Psychosurgery,* Washington, DC, 1977, U.S. Department of Health, Education, and Welfare.

Potter W, Rudorfer M: Electroconvulsive therapy: a modern medical procedure, *N Engl J Med* 328:12, 1993.

Rappaport ZH: Psychotherapy in the modern era: therapeutic and ethical aspects, *Med Law* 11(5-6):449, 1992.

Reese T: Obsessive-compulsive disorders: a treatment review, *J Clin Psychiatry* 49:48, 1988.

Roberts GW, Leigh PN, Weinberger DR: *Neuropsychiatric disorders,* London, 1993, Mosby.

Roose SP, Nobler M: ECT and onset of action, *J Clin Psychiatry* 62(suppl 4):24, 2001.

Sackeim HA et al: Effects of stimulus intensity and electrode placement on the efficacy and cognitive effects of electroconvulsive therapy, *N Engl J Med* 328(12):839, 1993.

Smith D: Shock and disbelief, *The Atlantic Monthly,* p. 79, February, 2001.

Swartz CM: ECT or programmed seizures? *Am J Psychiatry* 150(8):1274, 1993a.

Swartz CM: Seizure benefit: grand mal or grand bene? *Neurol Clin* 11(1):151, 1993b.

Tomac TA, Rummans TA, Pileggi TS: Safety and efficacy of electroconvulsive therapy in patients over age 85, *Am J Geriatr Psychiatry* 5(2):126, 1997.

Tueber HC, National Commission for the Protection of Human Subjects of Biomedical and Behavioral Sciences: *Psychosurgery,* Sec III, Washington, DC, 1977, U.S. Department of Health, Education, and Welfare.

Valenstein ES: *The psychosurgery debate,* San Francisco, 1980, WH Freeman.

Weinstein MD: Migraine occurring as sequela of electroconvulsive therapy, *Headache* 33(1):45, 1993.

Ziring B: Issues in the perioperative care of the patient with psychiatric illness, *Med Clin North Am* 77(2):443, 1993.

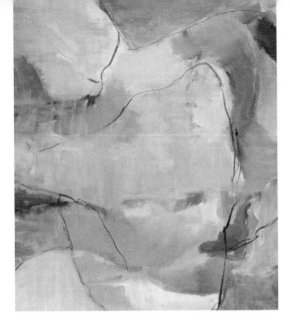

Chapter 40

Alternative and Complementary Therapies

Beverly K. Hogan

Learning Objectives

After reading this chapter, you should be able to:

- Define alternative therapy, and give three examples of categories of alternative therapy.
- Trace the historical use of alternative therapies to the current state of use.
- Define complementary therapy and give an example to illustrate what is meant by complementary versus alternative therapy.
- Name common alternative and complementary therapies used for psychiatric symptoms, and state the current research conclusions regarding their efficacy.
- Describe how various alternative and complementary therapies are regulated.
- Name three dangerous interactions with herbal therapies.
- Explain the role of the nurse in assessment and intervention with clients using alternative or complementary therapies.

Each year, nearly $1 trillion is spent on health care in the United States, with $22 billion spent on alternative therapies. This figure is remarkable considering most of this money is an out-of-pocket expense (Eisenberg et al, 1998; Snyder, Lindquist, 2001). Eighty percent of the world's population relies on therapies that are called *alternative* in the United States (Folks, Gabel, 2001). Estimates suggest that one out of three consumers in the United States use alternative therapies in one form or another. In a follow-up study of uses of alternative therapies, Eisenberg and colleagues (1998) found an almost 50% increase in alternative care visits from a previous survey (in 1990), a number *exceeding the total number of visits to all primary care physicians* in the United States. Clearly, the American health care consumer is willing to consider treatments offered outside mainstream medicine.

Among people using alternative therapies along with traditional medicine, less than one half disclose this use to their health care provider (Eisenberg et al, 1998). Because alternative therapies may interact with traditional therapies and may also have their own set of side effects, it is important to know whether the patient is using these therapies. Additionally, cultural competence requires that nurses be knowledgeable about "alternative" health care beliefs and practices. The nurse's ability to respond in an informed and open manner is essential for obtaining accurate information (Snyder, Lindquist, 2001).

Key Terms

Acupuncture An ancient Chinese health practice that involves puncturing the skin with hair-thin needles at particular locations, called acupuncture points, on the patient's body. Acupuncture is believed to help reduce pain or change a body function. Sometimes the needles are twirled or given a slight electric charge (http://nccam.nih.gov/fcp/factsheets/acupuncture/acupuncture.htm).

Alternative therapy Broad range of healing philosophies and approaches mainstream Western medicine does not commonly use, accept, study, understand, or make available.

Complementary therapy Same as alternative therapy but denotes therapy used as an adjunct to rather than as a replacement for conventional treatment.

Herbaceuticals Plant or plant part that produces and contains chemical substances that act on the body.

Homeopathy Unconventional Western system that is based on the principle that "like cures like" (i.e., the same substance that, in large doses, produces the symptoms of an illness, in very minute doses, cures it). Homeopathic physicians believe that the more dilute the remedy is, the greater its potency will be. Therefore these practitioners use small doses of specially prepared plant extracts and minerals to stimulate the body's defense mechanisms and healing processes to treat illness.

Naturopathic physician Alternative care practitioner who holds an naturopathic doctorate degree.

Naturopathy Views disease as a manifestation of alterations in the processes by which the body naturally heals itself and emphasizes health restoration rather than disease treatment. Naturopathic physicians employ an array of healing practices, including diet and clinical nutrition; homeopathy; acupuncture; herbal medicine; hydrotherapy (the use of water in a range of temperatures and methods of applications); spinal and soft-tissue manipulation; physical therapies involving electric currents, ultrasound, and light therapy; therapeutic counseling; and pharmacology.

Psychoneuroimmunology Field of research focusing on the interactions of mind, environment, and bodily function, particularly immune system function.

Western medicine Term conventional clinicians use to describe the medicine practiced by holders of medical doctor (MD) or doctor of osteopathy (DO) degrees, some of whom may also practice complementary and alternative medicine. Other terms for conventional medicine are allopathy; regular, mainstream medicine; and biomedicine.

Potential consumers of mental health services are also seeking alternative treatments. A study of alternative and complementary therapies revealed that the majority of people in the United States with self-defined anxiety attacks or severe depression use some form of alternative and complementary therapy to treat these conditions (Kessler et al, 2001).

This chapter will use the term *alternative* to refer to therapies that are *not generally accepted by* mainstream Western medicine. Complementary therapy will be used to refer to treatments used *in conjunction with* traditional or conventional Western medicine. The history and current status of alternative and complementary therapies will be explored in this chapter. Coverage of the entire field of alternative and complementary therapies is beyond the scope of this text. Therapies with some scientific support will be addressed, as will some of those with less rigorous support. Finally, the implications of this information and the consequent controversies will be examined within the context of nursing care.

HISTORIC PERSPECTIVE

In ancient times, the belief held that fate, evil spirits, or the gods caused illness. Hippocrates, the father of modern medicine, is credited with introducing beliefs suggesting that illness resulted from an interaction between the mind-body and the environment. Care of the whole person was considered central to the practice of medicine, and well into the 1800s, alternative therapies and conventional medicine peacefully coexisted. However, as surgical techniques improved and microbes came to be understood as disease-causing agents, a preference for more scientifically based therapies developed. By the 1900s, alternative therapy was dismissed as quackery. Medical advances continued throughout the twentieth century, but as early as the 1960s, a growing dissatisfaction with health care was becoming apparent. Not only had conventional medicine failed to live up to its promise, but it also created a cadre of chronic diseases and toxic medications with which its practitioners treated patients. Many consumers began the search for more palatable alternatives. Furthermore,

Resources for Learning More about Alternative
and Complementary Medicine

- American Botanical Council: www.herbalgram.org or
  www.herbs.org
- U.S. Food and Drug Administration: www.fda.gov
- National Center for Complementary and Alternative
  Medicine, National Institutes of Health:
  www.nccam.nih.gov
- *Physicians Desk Reference of Herbal Medicine*
- *Mosby's Handbook of Herbs and Natural Supplements*,
  Linda Skidmore-Roth, 2001

Alternative Therapies

Herbals
Homeopathic remedies
Acupuncture
Meditative practices
Massage therapy
Magnetic stimulation
Omega-3 fatty acids

conventional medicine with its reliance on scientific methodologies and single agent causation had created a dual system of care (i.e., not holistic) in which psychologic and spiritual issues were left to other disciplines. Although acute care medicine became good at keeping people from dying, it did little to enhance quality of life (Gaydos, 2001; Snyder, Lindquist, 2001). This growing dissatisfaction coupled with other events (see later discussion) formed the groundswell for this emerging field.

One of the events that gave credence to the alternative health movement arose from concerns about the effects of stress on health. A proliferation of research and the development of a new emerging field of psychoneuroimmunology resulted. These scientifically based findings brought about a renewed interest in mind-body interactions. Ironically, this holistic approach to medicine was similar to that which Hippocrates had envisioned. Modalities that had remained in mainstream medicine in the East were becoming popularized as alternative therapy in the West. A dissatisfied yet receptive consumer awaited.

The growing popularity of alternative treatments attracted the attention of many special-interest groups and eventually resulted in the federal government's creation of the Office of Alternative Medicine (OAM) in 1992. OAM's mission was to provide the public with *information* regarding the safety and efficacy of these therapies. The U.S. Food and Drug Administration (FDA) was unable to regulate herbals because herbs were classified as dietary and nutritional supplements. In 1994 the FDA, as a result of the Dietary Supplement and Health Education Act (DSHEA), was able to require labeling on herbals, stating there was *no proof of efficacy, safety, or standards for quality control*. In Germany, France, the United Kingdom, and Canada, quality and safety of herbs are enforced by the federal government (Folks, Gabel, 2001). As herbals and other alternative therapies continued to gain popularity in the United States, OAM, as a *division of the National Institutes of Health (NIH), broadened* its scope to include research as an objective. The National Center for Complementary and Alternative Medicine (NCCAM) became the new name for OAM in 1992. One of the directives of NCCAM is to fund research into the efficacy and safety of alternative treatments. Bastyr University, an accredited school for naturopathic medicine, has been the recipient of several NCCAM-funded NIH grants to study particular therapies for their safety and efficacy in mainstream medicine (http://nccam.nih.gov, 2001).

German Contributions

Alternative therapies are an integral part of the German health care system. For instance, St. John's wort, an herbal antidepressant, is prescribed by German doctors 20 times more often than is Prozac, a widely prescribed antidepressant in the United States. Many alternative therapies have been validated in Germany, where their use is widespread (NCCAM, 2001). In 1978 the German federal government established an expert committee, Commission E, to evaluate the safety and efficacy of over 300 herbals sold in Germany. Commission E was composed of 24 members recommended by associations of health professionals, nonmedical practitioners (called *heilpraktikers* in Germany), pharmacologists, toxicologists, biostatisticians, and by representatives of the pharmaceutical industry. The results of their investigation into the efficacy and safety of herbs has been published in monographs that are now known as the Commission E monographs. These monographs serve as the basis for the medical usage of herbs within the German health care system and outline acceptable manufacturing processes on the basis of available scientific and clinical evidence (http://www.herbalgram.org/browse.php/comm_e_int, 2001). This document has recently been translated into English and is no doubt being carefully reviewed by many interested groups at this very moment.

Alternative Therapy and Nursing Education

If Commission E studies are deemed methodologically sound, herbal medicine practice will be transformed. The double-blind study is the gold standard for Western medicine in which single causality is sought. Whether the scientific basis for herbs and other alternative therapies is understood, the fact remains that the American public is using these therapies. In 1996 the NIH office of alternative therapies convened with leaders in medicine and nursing to hold the first National Conference on Medical and Nursing Education in Complementary Medicine. The purpose of the conference was to address the need to include courses in alternative therapies in their respective curriculums. A consensus to include alternative therapies was reached, although many details have not been worked out (Gaydos, 2001; Wetzel, Eisenberg, Kaptchuk, 1998). The remainder of this chapter is devoted to providing an overview of alternative and complementary therapies applicable to psychiatry. Initially, a review of these therapies with support in the research literature will be presented.

HERBAL THERAPIES (HERBACEUTICALS)

Herbs include plant roots, tree barks, berries, leaves, resins, and flowers. Herbal therapy has been used for centuries and was referred to in the writings of Hippocrates. Although 30% of all modern drugs are derived from plants, only 1% of plants have been analyzed for their potential medicinal uses. As noted, medicinal uses for herbs have a long history, particularly in non-Western societies.

Twenty percent of people in the United States use herbs for chronic conditions. Most herbs are generally not recommended for use in pregnancy, and some are known abortifacients (Folks, Gabel,

2001). A common misconception associated with herbals is *natural equals not harmful*. There are numerous reports in medical and scientific journals of severe reactions to herbs, including hepatotoxicity, liver failure, renal failure, gastrointestinal (GI) tract obstruction, cardiac arrhythmias, seizure, exacerbation, development of psychiatric symptoms, and even fatalities (Ernst, 1998).

Four of the twelve most common herbs are used to treat or prevent psychiatric symptoms (Beaubrun, Gray, 2000). Treatment of depression is perhaps the most prominently mentioned use of these agents. Herbals are among the most frequently tried alternative therapy for depression (Ernst, 1998). Table 40-1 provides a summary of herbals used for psychiatric symptoms.

St. John's Wort

This herb is a popular treatment for mild to moderate depression; it is also used to treat anxiety, seasonal affective disorder, and sleep disorders. Extracts of the plant are sold as a nutritional supplement after being prepared with a powder or oil; the herb is available in capsule, tea, or tincture forms. St. John's wort is among the top-selling botanical products in the United States, with industry-estimated sales of $400 million in 1998. If efficacy is established, St John's wort is expected to be in even greater demand because of its having fewer and less severe side effects compared with traditional antidepressant drugs (Linde K, 1996; NCCAM, 2001).

Although no consensus exists regarding the mechanism of action for St. John's wort, it is thought to have an affinity for gamma-aminobutyric acid, both $GABA_A$ and $GABA_B$, serotonin, central benzodiazepine, and other receptors (Folks, Gabel, 2001). Several mechanisms of action of St. John's wort have been proposed, including the following:
- Inhibition of monoamine (serotonin, dopamine, and norepinephrine) reuptake (low serotonin, norepinephrine, and dopamine levels are associated with depression)
- Modulation of interleukin-6 (IL-6) activity: IL-6, a protein involved in intercellular communication in the immune system, may lead to increases in adrenal regulatory hormones, such as cortisol (elevated cortisol is associated with depression; see Chapter 29). St. John's wort may

|Table 40-1| Common Herbs Used to Treat Psychiatric Symptoms

Herbal Product	Contraindications	Adverse Side Effects	Drug Interactions
Angelica 1-2 g twice daily whole herb	Diabetes Peptic ulcer disease Bleeding disorders Pregnancy Breast-feeding	CV: decreased BP GI: anorexia, flatulence, spasms, dyspepsia Integumentary: photo-sensitivity, phototoxicity, dermatitis	Increased PTT with anticoagulants
Chamomile 300-400 mg up to 6 times/day	Known abortifacient Cross sensitivity to sunflowers, ragweed, and members of aster family (echinacea)	Hypersensitivity-allergic reactions Burning of face, mouth, eyes, and mucous membranes	Anticoagulants Increases effects of CNS drugs
Gingko biloba 120 mg/day	Pregnancy Breast-feeding Peptic ulcer disease and other bleeding problems	Headache, anxiety, and restlessness	Trazodone
Kava-kava 100-200 mg/day	?Liver disease	Scaling of skin overdose	Antiparkinsonian agents benzodiazepines CNS depressants
Melatonin			More data needed
St. John's wort 900 mg/day	Pregnancy Breast-feeding	Dizziness. insomnia, restless-ness, constipation, abdominal cramps, photosensitivity	Protease inhibitors olanzapine (Zyprexa) Oral contraceptives
Valerian officinalis 400-900 mg/day	Pregnancy Breast-feeding	Dependence	MAOIs, warfarin, phenytoin

BP, Blood pressure; *CNS*, central nervous system; *CV*, cardiovascular; *GI*, gastrointestinal; *PTT*, prothrombin time; *MAOIs*, monoamine oxidase inhibitors.
From Folks DE, Gabel T: Herbaceuticals in psychiatry. In Keltner N, Folks D, editors: *Psychotropic drugs*, ed 3, St Louis, 2001, Mosby.

reduce levels of IL-6 and thus causes an antidepressive effect (Linde et al, 1996; NCCAM, 2001).

An analysis of 23 European clinical studies of St. John's wort concluded that it has antidepressive effects in cases of mild to moderate depression (the dose varied considerably among the studies). These studies compared St. John's wort with tricyclic antidepressants (TCAs) but not the newer antidepressants. Studies regarding long-term use of St. John's wort are lacking at present. The first large-scale controlled clinical trial in the United States to assess whether this herb has significant therapeutic effect in patients with clinical depression is currently underway in a number of clinical sites across the United States (Beaubrun, Gray, 2000; NCCAM, 2001).

In a review of over two dozen clinical studies of St. John's wort, nine were considered "well controlled" at standardized doses of 900 mg per day. These nine studies demonstrated improvement on standard rating scales for depression. Overall, there were fewer side effects associated with St. John's wort

($\cong 20\%$) when compared with traditional antidepressant treatment ($\cong 50\%$) (Beaubrun, Gray, 2000).

St. John's wort is generally safe, with most side effects emerging at dose ranges exceeding those recommended for depression. Indications are that St. John's wort may interact with olanzapine (Zyprexa), preventing its metabolism and dramatically increasing blood levels. St. John's wort may also increase the risk for serotonin syndrome and should not be taken with other antidepressants, particularly selective serotonin reuptake inhibitors (SSRIs) (Beaubrun, Gray, 2000). Other reported side effects and adverse reactions to St. John's wort include dizziness, insomnia, restlessness, constipation, abdominal cramps, and photosensitivity (Skidmore-Roth, 2001). St John's wort is thought to induce cytochrome P450 3A4, thus potentially speeding the metabolism of many drugs. For example, St John's wort decreases blood levels of protease inhibitors, such as those used in treatment of human immunodeficiency virus (HIV) infection (Folks, Gabel, 2001; Skidmore-Roth, 2001). Some reports suggest that St. John's wort may reduce the effectiveness of oral contraceptives, thereby increasing the risk of pregnancy (Ayd, 2000). In summary, St. John's wort appears to be efficacious in the treatment of mild to moderate depression; but its use in severe depression cannot be recommended (Beaubrun, Gray, 2000).

CLINICAL EXAMPLE

Sam S. is a 47-year-old male Caucasian who has been treated for depression on several occasions in the past. Sam has had several recurrences of depression because he does not like taking "psychiatric drugs." Sam began taking St. John's wort made by Nature's Source, at a dose of 750 mg/day. Sam believes his depression is improved and feels better about taking a "natural" herb. Because Sam has never had an episode of severe depression and has never been suicidal, Sam's psychiatrist agrees with Sam's plan to continue St. John's wort and asks Sam to come in for psychiatric evaluation of his depression every 6 months.

Kava-Kava

Kava-kava is part of the traditional religious and social ceremonies in Polynesia and other Pacific islands. Kava-kava is prized for its ability to soothe the worried mind. Kava-kava is one of the few herbs in which the pharmacologically active ingredients are known. The active ingredients are kava-kava pyrones, which are thought to inhibit monoamine oxidase-B (Uebelhack, Franke, Schewe, 1998). Kava-kava does not appear to affect cognitive functioning, mental acuity, or coordination. Although high doses can be dangerous, there appears to be few side effects when taken in the recommended dose range (100 to 200 mg/day) (Beaubrun, Gray, 2000). There is a single report of coma associated with an overdose of kava-kava (Almeida, Grimsley, 1996). Kava-kava has an affinity for benzodiazepine receptors (Folks, Gabel, 2001) and acts directly on the limbic system. Kava-kava has been reported to produce electroencephalogram (EEG) changes similar to those seen with benzodiazepines (Wong, Smith, Boon, 1998). Several studies document its effectiveness in reducing anxiety. Kava-kava interacts with antiparkinson drugs, benzodiazepines, and other drugs that act on the central nervous system (CNS) (Skidmore-Roth, 2001). Long-term use can cause scaling of the skin (Folks, Gabel, 2001; McEnany, 2001.

CLINICAL EXAMPLE

Sherry S., a 26-year-old African-American woman was admitted to the psychiatric unit for depression with psychotic features. Sherry received a 1-mg injection of lorazepam (Ativan) in the emergency room. On admission to the unit, Sherry was noted to have slurred speech, poor coordination, and slow responses. Sherry has not been on any scheduled or prescribed medications, but the nurse found a bottle of kava-kava among Sherry's belongings. Sherry's excessive response to the lorazepam (Ativan) was most likely a result of her concomitant use of the herbal preparation, kava-kava.

Valerian

Over 250 different species of valerian are native to Europe and Asia. The one used for anxiety comes from the plant of the genus *Valerian officinalis*. Considerable difference exists in the potency of valerian, depending on the manufacturing process. The general dose range of 400 to 900 mg/day has been shown to be effective in decreasing sleep latency, nocturnal awakening, and a subjective sense of "good sleep" (Beaubrun, Gray, 2000). Valerian has an affinity for the $GABA_A$ and serotonoin$_{1a}$ receptors (Folks, Gabel, 2001). Valerian has also been extensively studied and is effective in relieving anxiety. Possible adverse effects include enhancing the effects of other CNS-acting drugs and negating the effects of other drugs including, monamine oxidase inhibitors (MAOIs), warfarin, and phenytoin (Skidmore-Roth, 2001). There has been a case report in the literature of cardiac complications apparently caused by a withdrawal phenomenon in a male patient taking 530 mg to 2 g per dose, five times a day (Garges, Varia, Doraiswamy, 1998; McEnany, 2001). A tea containing valerian, skullcap, and chaparral has been associated with acute hepatitis (Ernst, 1998).

In summary, *Valerian officinalis* appears to be useful for anxiety and insomnia; however, caution regarding dependence and withdrawal is in order.

Chamomile

Chamomile also has an affinity for benzodiazepine receptors and may interact with the histamine system as well (Folks, Gabel, 2001). Multiple studies have demonstrated the herb's ability to promote relaxation and sleep and to decrease anxiety. Side effects may involve a burning sensation of the face, eyes, and mucous membranes when using topical formulations. Chamomile may interfere with anticoagulants and probably increases the effects of other CNS-acting agents (Skidmore-Roth, 2001). More controlled studies are needed on the use of chamomile for specific psychiatric symptoms.

Angelica

Several studies have shown angelica to cause significant muscle relaxation without changes in level of consciousness. Angelica can cause hypotension, GI distress, photosensitivity, phototoxicity, and photodermatitis. Angelica should be used with caution in patients with diabetes, peptic ulcer, bleeding disorders, and with anticoagulant therapy (Skidmore-Roth, 2001). At present, studies on the use of angelica for specific psychiatric disorders are insufficient.

Ginkgo

One of the top-selling herbs in the United States, gingko has consistently demonstrated improvement in memory, concentration, and mood in patients with dementia. A 52-week double-blind, placebo-controlled study of participants who were given 120 mg of gingko per day showed an overall improvement in cognitive subscales of the Alzheimer Rating Scale (Beaubrun, Gray, 2000). Ginkgo has also proven useful in brain trauma and cerebral insufficiency. One to three months is required to achieve the full effect. Multicenter controlled studies have demonstrated the ability of ginkgo to improve memory and attention (Folks, Gabel, 2001). At least one trial has demonstrated improvement in depression when gingko is used to augment antidepressant therapy in medication refractory patients (Wong, Smith, Boon, 1998). Ginkgo has also been used as an antidote to erectile dysfunction caused by antidepressants. Random controlled trials of gingko and four standard cholinesterase inhibitors showed no difference in therapeutic effects (McEnany, 2001). Ginkgo helps to modulate vascular tone and decreases thrombosis by antagonizing the platelet-activating factor; it may increase the effects of anticoagulants and should be used with caution in patients with potential bleeding problems, such as peptic ulcer disease (Folks, Gabel, 2001; Skidmore-Roth, 2001). The pharmacologic action involves increased release of catecholamines. Side effects related to this action include headache, anxiety, and restlessness (Skidmore-Roth, 2001). Ginkgo should not be used concurrently with MAOIs (Skidmore-Roth, 2001). One case of coma possibly resulting from an interaction between gingko and trazodone (Desyrel) has been reported (McEnany, 2001).

CLINICAL EXAMPLE

Thomas J. is a 76-year-old African-American man who has been on maintenance doses of Coumadin after open-heart surgery 6 months ago. Thomas was admitted to the general medical unit with an abnormal prothrombin time. When assessing his medication adherence practices, Thomas tells the nurse practitioner that he takes gingko for his memory. The treatment team was able to make appropriate dose adjustments to Thomas's Coumadin and further evaluated his complaints about his memory.

Melatonin

Several studies demonstrate the efficacy of melatonin in reducing sleep onset latency and the number of nocturnal awakenings. Some promising studies have been conducted on the use of melatonin in resynchronizing the biologic clock and preventing "ICU syndrome" (i.e., delirium, psychosis) (McEnany, 2001).

Critical Thinking Questions

If asked to make recommendations about alternative therapies, what criteria should be used in making any recommendations or giving advice? What would you tell someone about alternative therapies? What cautions would you take about alternative therapies?

ACUPUNCTURE

Acupuncture is one of the most thoroughly researched and documented alternative practices. Many conventional therapies are not as thoroughly studied as is acupuncture. In its original form, acupuncture was based on the principle that the workings of the human body are controlled by a vital force or energy called *Qi* (pronounced "chee"), which circulates between the organs along channels called meridians. Acupuncture points are located along meridians, and fine needles are inserted through the skin and left in position briefly, sometimes with manual or electrical stimulation. Acupuncture is only one means in Chinese medicine of altering the flow of Qi. Acupuncture needles are extremely fine and do not hurt in the same way as, for instance, the needle used for an injection (Acupuncture Nitt Consensus Conference Statement, 1997).

Acupuncture has been used successfully for a variety of conditions (Vickers, Zollman, 1999). Several studies demonstrate the effectiveness of acupuncture for major depression, although repeated studies are needed to validate these findings. Combining acupuncture with mild electrical stimulation of the acupuncture needles has been found to influence norepinephrine metabolism in experimental animals. Clinical research suggests acupuncture to be equally effective as is amitriptyline (Elavil) when measuring treatment effects and rates of recurrence (Ernst, 1998; Luo et al, 1998). Acupuncture may be especially useful for patients who are unable to tolerate the anticholinergic side effects of TCAs.

Acupuncture is also useful as a *complementary* therapy in the treatment of substance abuse. Outpatient acupuncture programs were compared with residential detoxification programs with regard to relapse rates at 6 months after detoxification. Acupuncture patients were less likely to be readmitted by comparison (Shwartz et al, 1999). A 1997 consensus panel for the NIH, composed of 25 expert presenters and 12 panel members, evaluated the available literature on the efficacy of acupuncture for various conditions. The panel concluded sufficient evidence existed to support its endorsement as a complementary therapy for drug addiction (Acupuncture Nitt Consensus Conference Statement, 1997).

Although there have been reports of serious adverse events associated with acupuncture, such as pneumothorax, hepatitis, and other infections, these side effects are believed to be a result of poor technique by untrained acupuncturists. Side effects and risks associated with acupuncture are rare but may include contact dermatitis, pain in the puncture region, ecchymosis with or without pain, malaise, transient hypotension, forgotten needles, minor hemorrhage, or aggravation of the initial complaint (Yamashita et al, 1998).

Not surprisingly, Western medicine is not satisfied with the explanation of acupuncture's mechanism of action (i.e., restoring Qi). The search for more scientific explanations does suggest an alteration in neurotransmitters, neurohormonal mechanisms, and blood flow. Additional evidence substantiates an alteration of the sensory pathways affecting functions in the brain and the periphery (Acupuncture Nitt Consensus Conference Statement, 1997).

Critical Thinking Question

Acupuncture, which has traditionally been considered an alternative therapy, is now widely used by many people; several studies support its use for certain conditions. At what point does an alternative therapy become a conventional therapy?

MEDITATIVE AND SPIRITUAL PRACTICES

Yoga comes from Hindu and Buddhist traditions and emphasizes meditation and relaxation. One small study ($n = 5$) showed a 71% reduction in obsessive-compulsive disorder (OCD) symptoms for subjects practicing yoga (Shannahoff-Khalsa, Beckett, 1996). Five patients were well stabilized on fluoxetine (Prozac) before the study, three stopped medication after 7 months or less, and two experienced significantly reduced symptoms. Because of the limited number of subjects, however, these findings must be embraced with caution. Nonetheless, these techniques merit further investigation under controlled conditions, and these studies may lead to new approaches for the treatment of OCD and other anxiety-related disorders.

Several studies have been conducted over the last several decades on beneficial effects of relaxation and meditation for psychiatric conditions. One apparent effect is a modulation of sympathetic tone, suggesting increased resilience to daily stresses (Infante, 2001). In a study evaluating catecholamine levels in practitioners of transcendental meditation, catecholamine (epinephrine and norepinephrine) levels were found to be significantly lower compared with those in control groups. Normally, catecholamine levels follow a circadian rhythm, with increased levels during the morning followed by gradual decrease through the day. The authors believe a lack of rhythmic changes in catecholamine levels among these practitioners represents a lowered hormonal response to daily stress (Infante, 2001). Practitioners of transcendental meditation and yoga have also demonstrated significantly higher levels of melatonin following meditation. Numerous positive health benefits have been attributed to melatonin's functions, such as maintenance of biologic rhythms, augmentation of the immune system, and antiaging, anticancer, and antistress effects (Tooley et al, 2000). Other studies find a potential use of meditation for anxiety disorders (Kabat-Zinn et al, 1992; Miller, Fletcher, Kabat-Zinn, 1995).

Similar to meditative practices are spiritual therapies. The number one spiritual therapy used as an "alternative" or complementary health care practice is prayer. When used for health concerns, prayer is considered an alternative health practice. Studies suggest that many African Americans and women, in particular, are more likely to rely on community supports, particularly the church (Seniors Use Prayer to Cope with Stress).

MASSAGE THERAPY

Although studies reveal an immediate positive effect on the subjective sense of well being, few studies have demonstrated the usefulness of massage in psychiatric disorders. One study documented improvement in mood after a treatment period of 5 days in adolescents with adjustment disorder and depression. The treatment duration and sample size were insufficient to draw conclusions beyond this limited period (Ernst, 1998).

CLAIMS FOR ALTERNATIVE AND COMPLEMENTARY THERAPIES THAT ARE POTENTIALLY PROMISING FOR PSYCHIATRY

Omega-3 Fatty Acids for Bipolar Disorder and Schizophrenia

The source of omega-3 fatty acids is fish oil. The benefits of these particular fatty acids are currently being studied for several possible therapeutic uses. Biochemical studies of the white blood cells show high-dose omega-3 fatty acids incorporated into membrane phospholipids and appear to inhibit signal-transduction pathways. Omega-3 fatty acids are also incorporated into neuronal phospholipids in animal models, suggesting a possible similarity to the mechanisms of lithium and valproate (Depakene). Patients with subacute mania treated with omega-3 fatty acids had significantly longer periods of remis-

sion compared with the placebo group (Stoll et al, 1999). Early results from a few trials also suggest a positive effect of omega-3 fatty acids over placebo for scale-derived mental state outcomes in patients with schizophrenia (Joy, Mumby-Croft, Joy, 2000).

Rapid Transcranial Magnetic Stimulation for Depression, Mania, and Schizophrenia

Rapid transcranial magnetic stimulation (rTMS) has been proposed as a possible new treatment for refractory depression. The treatment involves the passage of magnetic waves through the skull using a special machine. Unlike electroconvulsive therapy (ECT), the patient does not have to undergo anesthesia, and no obvious major side effects occur from treatment.

Preliminary evidence suggests an improvement in symptoms of depression among patients with major depression and some possible benefit in reducing anxiety and restlessness in patients with schizophrenia (Feinsod et al, 1998) when these patients undergo rTMS.

Erfurth and colleagues (2000) describe a case of medication refractory mania responsive to rTMS as the only treatment. Prefrontal rTMS has also been shown to reduce symptoms in psychotic patients (Rollnik et al, 2000).

Lisanby and colleagues (2001) demonstrated that rTMS produces the same effect as does ECT, but without seizures. These authors reported one case of an ECT-like seizure using similar voltage equivalents to that of ECT, however. Additionally, verbal memory and reaction time are not impaired with rTMS as it is with ECT (Padberg et al, 1999). As the role and effectiveness of this treatment become better established, the possible use of rTMS across a broad range of psychiatric illnesses can be better evaluated.

Naturopathic and Homeopathic Remedies for Affective and Anxiety Disorders

Naturopathy encompasses many natural healing practices, including herbal and homeopathic preparations, nutritional counseling, light therapy, and several others. A naturopathic doctor (ND) is licensed to practice naturopathic healing methods, including the prescribing of homeopathic remedies.

Homeopathy is a system of care that attempts to stimulate the body to heal itself. Symptoms are believed to represent the body's attempt to restore itself to health, thus a homeopath will use a remedy to stimulate the body to move in the direction it is already going. For example, instead of trying to stop a cough with suppressants, as conventional medicine does, a homeopath will give a remedy that would cause a cough in a healthy person and thus stimulate the ill body to restore itself.

In conventional therapy, the goal is *control* of the illness through regular use of medical substances. Homeopathy's aim is the complete restoration of health. Symptoms are not seen as something wrong that must be corrected, but rather, as signs of the way in which the body is attempting to help itself. Although Hippocrates first postulated this principle of "likes curing like," Samuel Hahnemann established the first practical application in 1796 (National Center for Hoemopathy, 2001).

The exact nature of symptoms is important because even slightly different symptoms require different homeopathic treatments. Any substance may be considered a homeopathic medicine if it has known effects that mimic the symptoms, syndromes, or conditions that it is administered to treat and is manufactured according to the specifications of the Homeopathic Pharmacopoeia of the United States (HPUS) (National Center for Hoemopathy, 2001).

The HPUS is a standard reference text detailing the sources, composition, and preparation of the homeopathic drugs, which are prescribed on the basis of the "Law of Similars." An example of a homeopathic drug is aconite or wolf's bane, prescribed in any case in which the symptoms come on suddenly, especially if exposure to cold might be a causative factor. (National Center for Hoemopathy, 2001).

Few studies on homeopathic remedies for psychiatric symptoms have been done. One small study ($n = 12$) suggested the possible usefulness of homeopathy in the treatment of affective and anxiety disorders in patients with mild to severe symptomatic conditions (Davidson et al, 1997).

HERBALS THAT MAY BE PROBLEMATIC FOR PSYCHIATRIC PATIENTS

- Ginseng can exacerbate mania and precipitate acute anxiety and insomnia (Folks, Gabel, 2001).
- Evening primrose can exacerbate mania.
- Ephedra can cause nervousness, irritability, and insomnia.
- Yohimbine can cause nervousness irritability and insomnia. Yohimbine has been known to cause an allergic reaction culminating in a lupuslike syndrome (Ernst, 1998). Yohimbine can cause elevated blood pressure, which is pronounced if taken with TCAs (Ayd, 2000).
- Chaste tree may interact with dopaminergics (Wong, Smith, Boon, 1998).
- Reports suggest severe extrapyramidal symptoms following heavy betel nut consumption in patients on neuroleptics (Ayd, 2000).

Herbals are known to interact with certain drugs and raise a concern for patients taking drugs with a narrow therapeutic window (i.e., TCAs, lithium) (Hatcher, 2001).

GENERAL CONCERNS

Herbals

The method of manufacture of herbals determines the potency of an herb. Herbal concentration and dose potency are highly dependent on several factors for which there can be great variability (http://nccam.nih.gov/fcp/factsheets/stjohnswort/stjohnswort.htm, 2001). Although the American Herbal Association and the American Botanical Council have attempted to regulate safety, there is currently no guarantee of purity or standardization of herbal products. A *Los Angeles Times* survey indicated three of ten herbal products contained only one half the potency listed on the product label (Beaubrun, Gray, 2000; Hatcher, 2001; Snyder, Lindquist, 2001).

Another potential problem includes findings that many people using alternative remedies are doing so without any kind of supervision (Eisenberg et al, 1998). Potentially, this "self-medicating" may lead to a dangerous delay in seeking more efficacious care. Numerous people from ethnic minorities are likely to turn to alternative health practices for health care needs. When taking the initial history and performing a physical examination, it is important to ask patients not only about their symptoms, but also if they know what caused the illness. Patients' answers may reveal whether they subscribe to a folk or magical belief system (http://www.ncddr.org/du/researchexchange/v04n01/cultures.htmlfrican, 2002).

A concern about self-medication with herbals and other alternative therapies for psychiatric patients is that, if the treatment does not work, it may be difficult for the patient to judge the effects caused by increasingly impaired judgement as the illness symptoms progress. Box 40-1 provides a summary of general precautions regarding herbals.

> ### *Critical* Thinking Questions
>
> What are the implications of patients self-medicating with alternative therapies? Are there any dangers? What are the possible benefits? What conditions might a patient try an alternative therapy for that a clinician should evaluate immediately?

Competence of Practitioners

Training and credentialing of practitioners is important. There are opportunities, without regulation, for tremendous variation in the preparation and expertise of practitioners. The form of legislative authorization varies from state to state and includes licensure, certification, or registration. The best regulated alternative therapies are acupuncture and naturopathy. Box 40-2 lists helpful questions to ask alternative care practitioners.

Acupuncture is regulated by practice acts in 26 states. States not having practice acts limit the practice of acupuncture to designated medical providers or require medical supervision. Acupuncturists are held to the same standard of care as are licensed physicians (Sale, 2001). Professional acupuncturists train for up to 4 years full time and may acquire university degrees on completion of their training. Some acupuncturists have also completed training in the principles and practice of Chinese herbalism. Accredited acupuncture courses include conventional anatomy, physiology, pathology, and diagnosis. A national credentialing agency, the National Commission for Certification of Acupuncturists, provides examinations for entry-level practice. The agency also serves as a disciplinary and grievance board, giving consumers an avenue for holding practitioners accountable.

Nonphysicians, including nurses, may complete coursework, practicums, and examinations to receive credentialing for entry-level practice. The American Association of Medical Acupuncturists provides credentialing for physician-trained acupuncturists. State practice regulations vary greatly. For instance, some states require that a prospective patient with a serious disease first be diagnosed and referred by a medical physician.

Great variation also exists in the practice of NDs. Most definitions of what constitutes naturopathic practice place emphasis on the use of natural substances or methods that stimulate the body's natural capacity for healing. Naturopathic practice may include a variety of therapies, and naturopaths often prescribe homeopathic and herbal remedies, among others. In the United States, several universities offer the naturopathic doctorate. It should be noted that several correspondence schools also offer the natur-

Box 40-1	General Precautions for Consumers and Health Care Professionals Regarding Herbals

Avoid products with multiple herbs:
- Check the active and inactive ingredients for possible combinations and additives.
- Avoid imported herbs because of differences in dose effects.
- Buy only from reputable, established companies and with the United States Pharmacopoeia (USP) seal of approval.
- Always inform health care provider of any use of herbal products, including topicals.
- Discontinue if any unusual side effects occur and report adverse reactions to Medwatch at 1-800-322-1088.
- Avoid herbals during pregnancy, when attempting to get pregnant, and during breast-feeding.
- Avoid self medicating with herbals before a medical illness has been ruled out.

Box 40-2	Questions to Ask Alternative Care Practitioners

- Where did you receive your training or education to practice?
- Have you been certified to practice? By whom?
- Do you have a license?
- Have you treated other patients with conditions such as mine?
- What will be involved in my treatment?
- How many treatments will be necessary?
- How much will the treatment cost?
- How will you determine if I am responding to the treatment?
- Are you willing to send a report to my physician?

opathic doctorate. Many health care professionals do not view university and correspondence programs as equivalent. NDs are licensed to practice in 12 states. States without licensing may still have practitioners that practice under another professional license. Some states prohibit the practice of naturopathy, except by physicians. Wide arrays of natural therapies are generally under the scope of practice for naturopathy. Natural medicines, including homeopathy, herbal remedies, and vitamins, are usually included (Sale, 2001). Legally, practitioners are accountable under the law and may be sued for practicing outside the scope of their practice. The legal system expects a practitioner to make and document referrals for serious conditions. It is also reasonable to expect practitioners to encourage patients to inform their health care provider of their naturopathic therapy. Practice acts exist in some states, requiring licensure to practice homeopathy (Sale, 2001).

Nurses and Alternative Therapies

Many nurses have pursued education to prepare themselves to administer alternative therapies for which they have received specialized training or additional certifications or both (Frisch, 2001; Snyder, Lindquist, 2001). The American Holistic Nurses Association offers certification in holistic nursing, designated as registered nurse (RN); certified holistic nurse (HNC), for nurses meeting competency standards for integrating the body-mind-spirit connection into their own self-care and the care of their patients. The American Holistic Nurse Association requires completion of an examination and adherence to standards of practice that ensure nurses engaged in the practice of holistic nursing have integrated foundational concepts of holistic nursing into their lives and practice and demonstrate proficiency in the body of knowledge specific to holistic nursing. The HNC designation has more to do with the attitude of the practitioner than it does with specific techniques used (American Holistic Nurses Association, 2002).

Similar to all certifications, the HNC designation is a special recognition of excellence in a particular area. Many HNC nurses use complementary therapies in their everyday practice. It is generally recommended that nurses using alternative therapies in practice make sure that they are not violating agency policy, practicing outside the realm of what would be considered a nursing outcome, and that documentation should be done within a nursing context (Frisch, 2001).

Future Directions of Integrative Health Care

Many patients consider herbs to be natural and therefore "harmless." However, as previously noted, this view is not the case. This potential for adverse effects has to be considered in assessment and planning with patients. On the other hand, although some therapies probably do no harm, they do not help either. When considering alternative therapies, it is important to keep an open mind the following: some are helpful, some cause harm, and some, though harmless, probably offer no more than a placebo effect.

Many alternative practices have been handed down across generations and are an integral part of an individual's beliefs about health and illness. Some nurses tend to reject alternative therapies outright based on their own beliefs about health and illness. It is important for these nurses to remember that many conventional treatments are poorly understood and have been used because "they work" or because all other treatments have failed. Many people who use alternative or complementary therapies suffer from chronic illnesses, and conventional medicine has not helped (Astin, 1998; Gaydos, 2001).

Alternative Therapies and Culturally Competent Health Care

It is important to remember that mainstream medicine in the United States is geared to upper middle-class European Americans; as such, mainstream medicine may be difficult for members of other cultures to accept. Groups of people embracing beliefs about the integration of body, mind, and spirit may find the impersonal focus on disease of a single body system to be inadequate. Although most people of other ethnic minorities consult health care practitioners, especially for urgent care, many still hold to practices and beliefs that require the health care practitioner to be aware of the specific beliefs and practices relevant to the ethnocultural background of the person seeking help. Members of most ethnic minorities in the United States maintain at least some of their cultural practices. As the number of ethnic minorities continues to grow, health care practitioners are challenged to develop culturally competent health care systems. The following discussion does not intentionally omit any particular cultural group but focuses on the rapidly growing and marginalized minority groups in the United States: African Americans, Asian Americans, Hispanic Americans, and Native Americans. For a comprehensive discussion of cultural issues, the student is referred to the excellent text, *Transcultural Nursing: Assessment & Intervention,* by Giger, Davidhizar (1999).

African Americans

African Americans have historically been denied access to health care. Before the civil rights era, African Americans were prohibited from receiving treatment in "White" health care facilities. Since the civil rights era, African Americans have continued to suffer disparities in health care. Multiple factors influence these disparities: inadequate insurance coverage, mistrust of the health care system, discrimination, and social and psychologic factors. Regarding mental health care, compared with the general population, African Americans are frequently misdiagnosed and are more often prescribed higher potency medications with higher side-effect profiles, without regard to differences in metabolism. It is little wonder that African Americans have continued to turn to some of the folk healing practices and spiritual healing brought by their ancestors from Africa. Many of these remedies continue to be used by some African Americans. The root worker, an expert in various herbs, spices, and roots that are useful for healing, is an example of a folk practitioner within African-American communities.

Among African Americans, spirituality is the most often turned to relief from a variety of stresses, including illnesses. A study from the University of Florida and Wayne State University showed that African Americans rely more heavily on religion and prayer than do Caucasians in America (Seniors Use Prayer to Cope with Illness, 2000). The laying on of hands is an important aspect of spiritual healing in many African-American church communities. Failure to acknowledge the spiritual component of African-American communities omits a significant aspect of the basic, fundamental beliefs about health and illness among African Americans (Giger, Davidhizar, 1999).

Asian Americans

Asian Americans have a strong tradition in Eastern medicine practices. The ideas held by many Asian Americans are contrary to Westernized health care methods to the extent that it is difficult to imagine an Asian American seeking care from traditional Western medical practitioners. Chinese medicine, for instance, uses herbals and acupuncture to restore balance of the Qi, or life energy force. The concept of yin and yang are central to the traditional Eastern medical practice of acupuncture, herbal medicines, and massage. Yin and yang represent the powers that regulate all things in the universe, with yang representing the positive force and yin representing the negative force. Specific healing practices are geared toward restoring a balance between these two opposing and essential forces. Asian Americans are the least likely group to consult a mental health practitioner and the most likely to experience side effects to psychotropic medications (Giger, Davidhizar, 1999). According to Eastern health beliefs, treatments that focus only on symptoms are not addressing the underlying cause. It should be noted that the global term "Asian" encompasses a huge number of geographic regions and cultures, with major differences between region and countries.

Hispanic Americans

Hispanic Americans face particular difficulty accessing health care. Chief among these barriers is that, of all minority groups in the United States, Hispanic Americans are the least likely to be insured. Another major barrier is language. The majority of Hispanic Americans speak Spanish, yet few health care professionals speak second languages. Hispanic Americans are more likely to be misdiagnosed when speaking in English. Some Hispanic Americans subscribe to the hot-cold theory of health and illness whereby health is maintained through adherence to appropriate nutritional remedies classified as "hot" or "cold" foods. The hot or cold designation does not refer to the temperature; rather, it is based on other factors. For example, cancer and headaches are considered "cold" illnesses, whereas rashes and skin ailments are considered "hot" illnesses. Examples of cold foods would be fruits, fresh vegetables, dairy products, and some meats (e.g., goat, fish, chicken). Hot foods include some meats (e.g., beef, waterfowl, mutton), eggs, cereal grains, and aromatic beverages.

Similarly, treatments are also classified as "hot" and " cold." Penicillin would be a "hot" treatment to be administered with a "cold" illness, and milk of magnesia would be a "cold" treatment to be used with "hot" illnesses.

There are many folk practitioners in Hispanic cultures:

- Family folk healer, usually a woman within the family, is respected for his or her knowledge of folk remedies.
- Yerbero is a folk healer with a special knowledge of many healing practices using herbs and spices.
- The Curandero, who is believed to have the God-given gift of healing, deals with serious imbalances between God and man and between hot and cold.

It is important to consider that, with the Hispanic American, self-medication is a traditional practice. In Mexico, for example, many drugs available only by prescription in the United States are available over the counter (Giger, Davidhizar, 1999). It should also be noted that the global term "Hispanic" does not truly address the major differences between specific peoples and cultures that are linked by familial and patriotic ties to specific geographic regions and country.

Native Americans

Native Americans' access to health care is included as part of the treaties made with the United States government, which offers conventional Western medicine. However, Native Americans' beliefs and practices in dealing with health care involve the concept of a disharmony with "Mother Earth." Native healing ceremonies and the traditional medicine man are a most important part of Native-American culture. An example of a traditional Native-American practice is the jish, which are medicine bundles containing sacred and symbolic items used for healing and blessing and carried by the medicine man. A cooperative spirit has existed between the Native-American traditional healers and the conventional health care providers through the Indian Health Service (Giger, Davidhizar, 1999).

It might be said that conventional medicine is a significant factor contributing to the overall disharmony with Mother Earth. Given the history of the ousting of Native Americans, it is no wonder that they hold to many of their native traditions. Native Americans still practice the use of natural herbs and various rituals and ceremonies for healing. Each particular tribe of Native Americans engages in traditions specific to their tribe.

Nurse and Physician Education

Nurses and physicians can expect an increased emphasis on alternative therapies in their respective curricula. Surveys of medical schools indicate the vast majority offer coursework, practicums, or content on alternative and complementary medicine. Currently, significant variability and inconsistently defined learner objectives are present between and among existing programs. As alternative and complementary therapy education becomes more mainstream, curricula will be refined (Wetzel et al, 1998). Georgetown University, the University of California at San Francisco, and the University of Minnesota have fully developed programs on this content and are leaders in alternative approaches.

The NCCAM offers training grants for the purpose of integrating alternative and complementary therapies into the curricula of medical and nursing programs. Deciding which therapies to include in curricula will emerge as leaders continue to explore this aspect of education. Beyond the difficulty inherent with defining alternative and complementary therapy and the corresponding confusing terminology, a formidable challenge is the fact that these therapies arise out of belief systems that are quite different than those in Western values and beliefs (Gaydos, 2001). The most reasonable approach may be to focus on the theoretical underpinnings of particular treatment modalities and available scientific evidence supporting their use (Gaydos, 2001; Snyder, Lindquist, 2001; Wetzel, Eisenberg, Kaptchuk, 1998).

Because alternative treatment is potentially lucrative, many interested parties can be expected to appear at the political table to fight for their piece of this profitable pie. Should this battle become too intense, the values of alternative and naturopathic medicine run the risk of falling prey to the same ills afflicting traditional medicine.

Because nursing has always focused on holistic care of human beings, integrating this knowledge and these techniques into the practice of nursing can further enhance this focus (Frisch, 2001). The overarching philosophy present in most alternative practices is a respect for the individual's capacity for self-healing. This approach is very much in concert with traditional nursing and thus is not as foreign as some suggest. Rather than viewing alternative therapies as a threat, the authors recommend that nurses conceptualize alternative therapies as a challenge and strong nudge toward a paradigm shift in our current system of care (Astin, 1998).

Note to students: *One thing that has likely been crossing your mind as you read this chapter is that the very definition of what is alternative is itself quite controversial. By the strictest definition, anything that is not considered mainstream medicine with approved indications should be considered alternative. Whether something is considered alternative or complementary depends on the purpose of the treatment and who is recommending the treatment. Furthermore, what is alternative at the moment may be mainstream in the near future (Astin, 1998; Frisch, 2001). Perhaps alternative therapies are needed to stimulate this shift back to the original intent of patient care.*

Critical Thinking Question

What do you think about patients taking health into their own hands and engaging in practices not proven by the scientific method and the medical community?

Key Concepts

1. Alternative therapies are therapies that are used instead of mainstream medicine; complementary therapies are those outside of mainstream medicine that are used along with traditional medical therapies.
2. Increasing numbers of patients are using alternative or complementary therapies. The public is clearly more receptive to alternatives than it is to the traditional health care system.
3. Alternative health practices have been around for centuries but lost favor with the disease-based scientific model of care. A renewed interest in alternative health practices has emerged as dissatisfaction with our current system of care has grown.
4. The NIH has created an office of complementary and alternative medicine, initially called the OAM and renamed, in recent years, to NCCAM.

5. The FDA does not regulate herbal products but does require labeling that indicates lack of proven efficacy and quality control standards.
6. St. John's wort is the most widely used herbal for depression. Studies have generally demonstrated effectiveness of St. John's wort for mild to moderate depression. St. John's wort should not be taken with other antidepressants, especially SSRIs, and may interfere with the protease inhibitors often used for HIV-positive patients.
7. Kava-kava is an herbal anxiolytic without problems such as coordination and alertness associated with "normal" doses of the benzodiazepines. Problem can occur if taken with CNS-acting drugs, and overdose is possible.
8. Valerian is an herbal anxiolytic useful for anxiety and insomnia. Withdrawal syndromes similar to benzodiazepine withdrawal can occur, and valerian can increase the effects of other centrally acting drugs. Valerian may reduce the effectiveness of anticoagulants and antiseizure drugs.
9. Chamomile and angelica have also been used for anxiety but have fewer supporting studies compared with kava-kava and valerian.
10. Gingko is one of the top selling herbals in the United States and is effective for brain trauma, memory impairment, and cerebral insufficiency. Gingko should not be taken by anyone with a history of bleeding problems because it exacerbates the effects of anticoagulants.
11. Melatonin has been suggested as possibly useful for "ICU syndrome" and for sleep.
12. Acupuncture is one of the most thoroughly researched alternative therapies and shows evidence of effectiveness in the treatment of substance abuse when used in conjunction with traditional therapies.
13. Yoga, meditation, and other spiritual practices have been useful for regulating anxiety levels.
14. Omega-3 fatty acids, found in fish oils, have promise for improving clinical outcomes in many conditions, including mania and schizophrenia.
15. rTMS has been suggested as a promising treatment for depression and psychosis. rTMS apparently does not cause memory deficits, as sometimes occurs with ECT.
16. Homeopathy, which is a system and philosophy of care using "natural" remedies to stimulate the body to heal itself, is based on the Law of Similars or "like cures like." Approved homeopathic remedies may be found in the HPUS.

17. Some herbals are known to be problematic for psychiatric patients, particularly evening primrose, ephedra, yohimbine, ginseng, chaste tree, and bethel nut.

18. One concern about patients taking herbals without supervision is that the patients may delay seeking essential treatment.

19. Health care professionals should routinely question patients about the use of herbals or other alternative therapies.

20. The alternative therapies that are best regulated include acupuncture and homeopathy. States vary greatly in their individual regulation of alternative health care practitioners.

21. Nurses demonstrating the ability to integrate mind-body-spirit into their clinical practice may be certified through examination and adherence to standards of practice by the American Holistic Nurses Association, with the designation of HNC. Nurses possessing HNC credentials may also have been trained in alternative therapies through special education or credentialing.

22. It is important to address cultural and ethnic uses of alternative therapies and to respect the practices of patients.

23. African Americans are frequently misdiagnosed and have historically been marginalized by traditional medicine. Spirituality is the remedy and is the most often used among African Americans.

24. Asian Americans have beliefs about health and illness that are contrary to Westernized medicine and have traditionally used a number of alternative remedies, including herbals, acupuncture, and massage.

25. Hispanic Americans face particular difficulty accessing health care and hold a number of beliefs and traditions contrary to traditional medicine.

26. Native Americans have been successful at maintaining their rights to practice their traditional healing ceremonies and to seek help from a medicine man.

27. Nurse and physician education can be expected to include alternative and complementary medicine as part of their core curriculum in the future.

28. The concept of alternative versus complementary therapy, by definition, changes as the therapy becomes incorporated into mainstream medicine.

References

Acupuncture: National Institutes of Health Consensus Development Conference Statement, November 3-5, 1997. Available at URL: http://odp.od.nih.gov/consensus/cons/107/107_statement.htm Retrieved September 2001.

Almeida JC, Grimsley EW: Coma for the health food store: interaction between kava and alprazolam, *Ann Intern Med* 125(11):940, 1996.

American Holistic Nurses Association. Available at http:www.ahna.org/edu/certification.html, 2002

Astin JA: Why patients use alternative medicine: results of a national study, *JAMA* 279(19):1548, 1998.

Ayd F: Evaluating interactions between herbal and psychoactive medications, *Psychiatr Times* 17(12):45, 2000.

Beaubrun G, Gray G: A review of herbal medicines for psychiatric disorders, *Psychiatr Serv* 51:1130, 2000.

Commission E Monographs: Introduction. Available at URL: http://www.herbalgram.org/browse.php/comm_e_int Retrieved September 22, 2001.

Davidson JR et al: Homeopathic treatment of depression and anxiety, *Altern Ther Health Med* 3(1):46, 1997.

Eisenberg D et al: Trends in alternative medicine use in the United States, 1990-1997. Results of a follow-up national survey, *JAMA* 280:1569, 1998.

Erfurth A et al: Euphoric mania and rapid transcranial magnetic stimulation, *Am J Psychiatry* 157(5):835, 2000.

Ernst E: Harmless herbs? A review of the recent literature, *Am J Med* 104:170, 1998.

Feinsod M et al: Preliminary evidence for a beneficial effect of low-frequency, repetitive transcranial magnetic stimulation in patients with major depression and schizophrenia, *Depress Anxiety* 7(2):65, 1998.

Folks D, Gabel T: Herbaceuticals in psychiatry. In Keltner N, Folks D, editors: *Psychotropic drugs,* ed 3, St Louis, 2001, Mosby.

Frisch N: Nursing as a context for alternative/complementary modalities, May 31, 2001, *Online J Issues Nurs* 6(2), Manuscript 2. Available at URL: http://www.nursingworld.org/ojin/topic15/tpc15_2.htm Retrieved 2001.

Frisch N: Standards for holistic nursing practice: a way to think about our care that includes complementary and alternative modalities, May 31, 2001, *Online J Issues Nurs* 6(2), Manuscript 4. Available at URL: http://www.nursingworld.org/ojin/topic15/tpc15_4.htm Retrieved 2001.

Garges H, Varia I, Doraiswamy P: Cardiac complications and delirium associated with valerian root withdrawal, *JAMA* 280(11):1566, 1998.

Gaydos HL: Complementary and alternative therapies in nursing education: trends and issues, *Online J Issues Nurs* 6(2), Manuscript 5, 2001. Available at URL: http://www.nursingworld.org/ojin/topic15/tpc15_5.htm Retrieved 2001.

Giger J, Davidhizar R: *Transcultural nursing: assessment & intervention,* ed 3, St Louis, 1999, Mosby.

Goldman J, Nahas G, George MS: What is transcranial magnetic stimulation? *Harv Ment Health Lett* 17(2):8, 2000.

Hatcher T: The proverbial herb, *Am J Nurs* 101(2):36, 2001.

Infante JR et al: Catecholamine levels in practitioners of the transcendental meditation technique, *Physiol Behav* 72(1-2):141, 2001.

Joy CB, Mumby-Croft R, Joy LA: Polyunsaturated fatty acid (fish or evening primrose oil) for schizophrenia, [review] [7 refs], *Cochrane Database of Systematic Reviews* [computer file](2):CD001257, 2000.

Kabat-Zinn J et al: Effectiveness of a meditation-based stress reduction program in the treatment of anxiety disorders, *Am J Psychiatry* 149(7):936, 1992.

Kessler R et al: The use of complementary and alternative therapies to treat anxiety and depression in the United States, *Am J Psychiatry* 158:289, 2001.

Kirkcaldie M, Pridmore S: Transcranial magnetic stimulation in psychiatry. Available at URL: http://www.musc.edu/ tmsmirror/intro/layintro.html, 1999. Retrieved January 30, 2002.

Linde K et al: St. John's wort for depression-an overview and meta-analysis of randomized clinical trials, *BMJ* 313(7052):253, 1996.

Lisanby S et al: Magnetic seizure therapy of major depression, *Arch Gen Psychiatry* 58(3):303, 2001.

Luo H et al: Clinical research on the therapeutic effect of the electro-acupuncture treatment in patients with depression, *Psychiatry Clin Neurosci* 52(suppl):S338, 1998.

McEnany G: Herbal psychotropics part 3: focus on kava, valerian, and melatonin, *J Am Psychiatric Nurs Assoc* 6:126, 2001.

McEnany G: Herbal psychotropics part 4: focus on ginkgo biloba, l-carnitine, lactobacillus, acidophilus, and ginger root, *J Am Psychiatric Nurs Assoc* 7:22, 2001.

Miller JJ, Fletcher K, Kabat-Zinn J: Three-year follow-up and clinical implications of a mindfulness meditation-based stress reduction intervention in the treatment of anxiety disorders, *Gen Hosp Psychiatry* 17(3):192, 1995.

National Center for Complementary and Alternative Medicine Fact Sheets. St. John's Wort, 2001. Available at URL: http:// nccam.nih.gov/fcp/factsheets/stjohnswort/stjohnswort.htm Retrieved September 22, 2001.

National Center for the Dissemination of Disability Research (NCDDR): Cultural and other considerations that can influence effectiveness within the rehabilitation system, *Research Exchange* 4(1), 1999. Available at URL:http:// www.ncddr.org/du/research exchange/v04n01/cultures.htmlfrican Retrieved January 2002.

National Center for Homeopathy. Available at URL: http://www. homeopathic.org/introduction.htm. Retrieved October 2001.

Padberg F et al: Repetitive transcranial magnetic stimulation (rTMS) in pharmacotherapy refractory major depression: comparative study of fast, slow, and sham rTMS, *Psychiatry Res* 88:163, 1999.

Rollnik JD et al: High frequency repetitive transcranial magnetic stimulation (rTMS) of the dorsolateral prefrontal cortex in schizophrenic patients, *Neuroreport* 11(18):4013, 2000.

Sale D: Overview of legislative development concerning alternative health care in the United States, 2001. Available at URL: http://www.healthy.net/public/legal-lg/regulations/fetzer.htm. Retrieved: 2001.

Seniors use prayer to cope with stress, prayer no. 1, alternative remedy, Dec 28, 2000, *University of Florida News*. Available at URL: http://www.napa.ufl.edu/2000news/prayer.htm Retrieved January 30, 2002.

Shannahoff-Khalsa DS, Beckett LR: Clinical case report: efficacy of yogic techniques in the treatment of obsessive compulsive disorders, *Int J Neurosci* 85(1-2):1, 1996.

Shwartz M et al: The value of acupuncture detoxification programs in a substance abuse treatment system, *J Subst Abuse Treat* 17(4):305, 1999.

Skidmore-Roth L: *Handbook of herbs & natural supplements,* St Louis, 2001, Mosby.

Snyder M, Lindquist R: Issues in complementary therapies: how we got to where we are, May 31, 2001, *Online J Issues Nurs* 6(2), Manuscript 1. Available at URL: http://www.nursingworld.org/ ojin/topic15/tpc15_1.htm. Retrieved 2001.

Stoll A et al: Omega-3 fatty acids in bipolar disorder: a preliminary double-blind, placebo-controlled trial, *Arch Gen Psychiatry* 56:407, 1999.

Tooley G et al: Acute changes in night time plasma melatonin levels following a period of meditation, *Biological Psychology* 53:69, 2000.

Uebelhack R, Franke L, Schewe HJ: Inhibition of platelet MAO-B by kava pyrone enriched extract from Piper methysticum Forster (kava-kava), *Pharmacopsychiatry* 31(5):187, 1998.

Vickers A, Zollman C: ABC of complementary medicine acupuncture, *BMJ* 319:973, 1999.

Wetzel M, Eisenberg D, Kaptchuk T: Courses involving complementary and alternative medicine at US medical schools, *JAMA* 280:784, 1998.

Wilson J: What is homeopathy? Available at URL:http://www. homeopathicdoctor.com/page8.html. Retrieved October 2001.

Wong A, Smith M, Boon H: Herbal remedies in psychiatric practice, *Arch Gen Psychiatry* 55:1033, 1998.

Yamashita H et al: Adverse events related to acupuncture, *JAMA* 280(18):1563, 1998.

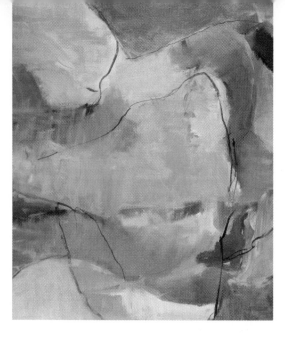

Chapter 41

Survivors of Violence and Trauma

Lee H. Schwecke

Learning Objectives

After reading this chapter, you should be able to:

- Recognize the seriousness of violence and trauma in the United States.
- Describe the emotional reactions of adult victims of crime, workplace violence, terrorism, torture, rape, childhood sexual abuse, and partner abuse.
- Recognize the dynamics involved in childhood sexual abuse.

- Analyze the way in which the cycle of violence inhibits individuals from leaving abusive relationships.
- Identify the needs of victims of violence and trauma.
- Describe strategies for facilitating the transition from "victim" to "survivor" of violence or trauma.
- Develop a nursing care plan for survivors of violence and trauma.

The victimization of any individual by another creates serious mental health, social, community, and legal problems. Violence in all forms is prevalent in this society. Nurses, regardless of their areas of practice, will come in contact with the victims—as inpatients, outpatients, home-care patients, emergency care patients, parents of patients, friends, and relatives. Although the victims are typically seen initially for physical injuries, their psychologic needs require attention if long-term mental health problems are to be prevented.

Forensic nursing is emerging as a vital aspect of the holistic care of victims and perpetrators of violent crimes and their families (Peternelj-Taylor, 2001). This care includes obtaining clinical histories, documenting evidence, including photographs of injuries, and quality nursing interventions in a holis-

tic care framework, which includes consideration of all the medical-legal aspects of the patient's problems (Hammer, 2000). The rights of the alleged perpetrators of crime, suspects, and victims must be protected so the legal case will not be jeopardized (Piercy, Greenwood, 2002).

This chapter focuses on victims of violence and trauma, beginning with a brief overview of general reactions to any crime, workplace violence, terrorism, torture, and ritual abuse, followed by a more in-depth look at rape, adult survivors of childhood sexual abuse, and individuals abused by their partners. A small number of perpetrators of rape, sexual abuse, and partner abuse are female, but the most common pattern of this victimization is by males against females (New, Berliner, 2000). The short- and long-term reactions of victims described in this chapter are generally true for both male and female victims; however, men sometimes have a more difficult time admitting to and dealing with their emotional victimization than women. The added impact on males of sexual violation by other males, both as children and as adults, is a result, in part, of their fears about homosexuality (Ray, 2001).

Beyond the scope of this chapter are the issues of peer victimization and crime and violence by children and adolescents, despite national attention to gangs, school shootings, dating violence (verbal, physical, and sexual), bullying, hate crimes against certain populations, property damage, and fighting (with or without weapons) (Bond et al, 2001; Cleary, 2000; James et al, 2000; Miller, 2001b). Also beyond the scope of the chapter is the issue of elder abuse. Unfortunately, older adults can be the victims of all the crimes discussed in this chapter, as well as the particular crimes in the category of "elder abuse," such as emotional and financial abuse and neglect and abandonment, despite their inability to provide for their own self-care (Bergeron, 2000; Hoban, 2000).

VIOLATION BY CRIME

Effects of Crimes

Not all crimes involve physical violence, injury, and threat to life; however, all crimes involve emotional violation and trauma. The victim's identity is affected even with the loss or destruction of possessions and property because these are a representation of an individual's identity and have personal significance. Crime undermines foundations formed in the first two stages of human development, regardless of the victim's age when the crime occurred (see Chapter 3). There is a loss of trust, not only in the criminal, but also to some degree in all other individuals. Victims also lose a sense of ability to control their own lives and themselves (autonomy issues).

The emotional reactions to crime vary greatly according to the individual, the situation, and the meaning of the crime to that person. However, typical reactions are denial, fear, anger, powerlessness, and depression. A sense of failure and guilt are common; victims wonder what they did to cause the crime and how they might have prevented or stopped it. Victims usually feel ashamed and unworthy, as well as contaminated or "dirty," whether or not they were physically touched by the perpetrator.

Fantasies of revenge or a wish for legal retribution are typical. The relationships of victims to family and friends can be disturbed, in part, because of the loss of trust, but also because of the response of others. Caring individuals often imply that the victim was responsible for the crime with questions such as, "Why were you there alone at night? Why were you carrying so much cash? Why didn't you install that burglar alarm?" The victim may feel alienated and isolated. Hospital personnel, the police, and the legal system may also convey a "blaming-the-victim" attitude in their manner of questioning and in focusing only on the "facts" without any emotional support or empathy.

Workplace violence is a particular crime that is getting increased employer and media attention recently and is included here because nurses are three times more likely to be the victims than are other professionals (Steelfel, 2001). This type of crime includes verbal abuse, sexual harassment, stalking, assault and battery, rape, and murder perpetrated by patients or their visitors, other employees, former or current partners of employees, and intruders from the outside looking for specific items, such as money or drugs (Farella, 2001; Gillmore-Hall, 2001). A 1999 study on workplace violence done by the National Institute for Occupational Safety and Health found that 38% of reported assaults took place in health care facilities and almost one half of these assaults were committed by patients (Worthington, Franklin, 2000).

Verbal abuse includes intimidation, ridicule, aggressive posturing, rude gestures, threats, ostracism, and offensive notes or e-mails (Steelfel, 2001). In a 1999 survey, 94% of the nurses reported verbal abuse, with an average of 5 to 6 incidents per month (Stringer, 2001). Verbal abuse, especially when the abusers are physicians, has been linked to the high turnover of nurses and, indirectly, to the nursing shortage (Parks, 2001; Stringer, 2001).

Sexual harassment is defined as "an unwelcomed sexual advance or conduct on the job that creates an intimidating, hostile, or offensive working environment...[ranging from]...repeated offensive or belittling jokes to pornography or outright sexual assault" (Farella, 2001, p. 14).

According to a 1988 survey of the federal workforce, 42% of all women and 15% of all men have experienced some form of harassment (Farella, 2001).

Stalking is a crime that can occur anywhere but often follows victims to their workplace.

> Stalking is obsessional pursuit, harassment, and intimidation by a person who has or believes he has a significant personal relationship with the object of his unwanted attention. Stalkers may send letters, packages, or e-mails, make harassing phone calls, or appear repeatedly at the victim's home or workplace. Sometimes they destroy property and assault or even murder their victims. In the spectrum of actions that lie between surveillance and physical harm, it is probably repeated harassment that defines the difference between stalking and unwanted courtship by a stranger, rejected suitor, or former lover. (Miller, 2001a, p. 5)

One survey indicated that 41% of all men and 12% of all women have been stalked at least once in their lifetimes. Men account for 80% to 90% of the stalkers, and women are their victims in 80% to 90% of the cases. However, some cases involve female-to-male, male-to-male, or female-to-female stalking (Miller, 2001a).

The media tends to focus on the stalking of celebrities and public officials. The stalkers in these cases tend to be psychotic or have delusions about their victims and the supposed love relationship. However, most cases of stalking occur as the victim is trying to end a casual, dating, or marital relationship. This pattern is more likely than is celebrity stalking to involve physical violence (80%) and sexual assault (30%) and to be carried out by nondelusional individuals. About 30% of all female homicides are by former partners (Miller, 2001a; Meloy, 1999).

The Occupational Safety and Health Administration encourages voluntary compliance by employers with their workplace violence guidelines published in 1998. Briefly, these guidelines suggest the following: (1) systematic education of all employees about verbal abuse, sexual harassment, and other forms of violence along with ways to prevent and deal with them; (2) development of corporate policies and procedures related to workplace violence and reporting procedures; (3) definition of roles for supervisors, employee health staff, and security personnel; and (4) provision for treatment and counseling for employee victims (Farella, 2001; Gilmore-Hall, 2001; Monarch, 2000; Trossman, 2001).

Recovery from Violence and Trauma

Many models have been formulated about the process of recovery from traumas such as crimes. Most researchers agree that the duration and severity of the trauma, the victim's resources, and the nature of help available during and immediately after the crime or trauma influence recovery. Typically, three stages of recovery are defined: initial disorganization (impact), a struggle to adapt (recoil), and reconstruction (reorganization). The brief summary here is derived from the views of Tynhurst (1951), Fox and Scherl (1972), Janoff-Bulman (1997), and Clark (1997). The stages are not clearly separated, and the readjustment process is not smooth. Vacillation among the stages may occur, and recovery may take months or years.

Impact

The initial reaction to a single event trauma usually lasts from a few minutes to a few days. Common responses are shock, denial, disbelief, and confusion. There may be paralyzing fear, hysteria, horror, anger, shame, a sense of helplessness and vulnerability, physiologic responses, and disturbed sleeping and eating. These reactions may occur for a longer time when the crime is ongoing, such as harassment or stalking. Some victims react less visibly or in a delayed manner; they look calm, organized, and rational, and take all the necessary actions initially needed. Later, the other reactions may occur. Occasionally, the victim's reaction may include dissociative symptoms (amnesia, depersonalization, numbing, detachment), intrusive memories (nightmares, flashbacks), and severe anxiety. These symptoms may indicate that the victim is experiencing acute stress disorder (ASD) (see Chapter 31).

Recoil

In the recoil stage, victims begin the struggle to adapt. The immediate danger may be over, but a great deal of emotional stress remains. In the beginning of this phase, there are periods in which victims look and act "normal" and are able to carry out daily routines at home and at work. Activity helps suppress fears, anger, and sadness. Later in the phase, there is a desire to talk about the details of and feelings about the trauma. Victims often feel a need for support and to be temporarily dependent. Fantasies of revenge are natural during this stage. In the weeks and months following crime trauma, victims gradually become aware of the full impact the event has had on their lives.

Reorganization

Reorganization may take months or years to accomplish. Although the crime trauma is not forgotten, the anxiety, fear, and anger diminish, and victims reconstruct their lives. The beginning of this phase includes reviewing and organizing what happened specifically and why ("Why me?"); attributing blame to self, others, or both; justifying one's own actions at the time and later; and regaining a sense of control and self-protection. Grief over losses resolves slowly. Lingering nightmares, frustrations, and disillusionment may occur; however, these subside as victims reengage in life and activities. If reorganization is not effective, victims may experience degrees of symptoms that, in some cases, are clinically diagnosable (e.g., posttraumatic stress disorder [PTSD]; see Chapter 31).

Even with satisfactory recovery, victims sense that they and their lives are, and always will be, different as a result of the crime. The goal of recovery is to move from victim status to survivor status by integrating the memories of the crime trauma and moving on in life with restored functioning, a reasonable sense of safety and security, healthy relationships, and improved self-esteem.

Psychotherapeutic Management

Nurse-patient relationship

Although empathy, emotional support, and a willingness to listen are important in all stages of recovery, specialized care is needed in each stage. During the impact stage, the focus is on the survivor's need for physical safety and emotional security (see Chapter 12 for these crisis intervention strategies).

Reassurance, protection from further harm, and sometimes medical care are needed. Survivors may need clear, simple directions on what to do, where to go, and what to avoid. It is crucial that nurses avoid accusations (blaming), intimidations, unnecessary intrusions, and invasion of privacy. In most instances, crisis intervention is face-to-face at the scene of the crime or in the emergency room. For survivors who are superficially calm and in control, the crisis inter-

vention may be needed a few hours or days later, when the trauma "reality hits." Phone numbers for crisis-phone or walk-in services can be given to survivors before they leave the emergency room.

During the recoil stage, survivors need validation of their worth and of their rights as victims. Referrals can be made to a victim's assistance program and for legal, insurance, or financial assistance if needed. If family and friends are not fully available during the episodes of emotional turmoil in the recoil phase, then short-term counseling may be beneficial. During the struggle to adjust, support groups with other survivors can be useful. Whether the group is short-term (6 to 8 weeks) or ongoing, and whether the group is professionally led or self-led, there is value in receiving information, encouragement, and companionship from others who "have been there."

In the reorganization stage, most survivors are able to recover and grow with minimal assistance. Long-term counseling is sometimes needed to overcome anxiety, phobias, depression, suicidal ideation, or other posttraumatic symptoms. It is uncommon for survivors to need hospitalization beyond initial medical care. Exceptions include survivors who are unable to function or meet basic needs or those who become suicidal.

Psychopharmacology

Survivors of crime do not generally need medications. Antianxiety agents (benzodiazepines) are prescribed occasionally for short-term use to decrease anxiety and facilitate sleep.

Milieu management

Many communities have temporary or ongoing groups for survivors of disasters, divorce, death of a loved one, sudden infant death syndrome (SIDS), rape, incest, and physical and emotional abuse, as well as for survivors of suicide, mass murders, torture, and abduction of children.

TERRORISM

Nature of the Problem

September 11, 2001 is the day that awakened the United States to the realities of terrorism—its unpredictability and devastation. Before this day, terrorism was a news story about terrible acts in foreign countries somewhere else in the world. Terrorism can be perpetrated under the "justification" of various military, political, social, cultural, or religious causes. The acts of terrorism can involve plane crashes, bombings, military warfare, biologic and chemical agents, trained or programmed assassins, and suicide bombers. Terrorism is a crime that rarely affects only a single individual; victimization can involve thousands who are injured or killed in a single event. The victims of terrorism include those who were injured or killed; police, fire, and rescue personnel; businesses and their employees; the friends and families of all the victims; and potentially anyone who witnessed (directly or via the media) the tragedy.

Effects of Terrorism

Terrorism can have more devastating results than natural disasters or major accidents because terrorism is not only "man-made," but it is also not accidental. The purpose of terrorism is to terrorize, kill, or injure targeted groups and to generate fear that it can or will happen again (Miller, 2002). The trauma of terrorism is more pervasive, lasting, and severe than are other violent crimes (Howard-Ruben, 2001). The survivors typically experience some degree of grief and mourning and acute stress or posttraumatic stress symptoms that are expected reactions to an abnormal and horrifying event. The reactions can include "shock, anger, grief, and fear...fatigue, headaches, indigestion, nightmares, and intrusive images" (Miller, 2002, p. 1). Feeling depressed and having trouble with concentration and sleep also occurs. Some individual experience prolonged grieving, ASD, PTSD, or other disorders triggered by the terrorist acts. The event may also retrigger memories of previous traumatic experiences or exacerbate pre-existing disorders (Miller, 2002).

Recovery from Terrorism

Most individuals will recover with the support of loved ones and friends, memorial or religious services, community meetings, and a return to their normal activities (Miller, 2002). Relaxation techniques and physical activities may be helpful. Critical incident stress-management strategies (described with PTSD in Chapter 31) can also facilitate recovery and prevent untoward consequences. A major goal of recovery is to regain some sense of trust, safe-

ty, and security while acknowledging that future terrorist attacks are possible. In general, recovery will parallel the stages of recovery described earlier (impact, recoil, and reorganization) but may be lengthier and more complicated, depending on the severity and duration of the trauma. On a larger scale, most cities and hospitals are reviewing their disaster plans for the capacity to respond to terrorist attacks, biologic and chemical warfare, and large-scale bombings. For many cities, an effort has been made to improve city-wide, coordinated plans among police, fire, and rescue agencies, as well as hospitals, mental health facilities, and local and state emergency management administrations. Psychiatric nurses and mental health personnel with mental health disaster-management skills are included in the planning.

TORTURE, RITUAL ABUSE, AND MIND CONTROL

Nature of the Problem

Public and professional attention to the effects of torture, serial ritual abuse (SRA), and mind control (MC) on mental health has waned in recent years, although the crimes have not, according to the victims. The effect of these crimes, whether perpetrated by individuals, relatives, gangs, cults (satanic or nonsatanic), hate groups, or military-political organizations, is more severe because they involve multiple, calculated, and organized crimes against each victim or group of victims. This type of crime is used to create fear, humiliation, and submission in individuals, communities, and societies (Indianapolis Anorexia Nervosa and other Disorders [ANAD], a support group for survivors who have developed eating disorders, 2002). Statistics on the prevalence of torture, SRA, and MC are not readily available because of the problems in acknowledging, reporting, and proving occurrences, but the rates may be similar to those of family child abuse (Valente, 2000). The threat of further harm to the self, pets, or family tends to keep victims silent. Especially in SRA and MC, perpetrators may use triggers to maintain victims' silence or to control their actions, such as special words, hand signals, or greeting cards (Indianapolis ANAD, 2002). Drug and MC experiments before the 1970s (e.g., covert military-political operations [MK-ULTRA] programming that trained or programmed assassins for U.S. security forces; MK-ULTRA was publically described in the movie, "Conspiracy Theory") are becoming more widely known as the "Freedom of Information Act," and have resulted in the declassification of military and political documents.

Torture, ritual abuse, and mind-control tactics

According to survivors, torture involves physical, psychologic, pharmacologic, MC, sexual tactics, or any combination aimed at damaging the victims' identity, personality, emotional stability, spirit, and physical integrity. Torture, SRA, and MC can begin with abduction and detention and end with execution, or it can be ongoing over time. Tactics can include using hot irons, electric shock, submersion, suffocation, large doses of drugs, beatings, physical restraint, confinement in cramped and buried containers, gang rape, sexual and physical mutilation, being tied or hung in the air (or both), being photographed during the abuse, starvation, sleep deprivation, brainwashing, indoctrination, MC, programming, threats to or lies about the safety of loved ones and pets, overstimulation, and threats with weapons (Indianapolis ANAD, 2002; Rockwell, 1994; Ross, 1995; Valente, 2000).

CLINICAL EXAMPLE
Children who were examined following ritual abuse in a day-care center reported being locked in a cage, put in a coffin, held underwater, injected with needles, tied and hung from hooks, sexually assaulted, and threatened with guns and knives. The children were told that if they told anyone about the abuse, their parents, siblings, or pets would be killed (Hudson, 1991).

Effects of Torture, Ritual Abuse, and Mind Control

Common outcomes of torture, SRA, and MC are injuries to the head, teeth, and genitals, as well as bone fractures, dislocations, scars, burns, pain, and chronic headaches. The emotional effects are more severe and longer-lasting than those caused by other crimes. Themes are a sense of violation, dehumanization, humiliation, and powerlessness; guilt about harming others or animals; loss of trust and self-esteem; identity and personality changes; terror and insecurity; and damaged social and family relationships (Bloom, 1994; Valente, 2000). Trauma specific fears (e.g., small dark spaces or nudity), hypersexuality, and obsessions with magic or devils are common. Physiologic changes similar to those found in PTSD are also evident. Victims may be forced or programmed to commit crimes against others. They may talk about topics that do not make sense to professionals, such as the Greek alphabet, sex trade, white slavery, drinking blood, and satanic rituals (Indianapolis ANAD, 2002). Other specific responses resulting from torture are listed in Box 41-1.

There is much controversy about assigning psychiatric diagnoses (e.g., PTSD, adjustment disorder, major depression, dysthymia, anxiety disorder, dissociative identity disorder, or other dissociative disorders) to victims who are having typical reactions to horrific crimes (Torem, 2000). The major concern is that diagnosis is another form of victimization, stigmatization, and discounting of the validity of reports of these crimes. Blaming the victim draws

---

Box 41-1 | Specific Responses Resulting from Torture, Serial Ritual Abuse, Mind Control

Anxiety-panic-terror
Anger-rage-aggression
Fatigue-insomnia
Guilt-shame-spiritual distress
Withdrawal-isolation
Denial-repression-suppression
Memory disturbances-amnesia
Nightmares-flashbacks
Body-kinesthetic memories
Hyperarousal-sensitivity to stress
Impulsiveness
Alienation-estrangement
Extreme passivity
Depression
Dissociation-numbing
Decreased concentration
Sexual dysfunctions
Mistrust-suspiciousness
Unresponsiveness
Suicidal-homicidal ideation
Emotional lability
Self-mutilation

Adapted from van der Kolk B, McFarlane AC, Weissaeth L: *Traumatic stress: the effects of overwhelming experience on mind, body, and society,* New York, 1996, Guilford Press; Turkus JA: The treatment challenge, *Many Voices* 12(6):6, 2000; Personal interviews: Indianapolis ANAD, 2002; Valente S: Controversies and challenges of ritual abuse, *J Psychosoc Nurs* 38(11):8, 2000.

attention away from the individual, social, cultural, and political variables creating and fostering torture, SRA, and MC and from research on strategies for prevention. Some professionals even view PTSD as insufficient for acknowledging the catastrophic effects experienced by victims and their families.

Recovery from Torture, Ritual Abuse, and Mind Control

Because torture, SRA, and MC tend to be ongoing, the impact stage of recovery persists but may wax and wane over the years. In the recoil stage, adaptation is difficult because of the severity of the emotional stress remaining after these crimes end. Although supportive, cognitive, behavioral, psychodynamic, and pharmacologic approaches are useful in helping these survivors reorganize their lives, this stage is likely to be prolonged with more relapses during other life crises. Admission to a specialized program or psychiatric unit may be needed during intense therapy periods when the risk of self-mutilation, suicide, or exacerbation of substance abuse is present (Courtois, Turkus, 1998). The major goals for recovery (Valente, 2000) are the following:

1. The decrease in, and eventual elimination of, self-destructive behaviors (self-mutilation, suicide, substance abuse, and manipulation)
2. Processing and integrating the memories of the experiences, often from the least to most bizarre experiences (as in the recovery from PTSD and the integration of multiple personalities)
3. Expressing and dealing with the intense emotions, especially anger and rage
4. Becoming aware of suppressed or repressed feelings and positive emotions
5. Developing or reestablishing healthy relationships with family, friends, and the community
6. Learning about boundaries, privacy, self-integrity, and empathy

The short- and long-term reactions of survivors described in this section are generally true for both males and females; however, men sometimes have a more difficult time admitting to and dealing with their emotional victimization than women. The added impact on males of sexual violation by other males, both as children and as adults, is a result, in part, of their fears about homosexuality (Ray, 2001).

Psychotherapeutic Management

Nurse–patient relationship

Conveying acceptance, caring, and support are crucial if survivors are going to trust enough to discuss their experiences. Survivors must have time and space to process the issues at their own pace. Survivors may need "prompting," which also conveys understanding, such as, "It sounds as if you have been traumatized or tortured" or "I wonder if you have experienced activities using the Greek alphabet." Strategies used with patients experiencing PTSD are particularly useful for survivors of torture and ritual abuse (see Chapter 31). Other models for trauma recovery are also available, such as those described by Miller and Guidry (2001) and Rothschild (2000).

Depending on the origin of the torture, SRA, or MC (individuals, relatives, gangs, hate groups, cults, military-political organizations), it may be crucial to understand the survivor's family, religious, cultural, and political background. Referrals for treatment or correction of physical injuries may be appropriate, such as dentists, plastic surgeons, gynecologists, neurologists, or gastroenterologists (Turkus, 2000).

Psychopharmacology

Using medication in treating survivors of torture, SRA, and MC is highly controversial, especially because drugs were often a part of the abuse as it occurred. Sometimes the medications used in treating PTSD, anxiety disorders, depression, and psychosis are effective.

Milieu management

Specialized treatment centers (e.g., Center for Victims of Torture in Minnesota, The Center: Post-Traumatic Disorders Program in Washington, DC) use a multidisciplinary approach in providing treatment and rehabilitation for survivors and their families. Some centers and programs use bicultural counselors to facilitate counseling with immigrants and former gang members. Self-help and therapy groups may be useful for survivors with similar experiences and needs, such as political refugees; rape, childhood sexual abuse, and partner abuse survivors; and former cult members and former gang members.

RAPE AND SEXUAL ASSAULT

Nature of the Problem

Statistics indicate that rape is an underreported crime in the United States; probably only 10% to 30% of rapes are reported. Valid statistics are not available for sexual assault and rape because of this lack of reporting. A woman may be raped at any age, but the highest risk occurs between the ages of 16 and 19 (Brown, 2001). Rape of men by men is increasing but is rarely reported. Of the reported sexual assaults and rapes, 90% involve a male perpetrator and a female victim (Brown, 2001).

One major problem in reporting rape is that laws and attitudes vary in different states and communities. In general, rape is considered forcible penetration of the victim's body by the perpetrator's penis, fingers, or objects without consent (Martin et al, 2000). Any other form of forced sexual contact (from touch to mutilation) is considered sexual assault. Despite sexual contact, it is generally acknowledged that rape is not sexually motivated, but involves a desire for power and control, a wish to humiliate the victim, and the playing out of a (sexual) fantasy (Brown, 2001). Some prosecutors still do not accept rape as a charge if the two individuals know each other (date rape), despite the fact that, in 90% of reported rapes, the victim knows the offender at least casually (Brown, 2001). Date or acquaintance rape may be complicated with the use of amnesics ("date rape drugs"), other drugs, and alcohol that interfere with the remembering of the rape (Osterman, Barbiaz, Johnson, 2001). Some states lack "marital rape" statutes, or prosecutors are reluctant to charge husbands with raping their wives. Unfortunately, many members of our society ignore rape or convey the message that anyone who is raped asked for it (blaming the victim).

Effects of Rape and Sexual Assault

Similar to all crime victims, the rape victim experiences a severe violation and all the possible emotions of the impact stage. In addition to internal and external bodily injuries, there may be a threat to life with weapons, a threat to return and rape again, to kill if the rape is reported, or the perpetrator may kill the victim during or after the rape (Brown,

2001). Victims usually live but wish they had died. The traumatic memories of the rape usually include the tastes, smells, sounds, and sights, as well tactile sensations and physical pain (Brown, 2001). These memories and the powerlessness, loss of control, fear, shame, guilt, humiliation, rage, and feelings of being contaminated or "dirty" may be overwhelming. A typical reaction of the victim is the wish to regain a sense of control and retreat to a safe place, take a thorough shower, and destroy any damaged belongings. To do so is to destroy most of the evidence that would be required if the victim later decides to report the rape and prosecute. Avoiding medical attention also places victims at risk for acquired immunodeficiency syndrome (AIDS), Hepatitis B, sexually transmitted diseases (STDs), pregnancy, and improper healing of any physical injuries (Piercy, Greenwood, 2002).

CLINICAL EXAMPLE

A 24-year-old woman called a rape crisis line complaining of anxiety at work, not sleeping, fear of being out at night, overwhelming anger, and feeling "dirty" and ashamed. For several weeks she felt that a co-worker was watching her. Last Friday, as she was leaving work late, the co-worker pushed her into her car and raped her. She did not report the rape and hid in her apartment all weekend. She forced herself to go to work on Monday. The man acted friendly toward her, as if nothing had happened.

Recovery from Rape and Sexual Assault

Despite an outward appearance of calm composure and a denial at times of the need for help, the rape survivor needs assistance, information, and support. It may not be until the survivor begins the up-and-down struggle of the recoil stage that the losses, anger, and needs are recognized. In an emergency department, collecting evidence may be a priority for staff, but for the survivor, it is perceived as further intrusion and violation. To staff, survivors may seem resistant and uncooperative, while survivors are trying to protect themselves and regain a sense of control (Brown, 2001). Box 41-2 lists some of the needs and rights of survivors.

Many communities have developed specialized services for rape survivors within clinics or hospitals

| Box 41-2 | Needs and Rights of Rape Survivors

1. Crisis intervention: information, counseling, and referrals
2. Help with basic needs: housing, transportation, child care, safety
3. Medical information and care: information about pregnancy prevention, testing for sexually transmitted diseases, follow-up care, and counseling
4. Advocacy for whatever choices are made about reporting or prosecuting
5. Protection of rights: to privacy, confidentiality, gentleness, sensitivity, and explanations of procedures and tests
6. Protection of rights: to refuse collection of evidence, to determine who will and will not be present during examinations, to get copies of all medical and legal reports, and to apply for reimbursement through victim's compensation
7. Fairness, information, and protection of legal rights during investigations, hearings, and trial, including not being asked about prior sexual experiences with anyone besides the suspect or defendant
8. Reasonable protection against further harm: escorts to court, restraining order, additional patrols, even relocation, if necessary

(as part of the emergency departments). Sexual assault nurse examiners have skills in collecting forensic evidence while providing empathy, support, and information. These nurses also encourage the beginning of the recovery process by challenging any myths held by the survivors, such as, "I should have fought him off" (Brown, 2001; Girardin, 2001; Piercy, Greenwood, 2002).

The specialized rape services have information packets prepared for rape survivors and staff in hospitals, counseling centers, and other crisis services. Survivors can be encouraged to keep the information sheets, as well as phone numbers of resources, for later use. The temporarily composed and calm victim who denies the need for help should be especially encouraged to take materials home. A sexual assault nurse examiner may also call a sexual assault advocate, an advocate from a victim's assistance program, or a rape crisis counselor to initiate contact with the survivor and make periodic follow-up contact days, weeks, and months later (Brown, 2001).

The ability to make follow-up contact with a rape survivor after the impact stage can be beneficial when the emotional, physical, or legal issues and

concerns arise (Brown, 2001). In the recoil stage, most survivors begin to react to the significant effect that rape has had on their lives; they may alternately deny and admit to experiencing turmoil. Fear and mistrust are major issues and may be directed toward individuals resembling the perpetrator or toward everyone around them (especially if others convey any hint of blaming the victim). Survivors may be afraid to leave the one place they designate as safe. Survivors are able to go out with family and friends, but they more often avoid strangers, places similar to the rape scene, and intimacy, especially sexual relationships. If the rapes occurred in their residence, survivors may move or at least make safety-related changes to prevent recurrence, or they may ask for someone to stay with them at night for a while. Being alone and unprotected is usually frightening, especially when nightmares and traumatic memories occur. Survivors need help in reaffirming that they are worthwhile individuals, with dignity and rights, who did not cause and did not deserve the rape. They need to know that their anger is natural, especially about the violation of person and privacy, the humiliation, and the sense of powerlessness. Survivors often question whether they might have fought off the attacker. Survival is most important; if the victim survived the rape, then he or she did exactly what was necessary to stay alive.

Rape Trauma Symptoms

One way to monitor and evaluate the rape survivor's responses to the trauma and recovery process through the recoil and reorganization stages is to assess periodically for improvements in the rape trauma symptoms (DiVasto, 1985) listed in Box 41-3. It is important to remember that survivors vacillate in the recoil stage between repression or suppression and dealing with the trauma. Even progress in the reorganization stage is not smooth; backslides occur at times, especially if new situations trigger memories of the rape. Survivors may avoid future routine gynecologic and rectal examinations to avoid reexperiencing the trauma (Osterman, Barbiaz, Johnson, 2001). The use of restraints during an inpatient stay may also reactivate the trauma symptoms. Survivors may need help in overcoming difficulties in sleeping and eating, relationship problems, lowered self-esteem, and depression. The goals of

Box 41-3 Rape Trauma Symptoms

- Sleep disturbances, nightmares
- Loss of appetite, somatic symptoms
- Fears, anxiety, phobias, suspicion
- Decrease in activities and motivation
- Disruptions in relationships with partner, family, friends
- Self-blame, guilt, shame
- Lowered self-esteem, feelings of worthlessness

recovery from rape and sexual assault are the same as those for all survivors of crime. In addition, rape survivors may need to develop or regain healthy sexual functioning and relationships (Osterman, Barbiaz, Johnson, 2001). Survivors need to transfer "traumatic" memories to narrative or "past" memories by processing the sensory memories and decreasing their strength and influence (Brown, 2001).

Psychotherapeutic Management

Nurse-patient relationship

The rape or sexual assault survivor needs continual empathy, support, and an opportunity to process the events and intense feelings, as well as to regain a sense of psychologic safety (Osterman, Barbiaz, Johnson, 2001). Although it is more time- and energy-consuming, the best approach in collecting evidence and providing nursing care is to move slowly and supportively at the individual survivor's pace and to give rationales for and descriptions of procedures and referrals. Nurses can be particularly helpful to rape survivors. Male and, especially, female survivors tend to feel safer with a woman and may refuse to talk to a man, especially alone. The presence of a nurse or sexual assault advocate through examinations and interrogations can be reassuring. Survivors may or may not choose to have a friend or family member stay with them for additional support. A sense of shame or guilt may interfere with reaching out for support (Osterman, Barbiaz, Johnson, 2001).

Crisis intervention is the most appropriate approach during the impact stage. Short-term counseling and a rape support group can be beneficial during the recoil stage. Long-term counseling may be needed during the reorganization stage, especially if the survivor decides to prosecute the perpetrator. The lengthy legal processes can seriously delay recovery. In many trial situations, the survivor is still treated as a criminal during cross-examinations. On the other hand, conviction and imprisonment of the perpetrator can help survivors feel vindicated, compensated, and safer in their environments.

If the symptoms of rape trauma do not gradually diminish and reorganization of lifestyle does not seem to occur, the survivor needs to be assessed for and helped with any new problems, such as posttraumatic stress, anxiety, excessive anger and guilt, depression, acting out, isolation, suicidal thoughts, self-destructive behaviors, substance abuse, phobias, negative or destructive relationships with others, and reactivation of childhood sexual abuse memories. With any of these behaviors, longer-term counseling is a necessity, and hospitalization may become essential.

Psychopharmacology

Although rarely prescribed to rape survivors, benzodiazepines to reduce anxiety and provide for sleep may be used on a temporary basis. Alternatively, an antidepressant taken at bedtime, especially trazodone (Desyrel), may be ordered if symptoms of depression exist with a sleep disturbance. If nightmares or traumatic memories are severe, a short course of an atypical antipsychotic such as risperidone (Risperdal) may be indicated.

Milieu management

Referral can be made to a rape support group or center, which encourages expressing anger safely, overcoming guilt and shame, building self-esteem and trust, and assisting in regaining control of the survivor's life and a sense of safety. Support groups are sometimes available for relatives, especially partners, of rape survivors to help them deal with the trauma, the stereotyping and myths, and the changes occurring in the survivors and themselves.

Critical Thinking Question

As an emergency room nurse, you are treating a 19-year-old male victim who was tortured and raped by a local gang. The victim refuses to give any details or to identify members of the gang. Describe what information you would give him about being a victim and the benefits of follow-up counseling.

ADULT SURVIVORS OF CHILDHOOD SEXUAL ABUSE

Nature of the Problem

The crimes of childhood sexual abuse (by nonrelatives) and incest (by relatives) are especially destructive for two major reasons: the crimes are not one-time occurrences, and the perpetrators are usually known and trusted. Unfortunately, these crimes are common. Studies suggest that 15% to 30% (an average of 22%) of all girls and 7% of all boys have experienced childhood sexual abuse (Roberts, 2000; Sappington, 2000). Sexual abuse of boys may be much higher. It is sometimes harder for men to reveal the abuse because of the fear of being seen as unable to protect themselves, weak, or gay (Ray, 2001; Romano, DeLuca, 2000). However, the number of children who have been sexually abused and never reported it, even when they became adults, is not actually known.

Sexual abuse and incest include voyeurism and exhibitionism, which can lead to intercourse and mutilation, but always involve a younger victim who is not capable of giving consent to the older, more powerful, individual. Male perpetrators are commonly fathers, uncles, stepfathers, older brothers, cousins, grandfathers, neighbors, scout leaders, camp counselors, coaches, and religious leaders. Less frequently, the perpetrators are females: mothers, older sisters, other relatives, day-care workers, teachers, coaches, neighbors, and babysitters. Victims are from every social, cultural, ethnic, and economic group.

Although sexual abuse can be violent, it typically is not. Coercion is possible because of the victim's dependent, trusting, or loving relationship with the perpetrator. The victim is urged to maintain the "secret" with various threats, such as the following: the victim will be taken away from the family; the perpetrator will be put in a mental hospital or jail; the parents will divorce; the other parent will get sick; there will be no abuse of siblings if the victim is compliant; love will be withdrawn; no one would believe the victim anyway; or there will be physical abuse if the victim does not comply. Even when no physical violence takes place, victims usually fear that it will occur if they resist the perpetrator. Factors such as family disorganization, economic instability, secrecy and communication difficulties, substance abuse, and other forms of abuse (emotional, verbal, physical, and so forth) and neglect seem to correlate with sexual abuse (Davis, Petretic-Jackson, 2000; Romano, DeLuca, 2000; Sappington, 2000; Young, Boyd, Hubbell, 2001).

Even if the young victims want to disclose the abuse, it is difficult for them because they lack the words and concepts to describe the event. An emotional reaction of fear and confusion usually occurs, and some physical pain, but not a moral, ethical, or legal concept of "wrong." Most victims who, as children, tried to tell a parent or other adults were met with disbelief, denial, or pressure to retract their accusations. It is difficult for anyone to believe that the partners they love or respected members of the community are capable of sexual abuse. Police, prosecutors, judges, mental health professionals, and the general public may discount a child's report as unreliable, a fantasy, distorted, or faked at the urging of a parent (Davis, Petretic-Jackson, 2000). There are also potential "benefits" from the sexual relationship; the child is made to feel special, with extra attention from and time with the perpetrator that other children do not enjoy. A certain power comes from trying to please the adult and from receiving a degree of affection (Davis, Petretic-Jackson, 2000). At times, the child may even have the physical experience of sensual pleasure. However, the emotional pleasure and concept of sexual love are absent. (All children make bids for attention and affection. Even if they are cute, coy, or flirtatious, these desires should not be viewed as seduction. Perpetrators of sexual abuse choose to misinterpret the child's behaviors to meet their own needs and should still be held responsible for the crime.)

Effects of Childhood Sexual Abuse on the Child

For the victim, the end result is disturbed growth and development (beginning with trust and autonomy issues), ambivalence about the experience (both the benefits and the pain), and denial of what is happening to protect the whole family or the community. The young child is fulfilling the roles of child and lover to the perpetrator, and roles of child and protector to the rest of the family or community (protecting them from the "horrible secret"). As a result, the child begins a long-term process of taking care of others to the exclusion of personal needs. Basically, the child wishes for love, not sex, but eventually feels guilty, exploited, betrayed, angry, "dirty," helpless, and responsible. Denial, repression, suppression, rationalization, and dissociation are mechanisms used by young victims to cope with this "no-win" situation. Sleep and eating disturbances, enuresis, anxiety, depression, aggression, an active fantasy life, masturbation, sexualized play, sexual aggression, poor impulse control, somatization, alienation, fear, shame, guilt, self-blame, self-destructive behaviors, running away, and truancy are common (Davis, Petretic-Jackson, 2000; Roberts, 2000; Young, Boyd, Hubbell, 2001). The more severe the abuse is, the more likely that repression will begin near puberty. If the sexual abuse continues through adolescence, repression is less likely. Repression normally lasts until victims are in their 20s or 30s and are having trouble with close relationships or parenting.

Effects of Childhood Sexual Abuse on the Adolescent

As adolescents, sexual abuse victims show mostly overt methods of dysfunctional coping, such as impulsive acting-out, violence toward others, self-destructive behaviors, self-mutilation, sleeping and eating disorders, suicide attempts, running away, truancy, delinquency, substance abuse, sexual acting out, prostitution, early pregnancy, and early marriage (Davis, Petretic-Jackson, 2000; Young, Boyd, Hubbell, 2001). For victims who cope through self-mutilation, these behaviors tend to begin between the ages of 13 and 15 (Machoian, 2001).

Adolescents may have fantasies of revenge and wish for the perpetrator's death. The anger toward the perpetrator and other adults (for not protecting them) approaches rage but is not directly expressed. Victims may not even be aware of the reason for their rage, shame, guilt, confusion, sense of alienation, and isolation and may not realize that their acting-out behaviors are related to the abuse. Regression, depersonalization, dissociation, manipulation, low self-esteem, impaired social skills, spiritual distress, thought and memory disturbances, self-neglect, aimlessness, and withdrawal are common. Sexual abuse survivors are also more likely than the general population to be raped and battered in adolescence and later in life (Davis, Petretic-Jackson, 2000; Kreidler et al, 2000; Sappington, 2000; Young, Boyd, Hubbell, 2001).

Effects of Childhood Sexual Abuse on the Adult

For many victims of childhood sexual abuse, the process of surviving childhood and adolescence and becoming an adult is similar to delayed PTSD: repression of memories (even nonsexual ones) followed by a breakthrough of unwanted, intrusive memories. The memories may begin as nightmares, kinesthetic sensations (such as flinching or vaginal pain when touched by a partner in the same way as did the perpetrator), or flashbacks. The memories may return gradually, in pieces, or in a sudden, overwhelming flood. Victims cannot be rushed to remember the abuse before they are ready to cope with it.

On the surface, adult victims may look relatively uninjured because of denial, dissociation, amnesia, emotional deadening, or repression. They enter counseling for manifestations of the abuse rather than for the incest or sexual abuse itself. The list of reactions in Box 41-4 can be used as a checklist to identify the issues to be addressed in counseling. Victims who see this checklist typically express amazement (that so much has resulted from the sexual abuse) and relief (that there is finally an explanation for all their "craziness"). Up to this point, victims tended to deny or minimize the relationship of the sexual abuse to any of their current problems. It then becomes evident to victims that the event has disturbed their whole growth and development process, their self-esteem, and has set them up for other abusive relationships. Until counseling finally focuses on the underlying cause of their reactions, victims tend to seek treatment repeatedly without relief.

The inability to handle the memories of abuse and the painful emotions, especially anger, often induces thoughts of suicide: to escape the pain and depression; to "die with the secret"; to avoid conflict with the family or perpetrator; to stop feeling "crazy"; and to end the nightmares and flashbacks that are so frightening. Self-harm or mutilation is a common way of dealing with the emotional pain, loss, rage, and abandonment. Victims describe various patterns of their mutilation (Alper, Peterson, 2001; ANAD, 2002; Dresser, 1999; Machoian, 2001):

1. When feeling overwhelmed, they inflict harm as a cry for help when they feel no one is listening or cares.

|Box 41-4| Adult Manifestations of Childhood Sexual Abuse

Memory Disturbances

Amnesia about the abuse
Memory gaps about childhood
Inability to think straight

Keeping Unnecessary Secrets

Relationship Issues

"Trouble connecting" with others
"Running away" from others
Fear of men/fear of women
Trouble trusting others and their
   motives
Fear of intimacy
Fear of abandonment/rejection
Unable to maintain intimacy
Trouble giving/receiving affection
Feeling alienated from others
Fear of being used/abused
Trouble saying "no"
Taking care of others
Trouble with parenting
Entering abusive relationships
Poor choices of partners

Body Symptoms

Vague/transient pains
Memories of physical pain
Chronic pain or migraine headaches
Gagging/nausea/vomiting
Unpleasant sensation when touched
Negative/distorted body image
Self-conscious about body
Overly conscious of appearance

Anger Issues

Fear of expressing anger
Holding anger in
Crying instead of being angry
Fantasies of revenge

Feeling violent/full of rage
Fear of violence
Homicidal thoughts

Anxiety Issues

Easily startled
Inability to relax
Fear of being attacked/exposed
Hypervigilance
Feeling like a frightened child
Fear of the dark
Panic attacks
Phobias/agoraphobia

Addiction Issues

Alcohol/drug abuse or dependence
Compulsive spending

Intrusive Thoughts and Memories

Intense nightmares, unwanted thoughts
Flashbacks: feeling, seeing, smelling, tasting, hearing

Detachment Issues

Feeling numb/unreal
Disconnected from feelings from body
Feeling as if there are "personalities"
   inside
"Out-of-body" experiences

Control Issues

Fear of authority/rules
Need to be in control/feeling out of con-
   trol
Pretending to be out of control (or
   helpless)
Fear of being vulnerable
Ambivalent about being taken care of
Letting others be in control
Trying to control others

Allowing children to be abused

Identity Issues

Confusion about identity or roles
Negative self-image
Need to be perfect or perfectly bad
Underachievement or overachievement
Need to be totally competent

Sexual Issues

Concealing sexual feelings
Discomfort with sexual touching
Feeling nonsexual
Lack of orgasms/sexual dysfunctions
Confusion about sexuality/sexual
   identity
Feeling "dirty"
Trading sex for favors
Promiscuity/prostitution
Wondering if one is gay

Self-Punishment

Suicidal thoughts/attempts
Wanting to die or to be dead
Self-mutilation
Compulsive eating or dieting
Bingeing/purging

Other Feelings

Low self-esteem/guilt/shame
Fear of feelings
Feeling stuck
Feeling like a failure
Chronic dissatisfaction
"Frozen" emotions
Lack of a sense of humor
Feeling inadequate
Feeling "walled in"
Feeling "crazy"

2. When emotions build up, they go numb or dissociate and have to inflict pain to make sure they can still feel.
3. When they are feeling unreal (depersonalization), they draw blood to make sure they are alive.
4. They cause physical pain so that they do not have to focus on the emotional pain.
5. They punish themselves when they are feeling self-loathing, guilt, shame, or fear.

6. They use the mutilation to relieve the anger or rage toward self and others.
7. They may use the mutilation as an attempt to manipulate others.
8. The mutilation may become chronic and addictive, especially if it produces a "high" (related to endogenous opiates).

Some evidence suggests that suicide attempts may have similar dynamics as self-mutilation and also may become a chronic pattern or addiction (Mynatt, 2000).

Alcohol and drugs are often used to avoid or numb the pain and memories and to bring fleeting pleasure that is otherwise elusive (Davis, Petretic-Jackson, 2000). Food may also provide brief pleasure or "fill an emptiness inside," but leads to feeling bloated and guilty and a need to purge. Although sex is not usually enjoyable, it can bring relief from loneliness, temporary attention, affection, and approval. On the other hand, sexual encounters may trigger traumatic flashbacks, anxiety, fear, shame, disgust, or a sense of helplessness. Healthy adult relationships and sexual intimacy are difficult because of problems in trusting anyone and the history of linking abuse and love. Victims have boundary issues, trouble setting limits with others, and difficulty with asking for what they really need (Davis, Petretic-Jackson, 2000). Victims also tend to be caretakers, rescuers, and co-dependents.

CLINICAL EXAMPLE

Jan Lester, 30 years of age, was admitted to a psychiatric unit as a result of suicidal ideations and 12 superficial cuts on her wrists. Nine months ago, she began having nightmares about being awakened at night as a child with someone on top of her. During the nightmares, she would wake up crying with strange body sensations, gagging, pressure on her chest, and vaginal pain. As the nightmares and memories became more complete and vivid, she realized her father had frequently had sex with her while her mother was asleep. As her father's fiftieth birthday approached, she felt as if she could not tolerate going to his party. She wanted to be dead but was unable to force herself to cut her wrists more deeply. She wanted help.

Victims' reactions to the trauma (see Box 41-4) often get labeled as clinical symptoms. When an axis I diagnosis is given to patients, it is commonly depression (atypical type), PTSD, substance-abuse disorder, eating disorder, anxiety disorder, somatoform disorder, dissociative disorder (including dissociative identity disorder), or impulse-control disorder. Axis II personality disorders are commonly given, such as borderline, narcissistic, histrionic, avoidant, dependent, atypical, or mixed disorders (Davis, Petretic-Jackson, 2000; Kreidler et al, 2000).

Receiving a diagnosis is a major problem, not only because of the stigma and blaming the victim, but also because the diagnosis often becomes the focus of treatment rather than the underlying issue. Lack of appropriate treatment carries a major risk not only for adult survivors, but also for their children, especially if the survivors are still in a stage of repression. Evidence suggests that untreated or improperly treated victims occasionally set up dysfunctional, disorganized families who contribute to the incestuous abuse of their children. With their own denial, repression, amnesia, or other mechanisms, survivors have trouble relating to their partners and are unable to "see" the partners' involvement with their children. Perpetrators may sexually abuse their younger siblings, children, grandchildren, nieces, nephews, and others. Examples of incest have surfaced within three and four generations of a family. Breaking this cycle is crucial.

Recovery from Childhood Sexual Abuse

In some ways, recovery from childhood sexual abuse or incest is similar to recovery from all crimes or from PTSD, but it tends to be more complex, difficult, and lengthy by comparison, especially if emotional abuse by the family is ongoing or the survivor still lives with the abuser. The memories and emotions are strong, painful, and confusing. The intense anger and ambivalence toward the perpetrator are hard for both the survivor and the nurse to handle. Survivors need to know in the beginning that the symptoms and emotional pain will probably worsen before they improve as the review of experiences occurs. Although outpatient counseling often takes 2 years or more, survivors tend to engage in treatment sporadically. It is common for survivors to initially disclose, discuss, vent, and feel "cured." Then, as new crises or relationship problems emerge, survivors return to counseling to deal with each issue and its possible connection to the original trauma. Getting a patient to commit to continuous, long-term counseling is sometimes difficult, but the nurse can emphasize the desirability and value of at least sporadic counseling.

The overall goals of recovery are safety and security, rebuilding trust, assertiveness skills, improved self-esteem and self-acceptance, forgiveness of self, adaptive coping with life and its stresses, the capacity for intimate relationships and genuine sexual pleasure, improvements in affect, and reduced anxiety, anger, shame, guilt, fear, and dissociation, as well as the prevention of sexual abuse of future generations (Davis, Petretic-Jackson, 2000; Kreidler et al, 2000; Sappington, 2000).

Psychotherapeutic Management

Nurse-patient relationship

Much depends on the nurse's ability to develop a trusting relationship with the survivor quickly. Empathy, active support, compassion, warmth, and being nonjudgmental are crucial. Survivors need to be calmly and matter-of-factly asked about childhood sexual abuse because they are not likely to reveal it spontaneously. The old and perhaps current coercions to "keep the secret" remain strong in the minds of survivors; they need to feel safe about confidentiality and the nurse's acceptance before disclosure will occur. How much detail is revealed and how soon depends, in part, on the nurse's ability to be receptive to the experiences without being critical of the perpetrator, of other adults in the family, or of the survivor's loyalty to them. The survivor needs to be reassured that all the experiences and emotions (positive, negative, and ambivalent) are valid and that exploring these is the beginning of the process of working through recovery (Davis, Petretic-Jackson, 2000). It is usually helpful for survivors to be reminded periodically that they were not responsible for and did not deserve the sexual abuse, are not to be blamed, were not in control of the situation, and that the way they coped with it in the past was the best they were able to do at the time. Cognitive-behavioral approaches and education about the dynamics of sexual abuse and reassurances about recovery can be useful in correcting faulty perceptions about the abuse, decreasing self-blame and guilt, and instilling hope for the future despite the inability to change the past. Nursing interventions for survivors are listed in the box below.

Mentally and emotionally reexperiencing traumatic events is disturbing; only periodic small doses may be tolerable. It is helpful to remind survivors that "they went through the abuse alone, but they do not have to remember it alone." If traumatic flashbacks or dissociation occurs, it is important to bring

---

Key Nursing Interventions   Survivors of Childhood Abuse

- Contract for safety and control of impulses to harm self or others.
- Set limits on self-destructive or self-harm patterns.
- Establish a trusting and supportive environment.
- Accept all feelings and reactions as normal responses.
- Ask permission before touching survivors.
- Reinforce that recovery is possible, even if it is difficult.
- Educate about the dynamics of abuse and recovery processes.
- Assist survivors in understanding current behaviors as reflections of survival strategies used in childhood.
- Facilitate reevaluation of the sexual abuse, its circumstances, and its effects, but without pressuring.
- Encourage coping choices that are in survivors' best interests.
- Discuss safeguarding other children if the perpetrator still poses a risk.
- Support choices about future disclosures, confrontation, or reporting.
- Be aware that family members and others may feel split loyalty and engage in dysfunctional roles and interaction patterns.
- Decrease feelings of isolation, shame, and stigma.

- Encourage self-acceptance.
- Facilitate acknowledgment, forgiveness, and love for the "child within."
- Teach and encourage stress management and anger reduction.
- Facilitate the transfer of responsibility and anger to the perpetrator but set limits on acting out fantasies of revenge.
- Foster separation and individuation from the family and its patterns.
- Help to find meaning in the experience and mourning of all the losses (grieving is a very painful experience).
- Facilitate the change from victim to survivor status (reexperiencing and integrating the positive, negative, and ambivalent feelings and memories).
- Facilitate reexperiencing and reworking of maturational tasks that were missed or experienced prematurely.
- Educate about life skills, communication skills, coping skills, assertiveness, decision making, conflict resolution, boundary setting, friendship, intimacy, sexuality, and parenting.
- Refer to outpatient counseling and appropriate support groups.

the survivors "back to the present" by reminding them where they are and that the nurse is with them now. The nurse and survivors can monitor their safety and tolerance of the process to prevent becoming overwhelmed, retreating, attempting suicide, or self-mutilating. Anger-release strategies, such as using a foam bat *(batacca)* while talking to a chair that represents the perpetrator or nonprotective adults, often help the survivor express thoughts and feelings that could not be expressed in childhood. Play therapy, therapeutic stories, and art therapy can be especially useful in helping children process their abuse (Bennett, 1997; Hinds, 1997). Writing memories and painful feelings in an ongoing journal and writing "letters" to the perpetrator and others that will not be sent can be useful (Day, 2001).

Confrontation of the family or perpetrator by the survivor is not necessarily a desired outcome or a safe option. Confrontation may be done symbolically with the nurse rather than directly with the perpetrator and other family members. If survivors choose to confront directly, much preparation is needed, even rehearsals with the nurse, before the event. Survivors need to consider, plan for, and rehearse their reactions to all the potential responses of family members. The most typical family responses are denial, rationalization, and blaming the victim; confessions and apologies are unlikely. (See Family Issues box.) Survivors can be helped to debate the benefits and risks of confrontation, as well as the degree and type of contact they want to have with the family, even if they do not confront them or if the survivors are to protect their own children. An important consideration for the nurse and the survivor to discuss is the mandatory reporting of child abuse if younger children are currently victims of abuse. This type of report is understandably difficult for both the nurse and the survivor and needs to be carefully but directly addressed.

When survivors are in outpatient counseling, it is important to consider priorities in each counseling session. Current crises and problems need to be addressed (instead of the sexual abuse) as they arise. For example, gynecologic and physical examinations may be distressing and trigger flashbacks (Roberts, 2000). This aspect is also critical for self-destructive behaviors that are heightened because of counseling, such as suicidal ideation, self-mutilation, and substance abuse. Hospitalization may be necessary if the crisis is severe. Although survivors view recovery as frightening and painful, they also experience relief that they are making progress.

Psychopharmacology

Medications are not always needed or desirable for adult survivors of childhood sexual abuse, especially if substance abuse is a problem or potential problem. For the small number of survivors with serious psychopathology, medications should be given according to the axis I diagnosis, such as depression. An antidepressant such as trazodone (Desyrel) may be used if the depressive symptoms are interfering with sleep. Benzodiazepines or Clonidine may be given on an as-needed basis to help control the emotional or autonomic arousal that occurs during the reexperiencing of traumatic memories. Occasionally, low doses of risperidone (Risperdal) are given for persistent and severely disturbing nightmares or flashbacks.

Milieu management

On an outpatient basis and during any brief hospitalizations, cognitive-behavioral and affect management groups can be a useful adjunct to nursing care (Kreidler et al, 2000). If available, a short-term or ongoing sexual abuse–incest recovery group is beneficial. Some self-help groups include Incest Survivors Anonymous, Survivors of Sexual Abuse, and Daughters and Sons United. Parents United for the nonperpetrator parent can be suggested, if appropriate. The perpetrator may also be referred to counseling. Family therapy is sometimes appropriate.

Other groups that may be recommended, depending on the symptoms and needs of the survivor, are Co-dependency Anonymous, Adult Children of Alcoholics, Alcoholics or Narcotics Anonymous, and Emotions Anonymous. Survivors may also be directed to classes or short-term groups on decision making or problem solving, communication or relationship skills, conflict resolution, parenting skills, and human sexuality.

Critical Thinking Question

You are working with a patient who was sexually abused as a child by her father. The father insists on visiting his daughter and telling you about her history of emotional problems and lying about the family. What is your approach in working with the father?

Family Issues | False Memories? False Allegations?

There are families, including members of the False Memory Syndrome Foundation, who claim they have been wrongly accused of sexual abuse by their children or adult children. These families and some professionals especially challenge the validity of the processes of repression and delayed recovery of memories of abuse. They warn that those who interview children, those who counsel children and adults, and members of support groups can implant false memories and provide support for false allegations. These families and professionals question the credentials and training of many who counsel children and adults who claim they were abused. They cite studies of recent and long-term memory to support their views about distorted and false memories. They sometimes question the claims of serious emotional damage to victims as a result of actual sexual abuse. They support the premise that false memories and false allegations are destroying the families of these children.

Other professionals and adult survivors of childhood sexual abuse maintain that the graphic details of children's traumatic memories and the use of sexual descriptions, very advanced for their ages at the time, support the credibility of the abuse charges. These professionals and survivors claim that denial, repression, amnesia, and dissociation are real phenomena used by children, adolescents, and adults to protect themselves emotionally from the abuse as it was happening and from the later realization of its moral, legal, ethical, and emotional significance. These individuals maintain that 75% or more of survivors are able to collect strong corroborating evidence of their abuse and recovered memories. They cite recent neurochemical studies of traumatic memory processes, stress, and PTSD (see Chapter 31) to support their view of the validity of repression, dissociation, and recovered memories. They acknowledge that 2% to 10% of claims of sexual abuse by children and divorcing

parents may be false, and then report that perhaps 75% to 90% of valid child abuse is *never* reported by children, agencies, and professionals. They point out that the False Memory Syndrome Foundation admits that it collects only information on denials of charges of abuse, but that it has no way of knowing if these denials are true or false. Survivors and professionals contend that those who molest children *typically* threaten the victims to "keep the secret" and use denial, minimization, and rationalization when charged with abuse. They also express concern that claims of false memories and false allegations are efforts to disconfirm and "blame the victim," protect abusers (and society), and minimize the severity of the short- and long-term effects of abuse. They contend that families are being destroyed by intrafamilial violence (not the reports of abuse) and that abused children suffer emotional pain and a wide variety of problems throughout childhood, adolescence, and adulthood.

As a result of this controversy, it is recommended that those working with possible survivors of childhood sexual abuse do the following:

1. Allow patients' memories to emerge without pressure and "leading" questions.
2. Avoid specific sexual abuse explanations for patients' symptoms.
3. Follow established guidelines for interviewing child victims and others to assess credibility of memories and testimony.
4. Interview anyone who might provide corroboration or disconfirming evidence.
5. Use established therapeutic techniques rather than nonestablished ones.
6. Avoid using hypnosis and sodium amytal injections as a way of recovering repressed memories.

Adapted from Gardner RA: *True and false accusations of child sex abuse*, New York, 1992; Leavitt F: Iatrogenic memory change: examining the empirical evidence, *Forensic Psychology* 19(2):21, 2001; Loftus EF, Potage DC: Repressed memories: when are they real? *Psychiatr Clin North Am* 22(1):61, 1999; Valente S: Controversies and challenges of ritual abuse, *J Psychosoc Nurs* 38(11):8, 2000; Satel SL: Who needs trauma initiatives? *Psychiatr Serv* 52(6):815, 2001; van der Kolk B, McFarlane AC, Weissaeth L: Traumatic stress: the effects of overwhelming experience on mind, body, and society, New York, 1996, Guilford Press; Personal interviews, Indianapolis ANAD, 2002.

VICTIMS OF PARTNER ABUSE

Nature of the Problem

An estimated one third of women (from adolescents to older adults) each year in the United States suffer from repeated physical abuse by a partner. More than one third to one half of women around the world have suffered partner assault at least once in their lifetimes (Evans, Helton, Blackburn, 2001; Hastings, 2001; Poirier, 2000). The number is even higher when psychologic abuse and other violations of rights are considered (Fig. 41-1). More than 90% to

95% of this abuse is by a man toward a woman (Gerard, 2000; Hastings, 2001). Every few seconds, a woman is abused, raped, tortured, or beaten by her husband, boyfriend, lover, former partner, or estranged partner, and most of this abuse goes unreported, even when injuries are severe enough to require treatment. Of female patients who visit emergency departments, 54% have been assaulted or battered by partners (Sappington, 2000). Prior partner abuse increases the risk of it occurring during pregnancy (Farella, 2000; Horon, Cheng, 2001).

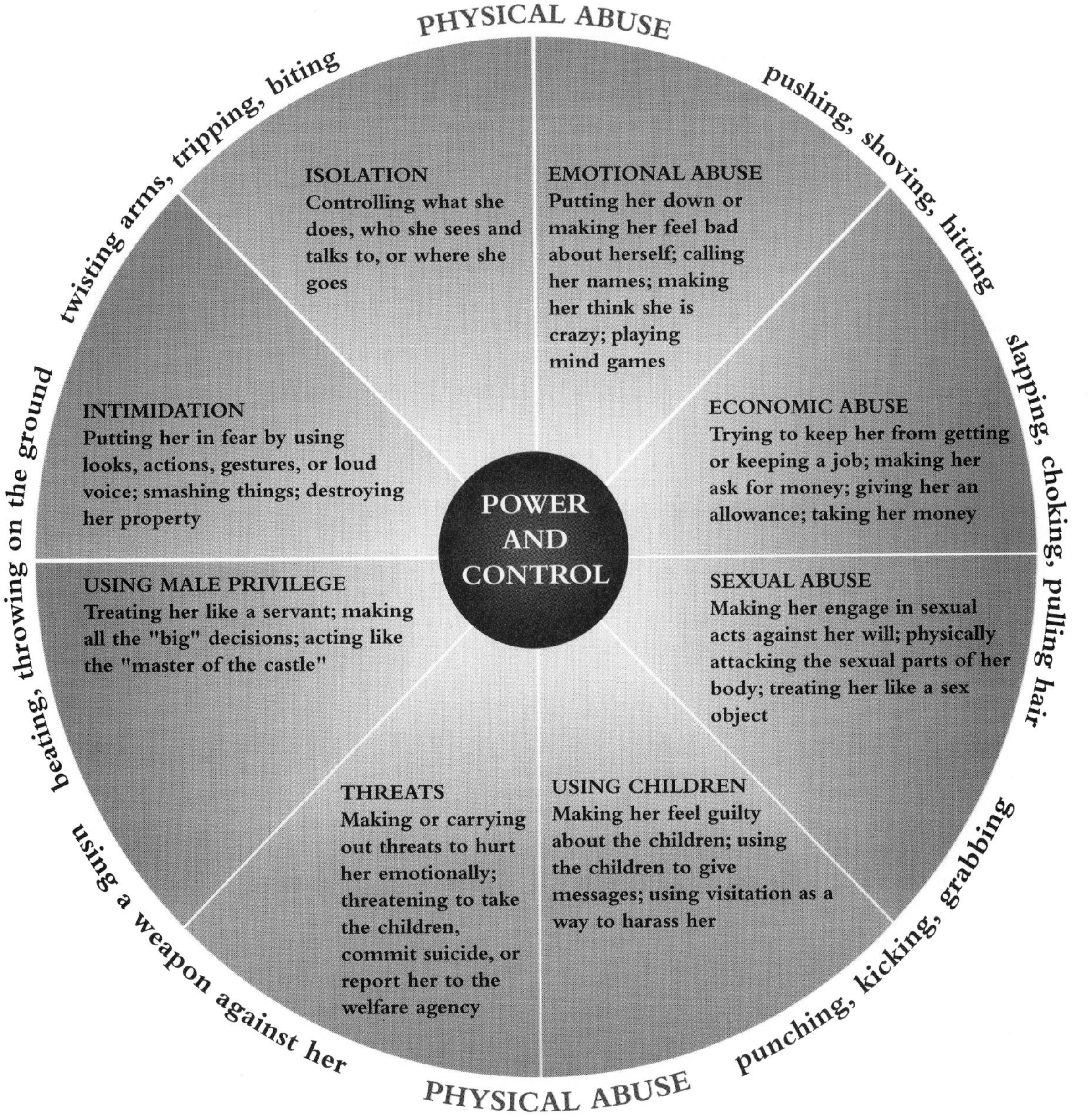

PHYSICAL ABUSE

twisting arms, tripping, biting

pushing, shoving, hitting

slapping, choking, pulling hair

beating, throwing on the ground

punching, kicking, grabbing

using a weapon against her

PHYSICAL ABUSE

ISOLATION
Controlling what she does, who she sees and talks to, or where she goes

EMOTIONAL ABUSE
Putting her down or making her feel bad about herself; calling her names; making her think she is crazy; playing mind games

INTIMIDATION
Putting her in fear by using looks, actions, gestures, or loud voice; smashing things; destroying her property

ECONOMIC ABUSE
Trying to keep her from getting or keeping a job; making her ask for money; giving her an allowance; taking her money

POWER AND CONTROL

USING MALE PRIVILEGE
Treating her like a servant; making all the "big" decisions; acting like the "master of the castle"

SEXUAL ABUSE
Making her engage in sexual acts against her will; physically attacking the sexual parts of her body; treating her like a sex object

THREATS
Making or carrying out threats to hurt her emotionally; threatening to take the children, commit suicide, or report her to the welfare agency

USING CHILDREN
Making her feel guilty about the children; using the children to give messages; using visitation as a way to harass her

Figure 41-1 The desire for power and control results in both psychologic and physical abuse. (From Domestic Abuse Intervention Project: *Power and control,* Duluth, Minn, 1987, The Project.)

Partner-abuse victims tend to conceal their victimization. They are acutely aware that disclosure of their plight will be met with denial or minimization by the partner, friends, and relatives and by increased abuse by their partners (Merrell, 2001). As abused women become more independent (both emotionally and financially), the incidence of violence by their partners increases as well. The fact that 30% to 50% of all women killed in the United States are killed by a partner as they tried to leave or had left supports women's fears (Gerard, 2000; Hastings, 2001; McClellan, Killeen, 2000). About 50% of victims murdered by partners were seen in the emergency departments for other injuries at other times before they died (Gerard, 2000). Women also kill their partners (3.9% of all male homicides), but mostly in self-defense after a history of beatings (McClellan, Killeen, 2000; Stith, 2000).

Studies show that partner abuse crosses all social, racial, cultural, and economic classes, including both homosexual and heterosexual relationships, but is more often reported by individuals on welfare. This tendency is because the victims are more likely to be in contact with reporting agencies such as public health nursing, welfare offices, public clinics, and emergency rooms. Individuals with higher incomes are likely to obtain private services that do not report the abuse (Poirier, 2000).

The relationship of alcohol and drug abuse to violent behavior has been the subject of many studies on partner abuse. Some abusers are abstainers, but more are substance abusers. The victims' view is that abusers use alcohol and drugs as an excuse for their violence and drink when they are about to become violent. Victims also report a correlation between alcohol or drugs and the severity of violence. The combination of substance abuse and violence encourages victims to blame the substance rather than to hold the batterers accountable for their violent behaviors. Women often describe their abusers as "Dr. Jekyll and Mr. Hyde," with changing personalities: gentle, loving, and kind at times; rude, uncaring, and violent at other times. This change is explained, in part, by the cycle of violence described later.

In some relationships, violence is mutual (but not necessarily equal) and is the result of efforts to resolve negative communications and escalating conflicts (McClellan, Killeen, 2000). These couples are often motivated to change and can be taught more effective skills for handling conflict and anger (Stith, 2000). This mutual-violence pattern differs from, but can become, the more common pattern of using violence to exploit and control a partner, often arising out of anger, fear of abandonment, jealousy, or any combination (McClellan, Killeen, 2000). This second pattern almost always involves a man abusing a woman, and the man has little motivation to change. Separate interventions and therapy with the man may interrupt the cycle of violence (Evans, Helton, Blackburn, 2001; Merrell, 2001).

The nature of modern society is a factor to be considered in partner abuse. The portrayal of physical and sexual violence in the media (television, music videos, and films) continues to increase in frequency and severity. Women are still portrayed by the media as second-class citizens at times. In addition, it is well documented that witnesses of family violence and victims of child abuse and neglect tend to become perpetrators of other violence or the abusers and partners of abusers (McClellan, Killeen, 2000; Sappington, 2000; Windom, Maxfield, 2001).

Effects of Partner Abuse

Most experts acknowledge the development of learned helplessness, hopelessness, isolation, and resignation in response to ongoing emotional and physical abuse. Abused women do not report that they enjoy the abuse, but they do have a tendency to believe their partners' view that they deserve the abuse. Box 41-5 presents common reasons why women endure long-term abuse. Another accepted view of why women endure abuse is the "cycle of violence" (Box 41-6). During the "honeymoon" stage, the "good side" of the men is evident, and the women are reminded of their love and the happy potential of the relationship (Farella, 2000; Gerard, 2000; Walker 1979). Women report feeling as if they want to and can help their partners overcome their problems and violent behaviors. There is still a shortage of safe places to go, as well as a shortage of services to help victims become independent. Many states still have outdated laws that indirectly perpetuate abuse rather than foster arrest of the abuser for assault and battery. Arrest is the major way that batterers will get the message that their violence is a crime and not their "right."

Battered woman syndrome has been suggested as a subclassification of PTSD because repetitive abuse is a serious threat to the victim's health and life. Victims often report nightmares, flashbacks, recurrent fears of more violence, emotional detachment, numbness, startle response, sleep problems, guilt, impaired concentration, and hypervigilance. Other symptoms of battered woman syndrome are not addressed by the PTSD criteria, such as depression, hostility, low self-esteem, self-blame, relative passivity, psychosomatic complaints, fatalism, and an unwillingness to seek help (Farella, 2000; Poirier,

Box 41-5 | Why Women Stay as Long as They Do

Situational Factors

- Economic dependence; lack of job skills
- Fear of greater physical danger to themselves and their children if they attempt to leave or have partner arrested
- Fear of emotional damage to children because of being without a father
- Fear of losing custody of children
- Lack of alternative housing
- Social isolation; lack of support from family or friends
- Lack of information regarding alternatives
- Fear of involvement in court processes
- Fear of retaliation from partner or partner's family

Emotional Factors

- Poor self-image; fear of being alone
- Being in a state of denial, and living a "secret"
- Personal embarrassment and protecting the image of husband and family

- Insecurity over potential independence and lack of emotional support
- Guilt about failure of marriage or relationship
- Fear that partner is not able to survive alone
- Belief that partner is "sick" and needs her help
- Belief that partner will change
- Ambivalence and fear over making formidable life changes and increased responsibility

Cultural Factors

- Knowing batterers are not held accountable for their violent actions
- Believing the abuse is her fault
- Being raised to be passive and submissive
- Developing survival skills instead of escape skills
- Recognizing that the legal system is a male-dominated system

Plus: She Still Loves Him

Adapted from Julian Center Shelter, Indianapolis, Ind., and Task Force on Families in Crisis, Nashville, TN.

2000). However, as with PTSD, battered women show typical reactions to a chronic trauma, not symptoms of psychopathology. Labeling and blaming the victims again shifts responsibility away from the perpetrators.

According to victims, it is unlikely that abused women will leave their partners until they realize that the cycle is not going to stop, that they have the emotional support to leave and a safe place to go. Fearing that the next beating may be fatal, finding that their partners are physically or sexually abusing their children, and realizing that their children are learning to be abusive are incentives for leaving permanently (Farella, 2000).

Recovery from Partner Abuse

Immediately preceding or at the beginning of a serious battering incident, the victims are frightened, amenable to crisis intervention, and more likely to call the police or a crisis service agency for help. Getting victims and their children to a shelter or other safe place (if they will go) is desirable when immediate danger of injury is present. If injuries have occurred, victims should be encouraged to go to an emergency department. In either case, crisis workers, shelter workers, or nurses can begin the

important process of assessment and giving information that can make a dent in the cycle of abuse. Even if the survivors are not yet ready to leave their partners, they can be given an easily concealed wallet-size card with telephone numbers of police, prosecutors, crisis services, victims' assistance, shelters, support groups, and perhaps a short message about the inevitability of the cycle of violence and the fact that no one deserves to be abused. If contact is only by phone or if they are worried that the abusers will find the card, they can be asked to write down the phone numbers on the back of a picture in their wallets. Survivors can also be given ideas for developing a safety or escape plan, such as packing a bag with medicines and clothes for them and their children, house and car keys, money and change for the pay telephone, and important phone numbers and papers (e.g., bank account numbers, birth certificates, social security numbers, medical insurance cards, "no contact orders"). They should also be informed of the protections afforded by legal statutes, protective orders, and the newer antistalking laws. Long-term goals for survivors of partner abuse are to develop self-confidence, self-respect, independence, healthy support systems, and a sense of freedom, safety, and empowerment.

| Box 41–6 | Cycle of Violence

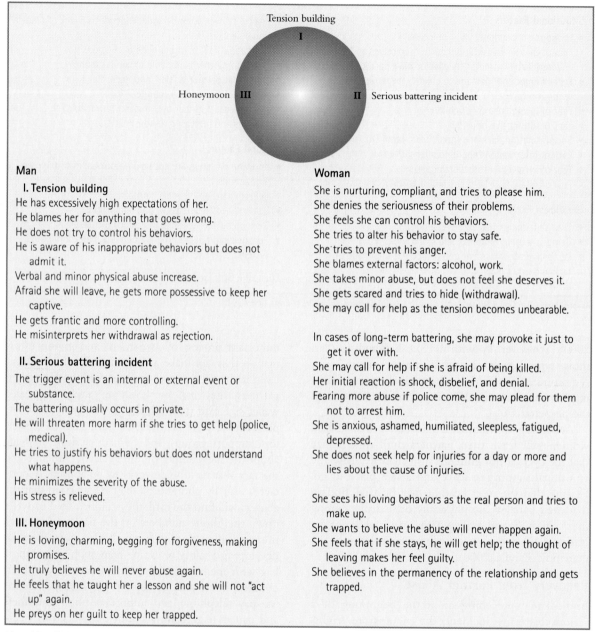

Man

I. Tension building

He has excessively high expectations of her.

He blames her for anything that goes wrong.

He does not try to control his behaviors.

He is aware of his inappropriate behaviors but does not admit it.

Verbal and minor physical abuse increase.

Afraid she will leave, he gets more possessive to keep her captive.

He gets frantic and more controlling.

He misinterprets her withdrawal as rejection.

II. Serious battering incident

The trigger event is an internal or external event or substance.

The battering usually occurs in private.

He will threaten more harm if she tries to get help (police, medical).

He tries to justify his behaviors but does not understand what happens.

He minimizes the severity of the abuse.

His stress is relieved.

III. Honeymoon

He is loving, charming, begging for forgiveness, making promises.

He truly believes he will never abuse again.

He feels that he taught her a lesson and she will not "act up" again.

He preys on her guilt to keep her trapped.

Woman

She is nurturing, compliant, and tries to please him.

She denies the seriousness of their problems.

She feels she can control his behaviors.

She tries to alter his behavior to stay safe.

She tries to prevent his anger.

She blames external factors: alcohol, work.

She takes minor abuse, but does not feel she deserves it.

She gets scared and tries to hide (withdrawal).

She may call for help as the tension becomes unbearable.

In cases of long-term battering, she may provoke it just to get it over with.

She may call for help if she is afraid of being killed.

Her initial reaction is shock, disbelief, and denial.

Fearing more abuse if police come, she may plead for them not to arrest him.

She is anxious, ashamed, humiliated, sleepless, fatigued, depressed.

She does not seek help for injuries for a day or more and lies about the cause of injuries.

She sees his loving behaviors as the real person and tries to make up.

She wants to believe the abuse will never happen again.

She feels that if she stays, he will get help; the thought of leaving makes her feel guilty.

She believes in the permanency of the relationship and gets trapped.

Adapted from Walker L: *The battered woman*, New York, 1979, Harper & Row; Gerard M: Domestic violence: how to screen and intervene, *RN* 63(12):52, 2000.

Psychotherapeutic Management

Nurse-patient relationship

Because most abused women seek help for their injuries at least once, nurses can be instrumental in offering information and assistance (Gerard, 2000). Nurses in emergency departments, clinics, physi-cians' offices, and community health agencies need to know particularly how to recognize a survivor, make an assessment, and refer them to available ser-vices. Some common cues to abuse are listed in Box 41-7. The assessment process is often difficult because survivors fear disclosure, are embarrassed about the situation, desire to be treated quickly and

| Box 41-7 | Common Cues to Partner Abuse

- Repeated, vague symptoms or illnesses that are not confirmed by tests, such as backache, abdominal pain, indigestion, headaches, hyperventilation, anxiety, insomnia, fatigue, anorexia, heart palpitations
- Unexplained injuries or ones with unlikely explanations and embarrassment about them
- Hidden injuries such as those in areas concealed by clothes or visible on physical or x-ray examination only; for example, head and neck injuries, internal injuries, genital injuries, scars, burns, joint pain or dislocations, numbness, hearing problems, or bald spots
- Injuries with recognizable marks such as those from a belt, iron, raised ring, teeth, fingertips, cigarette, gun, or knife
- Multiple fractures or bruises in various stages of healing
- Jumpiness or flinching in the presence of the abuser
- Substance abuse and suicidal thoughts or attempts

- Attempts to conceal fear of the partner
- Continual efforts to keep partner from getting angry
- Denial of any problems in the relationship
- Lack of relationships with family or friends
- Isolation or confinement to home
- Guilt, depression, anxiety, low self-esteem, sense of failure, concealed anger
- Continual justification of own actions and whereabouts to partner
- Continual justification of the abuser's actions in public; excusing or rationalizing the behaviors
- Believing in family unity at all costs and in traditional stereotypes
- Believing in managing alone, even when help is offered
- An oversolicitous partner who does not want to leave the victim alone with hospital or agency staff or even with family and friends

Adapted from Constantine RE, Bricker PL: Social support, stress, and depression among battered women in the judicial setting, *J Am Psychiatr Nurses Assoc* 3(3):81, 1997; Merrell J: Social support for victims of domestic violence, *J Psychosoc Nurs* 39(11):31, 2001.

leave, and sometimes the abusers are present. It is important to interview the victim privately and with sensitivity, empathy, and compassion. Box 41-8 describes other responses that survivors consider helpful.

The most crucial information to document in an initial contact is the following:

1. Identity and current location of the abuser
2. Location and safety of any children
3. Length and frequency of abuse
4. Types of abuse (physical, psychologic, sexual, financial) and use of weapons
5. Types and locations of injuries (photographs and body maps are preferred)
6. Availability of weapons at the place of residence
7. Use and abuse of substances and medications by victim and abuser
8. Types of service desired (police, legal, shelter, crisis counseling, knowledgeable clergy, social service agencies, and transportation)
9. Referrals made

Even if the initial contact is brief, it is important to convey to survivors that they are not alone in their abuse and that there are those willing to help when they are ready. Survivors also need to be told more than once that they do not cause and do not deserve the abuse. The nurse must convey to survivors that they are important and have dignity and worth. They

| Box 41-8 | Helpful Responses to Partner Abuse

- Be nonjudgmental, objective, and nonthreatening.
- Ask directly if abuse is occurring.
- Identify the abuser's behavior as abusive.
- Acknowledge the seriousness of the abuse.
- Assist the victim to assess internal strengths.
- Encourage the use of personal resources.
- Give the victim a list of resources: shelters, financial aid, police, and legal assistance.
- Allow victim to choose own options.
- Offer names of relevant support groups.
- Help victim to develop a safety or escape plan.
- Tell the abuser to stop the abuse and get help.
- Do not disbelieve or blame the victim.
- Do not get angry with the victim.
- Do not refuse to help if the victim is not ready to leave the abuser.
- Do not align with the abuser against the victim.
- Do not push the victim to leave the abuser before ready.

need acknowledgment of their mental and physical exhaustion, fears, ambivalence about the abusers and leaving and their wish to help the abuser, as well as themselves. It is difficult for nurses (and all professionals) to accept that survivors cannot be pushed, rushed, or coerced into leaving the abuser before they are ready. In fact, survivors may want to try couples counseling and even personal counseling (when the abuser refuses counseling) more than once before "giving up hope" of saving the relationship and of helping the ones they love. It is important to recognize and to acknowledge that it is common for survivors to leave and return several times. Survivors need not feel guilty or ashamed for trying to improve the relationship. In fact, the guilt of leaving will be lessened if they believe they have "tried everything" and are finally able to acknowledge that nothing will change because the abusers are the only one who can control the violence and stop the abuse.

When an abused woman does leave her partner, the problems are not over. "If You Have Left an Abusive Man" (Box 41-9) describes some of the common reactions the abuser may have and ways he may behave. Survivors frequently need longer-term counseling and social services to recover and become independent, especially if the abuser is unwilling to participate in couples counseling or an abusers' program (often a court-ordered program of group education and counseling lasting 26 weeks or more). Nursing interventions for survivors (individually or in groups) generally focus on the following:

1. Reiterating information about abuse, the cycle of violence, and the abuser's accountability
2. Building self-esteem and confidence
3. Sharing of feelings, especially anger, frustration, fear, and anxiety

| Box 41-9 | If You Have Left an Abusive Man...

1. Your problems are not over.
2. Your abuser will try to locate you through family and friends. He will play on their sympathy or intimidate them.
3. He will repeatedly apologize, make promises about changing, and give gifts.
4. Next, he will threaten or intimidate you, your children, family, and/or friends.
5. He may threaten to kill himself because of you.
6. He often threatens to take your children away.
7. In another step, he will enter counseling and/or will express religious fervor.
8. He may try to find a counselor or religious leader to try to convince you to return to him.
9. Next, he may harass and stalk (begging, crying, phone calls, written or verbal threats, legal actions, or following you from location to location).
Regardless of his tactics, take advantage of legal, community, and personal resources to protect yourself and your children.

Adapted from the Salvation Army Domestic Violence Program, Indianapolis, Ind.

4. Decreasing shame, guilt, embarrassment, manipulation, and isolation
5. Confirming personal rights, as well as legal rights
6. Teaching stress-management techniques
7. Teaching communication techniques
8. Teaching conflict-resolution techniques
9. Teaching assertiveness training
10. Teaching parenting techniques
11. Decreasing co-dependency behaviors
12. Building a new, improved support system
13. Setting goals, specific planning for immediate future
14. Resolving grief

Referrals may also be needed for job counseling or training, legal assistance, financial aid, and permanent housing. At any stage of working with survivors, brief hospitalization may be needed because of injuries, suicide attempts, or substance abuse and for treatment of serious problems such as depression, anxiety, or panic attacks.

Psychopharmacology

Medications normally are not needed but are commonly given to survivors. Often *mis*prescribed medications are antidepressants, benzodiazepines, and hypnotics. These same medications may be used appropriately if the survivor's symptoms of depression, anxiety, sleeplessness, or nightmares are severe. Continual assessment is needed to determine when medications are no longer needed to prevent abuse and addiction.

Milieu management

Groups in inpatient or outpatient settings that may be relevant for survivors are those focusing on self-esteem, problem solving, assertiveness, relationship issues, stress management, and co-dependency. Substance-abuse groups should be recommended if necessary. In the community, a group for abused women is desirable. Turning Point and Breaking Free are two of these groups.

Critical Thinking Question

Your co-worker is sharing with you that she is thinking about leaving her husband because of his drinking and long-term emotional abuse of her. She expresses a fear that he might try to kill her and a fear of raising her two children alone. What information would you offer her?

Case Study

Rachael Benton, a 26-year-old survivor of incest by her father, is married to Richard. She has an 8-year-old child, Matthew; Richard has three boys, Robert, James, and Daniel, ages 11, 8, and 7, who live with them. Angela, age 5, was born after Rachael and Richard were married. Matthew was removed from the home after being abused by Robert. Rachael sought help by attending a battered women's group.

Rachel's situation was difficult to resolve. Because of heavy drinking, Richard was missing work and changing jobs. His income declined and was sporadic but expenses did not decline. Without insurance, Rachel's repeated treatment of menstrual irregularities, back pain, chronic and severe headaches, and diarrhea were not paid for. She avoided treatment for bruises, a superficial knife wound, head cuts, and contusions. Richard repeatedly punched her stomach during a pregnancy, causing a miscarriage.

It was when Richard raped her that Rachael believed there was no hope of change and that she had to leave. As Rachael became more assertive and independent, Richard demanded that she stay home, bought a shotgun to convince her to stay, and took the starter off the car. He rode to work with co-workers. Rachael had not adopted Richard's boys, so she could not take them with her. She was afraid that his verbal abuse of them would turn to physical violence when she left. Richard knew about all the places she thought of going.

It took 4 months to develop, coordinate, and implement arrangements so that Rachael and Angela were safe in leaving Richard. Neighbors, friends, and teachers were warned of the potential abuse of the boys and given the phone number for anonymously reporting child abuse. Rachel's mother rented her a small trailer in a rural town and obtained forms for Aid to Families with Dependent Children. Rachael secretly and gradually packed clothes and important documents in the trunk of a group member's car.

One night (14 months after the group began) Richard got drunk, beat Rachael, and tried to rape her again. She fought him off and waited until he passed out. The member with the packed car drove her to the new trailer. As expected, Richard got his shotgun and went to every friend of Rachel's, but none knew where she was. He drove to Rachel's mother's home, and she called the sheriff when his car pulled into the driveway. Richard was escorted out of the county and warned not to return. Within a week, Daniel's teacher filed a child abuse report about bruises found on him. Within 2 weeks, the boys were removed from the home and returned to their natural mother.

Rachael has received proper medical treatment and feels healthier. She is now divorced, going through a job-training program, and maintaining her secret location. She feels safe but is still in counseling once a month to complete her emotional recovery. She attends a support group for battered women once a week.

Care Plan

Name: Rachael Benton   Admission Date: _____

DSM-IV-TR Diagnosis: Survivors of violence and trauma _____

Assessment	**Areas of strength:** Bright, articulate, and capable of problem solving; mother and one friend willing to help; developing trust in group and beginning to process her feelings and rights. **Problems:** Lack of safe housing and employment; inability to remove husband's children from the house and fear he will abuse them; fear of increased abuse of her, even death, if she tries to leave; severe headaches.
Diagnoses	• Decisional conflict related to dysfunctional marriage as evidenced by attendance in a battered women's support group. • Posttrauma syndrome related to physical, emotional, and economic abuse as evidenced by physical wounds, fear, and emotional trauma. • Fear (of leaving husband) related to potential abuse of sons as evidenced by reluctance to leave without stepsons.
Outcomes	*Short-term goals:* *Date met* • Patient will remove bullets from gun; design an escape plan. _____ • Patient will verbalize ability to survive on her own; confirm housing in rural county. _____

Continued

Care Plan—cont'd

Name: <u>Rachael Benton</u>   Admission Date: _____

DSM-IV-TR Diagnosis: <u>Survivors of violence and trauma</u>

Outcomes

Long-term goals:
- Patient will enroll in job-training program.
- Patient will obtain legal assistance for divorce.
- Patient will seek medical treatment for chronic problems.

Planning/ Interventions

Nurse-patient relationship: Listen nonjudgmentally and empathically; accept "strange" behaviors related to secrecy and self-protection; avoid disparaging spouse and pressuring to leave; locate resources for training, finances, counseling, and medical care in rural county.

Psychopharmacology: Desyrel, 50 mg at bedtime, to alleviate moderate depression and to improve sleep. Tylenol No. 3 prn for severe headaches.

Milieu management: Encourage continuing in local support group; locate support group in rural county; continue assessment of safety of patient and children.

Evaluation

Patient has moved to rural county and joined support group; is receiving counseling and medical care. Husband's children were removed and placed with natural mother.

Referrals

Has an appointment with a job-training program in the rural county.

Key Concepts

1. Not all crimes involve physical violence and injury; however, all crimes involve emotional violation and injury. Victims lose a sense of the ability to control their own lives, as well as losing trust in others.
2. Progression through the stages of recovery from a crime may take years. Crisis intervention and group meetings with other survivors can facilitate recovery.
3. In assisting survivors, sensitivity to their needs is crucial to build trust and to avoid blaming the victim.
4. Information about counseling resources and support groups can be given to the survivors of rape and partner abuse for later use, even if there is an initial denial of the need for help.
5. Adult survivors of childhood sexual abuse may repress the memories for years as a result of the emotional turmoil and sense of being betrayed by the abuser and others.
6. Adult survivors of childhood sexual abuse typically enter counseling for a variety of overt problems, unaware of how these are related to childhood trauma.
7. The reexperiencing and working through of traumatic torture, SRA, and MC memories is a painful, lengthy, and sometimes sporadic process that requires intense support and empathy.
8. The concepts of learned helplessness, the cycle of violence, and other situational, emotional, and cultural factors help explain why survivors often remain with their abusive partners.
9. Immediately preceding or at the beginning of a serious battering incident is when abuse victims are most amenable to crisis intervention and referrals for needed services.
10. Patience, support, and information are critical aspects of nursing interventions with all survivors.

References

Alper G, Peterson SJ: Dialectical behavior therapy for patients with borderline personality, *J Psychosoci Nurs* 39(10):38, 2001.

Bennett L: Projective methods in caring for sexually abused young people, *J Psychosoc Nurs Ment Health Serv* 35(4):18, 1997.

Bergeron LR: Servicing the needs of elder abuse victims, *Policy Pract Public Hum Serv* 4(9):40, 2000.

Bloom SL: Hearing the survivor's voice: sundering the wall of denial, *J Psychohistory* 21(4):461, 1994.

Bond L et al: Does bullying cause emotional problems? A prospective study of young teenagers, *BMJ* 323(7311):480, 2001.

Brown K: Rape and sexual assault: the nursing role, *Nursing Spectrum:* Metro Edition 29, August, 2001.

Clark CC: Post traumatic stress disorder: how to support healing, *AJN* 92(8):27, 1997.

Cleary SD: Adolescent victimization and subsequent suicidal and violent behaviors, *Adolescence* 35(140):671, 2000.

Courtois CA, Turkus JA: Hospitalization as part of the recovery process, *Many Voices* 10(2):8.1998.

Davis JL, Petretic-Jackson PA: The impact of child sexual abuse on adult interpersonal function: a review and synthesis of the empirical literature, *Aggression Violent Behav* 5(3):291, 2000.

Day AL: The journal as a guide for the healing journey, *Nurs Clin North Am* 36(1):131, 2001.

DiVasto P: Measuring the aftermath of rape, *J Psychosoc Nurs Ment Health Serv* 23(2):33, 1985.

Dresser JG: Wrapping: a technique for interrupting self-mutilation, *J Am Psychiatr Nurses Assoc* 5(2):67, 1999.

Evans GW, Helton SM, Blackburn LS: Students go to court: experiential learning about domestic violence, *J Am Psychiatr Nurses Assoc* 7(3):67, 2001.

Farella C: Hot and bothering: sexual harassment in the workplace is no joke, *Nursing Spectrum:* Metro Edition 14, September, 2001.

Farella C: Love shouldn't hurt: understanding domestic violence, *Nursing Spectrum:* Metro Edition 14, November, 2000.

Fox SS, Scherl DJ: Crisis intervention with rape victims, *Soc Work* 17:37, 1972.

Gerard M: Domestic violence: how to screen and intervene, *RN* 63(12):52, 2000.

Gillmore-Hall A: Violence in the workplace: are you prepared? *AJN* 101(7): 2001.

Girardin B: Is this forensic specialty for you? *RN* 64(12):37, 2001.

Hammer R: Caring in forensic nursing: expanding the holistic model, *J Psychosoc Nurs* 38(11):18, 2000.

Hastings DP: The New Hampshire health initiative on domestic violence, *Nursing Forum* 36(1):31, 2001.

Hinds J: Once upon a time: therapeutic stories as a psychiatric nursing intervention, *J Psychosoc Nurs Ment Health Serv* 35(5):46, 1997.

Hoban SS: Elder abuse and neglect, *AJN* 100(11):49, 2000.

Horon IL, Cheng D: Homicide: leading cause of death in pregnant women, *AJN* 101(6):20, 2001.

Howard-Ruben J: Defending our mental health: psychological warfare, *Nursing Spectrum:* Metro Edition 24, November, 2001.

Hudson PS: *Ritual child abuse: discovery, diagnosis and treatment,* Saratoga, Calif, 1991, R & E.

James WH et al: Youth dating violence, *Adolescence* 35(139):455, 2000.

Janoff-Bulman R: Understanding reactions to traumatic events, *Harv Ment Health Lett* 14(4):8, 1997.

Kreidler MC et al: Trauma and dissociation: treatment perspectives, *Perspect Psychiatr Care* 36(3):77, 2000.

Machoian L: Cutting voices: self injury in three adolescent girls, *J Psychoc Nurs* 39(11):22, 2001.

Martin L et al: Psychological and physical health effects of sexual assaults and nonsexual traumas among male and female United States Army soldiers, *Behav Med* 26:23, 2000.

McClellan AC, Killeen MR: Attachment theory and violence toward women by male intimate partners, *J Nurs Scholarship* Fourth Quarter:353, 2000.

Meloy JR: Stalking. An old behavior, a new crime, *Psychiatr Clin North Am* 22(1):85, 1999.

Merrell J: Social support for victims of domestic violence, *J Psychosoc Nurs* 39(11):30, 2001.

Miller D, Guidry L: *Addictions and trauma recovery: healing the body, mind and spirit,* New York, 2001, WW Norton.

Miller MC: Stalking, *Harv Ment Health Lett* 17(9):5, 2001a.

Miller MC: Bullies and their victims, *Harv Ment Health Lett* 18(5):4, 2001b.

Miller MC: Disaster and trauma, *Harv Ment Health Lett* 18(7):1, 2002.

Monarch K: Protect yourself from sexual harassment, *AJN* 100(5):75, 2000.

Mynatt S: Repeated suicide attempts, *J Psychosoc Nurs* 38(12):24. 2000.

New M, Berliner L: Mental health service utilization by victims of crime, *J Trauma Stress* 13(4):693, 2000.

Osterman JE, Barbiaz J, Johnson P: Emergency interventions for rape victims, *Psychiatr Serv* 52(6):733, 2001.

Parks S: Silence verbal abuse, *Nursing Spectrum:* Metro Edition 20, August, 2001.

Personal interviews: Indianapolis ANAD, 2002.

Peternelj-Taylor C: Forensic psychiatric nursing: a work in progress, *J Psychosoc Nurs* 39(9):8, 2001.

Piercy D, Greenwood M: DOVE program takes flight, *Nursing Spectrum:* Metro Edition 18, January, 2002.

Poirier N: Psychosocial characteristics discriminating between battered women and other women psychiatric inpatients, *J Am Psychiatr Nurs Assoc* 6(5):144, 2000.

Ray SL: Male survivors' perspectives of incest/sexual abuse, *Perspect Psychiatr Care* 37(2):49, 2001.

Roberts SJ: Primary health care of survivors of childhood sexual abuse: how can psychiatric nurses be helpful? *J Am Psychiatr Nurses Assoc* 6(6):191, 2000.

Rockwell RB: One psychiatrist's view of satanic ritual abuse, *J Psychohistory* 21(4):443, 1994.

Romano E, DeLuca RV: Male sexual abuse: a review of effects, abuse characteristics, and links with later psychological functioning, *Aggress Violent Behav* 6(1):55, 2000.

Ross C: *Satanic ritual abuse: principles of treatment,* Toronto, 1995, University of Toronto.

Rothschild B: *The body remembers: the psychophysiology of trauma and trauma treatment,* New York, 2000, WW Norton.

Sappington AA: Childhood abuse as a possible locus for early intervention into problems of violence and psychopathology, *Aggress Violent Behav* 5(3):255, 2000.

Steelfel L: ICN takes aim at violence, *Nursing Spectrum:* Metro Edition 11, May, 2001.

Stith SM: Prevalence and costs of domestic violence, *Am Assoc Marriage Fam Ther* 2(3):1, 2000.

Stringer H: Raging bullies, *Nurse Week* 10, February 12, 2001.

Torem MS: The role of medication in treatment of dissociative disorders, *Many Voices* 12(3):6, 2000.

Trossman S: Illinois RNs win workplace safety measures, *Am Nurse* 1, January/February, 2001.

Turkus JA: The treatment challenge, *Many Voices* 12(6):6, 2000.

Tynhurst JS: Individual reactions to community disaster, *Am J Psychiatry* 107:764, 1951.

Valente S: Controversies and challenges of ritual abuse, *J Psychosoc Nurs* 38(11):8. 2000.

van der Kolk B, McFarlane AC, Weissaeth L: *Traumatic stress: the effects of overwhelming experience on mind, body, and society,* New York, 1996, Guilford Press.

Walker L: *The battered woman,* New York, 1979, Harper & Row.

Windom CS, Maxfield MG: An update on the "cycle of violence," *National Institute of Justice* 1, February, 2001.

Worthington K: Violence in the health care workplace, *AJN* 100(11):69, 2000.

Worthington K, Franklin P: Workplace violence, *AJN* 100(12):73, 2000.

Young AM, Boyd C, Hubbell AA: Social isolation and sexual abuse among women who smoke crack, *J Psychosoc Nurs* 39(7):12, 2001.

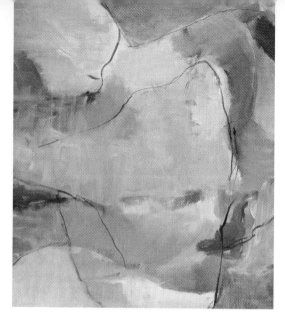

Chapter 42

Child and Adolescent Psychiatric Nursing

Larry Scahill, Eileen Hanrahan

Learning Objectives

After reading this chapter, you should be able to:
- Describe the major categories of child psychiatric disorders.
- Describe the frequency of serious psychiatric disorders in children and adolescents.
- Identify genetic and environmental factors that can elevate the risk of developing a psychiatric disorder.
- Describe the symptoms of the selected child and adolescent psychiatric disorders.
- Identify principles of nursing intervention with children and adolescents.

Recent contributions from several disciplines have increased our understanding of psychiatric disorders that occur in childhood. Through the field of epidemiology, appreciation for the frequency and distribution of child psychiatric disorders has increased. Dramatic developments in neuroscience have deepened our grasp of the biologic underpinnings of some psychiatric disorders, such as attention-deficit hyperactivity disorder (ADHD), autism, and Tourette's syndrome. Studies in behavioral genetics have shown that several psychiatric disorders of childhood have a strong genetic contribution, though environmental contributions should always be considered. Recent investigations in molecular genetics suggest that specific genes are associated with some psychiatric dis-

orders. Clinical research has provided information to guide both pharmacologic and behavioral approaches to treatment. Despite these advances, however, the etiologic factors of most childhood psychiatric disorders remain unknown, and many treatments lack empirical support.

This chapter reviews the major categories and frequency of child psychiatric disorders, as well as the factors that influence the probability of developing a psychiatric disorder. The clinical features of selected child psychiatric disorders are also described. The chapter concludes with a brief discussion of treatment issues, including psychopharmacologic and behavioral therapy, as well as a description of the treatment settings in child and adolescent psychiatry.

Key Terms

Attention-deficit hyperactivity disorder (ADHD) Relatively common disorder of childhood onset characterized by inattention, impulsiveness, and overactivity.

Child abuse Harmful physical, emotional, and/or sexual acts inflicted on a child.

Epidemiology The study of the frequency and distribution of disease conditions in the population.

Family system A field of influence exerted on each family member due to the complex interaction of all family members.

Genetic vulnerability Inherited liability that increases the risk of manifesting a psychiatric disorder.

Pervasive developmental disorder (PDD) Any one of several conditions that are characterized by multiple social and cognitive delays.

Prevalence Estimate of the frequency of a disease condition in the population (e.g., ADHD affects 5% to 11% of the school-aged children).

Psychosocial adversity Environmental conditions such as poverty, unemployment, or overcrowded living conditions that do not support optimal development of the child

Resilience Capacity to move forward with development despite psychosocial adversity or genetic vulnerability.

SCOPE OF THE PROBLEM

A report from the Surgeon General (Satcher, 1999) estimates that 10% of school-aged children have serious mental health problems. Another 10% has milder problems that may pose some interference with interpersonal relationships and adjustment to school. This percentage translates into an estimated 8 to 12 million youngsters with significant mental health problems in the United States. Despite the documented frequency of psychiatric disorders in children and adolescents, as few as one in five are using specialized mental health services (Burns et al, 1995; Satcher, 1999). In lieu of obtaining mental health services in child psychiatric clinics, children may receive mental health services in primary care settings and public schools (Briggs-Gowan et al, 2000; Satcher, 1999).

Epidemiology of Child Psychiatric Disorders

Epidemiology is the study of the frequency and distribution of disease conditions in the population. The primary concerns in epidemiology are how common a disorder is in a given population and whether particular subgroups are at increased risk for developing a specific disorder. For example, men are more likely to have a myocardial infarction than women, though women are at higher risk than are men for osteoporosis. Recently, methods of epidemiology have been applied to child psychiatry, resulting in a better understanding of both the frequency and the distribution of these disorders in the population. This effort has profited from recent

improvements in the operational criteria of psychiatric disorders and diagnostic interview methods built on these criteria.

Any number of genetic or environmental characteristics may influence the likelihood of developing a psychiatric disorder. Characteristics that increase the probability of having a psychiatric disorder are called risk factors. Although often described as separate, genetic influences and environmental conditions may interact to elevate the risk of a child psychiatric disorder. Thus risk factors for a psychiatric disorder can be additive. Examples of biologic risk factors include the inherited genetic abnormality seen in fragile X syndrome (which is among the most common genetic forms of mental retardation). Poverty, child abuse, overcrowded living conditions, and exposure to alcohol in utero are examples of environmental risk factors.

Genetic Factors

Several psychiatric disorders are presumed to have an important genetic component. Indeed, for depression, anxiety disorders, tic disorders, and ADHD, having a close family member with a specific disorder may be the single largest contributor to the likelihood of the same disorder in a child. Various methods are used to study the genetic contribution to psychiatric disorders, including twin, family, and adoption studies. More recently, powerful new molecular biologic techniques have also been applied to the study of psychiatric disorders (State et al, 2000). The first question to ask when considering the genetic contribution for a given disorder is whether the disorder recurs more frequently in families compared with the general population. However, simply showing that a disorder such as depression is more common in children who have a depressed parent does not prove that depression is inherited. The developmental impact of having a depressed parent may increase the risk of depression in a child through environmental influences.

To establish that genetic inheritance confers vulnerability for a psychiatric disorder, researchers turn to twin and adoption studies. Twin studies exploit the fact that identical (monozygotic) twins share 100% of their genes in common, whereas dizygotic twins share an average of 50% of their genes. Thus, if a disorder is truly genetic, it should be present in both identical twins, whereas the expected *concordance* in dizygotic twins would be significantly less. On the other hand, disorders that are caused by environmental influences exert similar impact on development regardless of whether the twins were genetically identical. Thus if a disorder were primarily due to environmental influences, there would be no difference in the concordance between monozygotic and dizygotic twins. Twin studies have demonstrated a strong genetic contribution in ADHD (Levy et al, 1997; Stevenson, 1992), obsessive-compulsive disorder (Carey, Gottesman, 1981), Tourette's syndrome (Price et al, 1985), and autism (Rutter et al, 1999). Although none of these disorders shows 100% concordance in monozygotic twins, the percentage of mutually affected monozygotic twins is significantly greater than it is in dizygotic twins for each of these disorders.

Although twins can provide strong support for a genetic factor, these methods do not elucidate the mode of inheritance (Box 42-1). If a disorder runs in families and is genetically inherited, it would be expected to recur in specific patterns within families. The formal method for evaluating the pattern of inheritance in families is called segregation analysis. Through segregation analysis, known models of inheritance can be compared with the observed pattern.

If a disorder is genetically inherited, it implies that the action of one or more genes is abnormal. Recently developed techniques in molecular biology may lead to the identification of a gene or genes that cause psychiatric disorder of childhood. The

---

| **Box 42-1** | Types of Inheritance |

Autosomal Dominant

One parent is affected with the disorder and passes on a single copy of the disease-causing gene to the affected offspring. Huntington's chorea is an example of a neuropsychiatric disorder that is inherited as an autosomal dominant condition.

Autosomal Recessive

To be affected, the child must have two copies of disease-causing gene. Each unaffected parent passes on one disease-causing gene to the affected offspring. Phenylketonuria is due to autosomal recessive inheritance.

Sex-Linked Inheritance

Recalling that women have an XX karyotype and men have an XY karotype, it is possible for a mother to carry a trait on one X chromosome without being affected. Although the gene is not expressed in the mother, the male offspring is affected. Some forms of hemophilia follow a sex-linked inheritance pattern.

Polygenetic Inheritance

Some disorders recur in higher-than-expected rates in families but follow more complex patterns than autosomal dominant or autosomal recessive inheritance. These disorders are presumed to be caused by several genes acting in combination. Schizophrenia, autism, and some forms of learning disability are believed to follow a polygenetic pattern.

---

primary function of genes is to encode for proteins in a series of carefully engineered steps from deoxyribonucleic acid (DNA) to ribonucleic acid (RNA) to a specific protein. Thus a genetically determined disorder is ultimately caused by a disruption in function of these molecular procedures, resulting in impaired function of the protein product (State et al, 2000). In fragile X syndrome, for example, the gene that regulates an early step in the process of protein manufacture (i.e., transcription of the DNA message to RNA) appears to be defective. The precise way in which this disruption in the molecular biology produces the physical characteristics and symptoms of fragile X syndrome remains unclear.

Environmental Factors

Broadly speaking, environmental factors are any and all nongenetic exposures, including intrauterine insults, adverse family conditions, poverty, unsupportive community circumstances, natural disasters, traumatic events, and toxic substances (e.g., ingesting lead paint). Ideally, genetic and environmental influences can be distinguished. In actuality, however, genetic and environmental factors interact in complex ways, making it difficult to attribute exclusive causality. For example, phenylketonuria (PKU) is a metabolic defect inherited in an autosomal recessive fashion that results in a toxic accumulation of phenylalanine in the brain. However, if PKU is detected, a low-phenylalanine diet will limit the negative impact of the inherited metabolic defect.

Psychosocial adversity

Several studies have shown that adverse psychosocial conditions such as poverty, family discord, overcrowded living conditions, sexual abuse, physical abuse, and a parent with a history of substance abuse or a psychiatric disorder are associated with psychiatric disorders in children and adolescents (Szatmari, Offord, Boyle, 1989; Biederman et al, 1995a; Scahill et al, 1999). Moreover, these risk factors appear to be additive. In a clinical sample of children with ADHD, Biederman and colleagues (1995a) found that, as the number of these adverse elements increases, the likelihood of ADHD also increases. As previously suggested, however, the association of these adverse psychosocial conditions with child psychiatric disorders does not preclude a genetic contribution.

On the other hand, it is clear that not all children who are exposed to psychosocial disadvantage develop a psychiatric disorder. Indeed, some children seem to grow and mature into well-adjusted individuals despite the presence of multiple environmental risk factors. The environmental and constitutional elements that account for these resilient children are poorly understood and deserve further investigation. It may be that a supportive relationship with a member of the extended family or a member of the community protects the child from the adverse of psychosocial conditions. Resilience can also be fostered within the environment such that the ill effects of a genetic vulnerability can be mitigated. For example, a child with an inherited vulnerability for ADHD is more likely to achieve an optimal outcome if reared in a predictable family environment than would a child with a similar vulnerability reared in a more chaotic family circumstance.

Family systems

Families develop in a manner that is analogous to child development. Although families come in several sizes and compositions, families typically begin with the formation of a couple. When the couple comes together, each individual makes a transition from single life to family life. This transition to family life takes a major step forward with conception and birth (or adoption) of a child. Each subsequent phase of the child's development—infancy, toddlerhood, elementary-school age, adolescence, and young adulthood—calls for an adjustment by the family unit. The rules, rituals, and communication patterns that define the family system have an impact on the child's development. Similarly, the child's development influences the family system.

DIAGNOSTIC CATEGORIES OF CHILD PSYCHIATRIC DISORDERS

The introduction of the *Diagnostic and Statistical Manual of Mental Disorders,* third edition (DSM-III) in 1980 (American Psychiatric Association [APA], 1980) represented an important milestone in the definition of mental illness. For the first time, psychiatric diagnoses were described in operational terms with clearly stated (though not necessarily empirically verified) criteria. The DSM-III also introduced a multiaxial diagnostic system that included not only the primary mental illness (Axis I), but also noted the presence of mental retardation (Axis II), medical illness (Axis III), psychosocial stressors (Axis IV), and assessment of functioning (Axis V). The DSM-IV (APA, 1994) contains several changes from DSM-III but retains the same essential features.

Childhood psychiatric disorders can be divided into several broad categories, such as developmental disorders, disruptive behavior disorders, internalizing disorders, tic disorders, psychotic disorders, and elimination disorders.

DEVELOPMENTAL DISORDERS

Mental Retardation

Mental retardation is defined by subaverage intelligence (intelligence quotient [IQ] below 70) that is accompanied by impairments in performing age-expected activities in daily living. Intelligence is

| Table 42-1 | DSM-IV Classification of Mental Retardation |

Severity	IQ Range
Mild	55-69
Moderate	40-54
Severe	25-39
Profound	Below 25

| Table 42-2 | Selected Pervasive Developmental Disorders in DSM-IV-TR |

Disorder	Prevalence
Autistic disorder	5 to 20 per 10,000
Asperger's disorder	1 to 10 per 10,000*
PDD-not otherwise specified	10 to 40 per 10,000*

*Accuracy of estimate is hampered by changes in definition.

measured by a standardized test and can be used to define the degree of mental retardation (Table 42-1). Impaired adaptive functioning is often a clinical judgment, but standardized assessments such as the Vineland Adaptive Behavior Scales (Sparrow, Balla, Cicchetti, 1983) are available.

The prevalence of mental retardation is estimated at 2.0%, with a range from 1.0% to 2.5%. Most of the mentally retarded (nearly 90%) are in the mildly retarded range. The causes of mental retardation vary from specific genetic abnormalities such as fragile X syndrome, trisomy 21 (Down syndrome), and phenylketonuria to "multifactorial" causes in which several genes are presumed to interact with environmental factors. In addition to intellectual handicap, mentally retarded children may also have a psychiatric disorder.

Pervasive Developmental Disorders

The pervasive developmental disorders (PDDs) are a group of disorders characterized by impairments across multiple domains of development. Although not a defining feature of PDDs, many of these children demonstrate varying degrees of mental retardation. Table 42-2 presents the more common forms of PDD described in DSM-IV.

These PDDs share several common features, including delayed socialization and stereotypical behaviors such as rocking, hand flapping, and peculiar preoccupations. These children are rigid and often intolerant of change in routines. These children also tend to perseverate on themes of idiosyncratic interest and are prone to behavioral outbursts in response to modest environmental demands.

Autistic disorder

Since the first description of autism by Leo Kanner over 50 years ago, several theories have been advanced concerning its cause. For example, in the 1950s and 1960s serious consideration was given to the notion that detached professional parents might be the cause of autism (Cohen, Volkmar, 1997). This explanation is no longer accepted and suggests a bias of ascertainment in that professional families were more likely to seek treatment from medical centers that evaluated children with profound developmental delays. In addition, this conceptualization fails to recognize that the parental indifference might have been rooted in the child's incapacity for reciprocal communication.

A recent epidemiologic study reported a prevalence of 20 per 10,000 for autistic disorder in children (Chakrabarti, Fombonne, 2001). This estimate, which is 2 to 4 times greater than previous estimates, may not reflect an increase in the prevalence of autistic disorder; rather, it probably reflects improved classification of children with developmental disorders. For example, a substantial percentage of children with autistic disorder are mentally retarded, and about 25% have seizure disorders. Prior studies may have classified these children as mentally retarded rather than children with autism. Family genetic and twin data suggest a strong genetic contribution to autism, but the specific cause remains unknown. Several studies have observed higher serum levels of serotonin in children with autism, resulting in considerable research interest in the serotonin system. However, the failure to replicate this finding in other studies suggests that hyperserotonemia may be true only for some autistic patients. Further evidence implicating the serotonin system comes from a study that observed an association between autism and the structure of the serotonin receptor (Cook et al, 1997). If this finding is replicated, it may have important implications for pharmacotherapy in autism.

Autism can be differentiated from the other forms of PDD because it has an early age of onset (before 30 months of age), social relatedness is profoundly disturbed, communication is delayed and deviant, and the delayed developmental profile is relatively constant (e.g., in Rett's disorder, a rare developmental disorder, previously acquired skills rapidly decline). Children with autism appear aloof and indifferent to others and seem to prefer inanimate objects to human contact. Language, if present, is characterized by abnormal intonation, pronoun reversals, and echolalia (repetition of words or phrases spoken by others). Other common features of autism, which may also be present in other variants of PDD, are stereotypical behaviors such as rocking and hand flapping, extraordinary insistence on sameness, and preoccupation with peculiar interests (e.g., fans, air conditioners, train schedules).

Asperger's disorder

Asperger's disorder was also described about 50 years ago, but it was not included in DSM-III or DSM-III-R (revised version). Compared with children with autism, children with Asperger's disorder are less likely to be mentally retarded, and their linguistic handicap is less severe. Indeed, these children often have normal intelligence, and verbal intelligence is typically higher than performance intelligence. The social deficits in Asperger's disorder include inept initiation of social interactions, impaired reading of social cues, and a tendency toward concrete interpretation of language. Speech tends to be stilted, and intonation is abnormal. These children tend to be clumsy, have difficulty managing transitions, and are preoccupied with matters of private interest.

The prevalence of Asperger's disorder is a matter of dispute because consensus about the diagnostic criteria has only recently been achieved (Cohen, Volkmar, 1997). Asperger's syndrome appears to be more common in boys than in girls. Although no genetic marker has been identified, the disorder often runs in families with high recurrence in fathers.

Pervasive developmental disorder— not otherwise specified

The classification of pervasive developmental disorder–not otherwise specified (PDD-NOS) is a residual category reserved for children who do not meet criteria for a more specific type of PDD such as autism or Asperger's syndrome. The prevalence is difficult to estimate with accuracy because of changes in the definition. For example, DSM-III and DSM-III-R do not include this category. Given the heterogeneity of PDD-NOS, it is unlikely that a single etiologic factor will ever be identified. Both genetic and environmental causes, particularly perinatal exposures, probably play a role in the cause of PDD-NOS.

Children with PDD-NOS exhibit traits that are similar to those described for autism and Asperger's disorder. Differential diagnosis is determined by age of onset, severity of speech and language deficit, degree of social impairment, and level of interest in interpersonal relationships (Koenig, Scahill, 2001). In general, these features are less severe in PDD-NOS than in autism.

Specific Developmental Disorders

Specific developmental disorders are characterized by a delay in a discrete domain of development. This section focuses on learning disorders and communication disorders.

Learning disorders

Learning disorder (also called learning disability) is characterized by a significant discrepancy between aptitude (IQ) and achievement in a particular area, such as reading or mathematics. The specificity of the delay is what differentiates learning disorders from the more global deficits observed in mental retardation and PDD.

The most common type of learning disorder is reading disability (also called dyslexia). Estimates range from 3% to 5% of school-age children with boys being affected more often than girls in most studies (Pennington, 1991). However, in a large community survey, no gender difference in reading disability was present (Shaywitz et al, 1990). In clinical samples, reading disability is associated with a range of psychiatric disorders, but whether this apparent association is caused by characteristics that are related to seeking treatment is unclear. Less is known about the prevalence of nonverbal learning disorder (mathematics disorder), with estimates ranging from 0.1% to 1.0% and no apparent difference between boys and girls.

Communication Disorders

Communication disorders involve speech (the motor aspects of speaking) or language, which refers to the formulation and comprehension of verbal communication. The prevalence of speech and language disorders was reported as 19% in one community study of 5-year-old children (Beitchman et al, 1986a). Communication deficits present early in childhood do resolve in some children. In both clinical and community samples, speech and language disorders have been shown to be strongly associated with psychiatric disorders (Beitchman et al, 1986b). Whether the psychiatric disorder and the communication disorder share an underlying cause or whether the prior presence of a communication disorder is a predisposing factor for development of a psychiatric disorder is unclear.

Theories suggest that language delay and reading disability may share the same underlying phonologic defect (Pennington, 1991). Both reading disability and a speech or language handicap can exert a negative impact on socialization and education. For example, peers may tease a child with an articulation defect or stuttering, causing withdrawal and a poor self-image. Because reading is a cornerstone of learning, children with reading disability may fall behind their age-mates in school—especially if the reading disability is undetected.

DISRUPTIVE BEHAVIOR DISORDERS

The disruptive behavior disorders include three relatively common child psychiatric disorders: ADHD, oppositional defiant disorder, and conduct disorder (Table 42-3). These disorders are more common in boys compared with girls and are associated with low socioeconomic status, urban living, single parenthood, family dysfunction, learning disabilities, language delay, and a positive family history of a disruptive behavior disorder (Biederman et al, 1992; Biederman et al, 1995a; Scahill et al, 1999; Szatmari, Offord, Boyle, 1989).

Table 42-3	Types and Prevalence of Disruptive Behavior Disorders
Disorder	**Range of Estimates (%)**
Attention-deficit hyper- activity disorder	2-11
Oppositional defiant disorder	5-10
Conduct disorder	4-10

Attention–Deficit Hyperactivity Disorder

ADHD is characterized by inattention, impulsiveness, and overactivity. DSM-IV represents another conceptualization of ADHD and allows the description of a primarily hyperactive-impulsive type, a primarily inattentive type, or a combined type (see box on page 583). Classically, children with ADHD are restless, overactive, distractible, reckless, and disruptive. ADHD is a relatively common disorder in school-age children, affecting an estimated 2% to 11% (Costello et al, 1996; Wolraich et al, 1996). ADHD is a frequent presenting complaint in child mental health clinics, and long-term disability is not uncommon (Barkley, 1998; Burns et al, 1995;). Thus ADHD is of significant public health importance.

Several environmental exposures have been proposed as potential causes of ADHD, including perinatal insults, head injury, psychosocial adversity, lead poisoning, and diet (e.g., food allergies, sensitivity to food additives). These hypotheses may explain some cases of ADHD; it is unlikely, however, that any one of these exposures alone will explain a significant portion of children with ADHD. Large community-based studies have confirmed that psychosocial adversity is highly associated with ADHD (Scahill, et al, 1999; Szatmari, Offord, Boyle, 1989). Whether these adverse psychosocial conditions are causal or contributing factors to other undetermined factors is unclear. The claim that food additives or allergies cause ADHD is supported largely by case reports, because most controlled studies fail to support a causative role for diet in ADHD (Scahill, DeGraft-Johnson, 1997).

Based on evidence from twin and family studies, clearly, genetic endowment plays a role in the cause of ADHD. Although identical twins were not fully concordant for ADHD, monozygotic twins are far more likely to be mutually affected than dizygotic twins (Levy et al, 1997; Stevenson, 1992). Family genetic studies have also shown that biologic relatives of children with ADHD are more likely to be affected by ADHD than biologic relatives of pediatric controls (Biederman et al, 1992).

The cause of ADHD remains unknown, but a growing body of evidence suggests that subtle dysfunction in the frontal lobe and functionally related subcortical structures play an essential role in the core symptoms of ADHD (Barkley, 1998). The frontal lobe, which is responsible for planning, attention, and regulation of motor activity, has been

---

DSM-IV-TR   Criteria for Attention-Deficit Hyperactivity Disorder

A. Either (1) or (2):
  1. Inattention: At least six of the following symptoms of inattention have persisted for at least 6 months and are maladaptive:
    a. Inattentive to details or makes careless mistakes in schoolwork.
    b. Difficulty sustaining attention in tasks or play.
    c. Does not seem to listen to what is being said.
    d. Poor follow-through on instructions and fails to finish schoolwork and chores.
    e. Difficulties with organizing tasks.
    f. Avoids or strongly dislikes sustained mental effort.
    g. Often loses things necessary for tasks or activities.
    h. Is often easily distracted by extraneous stimuli.
    i. Is often forgetful in daily activities.
  2. Hyperactivity-impulsivity: At least six symptoms of hyperactivity-impulsivity that are maladaptive and have persisted for at least 6 months:

  a. Hyperactivity
    i. Fidgety
    ii. Inappropriately leaves seat (in classroom)
    iii. Inappropriate running or climbing
    iv. Difficulty in playing or engaging in leisure activities quietly
    v. Often "on the go"
    vi. Talks excessively
  b. Impulsivity
    i. Blurts out answers to questions
    ii. Often has difficulty waiting in lines or awaiting turn
    iii. Often interrupts or intrudes on others
B. Onset no later than 7 years of age.
  1. Other criteria concern context of behavior, level of impairment, and the need to rule out other diagnoses.

Adapted from the American Psychiatric Association: *Diagnostic and statistical manual of mental disorders*, ed 4, text revision, Washington, DC, 2000, APA.

---

shown on volumetric magnetic resonance imaging (MRI) to be slightly smaller in boys with ADHD than it is in controls (Castellanos et al, 1996). Positron emission tomography (PET) also shows that adults with a history of ADHD have reduced metabolic activity (hypoperfusion) in the frontal lobe (Swanson, Volkow, 2001). Although not a consistent finding, structural MRI studies have also found small volumetric differences in the basal ganglia (Castellanos et al, 1996). These subcortical structures are highly connected to the frontal lobe and play a role in cognition and motor activity.

Oppositional Defiant Disorder

Oppositional defiant disorder (ODD) is defined by an enduring pattern of disobedience, argumentativeness, explosive angry outbursts, low frustration tolerance, and a tendency to blame others for quarrels or accidents. This pattern of behavior may begin early in development. Indeed, ODD is the most common psychiatric diagnosis of preschool children. As a child progresses through development, ODD tends to be associated with co-morbid diagnoses of anxiety and mood disorders and either a single or co-morbid diagnosis of ADHD (Lavigne et al, 2001).

By definition, children with ODD are frequently in conflict with adults. They may also have trouble maintaining friendships. In both clinical populations and community samples, substantial overlap with ADHD exists, though the two disorders do not always occur together.

Conduct Disorder

Conduct disorder is distinguishable from ODD because it is characterized by more serious violations of social standards, such as aggression, vandalism, cruelty to animals, stealing, lying, and truancy.

As with the other disruptive behavior disorders, co-morbidity is common in conduct disorder with higher-than-expected rates of ADHD, depression, and learning disorders. The relationship between ADHD and conduct disorder is intriguing and points out the potential contribution of family genetic studies. Faraone and colleagues (1991) showed that children with ADHD plus conduct disorder were more likely to have conduct disorder in their families than were children with ADHD alone. The rate of ADHD in the families of both subgroups was similar whether conduct disorder was present in the index child or not. As pointed out by the authors, these findings suggest ADHD plus conduct disorder may represent a particular form of ADHD that is distinguishable from ADHD alone.

INTERNALIZING DISORDERS

Anxiety Disorders

DSM-IV defines several anxiety disorders, including general anxiety disorder, separation anxiety, agoraphobia, panic disorder, posttraumatic stress disorder, and obsessive-compulsive disorder. This section focuses on separation anxiety and obsessive-compulsive disorder. Generalized anxiety disorder, agoraphobia, panic disorder, and posttraumatic stress disorder are described in Chapter 31.

Separation anxiety disorder

Many children experience some discomfort on separation from their mother or major attachment figure. For children with separation anxiety disorder, profound distress on entry to school may occur, and some children may refuse to go to school. In some cases, the child may "shadow" the mother around the house and not let the mother out of sight. When asked, most children with separation anxiety disorder will express worry about harm or permanent loss of the mother or major attachment figure.

The prevalence of separation anxiety disorder is estimated at 4% of school-aged children. The diagnosis of separation anxiety disorder in DSM-IV is based on childhood onset of excessive anxiety on separation from home or major attachment figure. The manifestations typically include acute distress accompanied by reluctance or refusal on separation and frequent nightmares about separation. The excessive anxiety must be present for at least a month and be the source of significant impairment at home, at school, or with friends.

Anxiety disorders recur in families at a much higher than expected rate, and it is likely that both environmental and genetic factors play an etiologic role in separation anxiety disorder. Life events, such as a family move, a change to a new school, or a death in the family, may predate the onset of separation anxiety. Additional evidence suggests that extreme shyness (fearfulness in new situations) is a heritable trait, and the presence of this trait in a child elevates the risk of an anxiety disorder (Biederman et al, 2001). Additional research is needed to determine the relative contribution of genetic and environmental factors in separation anxiety disorder.

Obsessive-compulsive disorder

Obsessive-compulsive disorder (OCD) is a heterogenous disorder affecting 2% to 3% of adolescents and adults (Karno et al, 1988; Valleni-Basile et al, 1994). Although the prevalence is probably lower in the prepubertal age group (Costello et al, 1996), OCD can be identified in children as young as 8 years of age (Riddle et al, 1990).

Obsessions are recurring thoughts or images that are disturbing and difficult to push out of the mind. Compulsions are repetitive behaviors that the person feels obliged to complete. Attempts to resist these ritualized behaviors typically increase anxiety and intensify the urge to perform the compulsion. In many cases, the reported purpose of the ritual is to prevent some dreaded event, whereas other patients state that the ritual is done to achieve a sense of completion. In either case, the performance of the compulsion achieves a momentary decrease in anxiety. This reduction in anxiety, albeit brief, reinforces the compulsive habit.

Common obsessions in children and adolescents such as contamination, fear of harm coming to self or family members, worry about acting on unwanted aggressive impulses, and concern about order and symmetry are similar to those reported by adults. Common compulsions include hand washing, cleaning rituals, requesting reassurance about matters of health and well-being, ordering and arranging objects, complex touching habits, checking, counting, and repetition of routine activities to achieve a sense of completion. To warrant a diagnosis of OCD, obsessional worries, compulsive habits, or both must waste time (at least an hour per day), must cause distress, and must interfere with daily activities.

Data from several lines of research have converged over the last two decades to clarify the neurobiologic factors of OCD. These data, derived primarily from neuroimaging studies, suggest that OCD is caused by dysregulation of brain circuits that connect the cortex, the basal ganglia, and the thalamus (Rauch et al, 2001). Another source of evidence is the replicated finding in both children and adults that antidepressant drugs that block serotonin at presynaptic reuptake sites are effective for a majority of patients with OCD (see Griest et al, 1995 and Grados, Scahill, Riddle, 1999 for reviews). By contrast, drugs that block the presynaptic reuptake of norepinephrine are not effective in OCD.

Mood Disorders

DSM-IV defines several mood disorders, including major depressive disorder, dysthymic disorder, bipolar I and bipolar II disorders, and cyclothymic disorder. Although these disorders can occur in children and adolescents, they are more common in adults (see Chapter 28). This section provides a brief discussion of major depressive disorder and bipolar disorder in children and adolescents.

Major depressive disorder

Depression is characterized by sadness, feelings of worthlessness, loss of interest in usual activities, sleep or appetite disturbance, loss of energy, diminished activity, decreased capacity to concentrate, and recurrent thoughts of death or suicide. At least five of these symptoms must be present on a daily basis and persist for at least 2 weeks (APA, 1994). The manifestations of depression in children are similar to those observed in adults. However, children may be less able to verbalize their feelings and irritability may be a predominant feature in children and adolescents (Box 42-2). Although these developmental differences have been observed in several studies, the symptoms listed are not unique to each age group (Kovacs, 1996). The prevalence of depression in children and adolescents ranges from 1% to 5%, with important differences by age and gender. Overall, depression is less common in prepubertal children, with boys at slightly higher risk than girls in the younger age group. During adolescence, depression is more common in girls.

As with other psychiatric disorders of childhood, co-morbid mental disorders are common in children with major depressive disorder (MDD). The most frequent co-morbid disorders in both children and adolescents include dysthymia, anxiety disorders, and disruptive behavior disorders. In adolescents, personality disorders such as borderline personality and substance abuse are of particular concern.

A large body of data shows that depression involves the hypothalamic-pituitary-adrenal axis, as well as the norepinephrine and serotonin systems in the brain, but the precise mechanism is not well understood. Family studies provide evidence that the risk for depression is substantially higher if a history of depression exists in an immediate family member (Klein et al, 2001; Merikangas, Angst, 1995).

Critical Thinking Question

A child with separation anxiety expresses recurring worry about a parent's safety. How is this different from obsessive-compulsive disorder?

Box 42-2 | Differences in the Manifestation of Depression in Children and Adolescents

Early Childhood
Anxiety symptoms
- Separation anxiety
- Excessive worry
Somatic complaints
Temper tantrums
Noncompliant behavior
Delusions
Auditory hallucinations (rare)

Middle and Late Childhood
Sleep and appetite disturbance
More verbal expression of:
- Depressed mood
- Worthlessness
- Guilt
- Hopelessness

Adolescents
Sleep disturbance
- Hypersomnia
Verbal expression of depressed mood
Appetite disturbance
- Weight loss or gain
Suicidal thoughts/plans
Poor self-care

Although these developmental differences have been observed, the symptoms listed are not unique to each age group.

Bipolar disorder

DSM-IV defines two major types of bipolar disorder: bipolar I and bipolar II. Bipolar I disorder is defined by mania with or without a history of depression. Bipolar II disorder is characterized by a history of major depression and hypomania, but not a full manic episode (Box 42-3) (APA, 1994).

The existence of bipolar illness in young children is a matter of current controversy. Some investigators suggest that bipolar illness is rare in prepubertal children, whereas others contend that it is simply underdiagnosed. This debate is further complicated by disagreement concerning whether bipolar illness in children has the same clinical features as those seen in adults (Giedd, 2000; Weller, Weller, Fristad, 1995). Using structured diagnostic interviews, Biederman and colleagues (1995b) identified 14% ($n = 43$) of children with bipolar disorder in their psychopharmacology specialty clinic. These children, some of whom had a history of depression, showed more severe psychopathology when compared with a group of children with ADHD.

|Box 42-3| Manic Episode

Persistent period (at least 1 week) of expansive or irritable mood accompanied by three or more of the following:
- Inflated self-esteem
- Decreased need for sleep
- Pressure of speech
- Racing thoughts
- Highly distractible
- Increase in goal-directed activity (or agitation)
- Unrestrained involvement in pleasurable activities

|Table 42-4| Types and Features of Tic Disorders in DSM-IV-TR

Tic Disorder	Clinical Features
Transient	Motor **and/or** phonic tics for at least 2 weeks, but less than 1 year
Chronic	Either motor **or** phonic tics for more than 1 year
Tourette's*	Both motor **and** phonic tics for more than 1 year

*In DSM-IV—Tourette's disorder, also called Tourette syndrome.

The prevalence of bipolar illness in adolescents is estimated at approximately 1% (Lewinsohn, Klein, Seeley, 1995). In this large community survey, girls were more frequently affected than boys. The mean age of onset for the whole group was about 12 years of age, with depression being the most common feature before onset. Another 5% in this large community sample showed *core* symptoms of bipolar illness without meeting the criteria for any specific disorder. This observation suggests that bipolar illness in children and adolescents may reside on a spectrum from mild to severe. Thus children and adolescents with mild symptoms may not meet the diagnostic criteria for the disorder, but they may be impaired.

TIC DISORDERS

Tic disorder is a general term used to describe several disorders that are characterized by motor or phonic tics or both. Motor tics are typically rapid, jerky movements of the eyes, face, neck, and shoulders, but other muscle groups may also be involved. Motor tics may also take the form of slower and more purposeful movements. The most common phonic tics are throat clearing, grunting, or other repetitive noises. More complex sounds such as words, parts of words, and obscenities occur in a minority of patients. Table 42-4 presents a list of tic disorders and their defining features.

As shown in Table 42-4, Tourette's syndrome (TS) is a chronic movement disorder that is defined by the presence of multiple motor and phonic tics. The prevalence of TS is estimated to be between 1 and 8 cases per 1000, with boys being affected 3 to 6 times more often than girls (Kurlan et al, 2001; Scahill, Tanner, Dure, 2001).

In the 1970s the potent dopamine postsynaptic blocker, haloperidol, was found to be helpful in reducing tic symptoms. This observation prompted speculation about the role of central dopamine systems in the cause of TS. Since then, several other neurochemical systems have been implicated in TS, including norepinephrine, endogenous opioids, serotonin, and androgens. Several family-genetic studies reported data consistent with autosomal-dominant inheritance. These studies also showed that the range of expression is variable and probably includes TS, chronic motor or chronic vocal tic disorder, and OCD as well (Pauls et al, 1991). Further support for a genetic hypothesis came from twin studies that showed monozygotic twins are far more likely to be concordant for TS than are dizygotic twins. In many cases, however, concordant monozygotic twins were not equally affected, suggesting that environmental factors also have an impact on the expression of the gene. More recent family-genetic studies suggest that the inheritance of TS may involve more than a single gene rather than a straightforward autosomal dominant pattern (Walkup, et al, 1996).

Although the cause of TS is unknown, several lines of evidence point to dysregulation of circuits that travel from the cortex through the basal ganglia (Peterson et al, 1999). The basal ganglia are a group of subcortical structures that play an important role in planning and executing movement, as well as higher cognitive functions. These circuits are organized into five parallel, minimally overlapping pathways, each of which appears to serve separate functions. Dysregulation of one or more of these circuits has been implicated in the pathophysiologic nature of several disorders, including OCD, schizophrenia, TS, Huntington's chorea, and Parkinson's disease (Mink, 2001; Peterson et al, 1999).

PSYCHOTIC DISORDERS

Psychotic symptoms may occur in the context of several disorders, such as bipolar illness, depression, and PDD. Psychotic disorders such as schizophrenia are defined using the same criteria as those for adults and are rare in children. For example, childhood-onset schizophrenia is estimated at 2 cases per 100,000 compared with 2 to 10 cases per 1000 in late teen years. The precise cause of schizophrenia is unknown, but as previously suggested, genetic influence is strongly implied. Neuroimaging data suggest a loss of inhibitory control in pathways connecting the frontal lobe to subcortical structures, including the basal ganglia and thalamus (Berman, Weinberger, 1999).

ELIMINATION DISORDERS

Enuresis

Enuresis usually refers to bed-wetting (nocturnal enuresis). However, enuresis can also be characterized by repeated urination on clothing during waking hours (diurnal enuresis). For nocturnal enuresis, DSM-IV specifies that bed-wetting occurs at least twice per week for a duration of 3 months and that the child be at least 5 years of age. Boys are more often affected than girls, and the prevalence goes down with age. An estimated 6.7% of 5-year-old boys, 3.0% of boys ages 9 to 11, and 1.0% of 14-year-old boys have nocturnal enuresis.

Encopresis

Encopresis is defined as soiling clothing with feces or depositing feces in inappropriate places in a child 4 years of age or older. Additional diagnostic criteria require that the soiling occur at least once per month and that it not be the result of a medical disorder such as aganglionic megacolon (Hirschsprung's disease). The most common cause of encopresis is leakage of stool around a fecal impaction. Fecal impaction may start because the child withholds in response to the urge to defecate. Over time, a loss of muscle tone may occur in the lower bowel, and the child loses the normal urge to defecate and may not even be aware of the leakage. Encopresis affects an estimated 1.5% of school-age children and is three to four times more common in boys than in girls. As with enuresis, the frequency of the condition goes down with age.

Treatment

CLINICAL EXAMPLE

Allan, a 9-year-old fourth grader, was referred by his pediatrician to the outpatient clinic for an evaluation of his overactivity, impulsiveness, poor concentration, and disruptive behavior in school. At the time of referral, he lived with his mother and younger sister in a small apartment after having moved from a neighboring town. His mother works part time as a waitress. The history revealed that he had been treated with methylphenidate (Ritalin) in the second grade with uncertain benefit. However, his mother was unable to recall the dose or the duration of treatment.

The developmental history was remarkable for significant marital discord during the pregnancy, resulting in the couple's first separation. This marital discord was characterized by the father's alcohol abuse, parental arguments, and occasional physical fights. The couple finally divorced 3 years later, just before the birth of Allan's younger sister. Allan achieved motor milestones early, but was late in speech and language acquisition. He had only a few words by 2 years of age and, when he entered preschool at the age of 3 years, his speech was poorly understood by nonfamily members.

Overactivity and inability to play with other children without fighting led to Allan's dismissal from the first preschool. His mother reported that Allan did better in the second preschool, which had a more structured program. He remained in this program until the first grade, when he entered the public school. In the first and second grades, Allan's teachers reported that he was hard to manage because of overactivity, calling out without permission, and interfering with the affairs of other children. Although generally good-natured, Allan's intrusive style and occasional aggressive behavior caused him to be rejected by his classmates. He was highly distractible and unable to stay on task. Not surprisingly, he fell behind academically and was barely able to read at the end of second grade. In his current school setting, Allan has been frequently ejected from the classroom for disruptive behavior. After instigating a fight in the schoolyard, he had been admonished to stay away from older boys during recess.

Allan was a healthy boy with no history of serious injuries or illnesses or hospitalizations. He had multiple middle-ear infections during the first 3 years of life, but had not had any since the age of 5 years. Review of body systems revealed a recent history of intermittent

Continued

constipation and soiling. According to Allan's mother, this problem had occurred in second grade, but resolved without intervention after 1 or 2 months. He had no known allergies to foods or medication; his last physical examination was before the start of fourth grade.

TREATMENT SETTINGS

Traditionally, there were two treatment settings for children and adolescents with psychiatric disorders: specialized inpatient units and outpatient services. Driven in part by the high cost of inpatient care, and by the recognition that the level of care should be congruent with symptom severity, a wider range of mental health services has emerged in recent years. It is now possible in some communities to receive mental health services in the home, in school-based clinics, in after-school programs, specialized educational programs, day hospitals, therapeutic foster homes, and residential treatment centers, as well as the traditional outpatient and inpatient settings. In all likelihood, this range of mental health services will expand.

PSYCHOPHARMACOLOGY

Several different classes of medications are used in the treatment of children and adolescents with psychiatric disorders (for a detailed review see Scahill, 2000). Many of the drugs used in the treatment of children and adolescents with serious psychiatric symptoms were developed for other purposes (Table 42-5). In addition, the same drug may be prescribed for any one of several problems. Unfortunately, many of these medications have entered clinical practice without the benefit of carefully controlled studies to guide their use. For example, clonidine was developed as an antihypertensive medication and is used in the treatment of ADHD and tics. Although studies have been conducted in both children and adults with tics, the data supporting its use in ADHD have been limited until recently (Tourette's Syndrome Study Group, 2002).

An important guiding principle in pediatric psychopharmacology is that children are physiologically different from adults. These differences can have an impact on dose, clinical response, and side effects. For example, children often require larger doses of psy-

| Table 42-5 | Classes of Medications Used in the Treatment of Children and Adolescents with Psychiatric Symptoms

Class	Purpose(s)	Empirical Support*
Stimulants	ADHD	Excellent
Tricyclic antidepressants	1. Depression	Fair
	2. ADHD	Good
	3. Enuresis	Good
	4. Separation anxiety	Fair
	5. OCD (clomipramine)	Excellent
Serotonin reuptake inhibitors	1. OCD	Excellent
	2. Depression	Good
	3. Anxiety	Good
Traditional neuroleptics	1. Psychosis	Excellent
	2. Tics (haloperidol and pimozide)	Excellent
	3. Severe impulsiveness in ADHD	Good
	4. Agitation in PDD	Good
Atypical neuroleptics (risperidone best studied to date)	1. Psychosis	Good
	2. Agitation in PDD	Fair
	3. Tics	Good
Alpha-2 agonists	1. Tics (clonidine)	Good
	2. ADHD (clonidine and guanfacine)	Good
Mood stabilizers	1. Mania (lithium)	Good
	2. Mania (valproate)	Poor

*Poor, No or few studies in pediatric populations or little support from existing studies; *fair,* few controlled studies in pediatric populations or concern about side effects; *good,* some data from controlled studies, but findings are inconsistent or only one study has positive results; *excellent,* consistent body of data from controlled studies showing both efficacy and safety (see text for more details).

ADHD, Attention-deficit hyperactivity disorder; *OCD,* obsessive-compulsive disorder; *PDD,* pervasive developmental disorder.

chotropic drugs, on a milligram-per-kilogram basis, than do adults to achieve beneficial effects. Although it is not completely clear why this is the case, the speculation is that more efficient liver metabolism and glomerular filtration in children plays some role (Vitiello, 1998). Because of developmental differences in neural pathways, drug effects (pharmacodynamics) may be different in children compared with adults. For example, norepinephrine, dopamine, and serotonin systems all undergo developmental changes in childhood (Vitiello, 1998). These developmental differences may explain the inconsistent results of the tricyclic antidepressants (TCAs) in children with depression compared with adults and the more frequently observed activating side effects of selective serotonin reuptake inhibitors (SSRIs) in children (Martin, Kaufman, Charney, 2000).

Stimulants

The most frequently used stimulants are methylphenidate (Ritalin) and dextroamphetamine (Dexedrine) and the mixed amphetamine compound (d,l-amphetamine) Adderall. Of these various preparations, methylphenidate is by far the most common, being used by approximately 3% of school-aged children. The preference for methylphenidate over the other stimulants is probably because of its familiarity (Greenhill et al, 1996). Another less commonly used stimulant is pemoline (Cylert). Because of concern about the risk of hepatic failure, this medication is falling out of use.

A recent federally funded, multisite study enrolled 576 children and randomly assigned them to one of four groups: expert medication management (from one of the research centers), expert medication management with behavioral treatment, behavioral treatment alone, or treatment in the community. In this design, treatment in the community was the control condition. The behavior-therapy program in the behavior treatment–only group and the combined treatment group was the same and was delivered in structured fashion to ensure consistency across sites. Important questions for the study included whether expert medication management would be superior to treatment obtained in the community and whether behavior therapy would show additive benefit when combined with medication treatment. Subjects were reassessed at 14 months. Compared with the community controls,

the group who received expert medication management and the group that received expert medication management with behavior therapy did significantly better when rated by teachers and parents. No difference occurred between the behavior treatment only and community controls (MTA Group, 1999). In both the expertly managed medication groups and the community control group, methylphenidate was the most commonly used drug. The medication management at the research centers tended to involve higher doses on average and to use three doses per day rather than two, which was the norm in the community sample.

The optimal daily dose of methylphenidate ranges between 0.6 mg and 1.5 mg/kg of body weight per day in three divided doses. This level translates into roughly 10 mg, two times daily (breakfast and lunch) and 5 mg at 4:00 PM for a 45-pound (20-kg) child. Slightly higher doses may be tried in cases showing equivocal response, but doses above 60 mg per day are not recommended. The usual dose of dextroamphetamine (or d,l-amphetamine) is lower than that of methylphenidate and is rarely given more than twice a day. The total daily dose is typically in the range of 15 to 20 mg per day in younger children and 40 mg per day in older children (i.e., for a total dose of 0.3 mg and 1.0 mg/kg per day).

Immediate release methylphenidate and the amphetamines are given just before or with meals to prevent loss of appetite. Other side effects of the stimulants include insomnia, mood lability, tics, and abnormal movements; a tendency to become overfocused on details; and, rarely, agitation and psychotic symptoms. In the usual short-acting form, methylphenidate and the amphetamines have a duration of action of about 4 and 6 hours, respectively. As the medication effects wear off, a behavioral rebound can occur. To soften the rebound effect later in the day, the third dose of methylphenidate or the second dose of amphetamine is typically lower than the previous dose. Recently, several new long-acting stimulant preparations of methylphenidate (Concerta, Metadate) and d,l-amphetamine (Adderall-XR) have entered the marketplace. The primary advantages of these long-acting preparations is that the child does not have to take a second dose of the medication in school and the drug dose across the day may be more even. One drawback of the long-acting preparations is that they often provide less flexibility in dosing.

Tricyclic Antidepressants

TCAs, including imipramine, desipramine, nortriptyline, and clomipramine, are a group of chemically related compounds that have been used in children and adolescents for over 30 years. As suggested in Table 42-5, these agents have been used in the treatment of depression, enuresis, separation anxiety, ADHD, and OCD with mixed results, depending on the specific agent and the disorder in question.

To date, the efficacy of the TCAs in the treatment of children with depression has not been demonstrated (Martin et al, 2000). Apparently, however, at least some children with depression do benefit from nortriptyline at daily doses in the range of 0.64 to 1.57 mg/kg per day.

Placebo-controlled studies have demonstrated the effectiveness of desipramine in the treatment of ADHD (Biederman et al, 1989; Singer et al, 1995). However, concern about alterations in cardiac conduction has decreased enthusiasm for the use of desipramine in pediatric populations. Imipramine has been studied in several controlled trials for separation anxiety with inconsistent results. The most recent study failed to show that imipramine was better than placebo (Klein, Koplewicz, Kanner, 1992). Imipramine has also demonstrated efficacy in the treatment of enuresis. However, since the introduction of the synthetic antidiuretic hormone, desmopressin (DDAVP), use of imipramine for enuresis has declined.

Clomipramine is unique in that, in addition to the norepinephrine reuptake properties common to the other TCAs, it also has serotonin reuptake properties (Grados, Scahill, Riddle, 1999). This mechanism is believed to be the explanation for its effectiveness in the treatment of OCD. In a multicenter trial, clomipramine was superior to placebo in adolescents with OCD (DeVeaugh-Geiss et al, 1992). The typical dose of clomipramine ranges from 75 mg to 250 mg, depending on the age of the child, with younger children on the lower end of the range.

The side effects of the TCAs include dry mouth, fatigue, dizziness, sweating, weight gain, urinary retention, tremor, tachycardia, and agitation. These side effects can often be managed by lowering the dose or changing the dose schedule (e.g., splitting into two doses per day). All of the TCAs have the capacity to change cardiac conduction. Therefore children and adolescents treated with any of the TCAs should receive a cardiogram at baseline and periodically during treatment. Resting heart rate over 120 bpm is cause for concern.

Selective Serotonin Reuptake Inhibitors

SSRIs is a group of chemically unrelated compounds that was originally developed as antidepressants. The success of clomipramine in the treatment of OCD prompted great interest in these drugs for the treatment of OCD, as well as depression. Currently, five SSRIs are marketed in the United States, including fluoxetine (Prozac), sertraline (Zoloft), paroxetine (Paxil), fluvoxamine (Luvox), and citalopram (Celexa). Each of these has shown efficacy in the treatment of depression in adults. Fluoxetine, sertraline, and fluvoxamine have also demonstrated efficacy for OCD in controlled trials in both children and adults (see Griest et al, 1995 and Grados, Scahill, Riddle, 1999 for reviews).

The precise mechanism of the SSRIs is not completely understood. It is known that SSRIs block the return of serotonin into the presynaptic neuron—hence the term reuptake inhibitors. All five of the SSRIs have relatively long half-lives, permitting single daily dosing, with the exception of fluvoxamine, which is often given twice daily (Box 42-4).

Side effects of the SSRIs

The most common side effect of the SSRIs in children and adolescents is behavioral activation, which may be characterized by motor restlessness, insomnia, hypomania, and disinhibition. Behavioral activation is most likely to occur early in treatment but may also be seen with dose increases (Grados, Scahill, Riddle, 1999). Other side effects include abdominal pain, heartburn, diarrhea, and decreased appetite. Case reports indicate suicidal ideation and self-injurious behavior with fluoxetine (King et al, 1991), but whether this reaction is attributable to fluoxetine alone or all SSRIs is unclear.

When a child is placed on an SSRI for OCD or depression and has a positive response, parents frequently inquire about the duration of treatment. In the absence of clear evidence to guide the decision, most clinicians suggest discontinuation after a symptom-free period of 8 to 12 months (Birmaher, Brent, Benson, 1998). Parents should be discouraged from abrupt withdrawal because of several reports of

Fluoxetine

Fluoxetine (Prozac) comes in a 10- or 20-mg capsule, a liquid form, and a weekly dose formulation. Because of the long half-life (fluoxetine also has an active metabolite with an even longer half-life), the dose is typically increased slowly to avoid overshooting the optimal dose. The typical starting dose is 5 to 10 mg per day, and the dose range for most children and adolescents will be between 10 and 40 mg per day. Fluoxetine has been shown to be effective in the treatment of depression and OCD in pediatric studies.

Sertraline

Sertraline (Zoloft) has shown superiority to placebo in large-scale study in OCD and is available in 50- and 100-mg tablets that can easily be broken in half. The starting dose might be 25 mg with gradual increases to a range of 25 to 150 mg in children. Adolescents may receive slightly higher doses. Some patients respond at lower doses, hence dosing should be individualized.

Fluvoxamine

Fluvoxamine (Luvox) has been evaluated in a large multi-center study in children and adolescents with OCD and now has approval from the Food and Drug Administration for use in pediatric populations. The medication comes in a 25-, 50-, and 100-mg tablets—each of which can be broken in half. Treatment may begin with 12.5 to 25 mg per day and may be increased by 25 mg every 5 to 7 days as tolerated. The typical dose range is 50 to 200 mg per day in children. It is often administered in two divided doses.

Paroxetine

Paroxetine (Paxil) comes in 20- and 30-mg tablets that can be broken in half. To date, paroxetine has been studied in depression and OCD in pediatric populations. A reasonable starting dose would be 10 mg per day to a total dose of 10 to 40 mg in a single daily dose.

emotional instability, dizziness, nausea, nervousness, and confusion on abrupt withdrawal of sertraline and paroxetine (Rosenbaum et al, 1998). Fluoxetine, which has a longer half-life, was not associated with these complaints. Fluvoxamine was not evaluated in this study. However, because fluvoxamine is also relatively short acting compared with fluoxetine, abrupt withdrawal of fluvoxamine should be avoided. Children and parents should also be informed that symptoms of OCD or depression may return after planned discontinuation of an SSRI.

A recent multisite study conducted by the Research Unit on Pediatric Psychopharmacology Anxiety Group evaluated the efficacy and safety of fluvoxamine in childhood-onset anxiety disorders (RUPP Anxiety Group, 2001). The study included 128 children and adolescents (age range, 6 to 17 years) with generalized anxiety disorder, separation anxiety disorder, social phobia, or any combination. Before randomization, eligible subjects were given 4 weeks of cognitive psychotherapy. Subjects who remained symptomatic after the 4-week psychotherapy were randomized to fluvoxamine or a placebo for 8 weeks under double-blind conditions. After 8 weeks of treatment at an average dose of 4.4 ± 2.2 mg/kg, a 52% improvement was noted on the Pediatric Anxiety Rating Scale (PARS) in the fluvoxamine group compared with a 16% improvement in the placebo group. The side effects observed in this study were similar to those reported in pediatric samples with OCD. The most common adverse effects included abdominal discomfort, behavioral activation, headache, and drowsiness (greater than 20% for each).

Traditional Antipsychotics

Traditional neuroleptics, such as the phenothiazines and haloperidol, primarily block D_2 dopamine receptors. The newer, atypical neuroleptics such as olanzapine and risperidone not only block dopamine receptors, but are potent antagonists of specific serotonin receptors as well. This pharmacologic property appears to be protective against extrapyramidal side effects (EPSEs).

In children, neuroleptics are used to treat both psychotic and nonpsychotic symptoms, including stereotypies and agitation, severe hyperactivity, aggressive or self-injurious behavior, and tics (Scahill, Skrypeck, 1997) (Box 42-5). These target symptoms are associated with disorders such as PDD, refractory ADHD, bipolar disorder, severe conduct disorder, and TS.

Side effects of the traditional antipsychotics

Low-potency neuroleptics are associated with sedation and orthostatic hypotension. By contrast, the higher-potency agents are associated with EPSEs, such as dystonia, dyskinesia, akathisia (subjective feeling of restlessness), and parkinsonism. In some cases, the dystonia is pronounced and is exhibited by

| Box 42–5 | Traditional Antipsychotics

Thioridazine

Thioridazine (Mellaril) is a low-potency neuroleptic in the phenothiazine chemical family. It has been used for the treatment of severe hyperactivity and/or agitation. The introduction of the atypical antipsychotics and concern about the potential for inducing cardiac arrhythmias have contributed to the decline in the use of thioridazine.

Thiothixene

Thiothixene (Navane) is a neuroleptic of intermediate potency that is used primarily for psychosis or severe agitation. In children, treatment typically begins with 2 mg twice to three times per day with gradual increases to 5 mg two to three times daily. This schedule may be more aggressive, and higher dose levels may be used in acute psychotic states.

Haloperidol

Haloperidol (Haldol) is a high-potency neuroleptic that is unrelated to the phenothiazines. It has been studied in pediatric populations for the treatment of psychosis, PDD, conduct disorder, and tic disorders. The typical dose ranges from 1 to 2 mg per day for the treatment of tics to 10 mg per day for the management of acute psychosis.

Pimozide

Pimozide (Orap) is another high-potency neuroleptic that is used specifically for the treatment of tics. It comes in 1-mg and 2-mg tablets; the typical dose range is 1 to 4 mg per day.

Risperidone

Risperidone (Risperdal) is a newer atypical antipsychotic medication that has potent dopamine- and serotonin-blocking properties. Emerging data suggest that risperidone is effective for the treatment of tics, as well as aggression, agitation, and self-injury in children with autism.

torticollis and rolling of the eyes upward (i.e., oculogyric crisis). Treatment of acute dystonia includes immediate injection of an anticholinergic medication such as benztropine (Cogentin) and slowing down the rate of increase of the neuroleptic. Other side effects of the traditional antipsychotics include cognitive blunting, irritability, depressed mood, blurred vision, dry mouth, and weight gain. Finally, long-term treatment with a neuroleptic places the patient at increased risk for tardive dyskinesia (Campbell et al, 1997), which is a chronic neurologic condition involving abnormal movements of the face, mouth, and sometimes the arms. These poten-

tial short- and long-term side effects should be discussed with the child and family before and during treatment with this group of medications.

Atypical Antipsychotics

Concerns about the potential long- and short-term adverse effects of the traditional neuroleptics have prompted the development of a new class of neuroleptics. The first medication of this new class was clozapine, which was introduced in the 1960s. Although early results were encouraging, clozapine was nearly withdrawn from use because of concerns about agranulocytosis. Currently, clozapine is reserved for cases of treatment-refractory schizophrenia. The atypical neuroleptics block both serotonin and, to some extent, dopamine receptors. Over the last few years, several agents with this dual action have been introduced, such as risperidone (Risperdal), olanzapine (Zyprexa), quetiapine (Seroquel), and ziprasidone (Geodon). This section focuses on risperidone because the other agents listed have little or no data concerning their use in children and adolescents (see Scahill, Lynch, 1998 for a review).

Risperidone came on the market in early 1994. Since then, risperidone has been used in several open-label studies in children and adolescents with a wide range of problems, including tic disorders, PDD, schizophrenia, and severe disruptive behavior. The dose levels ranged from 0.5 mg per day to 10.0 mg per day. Careful review of these studies suggests that extrapyramidal symptoms are infrequent and clearly related to the rate of dose increase. In studies that used a slow upward dose schedule, extrapyramidal symptoms were not observed (Scahill, Lynch, 1998). The most common side effect across these studies was weight gain. Children who are placed on this drug should be weighed at baseline and periodically during treatment. One case of elevated liver function tests accompanied by fatty infiltration also occurred (Kumra et al, 1997). A recent placebo-controlled study of 101 children with autism showed that 2 mg risperidone per day was superior to placebo for reducing aggression, tantrums, and self-injury (RUPP Autism Network, in press).

Alpha-2 Agonists

The alpha-2 agonists, clonidine (Catapres) and guanfacine (Tenex), were developed as antihypertensive agents. These drugs turn down norepinephrine activity in the brain. Clonidine can be useful for the treatment of tics as shown in a recent double-blind study (Leckman et al, 1991). Support for the use of clonidine in the treatment of ADHD is less consistent, though a recent placebo-controlled study showed that it was superior to the placebo in a sample of children with tic disorders and ADHD. In addition, the combination of clonidine and methylphenidate provided additional benefits (Tourette Study Group, 2002). The typical daily dose of clonidine ranges from 0.15 to 0.25 mg per day divided into three or four doses. The most common side effect of clonidine is sedation. Dry mouth, headache, irritability, and sleep disturbance may also occur. Although rarely a problem, blood pressure should be monitored during treatment, especially when starting the medication. Abrupt discontinuation, however, can cause a rebound in blood pressure and should be avoided.

In doses ranging from 1.0 to 4.0 mg per day in three divided doses, guanfacine has been evaluated in preliminary studies, including one placebo-controlled study. In the study, 17 children with ADHD and a tic disorder were randomly assigned to receive guanfacine and 17 received placebo. After 8 weeks of treatment, the guanfacine group showed improvements in ADHD symptoms and tics compared with the placebo group (Scahill et al, 2001). Because guanfacine has a longer duration of action and is less sedating than is clonidine, it is of increasing interest in ADHD, but more study is needed.

COGNITIVE-BEHAVIORAL THERAPY

Contemporary treatment of children and adolescents often involves a multimodal approach, which may include medication, family treatment, group therapy, and individual therapy for the child. Cognitive-behavioral therapy is a form of individual therapy that has been successfully applied to children with disruptive behavior disorders and anxiety disorders. Other psychotherapeutic interventions such as interpersonal therapy (IPT) have been shown to be effective in adults and adolescents (Mufson et al, 1999). This section focuses on cognitive-behavioral techniques that are used in the treatment of ADHD and OCD.

Cognitive-Behavioral Therapy in ADHD

Recalling that the hallmark features of ADHD are inattention, overactivity, and impulsiveness, the goal of cognitive-behavioral therapy in ADHD is to improve the child's ability to "stop, look, and listen" before acting. Several approaches have been developed to accomplish this overall aim.

Social skills training

Social skills training teaches the child to recognize the impact of his or her behavior on others. Because impulsive children and adolescents often fail to recognize the adverse effects of their verbal and nonverbal behavior, social skills training uses instruction, role playing, and positive reinforcement to improve interpersonal relationships and to enhance social outcomes.

Problem-solving skills training

Problem-solving skills training focuses on defective cognitive processes such as assessment of situations, as well as interpretation of events and expectations of others. Children with disruptive behavior problems often misinterpret the intentions of others, for example, perceiving hostility when none was intended. Through instruction and role-playing, problem-solving skills training teaches the child to generate alternative interpretations for the behavior of others and options for a response. These options are then evaluated for their likely consequences on the situation and on interpersonal relationships.

Parent training

The reckless and impulsive behavior of children with ADHD and other disruptive behavior disorders often elicit punitive responses from their parents. Parent training attempts to provide parents with a new understanding of their child's behavior and new ways of responding to it. These programs emphasize the importance of clear limits concerning unwanted behavior and positive reinforcement (praise and tangible rewards) for desired behaviors. The use of point systems and mild punishments such as time-out are also presented. Parent training programs may be offered in a group format or in a family therapy setting (Barkley, 1998).

Cognitive-Behavioral Therapy in OCD

Cognitive behavior therapy for OCD is based on exposure and response prevention. Exposure refers to deliberate confrontation of a situation or event that triggers anxiety or the urge to perform the rit-

|Box 42–6| Treatment Plan: Allan

Diagnosis

Axis I   ADHD: combined type
         Encopresis
         Reading disorder
Axis II None
Axis III None
Axis IV Academic problems
         Inadequate finances
         Family dysfunction
Axis V   Global assessment of functioning: 50

Goals

1. Reduce overactivity and impulsive behavior.
2. Improve social judgment.
3. Remediate delayed reading skills.
4. Restore normal bowel function.

Placement

The treatment plan includes placement in a day treatment program due to degree of impulsiveness and tendency to provoke retaliation from others. This placement will also permit the application of multiple treatments, including social skills training, parent training for Allan's mother, and close monitoring of pharmacotherapy. The day hospital program will also include a psychoeducational evaluation to clarify his reading disability and generate remediation strategies.

Medication

After a 2-week observation period, a trial of methylphenidate will be initiated. Despite report of a previous unsuccessful trial, available evidence suggests that the trial was inadequate. Therefore, before moving on to another stimulant or to a nonstimulant alternative, response to methylphenidate in a carefully monitored trial is appropriate. The medication will be started at 5 mg per day and increased to 5 mg tid (8 AM, 12 noon, and 4 PM) after 4 days. If well tolerated, dose will be increased 4 days later to 10 mg in the morning, 10 mg at noon, and 5 mg at 4 PM. Thereafter, dose will be increased depending on response, with a maximum dose of 30 to 40 mg per day in three divided doses with the third dose roughly half the dose of the morning and noon doses.

Bowel Retraining Program

In collaboration with his primary care providers, will initiate a bowel retraining program. Step 1 is educating the mother and Allan about normal bowel function and the vicious cycle of fecal impaction and leakage of stool around the hardened mass of stool. This educational effort should help to decrease the mother's anger at Allan for this problem and will help motivate Allan to engage in solving the problem. Step 2 is to clean out the bowel (e.g., with a laxative and mineral oil). Step 3 is the behavioral treatment program, which typically involves daily sitting on the toilet after each meal for 10 minutes. Rewards in the form of stickers or points will be given at school and at home for participating in the program. Special bonuses can be awarded for successful defecation. The stickers or points can be "cashed in" for small prizes at the end of each week.

ual. Response prevention consists of blocking the compulsive behavior despite the presence of the urge to complete it. For example, if the patient feared contamination and felt the need to wash after touching sticky materials, the patient might be encouraged to touch a sticky counter and then refrain from washing. These techniques have clearly demonstrated their usefulness in the treatment of adults with OCD and recently have been applied to children (see Piacentini, 1999, for a review).

The theory behind exposure and response prevention is that rising anxiety occurs in response to external events (a trigger). Second, the anxiety associated with the triggering event or situation is exaggerated. Third, because the performance of the ritual results in a rapid decline in anxiety, it reinforces the idea that the compulsive behavior is a useful strategy for managing anxiety. Unfortunately, the success of the ritualized behavior is typically short-lived. Finally, systematic confrontation of the triggering event or situation results in decreased anxiety even if the ritual is not performed. Box 42-6 presents a traditional treatment plan for the case presented earlier in this section.

Critical Thinking Question

When working with a parent of a child with ADHD, how might a nurse explain the child's need for structure in the home without seeming to blame the parent for the child's problem behavior?

Key Concepts

1. Current prevalence estimates of psychiatric disorders in children indicate that they are relatively common, but only a small percentage of children are receiving appropriate treatment.

2. Risk factors for childhood psychiatric disorders include genetic factors and adverse environmental influences such as perinatal complications and psychosocial adversities, such as poverty, single parent family, family conflict, and a parent with a mental illness.

3. The presence of a risk factor increases the likelihood of developing a mental illness.

4. Children can be motivated by their peers. Psychotherapeutic management of children in the psychiatric inpatient setting is most effective when nurse-patient relationship and milieu issues are considered jointly.

5. Resilience is the ability of a child to maintain an optimal development course despite exposure to undesirable environmental conditions.

6. ADHD is the most common pediatric behavioral disorder. Central nervous system stimulants are the drugs most frequently used to treat children with ADHD.

7. Symptoms of autism include significant delays in socialization and communication, as well as repetitive behavior and restricted patterns of behavior.

8. Depression is uncommon in young children, but the prevalence increases in adolescents. Until recently, no antidepressant had been shown to be superior to a placebo in children and adolescents.

References

American Psychiatric Association: *Diagnostic and statistical manual of mental disorders,* ed 4, text revision, Washington, DC, 2000, APA.

American Psychiatric Association: *Diagnostic and statistical manual of mental disorders,* ed 4, Washington, DC, 1994, APA.

American Psychiatric Association: *Diagnostic and statistical manual of mental disorders,* ed 3, Washington, DC, 1980, APA.

Barkley RA: *Attention deficit hyperactivity disorder: a handbook for diagnosis and treatment,* New York, 1998, Guilford Press.

Beitchman JH et al: Prevalence of speech and language disorders in 5-year-old kindergarten children in the Ottawa-Carleton region, *J Speech Hear Disord* 51:98, 1986a.

Beitchman JH et al: Prevalence of psychiatric disorders in children with speech and language disorders, *J Am Acad Child Adolesc Psychiatry* 25:528, 1986b.

Berman KF, Weinberger DR: Neuroimaging studies of schizophrenia. In Charney DS, Nestler EJ, Bunney BS editors: *Neurobiology of mental illness,* New York, 1999, Oxford, University Press.

Biederman J et al: A double-blind placebo controlled study of desipramine in the treatment of ADD, Part I: efficacy, *J Am Acad Child Adolesc Psychiatry* 28(5):777, 1989.

Biederman J et al: Further evidence for family-genetic risk factors in attention deficit hyperactivity disorder, *Arch Gen Psychiatry* 49:728, 1992.

Biederman J et al: Family-environmental risk factors for attention-deficit hyperactivity disorder, *Arch Gen Psychiatry* 52:464, 1995a.

Biederman J et al: CBCL clinical scales discriminate prepubertal children with structured interview-derived diagnosis of mania from those with ADHD, *J Am Acad Child Adolesc Psychiatry* 34(4):464, 1995b.

Biederman J et al: Further evidence of association between behavioral inhibition and social anxiety in children, *Am J Psychiatry* 158(10):1673, 2001.

Birmaher B, Brent DA, Benson RS: Summary of the practice parameters for the assessment and treatment of children and adolescents with depressive disorders, *J Am Acad Child Adolesc Psychiatry* 37:1234, 1998.

Briggs-Gowan M et al: Mental health in pediatric settings: distribution of disorders and factors related to service use, *J Am Acad Child Psychiatry* 39(7):841, 2000.

Burns BJ et al: Children's mental health service use across service sectors, *Health Aff* 14(3):147, 1995.

Campbell M et al: Neuroleptic-related dyskinesias in autistic children: a prospective, longitudinal study, *J Am Acad Child Adolesc Psychiatry* 36:835, 1997.

Carey G, Gottesman II: Twin and family studies of anxiety, phobic, and obsessive-compulsive disorders. In Klein DF, Rabkin J, editors: *Anxiety: new research and changing concepts,* New York, 1981, Raven.

Castellanos FX et al: Quantitative brain magnetic resonance imaging in attention-deficit hyperactivity disorder, *Arch Gen Psychiatry* 53:607, 1996.

Chakrabarti S, Fombonne E: Pervasive developmental disorders in preschool children, *JAMA* 285(24):3093, 2001.

Cohen DJ, Volkmar FR: *Handbook of autism and pervasive developmental disorders,* ed 2, New York, 1997, Wiley.

Cook EH et al: Evidence of linkage between the serotonin transporter and autistic disorder, *Mol Psychiatry* 2:247, 1997.

Costello EJ et al: The Great Smoky Mountains study of youth: goals, design, methods, and the prevalence of DSM-III-R disorders, *Arch Gen Psychiatry* 53:1129, 1996.

DeVeaugh-Geiss J et al: Clomipramine hydrochloride in childhood and adolescent obsessive-compulsive disorder: a multicenter trial, *J Am Acad Child Adolesc Psychiatry* 31:45, 1992.

Faraone SV et al: Separation of DSM-III attention deficit disorder and conduct disorder: evidence from a family-genetic study of American child psychiatric patients, *Psychol Med* 21:109, 1991.

Giedd JN: Bipolar disorder attention-deficit/hyperactivity disorder in children and adolescents, *J Clin Psychiatry* 61:31, 2000.

Grados M, Scahill L, Riddle MA: Pharmacotherapy in children and adolescents with obsessive-compulsive disorder, *Child Adolesc Psychiatr Clin N Am* 8(3):617, 1999.

Greenhill LL et al: Medication treatment strategies in the MTA study: relevance to clinicians and researchers, *J Am Acad Child Adolesc Psychiatry* 35(10):1304, 1996.

Griest JH et al: Efficacy and tolerability of serotonin transport inhibitors in obsessive-compulsive disorder, *Arch Gen Psychiatry* 52:53, 1995.

Karno M et al: The epidemiology of obsessive-compulsive disorder in five US communities, *Arch Gen Psychiatry* 45:1094, 1988.

King RA et al: Emergence of self-destructive phenomena in children and adolescents during fluoxetine treatment, *J Am Acad Child Adolesc Psychiatry* 30:179, 1991.

Klein DN et al: A family study of major depressive disorder in a community sample of adolescents, *Arch Gen Psychiatry* 58(1):13, 2001.

Klein RG, Koplewicz HS, Kanner A: Imipramine treatment of children with separation anxiety, *J Am Acad Child Adolesc Psychiatry* 31:21, 1992.

Koenig K, Scahill L: Assessment of children with pervasive developmental disorders, *J Child Adolesc Psychiatr Nurs* 14(4):159, 2001.

Kovacs M: Presentation and course of major depressive disorder during childhood and later years of the life span, *J Amer Acad Child Adolesc Psychiatry* 35:705, 1996.

Kumra S et al: Case study: risperidone-induced hepatoxicity in pediatric patients, *J Am Acad Child Adolesc Psychiatry* 36:701, 1997.

Kurlan R et al: Prevalence of tics in schoolchildren and association with placement in special education, *Neurology* 57(8):1383, 2001.

Lavigne JV et al: Oppositional defiant disorder with onset in preschool years: longitudinal stability and pathways to other disorders. *J Am Acad Child Adolesc Psychiatry* 40:1393, 2001.

Leckman JF et al: Clonidine treatment of Gilles de la Tourette's syndrome, *Arch Gen Psychiatry* 48:324, 1991.

Levy F et al: Attention-deficit hyperactivity disorder: a category or a continuum? Genetic analysis of a large-scale twin study, *J Am Acad Child Adolesc Psychiatry* 36(6):737, 1997.

Lewinsohn PM, Klein DN, Seeley JR: Bipolar disorders in a community sample of older adolescents: prevalence, phenomenology, co-morbidity, and course, *J Am Acad Child Adolesc Psychiatry* 34:454, 1995.

Martin A, Kaufman J, Charney D: Pharmacotherapy of early-onset depression. Update and new directions, *Child Adolesc Psychiatric Clin of N Am* 9(1):135, 2000.

Merikangas KR, Angst J: The challenge of depressive disorders in adolescence. In Rutter M, editor: *Youth in the year 2000: psychological issues and interventions,* Cambridge, Mass, 1995, Cambridge University Press.

Mink JW: Neurobiology of basal ganglia circuits in Tourette syndrome: faulty inhibition of unwanted motor patterns? *Adv Neurol* 85:113, 2001.

The MTA Cooperative Group, Multimodal Treatment Study of Children with ADHD: A 14-month randomized clinical trial of treatment strategies for attention-deficit/hyperactivity disorder, *Arch Gen Psychiatry* 56(12):1073, 1999.

Mufson L et al: Efficacy of interpersonal psychotherapy for depressed adolescents, *Arch Gen Psychiatry* 56(6):573, 1999.

Pauls DL et al: A family study of Gilles de la Tourette syndrome, *Am J Hum Genet* 48:154, 1991.

Pennington BF: *Diagnosing learning disorders: a neuropsychological framework,* New York, 1991, Guilford Press.

Peterson BS et al: Tourette syndrome, tics, obsessions, and compulsions. In Leckman JF, Cohen DJ, editors: *Neuroanatomical circuitry tics, obsessions and compulsions, developmental psychopathology and clinical care,* New York: 1999, John Wiley & Sons.

Piacentini J: Cognitive behavioral therapy of childhood OCD, *Child Adolesc Psychiatr Clin N Am* 8(3):599, 1999.

Price RA et al: A twin study of Tourette syndrome, *Arch Gen Psychiatry* 42:815, 1985.

Rauch SL et al: Probing striato-thalamic function in obsessive-compulsive disorder and Tourette syndrome using neuroimaging methods, *Adv Neurol* 85:207, 2001.

Riddle MA et al: Obsessive-compulsive disorder in children and adolescents: phenomenology and family history, *J Am Acad Child Adolesc Psychiatry* 29(5):766, 1990.

Rosenbaum JF et al: Selective serotonin reuptake inhibitor discontinuation syndrome: a randomized clinical trial, *Biol Psychiatry* 44:77, 1998.

RUPP Anxiety Group: Fluvoxamine in the treatment of children and adolescents with anxiety disorders, *N Engl J Med,* 344(17):1279, 2001.

RUPP Autism Network: Risperidone in children with autism and serious behavior problems, *N Engl J Med,* in press.

Rutter M et al: Genetics and child psychiatry: II. Empirical research findings, *J Child Psychol Psychiatry* 40:19, 1999.

Satcher D: The history of the Public Health Service and the Surgeon General's priorities, *Food Drug Law J* 54(1):13, 1999.

Scahill L et al: A placebo-controlled study of guanfacine in the treatment of children with tic disorders and attention deficit hyperactivity disorder, *Am J Psychiatry* 158(7):1067, 2001.

Scahill L: Psychopharmacology for children. In Keltner NL, Folks DG, editors: *Psychotropic drugs,* ed 3, St Louis, 2000, Mosby.

Scahill L, DeGraft-Johnson A: Food allergies, asthma, and attention deficit hyperactivity disorder, *J Child Adolesc Psychiatr Nurs* 10(2):36, 1997.

Scahill L, Lynch KA: Atypical neuroleptics in children and adolescents, *J Child Adolesc Psychiatr Nurs* 11(1):38, 1998.

Scahill L, Skrypeck A: Traditional neuroleptics in children and adolescents, *J Child Adolesc Psychiatr Nurs* 10(3):41, 1997.

Scahill L, Tanner C, Dure L: Emotional and behavioral difficulties associated with Tourette syndrome, *Adv Neurol* 85:79, 2001.

Scahill L et al: Psychosocial and clinical correlates of ADHD in a community sample of young children, *J Am Acad Child Adolesc Psychiatry* 38(8):976, 1999.

Shaywitz SE et al: Prevalence of reading disability in boys and girls: results of the Connecticut longitudinal study, *JAMA* 264:998, 1990.

Singer HS et al: The treatment of attention-deficit hyperactivity disorder in Tourette's syndrome: a double-blind placebo-controlled study with clonidine and desipramine, *Pediatrics* 95:74, 1995.

Sparrow SS, Balla DA, Cicchetti DV: *Vineland adaptive behavior scales,* Circle Pines, Minn, 1983, American Guidance Clinic.

State MW et al: The genetics of childhood psychiatric disorders: a decade of progress, *J Am Acad Child Adolesc Psychiatry* 39(8):946, 2000.

Stevenson J: Evidence for a genetic etiology in hyperactivity in children, *Behav Genet* 22(3):337, 1992.

Swanson J, Volkow N: Pharmacokinetic and pharmacodynamic properties of methylphenidate in humans. In Solanto MV, Arnsten AFT, Castellanos FX, editors: *Stimulant drugs and ADHD. Basic and clinical neuroscience*, New York, 2001, Oxford University Press.

Szatmari P, Offord DR, Boyle MH: Correlates, associated impairments and patterns of service utilization of children with attention deficit disorder: findings from the Ontario Child Health Study, *J Child Psychol Psychiatry* 30:205, 1989.

Tourette's Syndrome Study Group: Treatment of ADHD in children with tics: a randomized controlled trial, *Neurology* 58:527, 2002.

Valleni-Basile LA et al: Frequency of obsessive-compulsive disorder in a community sample of young adolescents, *J Am Acad Child Adolesc Psychiatry* 33(6):782, 1994.

Vitiello B: Pediatric psychopharmacology and the interaction between drugs and the developing brain, *Can J Psychiatry* 43(6):582, 1998.

Walkup JT et al: Family study and segregation analysis of Tourette syndrome: evidence for a mixed model of inheritance, *Am J Hum Genet* 59:684, 1996.

Weller EB, Weller RA, Fristad MA: Bipolar disorder in children: misdiagnosis, underdiagnosis, and future directions, *J Am Acad Child Adolesc Psychiatry* 34:709, 1995.

Wolraich M et al: Comparison of diagnostic criteria for attention-deficit hyperactivity disorder, *J Am Acad Child Adolesc Psychiatry* 35:319, 1996.

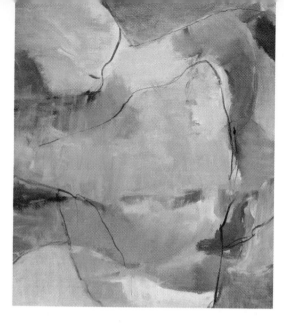

Chapter 43

Mental Disorders in Older Adults

Catherine S. Childers, MSN, RN

Learning Objectives

After reading this chapter, you should be able to:

- Describe the barriers to mental health care that exist for older adults.
- Describe the various treatment options and care settings available to older Americans.
- Identify the unique variations in symptoms of mental disorders evidenced by older adults.

- Identify major substance abuse issues in older adults.
- Recognize pharmacokinetic and pharmacodynamic changes in older adults that impact pharmacotherapy.
- Describe the psychologic assessment of older adults.
- Identify therapeutic goals for older adults.

INTRODUCTION

The U.S. Surgeon General warns that a crisis in geriatric mental health care is looming (U.S. Department of Health and Human Services [USDHHS], 1999). Currently, approximately 20% of older Americans experience mental disorders, and the National Institute of Mental Health (NIMH) projects 15 million older adults will need mental health services by the year 2030 (Administration on Aging [AoA], 2001c; NIMH, 1999a; USDHHS, 1999). This number includes individuals who experience mental disorders for the first time in late life and those whose early-onset psychiatric disorders persist as chronic or recurrent conditions. Mental disorders in older adults may have a clear biochemical basis or may be a reaction to stressors commonly occurring

in late adulthood. Regardless of cause, mental illness exacts a high toll in excess disability and disproportionate use of health care services.

Rapid growth in the older population is fueling interest in issues surrounding mental health and aging. In 1998, 12.7% of the U.S. population was over the age of 65. By the year 2030, the number of Americans over age 65 will account for 20% of the population. This segment will include 76 million aging members of the "baby boom" generation, a group that already has relatively high rates of anxiety, depression, schizophrenia, and substance abuse (AoA, 2001c). Life expectancy is also lengthening. By 2050, the number of Americans over age 85, known as the *old-old*, will increase fourfold or more, placing a significantly greater number of people at risk for mental disorders (National Institute on Aging [NIA], 2001). Box 43-1 provides an overview of the prevalence rates of selected psychiatric diagnoses in the current older population. The personal and economic consequences of mental disorders in this rapidly expanding cohort require heightened attention to the special mental health needs of older adults.

Modern culture, which tends to celebrate youth, has placed little emphasis on understanding old age. This unfortunate bias has contributed to insufficient knowledge about mental health disorders in the older population, as well as public policies that adversely affect access to care. Recent research has increased the ability of health care providers to dif-

ferentiate illness from normal aging and to identify differences between the clinical presentation and course of mental disorders in older adults and other age groups. Government agencies have joined together to investigate factors that influence older adults. A better understanding of the complex interplay of physical health, social factors, and emotional well being in older adults is leading to mental health strategies tailored for the special needs of this group.

Nurses involved in the care of older adults should be familiar with prevention, detection, and treatment strategies for mental disorders throughout the continuum of care. This chapter presents an overview of mental health issues in older adults that are different from those of other age groups. Stressors, policy issues, barriers to mental health care, and common mental disorders occurring in older adults are discussed along with assessment and psychotherapeutic management. Cognitive disorders, which account for some of the most frequently occurring mental disorders in older adults, are covered in Chapter 32.

Barriers

Psychiatric disorders may lead to or exacerbate coexisting physical conditions by impairing older adults' physiologic function, independence, and ability to rally social support (USDHHS, 1999). Studies indicate that only one half of older adults who acknowledge mental health problems receive any treatment, and only a fraction of those treated receive specialty mental health services (AoA, 2001c). The unmet treatment needs result from *patient barriers*, *provider barriers*, and *system-economic barriers*.

Patient barriers

Attitudes of older adults themselves serve as a barrier to seeking mental health care. Patients and families who subscribe to stereotypes about normal aging may delay seeking care if they believe that conditions such as depression or memory loss are a normal part of aging (USDHHS, 1999). Additionally, older individuals may be reluctant to seek psychiatric care because admitting mental health problems is seen as a weakness and is more stigmatizing than it might be for a younger person. Seeking psychiatric care may also represent a loss of control and elicit fear of institutionalization. Furthermore, when outside help is required, people who grew up in an

Box 43-1 | One-Year Prevalence Rates Age 55+ Based on Data from Epidemiologic Catchment Area

	Prevalence (%)
Any Anxiety Disorder	11.4
Simple Phobia	7.3
Social Phobia	1.0
Agoraphobia	4.1
Panic Disorder	0.5
Obsessive-Compulsive Disorder	1.5
Any Mood Disorder	4.4
Major Depressive Episode	3.8
Unipolar Major Depression	3.7
Dysthymia	1.6
Bipolar I	0.2
Bipolar II	0.1
Schizophrenia	0.6
Somatization	0.3

Adapted from U.S. Department of Health and Human Services: *Mental health: a report of the Surgeon General*, Rockville, MD, 1999; U.S. Department of Health and Human Services, Substance Abuse and Mental Health Services Administration, Center for Mental Health Services, National Institutes of Health, National Institute of Mental Health.

era that emphasized self-reliance are more likely to rely on family, friends, and other informal supports than they are on mental health professionals who are often viewed with skepticism.

Provider barriers

Older adults are more likely to receive care from primary care physicians than they are from geriatric specialty providers. Despite the rapid growth in the over-65 population and recognition of their unique needs, geriatric specialists (e.g., geriatricians, geropsychiatrists, geriatric nurse specialists) are scarce. Only 23% of baccalaureate nursing programs incorporate a required course in geriatric nursing, limiting nurses' preparation for providing care to older adults (American Association of Colleges of Nursing [AACN], 2000; Rosenfeld et al, 1999). Nurses and other health care providers who are not attuned to the complexities of geriatric care may miss opportunities to identify mental health disorders or predisposing factors.

Accurate assessment and diagnosis requires familiarity with diagnostic tools such as the Geriatric Depression Scale found in this text. Furthermore, individuals working with older adults must recognize that mental disorders may be expressed through somatic complaints and that symptoms of co-morbid physical problems may compound the difficulty of diagnosing a mental disorder. An additional complication is physician reluctance to diagnose those mental disorders identified for fear of stigmatizing their geriatric patients (Tune, 2001).

Ageism, the negative stereotyping and devaluation of people solely because of their age, is also a significant barrier. The National Coalition on Mental Health and Aging (1994) defines ageism as the stereotypical view that mental health problems are part of the aging process. To serve older adults effectively, professionals must be attentive to their biases and stereotypes and increase their geriatric-specific knowledge.

System-economic barriers

Diagnosis of psychiatric disorders in geriatric patients consumes time and resources not covered by reimbursement rates. This and other funding issues, along with a lack of collaboration and coordination among primary care, mental health, and aging services providers, thwart the provision and receipt of adequate mental health care for older adults (AoA, 2001c). The cost of mental health care has been a major disincentive to providers, as well as older adults who might otherwise seek psychiatric assistance. Historically, insurers, including federally funded Medicare and Medicaid, have placed severe limits on reimbursement for mental health care. Some insurers, including the growing number of Medicare replacement Health Maintenance Organizations (HMOs), exclude mental health and substance-abuse treatment altogether. Only in the last few years has legislative effort addressed parity in mental health coverage. Nonetheless, financing policies furnish incentives that favor use of some services over others or preclude the provision of needed services (USDHHS, 1999). Mental health services are highly fragmented, and individuals who seek treatment are stymied by a lack of information about where to go for effective and affordable services. Case management programs are being introduced to coordinate services and reduce costs.

> **Critical Thinking Question**
>
> Many older adults have no insurance coverage to offset the high cost of prescription medications. How might this affect compliance?

CONTINUUM OF CARE

Because of the prevalence and profound negative consequences of mental disorders in late life, nurses who encounter older adults in any setting should consider their physical, social, and emotional needs. Whenever possible, factors that place older adults at risk for mental disorders or problems stemming from mental illness should be identified and plans developed to meet the needs.

Prevention

A balance of physical, social, and emotional functioning contributes to mental health. Many of the changes that accompany advancing age affect this balance, increasing older adults' vulnerability to mental disorders. A primary stressful event (e.g., broken hip [physical]) may lead to secondary stressors (e.g., emotional isolation). Health problems, acute and chronic, may lead to dependence, relocation, isolation, and financial hardship. A closer examination of these consequences may prove enlightening.

Dependence: Loss of independence, even temporarily, is terribly threatening in a person's later years because having to rely on others might signal a continued dependency.

Relocation: Moving from familiar surroundings to a new environment is also threatening. To many older individuals, familiar surroundings represent a connection to all that is important in life. Additionally, the related changes can be overwhelming for some individuals with limited adaptive capacity.

Isolation: Most older individuals have fewer meaningful connections than they had in earlier life. Death, a mobile society, and estrangements are but a few reasons for this reality. Health care–related isolation can be particularly devastating for some older adults.

Financial hardship: Although many older individuals are financially secure, a significant number find unexpected medical expenses to be difficult or even impossible to meet on a fixed income. Most older adults have little, if any, ability to increase their income to meet additional unplanned expenses.

Adaptive mechanisms: Meaning, control, support

Losses common in the late years of life are listed in Box 43-2 and often precede the onset of mental disorders in older adults. Despite numerous inevitable changes, the majority of older adults adjust well and express a high degree of satisfaction with life (USDHHS, 1999). Exposure and adaptation to stressors varies with each older adult's economic and social resources, physical status, ethnicity, gender, and life experiences (AoA, 2001c). Successful adaptation is enhanced by the ability to give meaning to experiences. Part of this process is comparing problems with

| Box 43-2 | Losses that Occur More Frequently Among Older Adults |

Loss of health
Loss of loved ones
Loss of hearing and vision
Loss of status
Loss of work
Loss of income
Loss of friends
Loss of cognitive skills
Loss of home and community
Loss of mobility

what is experienced and expected by others who are the same age (Federal Interagency Forum on Aging [FIFA], 2000). This observation may account for 72% of older Americans reporting their health as good to excellent despite multiple coexisting medical conditions and impairments (FIFA, 2000). As one sage elder noted, at some point, simply being alive can be seen as a sign of good health. This coping skill is especially helpful when the stressor, such as a chronic health problem, is not easily modified.

Another adaptive mechanism that assists older adults to cope with stressful events is the use of mastery—the sense of ability to exercise control over circumstances. For this reason, unplanned stressors may be experienced as more negative than are planned ones. For example, adequate planning for the social and financial implications of retirement significantly affects adjustment to this major life change. Nurses can reinforce mastery by encouraging the older person's participation in care decisions.

Support systems (i.e., family, friends, private and government organizations) are valuable sources of emotional support and aid and are important predictors of physical and mental health and delayed institutionalization (FIFA, 2000). Measures that contribute to physical health and promote social functioning are important components of preventing mental disorders in older adults. Improved health care and programs developed to target older adults' needs have resulted in declines in the rates of disability and poverty, which are key indicators of well being in older adults, reported by the AoA.

Caregiver training and transportation

Enactment of the Older Americans Act Amendments of 2000 led to funding of programs to meet the special needs of an aging population. For example, The National Family Caregiver Support Program provides training, counseling, and respite for the caregivers of older adults, a group at risk for depression (AoA, 2001a). Another example is The National Aging Network and Transportation Assistance program, established to address transportation needs (AoA, 2001b). Lack of transportation has been cited as a factor in isolation and is a barrier to accessing health care. Nurses play a key role in illness prevention by providing information about mental health and available resources at sites where older adults are likely to visit.

Local Area Agency on Aging

The government section of the telephone book contains the number for a local Area Agency on Aging (AAA). This organization is a valuable resource for older adults and their caregivers who often have difficulty initiating a search or negotiating access to care.

Critical Thinking Questions

If you have had the opportunity to meet the caregiver of an older person with a mental disorder, were both the patient and the caregiver participants in decision making? Did the caregiver treat the patient in the way you would want to be treated in that situation? Describe both the positive and the negative aspects of nurse-patient-caregiver interactions.

Detection

Measures that promote early detection of mental disorders in older adults include increasing public awareness of mental health issues, encouraging collaboration among service providers, and increased training of health professionals. Public education that emphasizes symptoms of mental disorders and treatment options does much to dispel the myths and stigma surrounding mental illness and empowers older adults to seek treatment. The gatekeeper program is an example of the effectiveness of enhanced community involvement. Public service workers such as grocery clerks, postal employees, and public utility workers are recruited and trained to identify and report vulnerable elders (Warren, 1999). Nurses in all settings can contribute to early detection by assessing and reporting stressors and symptoms.

Treatment Sites

Federal legislation has strongly influenced care of older adults who have mental disorders. The Community Mental Health Act of 1963 initiated deinstitutionalization, resulting in a large number of individuals with severe and persistent mental disorders (SPMD) being discharged from state and county mental hospitals to less restrictive settings. Many discharged older adults were placed in nursing homes where inappropriate and inadequate care, including excessive use of physical and chemical restraints, led to the passage of the Nursing Home Reform Act, known as the Omnibus Reconciliation Act of 1987

(OBRA). This legislation set stringent limits on the use of physical restraints and established guidelines for psychotropic drug use that influence drug selection, dosing, and duration of treatment. In addition, to prevent nursing home placement for those who need psychiatric care in hospital or community programs, OBRA requires preadmission screening for all individuals with suspected mental disorders. Nursing home residents whose only need for nursing care stems from mental disorders are discharged. Nonetheless, 89% of institutionalized older people with SPMD now live in nursing homes (USDHHS, 1999). Most of these residents do not receive adequate psychiatric treatment because of a lack of mental health training for nursing home staff and inadequate Medicare and Medicaid funding to cover behavioral health care (AoA, 2001c; Shea, Russo, Smyer, 2000).

The majority of older adults with SPMD live in the community, also with unmet needs. Currently, only a small percentage of community mental health centers have staff or services that target the needs of older adults, and primary care physicians are ill prepared and typically too rushed to treat mental disorders adequately (USDDHS, 1999). When care is provided, it is not uncommon for older adults to receive inappropriate psychotropic medication (USDHHS, 1999). Community-based mental health service needs will continue to increase as institutionalization continues to decline. The AoA (2001c) has identified numerous opportunities for improvement in community services and stresses the need for enhanced collaboration among the mental health system, primary care providers, and the aging network. Among the service needs are *mental health outreach programs* to identify high-risk individuals, ensure appropriate referrals, and provide supportive services to increase functioning. *Adult day services* designed for functionally impaired older adults provide opportunities for health monitoring and intensive intervention. *Respite care and caregiver programs* benefit both patients and their families. Professionally guided *support groups* and *self-help groups* led by mental health consumers or family members may also be beneficial for older adults and their caregivers. Participation reduces feelings of isolation, increases knowledge, and promotes coping efforts (USDHHS, 1999). Opportunities for nursing involvement abound.

PSYCHOPATHOLOGY IN OLDER ADULTS

Unit Six of this text provides an in-depth review of diagnostic classifications. This section is meant to supplement this information by detailing unique information on the presentation, course, and treatment of mental disorders in older adults. It is important for nurses in all practice areas to note that treating older adults with mental disorders benefits overall health by improving functional ability and compliance with health care instructions.

DEPRESSION

As in other age groups, depression in older adults may result from psychosocial stress, biochemical changes, co-morbid medical conditions, pharmaceutical agents, or a combination of factors. The effects of depression extend beyond well-known and emotionally distressing symptoms such as sadness, worthlessness, hopelessness, helplessness, fear, shame, and guilt. Less obvious effects include diminished social, cognitive, and physical functioning along with increased mortality. This constellation of effects exacts an enormous personal and economic toll. Inadequate detection and treatment adds to the burden.

Despite the fact that depression in older adults responds to the same interventions as those used in other age groups, nearly two thirds of older adults with depression do not get treatment, and treatment is thought to be adequate for only 11% of those who do receive care (NIMH, 2001; USDHHS, 1999). The cost of health care for depressed patients is up to twice that of their elderly undepressed counterparts, the result of more medical hospitalizations, physician and emergency room visits, drug use, and often unnecessary tests and procedures (Campbell et al, 2000). In a global comparison of disease burden, depression ranked second only to ischemic heart disease in years of life lost to disability or death. In other words, depression has a disabling effect equivalent to blindness or paraplegia (National Institutes of Health [NIH], 2001).

Incidence

The prevalence of late-life depression varies tremendously among reported studies. The rate of major depression diagnosed using the *Diagnostic and Statistical Manual of Mental Disorders-fourth edition, text revision* (DSM-IV-TR) criteria declines with age, but depressive symptoms increase (Forsell, Winblad, 1999). Table 43-1 demonstrates this trend and the increased risk for women over men. Rates for major depression increase in a linear fashion from 2% to 5% in community dwellers, to 5% to 10% in primary care settings, to 6% to 14% of medically ill elders (Kayton, 2001). The co-occurrence of depression exacerbates the course of other diagnoses.

Presentation

Many factors complicate the detection of depression. Depression in older adults frequently does not align neatly with current DSM-IV-TR criteria, and many depressive symptoms can be attributed to physical causes in individuals with concurrent medical illnesses. Older adults are more likely to present with memory disturbance or somatic complaints than they are with the feelings associated with depression for which younger patients seek care. Older adults also may lack the range of vocabulary younger individuals commonly possess to describe emotions. Rather than expressions of sadness, diminished self-esteem, irritability, or apathy, for example, older adults are more likely to complain of "having the blues" or "feeling worthless." Cultural

| Table 43-1 | Percentage of Noninstitutionalized Persons, Age 65 and Older, with Severe Depressive Symptoms (1998) |

	Total	Men	Women
65 to 69	15.4	12.1	18.0
70 to 74	14.3	10.3	17.2
75 to 79	14.6	10.4	17.4
80 to 84	20.5	17.1	22.4
85 or older	22.8	22.5	23.0

Source: Federal Interagency Forum on Aging-Related Statistics: *Older Americans 2000: key indicators of well-being Appendix A: detailed tables.* Available at http:www.agingstats.gov/tables%202001/tables-healthstatus. html#Indicator%2016

competence demands that professionals recognize differences in expression common to ethnic and cultural subgroups within the older population as well.

In addition to diagnostic barriers already discussed, the connection between medical conditions and depression complicates diagnosis. It is difficult to determine whether common physical indicators of depression in older adults, including weight loss, fatigue, insomnia, constipation, and multiple vague aches and pains, are the result of a mood disorder or symptoms of a medical problem. The DSM-IV-TR diagnosis of "Mood Disorder Due to a General Medical" can be given when mood symptoms are a direct physiologic consequence of medical conditions (American Psychiatric Association [APA], 2000). For example, depression coexists in 11% to 57% of patients with dementia and accounts for greater deficits than can be attributed to the primary diagnosis alone (Kales et al, 1999). If depression *followed* the diagnosis of a catastrophic illness such as Parkinson's disease, however, another DSM-IV-TR diagnosis would be pursued.

Although depression is caused by a medical illness in some cases, in other cases depression causes physiologic changes that enhance susceptibility to disease. (See Chapter 29 for tables detailing drugs and physical illnesses commonly associated with depression.) Depression adversely affects endocrine, neurologic, and immune processes by increasing sympathetic tone, decreasing vagal tone, and causing immunosuppression (Penninx et al, 1999). People with depression are more likely to smoke, drink alcohol excessively, be physically inactive, and have poorer eating habits than those who are not depressed. These changes and health habits may be factors in depression as a predictor of coronary artery disease and diabetes and the increased risk of death following myocardial infarctions (Creed, 1999; Kayton, 2001).

Because of the shared cognitive symptoms of depression and dementia, misdiagnosis of dementia occurs frequently. Depression that mimics dementia is termed *pseudodementia*. Shared symptoms include poor memory, disorientation, poor judgment, and agitation or motor retardation. In addition to psychologic tests, nursing observations can be critical to correcting misdiagnosis. Nurses should assess for higher functioning than that expected in dementia and can also look for a downcast mood that can help distinguish depression from the blander affect of true dementia. Differentiating these disorders is important for treatment. Psychotic depression may also be confused with cognitive or other psychiatric disorders. When depression occurs for the first time after age 60, delusions are more common than they are with early-onset depression. Delusions of persecution or of having an incurable illness, as well as nihilistic delusions, are more frequent than are delusions associated with guilt (Blazer, Koenig, 1996). Hallucinations, however, are an uncommon feature of psychotic depression. Many older adults with psychotic depression may ruminate, express suspiciousness, and voice multiple physical complaints. Psychotic depression is often resistant to traditional antidepressant medications and psychotherapy. As a result, electroconvulsive therapy (ECT) is frequently used in treatment.

Electroconvulsive Therapy

ECT is often the treatment of choice for severe depression in older adults, especially those who are poor candidates for drug therapy or have failed to respond to other treatments. ECT offers a rapid response that is necessary when patients are suicidal or in danger of medical crisis. The safety and efficacy of ECT have been demonstrated for all age groups, including the old-old (Tew et al, 1999). Chapter 39 provides a thorough review of the topic.

Misinformation and the sigma of ECT may discourage patients and their families from providing consent. Nurses should be sensitive to this barrier and provide factual information to dispel myths. After ECT, some older adults, particularly those with cognitive disorders, develop delirium or exhibit persistent confusion (Kelly, Zisselman, 2000). During this time, the nurse must take precautions to promote physical and emotional well being.

Suicide

Older Americans are disproportionately more likely to commit suicide, the most serious and tragic consequence of missed or under-treated depression. Several studies have found that 70% of older adults who commit suicide have visited a primary care physician within a month (NIMH, 2001). Older adults comprise only 13% of the population but account for 19% of reported suicides. Table 43-2 demonstrates that the incidence of suicide increases

Table 43-2	Rate of Suicide Among Older Adults (Rates per 100,000 Population Based on 1997 Data)
55-64 years old	13.5
65-74 years old	14.4
75-84 years old	19.3
85 years old and over	20.8
White men over 85 years old	65.0
Average rate across the life span	10.6

Hoyert DL, Kochanek KD, Murphey SL: Deaths: final data for 1997, *National Vital Statistical Report* 47(19), USDHHS Publication no. 99-1120, Hyattsville, Md, 1999, National Center for Health Statistics.

with age and that Caucasian men over age 65 have the highest rate of all. Suicidal gestures and impulsiveness, more common among young adults, are rare in older adults. Although women attempt suicide more frequently than do men, men have a higher suicide attempt-to-completion ratio. Women are more likely than are men to attempt suicide by overdose, while men are more likely than women to use highly lethal means. Despite these statistics, firearms were the most common method of suicide by both men and women 65 years and older, accounting for 78.0% of male and 34.8% of female suicides (NIMH, 1999b). In older adults, failed attempts are usually not a "cry for help"; rather, they are a serious yet unsuccessful suicide bid.

The rate of suicide may be even higher than is reported because statistics do not include chronic suicide. This term characterizes death caused by slower, less obvious means than are the abrupt acts usually associated with suicide. Refusing to eat, noncompliance with medication, excessive alcohol intake, and physical risk taking may result in death but are not recorded as suicide (Butler, Lewis, 1995). Depression is a strong predictor of patients' decisions to support euthanasia or forego life-sustaining treatment (Blank et al, 2001). Suicide does not always arise from depression. For some individuals who face life-threatening illness, suicide is the ultimate means of exercising control over the situation. "Rational" or physician-assisted suicide is an area of great concern to society, practitioners, and legal decision-makers.

Suicide prevention begins with the detection of risk (Box 43-3). It is important for nurses to listen to the themes of conversation and observe for signs that may signal suicidal risk or thoughts. Particular attention should be given to older individuals who are beginning to recover from depression: as energy

Box 43-3	Predictors of Suicide Risk in Older Adults
Over 65 years of age
Male
White
Chronic or uncontrolled pain
Bereavement
Unmarried (widowed or divorced)
Social isolation
Retirement
Financial difficulty
Hopeless or helpless
Alcohol or drug abuse
History of previous attempt
Major depressive disorder, particularly psychotic depression or depression that is due to a general medical condition

returns, the risk of suicide increases. Intent might be signaled by a new preoccupation with religious issues, giving away possessions, changing a will, or other new behaviors. People may feel ashamed to plainly voice ideas of self-harm, so if negative statements or behaviors are detected, it is essential to ask directly about any intentions. The notion that these discussions can stir suicidal thought is a myth.

CLINICAL EXAMPLE
Mr. White is an 86-year-old Caucasian who has outlived two wives. Mr. White has remained sexually active into his 80s, but within the last 2 years, he has had difficulty attaining an erection. Mr. White relates that a younger woman (mid-50s) recently asked about spending the night. She did, and Mr. White was unable to perform sexually. He said, "I'm just no good anymore." Mr. White said he was embarrassed by his sexual dysfunction. He states that he has had thoughts of suicide but would not act on them. He promises the nurse that he will call if he has an urge to harm himself.

CLINICAL EXAMPLE
Mr. Timchuk is a 77-year-old Caucasian with chronic obstructive pulmonary disease (COPD). He has great difficulty doing any physical activity. Mr. Timchuk is very despondent over his condition, and there is little hope that he will improve. Although he has not verbalized a desire to "end it all," he states that he would be better off dead. The nurse understands that he is at great risk for self-harm.

MANIC EPISODES

Manic symptoms in older adults may be associated with bipolar disorder, medical and neurologic conditions, substance abuse, or medication. In older adults, bipolar disorder accounts for 5% to 19% of mood disorders, most often as a recurrence of an existing disorder (Cassano et al, 2000). Late-onset bipolar disorder is defined as cases in which symptoms first occur after age 40. Differences between early- and late-onset bipolar disorder suggest that they may be different subforms of manic-depressive illness (Schurhoff et al, 2000). Affective disorders are less common in first-degree relatives of those with late onset than in those with earlier onset (Cassano et al, 2000; Schurhoff et al, 2000). Late-onset bipolar disorder is generally less severe with fewer and milder manic symptoms compared with early-onset bipolar disorder. Features may include grandiosity, disorientation, euphoria, or irritability. Secondary mania is the term used to describe manic symptoms associated with medical conditions or drugs. A substantial proportion of new-onset manic symptoms in older adults is associated with cerebral disorders or injuries and may run a bipolar course, with intervening periods of euthymia (Snowdon, 2000). Nursing interventions must address the negative impact of agitation and distractibility on self-care and self-protection in older adults.

CLINICAL EXAMPLE

The local police department's community service officer brought Ms. Ellington, a 72-year-old Caucasian, to the hospital. She was found sitting outside a homeless shelter surrounded by boxes of personal belongings, drinking orange juice that had a strong odor of alcohol. She wore tight animal print leggings, a transparent blouse, and thigh-high white boots. A decorated wide-brim hat covered her sparse flame-red hair. On admission, Ms. Ellington was cursing loudly and threw her dentures at the first staff person who approached. Although she was well known to the staff, Ms. Ellington claimed that she was a Hollywood star who had been kicked out of her own mansion by friends, robbed of identification, and shipped to this city where she would be unknown. In fact, according to police, she had been evicted from several shelters for disruptive behavior. An empty bottle of lithium and an unfilled prescription for more were found in her purse.

PSYCHOTIC DISORDERS

Psychotic disorders, characterized by delusions, hallucinations, disordered thoughts, bizarre behavior, or other evidence of impaired reality testing, are among the most severe psychiatric disorders. Symptoms often contribute to the institutionalization of older adults. Active psychosis is as disabling as quadriplegia on the disability component of the Disability Adjusted Life Years (DALYs) measure (NIMH, 2001). Nurses should be familiar with the numerous physical conditions and medications associated with psychosis in older adults (Box 43-4). A comprehensive assessment, including the nature and content of delusions and hallucinations, can facilitate identification of reversible causes and contribute to the accurate diagnosis necessary for determining the most effective course of treatment.

Schizophrenia

Although generally regarded as an illness with onset in late adolescence or early adulthood, symptoms first occur after age 40 in approximately 23.5% of all patients with schizophrenia, with a high female-to-male ratio (Howard et al, 2000). Two classifications are being investigated: *late-onset* schizophrenia (after age 40) and *very-late-onset* (after age 60) (Howard et al, 2000). Late-onset and typical early-onset schizophrenia share some characteristics, including severe positive symptoms (delusions, hallucinations, bizarre or disorganized behavior, impaired communication) and a chronic course. Late-onset patients are more likely than their earlier-onset counterparts to present with bizarre, persecutory delusions; visual, tactile, and olfactory hallucinations; and accusatory or abusive auditory hallucinations (Howard et al, 2000; McClure, Gladsjo, Jeste, 1999). Disorganization and negative symptoms (withdrawal, apathy, and anhedonia) are less prominent than they are in early onset. A majority of individuals diagnosed with schizophrenia late in life have abnormal premorbid personality traits but, compared with persons with early-onset schizophrenia, are more likely to have better employment and marital histories. For many individuals, late-onset schizophrenia marks the beginning of a chronic disorder with periods of remission and symptom recurrence. The insidious deterioration of personality and social adjustment characteristic of early-onset schizophrenia also occurs; however, cognitive declines are no faster in

| Box 43-4 | Disorders Associated with Psychosis in the Older Adult Population

Neurological disorders	**Endocrinopathies**	**Differential diagnosis**
Parkinson's disease	Hyper/hypothyroidism	Psychotic disorder that is due to a general medical condition
Alzheimer's disease	Hyper/hypoparathyroidism	Delirium
Pick's disease	Addison's disease	Dementia with delusions and hallucinations
Diffuse Lewy body disease	Cushing's disease	Mood disorder with psychotic features
Vascular dementia	Hypoglycemia	Delusional disorder
Seizure disorders		Psychosis secondary to substance abuse or dependence
Hydrocephalus	**Vitamin deficiencies**	Brief reactive psychosis
Demyelinating diseases	Thiamine, niacin, B_{12}, folate	Psychosis not otherwise specified or schizophreniform disorder
Neoplasms		Schizophrenia
Encephalopathies	**Other conditions**	
Neurosyphyllis	Iatrogenic (secondary to drugs)	
Spinocerebellar degeneration	Lupus	
	Alcohol intake or withdrawal	
	Temporal arteritis	
	Hyponatremia	
	Delirium	

Jeste DV, Harris MJ, and Paulsen JS: Psychosis. In Sadavoy J et al, editors: *Comprehensive review of geriatric psychiatry-II*, ed 2, Washington, DC, 1996, American Psychiatric Press; McClure FS, Gladsjo JA, Jeste DV: Late-onset psychosis: clinical, research, and ethical considerations, *Am J Psychiatry* 156(6):935, 1999.

older noninstitutionalized patients with schizophrenia than they are in normal comparison subjects (Zorrilla et al, 2000). In all age groups, antipsychotic medications are an effective treatment for many of the positive symptoms, especially when coupled with a structured environment (milieu), including social skills training and supportive nurse-patient interactions. Very late–onset cases of schizophrenia may arise in the context of sensory impairment and social isolation, thus nursing actions aimed at remediation in these areas is essential (Howard, 2000).

Research documenting the long-term course of schizophrenia is extremely limited, however, many chronic schizophrenic patients reach late life in spite of the high mortality associated with chronic early-onset schizophrenia. Mortality is associated with a high risk of suicide and medical problems, often related to co-morbid substance abuse—especially nicotine dependence. Emphysema and other pulmonary and cardiac problems are common. The increase of movement disorders in older patients treated with traditional antipsychotics complicates medical management, increases the degree of disability associated with the disorder, and contributes to the high cost of services for elderly patients with schizophrenia.

A study of treatment costs and mental health service use by age cohorts suggests that older people with schizophrenia continue to use inpatient or institutional services more than they do community mental health organizations (Cuffel et al, 1996). Long-term institutionalization poses problems of learned dependence and decreases in problem-solving and coping skills. The negative symptoms of schizophrenia also contribute to impaired social functioning, which includes areas such as social appropriateness and grooming (Patterson et al, 2001). Nurses should note that older schizophrenic patients, especially those who are returned to the community after long-term institutionalization, might have significant deficits in daily living skills and lack the social networks that are important to successful adaptation. Thus these individuals have a high need for daily living services. Caregivers should emphasize problem-solving skills and interventions that promote social functioning.

CLINICAL EXAMPLE

Ms. Auger is a 68-year-old Caucasian brought to the hospital by her sister with whom she lives. She accuses her sister of forcing her into the hospital so the sister can steal her money and car. The sister can recall no recent major stressor or signs of physical illness. She states that Ms. Auger has no history of psychiatric symptoms, but has always been a "loner." Despite

Continued

obtaining a college degree, she had a stormy employment history because she was "unable to get along" with co-workers. She also was unable to sustain a long-term relationship with any man she dated. Ms. Auger's appearance is evidence of her inattention to dress and grooming. Although cooperative with examination, her mood is dysphoric, and she has a flat affect. She admits to auditory hallucinations, particularly voices of people she knows, often conversing with each other. The voices tell her they will steal from her, and they sometimes tell her to hurt herself.

A complete evaluation resulted in a diagnosis of schizophrenia. The geropsychiatrist ordered Zyprexa (olanzapine) 2.5 mg q hs.

Paranoid Thinking

Paranoid symptoms are not uncommon in older adults. Delusions are generally chronic and well systematized and, unless associated with dementia or delirium, are not associated with memory loss, disorientation, or diminished cognitive function (Koenig et al, 1996). Paranoia may be a feature of depression, occur after a stressful life event, or result from delirium or some other mental disorder. The content often involves persecution, jealousy, or unusual situations that may conceivably occur in real life. For example, delusional jealousy, often involving allegations of infidelity, is strongly associated with dementia (Sibisi, 1999). It is important to investigate actual facts before labeling beliefs as delusional because patients may relate bizarre tales that have a basis in reality. Because coping behaviors are compromised with age, paranoid thinking often emerges as a defense mechanism against a potentially hostile environment. Walking to the corner store in some neighborhoods may be perilous for older individuals because they are less able than are younger people to fend off aggressors. A retreat into an environment that the fearful elder can control results in increasing isolation. Although the threat may be based on reality, the resulting isolation and decrease in external stimuli, along with suspicious behaviors, can lead to paranoid thinking.

CLINICAL EXAMPLE

Mrs. Justice is a 81-year-old African American referred to the community mental health center by her primary care physician for treatment of psychosis. The neatly attired and spry woman tearfully relates that "haunts" have been breaking into her house at night, stealing money and other possessions. She sees the ghostly apparitions at least once a month, and when they appear, they speak to her, most often saying, "You stay out of the way, old woman, or we'll get you!" Before initiating pharmacologic intervention, a nurse practitioner conducted a home visit and found Mrs. Justice's home in disarray. Broken windows, gaps where kitchen appliances had been removed, and other findings led the nurse to request a police investigation. On the first night of their home surveillance, police arrested two young men dressed in white sheets who were hiding behind high shrubbery in front of the house. Interventions that were social rather than pharmacologic were instituted. (This actual case is an example of the way in which cultural awareness and careful investigation prevented subsequent inappropriate diagnosis and treatment.)

ANXIETY DISORDERS

The prevalence of anxiety disorders is the highest of all mental disorders in older adults. Little research specifically addresses anxiety symptoms and syndromes in older adults, perhaps because epidemiologic data reveal lower rates of anxiety disorders in community-dwelling older adults compared with younger groups (Lenze et al, 2000; USDHHS, 1999). As with other mental disorders, most anxiety disorders do not begin in later life but are a recurrence or worsening of a preexisting condition (Lang, Stein, 2001). Cognitive, behavioral, somatic, and physiologic symptoms are similar to those of other age groups (Box 43-5).

Many older adults have symptoms of anxiety that fail to meet diagnostic criteria for an anxiety disorder. As many as 23% to 38% of older adults with depression also experience anxiety, sometimes at a level that meets DSM-IV-TR criteria for generalized anxiety disorder, panic disorder, or a phobia (Lenze et al, 2000). Generalized anxiety disorder in conjunction with depression results in increased severe depressive symptoms, including suicidal ideation. As with other disorders, an increase in somatic symptoms and a decrease in social functioning may occur (Lenze et al, 2000). Two anxiety disorders defined in the DSM-IV-TR may be overrepresented in older adults. *Anxiety Due to a General Medical Condition* is a commonly used diagnosis resulting from the frequency of anxiety related cardiovascular, endocrine, respiratory, and neurologic

| Box 43-5 | Signs and Symptoms of Anxiety

Gastrointestinal or genitourinary symptoms	Musculoskeletal
Abdominal Pain	Backache
Anorexia	Fatigue
"Butterflies"	Muscle tension
Dry mouth	Tremulous
Diarrhea	**Neurologic**
Nausea	Dizziness or faintness
Urinary frequency	Parasthesia
Vomiting	**Psychologic**
Cardiovascular symptoms	Apprehensive
Chest discomfort	Compulsive
Diaphoresis	Fearful
Dyspnea	Feelings of dread
Flushing	Irritable
Hyperventilation	Intolerant
Pallor	Panicky
Palpitations	Phobic
Tachycardia	Preoccupied
	Tense or worried

Adapted from Keltner N, Folks D: *Psychotropic drugs*, ed 3, St Louis, 2001, Mosby.

disorders in this age group (Keltner, Folks, 2001). *Substance-induced anxiety disorder* may be present in as many as 10% of community-dwelling older adults and 40% of nursing home residents, a consequence of substance abuse and dependence, as well as toxicity from prescription drugs (Folks, Fuller, 1997). The relationship between stressful life events and losses are unknown at this time; however, they may play a significant role in late-life anxiety. For example, fear of crime and fear of dying are two specific phobias that are likely to occur in older adults. Although anxiety is a normal emotion that alerts a person to impending danger or an unpleasant event, it can be considered maladaptive when it interferes with functioning (Sheikh, 1996).

SUBSTANCE ABUSE

Substance abuse and dependence place older adults at tremendous risk of negative physical, psychologic, and social consequences but often goes undetected. Late-life alcohol and drug use and dependence are problems that have received little attention until recent years, thus a great deal is yet to be learned about geriatric specific prevention, detection, and treatment options. Estimates of the current prevalence of alcohol abuse in older adults vary widely

from 1% to 15% (Blow, 2000; USDHHS, 1999). These numbers are expected to increase rapidly as a result of aging "baby boomers" who have a greater history of alcohol abuse than do the current older cohort. Similar expansion is expected with illicit drug use, currently a problem for only 0.1% of older adults (USDDH, 1999). A larger problem is the frequent misuse of prescription and over-the-counter (OTC) drugs, sometimes to the point that it can be characterized as drug abuse. It is important for nurses to understand factors that contribute to substance abuse and recognize presenting symptoms and potential consequences. Unless nurses and other health care providers recognize the serious problems that alcohol and prescription drugs pose for older adults and take measures to intervene, quality of life is diminished, independence compromised, and physical deterioration is accelerated.

Alcohol Abuse and Dependence

Alcohol abuse and dependence may occur for the first time in late life or may represent an unresolved problem from earlier life. More men than women approach late life with problem drinking, and although men represent the majority of older people who abuse alcohol, late-onset alcohol abuse is more common in women than it is in men (Blow, 2000; Ludwick et al, 2000). A number of risk factors have been identified for late-onset problematic drinking. The presence of chronic medical disorders and sleep disturbances may lead some older people to self-medicate with alcohol to control pain or induce sleep. Some isolated older adults or those with excessive leisure time use drinking to combat boredom or loneliness. Individuals who have lost a spouse are particularly at risk (Byrne, Raphael, Arnold, 1999). For some individuals, alcohol is seen as a means of decreasing or escaping the emotional distress of psychiatric disorders. When an alcohol-use disorder is associated with another mental disorder, the term *dual diagnosis* is used. Affective and organic mental disorders most frequently coexist with alcoholism in older adults, however, anxiety disorders and schizophrenia are also related.

Older adults' problematic alcohol use is often minimized or undetected by health care providers. Older adults often under report consumption, the result of impaired recall, guilt, or shame. Social stigma is especially strong in older women who are more likely than men to drink secretly at home and make efforts to conceal their drinking behavior (Ludwick et al, 2000). Along with assessment of the quantity of alcohol consumed, physiologic changes that occur with aging, medications, and certain conditions (e.g., cognitive disorders) that intensify alcohol's effects must be considered. Older people show greater central nervous system sensitivity to alcohol than younger drinkers, thus adverse effects on cognition and coordination will be more pronounced by comparison. Because of age-related changes, the same amount of alcohol will produce a blood alcohol level about 20% higher in a 65-year-old person than in a 30-year-old individual (Ganzini, Atkinson, 1996). Thus even if older adults do not increase the level of alcohol consumption over that of earlier years, problems may result.

DSM-IV-TR indicators for diagnosis of substance abuse are geared toward the impact of alcohol use on employment and driving, often irrelevant for older adults. Screening tools such as the CAGE test and the Geriatric Michigan Alcohol Screening Test (G-MAST) can assist identification of at-risk drinkers but are not routinely included in elders' health assessments (Conigliaro, Kraemer, McNeil, 2000). It is important to ask questions about alcohol consumption and its effects on life.

| Box 43-6 | Potential Alcohol-Related Problems in the Older Adult Population

Fluctuations in activities of daily living and instrumental activities of daily living
Self-neglect
Trauma (e.g., falls, burns, accidents)
Weight loss
Dehydration
Gastrointestinal complaints (e.g., pain, bleeding, chronic diarrhea)
Incontinence
Increased medical complaints
Neuropathy
Jaundice
Ascites
Unexpected drug effects
Confusion or Delirium
Dementia (Wernicke-Korsakoff syndrome)
Depression
Sleep disturbance
Family discord
Legal trouble (especially driving under the influence)

Nurses should also be attuned to the possibility of alcohol as a contributing factor in many problems seen in elderly medical and psychiatric patients. Box 43-6 lists some of the presenting features of elderly problem drinkers. Problem drinkers generally have more health-related complaints than their peers, and older women are particularly susceptible to alcohol's toxic effects (Ludwick et al, 2000). Unfortunately, withdrawal symptoms may be the first indication of alcohol dependence. Alcohol withdrawal includes a broad spectrum of symptoms, and although the severity of withdrawal symptoms are not appreciably different across age groups (Wetterling et al, 2001), physiologic changes and co-morbid physical conditions place older adults at an increased risk. Nurses have a significant role in the management of alcohol withdrawal (Box 43-7).

A variety of interventions are available to support continued abstinence after withdrawal. For some late-onset drinkers, education and abstinence advice is effective (Blow, 2000). For other drinkers, including long-term alcohol abusers, formal programs are necessary. Greatest success is achieved when the program is geared specifically for older adults. Three important differences from the usual approach used by one successful program include outreach with counselors going to the individual's home, lack of confrontation about addiction, and an overall focus on quality of life and maintenance of independent living (Graham et al, 1995). Programs for older adults emphasize peer bonding and shared reminiscing in addition to cognitive-behavioral training that addresses themes such as self-efficacy, self-esteem, and relapse-prevention strategies. Whenever possible, it is of paramount importance to address the factors that initially led to problem drinking.

| Box 43-7 | Nursing Care of Alcohol-Withdrawal Syndrome in the Older Adult Population

Assess withdrawal symptoms
Assess vital signs
Educate about withdrawal process
Assist with activities of daily living
Reduce environmental stimuli
Supplement diet to meet nutritional needs
Reorient
Provide relaxation exercises

Drug Misuse and Abuse

Although older adults do not have a significant problem with illicit drug use, problems result from the overuse and misuse of prescription and OTC medications. Older adults use 25% to 30% of all prescription drugs and an even larger share of OTC agents (Substance Abuse and Mental Health Service Administration [SAMHSA], 2001). A large portion of prescriptions for this age group is for psychoactive, mood-changing drugs that carry the potential for misuse, abuse, or dependency. Box 43-8 provides guidelines for the use of psychotropic drugs in older adults. Benzodiazepines, used for treatment of anxiety and insomnia, are of particular concern because they are frequently prescribed at inappropriately high doses and for excessive periods (USDHHS, 1999). This practice may lead to tolerance, physiologic dependence, and psychologic dependence. Women are more likely to receive and abuse psychoactive drugs than are men (Blow, 2000; USDHHS, 1999).

Intentional and accidental misuse of drugs contributes to adverse health problems in older adults. An estimated 83% of adults over age 65 take at least one prescription drug, and 30% of adults take eight or more prescription drugs each day (SAMHSA, 2001). Compliance is a significant problem, exacerbated by poor vision and hearing, physical deficits, confusion, mental disorders, and inadequate instructions. Drug costs and packaging should also be considered as factors that promote noncompliance. Further complicating the situation, older adults may add several OTC agents, combine medications with alcohol, or take medication prescribed for others without notifying their physician. Many older adults see multiple physicians, each of whom may prescribe drugs without reliable information about medications that the others prescribe. Confusion caused by generic and trade names can result in older adults taking the same medication under two names at the same time. Polypharmacy is common, thus the nurse should be aware of potential complications and encourage patients to "brown bag" all medications for cataloging. Drug regimens should be simplified and carefully explained.

| Box 43-8 | Guidelines for Psychotropic Drug Use in Older Adults |

Initial dose (start low—go slow)

- Usually one-third to one-half of dose used for younger adults is effective.
- Start with a small dose and gradually increase until therapeutic effect or adverse side effects occur.

Daily Dose

- Use the smallest dose that produces relief.
- Simplify dosing schedule.

Individualization

- Monitor blood levels when possible.
- Consider effect of other drugs and conditions.
- Partial symptom relief may be the most judicious and realistic goal.

Discontinuation

- Gradually taper off psychotropic drugs.
- If patients can manage without drug therapy, they should be allowed to do so.

Critical Thinking Questions

Do nurses at the facility where you have clinical rotations routinely include the same questions for alcohol and substance abuse in their assessments of geriatric patients as they do for younger adults? Do you feel comfortable asking your patients' questions about the alcohol or drugs they ingest?

ASSESSMENT OF OLDER ADULTS WITH MENTAL DISORDERS

Mental disorders are not isolated phenomena in older adults. Therefore comprehensive psychosocial and physical assessments are required to determine factors that influence the older adult's level of function. Family members or other caregivers, who often play a pivotal role in the function of older adults, should be included in the assessment process whenever possible. The goals of the initial assessment and subsequent reassessments are to collect accurate information, identify problems and assets, plan interventions, predict outcomes, and measure changes over time. Because of the volume and depth of information needed, the nurse often works collaboratively with other disciplines to complete the assessment and contribute findings to an interdisciplinary team. Input from all disciplines, the patient, and caregivers is used to develop goals and methods for care.

| Box 43-9 | Enhancing Communication with Older Adults

Considerations	Nursing Implications
Slowed information processing	Do not rush; allow adequate time for questions to be answered.
	Avoid unnecessary interruptions.
Establish rapport	Offer a handshake.
	Make eye contact.
	Position at equal or lower level than patient.
	Address by title and last name unless asked to use another name.
Hearing deficits	Articulate words clearly.
	Face patient when speaking.
	Adjust volume of speech to patient's need; do not shout.
	Ensure use of hearing aid or amplifier.
	Use complementary nonverbal strategies (e.g., facial expressions, gestures).
Visual deficits	Provide adequate non-glare lighting.
	Ensure use of corrective lens.
Competing stimuli	Minimize background noise.
	Avoid times when patient is excessively tired, hurting, hungry, or has toileting needs.
	Provide privacy.
Education level	Match vocabulary to patient's level of use.
Decreased physical tolerance	Avoid overtiring.

Nurses who are sensitive to the unique psychosocial and physical needs of older adults and adapt the assessment to accommodate these needs will increase the chances of obtaining data that accurately represent the patient. Interviews might produce anxiety because older adults are often reluctant to discuss problems with a stranger, especially a young one. Older patients may be irritated by direct questions and view them as intrusive. Open-ended questions, which provide an opportunity for the patient to vent feelings and describe concerns and problems, often foster a healthy understanding of the patient's perspective of life and functioning. Strategies such as giving older people a measure of control, increasing self-esteem, using nonjudgmental wording, and providing positive reinforcement facilitate truthful information. Other strategies to enhance communication with older adults are listed in Box 43-9.

PSYCHOSOCIAL ASSESSMENT

A wealth of clinical data can be obtained by listening to the stories many older adults love to tell. Listening not only conveys a sense of appreciation for the individual's contributions across the life span, but also provides the patient a nonthreatening means of communicating pertinent information. The nurse should listen carefully during these conversations for persistent themes such as a guilt, stress, grief, fear, or despair (Cully, LaVoie, Gfeller, 2001). By accepting expressed fears and concerns, the nurse assures the patient that these expressions will not result in rejection. Information about past experiences and coping strategies, along with personal strengths and weaknesses, may also be revealed. Formal assessment tools previously described may also be used to assess mental status, depression, and problem alcohol consumption. Box 43-10 lists information to obtain during the initial assessment.

Caregivers should be included in the assessment process. Not only can they provide information to clarify or expand that given by the patient, their perspective of problems is also important for inclusion in a plan of care. Family members might be embarrassed to contradict information given by the patient in a joint interview. Because assessing family interaction is important, time should be spent interviewing the patient and family members, both separately and together. Nurses should use time with caregivers to assess ability and willingness to provide care and support for the patient. Many caregivers, often spouses or children, fail to take care of their own needs and lack information about support services and respite care. Helping family members deal with the stressors of caregiving increases family and patient adjustment.

| Box 43-10 | Assessment Information

Demographics (age, marital status)
Spiritual and cultural values
Personal and family history
History of legal difficulties
Economic status and sources of income
Education and work history
Lifestyle and perception of current life situation
Current living arrangements
Interests, pleasures, and activities
Friendship and social interactions
Sexual functioning
Medical information and history
Prescription and over-the-counter drugs
Alcohol, tobacco, and other chemical use
Cognitive, behavioral, and emotional status
Goals and plans for the future

| Box 43-11 | Functional Assessment

PADLs	IADLs
Bathing	Preparing meals
Dressing	Shopping
Eating	Managing money
Transferring	Using telephone
Walking	Using transportation
Toileting	Doing housework

PADLs, Physical activities of daily living; *IADLs*, instrumental activities of daily living.

PHYSICAL ASSESSMENT

Throughout this chapter, the connection between physical conditions and mental disorders has been stressed. Therefore a complete physical examination is an essential component in the assessment of any older adult presenting with symptoms of mental disorders. The examination techniques for each subsystem do not differ substantially from the examination of younger adults. Numerous texts detail findings expected as a result of "normal" aging. Adaptations for decreased mobility and obvious impairments must be made. Careful attention to every subsystem is required because, in older adults, examination might reveal abnormalities in a system not suggested by the presenting symptoms. For example, ataxia may result from fecal impaction; or subtle hearing loss can result in bizarre or incorrect responses, leading to erroneous assumptions about psychopathologic conditions. The nurse should use all senses during the examination, attending to the patient's visual presentation, odors, voice tone, and content. Blood tests, electroencephalograms, and neuroimaging studies may be ordered to identify conditions that contribute to symptoms of mental disorders.

Special attention should be given to defining the way physical problems interfere with the patient's functional ability. Older individuals assign a great value to independence, and its loss can contribute to lower self-esteem and declines in mental health. The loss of key abilities may result in shame and frustration. Older adults who are dependent on others may resent the idea that others have to provide care and may believe that they have become a burden. The resulting anger can be directed internally and result in depression or withdrawal, or it may be directed at caregivers. Assessment of physical activities of daily living (PADLs) and instrumental activities of daily living (IADLs) provides a measure of the older adult's functional ability and guides the selection of interventions and services to meet identified needs (Box 43-11). Patients, and sometimes their families, are often unable or unwilling to describe functional difficulties because of the threat to established patterns of lifestyle and interactions. According to the AoA (2000), 14% of older adults have difficulty carrying out PADLs and 21% report difficulties with IADLs. Observing task performance and carefully listening to both the patient and the collateral sources (e.g., family) describe daily activities may provide a more accurate picture of functional ability than direct questioning.

The physical examination should be used as an opportunity to assess for signs of abuse or neglect. Each state has laws that specify reporting requirements for intentional abuse, neglect, and exploitation of older adults. Laws also cover endangerment resulting from mental disorders. Chapter 4 details some of the legal issues that may stem from abuse or neglect.

Psychotherapeutic Management

Nurse-patient relationship

Ageist attitudes, intergenerational differences, communication deficits, and the multiple problems of older adults can pose significant obstacles to developing a therapeutic nurse-patient relationship. Nurses who are aware of their own feelings and reactions are able to focus on patients and their significant

Case Study

Ms. Othelia Thatcher, a 78-year-old Caucasian with a 10-year history of severe depression, has been hospitalized twice in the last 2 years. She received a series of electroconvulsive therapy (ECT) treatments during each stay, the last treatment received 11 months ago. Ms. Thatcher's cousin, a woman about 60 years old, brought the patient to the hospital emergency department this morning. The cousin described a gradual worsening of depressive symptoms over the past few months and says Ms. Thatcher seems to need ECT approximately once a year. About 6 or 7 months after a course of ECT is completed, the patient "goes bad again."

Ms. Thatcher complains of erratic sleep patterns and decreased appetite. She will not eat unless her cousin spoon-feeds her. The cousin reports that after a series of ECT, the patient is "easier to live with", plays with children, takes care of herself, helps with household tasks, and will "eat anything not nailed down."

The cousin estimates that the patient's depression began in the 1990s when "her only son, to whom she was very devoted," abandoned Ms. Thatcher to the welfare of the state and sold all of her furniture. This event occurred after the patient's extended hospitalization for treatment of pneumonia and a urinary tract infection. Since that time, Ms. Thatcher reportedly lived in five different boarding homes before her cousin took her to the hospital 3 years ago.

The cousin states that Ms. Thatcher has never verbalized suicidal or homicidal thoughts, but she has a basically "paranoid view of life." The cousin cannot recall Ms. Thatcher ever having hallucinations.

Care Plan

Name: <u>Ms. Othelia Thatcher</u>　　　　　　Admission Date: _____

DSM-IV-TR Diagnosis: <u>Major Depression</u>

Assessment	**Areas of strength:** Willingness to be treated; cooperative, good support system (cousin very concerned and wants patient back in home). **Problems:** Withdrawn, decreased interest in interactions and activities, decreased self-esteem, decreased energy, hopelessness, poor judgment.
Diagnoses	• Ineffective coping, disturbed sleep pattern, imbalanced nutrition: less than body requirements, impaired social interaction, self-care deficits
Outcomes	*Short-term goals:* • Maintain safety • Express feelings verbally • Increased energy for self care *Long-term goals:* • Able to talk about anger and disappointment related to son • Increase in self concept • Maintain independence though living in cousin's home

Date met
 _____
 _____
 _____

 _____
 _____
 _____

Planning/ Interventions	**Nurse-patient relationship:** Convey concern and acceptance without sympathy, encourage expression of feelings, interactions with others as tolerated, help patient explore anger with son. **Psychopharmacology:** Fluoxetine (Prozac) 20 mg q AM; risperidone (Risperdal) 0.5 mg q 12 hr; docusate sodium 100 mg bid. **Milieu management:** Provide adequate nutrition and hydration. Monitor patient for safety issues. Keep patient around others (not in room by self) as much as is reasonable. Keep naps short to facilitate sleep at night.
Evaluation	Patient expressed feelings of anger at being abandoned by son. Activity level increased. Minimal confusion post ECT. Medication maintained. Will be discharged to return to cousin's home.
Referrals	Schedule visit with home health nurse for follow-up care. Schedule appointment with outpatient program coordinator within 7 days.

others in a therapeutic manner. By empathizing with the patient and caregivers and focusing on the patient's needs, the nurse can assist patients and their families manage the activities and demands of daily living and improve the overall quality of both physical and mental health.

Mental disorders have a significant effect on a patient's abilities to manage even the simplest of cognitive and physical tasks. Depression, psychosis, anxiety, and other disorders can result in inattention or inability to perform routine ADLs. Therefore it is essential for geropsychiatric nurses to ensure adequate fluid and nutritional intake, monitor elimination and hygiene, take protective measures in the face of impaired judgment, and remain vigilant for symptoms of physical illness and treatment complications. Some older adults have multiple physical complaints, the result of illness or psychologic distress. The nurse should listen to complaints and evaluate potential causes. Summarizing and restating the patient's concerns out loud reinforces that the concerns have been heard. Interaction itself may be the real but unexpressed need of patients with persistent physical complaints (McCahill, Brunton, 1995).

Communicating a sense of unconditional acceptance of the patient as a fellow human being may be the most important intervention the nurse can provide. Spending time with the patient outside that required for tasks such as medication administration and ADLs communicates an appreciation for the patient as a person of worth. Providing opportunities for the patient to participate in care decisions and control the sequence of events, such as allowing the patient to choose when to bathe, enhances self-esteem, self-worth, and decision-making skills. The nurse must be aware of problems and unspoken needs and incorporate them into the plan of care.

Realistic goals

Establishing both short-term and long-range goals is important for nurses and patients. Discussions should be held with patients to stress the importance of goal setting. Often, ADLs can be a challenge, and developing a schedule of the day's activities with goals can help patients make decisions and cope with demands. Simple decisions may be difficult for older adults with mental disorders. Reducing the options available before allowing the patient choices can diminish frustration. For example, when it is time to dress, the nurse may restrict the choices of attire to two rather than offering an entire closet of options. The caregiver must be gentle and supportive because additional time may be needed to achieve goals. Caregivers who base care decisions on the goal of restoring the patient to maximal independent function are likely to resist the urge to save time and energy by taking over tasks. Nurses should provide information on self-care and disease management at a pace that facilitates understanding. Patience, positive reinforcement, and consistency by nurses benefit the patient.

Psychopharmacology

Polypharmacy, physiologic changes, and co-morbid physical disorders combine to increase the risk of unexpected drug effects in older adults. The negative impact of typical side effects is also exacerbated. Thus the pharmacologic management of psychiatric symptoms in older adults requires special consideration. Age-related changes that affect drug absorption, distribution, metabolism, and elimination are listed in Table 43-3. Co-administered drugs also affect *pharmacokinetics*. For example, antacids may delay absorption; proximal loop and potassium-sparing diuretics effect lithium excretion. *Pharmacodynamics* is the study of the actions and effects of drugs on organ tissue that bring about both intended effects and side effects. Knowledge of drugs' characteristics and their site and mechanism of action is important to understanding the sensitivity that older adults exhibit. For example, antipsychotic medications that act by blocking dopamine receptors have an increased likelihood of causing extrapyramidal side effects (EPSEs) in older adults who already have diminished dopamine concentrations. Nurses must observe and report both expected therapeutic and adverse medication reactions, as well as plan interventions to minimize the negative consequences of drug therapy. More extensive information is offered in the psychopharmacology unit of this text.

Antidepressants

Target symptoms of depression, side-effect profiles, dose schedules, and cost are factors in antidepressant drug selection. The selective serotonin reuptake inhibitors (SSRIs), which are generally favored for older adults, are effective, have a favorable side-effect profile, and are not lethal in overdose. SSRIs such as fluoxetine (Prozac), paroxetine (Paxil), sertraline

|Table 43-3 | Age-Related Changes: Effects on Pharmacokinetics

Physiologic Change	Effects	Special Considerations
• ↑ Gastric pH • ↓ Absorptive surface • ↓ Splanchnic blood flow • ↓ Gastrointestinal motility • ↓ Gastric emptying	Absorption	• Delayed absorption of oral medication. Acid drugs more rapidly absorbed than base drugs
• ↑ Body fat • ↓ Lean body mass • ↓ Total body water • ↓ Serum albumin • ↓ Cardiac output	Distribution	• Extended half-life of lipid soluble drugs which accumulate in adipose tissue (i.e., barbiturates, phenothiazines, benzodiazepines, phenytoin, TCAs) • ↓ Total plasma albumin = ↓ binding sites for protein bound drugs resulting in ↑ amount of free or active drug
• ↓ Hepatic blood flow • ↓ Hepatic mass • ↓ Hepatic enzyme activity	Metabolism	• Multiple drugs competing for same enzyme may ↓ liver metabolism. • There is a high degree of genetic variability in available hepatic enzymes
• ↓ Renal blood flow • ↓ Glomerular filtration rate • ↓ Tubular secretion • ↓ Number of nephrons • ↓ Creatinine production • ↓ Creatinine clearance	Elimination	• Creatinine clearance can be reduced despite normal serum creatinine levels due to ↓ lean body weight and ↓ creatinine production • Reduction in renal clearance may reduce dose requirements

Keltner N, Folks D: *Psychotropic drugs,* ed 3, St Louis, 2001, Mosby; Gareri P et al: Conventional and new antidepressant drugs in the elderly, *Prog Neurobiol* 61(4):353, 2000.

(Zoloft), fluvoxamine (Luvox), and citalopram (Celexa) are also used to treat primary anxiety disorders common to older adults (Compton, Nemeroff, 2001). Tricyclic antidepressants (TCAs) can be used in older adults, but their anticholinergic, antiadrenergic, and antihistaminic properties cause side effects that are particularly problematic for elderly patients. Typical anticholinergic side effects include dry mouth, blurred vision, tachycardia, urinary retention, and constipation. Although uncomfortable for young adults, these side effects may result in serious consequences for older adults. Amitriptyline (Elavil) has the highest anticholinergic profile of the TCA group and is typically a poor choice. Nortriptyline (Pamelor) and desipramine (Norpramin), on the other hand, have lower anticholinergic and sedative effects (Heffern, 2000). Novel antidepressant agents, such as bupropion (Wellbutrin) and trazodone (Desyrel), have a better side-effect profile than TCAs and are widely used. Bupropion causes little sedation, hypotension, anticholinergic response, or cardiotoxicity. Trazodone does not have anticholinergic effects but is sedating. The sedation distinction between antidepressants is important because depression is sometimes exhibited by agitation or sleep disturbance, and affected patients may benefit from the sedating properties of an antide-

pressant. When depression is exhibited by lethargy and excessive sleep, a more "activating" antidepressant is in order (e.g., bupropion, SSRIs). TCAs are not recommended for patients with known cardiac problems because of their association with changes in cardiac conduction, arrhythmias, and orthostatic hypotension. Patients should be carefully monitored for orthostatic changes, especially individuals who are also taking diuretics or vasodilators. Monoamine oxidase inhibitors (MAOIs) are rarely used in older adults because these medications have potentially serious side effects and require dietary restrictions (Compton, Nemeroff, 2001). Similar to most TCAs, MAOIs are lethal in overdose.

Full therapeutic response takes at least 2 to 4 weeks for most antidepressants. Many patients fail to respond to the first antidepressant prescribed. When this failure occurs, the nurse can reassure patients that this is not uncommon and that other drugs can be effective. Education on the importance of compliance and the need to continue antidepressant therapy, even when depressive symptoms resolve, is important. In most cases, antidepressants are continued for at least 6 months following symptom resolution to prevent relapse. Patients who are at high risk of relapse are maintained on antidepressants for longer periods (Whooley, Simon, 2000).

Antipsychotics

Antipsychotic drugs are used in the treatment of schizophrenia, acute psychosis, aggressive behavior, and agitation. Atypical antipsychotics such as olanzapine (Zyprexa) and risperidone (Risperdal) are regarded as the drugs of choice for treatment of older adults because of the favorable side-effect profiles and efficacy of these drugs (Maixner, 1999). The term "atypical" was introduced to describe the low propensity of these agents to cause EPSEs and tardive dyskinesia (TD), a significant advantage for older adults who, because of neurodegenerative processes, are at risk for developing disabling and stigmatizing movement disorders. As compared with traditional antipsychotics, atypicals also show greater efficacy for both the positive and negative symptoms of schizophrenia, lower cardiac effects, and reduced sedative effects. Drugs within this class vary widely in the site of action and side-effect profile.

Traditional antipsychotic drugs are categorized as high potency or low potency. The high-potency drugs, such as haloperidol (Haldol) and fluphenazine (Prolixin), are associated with EPSEs. The low-potency antipsychotics such as chlorpromazine (Thorazine) and thioridazine (Mellaril) cause sedation, anticholinergic, and cardiovascular side effects (particularly orthostatic hypotension) that make their use more problematic for older adults compared with high-potency agents. Antipsychotic drug doses for older adults tend to be one half or less than one half of those given to younger patients. Nurses must carefully monitor patients for side effects. Assessment tools, for example, the Abnormal Involuntary Movement Scale (AIMS), can be used to identify EPSEs and TD.

Antianxiety agents

Anxiety is a common late-life problem, and its management often involves benzodiazepines, buspirone (BuSpar), and antidepressants (Keltner, Folks, 2001). A disproportionate share of prescriptions for benzodiazepines are written for older adults despite the fact this age group is particularly vulnerable to common side effects such as drowsiness, cognitive suppression, and ataxia (Heffern, 2000). An increased risk of falls, disinhibition characterized by violence or agitation, and retrograde amnesia are additional related concerns (Keltner, Folks, 2001). Federal

guidelines along with improved practice guidelines for management of anxiety in older adults have encouraged the use of benzodiazepines, which are metabolized by phase II mechanisms (i.e., nonoxidative) such as lorazepam (Ativan) and oxazepam (Serax). Benzodiazepines are recommended only for short-term management of anxiety. Because withdrawal syndrome (including withdrawal seizure) can occur when benzodiazepines are removed after 30 or more days of use, they should be withdrawn slowly over several weeks or longer. Benzodiazepines are relatively safe drugs when taken alone but can cause severe sedation and respiratory suppression when combined with alcohol or other sedatives. Buspirone (BuSpar), a nonbenzodiazepine antianxiety agent, effectively manages anxiety without concerns for physical or psychologic dependence. Furthermore, buspirone is not sedating and has no an additive effect with alcohol. Its chief disadvantage is that full therapeutic effects are delayed for 3 to 6 weeks (Keltner, Folks, 2001).

Mood stabilizers

Mood-stabilizing drugs used for treating bipolar disorders and mixed depressive episodes include lithium, valproic acid (Depakote, Depakene), and the anticonvulsant carbamazepine (Tegretol). Lithium has long been the drug of choice for manic symptoms in people of all ages. Older adults have a therapeutic response at lower serum levels (0.4 to 0.8 mEq/L) and are at higher risk for toxic reactions related to altered fluid and electrolyte balance and co-administered medications, especially diuretics (Keltner, Folks, 2001; Snowdon, 2000). Valproic acid is gaining favor as a first-line agent because of its favorable side-effect profile. Systemic evidence is lacking on the use of carbamazepine in older adults with manic symptoms (Snowdon, 2000). Because therapeutic effects of mood stabilizers take weeks, neuroleptics and short-acting benzodiazepines are often considered as adjuncts to manage dangerous behaviors in the interval (Snowdon, 2000).

Milieu management

Nurses responsible for older adults with mental disorders in inpatient or day-care settings have a therapeutic responsibility to facilitate optimal function. Attention to all elements of the milieu can increase psychologic functioning and prevent the deterioration resulting from withdrawal and disuse of skills so well documented in institutionalized elders.

Effective milieu management changes the quality of life in institutional environments by working with residents to normalize the environment to the maximum degree possible. The traditional associations of "home" involve control over people who come and go, as well as control of personal spaces, furnishings, and accessories (Katz, 1995). Furniture, at a height that facilitates independent mobility, can be placed in conversational groupings. Common rooms are best equipped with large-print books, games with large print and pieces, and stimulating pictures. Individual rooms can be deinstitutionalized by encouraging residents to use their own bedspreads, family pictures, favorite calendars, and other personal items. This same strategy, even in acute-care settings, has the added benefit of providing orientation cues. Staff members often wear street clothes rather than traditional uniforms to encourage social interaction with residents and eliminate artificial barriers. It is important to remember privacy needs and respect personal space. Environmental adaptations that promote safety and independence for older adults are listed in Table 43-4.

Controlling aggression is a major component of maintaining individual and environmental safety. Violent or agitated behavior may be the result of poor frustration tolerance, ineffective coping strategies, impulsivity, or real or imagined threats to personal space. Nurses must look at the environment and develop strategies to minimize precipitating factors. Careful attention should be paid to the potential for background stimuli such as constant music or television to cause distress. Physical and chemical restraints to control behavior have numerous negative consequences, and alternative interventions should be attempted before use. Managing environmental stimuli, providing productive outlets for energy, and practicing redirection and diversion are important for reducing outbursts.

Therapeutic approaches should be based on the concept that all individuals have a need for human contact, social participation, and meaningful activity to maintain function. Individual and group interactions and activities should be planned to foster the greatest degree of independence and develop interpersonal and communication skills. A variety of activities can be tailored to match individual levels of physical and psychologic function. Pet therapy helps fulfill patients' needs to give and receive affection through supervised sessions of holding, stroking, and playing with specially screened animals. Exercise therapy, tailored to the needs of even people with limited physical ability, provides outlets for the excess energy of anxiety and provides stimulation and socialization opportunities. Music is also an effective way to make contact with patients. Songbooks, hymnals, and records offer an array of music choices familiar to older adults who often enjoy "sing-alongs" or simply listening to familiar and comfortable tunes. Planting and tending to plants can enhance physical function, relieve tension, and provide a sense of responsibility and accomplishment. These therapeutic activities and others are important opportunities to provide patients positive experiences and attain realistic goals.

|Table 43-4| Environmental Adaptations

Considerations	Interventions
Decreased ability to distinguish colors	• Use high-contrast colors in vivid hues
Mobility impairments	• Ensure nonslip floor surfaces
	• Provide adequate, nonglare lighting
	• Ensure well-fitting footwear
	• Provide chairs and toilets at comfortable height with armrests or handrails
	• Avoid placing rolling tables where patients might attempt to use for stability
	• Provide shower stools, nonskid tub guards, and grab bars
	• Provide ambulation rails
	• Remove obstacles, clutter, and spills promptly
Inability to read	• Mark spaces with pictures or universal symbols
Decreased thermoregulation	• Ensure comfortable temperature
	• Observe for signs of hypothermia or hyperthermia
	• Provide sweaters, blankets
	• Ensure safe water temperature

Selected Nursing Interventions for Assisting Older Adults with Depression
Assess and meet physical needs
Promote healthy behavior
Maximize independence
Promote sense of control
Provide consistency
Reinforce self-esteem
Acknowledge individual's feelings
Appreciate individual's uniqueness in context of entire life span and culture
Reinforce genuine hope
Identify available supports
Consider family and caregivers

Reminiscence

Older adults have a wealth of experiences that can be shared through storytelling. The nurse can use these memories to provide opportunities for pleasurable interaction and therapeutic gain. Reminiscence is the process of recalling past experiences, which allows the listener insight into the patient's history and perspective. Patients can benefit from multiple dimensions of reminiscence, including clarifying their sense of self, connecting with others, providing instruction, restructuring recalled events, recalling previously used problem-solving strategies, and bringing closure and calmness in death preparation (Cully, LaVoie, Gfeller, 2001). Reminiscence may occur in group or one-to-one interactions. In groups, participants are encouraged to share life experiences such as vacations, holidays, milestones, and family events. Leaders may stimulate memories by using pictures, music, and memorabilia. Reminiscence groups can provide validation for each member and help participants establish new relationships while enhancing valuable communication and socialization skills. Life review is a mechanism that uses reminiscence but is a different process. Evaluation of the entire life span through telling or writing a personal story is difficult work for the patient. In one-to-one interaction, the patient relates fears, conflicts, unresolved feelings, and unresolved losses, providing opportunities for therapeutic intervention.

Key Concepts

1. Despite the increase in the population of individuals 65 years of age and older, this group experiences major barriers to obtaining quality mental health care because of issues such as ageism, their own attitudes, and cost of care.
2. Depression is a common mental disorder among older adults, but it is often overlooked, misdiagnosed, and inadequately treated.
3. Symptoms of other illnesses may mask depression because older adults may be preoccupied with physical rather than emotional symptoms.
4. Age-related life events, losses, changes, and physical decline are associated with the onset of depression.
5. The nurse-patient relationship focuses on helping patients achieve their highest level of function. Caregivers, when available, should be included in planning strategies to manage the activities and demands of daily living.
6. Adequate nutrition, socialization, and achievement of small realistic goals in daily living activities help reduce anxiety and maintain or restore psychologic functioning.
7. Use of medications with older adults involves risks associated with polypharmacy, noncompliance, and altered pharmacokinetics.
8. SSRIs, bupropion, trazodone, and secondary TCAs are the recommended agents for treating depression in the older adult population.
9. When treating psychotic disorders, high-potency antipsychotics, such as haloperidol, are used more often than low-potency antipsychotics. New atypical agents are also first-line agents.
10. Antianxiety agents such as lorazepam and oxazepam, along with the nonbenzodiazepine anxiety agents are prescribed most often for this age group.
11. ECT can be effective treatment for older adults suffering from depression.

References

Administration on Aging: *A profile of older Americans: 2000,* Washington, DC, 2000, US Department of Health and Human Services.

Administration on Aging: *Family caregiving—fact sheet,* 2001a. Available at URL: www.aoa.dhhs.gov/may2001/factsheets/family-caregiving Accessed 7/14/01.

Administration on Aging: *Older adults, transportation and longevity—fact sheet,* 2001b. Available at URL: www.aoa.gov/factsheets/transportation Accessed 8/19/01.

Administration on Aging: *Older adults and mental health: issues and opportunities,* 2001c, Halpern PL. Available at URL: www.aoa.dhhs. gov/mh/report2001/exesum.html Accessed 7/15/01.

American Association of Colleges of Nursing (AACN) and the John A. Hartford Foundation Institute for Geriatric Nursing: *Older adults: recommended baccalaureate competencies and curricular guidelines for geriatric nursing care,* Washington, DC, 2000, AACN.

American Psychiatric Association: Mood disorders. In *Diagnostic and Statistical Manual of Mental Disorders, text revision,* ed 4, Washington, DC, 2000, The Association.

Blank K et al: Life-sustaining treatment and assisted death choices in depressed older patients, *J Am Geriatr Soc* 49(2):153, 2001.

Blazer DG, Koenig HG: Mood disorders. In Busse E, Blazer D, editors: *Textbook of geriatric psychiatry,* ed 2, Washington, DC, 1996, American Psychiatric Press.

Blow F: Treatment of older women with alcohol problems: meeting the challenge for a special population, *Alcohol Clin Exp Res* 24(8):1257, 2000.

Butler RN, Lewis ML: Late-life depression: when and how to intervene, *Geriatrics* 50(8):44, 1995.

Byrne G, Raphael B, Arnold E: Alcohol consumption and psychological distress in recently widowed older men, *Aust NZ J Psychiatry* 33(5):740, 1999.

Campbell T et al: Do physicians who diagnose more mental health disorders generate lower healthcare costs? *J Fam Prac* 49(4):305, 2000.

Cassano G et al: Current issues in the identification and management of bipolar spectrum disorders in "special populations," *J Aff Disorders* 59:S69, 2000.

Compton M, Nemeroff C: The evaluation and treatment of depression in primary care, *Clin Cornerstone* 3(3):10, 2001.

Conigliaro J, Kraemer K, McNeil M: Screening and identification of older adults with alcohol problems in primary care, *J Geriatr Psychiatry Neurol* 13(3):106, 2000.

Creed F: The importance of depression following myocardial infarction, *Heart* 82(4):406, 1999.

Cuffel B et al: Treatment costs and use of community mental health services for schizophrenia by age, cohort, *Am J Psychiatry* 153(7):870, 1996.

Cully J, LaVoie D, Gfeller J: Reminiscence, personality, and psychological functioning in older adults, *Gerontologist* 41(1):89, 2001.

Federal Interagency Forum on Aging-Related Statistics: *Older Americans 2000: key indicators of well-being,* Federal Interagency Forum on Aging-Related Statistics, Washington, DC, 2000, U.S. Government Printing Office. Also available at URL: www. agingstats.gov/chartbook2000/

Folks D, Fuller W: Anxiety disorders and insomnia in geriatric patients, *Psychiatr Clin North Am* 20(1):137, 1997.

Forsell Y, Winblad B: Incidence of major depression in a very elderly population, *Intl J Geriatr Psychiatry* 14(5)368, 1999.

Ganzini L, Atkinson R: Substance abuse. In Sadavoy J et al, editors: *Comprehensive review of geriatric psychiatry-II,* ed 2, Washington, DC, 1996, American Psychiatric Press.

Gareri P et al: Conventional and new antidepressant drugs in the elderly, *Prog Neurobiol* 61:354, 2000.

Graham K et al: Addictions treatment for older adults: evaluation of an innovative client-centered approach, New York, 1995, The Haworth Press.

Heffern W: Psychopharmacological and electroconvulsive treatment of anxiety and depression in the elderly, *J Psychiatr Ment Health Nurs* 7(3):199, 2000.

Howard R et al: Late-onset schizophrenia and very-late onset schizophrenia-like psychosis: an international consensus, *Am J Psychiatry* 157(2):172, 2000.

Hoyert DL, Kochanek KD, Murphey SL: Deaths: final data for 1997, *National Vital Statistics Report,* 47(19) DHHS Publication No. 99-1120, Hyattsville Md, 1999, National Center for Health Statistics. Jeste DV, Harris MJ, Paulsen JS: Psychosis. In Sadavoy J et al, editors: *Comprehensive review of geriatric psychiatry-II,* ed 2, Washington, DC, 1996, American Psychiatric Press.

Kales H et al: Health care utilization by older patients with coexisting dementia and depression, *Am J Psychiatry* 156(4):550, 1999.

Katz IR: Infrastructure requirements for research in late-life mental disorders. In Gatz M, editor: *Emerging issues in mental health and aging,* Washington, DC, 1995, American Psychiatric Press.

Kayton W: *The impact of major depression in patients with chronic medical illness.* Proceedings of the 154th Annual Meeting of the American Psychiatric Association, 2001.

Kelly K, Zisselman M: Update on electroconvulsive therapy (ECT) in older adults, *J Am Geriatr* 45(5):560, 2000.

Keltner N, Folks D: *Psychotropic drugs,* ed 3, St Louis, 2001, Mosby.

Koenig H et al: Schizophrenia and paranoid disorders. In Busse E, Blazer D, editors: *Textbook of geriatric psychiatry,* ed 2, Washington, DC, 1996, American Psychiatric Press.

Lang A, Stein M: Anxiety disorders. How to recognize and treat the medical symptoms of emotional illness, *Geriatrics* 56(5):24, 2001.

Lenze E et al: Co-morbid anxiety disorders in depressed elderly patients, *Am J Psychiatry* 157(5):722, 2000.

Ludwick R et al: Alcohol use in elderly women: nursing considerations in community settings, *J Gerontol Nurs* 26(2):44, 2000.

Maixner S et al: The efficacy, safety and tolerability of anti-psychotics in the elderly, *J Clin Psychiatry* 60(suppl 8):29, 1999.

McCahill M, Brunton S: The elderly patient with multiple complaints, *Hosp Pract* 30(12): 49, 1995.

McClure FS, Gladsjo JA, Jeste DV: Late-onset psychosis: clinical, research, and ethical considerations, *Am J Psychiatry* 156(6): 935, 1999.

National Coalition on Mental Health and Aging: *Building state and community mental health and aging coalitions: a "how-to" guide,* Dec 1994. Available at URL: http://www.mentalhealth.org/ resource/how1.htm. Accessed 7/31/97.

National Institute on Aging: *Strategic Plan for Fiscal Years 2001-2005.* Available at URL: www.nih.gov/nia/strat.plan/2001-2005 Accessed 8/31/01.

National Institute of Mental Health: *Crisis in Geriatric Mental Health,* 1999a. Available at URL: www.nimh.nih.gov/litalert/ geriatriccrisis.cfm Accessed 8/18/01.

National Institute of Mental Health: *Suicide Facts,* 1999b. Available at URL: www.nimh.nih.gov/research/suifact.htm Accessed 8/29/01.

National Institute of Mental Health: *Older adults: depression and suicide facts.* NIMH Publication no. 01-4593. 2001. Available at URL: www.nimh.nih.gov/publicat/elderlydepsuicide.cfm Accessed 8/19/01.

National Institutes of Health: *The impact of mental illness on society,* NIH Publication No. 01-4586, 2001. Available at URL: www. nimh nih.gov Accessed 8/29/01.

Patterson T et al: Social skills performance assessment among older patients with schizophrenia, *Schizophr Res* 48(2-3):351, 2001.

Penninx B et al: Minor and major depression and the risk of death in older persons, *Arch Gen Psychiatry* 56(10):889, 1999.

Rosenfeld P et al: Gerontological nursing content in baccalaureate nursing programs: findings from a national survey, *J Prof Nurs* 15(2):84, 1999.

Schurhoff F et al: Early and late onset bipolar disorders: two different forms of manic depressive illness? *J of Affect Disord* 58:S69, 2000.

Shea D, Russo P, Smyer M: Use of mental health services by persons with a mental illness in nursing facilities: initial impacts of OBRA 87, *J Aging Health* 12(4):560, 2000.

Sheikh J: Anxiety disorders. In Sadavoy J et al, editors: *Comprehensive review of geriatric psychiatry,* ed 2, Washington DC, 1996, American Psychiatric Press.

Sibisi C: The phenomenology of delusional jealousy in late life, *Int J Geriatr Psychiatry* 14:389, 1999.

Snowdon J: The relevance of guidelines for treatment mania in old age, *Int J Geriatr Psychiatry* 15:779, 2000.

Substance Abuse and Mental Health Service Administration (SAMHSA), The National Clearinghouse for Alcohol and Drug Information: *Use and abuse of psychoactive prescription drugs and over the counter medications,* 2001. Available at URL: www.health.org/govpubs/BKD250/26f.htm Accessed 9/18/01.

Tew J et al: Acute efficacy of ECT in the treatment of major depression in the old-old, *Am J Psychiatry* 156(12):1865, 1999.

Tune L: Assessing psychiatric illness in geriatric patients, *Clin Cornerstone* 3(3):23, 2001.

U.S. Department of Health and Human Services: *Mental health: a report of the Surgeon General,* Rockville, MD, 1999, U.S. Department of Health and Human Services, Substance Abuse and Mental Health Services Administration, Center for Mental Health Services, National Institutes of Health, National Institute of Mental Health. Also available at URL: www.sg.gov/library/mentalhealth/ Accessed 8/19/01.

Warren J: *Elderly drug abuse. PEN pages,* document 285071995, College of Agricultural Sciences, Penn State University, May 3, 1999.

Wetterling T et al: The severity of alcohol withdrawal is not age dependent, *Alcohol Alcohol* 36(1):75, 2001.

Whooley M, Simon G: Managing depression in medical outpatients, *N Engl J Med* 343(26):1942, 2000.

Zorrilla L et al: Cross-sectional study of older outpatients with schizophrenia and healthy comparison subjects: no differences in age-related cognitive declines, *Am J Psychiatry* 157(8):1324, 2000.

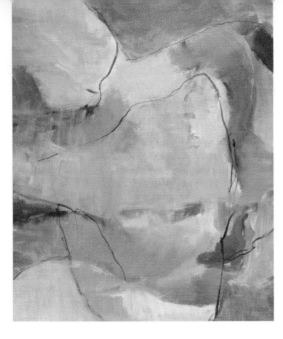

Chapter 44

Working with Patients with HIV Infection

James L. Raper; Katharine E. Stewart

Learning Objectives

After reading this chapter, you should be able to:

- Identify the groups most at risk for human immunodeficiency virus (HIV) transmission.
- Identify neurologic and neuropsychiatric complications for individuals with HIV.
- Identify psychiatric diagnoses associated with HIV.
- Discuss patient concerns related to HIV disclosure in a variety of settings.
- Identify issues of HIV-related discrimination in areas such as housing, employment, and health care.

- Describe the wide range of effects that substance use may have on people with HIV.
- Describe the principles of harm reduction as they apply to people with HIV who are abusing medications.
- Apply concepts of contracting to develop, implement, and maintain a narcotic management program.
- Identify common side effects associated with the medical treatment of HIV.
- Describe the way in which issues related to "quality of life" factor into treatment decisions.

INTRODUCTION

Over 430,000 people in the United States are currently living with diagnosed human immunodeficiency virus (HIV), and the Center for Disease Control and Prevention (CDC) estimates that almost as many individuals may be undiagnosed (CDC, 2000). Because the social and psychologic issues associated with HIV infection are often as significant as the physical issues, management of HIV-positive individuals is often a very complex process, requiring assessment and treatment across multiple levels. The process of working with patients with HIV infection can be examined from three perspectives. Intrapersonally, individuals with HIV disease often

face a long process of adjustment and adaptation to their diagnosis and, eventually, to the symptoms of the disease. This adjustment may be complicated by the interpersonal issues that can arise in the context of HIV, such as family conflict over disclosure of HIV status, sexual relationships, or stigmatization. Finally, complex social concerns exist for many HIV-infected individuals, who are frequently members of minority groups experiencing discrimination, are often living in poverty, or are coping with challenging life situations because of histories of abuse, psychiatric disorder, or substance abuse. Any or all of these three domains may influence the experience of the person living with HIV. The

Key Terms

Acquired immunodeficiency syndrome Term initially used to diagnose those with specific symptoms and opportunistic infections indicating a more advanced progression of HIV infection.

Enzyme-linked immunosorbent assay Most commonly used test to screen for the presence of antibodies to HIV-1 because of its low cost, standardized procedure, and high reliability.

Highly active antiretroviral therapy Drug therapy whereby three antiretroviral medications are used in combination to reduce the replication of HIV.

Human immunodeficiency infection Spectrum of illness caused by HIV that ranges from acutely or chronically HIV-infected adults to infants in the neonatal period.

Human immunodeficiency virus, type 1 Retrovirus identified as the cause of AIDS.

Kaposi's sarcoma One of the first opportunistic diseases described in association with AIDS and remains the most frequent malignancy associated with HIV infections.

Opportunistic illness Disease state that develops when the immune system is inactive or suppressed.

Pneumocystis carinii pneumonia Common presenting clinical manifestation of AIDS caused by *Pneumocystis carinii*, a fungal protozoan.

Polymerase chain reaction Relatively new laboratory technique developed for in vitro amplification of deoxyribonucleic acid (DNA) or ribonucleic acid RNA of an organism; commonly used to quantify the number of copies of HIV per cubic milliliter of blood.

---

mental health nurse who is cognizant of all three perspectives may be able to provide care with a greater understanding and an enhanced appreciation of the patient's struggle with the disease.

HIV disease can be categorized into roughly three stages:

- Asymptomatic
- Symptomatic
- End-stage disease

The experience of the asymptomatic phase of HIV is predominantly emotional and psychologic rather than characterized by physical signs and symptoms. The asymptomatic phase can be a period of significant psychologic disturbance or distress, ranging from individual fears of stigma, shame, and suffering, to common concerns about rejection and abandonment by a partner, to a deep feeling about HIV as further victimization in the context of daily concerns about survival.

The symptomatic phase of HIV is often marked by another period of adjustment, particularly among individuals who have become accustomed to coping with HIV as an "invisible" or asymptomatic illness. The appearance of symptoms may elicit fears of death and dying and may raise complicated issues regarding work, family, and social responsibilities. Depending on the type of opportunistic infection that the patient experiences, quality-of-life issues may be particularly salient, because many treatment regimens are invasive, painful, or disruptive. The

demands of adhering to complex medication regimens, increasingly frequent medical appointments, and lifestyle changes can be frustrating to many patients as well.

In end-stage HIV disease, which is characterized by more losses in quality of life and more serious opportunistic infections, patients may be faced with becoming dependent on others for care. Dementia is relatively common in end-stage HIV patients and may require intensive care and supervision. Existential concerns and end-of-life planning become central concerns for patients in this stage, and family relationships may as a result be particularly strained.

Thus addressing mental health concerns is of critical concern for many individuals with HIV. However, medical needs may at times take priority over important mental health issues. Even when the need for mental health assistance is recognized, many patients lack the energy to negotiate yet another treatment system. For many, HIV disease is just one problem among many others, such as diabetes, asthma, and hypertension; emotional disturbances and chronic mental illness; substance abuse and dependence; and chaotic or violent living conditions. Patients living with HIV, who also have other physical illnesses, substance abuse concerns, or mental health problems, may find themselves in fragmented systems of care in which providers with different treatment priorities and philosophies must work in concert to address the complexity of treatment issues.

All patients should be interviewed and assessed by a qualified health care professional to assist the patient in meeting his or her individual needs and to establish a baseline assessment of mental status and level of social functioning. Mental health care providers can, as part of their assessment process, serve as an important bridge between the patient and the multiple domains of treatment required by the patient's presentation. Many HIV-positive individuals, who often feel isolated and stigmatized both by medical providers and by people in their community, report that their most positive health care experiences were episodes in which the health care provider simply provided skilled emotional support, attentive listening, education, and empathy.

Assessment may also indicate the need for referral to a substance treatment program or psychologic-psychiatric evaluation, in addition to referral to programs of social support, housing, case management, and concrete services, depending on the needs of the individual. The mental health nurse who focuses, for example, on medication adherence without a comprehensive treatment plan addressing harm reduction or treatment for illicit drug use, psychiatric treatment for co-morbid psychiatric conditions, and a full range of support services is likely to fail. This leaves the HIV-infected patient with the feeling that the real sources of pain and suffering have been left unrecognized. When normal adjustment issues give way to formal psychologic disorders, accurate diagnosis is essential, as are knowledge of appropriate treatment, risks of harmful behaviors, and awareness of potential drug-drug interactions. This chapter addresses the demographic changes in the HIV or acquired immunodeficiency syndrome (AIDS) epidemic and reviews the intrapersonal, interpersonal, and social issues that may affect patients' mental and physical health. Specific recommendations are made for mental health nursing providers.

POPULATIONS AT RISK

When the epidemic began in the United States, HIV was primarily a disease of gay Caucasian men from a broad range of socioeconomic strata. However, since the early to mid-1990s, HIV rates have increased rapidly among women and men of color, and heterosexual transmission rates have increased as well. HIV is increasingly devastating African-American and Hispanic communities in the United States.

More than one half of the 40,000 new cases of HIV reported from July 1999 through June 2000 were among African Americans, and more than two thirds of children with AIDS in the United States are African American. Today, people infected with HIV are frequently from communities of poverty in which factors of intravenous drug use, incarceration, serious mental illness, and homelessness are common; many are engaged in sex work as a means to survive. Recent estimates indicate that 25% of people living with HIV in the United States were infected through unsafe injection drug use, and 15% were infected through unsafe heterosexual sex (Table 44-1).

Acquisition of HIV disease through transfusion of infected blood products has become extremely rare in the United States (see Table 44-1). Additionally, the risk of patients receiving blood components containing HIV has decreased markedly through the introduction of donor self-exclusion, HIV antibody screening of blood products, and heat treatment of coagulation factors. It is important to remember that there should be no donor-associated risk when donating blood because individual sterile equipment is used for each donor.

Health care workers have been identified as another group at potential risk for HIV infection related to exposure to blood or other infectious body fluids from patients. The risk of transmission in a specific situation is likely to vary, depending on the circulating viral titer in the source patient, the volume of blood injected, and the immune status of the exposed person. As with any blood-borne pathogen, there is occupational risk of HIV infection for health care workers (Table 44-2). The occupational risk for health care workers can be reduced by implementing and vigorously enforcing universal precautions and infection-control procedures, such as needleless equipment, protected needles, and goggles, regardless of the HIV status of the patient.

Critical Thinking Question

What should the nurse discuss concerning the establishment of realistic goals, expectations, advance care directives, and disability entitlements?

Although HIV clearly is not transmitted by casual exposure, there have been occasional reports of transmission among household contacts who experienced unprotected exposure to blood or bloody

|Table 44-1| US Adult-Adolescent AIDS Cases by Exposure Category (Cumulative Total)

MODE OF EXPOSURE	NO. OF CASES	PERCENTAGE
Single mode of exposure subtotal	571,667	77
Men who have sex with men	333,098	45
Injecting drug use	149,148	20
Hemophilia-coagulation disorder	4,156	1
Heterosexual contact	76,400	10
Receipt of transfusion[1]	8,653	1
Receipt of transplant of tissues, organs, or artificial insemination[2]	13	0
Other[3]	199	0
Multiple modes of exposure subtotal	106,248	14
Injecting drug use; heterosexual contact		
Men who have sex with men; injecting drug use		
Risk not reported or identified	67,188	9
TOTAL	745,103	100

From Centers for Disease Control and Prevention: *HIV/AIDS surveillance report* 12(1), Atlanta, 2000, US Department of Health and Human Services.
[1]Includes 37 adult-adolescents who developed AIDS after receiving blood that was screened negative for HIV antibody.
[2]After receiving tissue, organs, or artificial insemination from HIV-infected donors, 13 adults developed AIDS. Of these 13 adults, 4 received tissue or organs from a donor who was negative for HIV antibody at the time of donation (see *N Engl J Med* 326:726, 1992).
[3]Includes 162 people who acquired HIV infection perinatally but were diagnosed with AIDS after age 13.

|Table 44-2| Health Care Workers with Documented and Possible Occupationally Acquired AIDS-HIV Infection by Occupation (reported through June 2000, United States[1])

Occupation	DOCUMENTED OCCUPATIONAL TRANSMISSION[2] Number	POSSIBLE OCCUPATIONAL TRANSMISSION[3] Number
Dental worker, including dentist	0	6
Embalmer-morgue technician	1	2
Emergency medical technician-paramedic	0	12
Health aids–attendant	1	15
Housekeeper-maintenance worker	2	13
Laboratory technician, clinical	16	17
Laboratory technician, nonclinical	3	0
Nurse	23	35
Physician, nonsurgical	6	12
Physician, surgical	0	6
Respiratory therapist	1	2
Technician, dialysis	1	3
Technician, surgical	2	2
Technician-therapist, other than those listed	0	9
Other health care occupations	0	4
Total	56	138

From Centers for Disease Control and Prevention: *HIV/AIDS surveillance report* 12(1), Atlanta, 2000, US Department of Health and Human Services.
[1]Health care workers are defined as people, including students and trainees, who have worked in a health care clinical or an HIV laboratory setting at any time since 1978 (see CDC: *MMWR* 41:823, 1992).
[2]Health care workers who had documented HIV seroconversion after occupational exposure or who had other laboratory evidence of occupational infection: 48 had percutaneous exposure, 5 had mucocutaneous exposure, 2 had both percutaneous and mucocutaneous exposure, and 1 had an unknown route of exposure; 49 health care workers were exposed to blood from an HIV-infected person, 1 to visibly bloody fluid, 3 to an unspecified fluid, and 3 to concentrated virus in a laboratory; 25 of these health care workers developed AIDS.
[3]These health care workers have been investigated and are without identifiable behavioral or transfusion risks; each reported percutaneous or mucocutaneous occupational exposures to blood or body fluids, or to laboratory solutions containing HIV, but HIV seroconversion specifically resulting from an occupational exposure was not documented.

body fluids from HIV-infected patients receiving care at home. These instances further emphasize the importance of using appropriate precautions to minimize risk and of patient and family education. It is believed that risk of transmission in schools and the workplace is even more remote than it is in the home.

INTRAPERSONAL ISSUES

Patients with HIV disease often present with psychiatric or psychologic symptoms. These issues include both mild and severe mental illness (e.g., major depression, anxiety disorder, psychosis), substance abuse or dependence, difficulties adjusting to the HIV diagnosis, shame or guilt, and end-of-life concerns. Differential diagnosis of these symptoms is often a complex process, because many syndromes have similar symptom profiles. For example, dementia, depression, severe adjustment problems, or substance use may all cause the symptom of psychomotor slowing. Thus nurses may wish to familiarize themselves with some of the most common intrapersonal problems faced by patients with HIV to assist in diagnosis and treatment.

CLINICAL EXAMPLE

Marcus Matthews, a 32-year-old married African-American man, presents to clinic complaining of sleep difficulties, crying spells, difficulties with concentration and memory, and agitation. He was diagnosed with HIV disease approximately 10 months ago during a hospitalization for pneumocystis pneumonia. His CD4 cell count is 74/mm^3. He is currently taking zidovudine, stavudine, and indinavir for HIV, as well as trimethoprim-sulfamethoxazole, fluconazole, and paroxetine hydrochloride. Marcus has a history of depression and reports that at age 26 he was hospitalized for "manic depression." He admits that he began drinking after learning of his diagnosis and reports that he currently drinks about a 12-pack of beer per week. He had previously been abstinent from alcohol for nearly 2 years and denies other drug use. When asked about his understanding of his HIV disease, Mr. Matthews becomes very tearful. He states that he cannot understand why God wants him to die so young and that he is afraid now to hug and play with his 8-year-old son because "I would die if he got this horrible thing from me."

Neuropsychiatric Concerns

Up to 70% of patients with HIV disease are diagnosed with a psychiatric disorder at some point during their illness. Diagnoses may range from mild (e.g., mild depressive disorders, adjustment disorders, anxiety) to severe (e.g., bipolar disorder, borderline personality disorder). Adjustment disorder is the most common psychiatric disorder among patients with HIV infection, with up to two thirds of patients experiencing adjustment disorder with anxious, depressed, or mixed mood at some point during their illness (Bing et al, 2001; O'Dowd, Biderman, McKegney, 1993). Individuals with preexisting psychiatric disturbances may be at an increased risk for contracting or transmitting HIV because of increased risk behaviors such as multiple sexual partners or injection drug use, which may partially account for the relatively high prevalence of psychiatric illness in the HIV population (Kalichman et al, 1994).

It is critical for health care professionals to obtain a thorough psychiatric history from a patient who is experiencing any psychiatric symptoms, regardless of severity. This assessment is especially important because many psychiatric disorders (e.g., depression, bipolar disorder) may be exacerbated or may recur in the presence of the psychologic stress associated with diagnosis of HIV (Kelly et al, 1993). In addition, some medications commonly prescribed for HIV disease or its sequelae may have significant neuropsychiatric side effects, which exacerbate premorbid psychiatric symptoms.

HIV disease also is associated with multiple types of dementing processes (Table 44-3). The most common of these processes is direct HIV infection of the

---

Table 44-3	Syndromes Associated with CNS Dysfunction in HIV Disease

I. Direct HIV infection (HIV-associated dementia)
II. Opportunistic infection of CNS
   a. Cytomegalovirus (CMV) encephalitis
   b. Progressive multifocal leukoencephalopathy (PML)
   c. Cerebral toxoplasmosis
   d. Cryptococcal meningitis
   e. Tuberculosis brain abscess
   f. Varicella-zoster virus (VZV) encephalitis
III. Cancer-associated dementia
   a. CNS lymphoma
   b. Disseminated Kaposi's sarcoma

central nervous system (CNS) or HIV-associated dementia (HAD). A large proportion of patients develop signs of HAD at some point during the course of their disease (Grant et al, 1993), although antiretroviral treatment may reduce the incidence of symptoms (cited from Wesselingh, Thompson, 2001). HAD in its early stages is characterized by psychomotor slowing, delayed reaction times, and decreased concentration or attention. Apathy, social withdrawal, and loss of libido are also common.

Other opportunistic infections may affect the CNS, including bacterial, fungal, and viral infections in the brain and cancer-associated CNS disorders. Among the infections that are more common are progressive multifocal leukoencephalopathy (PML), CNS lymphoma, *Toxoplasma gondii* encephalitis, and cryptococcal meningitis. Many of these infections are associated with focal cognitive deficits and may develop quickly over a period of days or weeks (McArthur, 1994). Thus rapid assessment and diagnosis of neurologic symptoms are critical for HIV-positive patients.

In the clinical example of Mr. Matthews, the presenting symptoms are consistent with a recurrence of either major depression or bipolar disorder, both of which he had experienced before his diagnosis of HIV. However, evaluation may be necessary to rule out dementia, which is generally associated with low CD4 cell counts and often presents similarly to depression with cognitive disturbance (Stern et al, 2001). Neuroimaging (such as computed tomography [CT] and magnetic resonance imaging [MRI]) procedures may be required to determine which, if any, CNS infection or syndrome is present. Neuropsychologic testing can provide a useful adjunct to neuroimaging studies, because early stages of some dementing disorders may not be evident on CT or MRI but may be detectable through tests of memory, attention, or reaction time (Kent et al, 1994). In addition, the possibility of neuropsychiatric side effects associated with Mr. Matthews' complex medication regimen should be considered.

Substance Use

Substance use may either exacerbate or be exacerbated by psychiatric symptoms. Among individuals with HIV disease, substance use is quite common, with a significant proportion meeting the *Diagnostic and Statistical Manual of Mental Disorders* (DSM) criteria for substance abuse or dependence (Ferrando, Batki, 2000). Because substance abuse is associated with increased risk of HIV transmission or reinfection, patients with HIV and concomitant substance-use disorders should be offered treatment for substance use and counseled regarding risk reduction. Even if patients do not wish to pursue treatment for their substance use, they may benefit from counseling to teach risk-reduction strategies and to enhance adherence to antiretroviral medication regimens (Reiter et al, 2000).

Often, patients who have maintained abstinence from substance abuse can experience a relapse when they are diagnosed with HIV. In the case of Mr. Matthews, it appears that this relapse may have occurred. Even if Mr. Matthews does not currently meet criteria for substance abuse or dependence, his substance abuse may continue to worsen if he does not receive treatment. A thorough evaluation of Mr. Matthews' substance use and education regarding the effects of substance use on his medical and psychologic condition may be helpful in increasing his motivation to reduce his use or seek treatment.

Psychologic Issues

The experience of living with HIV disease may result in a variety of psychologic reactions. Although these reactions may occur at any time during the course of the disease, the periods immediately after learning of an HIV-positive test result, being diagnosed with an opportunistic infection or AIDS, or learning that one's prognosis is very poor are particularly likely to be associated with psychologic distress (DiClemente et al, 1996; Kalichman, 1998).

Many people with HIV experience anger, shame, or guilt when first informed of their HIV diagnosis. Although they may express suicidal ideation, relatively few individuals actually complete a suicidal attempt, and this risk is reduced if patients are provided appropriate support and counseling (Marzuk et al, 1997). Regular assessment for suicidal ideation or plan is appropriate in people with HIV, especially among patients who have a history of depression, substance use, impulsive behavior, or, of course, previous suicide attempts.

More often, individuals with HIV experience feelings of shame and guilt, which may be worse among those with strong moral or religious beliefs about risky sexual or illicit drug-related behavior.

Individuals may also experience what might be termed "contamination syndrome," which can be characterized by feelings of isolation, anticipation of global rejection by others, and fears of infecting others. These symptoms may be exacerbated by a lack of knowledge about HIV, its transmission, and the course of the disease, including the beliefs that casual contact may transmit HIV or that all patients with HIV will die within a very short time. Not only can these symptoms cause considerable distress and functional impairment (Kemppaineen, 2001), but they may also increase the risk of psychiatric or substance use problems and, paradoxically, the possibility of risky sexual behaviors. Supportive education about HIV and psychotherapy may help patients adjust to their diagnosis, engage in more adaptive behavior, and reduce inaccurate fears about their infection.

In the previous clinical example, Mr. Matthews exhibits shame, fears of premature death, and fears of infecting his child through casual contact. It is unclear whether his shame and fear are a result of his depression or substance use or, conversely, whether these issues are exacerbating the depression or substance use or both. However, education about the safety of casual contact with his son, education about the course of HIV infection and the life-prolonging benefits of antiretroviral therapy, and psychotherapy to allow him to work through his shame and feelings of being punished or persecuted would all be beneficial and would support any additional treatment for psychiatric or substance-use disorders. Because he expresses a religious component to his feelings of being punished or persecuted, Mr. Matthews may also benefit from a consultation with a chaplain who has experience working with HIV-positive patients.

Summary

Psychologic or psychiatric symptomatology in people with HIV disease is common. The complexity of most cases requires thorough assessment and evaluation so that the most appropriate and targeted treatment plan may be developed. This evaluation requires careful attention to the possibility of psychiatric illness, CNS disease, substance abuse or dependence, psychologic symptoms or adjustment problems, and misinformation or fears regarding HIV. Reassurance and support from medical team members is a critical part of helping patients adjust to an HIV diagnosis and ensuring proper treatment. Development of trust

and rapport with patients can facilitate history taking and can provide nurses with opportunities for brief educational or supportive interventions.

INTERPERSONAL ISSUES

HIV disease does not affect only the infected person. Rather, HIV can have a significant impact on personal relationships across a variety of domains. Family, social, and sexual relationships may be affected by the patient's diagnosis. Concerns about issues such as disclosure of HIV status, transmission risk to sexual partners, guardianship of one's children, or end-of-life planning may all be of critical importance in the overall management of people living with HIV.

CLINICAL EXAMPLE

Ms. Marie Simon, a 36-year-old divorced Caucasian woman, was diagnosed with HIV about 8 years ago and is currently quite ill, with liver failure secondary to hepatitis C infection and the long-term effects of antiretroviral medications. Her two children, sons ages 7 and 10 years, are uninfected. Ms. Simon's boyfriend of 3 years is HIV-negative and is aware of her diagnosis. He has stated that, should Ms. Simon die, he would be unable to take care of her sons but would like to be able to see them regularly. Ms. Simon's mother and sister are aware that Ms. Simon is very ill and have been caring for her children during her frequent hospitalizations. Both family members are unaware of her HIV diagnosis because Ms. Simon has told them that she has cancer. Ms. Simon is very worried about what will happen to her children if she dies but has resisted telling her family the truth about her diagnosis or enlisting their support in planning for the future. Ms. Simon states that she has no one except her boyfriend to talk with about her HIV-related concerns, because she is certain that if people in her small town knew of her HIV status, including her family, she and her children would be rejected. However, she also believes that her boyfriend gets tired of listening to her concerns, so she often does not express her feelings to him for fear of antagonizing him.

Sexual Relationships

Because one of the primary modes of HIV transmission is sexual activity, sexual and romantic relationships are almost always dramatically affected by an HIV diagnosis. Regardless of whether the

HIV-positive person is in a seroconcordant relationship (both partners are HIV-positive) or a serodiscordant relationship (only one partner is HIV-positive), the diagnosis may create considerable stress between the partners. In seroconcordant relationships, there may be questions or suspicions about whether one partner infected the other, concern about caring for the partner who is more physically ill, or conflict arising from partners' differing attitudes about disclosing to others outside the relationship. In serodiscordant relationships, the HIV-positive partner may feel responsible for protecting the other from HIV infection, or the HIV-negative partner may feel anxiety about contracting HIV. Partners may find these issues difficult to discuss, however. The HIV-negative partner may also worry about his or her ability to care for the HIV-positive partner during times of illness. Anxiety about transmission or disclosure, discomfort with barrier methods of safer sex, guilt or shame about HIV infection, or physical effects of HIV or its treatment may all affect sexual functioning in relationships. Deficits in communication or conflict resolution skills, unexpressed fears and expectations, or previously unresolved relationship issues may also contribute to relationship problems.

In Ms. Simon's clinical example, her initial presentation does not suggest that she and her partner are experiencing considerable distress. However, her partner's statement that he will be unable to care for her sons may suggest that he is becoming increasingly uncomfortable with Ms. Simon's illness and disability. In the late stages of HIV disease, partners often require as much reassurance and support as do the patients themselves as they cope with the challenges of living with a seriously ill loved one and experience anticipatory grief. Nurses caring for Ms. Simon may wish to talk with her about her opinions regarding her partner's functioning and offer support and encouragement to him when he attends medical appointments with her. If it appears warranted, individual or couples counseling may be offered to them.

Family Relationships

Relationships with family members, including parents, children, siblings, or others, may be affected by HIV whether or not the HIV-positive patient discloses his or her status to anyone in the family. Disclosure of HIV status is often a primary concern of newly diagnosed individuals, and disclosure to family members can be particularly stressful. Patients may feel isolated from family members who are unaware of their diagnosis but may fear rejection or other consequences if they do disclose. Disclosure issues become increasingly complicated during the symptomatic and end-stage phases of the disease, when patients who do not wish to disclose their diagnosis must often explain their symptoms using another "cover story," which may ultimately fail as family members interact with health care providers. Many patients benefit from empathy, support, and encouragement as they prepare to disclose their diagnosis to family members. Others may appreciate an opportunity either to practice disclosure with a supportive health care provider or to include the provider in a family meeting in which disclosure occurs.

For HIV-positive patients with children, guardianship and permanency planning may be of particular concern. Although these issues are not as pressing during the asymptomatic phase of the disease, many parents with HIV, while they are still quite healthy, begin considering the question of who will care for their children after the death of the parent. Patients should be encouraged to evaluate their options and, when possible, meet with an attorney who has experience dealing with HIV-positive parents. Patients will also need to make decisions about how and when to discuss their plans with their children and how to help their children cope with changes in the family, particularly as patients experience more symptoms or become seriously ill. Nurses, counselors, or other health professionals experienced in working with families affected by serious illness may be able to provide critically needed support during this process.

In Ms. Simon's case, disclosure and permanency planning issues are of particular concern. Because her family has been caring for her children during her illness, it is likely that they would be appropriate guardians after her death. However, the fact that family members are unaware of her diagnosis makes the process of planning for this transfer of care much more difficult. Nurses working with Ms. Simon may help her by exploring Ms. Simon's fears about disclosure to her family, the benefits of planning openly with her family about her needs and those of her children, and the possibility of helping her children understand to the best of their abilities her illness and possible death. Ms. Simon may need considerable support during disclosure to her family, as may her family members. Adequate support and counseling resources should be made available as needed to enhance the likelihood that Ms. Simon and her family will adapt to the stresses that will occur with the disclosure of her serostatus.

> ### *Critical* Thinking Question
>
> What are the issues regarding permanency planning, prognosis, likely course of disease, and palliative measures?

Social Support and Isolation

HIV-positive patients with higher levels of social support tend to have higher quality of life and, some studies suggest, longer life spans. However, fear of social conflict, rejection, or discrimination may make some individuals with HIV unwilling to avail themselves of supportive relationships that may be available to them. Although relationships may be supportive even without disclosure, patients may feel particularly isolated if there is no one with whom they may discuss the concerns and issues related to HIV. Friends or loved ones who are aware of the patient's diagnosis may provide a supportive environment that will help alleviate feelings of shame or contamination experienced by many people living with the virus.

However, disclosure of an individual's HIV status to friends or loved ones risks a loss of control over potentially damaging confidential information. Friends or loved ones may not appreciate the patient's desire for confidentiality or may seek support for themselves in coping with the stress of a friend's illness. Thus a person who discloses his or her HIV status to friends risks the possibility of their diagnosis becoming more widely known than they desire, in addition to the possible benefits of social support.

In Ms. Simon's case, the tendency to self-isolate because of fear that her HIV diagnosis would become widely known is quite evident. She is experiencing considerable distress because of her isolation and does not have any idea about where to seek support. Nurses working with Ms. Simon may help introduce her to support groups in her community or surrounding communities that are specifically for persons with HIV. In some larger communities, support groups specifically for HIV-positive women

may exist, which would provide opportunities for Ms. Simon to share and problem-solve with women in similar circumstances. HIV support organizations or agencies may have "buddy programs," which pair HIV-positive individuals with a volunteer (who may have HIV or not) for social support and companionship. Other communities may have church-based programs, such as care teams, that are accepting and supportive of people with HIV. Ms. Simon's health care providers can be invaluable in helping her identify one or more of these types of support and relieving her feelings of isolation.

Summary

All types of interpersonal relationships, from the close relationships with sexual partners, family members, and loved ones to less intimate relationships with other social contacts, may be affected by HIV disease. Individuals living with HIV may need assistance in coping with the fear and vulnerability associated with disclosing their status to their social network and managing interpersonal conflicts that may occur. In addition, any psychologic or psychiatric problems that the patient is experiencing may complicate their interpersonal relationships and make problem solving more challenging both for the patient and for their health care providers. Nurses working with HIV-positive patients may be able to offer an initial source of much-needed support and acceptance and then facilitate the process of either disclosing to family and friends or developing new support systems.

SOCIAL ISSUES

Most infectious epidemics have been associated with great fear or rejection of its victims, and HIV is no exception. Individuals living with HIV often experience a variety of social sequelae commonly related to stigmatization and discrimination. Several case examples are presented to illustrate common social consequences of HIV infection and its treatment.

> ### CLINICAL EXAMPLE
> Mr. Henry Carson, an attractive 39-year-old homosexual man, had a successful accounting practice when he developed *Pneumocystis carinii* pneumonia (PCP) that required hospitalization. Although he generally used safe-sex practices, he has admitted that he did not always use available protection during sexual activity. In the months before developing PCP, Mr. Carson

noticed several less serious health problems, including unintentional weight loss, toenail infection, and a persistent facial rash. When they were brought to his physician's attention, the conditions were dismissed, being related to excessive work and stress or common to people who exercise and use a public shower. Mr. Carson had never discussed his homosexuality with his physician. Mr. Carson's recuperation was complicated by a concomitant case of cytomegalovirus (CMV) colitis, a viral condition of the colon resulting in frequent bloody diarrhea. On his first clinic visit following a 2-week hospitalization, Mr. Carson was much improved and glad to be able to breathe without difficulty and experiencing normal bowel movements but was still quite weak and debilitated. A trusted friend had temporarily moved in to assist in managing the intravenous infusions for the CMV and the activities of maintaining a home. Mr. Carson was very concerned about his inability to return to work immediately, his appearance, and his inability to care for himself. He lacked the strength to work and feared that his mere appearance would discourage clients. To explain his absence from the office, he told his secretary that he had a family emergency that required him to be away. No family member or friend, with the lone exception of his trusted friend currently caring for him, was aware of his recently diagnosed illnesses.

Stigma

People living with HIV-AIDS are often victims of prejudice based on fear and misunderstanding. Similarly, the prejudice surrounding mental illness often results in unnecessary additional stigma for people living with HIV and mental illness. Important to an understanding of the individual with HIV who seeks mental health services is an understanding of the concept of stigma and its corrosive and debilitating effects.

The social construction of HIV has made it among the most stigmatized medical condition in modern history. HIV is viewed as much more than a transmissible and lethal condition. HIV stigmatization is fueled by misinformation about risks of HIV transmission, as well as by prejudicial attitudes against groups most affected by the epidemic or the sexual and drug-using behaviors that transmit HIV, and fears more generally associated with sickness and death. The social idiom of HIV can be illustrated by applying six general dimensions of social stigmas:

1. Although concealable early in its course, later stages of HIV infection are rarely hidden from others.
2. HIV infection interferes with social relationships.
3. The disease physically disables and disfigures and is therefore aesthetically unpleasant.
4. The origin of HIV infection is often, although not always, blamed on behaviors and choices.
5. The course of HIV infection is degenerative and not always alterable.
6. HIV is a high-peril condition in that it poses risks to others.

People infected with HIV suffer countless social repercussions. The fear of being stigmatized keeps many from seeking help. Family, friends, employers, coworkers, and health care providers can all contribute to social prejudice, discrimination, and isolation. Many infected individuals conceal their HIV status from others, often at the cost of their personal welfare. To these people, the social stigmas can become a source of chronic stress. People who experience repeated acts of discrimination can become bitter, hostile, suspicious, and alienated. HIV-related stigmas therefore contribute to the anxiety, depression, and interpersonal distrust experienced by so many people living with HIV.

Stigmatization can occur during any phase of HIV disease and interfere with coping and adjustment. Threats of social isolation and discrimination may keep patients from disclosing their HIV infection, thereby cutting off potential sources of social support. Depression and anxiety are common for people who do not disclose their HIV status to anyone. On the other hand, people who go totally public with their HIV status may also be highly distressed. Selective disclosure of HIV seropositivity to close and trusted confidants is related to the greatest degree of emotional adjustment.

Stigmas present several potential adverse health-related outcomes. Concerns about discrimination and stigmatization are among the most commonly cited reasons people avoid HIV testing. Fears of harassment and job discrimination may preclude opportunities for early medical interventions. HIV infection can result in loss of health insurance when it is deemed a preexisting condition. Although not entirely the result of social perceptions of HIV, discontinued health insurance benefits occur in a stigmatizing context and therefore join an accumulating array of adverse experiences for the patient. Stigmatization also originates from within the health profession, directly affecting the delivery of medical and mental health services. People with HIV often compare themselves with lepers in the health care system, facing impersonal attitudes of hospital staff and isolation within health care facilities.

In Mr. Carson's clinical example, even though he knew he was at risk, his concerns about stigmatization caused him to avoid being tested for HIV until he was severely ill and his life was in danger. He failed to discuss his homosexuality with his physician, an important piece of information that may well have prompted his physician to advise HIV testing, given the aforementioned constellation of minor complaints. The nurse providing care to Mr. Carson should focus on the improvement in his health status by consolidating lessons learned from illness and encouraging health-promotion behaviors such as adherence to highly active antiretroviral therapy (HAART) and secondary PCP prophylaxis. It will be important to help Mr. Carson develop realistic expectations in reassessing his work limitations. The nurse should also show empathy for unrealistic expectations and any return of denial of his compromised health status.

Treatment-Related Concerns and Discrimination

There are many side effects and complications associated with the medical management of HIV. For most patients with HIV, the benefits of HAART outweigh the risks. However, all available antiretroviral agents have the potential for causing side effects, and these side effects may lead to diminished quality of life or cause changes in patients' appearance or behavior that places them at risk for discrimination. Although the side effects may range from mild to severe, all patients should be warned and educated about the side effects that may occur with HAART.

CLINICAL EXAMPLE

Michael Barbie, a 28-year-old Caucasian homosexual male, had been taking the same three-drug HAART regimen of stavudine, lamivudine, and indinavir since 1997. His CD4 count was 431/mm^3 and his HIV ribonucleic acid (RNA) by polymerase chain reaction (PCR) was less than 50 copies per ml. Although very

pleased with his sustained response to medications, Mr. Barbie had noticed a 10-pound weight gain over the last 6 months. He was increasingly fatigued, had noticed problems with libido and erectile function and was increasingly sad most of the time. At the same time, his arms and legs seemed to be thinning, and he was losing weight in his face. More than one person had commented that he seemed thin. At his next clinic visit, he discussed his concerns with his physician, who reassured him and encouraged Mr. Barbie to continue his medicine because his overall health was good, and the prognosis continued to be excellent.

Mr. Barbie also experienced bouts of indinavir-related diarrhea. At least two or three times a day, it was necessary for him to leave his workstation to use the restroom. One day, he overheard two co-workers talking about him. During the conversation, one of the co-workers said that she knew a man with AIDS who had a body shape similar to Mr. Barbie's and that she had seen Mr. Barbie taking medicine. She went on to say that she thought Mr. Barbie had AIDS. The other co-worker said she was afraid to be around him. Soon after the day he overheard his co-workers' conversation, the store manager began criticizing Mr. Barbie's work performance, despite his 3-year history of above-average performance appraisals, a promotion to assistant manager, and a stellar attendance record. Eventually his employment was terminated.

Although he made several attempts to find other employment, Mr. Barbie had been unsuccessful. He was afraid to list his previous employer as a reference for fear that his HIV status would be disclosed. Under federal law, Mr. Barbie had the option of maintaining his health insurance by paying the premiums. However, without a paycheck he was unable to do so. He became increasingly depressed and hopeless and stopped looking for employment.

At his next clinic appointment, Mr. Barbie was tearful, unshaven, and wearing soiled clothing. He had stopped taking his medicine since he lost his job and insurance. His uninfected partner was paying all their bills as best as he was able. However, they were unable to afford the $1100 a month required for Mr. Barbie's medicine. Mr. Barbie explained that he feared that eventually his partner would leave him or kick him out of the apartment if he was not able to find work. He seemed hopeless and had no idea of what he was going to do.

Discrimination

Discrimination against people with HIV originates from the same fears and prejudices that give rise to other forms of stigma. Ridicule, violence, housing eviction, loss of insurance, denial of health and dental care, loss of supportive services, and loss of employment are also very real consequences for those who get HIV or get too close to HIV. Discrimination is a common experience for many HIV-infected gay men, injection drug users, school-age children, and commercial sex workers. It is not uncommon for HIV-infected people to be denied services by rental agents or bankers, to be harassed by the police, or to experience physical violence or attempted violence and work-related discrimination. A survey of people with HIV showed that people who experienced more acts of HIV discrimination reported significantly less general life satisfaction (Heckman et al, 1997). The most destructive forms of discrimination involve employment, health care, and mental health services.

It might be expected that HIV infection be concealed from employers. Discrimination in the workplace against people living with HIV can include reduced responsibilities, isolation from co-workers and the public, or termination. Although job termination on the basis of illness is legal when physical limitations prohibit the performance of required duties, there is protection against discrimination for the disabled if a worker's HIV status is declared. HIV is included under the Americans with Disabilities Act, which prohibits discrimination against otherwise qualified disabled individuals. However, laws and employment practices vary across states, and workers who suffer illegal terminations outside of high HIV-incidence areas may lack adequate representation and advocacy.

HIV-infected people who work in service occupations are especially vulnerable to discrimination. Employers are no different from the general public and often hold irrational beliefs that employees with HIV will threaten the health of customers. Even employers who know that HIV is not transmitted on the job may fear that the public will not understand and that their business might be adversely affected if it became known that an HIV-positive person was employed at their worksite. Similar to family members and friends, employers may fear HIV-related stigmas being displaced onto them.

HIV-positive health care professionals must limit themselves to noninvasive procedures; and for some, such as dentists, this is the equivalent of closing their practice. Despite universal precautions against HIV transmission and the fact that only a few providers have ever infected patients, the public fears health care services from HIV-infected practitioners. Interestingly, discrimination runs in the opposite direction as well, with health-care providers expressing discomfort about working with HIV-infected patients.

In Mr. Barbie's example, he has a multitude of social concerns related to discrimination. First, the nurse working with Mr. Barbie should help him identify harmful behaviors such as stopping his medications without consulting with his health care provider. The nurse must also be able to discuss decisions about whom Mr. Barbie should tell and when he should tell others about being HIV-infected. It is important for the nurse to show empathy for Mr. Barbie's conflicts about disclosure and fears of being rejected because of being HIV-infected. It may be beneficial to refer Mr. Barbie to a social support group to help him overcome the effects of stigmatization. Additionally, Mr. Barbie's lack of trust in his partner and fears that his partner will abandon him appear to be related to his loss of gainful employment. A nonjudgmental attitude, coupled with patience and continuity of care, would be important clinical responses for the nurse working with Mr. Barbie. Many individuals lose self-esteem if they are not able to continue working, or they feel anger and may wish to distance themselves from others whom they feel obligated to support. This tendency is particularly likely for men, who are often socialized to believe that caring for others is primarily a financial responsibility. If Mr. Barbie's situation further deteriorates, it may be necessary for the nurse to arrange for multiservice coordination, including housing and transportation assistance, vocational rehabilitation and education, and linkage to entitlement programs.

Mr. Barbie's concerns about a 10-pound weight gain while experiencing thinning of his arms and legs, coupled with a loss of weight in his face, indicate that he may be developing HIV-related lipodystrophy (HRL). Although the physical changes related to HRL have been identified, little attention has been focused on the potential psychologic effects of

HRL on individuals living with HIV and AIDS. There are profound psychosocial and social implications of living with bodily dysmorphism (Lyon, Turban, 2000). There have been reports of persons being identified as HIV-positive because of changes in their physique. HRL may result in lack of privacy in addition to the potential psychologic distress related to changes in body image. The nurse should assess for psychologic distress related to both body dysmorphism and concerns about potential long-term cardiovascular consequences of HRL. The nurse should provide the patient an opportunity to voice concerns about taking medications that, although life promoting, may be associated with significant social and psychologic implications.

Quality-of-Life Issues in Treatment

Morbidity and mortality associated with AIDS have declined dramatically in the last few years, in large part because of the efficacy of HAART. The extended life expectancy for most HIV-positive patients increases the need to strive to maintain the quality of their lives. There are six key impediments to quality of life for HIV-infected patients: anemia, malnutrition, sexual dysfunction, pain, cognitive dysfunction, and depression. Most HIV health care providers focus their attention on HAART, prophylaxis for opportunistic infections, drug toxicities, and viral resistance; however, patients focus most of their attention on their symptoms and how they feel. Fatigue, pain, and other symptoms associated with HIV infection and its treatment often impair patients' abilities to carry out the activities of daily living, decreasing not only their enjoyment of life, but also their ability to work, take care of their families, and care for themselves.

Because Mr. Barbie's quality of life is increasingly impaired by his physical symptoms, they require investigation. Fatigue, the primary symptom of anemia, adversely affects quality of life in HIV-infected patients as much as pain and nausea. Sexual dysfunction is a common complaint of men infected with HIV. Although psychosexual dysfunction in HIV-infected patients is not surprising in view of the strong sexual and social stigma associated with HIV infection and the risk of transmission of infection to sexual partners, there are physical causes of sexual dysfunction that should be investigated as well. In evaluating Mr. Barbie's sexual dysfunction,

the nurse will need to ask him about any changes in libido or orgasmic ability, in the quality and frequency of erections, or in the ability to ejaculate. Altered sexual function may be an obvious early indicator of testosterone deficiency. Testosterone replacement therapy is commonly used to treat hypogonadism in HIV-positive men.

As discussed under intrapersonal issues in this chapter, depression is common among HIV-infected individuals. Younger age, unemployment, lack of health insurance, lower CD4 counts, HIV-related symptoms, not having a partner, lower social support, and use of noninjection drugs have been identified as predictors of depression (Katz et al, 1966). If Mr. Barbie has a major depressive disorder, management should include antidepressant medication, counseling, education, assessment of suicide risk, and cognitive strategies.

Finally, Mr. Barbie's nonadherence to HAART is a significant issue in the treatment of his HIV infection, because suboptimal adherence can promote virologic failure and the development of antiretroviral drug resistance. Despite the importance of adherence, up to 50% of patients receiving HAART are nonadherent (Reiter et al, 2000). This failure may be a result of the complex dosing schedules and side effects associated with HAART, as well as conflicting expectations about treatment efficacy and low self-efficacy in correctly adhering to the regimen.

Substance Abuse

Although substance use has been discussed previously in this chapter as an intrapersonal issue to be assessed and treated, the social issues associated with substance abuse warrant further discussion. In particular, individuals with substance use problems may interact with the health care system in a way that demands particular care and attention by skilled providers.

CLINICAL EXAMPLE

Kyle Jewel is a 46-year-old gay man who recently closed a successful independent insurance brokerage company to assume primary care responsibilities to an aging and previously abusive mother. Mr. Jewel was infected with HIV in 1992. During the time since his infection, he has taken a number of HIV medications with limited success, primarily related to nonadherence. His nonadherence is primarily related to Mr. Jewel's self-described enjoyment of "partying." These parties can last for days or weeks and are characterized by high levels of alcohol and drug consumption. Mr. Jewel frequently complains to his health care providers of sinus headaches and pain in his extremities. He has received opioid analgesics (e.g., oxycodone, codeine, hydrocodone bitartrate) to control the more intense pain in the past. He requests pain medication at every clinic visit and calls between visits for refills. It is not uncommon for Mr. Jewel to report that he lost his pain medicines or that someone either borrowed or stole them. He also complains of nervousness, an inability to sleep, and difficulty concentrating. He inconsistently sees a psychotherapist for issues related to his family conflict, failed sexual relationships, and depression. In addition to his HIV medications, Mr. Jewel also takes alprazolam for anxiety and sertraline for depression. Recently, a local pharmacist called the clinic to request a hydrocodone bitartrate refill for Mr. Jewel. Investigation into the situation leads to the finding that Mr. Jewel receives opioid prescriptions from at least three physicians. His record reveals that he has undergone evaluation for a chronic pain syndrome by two pain specialists who were unable to determine the source of his pain and discharged him from their care.

One of the most challenging aspects of patient care in the context of HIV is the question of how to treat patients who need treatment for substance abuse but refuse to acknowledge their addiction. Harm reduction offers a means of conceptualizing and designing treatment that reaches vulnerable individuals who are unsure of what to do about their drug and alcohol use or who have complicating factors such as mental illness. The goals of harm reduction–based treatments are flexible and are established in collaboration between the patient and provider. Abstinence is never a condition of harm reduction–oriented treatment and may or may not be a goal.

Harm-reduction principles demand that the patient and provider negotiate a treatment plan that is congruent with what a patient perceives his or her needs to be. Expecting abstinence or change in drug use may not be appropriate until there is something to replace the function of drugs and alcohol, whether it is more effective psychiatric medication, a therapeutic relationship, or relief from social or economic distress. It is important to respond to the problems that a patient identifies as priorities, rather than to define all of a patient's life problems in terms of addiction. In other words, one must understand and attend to the patient's "hierarchy of needs."

The best treatment strategy also includes addressing ambivalence or the patient's mixed feelings about giving up his or her drug of choice, which is the core of harm-reduction therapy—the work that focuses on helping someone resolve ambivalence and make a decision. The decisions might range from using sterile syringes at all times, to using condoms in some sexual encounters, to quitting alcohol and smoking marijuana instead.

In Mr. Jewel's case, after long discussion, he decided that he would enter into a "controlled-substance management agreement" (Box 44-1) with his physician. Under the terms of the agreement, Mr. Jewel would receive a predetermined number of sustained-release analgesics each month. In turn, he would not seek prescription drugs from other providers or illegally. Mr. Jewel was also referred to a psychologist who was familiar with the care of patients with HIV, mental illness, and substance-use disorders.

Mr. Jewel's primary psychologic task is related to his inability to cope effectively with physical symptoms. The nurse must be able to help him not only identify his symptoms, but also learn to accurately describe them to the appropriate members of the health care team who may be able to provide relief. The provision of emotional support and compassion for his distress are important skills for the nurse. It may be helpful to educate Mr. Jewel about the causes of his symptoms of pain, the limitations of treatment, and the risks and benefits of using controlled substances. Showing empathy for Mr. Jewel's discomfort, distress, impatience, and fear of progression of his illness may be helpful in working with him. Mr. Jewel may, as his ambivalence about substance abuse issues resolves, benefit from referral to an abuse treatment program integrated with his medical care.

Disability and Returning to Work

The Social Security Act (SSA) helps people with disabilities by providing monetary benefits to the insured individual who "is under a disability" (42 U.S.C. §423[a][1]). The Act defines "disability" as an "inability to engage in any substantial gainful activity by reason of any physical or mental impairment which can be expected to result in death or which

| Box 44–1 | Controlled-Substance Management Agreement

Controlled-substance medications (i.e., opioids, tranquilizers and barbiturates) are very useful, but have a high potential for misuse and are therefore closely regulated by the local, state and federal government. Controlled-substance medications are intended to *relieve* or treat symptoms (or both) of various illnesses (i.e., insomnia, anxiety, inattentiveness), *not* simply to feel good.

The purpose of this Agreement is to prevent misunderstanding about certain medicines you will be taking and to help you and your physician comply with the laws regarding controlled medications. You are being asked to sign this Agreement with the following stipulations:

- I understand that this Agreement is essential to the trust and confidence necessary in a physician-patient relationship and that my physician undertakes to treat me based on this Agreement.
- I understand that if I break this Agreement, my physician will stop prescribing these controlled-substance medications.
- If that should happen, my physician will taper me off the medicine over a period of several days, as necessary, to avoid withdrawal symptoms. In addition, a drug-dependence treatment program or assessment may be recommended.
- I will communicate fully with my physician about the effectiveness or ineffectiveness of any prescribed medication.
- I will not use any illegal substances, including marijuana, cocaine, and others.
- I will not share, sell, or trade my medication with anyone or for any reason.
- I will not attempt to obtain any controlled medicines, including opioid pain medicines, controlled stimulants, or antianxiety medicines, from any other physician or individual.
- I am responsible for my controlled-substance medications. If the prescription of medication is lost, misplaced, or stolen, or if I use it up sooner than was prescribed, I understand IT WILL NOT BE REPLACED until the next scheduled visit.
- I agree that refills of my prescriptions for controlled-substance medications will be made only at the time of an office appointment or during regular office hours. No refills will be available during evenings, weekends, or holidays. I agree to call at least 24 hours ahead for refills of controlled substances.
- I agree to use _____ pharmacy, located at _____, telephone number _____, for filling prescriptions for all of my controlled-substance medications.

- I authorized the physician and my pharmacy to cooperate fully with any city, state, or federal law enforcement agency, including Alabama's Board of Pharmacy, in the investigation of any possible misuse, sale, or other diversion of my controlled-substance medications. I authorize my physician to provide a copy of this Agreement to my pharmacy. I agree to waive any applicable privilege or right of privacy or confidentiality with respect to these authorizations.
- I agree that I will submit to blood or urine tests if requested by my physician to determine my compliance with my treatment plan.
- I agree that I will use my controlled-substance medication exactly as prescribed and that use of my medicine at a greater rate will result in my being without medication for a period.
- I will bring all unused controlled-substance medication to every office visit.
- I agree to make and keep regularly scheduled appointments and understand that if I miss an appointment my controlled-substance medication will not be renewed until I am seen and evaluated by my physician.
- I understand that the main treatment goal is to improve my ability to function or work and reduce pain. In consideration of that goal and the fact that I am given potent medication to help me reach that goal, I agree to help myself by following a healthy lifestyle that includes exercise, proper nutrition, good sleep hygiene, and smoking and alcohol cessation (if recommended). I understand that only through following a healthier lifestyle can I hope to have the most successful outcome to my treatment.
- I agree to follow these guidelines and the treatment plan as prescribed by my physician. All of my questions and concerns regarding treatment have been adequately addressed and a copy of this document has been given to me.

This Agreement is entered into on this _____ day of _____, 20 ___.

Patient Signature: _____

Print Name: _____

Physician Signature: _____

Print Name: _____

Witnessed by: _____

Print Name: _____

has lasted or can be expected to last for a continuous period of not less than 12 months" (42 U.S.C. § 423 [d][1][A]). The impairment must be of such "severity that she is not only unable to do her previous work but cannot, considering her age, education, and work experience, engage in any other kind of substantial gainful work which exists in the national economy" (42 U.S.C. §423 [d][2][A]).

CLINICAL EXAMPLE

Terry Long is a 45-year-old woman who was diagnosed with HIV in 1992. Shortly thereafter, she developed tuberculosis and was not able to work in her job as a physical therapist. Her condition was very slow to respond to treatment. In the era of HIV care before HAART, Ms. Long's prognosis was very poor. In consultation with her employer, the decision was made that Ms. Long would apply for Social Security Disability Insurance (SSDI) benefits. The disability determination was made in her favor and she began to receive monthly disability payments.

In 1996 Ms. Long's HIV treatment was switched to a HAART regimen that included zidovudine, lamivudine, and indinavir. She had both an excellent virologic and immunologic response. Her HIV RNA by PCR currently remains below 50 copies/ml, and her CD4 count remains above 600/mm^3. She has experienced no signs of toxicity or clinical symptoms. In addition, over the last several years, Ms. Long has experienced many positive changes in her life. She no longer uses illicit drugs and incorporates many complementary therapies (including meditation, yoga, and exercise) into her overall treatment plan. She developed a relationship with a wealthy executive with whom she has lived for the last 5 years. They have traveled extensively both within the United States and abroad. In addition, she earns "spending money" as a local fashion model. After more than 5 years, Ms. Long was notified that continuation of her SSDI benefits were under review. At the same time, her boyfriend stated that he wanted to end their relationship.

When Ms. Long comes for her clinic appointment, she cannot stop crying. She explains that there is no way she can go back to work because, in her words, "it's been too long," "things have changed in the profession," and "I won't have time to stay healthy doing the things I usually do for myself." She is terrified that she will not be able to manage financially if she is living alone.

Ms. Long's situation is not uncommon. The provisions of case management, outreach support, patient education, and new skills training will be important in working with Ms. Long. Some of these services may be available through community-based AIDS service organizations and require close coordination with medical care. In addition, it would be important to explain to Ms. Long that the SSA sometimes grants SSDI benefits to individuals who not only can work, but also are working. For example, to facilitate a disabled person's reentry into the workforce, the SSA authorizes a 9-month trial work period during which SSDI recipients may receive full benefits. Improvement in a totally disabled person's physical condition, while permitting that person to work, will not necessarily or immediately lead the SSA to terminate SSDI benefits.

CONCLUSION

HIV disease has long-term and far-reaching effects on all aspects of affected patients' lives, as well as the lives of their families, friends, and social network members. Complex interactions between physical symptoms, psychologic or psychiatric functioning, interpersonal relationships, social interactions, stigma, discrimination, and social services may all exist. This complexity can complicate the process of assessment, diagnosis, and treatment of HIV-positive patients. However, nurses who are aware of the multiple domains that may affect patients' quality of life or treatment plan may be able to provide an invaluable service to patients by helping them and their other health care providers to be aware of multiple needs and to gain access to supportive resources.

Critical **Thinking Question**

What are the issues related to physical, emotional, and spiritual status of someone facing the end-stage of a life-threatening illness?

Key Concepts

1. Acquired immunodeficiency syndrome (AIDS) is the term initially used to describe the effects of a set of rare symptoms occurring in young homosexual men.
2. The human immunodeficiency virus (HIV) was isolated in 1983 from patients with AIDS.

3. HIV enters the body from the T4 lymphocyte of an infected person. The normal range of T4 cells is 600 to 1200/mm³. With HIV infection, the range is 0 to 200/mm³. The number of T4 cells correlates with symptoms and clinical course. The normal T4 to T8 ratio is 2:1. This ratio is often inverse with AIDS. The normal function of the T4 cell is absent or depressed in HIV infection.

4. Opportunistic infections are those the person would normally resist when the immune system is functional and healthy. Many of the opportunistic diseases are commonly found in the environment and were rarely seen before the HIV epidemic.

5. Health care providers are not in a high-risk category but do need to be aware of special precautions to avoid exposure. The potential for occupational transmission of HIV can be reduced by implementing and vigorously enforcing infection-control procedures, such as universal precautions.

6. Populations at risk for HIV infection are identified based on specific behaviors that are practiced by individuals within the population. The three main means of transmission are: (1) men who have sex with men, (2) injecting drug use, and (3) heterosexual contact, including sex with bisexual men and drug-injecting partners.

7. AIDS dementia, the most common late CNS dysfunction, is characterized by cognitive, motor, and behavioral dysfunction.

8. Most states have enacted laws to promote health care provider compliance with diagnostic confidentiality. Confidentiality is an ethical responsibility.

9. For the patient with AIDS dementia, the nurse can maintain a therapeutic milieu by ensuring that measures to safeguard the patient, staff, and other patients are used. These measures include universal precautions, one-to-one supervision, reality orientation, use of daily routine, posted schedules, clocks, and calendars to minimize confusion.

References

Bing EG et al: Psychiatric disorders and drug use among human immunodeficiency virus-infected adults in the United States, *Arch Gen Psychiatry* 58(8):71, 2001.

Centers for Disease Control and Prevention (CDC): *HIV/AIDS Surveillance Report* 12(1), 2000.

DiClemente et al: Adolescents and acquired immune deficiency syndrome (AIDS): epidemiology, prevention, and psychological response. In Corr CA, Balk DE, editors: *Handbook of adolescent death and bereavement*, New York, 1996, Springer.

Ferrando SJ, Batki SL: Substance use and HIV infection, *New Dir Ment Health Serv* 87:57, 2000.

Grant I et al: Depressed mood does not explain neuropsychological deficits in HIV-infected persons, *Neuropsychology* 7:53, 1993.

Heckman TG et al: Psychosocial predictors of life satisfaction among persons living with HIV infection and AIDS, *J Assoc Nurses AIDS Care* 3:21, 1997.

Kalichman et al: Factors associated with risk for human immunodeficiency virus (HIV) infection among chronic mentally ill adults, *Am J Psychiatry* 151:221, 1994.

Kalichman SC: *Understanding AIDS: advances in research and treatment*, ed 2, Washington, DC, 1998, American Psychological Association.

Katz MH et al: Depression and use of mental health services among HIV-infected men, *AIDS Care* 8(4):433, 1966.

Kelly JA et al: Factors associated with severity of depression and high-risk sexual behavior among persons diagnosed with human immunodeficiency virus (HIV) infection, *Health Psychol* 12:215, 1993.

Kent TA et al: Neuroimaging in HIV infection: neuropsychological and pathological correlation. In Grant I, Martin A, editors: *Neuropsychology of HIV infection*, New York, 1994, Oxford University Press.

Kemppaineen JK: Predictors of quality of life in AIDS patients, *J Assoc Nurses AIDS Care* 12(1):61, 2001.

Lyon DE, Turban E: HIV-related lipodystrophy: a clinical syndrome with implications for nursing practice, *J Assoc Nurses AIDS Care* 11(2):36, 2000.

Marzuk PM et al: HIV seroprevalence among suicide victims in New York City, 1991-1993, *Am J Psychiatry* 154:1720, 1997.

McArthur JC: Neurological and neuropathological manifestations of HIV infection. In Grant I, Martin A, editors: *Neuropsychology of HIV infection*, New York, 1994, Oxford University Press.

O'Dowd MA, Biderman DJ, McKegney FP: Incidence of suicidality in AIDS and HIV-positive patients attending a psychiatry outpatient program, *Psychosomatics* 34:33, 1993.

Reiter GS et al: Elements of success in HIV clinical care: multiple interventions that promote adherence, *Topics in HIV Medicine* 8(5):21, 2000.

Stern Y et al: Dana consortium on the therapy of HIV-dementia and related cognitive disorders. Factors associated with incident human immunodeficiency virus-dementia, *Arch Neurol*, 58(3):473, 2001.

Wesselingh SL, Thompson KA: Immunopathogenesis of HIV-associated dementia, *Curr Opin Neurol* 14(3):375, 2001.

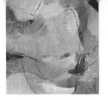

Diagnostic Criteria for Mental Disorders, Text Revision (DSM-IV-TR)*

The following text represents the complete list of diagnoses found in the DSM-IV-TR. Many diagnoses have notations that increase specificity. These notations are not always included here. The following clarifications are made to assist you in understanding this material: *NOS* = not otherwise specified; *X* = a specific code number is required.

Note to students: This list represents all DSM-IV-TR diagnoses. It does not, however, reflect some of the subtleties of coding found in the DSM-IV-TR manual. The student is directed to the manual should finer discrimination be sought.

Disorders Usually First Diagnosed in Infancy, Childhood, or Adolescence

Mental retardation

Note: *These are coded on Axis II.*

317	Mild Mental Retardation
318.0	Moderate Mental Retardation
318.1	Severe Mental Retardation
318.2	Profound Mental Retardation
319	Mental Retardation, Unspecified

Learning disorders

315.00	Reading Disorder
315.1	Mathematics Disorder
315.2	Disorder of Written Expression
315.9	Learning Disorder NOS

Motor skills disorder

315.4	Developmental Coordination Disorder

Communication disorders

315.31	Expressive Language Disorder
315.31	Mixed Receptive-Expressive Language Disorder
315.39	Phonological Disorder
307.0	Stuttering
307.9	Communication Disorder NOS

Pervasive developmental disorders

299.00	Autistic Disorder
299.80	Rett's Disorder
299.10	Childhood Disintegrative Disorder
299.80	Asperger's Disorder
299.80	Pervasive Developmental Disorder NOS

Attention-deficit and disruptive behavior disorders

314.xx	Attention-Deficit/Hyperactivity Disorder
.01	Combined Type
.00	Predominantly Inattentive Type
.01	Predominantly Hyperactive-Impulsive Type
314.9	Attention-Deficit/Hyperactivity Disorder NOS
312.8	Conduct Disorder
313.81	Oppositional Defiant Disorder
312.9	Disruptive Behavior Disorder NOS

Feeding and eating disorders of infancy or early childhood

307.52	Pica
307.53	Rumination Disorder
307.59	Feeding Disorder of Infancy or Early Childhood

Tic disorders

307.23	Tourette's Disorder
307.22	Chronic Motor or Vocal Tic Disorder

*Reprinted with permission from the American Psychiatric Association: *Diagnostic and statistical manual of mental disorders, text revision,* ed 4, Washington, DC, 2000, APA.

307.21 Transient Tic Disorder
307.20 Tic Disorder NOS

Elimination disorders

___.__ Encopresis
787.6   With Constipation and Overflow Incontinence
307.7   Without Constipation and Overflow Incontinence
307.6   Enuresis (Not Due to a General Medical Condition)

Other disorders of infancy, childhood, or adolescence

309.21 Separation Anxiety Disorder
313.23 Selective Mutism
313.89 Reactive Attachment Disorder of Infancy or Early Childhood
307.3 Stereotypic Movement Disorder
313.9 Disorder of Infancy, Childhood, or Adolescence NOS

Delirium, Dementia, and Amnestic and Other Cognitive Disorders

Delirium

293.0 Delirium Due to…
___.__ Substance Intoxication Delirium
___.__ Substance Withdrawal Delirium
___.__ Delirium Due to Multiple Etiologies
780.09 Delirium NOS

Dementia

290.xx Dementia of the Alzheimer's Type, With Early Onset (also code 331.0 Alzheimer's disease on Axis III)
  .10   Without behavioral disturbances
  .11   With behavioral disturbances
290.xx Dementia of the Alzheimer's Type, With Late Onset (also code 331.0 Alzheimer's disease on Axis III)
  .10   Without behavioral disturbances
  .11   With behavioral disturbances
290.xx Vascular Dementia
  .40   Uncomplicated
  .41   With Delirium
  .42   With Delusions
  .43   With Depressed Mood
294.1x Dementia Due to HIV Disease
294.1x Dementia Due to Head Trauma

294.1x Dementia Due to Parkinson's Disease
294.1x Dementia Due to Huntington's Disease
294.1x Dementia Due to Pick's Disease
294.1x Dementia Due to Creutzfeldt-Jakob Disease
294.1x Dementia Due to…
___.__ Substance-Induced Persisting Dementia
___.__ Dementia Due to Multiple Etiologies
294.8 Dementia NOS

Amnestic disorders

294.0 Amnestic Disorder Due to…
___.__ Substance-Induced Persisting Amnestic Disorder
294.8 Amnestic Disorder NOS

Other cognitive disorders

294.9 Cognitive Disorder NOS

Mental Disorders Due to a General Medical Condition not Elsewhere Classified

293.89 Catatonic Disorder Due to…
310.1 Personality Change Due to…
293.9 Mental Disorder NOS Due to…

Substance-Related Disorders

Alcohol-related disorders

Alcohol Use Disorders

303.90 Alcohol Dependence
305.00 Alcohol Abuse

Alcohol-Induced Disorders

303.00 Alcohol Intoxication
291.81 Alcohol Withdrawal
291.0 Alcohol Intoxication Delirium
291.0 Alcohol Withdrawal Delirium
291.2 Alcohol-Induced Persisting Dementia
291.1 Alcohol-Induced Persisting Amnestic Dementia
291.x Alcohol-Induced Psychotic Disorder
  .5   With Delusions
  .3   With Hallucinations
291.89 Alcohol-Induced Mood Disorder
291.89 Alcohol-Induced Anxiety Disorder
291.89 Alcohol-Induced Sexual Dysfunction
291.89 Alcohol-Induced Sleep Disorder
291.9 Alcohol-Related Disorder NOS

Amphetamine (or amphetamine-like)-related disorders

Amphetamine Use Disorders

304.40 Amphetamine Dependence
305.70 Amphetamine Abuse

Amphetamine-Induced Disorders

292.89 Amphetamine Intoxication
292.0   Amphetamine Withdrawal
292.81 Amphetamine Intoxication Delirium
292.xx Amphetamine-Induced Psychotic Disorder
  .11   With Delusions
  .12   With Hallucinations
292.84 Amphetamine-Induced Mood Disorder
292.89 Amphetamine-Induced Anxiety Disorder
292.89 Amphetamine-Induced Sexual Dysfunction
292.89 Amphetamine-Induced Sleep Disorder
292.9   Amphetamine-Related Disorder NOS

Caffeine-related disorders

Caffeine-Induced Disorders

305.90 Caffeine Intoxication
292.89 Caffeine-Induced Anxiety Disorder
292.89 Caffeine-Induced Sleep Disorder
292.9   Caffeine-Related Disorder NOS

Cannabis-related disorders

Cannabis Use Disorders

304.30 Cannabis Dependence
305.20 Cannabis Abuse

Cannabis-Induced Disorders

292.89 Cannabis Intoxication
292.81 Cannabis Intoxication Delirium
292.xx Cannabis-Induced Psychotic Disorder
  .11   With Delusions
  .12   With Hallucinations
292.89 Cannabis-Induced Anxiety Disorder
292.9   Cannabis-Related Disorder NOS

Cocaine-related disorders

Cocaine Use Disorders

304.20 Cocaine Dependence
305.60 Cocaine Abuse

Cocaine-Induced Disorders

292.89 Cocaine Intoxication
292.0   Cocaine Withdrawal
292.81 Cocaine Intoxication Delirium

292.xx Cocaine-Induced Psychotic Disorder
  .11   With Delusions
  .12   With Hallucinations
292.84 Cocaine-Induced Mood Disorder
292.89 Cocaine-Induced Anxiety Disorder
292.89 Cocaine-Induced Sexual Dysfunction
292.89 Cocaine-Induced Sleep Disorder
292.9   Cocaine-Related Disorder NOS

Hallucinogen-related disorders

Hallucinogen Use Disorders

304.50 Hallucinogen Dependence
305.30 Hallucinogen Abuse

Hallucinogen-Induced Disorders

292.89 Hallucinogen Intoxication
292.89 Hallucinogen Persisting Perception
       Disorder (Flashbacks)
292.81 Hallucinogen Intoxication Delirium
292.xx Hallucinogen-Induced Psychotic Disorder
  .11   With Delusions
  .12   With Hallucinations
292.84 Hallucinogen-Induced Mood Disorder
292.89 Hallucinogen-Induced Anxiety Disorder
292.9   Hallucinogen-Related Disorder NOS

Inhalant-related disorders

Inhalant Use Disorders

304.60 Inhalant Dependence
305.90 Inhalant Abuse

Inhalant-Induced Disorders

292.89 Inhalant Intoxication
292.81 Inhalant Intoxication Delirium
292.82 Inhalant-Induced Persisting Dementia
292.xx Inhalant-Induced Psychotic Disorder
  .11   With Delusions
  .12   With Hallucinations
292.84 Inhalant-Induced Mood Disorder
292.89 Inhalant-Induced Anxiety Disorder
292.9   Inhalant-Related Disorder NOS

Nicotine-induced disorder

Nicotine Use Disorder

305.10 Nicotine Dependence

Nicotine-Induced Disorder

292.0   Nicotine Withdrawal
292.9   Nicotine-Related Disorder NOS

Opioid-related disorders

Opioid Use Disorders

304.00 Opioid Dependence
305.50 Opioid Abuse

Opioid-Induced Disorders

292.89 Opioid Intoxication
292.0   Opioid Withdrawal
292.81 Opioid Intoxication Delirium
292.xx Opioid-Induced Psychotic Disorder
 .11   With Delusions
 .12   With Hallucinations
292.84 Opioid-Induced Mood Disorder
292.89 Opioid-Induced Sexual Dysfunction
292.89 Opioid-Induced Sleep Disorder
292.9   Opioid-Related Disorder NOS

Phencyclidine (or phencyclidine-like)–related disorders

Phencyclidine Use Disorders

304.90 Phencyclidine Dependence
305.90 Phencyclidine Abuse

Phencyclidine-Induced Disorders

292.89 Phencyclidine Intoxication
292.81 Phencyclidine Intoxication Delirium
292.xx Phencyclidine-Induced Psychotic Disorder
 .11   With Delusions
 .12   With Hallucinations
292.84 Phencyclidine-Induced Mood Disorder
292.89 Phencyclidine-Induced Anxiety Disorder
292.9   Phencyclidine-Related Disorder NOS

Sedative-, hypnotic-, or anxiolytic-related disorders

Sedative, Hypnotic, or Anxiolytic Use Disorders

304.10 Sedative, Hypnotic, or Anxiolytic Dependence
305.40 Sedative, Hypnotic, or Anxiolytic Abuse

Sedative-, Hypnotic-, or Anxiolytic-Induced Disorders

292.89 Sedative, Hypnotic, or Anxiolytic Intoxication
292.0   Sedative, Hypnotic, or Anxiolytic Withdrawal
292.81 Sedative, Hypnotic, or Anxiolytic Intoxication Delirium
292.81 Sedative, Hypnotic, or Anxiolytic Withdrawal Delirium

292.82 Sedative-, Hypnotic-, or Anxiolytic-Induced Persisting Dementia
292.83 Sedative-, Hypnotic-, or Anxiolytic-Induced Persisting Amnestic Disorder
292.xx Sedative-, Hypnotic-, or Anxiolytic-Induced Psychotic Disorder
 .11   With Delusions
 .12   With Hallucinations
292.84 Sedative-, Hypnotic-, or Anxiolytic-Induced Mood Disorder
292.89 Sedative-, Hypnotic-, or Anxiolytic-Induced Anxiety Disorder
292.89 Sedative-, Hypnotic-, or Anxiolytic-Induced Sexual Dysfunction
292.89 Sedative-, Hypnotic-, or Anxiolytic-Induced Sleep Disorder
292.9   Sedative-, Hypnotic-, or Anxiolytic-Related Disorder NOS

Polysubstance-related disorder

304.80 Polysubstance Dependence

Other (or unknown) substance-related disorders

Other (or Unknown) Substance Use Disorders

304.90 Other (or Unknown) Substance Dependence
305.90 Other (or Unknown) Substance Abuse

Other (or Unknown) Substance-Induced Disorders

292.89 Other (or Unknown) Substance Intoxication
292.0   Other (or Unknown) Substance Withdrawal
292.81 Other (or Unknown) Substance-Induced Delirium
292.82 Other (or Unknown) Substance-Induced Persisting Dementia
292.83 Other (or Unknown) Substance-Induced Persisting Amnestic Disorder
292.xx Other (or Unknown) Substance-Induced Psychotic Disorder
 .11   With Delusions
 .12   With Hallucinations
292.84 Other (or Unknown) Substance-Induced Mood Disorder
292.89 Other (or Unknown) Substance-Induced Anxiety Disorder
292.89 Other (or Unknown) Substance-Induced Sexual Dysfunction

292.89   Other (or Unknown) Substance-Induced
Sleep Disorder
292.9   Other (or Unknown) Substance-Related
Disorder NOS

Schizophrenia and Other Psychotic Disorders

295.xx   Schizophrenia
.30   Paranoid Type
.10   Disorganized Type
.20   Catatonic Type
.90   Undifferentiated Type
.60   Residual Type
295.40   Schizophreniform Disorder
295.70   Schizoaffective Disorder
297.1   Delusional Disorder
298.8   Brief Psychotic Disorder
297.3   Shared Psychotic Disorder
293.xx   Psychotic Disorder Due to…
.81   With Delusions
.82   With Hallucinations
___.__   Substance-Induced Psychotic Disorder
298.9   Psychotic Disorder NOS

Mood Disorders

Depressive disorders

296.xx   Major Depressive Disorder
.2x   Single Episode
.3x   Recurrent
300.4   Dysthymic Disorder
311   Depressive Disorder NOS

Bipolar disorders

296.xx   Bipolar I Disorder
.0x   Single Manic Episode
.40   Most Recent Episode Hypomanic
.4x   Most Recent Episode Manic
.6x   Most Recent Episode Mixed
.5x   Most Recent Episode Depressed
.7   Most Recent Episode Unspecified
296.89   Bipolar II Disorder
301.13   Cyclothymic Disorder
296.80   Bipolar Disorder NOS
293.83   Mood Disorder Due to…
___.__   Substance-Induced Mood Disorder
296.90   Mood Disorder NOS

Anxiety Disorders

300.01   Panic Disorder Without Agoraphobia
300.21   Panic Disorder With Agoraphobia

300.22   Agoraphobia Without History of Panic
Disorder
300.29   Specific Phobia
300.23   Social Phobia
300.3   Obsessive-Compulsive Disorder
309.81   Posttraumatic Stress Disorder
308.3   Acute Stress Disorder
300.02   Generalized Anxiety Disorder
293.89   Anxiety Disorder Due to…
___.__   Substance-Induced Anxiety Disorder
300.00   Anxiety Disorder NOS

Somatoform Disorders

300.81   Somatization Disorder
300.81   Undifferentiated Somatoform Disorder
300.11   Conversion Disorder
307.xx   Pain Disorder
.80   Associated With Psychological Factors
.89   Associated With Both Psychological
Factors and a General Medical Condition
300.7   Hypochondriasis
300.7   Body Dysmorphic Disorder
300.81   Somatoform Disorder NOS

Factitious Disorders

300.xx   Factitious Disorder
.16   With Predominantly Psychological Signs
and Symptoms
.19   With Predominantly Physical Signs and
Symptoms
.19   With Combined Psychological and
Physical Signs and Symptoms
300.19   Factitious Disorder NOS

Dissociative Disorders

300.12   Dissociative Amnesia
300.13   Dissociative Fugue
300.14   Dissociative Identity Disorder
300.6   Depersonalization Disorder
300.15   Dissociative Disorder NOS

Sexual and Gender Identity Disorders
Sexual dysfunctions
Sexual Desire Disorders

302.71   Hypoactive Sexual Desire Disorder
302.79   Sexual Aversion Disorder

Sexual Arousal Disorders

302.72   Female Sexual Arousal Disorder
302.72   Male Erectile Disorder

Orgasmic Disorders

302.73 Female Orgasmic Disorder
302.74 Male Orgasmic Disorder
302.75 Premature Ejaculation

Sexual Pain Disorders

302.76 Dyspareunia (Not Due to a General Medical Condition)
306.51 Vaginismus (Not Due to a General Medical Condition)

Sexual dysfunction due to a general medical condition

625.8   Female Hypoactive Sexual Desire Disorder Due to…
608.89 Male Hypoactive Sexual Desire Disorder Due to…
607.84 Male Erectile Disorder Due to…
625.0   Female Dyspareunia Due to…
608.89 Male Dyspareunia Due to…
625.8   Other Female Sexual Dysfunction Due to…
608.89 Other Male Sexual Dysfunction Due to…
___._   Substance-Induced Sexual Dysfunction
302.70 Sexual Dysfunction NOS

Paraphilias

302.4   Exhibitionism
302.81 Fetishism
302.89 Frotteurism
302.2   Pedophilia
302.83 Sexual Masochism
302.84 Sexual Sadism
302.3   Transvestic Fetishism
302.82 Voyeurism
302.9   Paraphilia NOS

Gender identity disorders

302.xx Gender Identity Disorder
   .6   in Children
   .85   in Adolescents or Adults
302.6   Gender Identity Disorder NOS
302.9   Sexual Disorder NOS

Eating Disorders

307.1   Anorexia Nervosa
307.51 Bulimia Nervosa
307.50 Eating Disorder NOS

Sleep Disorders

Primary sleep disorders

Dyssomnias

307.42 Primary Insomnia
307.44 Primary Hypersomnia
347   Narcolepsy
780.59 Breathing-Related Sleep Disorder
307.45 Circadian Rhythm Sleep Disorder
307.47 Dyssomnia NOS

Parasomnias

307.47 Nightmare Disorder
307.46 Sleep Terror Disorder
307.46 Sleepwalking Disorder
307.47 Parasomnia NOS

Sleep disorders related to another mental disorder

307.42 Insomnia Related to…
307.44 Hypersomnia Related to…

Other sleep disorder

780.xx Sleep Disorder Due to…
   .52   Insomnia Type
   .54   Hypersomnia Type
   .59   Parasomnia Type
   .59   Mixed Type
___._   Substance-Induced Sleep Disorder

Impulse-Control Disorders Not Elsewhere Classified

312.34 Intermittent Explosive Disorder
312.32 Kleptomania
312.33 Pyromania
312.31 Pathological Gambling
312.39 Trichotillomania
312.30 Impulse-Control Disorder NOS

Adjustment Disorders

309.xx Adjustment Disorder
   .0   With Depressed Mood
   .24   With Anxiety
   .28   With Mixed Anxiety and Depressed Mood
   .3   With Disturbance of Conduct
   .4   With Mixed Disturbance of Emotions and Conduct
   .9   Unspecified

Personality Disorders

Note: *These are coded on Axis II.*
301.0 Paranoid Personality Disorder
301.20 Schizoid Personality Disorder
301.22 Schizotypal Personality Disorder
301.7 Antisocial Personality Disorder
301.83 Borderline Personality Disorder
301.50 Histrionic Personality Disorder
301.81 Narcissistic Personality Disorder
301.82 Avoidant Personality Disorder
301.6 Dependent Personality Disorder
301.4 Obsessive-Compulsive Personality Disorder
301.9 Personality Disorder NOS

Other Conditions that May Be a Focus of Clinical Attention

Psychological factors affecting medical condition

316 ...*[Specified Psychological Factor] Affecting...[Indicate the General Medical Condition] Choose name based on nature of factors:*
  Mental Disorder Affecting Medical Condition
  Psychological Symptoms Affecting Medical Condition
  Personality Traits or Coping Style Affecting Medical Condition
  Maladaptive Health Behaviors Affecting Medical Condition
  Stress-Related Physiological Response Affecting Medical Condition
  Other or Unspecified Psychological Factors Affecting Medical Condition

Medication-induced movement disorders

332.1 Neuroleptic-Induced Parkinsonism
333.92 Neuroleptic-Malignant Syndrome
333.7 Neuroleptic-Induced Acute Dystonia
333.99 Neuroleptic-Induced Acute Akathisia
333.82 Neuroleptic-Induced Tardive Dyskinesia
333.1 Medication-Induced Postural Tremor
333.90 Medication-Induced Movement Disorder NOS

Other medication-induced disorder

995.2 Adverse Effects of Medication NOS

Relational problems

V61.9 Relational Problem Related to a Mental Disorder or General Medical Condition
V61.20 Parent-Child Relational Problem
V61.1 Partner Relational Problem
V61.8 Sibling Relational Problem
V62.81 Relational Problem NOS

Problems related to abuse or neglect

V61.21 Physical Abuse of Child
V61.21 Sexual Abuse of Child
V61.21 Neglect of Child
___.__ Physical Abuse of Adult
V61.12 If by partner
V62.83 If by a person other than partner
___.__ Sexual Abuse of Adult
V61.12 If by partner
V62.83 If by a person other than partner

Additional conditions that may be a focus of clinical attention

V15.81 Noncompliance with Treatment
V65.2 Malingering
V71.01 Adult Antisocial Behavior
V71.02 Child or Adolescent Antisocial Behavior
V62.89 Borderline Intellectual Functioning
  Note: *This is coded on Axis II.*
780.9 Age-Related Cognitive Decline
V62.82 Bereavement
V62.3 Academic Problem
V62.2 Occupational Problem
313.82 Identity Problem
V62.89 Religious or Spiritual Problem
V62.4 Acculturation Problem
V62.89 Phase of Life Problem

Additional Codes

300.9 Unspecified Mental Disorder (nonpsychotic)
V71.09 No Diagnosis or Condition on Axis I
799.9 Diagnosis or Condition Deferred on Axis I
V71.09 No Diagnosis on Axis II
799.9 Diagnosis Deferred on Axis II

Multiaxial System

Axis I Clinical Disorders
  Other Conditions that May Be a Focus of Clinical Attention
Axis II Personality Disorders (see above)
  Mental Retardation (see page 639)
Axis III General Medical Conditions
Axis IV Psychosocial and Environmental Problems
Axis V Global Assessment of Functioning

Axis III: General Medical Conditions (with ICD-9-CM Codes)

Infectious and Parasitic Diseases (001-139)

Neoplasms (140-239)

Endocrine, Nutritional, and Metabolic Diseases and Immunity Disorders (240-279)

Diseases of the Blood and Blood-Forming Organs (280-289)

Diseases of the Nervous System and Sense Organs (320-389)

Diseases of the Circulatory System (390-459)

Diseases of the Respiratory System (460-519)

Diseases of the Digestive System (520-579)

Diseases of the Genitourinary System (580-629)

Complications of Pregnancy, Childbirth, and the Puerperium (630-676)

Diseases of the Skin and Subcutaneous Tissue (680-709)

Diseases of the Musculoskeletal System and Connective Tissue (710-739)

Congenital Anomalies (740-759)

Certain Conditions Originating in the Perinatal Period (760-779)

Symptoms, Signs, and Ill-Defined Conditions (780-799)

Injury and Poisoning (800-999)

Axis IV: Psychosocial and Environmental Problems

Problems with primary support group

Problems related to the social environment

Educational problems

Occupational problems

Housing problems

Economic problems

Problems with access to health care services

Problems related to interaction with the legal system/crime

Other psychosocial and environmental problems

Axis V: Global Assessment of Functioning (GAF) Scale

Consider psychological, social, and occupational functioning on a hypothetical continuum of mental health–illness. Do not include impairment in functioning due to physical (or environmental) limitations.

Code   (Note: Use intermediate codes when appropriate (e.g., 45, 68, 72).

Code	
100 | 91	**Superior functioning in a wide range of activities, life's problems never seem to get out of hand, is sought out by others because of his or her many positive qualities. No symptoms.**
90 | 81	**Absent or minimal symptoms** (e.g., mild anxiety before an exam), **good functioning in all areas, interested and involved in a wide range of activities, socially effective, generally satisfied with life, no more than everyday problems or concerns** (e.g., an occasional argument with family members).
80 | 71	**If symptoms are present, they are transient and expectable reactions to psychosocial stressors** (e.g., difficulty concentrating after family argument); **no more than slight impairment in social, occupational, or school functioning** (e.g., temporarily falling behind in schoolwork).
70 | 61	**Some mild symptoms** (e.g., depressed mood and mild insomnia) **OR some difficulty in social, occupational, or school functioning** (e.g., occasional truancy or theft within the household), **but generally functioning pretty well, has some meaningful interpersonal relationships.**

60
|
51

Moderate symptoms (e.g., flat affect and circumstantial speech, occasional panic attacks) **OR moderate difficulty in social, occupational, or school functioning** (e.g., few friends, conflicts with peers or co-workers).

50
|
41

Serious symptoms (e.g., suicidal ideation, severe obsessional rituals, frequent shoplifting) **OR any serious impairment in social, occupational, or school functioning** (e.g., no friends, unable to keep a job).

40
|
31

Some impairment in reality testing or communication (e.g., speech is at times illogical, obscure, or irrelevant) **OR major impairment in several areas, such as work or school, family relations, judgment, thinking, or mood** (e.g., depressed man avoids friends, neglects family, and is unable to work; child frequently beats up younger children, is defiant at home, and is failing at school).

30
|
21

Behavior is considerably influenced by delusions or hallucinations OR serious impairment in communication or judgment (e.g., sometimes incoherent, acts grossly inappropriately, suicidal preoccupation) **OR inability to function in almost all areas** (e.g., stays in bed all day; no job, home, or friends).

20
|
11

Some danger of hurting self or others (e.g., suicide attempts without clear expectation of death; frequently violent; manic excitement) **OR occasionally fails to maintain minimal personal hygiene** (e.g., smears feces) **OR gross impairment in communication** (e.g., largely incoherent or mute).

10
|
1

Persistent danger of severely hurting self or others (e.g., recurrent violence) **OR persistent inability to maintain minimal personal hygiene OR serious suicidal act with clear expectation of death.**

0

Inadequate information.

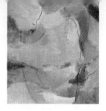

North American Nursing Diagnosis Association—Approved Nursing Diagnoses, 2001

Activity intolerance
Activity intolerance, Risk for
Adjustment, Impaired
Airway clearance, Ineffective
Allergy response, Latex
Allergy response, Risk for latex
Anxiety
Anxiety, Death
Aspiration, Risk for
Attachment, Risk for impaired parent/infant/child
Autonomic dysreflexia
Autonomic dysreflexia, Risk for

Body image, Disturbed
Body temperature, Risk for imbalanced
Bowel incontinence
Breast-feeding, Effective
Breast-feeding, Ineffective
Breast-feeding, Interrupted
Breathing pattern, Ineffective

Cardiac output, Decreased
Caregiver role strain
Caregiver role strain, Risk for
Comfort, Impaired
Communication, Impaired verbal
Conflict, Decisional
Conflict, Parental role
Confusion, Acute
Confusion, Chronic
Constipation
Constipation, Perceived
Constipation, Risk for
Coping, Compromised family
Coping, Defensive
Coping, Disabled family
Coping, Ineffective
Coping, Ineffective community
Coping, Readiness for enhanced community
Coping, Readiness for enhanced family

Denial, Ineffective
Dentition, Impaired
Development, Risk for delayed
Diarrhea
Disuse syndrome, Risk for
Diversional activity, Deficient

Energy field, Disturbed
Environmental interpretation syndrome, Impaired

Failure to thrive, Adult
Falls, Risk for
Family processes: alcoholism, Dysfunctional
Family processes, Interrupted
Fatigue
Fear
Fluid volume, Deficient
Fluid volume, Excess
Fluid volume, Risk for deficient
Fluid volume, Risk for imbalanced

Gas exchange, Impaired
Grieving
Grieving, Anticipatory
Grieving, Dysfunctional
Growth and development, Delayed
Growth, Risk for disproportionate

Health maintenance, Ineffective
Health-seeking behaviors
Home maintenance, Impaired
Hopelessness
Hyperthermia
Hypothermia

Identity, Disturbed personal
Incontinence, Functional urinary
Incontinence, Reflex urinary
Incontinence, Stress urinary
Incontinence, Total urinary

Diagnoses in *italics* are the ones most recently added to the list. Copyright © 2001 by the North American Nursing Diagnosis Association.

Incontinence, Urge urinary
Infant behavior, Disorganized
Infant behavior, Readiness for enhanced organized
Infant behavior, Risk for disorganized
Infant feeding pattern, Ineffective
Infection, Risk for
Injury, Risk for
Injury, Risk for perioperative positioning
Intracranial, adaptive capacity, Decreased

Knowledge, Deficient

Loneliness, Risk for

Memory, Impaired
Mobility, Impaired bed
Mobility, Impaired physical
Mobility, Impaired wheelchair

Nausea
Neglect, Unilateral
Noncompliance
Nutrition: less than body requirements,
    Imbalanced
Nutrition: more than body requirements,
    Imbalanced
Nutrition: more than body requirements, Risk for
    imbalanced

Oral mucous membrane, Impaired

Pain, Acute
Pain, Chronic
Parenting, Impaired
Parenting, Risk for impaired
Peripheral neurovascular dysfunction, Risk for
Poisoning, Risk for
Posttrauma syndrome
Posttrauma syndrome, Risk for
Powerlessness
Powerlessness, Risk for
Protection, Ineffective

Rape-trauma syndrome
Rape-trauma syndrome, compound reaction
Rape-trauma syndrome, silent reaction
Relocation stress syndrome
Relocation stress syndrome, Risk for
Role performance, Ineffective

Self-care deficit, Dressing/grooming
Self-care deficit, Bathing/hygiene
Self-care deficit, Feeding
Self-care deficit, Toileting
Self-esteem, Chronic low
Self-esteem, Situational low
Self-esteem, Risk for situational low
Self-mutilation
Self-mutilation, Risk for
Sensory perception, Disturbed
Sexual dysfunction
Sexuality patterns, Ineffective
Skin integrity, Impaired
Skin integrity, Risk for impaired
Sleep deprivation
Sleep pattern, Disturbed
Social interaction, Impaired
Social isolation
Sorrow, Chronic
Spiritual distress
Spiritual distress, Risk for
Spiritual well-being, Readiness for enhanced
Suffocation, Risk for
Suicide, Risk for
Surgical recovery, Delayed
Swallowing, Impaired

Therapeutic regimen management, Effective
Therapeutic regimen management, Ineffective
Therapeutic regimen management, Ineffective
    community
Therapeutic regimen management, Ineffective family
Thermoregulation, Ineffective
Thought processes, Disturbed
Tissue integrity, Impaired
Tissue perfusion, Ineffective
Transfer ability, Impaired
Trauma, Risk for

Urinary elimination, Impaired
Urinary retention

Ventilation, Impaired spontaneous
Ventilatory weaning response, Dysfunctional
Violence, Risk for other-directed
Violence, Risk for self-directed

Walking, Impaired
Wandering

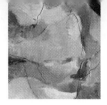

Geriatric Depression Scale

Choose the best answer for how you felt over the past week.

1.	Are you basically satisfied with your life?	Yes/No
2.	Have you dropped many of your activities and interests?	Yes/No
3.	Do you feel that your life is empty?	Yes/No
4.	Do you often get bored?	Yes/No
5.	Are you hopeful about the future?	Yes/No
6.	Are you bothered by thoughts you cannot get out of your head?	Yes/No
7.	Are you in good spirits most of the time?	Yes/No
8.	Are you afraid that something bad is going to happen to you?	Yes/No
9.	Do you feel happy most of the time?	Yes/No
10.	Do you often feel helpless?	Yes/No
11.	Do you often get restless and fidgety?	Yes/No
12.	Do you prefer to stay at home, rather than going out and doing new things?	Yes/No
13.	Do you frequently worry about the future?	Yes/No
14.	Do you feel you have more problems with memory than most?	Yes/No
15.	Do you think it is wonderful to be alive right now?	Yes/No
16.	Do you often feel downhearted and blue?	Yes/No
17.	Do you feel pretty worthless the way you are now?	Yes/No
18.	Do you worry a lot about the past?	Yes/No
19.	Do you find life very exciting?	Yes/No
20.	Is it hard for you to get started on new projects?	Yes/No
21.	Do you feel full of energy?	Yes/No
22.	Do you feel that your situation is hopeless?	Yes/No
23.	Do you think that more people are better off than you are?	Yes/No
24.	Do you frequently get upset over little things?	Yes/No
25.	Do you frequently feel like crying?	Yes/No
26.	Do you have trouble concentrating?	Yes/No
27.	Do you enjoy getting up in the morning?	Yes/No
28.	Do you prefer to avoid social gatherings?	Yes/No
29.	Is it easy for you to make decisions?	Yes/No
30.	Is your mind as clear as it used to be?	Yes/No

A score of 14 points or more suggests the presence of depression, which needs to be confirmed by clinical evaluation. From Yesavage JA, et al: Development and validation of a geriatric depression screening scale: a preliminary report, *J Psychiatr Res* 17:37, 1983. By permission. Count one point for a "yes" answer to questions 2, 3, 4, 6, 8, 10, 11, 12, 13, 14, 16, 17, 18, 20, 22, 23, 24, 25, 26, and 28 and one point for a "no" answer to questions 1, 5, 7, 9, 15, 19, 21, 27, 29, and 30.

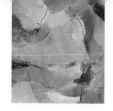

Simple Method to Determine Tardive Dyskinesia Symptoms: AIMS* Examination Procedure

PATIENT IDENTIFICATION _____ DATE _____

Rated by _____

Either before or after completing the examination procedure, observe the patient unobtrusively at rest (e.g., in waiting room).

The chair to be used in this examination should be a hard, firm one without arms.

After observing the patient, he or she may be rated on a scale of 0 (none), 1 (minimal), 2 (mild), 3 (moderate), and 4 (severe), according to the severity of symptoms.

Ask the patient whether there is anything in his or her mouth (e.g., gum, candy) and whether he or she can remove it.

Ask the patient about the *current* condition of his or her teeth. Ask the patient whether he or she wears dentures. Do teeth or dentures bother the patient *now?*

Ask the patient whether he or she notices any movement in the mouth, face, hands or feet. If yes, ask to describe and to what extent they *currently* bother the patient or interfere with his or her activities.

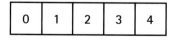

Have the patient sit in a chair with hands on knees, legs slightly apart, and feet flat on the floor. (Look at entire body for movements while in this position.)

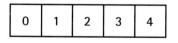

Ask the patient to sit with hands hanging unsupported. If a man, between his legs, if a woman and wearing a dress, hanging over her knees. (Observe hands and other body areas.)

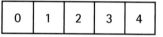

Ask the patient to open mouth. (Observe tongue at rest within the mouth.) Do this twice.

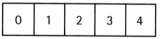

Ask the patient to protrude tongue. (Observe abnormalities of tongue movement.) Do this twice.

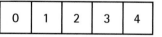

Ask the patient to tap thumb with each finger as rapidly as possible for 10 to 15 seconds; separately with the right hand and then with the left hand. (Observe facial and leg movements.)

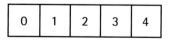

Flex and extend the patient's left and right arms (one at a time).

0 1 2 3 4

*Abnormal Involuntary Movement Scale
From Sandoz Pharmaceuticals, East Hanover, NJ 07936.

Ask the patient to stand up. (Observe in profile. Observe all body areas again, hips included.)

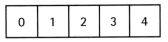

Ask patient to extend both arms outstretched in front with palms down. (Observe trunk, legs and mouth.)

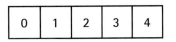

Have the patient walk a few paces, turn, and walk back to chair. (Observe hands and gait.) Do this twice.

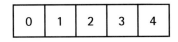

Appendix E

Rating Scale for Extrapyramidal Side Effects

1. **Gait**—The patient is examined as he or she walks into the examining room; his or her gait, the swing of the arms, and the general posture all form the basis for an overall score for this item. This is rated as follows:
   0–Normal
   1–Diminution in swing while the patient is walking
   2–Marked diminution in swing with obvious rigidity in the arm
   3–Stiff gait with arms held rigidly before the abdomen
   4–Stooped, shuffling gait with propulsion and retropulsion
2. **Arm dropping**—The patient and the examiner both raise their arms to shoulder height and let them fall to their sides. In a normal subject, a stout slap is heard as the arms hit the sides. In the patient with extreme Parkinson's syndrome, the arms fall very slowly. This is rated as follows:
   0–Normal, free fall with loud slap and rebound
   1–Fall slowed slightly with less audible contact and little rebound
   2–Fall slowed, no rebound

   3–Marked slowing, no slap at all
   4–Arms fall as though against resistance, as though through glue
3. **Shoulder shaking**—The subject's arms are bent at a right angle at the elbow and are taken one at a time by the examiner, who grasps one hand and also clasps the other around the patient's elbow. The subject's upper arm is pushed to and fro, and the humerus is externally rotated. The degree of resistance from normal to extreme rigidity is scored as follows:
   0–Normal
   1–Slight stiffness and resistance
   2–Moderate stiffness and resistance
   3–Marked rigidity with difficulty in passive movement
   4–Extreme stiffness and rigidity with almost a frozen shoulder
4. **Elbow rigidity**—The elbow joints are separately bent at right angles and passively extended and flexed, with the subject's biceps observed and simultaneously palpated. The resistance to this procedure is rated. (The presence of cogwheel rigidity is noted separately.) Scoring is from 0 to 4 as in shoulder shaking test.

5. **Fixation of position or wrist rigidity—** The wrist is held in one hand and the fingers are held by the examiner's other hand, with the wrist moved to extension flexion and both ulner and radial deviation. The resistance to this procedure is rated as in Items 3 and 4.

6. **Leg pendulousness—**The patient sits on a table with his or her legs hanging down and swinging free. The ankle is grasped by the examiner and raised until the knee is partially extended. It is then allowed to fall. The resistance to falling and the lack of swinging form the basis for the score on this item:

    0–Legs swing freely
    1–Slight diminution in the swing of the legs
    2–Moderate resistance to swing
    3–Marked resistance and damping of swing
    4–Complete absence of swing

7. **Head dropping—**The patient lies on a well-padded examining table, and his head is raised by the examiner's hand. The hand is then withdrawn and the head is allowed to drop. In the normal subject, the head will fall on the table. The movement is delayed in extrapyramidal system disorder, and in extreme parkinsonism it is absent. The neck muscles are rigid, and the head does not reach the examining table. Scoring is as follows:

    0–Head falls completely with a good thump as it hits the table
    1–Slight slowing in fall, mainly noted by lack of slap as the head meets the table
    2–Moderate slowing in the fall quite noticeable to the eye

    3–Head falls stiffly and slowly
    4–Head does not reach examining table

8. **Glabella tap—**Subject is told to open his eyes wide and not to blink. The glabella region is tapped at a steady, rapid speed. The number of times the patient blinks in succession is noted:

    0–0 to 5 blinks
    1–6 to 10 blinks
    2–11 to 15 blinks
    3–16 to 20 blinks
    4–21 or more blinks

9. **Tremor—**The patient is observed walking into examining room and then is reexamined for this item:

    0–Normal
    1–Mild finger tremor, obvious to sight and touch
    2–Tremor of hand or arm occurring spasmodically
    3–Persistent tremor of one or more limbs
    4–Whole body tremor

10. **Salivation—**Patient is observed while talking and is then asked to open his or her mouth and elevate the tongue. The following ratings are given:

    0–Normal
    1–Excess salivation to the extent that pooling takes place if the mouth is open and the tongue is raised
    2–Excess salivation is present and might occasionally result in difficulty speaking
    3–Speaking with difficulty because of excess salivation
    4–Frank drooling

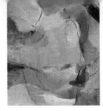

Appendix **F**

Controlled Substances: Uses and Effects

Drugs	Schedules	Trade or Other Names	Medical Uses	DEPENDENCE Physical	DEPENDENCE Psychological
Narcotics					
Opium	II III V	Dover's Powder, Paregoric Parapectolin	Analgesic, antidiarrheal	High	High
Morphine	II III	Morphine, MS Contin, Roxanol, Roxanol-SR	Analgesic, antitussive	High	High
Codeine	II III V	Tylenol w/Codeine, Empirin w/Codeine, Robitussin A-C, Fiorinal w/Codeine	Analgesic, antitussive	Moderate	Moderate
Heroin	I	Diacetylmorphine, horse, smack	None	High	High
Hydromorphone	II	Dilaudid	Analgesic	High	High
Meperidine	II	Demerol, Mepergan	Analgesic	High	High
Methadone	II	Dolophine, methadone, Methadose	Analgesic	High	High-low
Other narcotics	I II III IV V	Numorphan, Percodan, Percocet, Tylox, Tussionex, fentanyl, Darvon, Lomotil, Talwin*	Analgesic, antidiarrheal, antitussive	High-low	High-low
Depressants					
Chloral hydrate	IV	Noctec	Hypnotic	Moderate	Moderate
Barbiturates	II II IV	Amytal, Butisol, Florinal, Lotusate, Nembutal, Seconal, Tuinal, phenobarbital	Anesthetic, anticonvulsant, sedative, hypnotic, veterinary euthanasia agent	High-moderate	High-moderate
Benzodiazepines	IV	Ativan, Dalmane, diazepam, Librium, Xanax, Serax, Valium, Tranxene, Verstran, Versed, Halcion, Paxipam, Restoril	Antianxiety, anticonvulsant, sedative, hypnotic	Low	Low
Methaqualone	I	Quaalude	Sedative, hypnotic	High	High
Glutethimide	III	Doriden	Sedative, hypnotic	High	Moderate
Other depressants	III IV	Equanil, Miltown, Noludar, Placidyl, Valmid	Antianxiety, sedative, hypnotic	Moderate	Moderate
Stimulants					
Cocaine	II	Coke, flake, snow, crack	Local anesthetic	Possible	High
Amphetamines	II	Biphetamine, Delcobese, Desoxyn, Dexedrine, Obetrol	Attention deficit disorders, narcolepsy, weight control	Possible	High
Phenmetrazine	II	Preludin	Weight control	Possible	High
Methylphenidate	II	Ritalin	Attention deficit disorders, narcolepsy	Possible	Moderate
Other stimulants	III IV	Adipex, Cylert, Didrex, Ionamin, Melfiat, Plegine, Sanorex, Tenuate, Tepanil, Prelu-2	Weight control	Possible	High
Hallucinogens					
LSD	I	Acid, microdot	None	None	Unknown
Mescaline and peyote	I	Mexc, buttons, cactus	None	None	Unknown
Amphetamine variants	I	2.5-DMA, PMA, STP, MDA, MDMA, TMA, DOM, DOB	None	Unknown	Unknown
Phencyclidine	II	PCP, angel dust, hog	None	Unknown	High
Phencyclidine analogues	I	PCE, PCPy, TCP	None	Unknown	High
Other hallucinogens	I	Bufotenine, ibogaine, DMT, DET, psilocybin, psilocin	None	None	Unknown
Cannabis					
Marijuana	I	Pot, Acapulco Gold, grass, reefer, Sinsemilla, Thai sticks	None	Unknown	Moderate
Tetrahydrocannabinol	I II	THC, Marinol	Cancer chemotherapy antinauseant	Unknown	Moderate
Hashish	I	Hash	None	Unknown	Moderate
Hashish oil	I	Hash oil	None	Unknown	Moderate

From *Federal Register* 55(159):33590, Washington, D.C., Aug.16, 1990.

Tolerance	Duration (hrs)	Usual Method of Administration	Possible Effects	Effects of Overdose	Withdrawal Syndrome
Yes	3-6	Oral, smoked	Euphoria, drowsiness, respiratory depression, constricted pupils, nausea	Slow and shallow breathing, clammy skin, convulsions, coma, possible death	Watery eyes, runny nose, yawning, loss of appetite, irritability, tremors, panic, cramps, nausea, chills and sweating
Yes	3-6	Oral, smoked, injected			
Yes	3-6	Oral, injected			
Yes	3-6	Injected, sniffed, smoked			
Yes	3-6	Oral, injected			
Yes	3-6	Oral, injected			
Yes	12-24	Oral, injected			
Yes	Variable	Oral, injected			
Yes	5-8	Oral	Slurred speech, disorientation, drunken behavior without odor of alcohol	Shallow respiration, clammy skin, dilated pupils, weak and rapid pulse, coma, possible death	Anxiety, insomnia, tremors, delirium, convulsions, possible death
Yes	1-16	Oral			
Yes	4-8	Oral			
Yes	4-8	Oral			
Yes	4-8	Oral			
Yes	4-8	Oral			
Yes	1-2	Sniffed, smoked, injected	Increased alertness, excitation, euphoria, increased pulse rate and blood pressure, insomnia, loss of appetite	Agitation, increase in body temperature, hallucinations, convulsions, possible death	Apathy, long periods of sleep, irritability, depression, disorientation
Yes	2-4	Oral, injected			
Yes	2-4	Oral, injected			
Yes	2-4	Oral, injected			
Yes	2-4	Oral, injected			
Yes	8-12	Oral	Illusions and hallucinations, poor perception of time and distance	Longer, more intense "trip" episodes, psychosis, possible death	Withdrawal syndrome not reported
Yes	8-12	Oral			
Yes	Variable	Oral, injected			
Yes	Days	Smoked, oral, injected			
Yes	Days	Smoked, oral, injected			
Possible	Variable	Smoked, oral, injected, sniffed			
Yes	2-4	Smoked, oral	Euphoria, relaxed inhibitions, increased appetite, disoriented behavior	Fatigue, paranoia, possible psychosis	Insomnia, hyperactivity, and decreased appetite occasionally reported
Yes	2-4	Smoked, oral			
Yes	2-4	Smoked, oral			
Yes	2-4	Smoked, oral			

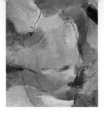

Glossary

absence seizure A type of generalized seizure in which there is an abrupt loss of consciousness (usually lasting less than 10 seconds); these seizures are nonconvulsive in nature and may not be noticed by others.

abstinence syndrome Physical signs and symptoms that occur when the addictive substance is reduced or withheld; also referred to as withdrawal.

abstract thinking The ability to find meaning in proverbs; the ability to conceptualize.

abuse Excessive use of a substance that differs from societal norms and causes clinically significant impairment.

acceptance The allowance of respect of individuality.

acetylcholine (ACh) A neurotransmitter synthesized by choline acetyltransferase from acetyl coenzyme A and choline. It is found in the peripheral nervous system at the myoneural junction, in the autonomic ganglia for parasympathetic or sympathetic systems, and in the parasympathetic postganglionic synapses, including cranial nerves (CNs) III, VII, IX, and X. Acetylcholine is found in the spinal cord, basal ganglia, and numerous sites within the cerebral cortex. Cortical acetylcholine is synthesized primarily in the nucleus basalis of Meynert and in the septal area near the hypothalamus.

acquired immunodeficiency syndrome (AIDS) Term initially used to diagnose those with specific symptoms and opportunistic infections indicating a more advanced progression of human immunodeficiency virus (HIV) infection.

acrophobia Dread of high places.

active listening Verbal and nonverbal skills used by the examiner to demonstrate interest and concern to the patient.

acupressure Meridians are stimulated by use of pressure to restore balance.

acupuncture Ancient Chinese health practice that involves puncturing the skin with hair-thin needles at particular locations called acupuncture points on the patient's body. Acupuncture is believed to help reduce pain or change a body function. Sometimes the needles are twirled, given a slight electric charge.

addiction Psychologic and physiologic symptoms indicating that an individual cannot control his or her use of psychoactive substances; termed substance dependence in the DSM-IV-TR.

advocacy Negotiating with others to develop, improve, and provide services for a patient.

affect Emotional range attached to ideas; outwardly demonstrated.

appropriate a. Emotional tone in harmony with the accompanying idea, thought, or verbalization.

blunted a. Disturbance manifested by a severe reduction in the intensity of affect.

flat a. Absence or near absence of any signs of affective expression.

inappropriate a. Incongruence between the emotional feeling tone and the idea, thought or speech accompanying it.

labile a. Rapid changes in emotional feeling tone, unrelated to external stimuli.

affective disorders Group of psychiatric diagnoses characterized by mood disturbances on a continuum of depression to mania; termed mood disorders in the DSM-IV-TR.

aggression Forceful verbal or physical action; that is, the motor counterpart of the affect of anger, rage, or hostility.

agitation Anxiety associated with severe motor restlessness.

agnosia Difficulty in recognizing familiar objects; a symptom of organic brain disease.

agnostic One who is uncertain about whether there is a god. (Greek *a,* no and *gnosis,* knowledge)

agoraphobia Fear of being in a place or situation in which escape might be difficult or embarrassing, or in which help might not be available in case of a panic attack.

agraphia Loss of the ability to write.

akathisia Motor restlessness generally expressed as the inability to sit still. Caused by the dopamine blockade by certain types of neuroleptic medications. An extrapyramidal side effect (EPSE).

alcoholic Individual whose compulsive use of alcohol causes problems at home, at work, or socially and who continues to use alcohol despite these adverse consequences.

Alcoholics Anonymous (AA) Self-help organization that uses a 12-step program to assist alcoholics to achieve and maintain sobriety; Al-Anon is concerned with the spouses of alcoholics; Alateen is concerned with the teenage children of alcoholics.

alertness Awareness and attentiveness to surroundings.

alternative therapy Broad range of healing philosophies and approaches mainstream Western medicine does not commonly use, accept, study, understand, or make available.

Alzheimer's disease More correctly referred to as dementia of the Alzheimer type (DAT). DAT is the most common type of dementia. The characteristic symptoms are amnesia, aphasia, apraxia, and agnosia. It is a cognitive mental disorder resulting in dementia that is related to a progressive deterioration of brain tissue, described as plaques and neurofibrillary tangles.

ambivalence Opposing impulses or feelings directed toward the same person or object at the same time.

amenorrhea Absence of menstruation.

amnesia Partial or total inability to recall past information.

anterograde a. Recent memory loss, as in the early stages of Alzheimer's disease.

global a. Total memory loss, as in advanced stages of Alzheimer's disease.

retrograde a. Remote memory loss, as in later stages of Alzheimer's disease

short-term a. Memory loss observed in alcoholic blackouts

amygdala Cluster of nuclei in the medial temporal lobe that is concerned with endocrine and behavioral functions and plays a role in food and water intake, drive behavior, and emotions connected with those behaviors. In animal studies, electrical stimulation of the amygdala causes defensiveness, rage, and/or aggression.

analytic worldview Values detail to time, individuality, and possessions.

anergia Absence of energy caused by changes in brain chemistry or anatomy or both.

anger Normal emotional response to the perception of a frustration of desires or threat to one's needs.

anhedonia Loss of pleasure in activities or interests previously enjoyed. A symptom noted in depression and schizophrenia.

anorexia nervosa Disorder characterized by a refusal to eat over a long period, resulting in emaciation, amenorrhea, disturbance in body image, and intense fear of becoming obese.

Antabuse (disulfiram) Drug given to alcoholics that blocks the breakdown of acetylaldehyde, producing nausea, vomiting, dizziness, flushing, and tachycardia if alcohol is consumed.

anterior commissure White matter tract that connects the olfactory structures bilaterally, as well as the temporal lobes and the amygdala.

anticholinergic effect Effect caused by drugs that block acetylcholine receptors. Common anticholinergic effects include dry mouth, blurred vision, constipation, and urinary hesitancy.

antisocial personality Personality disorder characterized by blatant disregard for social norms. Behavior is demonstrated on a continuum of mild to pathologic. Psychoanalytic theory attributes this disorder to an underdeveloped superego.

anxiety Nonspecific, unpleasant feeling of discomfort, with physiological and psychological symptoms that generally results from a perception of a threat to safety and security.

anxiety disorders Patterns of symptoms and behaviors in which anxiety is either the primary disturbance or a secondary problem that is recognized when the primary symptoms are removed.

anxiolytic Antianxiety drug.

apathy Lack of feeling, interest, or emotion; indifference that is occasionally a mechanism for avoiding intense emotion.

aphasia Difficulty in searching for words.

motor a. Impaired speech as a result of organic brain disorder in which understanding remains.

nominal a. Difficulty in finding the correct words in their appropriate sequence.

sensory a. Loss of ability to comprehend the meaning of words.

appropriate Suitable or fitting for a particular person, purpose, occasion, or situation. Examples include appropriate affect, response, and attire.

apraxia Inability to perform once known, purposeful, skilled activities in the absence of loss of motor function.

assault Legally, any behavior that physically or verbally presents an immediate threat of physical injury to another individual.

assertiveness Direct expression of feelings and needs in a way that respects the rights of others and self.

asylum (1) Place of safety or sanctuary; a refuge. (2) Institution for the care of the mentally ill; often associated with mistreatment and callousness.

atheist One who believes there is no god. (Greek *a*, no; *theos,* God)

attention-deficit hyperactivity disorder (ADHD) Relatively common disorder of childhood onset characterized by inattention, impulsiveness, and overactivity.

attitude Pattern of mental views and feelings accumulated through past experiences and affected by present stimuli. A manner, disposition, tendency, or orientation with regard to a person or situation.

atypical depression Subtype of depression occurring more often in younger individuals and is expressed by atypical symptoms; for example, increased appetite, weight gain, hypersomnia.

autism Preoccupation with self without concern for external reality. A self-made private world of the schizophrenic.

autistic thinking Thoughts, ideas, or desires derived from internal, private stimuli or drives that are often incongruent with reality; most often it is applied to persons with schizophrenia.

autonomic nervous system Division of the peripheral nervous system that is involuntary and innervates the viscera, heart, blood vessels, smooth muscle, and glands. It is divided into the parasympathetic (craniosacral system) and sympathetic (thoracolumbar system).

avolition Lack of motivation.

axon Long process from the neuronal cell body that transmits impulses away from the cell.

balance Process by which patients are helped to reach for independence while conforming to norms.

basal ganglia Large nuclei including the caudate nucleus, putamen, and globus pallidus, which are responsible for modulating voluntary movement.

battery Touching of the person of another, of his or her clothes, or anything else attached to his or her person without consent.

behavior Any observable, recordable, and measurable movement, response, or act of an individual (verbal and nonverbal).

behavior therapy Therapeutic approach that helps the patient modify behavior by modifying or changing old patterns of behavior.

binge Eating an unusually large amount of food in a relatively short period.

binge eating Disorder in which bingeing occurs without purging. Victims are generally overweight since they do not purge.

biological variations Physical differences between individuals or body structure, skin color, other visible characteristics, enzymatic and genetic variations, electrocardiographic patterns, susceptibility to disease, nutritional preferences and deficiencies, and psychologic characteristics.

bipolar disorder Affective or mood disorder characterized by at least one episode of mania with or without a history of depression.

biracial Individual who crosses two racial and cultural groups.

bizarre Markedly unusual in appearance, thought, style, character, or behavior. Absurd.

blackout Period in which the drinker functions socially for which there is no memory.

blocking Unconscious interruption in train of thought.

blood-brain barrier Guards the brain from fluctuations in body chemistry. Regulates the amount and speed with which substances in the blood enter the brain.

borderline personality disorder Disorder with the essential feature of a pervasive pattern of unstable self-image, interpersonal relations, and mood.

bradykinesia Slow or retarded movement.

brain stem Vital structure that carries all information to and from the cerebral cortex and spinal cord. Because the brain stem is also responsible for respiration, its function is essential for life. It consists of the midbrain, pons, and medulla.

bulimia Compulsive binge eating accompanied by purging and an overconcern with body shape and weight. It is characterized by an insatiable craving for food, resulting in episodes of continuous eating and often followed by purging, depression, and self-deprivation.

bulimia nervosa Disorder characterized by binge eating, compensatory behavior, and over-concern with body shape and weight.

bureaucracy Excessive rules and structure that get in the way of efficient, responsive, and creative nursing care solutions.

burnout Spiraling process of decreased effectiveness.

case management Collaborative process for meeting health needs through the use of a variety of services in a cost-effective manner.

catalepsy State of unconsciousness in which immobility is constantly maintained.

catatonia Immobility as a result of psychologic causes.

catatonic behavior Motor anomalies in nonorganic disorders such as schizophrenia.

catecholamines Derived from the amino acid tyrosine, these substances include dopamine, norepinephrine, and epinephrine. Catecholamines are a subcategory of the monoamines, which also include serotonin and histamine. Catecholamines and their synthesis products are widely distributed in the central and peripheral nervous systems.

caudate Basal ganglia nucleus that protrudes into the anterior horn of the lateral ventricle.

cerebral cortex Narrow ribbon of gray matter that lies on the surface of the cerebrum. The gray matter lies "on top of" the white matter. The reverse is true in the spinal cord.

child abuse Harmful physical, emotional, sexual, and/or verbal behavior inflicted on a child.

cholinergics Substances that stimulate the cholinergic system. In the peripheral nervous system, cholinergic drugs constrict the pupil, increase the production of saliva and respiratory secretions, slow the heart, and increase gastrointestinal peristalsis and urinary output.

chorea Greek term for *dance*. The choreas are demonstrated as hyperkinetic disorders characterized by involuntary, unpredictable, and random movements of the trunk, head, face, and limbs.

circumstantiality Digression of inappropriate thoughts into ideas, eventually reaching the desired goal.

cirrhosis Disease of the liver characterized by the development of scar tissue in the liver.

civil law Part of the legal system that is concerned with the legal rights and duties of private persons. Civil lawsuits can recapture monetary loss from professionals who have been guilty of false imprisonment, defamation of character, assault and battery, or negligence.

clang associations Words similar in sound but not in meaning that conjure up new thoughts.

clarification Communication skill that helps define a patient's responses through the use of direct questions.

claustrophobia Dread of closed places.

clinical depression Another term for major depressive disorder that defines the disturbance of a person's mood according to DSM-IV-TR criteria.

clinical supervision Formal meeting among psychiatric nursing peers whose purpose is to provide a place for nurses caring for patients to examine attitudes, reactions, and conflicts with patients on the unit and to find new ways of approaching patient problems.

clonic State in which rigidity and relaxation succeed each other.

closed-ended questions Questions that generally elicit a "yes" or "no" response. Useful in gathering factual data.

clouding of consciousness Incomplete clear-mindedness, with disturbance in perception and attitude. Example: stupor.

co-dependency Stress-related preoccupation with an addicted person's life, leading to extreme dependence on that person.

cognition Act or process of knowing and perceiving.

cognitive disorders Those that affect consciousness, memory, and other cognitive processes.

cognitive processes Pertaining to perception, judgment, memory, and reasoning.

coma Depressed consciousness wherein even extreme stimulation of the reticular activating system will not cause a response.

common law/case law Term *common law* is applied to the body of principles that has evolved and continues to evolve and expand from judicial decisions that arise during the trial of actual court cases. Law based on the outcome of cases.

communication Process that is the matrix for thought and relationships among all people regardless of cultural heritage.

community meeting Occurs within the therapeutic milieu and in which joint problem solving by community members is encouraged.

community mental health Application of the principles of psychiatric care to communities and groups of people. The goal of this effort is to maintain health, to prevent mental illness when possible, and, if treatment is indicated, to treat the individual closer to his or her support systems.

Community Mental Health Centers Act 1963 legislation authorizing federal funds for the construction of comprehensive mental health centers.

community worldview Community needs and concerns are more important than individual ones. Quiet respectful communication is valued, as well as meditation and reading as a learning style.

co-morbidity Simultaneous existence of medical and psychiatric problems, each complicating the other.

complementary therapy Same as alternative therapy but denotes therapy used as an adjunct to rather than as a replacement for conventional treatment.

complex partial seizure Formerly referred to as temporal lobe or psychomotor seizure; this seizure typically begins with a clouding of consciousness followed by some meaningless movement such as lip smacking or hand clapping; brief periods of forgetfulness are common.

comprehension Capacity to perceive and understand.

compulsion Uncontrollable impulse to perform an act or ritual repeatedly; may be in response to an obsession (unwilled, persistent thought), as in obsessive-compulsive disorder. The act or ritual serves to decrease anxiety. Examples of rituals include hand washing, cleaning, and checking (e.g., checking to see if door is locked).

concrete communication Inability to think and communicate abstractly.

concrete thinking Use of literal meaning without ability to consider abstract meaning (e.g., "don't cry over spilt milk" might be interpreted as meaning, "Okay, I'll cry over the sink.")

confabulation Unconscious filling of gaps in memory with imagined or untrue experiences that the person believes but has no basis in reality.

confidentiality Treating the information about and from patients in a private manner; information about patients is "confidential" and requires patient approval before disclosure.

conflict Differing perspectives among staff or patients regarding various aspects of treatment.

confused state Bewildered, perplexed, or unclear. The type and degree of confusion should be specified.

congruence Accordant states. Example includes mood-congruence, in which the person's visible emotional state correlates with his or her mood or feeling state.

consciousness State of awareness.

conservator Guardian; a legally appointed person who controls the affairs of a gravely disabled person, including the right to consent to or refuse psychiatric treatment.

consultant-liaison nurse Psychiatric mental health nurse who provides expert consultation for patients and staff in other parts of the hospital agency.

consumer Patient in treatment for psychiatric services.

continuum of care Levels of care through which an individual can move depending upon his or her needs at a given point in time.

contralateral Opposite side of the body.

conversion Process by which a psychic event, an idea, a memory, or an impulse is represented by a bodily change or symptom such as blindness or paralysis.

corporate compliance Health care provider's responsibility to comply with governmental laws and regulations.

corpus callosum Major connecting and communicating pathway between the hemispheres.

cortisol Glucocorticoid hormone found in the adrenal cortex that participates in carbohydrate and protein metabolism. Cortisol hypersecretion occurs in many depressed individuals. Excretion of this hormone is not suppressed in a significant number of persons with major depression after an injection of dexamethasone.

creed Set formula that states the religious and spiritual beliefs of a community of faith (Latin, *credo, I trust, believe*).

criminal law Part of the legal system concerned with crime that is defined in state and federal statutes.

crisis A 4- to 6-week period of severe emotional disorganization as a result of the failure of coping mechanisms or lack of support or both.

cultural awareness Process whereby the nurse acknowledges his or her cultural biases and recognizes that other individuals, groups or communities have their unique cultural similarities and differences.

cultural competence Process whereby the nurse has developed cultural awareness, knowledge, and skills to promote effective and quality health care for patients.

cultural diversity Variety of cultural groupings. These groups may include age, gender, socioeconomic status, religion, race, and ethnicity.

cultural negotiation Nurse's ability to work with a patient's cultural belief system in order to develop culturally appropriate interventions.

cultural preservation Nurse's ability to acknowledge, value, and accept a patient's cultural beliefs.

cultural repatterning Nurse's ability to incorporate cultural preservation and negotiation in order to identify patient needs, develop expected outcomes, and evaluate outcome plans.

cultural values Unique, individual expressions of belief related to culture that have been accepted as appropriate over time for persons in that culture.

culturally diverse nursing care Modification of nursing approaches to provide culturally competent care.

culture The internal and external manifestation of an individual, a group, or a community's beliefs, values, and norms that are used as premises for everyday life and functioning.

cupping Alternative, cultural, or medical treatment that uses a small glass or cup to conduct the moxibustion treatment.

custodial care Process of caring for hygienic and nutritional needs in an institution but not providing treatment for mental disorder.

cyclothymia Chronic mood disturbance of at least 2 years' duration involving numerous hypomanic episodes and numerous periods of depression. Cyclothymia does not meet the criteria for a manic episode or major depression.

deinstitutionalization Shift in treatment location from large public hospitals to community settings.

delirium Disorder with alterations in consciousness and changes in cognition, which is usually caused by a general medical condition or is substance-induced. Typically, deliria develop over a short period and are treatable. It is (usually) a reversible bewildered state of clouded consciousness, generally accompanied by restlessness, disorientation, and fear. May include periods of hallucinations.

delusion Fixed, false belief, not consistent with the person's intelligence and culture; unamenable to reason.
bizarre d. Absurd belief.
nihilistic d. False belief that the self, part of the self, or another object has ceased to exist.
paranoid d. Oversuspiciousness leading to persecutory delusions.
persecution d. False belief that one is being persecuted.
reference d. False belief that the behavior of others in the environment refers to oneself; derived from ideas of reference in which one falsely feels he or she is being talked about.
somatic d. False belief involving functioning of one's body

dementia Disorder that causes pronounced memory and cognitive disturbances. Typically, dementias are gradual in onset and progressive in course.

dendrites Many projections from the neuron that transmit impulses to the cell body.

denial Avoidance of disagreeable realities or threats by ignoring or refusing to recognize them. An unconscious defense mechanism that may or may not be adaptive.

dependence State in which a drug user must take a usual or an increasing dose of a drug to prevent the onset of abstinence symptoms or withdrawal or both.

depersonalization Feeling of unreality or strangeness related to one's self, body parts, bodily functions, or external environment.

depression Lowered or saddened mood state or major affective disorder, listed as a mood disorder in the DSM-IV-TR.

derailment Gradual or sudden deviation in train of thought without blocking.

derealization Distortion of spatial relationships so that the environment becomes unfamiliar.

devaluation Criticism of others that defends against one's own feelings of inadequacy.

dexamethasone suppression test (DST) Diagnostic test for clinical depression that measures the function of the hypothalmic-pituitary axis (HPA).

diencephalon Thalamus, hypothalamus, epithalamus, and metathalamus.

disinhibition State in which a person is unable to suppress urges or statements that may be socially unacceptable (e.g., telling a dirty joke in an inappropriate situation).

disoriented Disturbance in orientation of time, place, or person.

displacement Shift of emotion from an object or a person who incites the emotion to a less threatening source. An unconscious defense mechanism that may or may not be adaptive.

dissociation (1) Removal from conscious awareness of painful feelings, memories, thoughts, or aspects of identity. (2) Separation of mental or behavioral processes from the rest of the person's consciousness or identity. (3) Splitting or separation of any group of mental or behavioral processes from the rest of the person's consciousness or identity.

dissociative reaction Process by which an individual blocks off a part of his or her life from conscious recognition because of severe anxiety.

distractibility Inability to concentrate attention.

dopamine Brain neurotransmitter that influences muscle movement and emotions. The "dopamine theory" states that individuals with schizophrenia may have too much dopamine, which may account for their sensory-perceptual alterations. Research has refined this theory.

double bind Conflicting demands by significant individuals in a person's life. Cannot meet both demands, so person is doomed to failure.

dysarthria Difficulty in articulating.

dyskinesia Disturbed coordination and motor activity, usually producing a jerky motion. An EPSE of neuroleptic medications related to their effect on dopamine receptors. *See also* tardive dyskinesia.

dyslexia Difficulty in reading.

dysphagia Difficulty in swallowing.

dysphoria Disorder of affect characterized by depression, malaise, and anguish. Unpleasant mood state.

dysthymia Chronic mood disturbance involving a depressed mood for least 2 years, more days than not.

dysthymic disorder Results in depressed mood with a duration of at least 2 years, more days than not.

dystonia Rigidity in muscles that control posture, gait, or ocular movement. An EPSE of neuroleptic medications that block dopamine.

echolalia Psychopathologic repeating of words of one person by another. Noted in types of schizophrenia.

echopraxia Imitation of the body position of another.

ecologic worldview Based in the belief that there is interconnectedness between a person and the earth and that people have a responsibility to take care of the earth.

ego Personality process that focuses on reality, while striving to meet the needs of the id. The ego experiences anxiety and uses defense mechanisms for protection.

electroconvulsive therapy (ECT) Form of somatic therapy that uses electrical-induced seizures to relieve a person's intractable depressive symptoms.

ELISA test Used to detect specific antibodies. It is used to assist in the diagnosis of HIV infection through the identification of antibodies to HIV. *See also* enzyme-linked immunosorbent assay.

emaciated Made excessively thin by lack of nutrition.

emotion Complex feeling state with psychic, somatic, and behavioral components related to affect and mood.

empathy Objective understanding of how patients feel or how they see their situations.

enkephalins Widely distributed opioid-like neuropeptides that are part of the endorphin family. These substances mediate pain perception, taste, olfaction, arousal, emotional behavior, vision, hearing, neurohormone secretion, motor coordination, and water balance.

environmental control Ability of an individual to control nature by planning activities and tasks to assist in maintaining optimal balance in life.

enzyme-linked immunosorbent assay (ELISA) Most commonly used test to screen for the presence of antibodies to HIV-1 because of its low cost, standardized procedure and its high reliability.

epidemiology Study of the frequency and distribution of disease conditions in the population.

epilepsy Disorder of the central nervous system (CNS) in which the major symptom is a seizure. The seizure is caused by a temporary disturbance of brain impulses.

ethnicity Refers to groups whose members share a common social and cultural heritage passed on to each successive generation.

ethnocentrism Acknowledging and valuing only one's own culture.

ethnopharmacology Study of pharmacogenetic, pharmacodynamic, and pharmacokinetic influences based on different ethnic, racial, and cultural groups.

etiology Study of the causes of diseases, including both direct and predisposing causes.

euphoria False sense of elation or well being; pathologic elevation of mood; complete lack of tension. Most notable in the manic phase of bipolar disorder.

euthymia Normal, homeostatic mood state.

excitement Excited motor activity.

existentialism Philosophy that emphasizes the individual's ability and responsibility to make one's existence meaningful by making choices in the face of life's deep pain and uncertainty.

expansive mood Unrestrained expression of feelings.

extrapyramidal side effects (EPSEs) Involuntary muscle movements resulting from the effects of neuroleptic drugs on the extrapyramidal system. These drugs cause a dopamine blockade that creates a dopamine-ACh imbalance. EPSEs include akathisia, akinesia, dystonia, drug-induced parkinsonism, and neuroleptic malignant syndrome (NMS).

extrapyramidal system Outside the pyramidal (voluntary) tract. Coordinates involuntary movements.

eye contact Occasional glancing into the patient's eyes to demonstrate interest during an interaction.

faith Traditionally, the creed to which one assents within one's religious community, but the term can be used more broadly to describe one's total life view, religiously based or not.

family system Field of influence exerted on one another by family members because of the complex interaction of all family members.

fantasy Imaginary sequence of events. Common in childhood. Appropriate as long as the person is aware of reality.

fear Anxiety as a result of consciously recognized and realistic danger.

feedback Articulation of one's perception of what another person has said or meant. This process requires at least two people.

flashbacks Cognitive, emotional, and physical reexperiencing of traumatic events.

flight of ideas Speech pattern demonstrated by a rapid transition from topic to topic, frequently without completing any of the preceding ideas. Prominent in manic states.

free association In a therapeutic context, saying anything that comes to mind.

fugue Period of personality dissociation with memory loss.

gait Manner of progression in walking. Example: ataxic gait, in which the foot is raised high and the sole strikes down suddenly.

gamma-aminobutyric acid (GABA) Inhibitory amino acid neurotransmitter formed during the citric acid cycle from its precursor, glutamic acid. GABA receptors are widely distributed in the CNS and produce neuronal hyperpolarization through an influx of chloride ions. Drugs that increase GABA reduce anxiety and seizures.

general leads Interactive skills that facilitate the communication process by encouraging the patient to continue.

generalized seizure Involves both hemispheres of the brain at the onset of the seizure. Consciousness is usually impaired.

genetic vulnerability (1) Tendency to inherent traits, behaviors, and biological characteristics of one's ancestors. (2) Inherited liability that increases the risk of exhibiting a psychiatric disorder.

global Total memory loss, as in advanced stages of Alzheimer's disease.

globus pallidus Gray matter structure located medial to the putamen. This portion of the basal ganglia is smaller and triangular in shape. It is subdivided into the *globus pallidus externa* and *globus pallidus interna*.

glutamate Major excitatory transmitter in the CNS with receptors throughout the brain. Glutamate stimulation of N-methyl-D-aspartate (NMDA)–activated channels permits excessive inflow of calcium ions and production of free radicals that may cause neuronal death.

grand mal seizure Type of generalized seizure in which there is loss of consciousness and convulsions. This type of seizure is most frequently associated with epilepsy by laypersons.

gravely disabled Person who is unable to provide food, clothing, or shelter for himself or herself because of a mental illness.

gray matter Composed of the cell bodies and dendrites of neurons.

grimacing Contortion of facial muscles; may be EPSE.

gyri Convolutions of gray matter on the cerebrum.

hallucination False sensory perceptions not associated with real external stimuli. May involve any of the five senses: auditory, visual, olfactory, gustatory, or tactile.
  auditory h. Most prevalent in schizophrenia. The sounds may be perceived as thoughts or voices coming from any type of transmitter or from the patient's mind. The messages may be condemning or accusatory, or complimentary and encouraging. It is critical that the examiner be aware that the messages may be directing the patient toward harming self or others, so the message content cannot be ignored.
  tactile h. Common in alcohol withdrawal. Hallucinations may also be an effect of certain types of drugs, such as amphetamines, hallucinogens, and cannabis.
  visual h. Often associated with organic conditions.

hebephrenia Outdated schizophrenic subtype characterized by silliness, delusions, hallucinations, and regression.

herbaceutical Plant or plant part that produces and contains chemical substances that act on the body.

here-and-now focus Assisting patients to understand how their current behaviors influence daily living.

highly active antiretroviral therapy (HAART) Drug therapy in which three antiretroviral medications are used in combination to reduce the replication of HIV.

HIV antibody Specific to HIV; usually appears within 6 weeks after infection.

holistic Pertaining to totality or the whole (holistic care).

homelessness Without a home. Homeless individuals, including whole families, may live on the street exclusively or may make use of community shelters, halfway houses, cheap hotels, or board-and-care homes.

homeopathy Unconventional Western medicine system that is based on the principle that "like cures like," (i.e., that the same substance in large doses produces the symptoms of an illness, in very minute doses cures it). Homeopathic physicians believe that the more dilute the remedy, the greater its potency. Therefore homeopathic practitioners use small doses of specially prepared plant extracts and minerals to stimulate the body's defense mechanisms and healing processes to treat illness.

hostile Feeling intense anger and resentment, exhibited by destructive behavior.

hot or cold treatments Cultural-medical approaches to maintaining or returning a person to a state of wellness.

These approaches do not refer to the temperature of a treatment but to the fact that a specific, defined approach is appropriate for each state of wellness or illness.

human immunodeficiency infection Spectrum of illness caused by HIV that ranges from acutely or chronically HIV-infected adults to infants in the neonatal period.

human immunodeficiency virus (HIV) Isolated and recognized as the etiologic agent of acquired immunodeficiency syndrome (AIDS). HIV is classified as a lentivirus in a subgroup of the retrovirus.

human immunodeficiency virus, type 1 (HIV-1) Retrovirus identified to be the cause of AIDS.

humanist Individual who emphasizes people rather than the other parts of the observable world or religion.

Huntington's disease Genetically transmitted disease that includes motor and cognitive changes.

hydrotherapy Use of water (wet sheetpacks, 2- to 10-hour baths) for psychotherapeutic purposes.

hyperactivity (hyperkinesis) Restless, aggressive, often destructive activity. Prominent in manic states.

hypersomnia Increased and prolonged sleeping.

hypoactivity (hypokinesis) Decreased activity or retardation (psychomotor retardation); slowing of psychologic and physical functions.

hypomania Clinical syndrome similar to but less severe than that demonstrated in a full-blown manic episode.

hypothalamus Group of nuclei in the diencephalon that influences eating behavior, temperature regulation, emotional expression, and autonomic system. Dopaminergic neurons in the hypothalamus control lactation.

id Personality process that wants to experience only pleasure; is impulsive and without morals.

idealization Viewing others as perfect; exalting others.

ideas of reference Belief that some events have a special meaning (e.g., people laughing are perceived as laughing at the patient).

idiopathic Without known cause.

illogical (thinking) Contains erroneous conclusions or internal contradictions (irrational thoughts).

illusion Misinterpretation of a sensory input. Observed in alcoholic withdrawal and delirious states.

impaired parent Parent whose nurturing capabilities are compromised or absent, related to psychiatric or substance abuse disorders.

independence Taking actions for one's behalf, rather than asking others to do so.

individual responsibility Owning one's tasks, needs, feelings, and thoughts, and taking action to address these responsibilities and needs.

indoklon therapy Convulsive therapy–like electroconvulsive therapy (ECT); however, convulsions are induced by ether rather than by electrical stimulus.

informed consent Providing the patient with information about a specific treatment, including its benefits, side effects, and possible risks, that will enable him or her to make a competent and voluntary decision.

insight Recognition of motivational sources behind one's thoughts, actions, or behavior.

insomnia Inability to sleep or disrupted sleep patterns.

intellectual functioning Individual's general fund of knowledge, orientation, memory, mastery of simple mathematical equations, and capacity for abstract thinking.

intellectualization One of the (unconscious) defense mechanisms. A process of thinking excessively about the philosophic or theoretic basis to the extent that the anxiety-provoking issues are avoided.

internal capsule Broad band of myelinated fibers that separate the lentiform nuclei from the caudate nucleus and thalamus. Corticospinal (motor or pyramidal) tracts travel through the internal capsule, cerebral peduncles, and cerebral pyramids into the spinal cord, where they constitute the lateral corticospinal pathway. Damage to any of these structures can result in hemiparesis or hemiplegia.

involuntary commitment Commitment status in which a person who has the legal capacity to consent to mental health treatment refuses to do so and is involuntarily detained for treatment by the state.

ipsilateral Same side of body.

irrational beliefs Beliefs that are not logical but influence feelings and behaviors.

judgment and comprehension Ability to understand, recall, mobilize, and constructively integrate previous learning in meeting new situations.

Kaposi's syndrome (KS) Form of cancer that exhibits with pink-purple spots on the skin and mouth as a painless tumor.

kinesics Study of body movements.

Korsakoff's psychosis (Korsakov) Organic mental disorder with memory loss related to alcohol abuse.

Kraepelin German psychiatrist who initiated a classification system for psychiatry in 1896. He used the term *dementia praecox*.

labile Mood, affect, or behavior that is subject to frequent or unpredictable changes.

least restrictive alternative Environment that provides the necessary treatment requirements in the least restrictive setting possible. For example, a hospital setting is more restrictive than a board-and-care setting. If the board-and-care setting provides the necessary treatment requirements for a person, then that environment would represent the least restrictive alternative.

lentiform nuclei Putamen and globus pallidus of the basal ganglia.

lesion Injury to tissue.

lewy bodies Eosinophilic cytoplasmic inclusions seen in neuromelanin-containing neurons in Parkinson's disease.

limit setting Holding individuals to established norms with the intent of assisting them to function more constructively.

limited or special power of attorney Written document in which one person, the principal, authorizes another person, the attorney-in-fact, to act on the principal's behalf. In a limited power of attorney, the attorney-in-fact is granted only those powers specifically defined in the document.

lipid solubility Ability of a substance to dissolve in fat.

lithium Element or salt used in the treatment and prevention of manic episodes.

locus ceruleus Small nucleus ("blue spot") in the pontine tegmentum whose neurons are the major source of norepinephrine in the brain; present bilaterally.

loose association Pattern of speech in which a person's ideas slip off track onto another that is completely unrelated or only slightly related.

looseness of associations Vague, unfocused, illogical flow or stream of thought. Notable in schizophrenia.

magical thinking Belief that thoughts, words, or actions can cause or prevent an occurrence by some magical means.

malpractice Negligence by a professional. Malpractice is a civil action that can be brought against a nurse if he or she has breached a standard of care that a reasonably prudent nurse would meet.

managed care System of entities that arranges the relationship among payers, providers, and consumers; monitors and influences the behavior of the mental health providers and the outcomes of care; and reimburses for services.

mania Disordered mental state of extreme excitement, hyperactivity, euphoria, and hyperverbal behavior.

master-servant rule As applied to the employer-employee relationship, this rule holds the employer responsible for the acts of employees as long as the employees are acting within the scope of their employment or authority.

medially Toward the midline.

medulla Approximately 3 cm long and the most caudal portion of the brain stem. It controls respiration and supplies innervation to the tongue and palate.

melancholic depression Subgroup generally occurring in older individuals, often misdiagnosed as dementia; more often associated with dexamethasone nonsuppression. Depression usually worse in the morning, early morning awakening occurs, psychomotor retardation or agitation, excessive or inappropriate guilt, and significant anorexia or weight loss are symptoms of melancholia.

memory Function by which information stored in the brain is later recalled to the conscious mind.

meninges Outer lining of the CNS composed of the dura mater, arachnoid, and pia mater.

mental disorder "A clinically significant behavioral or psychological syndrome or pattern…associated with present distress or disability" (DSM-IV-TR, 2000).

mental retardation Lack of intelligence so great that it interferes with social and occupational performance.

mental status examination (MSE) Record of current findings that includes a description of patient's appearance, behavior, motor activity, speech, alertness, mood, cognition, intelligence, reactions, views, and attitudes.

meridian Lines in a body that are representative of psychologic or physical body functions. Cultural healers stimulate meridians and release harmful toxins or illness-producing spirits through the use of alternative treatment approaches such as moxibustion, cupping, coining, or skin scraping.

mesocortical tract Dopaminergic tract that projects from the ventral tegmental area near the substantia nigra to the neocortex, particularly the prefrontal cortex; involved in motivation, planning, behavior, attention, and social behavior.

mesolimbic tract Catecholaminergic neuronal tract (mostly dopaminergic) with cell bodies located in the ventral tegmental area of the midbrain and axons that project to the hippocampus, entorhinal cortex, amygdala, anterior cingulate gyrus, nucleus accumbens, and other limbic regions.

metabolic tolerance Occurs when the body is more efficient at metabolizing the substance.

midbrain Most rostral division of the brain stem. It contains important structures such as the cerebral aqueduct, superior and inferior colliculi, red nuclei, substantia nigra, cerebral peduncles, and oculomotor and trochlear cranial nerve nuclei.

milieu Environment or setting.

milieu management Purposeful manipulation of the environment to promote a therapeutic atmosphere.

milieu therapy Use of the environment to promote optimal functioning in a group or individual.

minority Social, religious, ethnic, or occupational group that constitutes less than a numerical majority of the population.

model of care Philosophy of causative and curative factors of mental illness, which drives the nature of the care activities offered.

monoamine oxidase Enzyme that metabolizes monoamines such as dopamine, norepinephrine, and serotonin.

monoamine oxidase inhibitors (MAOIs) Antidepressant drugs that increase the bioavailability of certain neurotransmitters by interfering with their metabolism.

monoamine(s) Category of neurotransmitters that contain one amino group and are derived from amino acids. Subcategories of monoamines include the catecholamines (dopamine, norepinephrine, epinephrine), which are derived from tyrosine, and the indolamine serotonin, which is derived from tryptophan. Histamine is categorized as a monoamine but is biochemically different. Monoamine-synthesizing neurons are primarily found in the brain stem but have a wide net of influence because of the ubiquitous distribution of their axonal projections.

mood Individual's internal state of mind that is exhibited through feelings and emotions.

mood disorder Diagnostic category in the DSM-IV-TR that includes the affective disorders.

mood disorder as a result of a general medical condition Disorder resulting in a disturbance or alteration of a person's mood that is the result of a specific medical and/or physiologic consequence.

moxibustion Alternative cultural medical treatment approach that used moxi and heat to release illness-producing spirits from the body, mind, or spirit.

mutism Refusal to speak.

NANDA North American Nursing Diagnosis Association.

narcissism Extreme self-centeredness and self-absorption (narcissistic personality disorder).

narcotherapy Induction of a state of sedation by intravenous administration of sedatives (e.g., amobarbital) or stimulants (e.g., methylphenidate).

National Institute of Mental Health Government organization in the National Institutes of Health concerned with mental health issues in the United States.

natural cause of illness Belief that everyone and everything in the world is interrelated and that a disruption of this connectedness causes illness or disease.

nature argument Etiology as related to biology.

naturopathic physician Alternative care practitioner who holds a Doctor of naturopathy (ND) degree.

naturopathy Views disease as a manifestation of alterations in the processes by which the body naturally heals itself and emphasizes health restoration rather than disease treatment. Naturopathic physicians use an array of healing practices that include diet and clinical nutrition; homeopathy; acupuncture; herbal medicine; hydrotherapy (use of water in a range of temperatures and methods of applications); spinal and soft-tissue manipulation; physical therapies involving electric currents; ultrasound and light therapies; therapeutic counseling; and pharmacology.

negativism Motiveless resistance to all instruction.

negligence Failure to do that which a reasonably prudent and careful person would do under the circumstances, or the doing of that which a reasonable and prudent person would not do.

neologism New word created by the patient for psychologic reasons. Noted in some types of schizophrenia.

neurofibrillary tangle Mass of abnormal filamentous material located within the cell body of neurons. These tangles occur in several brain disorders, such as Alzheimer's disease and are composed of cytoskeletal components.

neuroleptic Antipsychotic medication.

neuron Nerve cell.

neurotransmitter Chemical found in the nervous system (e.g., norepinephrine, serotonin, dopamine) that facilitates the transmission of nerve impulses across synapses between neurons.

noncompliance Failure to take medication as prescribed.

nonviolence Solving conflictual situations by methods other than verbal or physical aggression.

norepinephrine Catecholamine neurotransmitter that is primarily synthesized in neurons of the locus ceruleus in the pons. Deficiencies of norepinephrine are linked to depression.

norm Expected behavior for a given therapeutic setting.

nucleus accumbens This nucleus is adjacent to the medial and ventral portions of the caudate and putamen. The neurons in this nucleus project to both the globus pallidus and the substantia nigra; a major component of the "reward pathway."

nucleus basalis of Meynart Located bilaterally directly beneath the anterior commissure, it is the major brain site for the production of acetylcholine. Fibers from this nucleus project diffusely to the cerebral cortex.

nurse-patient interaction Purposeful use of the relationship between the patient and nurse for achieving patient treatment goals.

nursing diagnosis Statement that describes a patient's potential or actual problem or response to illness treatable by nurses.

nurture argument Etiology, as related to upbringing, life events, or other stressors.

obesity Abnormal increase in the proportion of fat cells, mainly in the viscera and subcutaneous tissues of the body.

objectivity Process of remaining open, unbiased, and emotionally separate from a patient.

obsession Pathologic persistence of an unwilled thought, feeling, or impulse to the extent that it cannot be eliminated from consciousness by logical effort.

obsessive-compulsive disorder Recurrent obsessions (thoughts) alternating with compulsions (behaviors). Both are unwilled.

occupational therapy Uses the activities of everyday living to help people with mental disabilities achieve maximum functioning and independence at home and in the workplace.

oculogyric crisis Involuntary tonic muscle spasms of the eye. The eyes usually roll upward in a fixed stare. This very frightening dystonic reaction is caused by antipsychotic drugs.

olfactory Pertaining to the sense of smell.

open posture Relaxed, yet attentive position with arms uncrossed. Enhances patient's trust in the examiner.

open-ended statement Statement that elicits further exploration of the patient's problem by encouraging communication; can also be in the form of a question.

openness Atmosphere in which people are free to express their thoughts and feelings without fear of ridicule or censure.

opportunistic illnesses Those that develop when the immune system is inactive or suppressed.

organic mental disorders Class of disorders of mental functioning caused by permanent brain damage or temporary brain dysfunction. The cause is known and may be primary (originating in the brain) or secondary to systemic disease. Cognition, emotions, and motivation are affected. The DSM-IV-TR uses the term cognitive disorder.

orientation Conscious awareness of person, place, and time.

panic State of extreme, acute, intense anxiety, accompanied by disorganization of personality and function.

paranoia Extreme suspiciousness of others and their actions.

paranoid thinking Oversuspiciousness thinking that may lead to persecutory delusions or projectile behavior patterns.

parkinsonism Causes of the disease are known, such as brain injury, antipsychotic drugs, carbon monoxide.

parkinsonism symptoms Masked faces, muscle rigidity, and shuffling gait. Symptoms are common in patients taking neuroleptic drugs; EPSE related to dopamine blockade.

Parkinson's disease Or idiopathic parkinsonism, where the cause is unknown. It pathologically presents a loss of dopaminergic neurons in substantia nigra and clinically exhibits a variety of motor and nonmotor signs and symptoms.

partial seizure Usually involves one hemisphere of the brain at the onset of the seizure.

passive aggression Anger expressed indirectly through subtle and evasive ways.

perception Awareness of objects and relations that follows stimulation of peripheral sense organs.

perseveration Psychopathologic repetition of the same word or idea in response to different questions.

personal control Exerting limits on one's own impulses to act in a manner that is contrary to one's best interests, treatment goals, or personal needs.

personality disorder Exaggerated, pathologic behavior patterns destructive to the individual and others.

pervasive developmental disorder (PDD) Any one of several conditions that are characterized by multiple social and cognitive delays.

petit mal seizure Variant of absence seizures that is characterized by a three-per-second spike and wave electro-encephalographic (EEG) pattern.

pharmacodynamic tolerance Occurs when higher blood levels are required to produce a given effect.

phobia Exaggerated, pathologic dread or fear of some specific type of stimulus or situation.

phobic disorder Severe phobic behavior patterns that render the individual dysfunctional. Avoidance of the feared object or situation serves to assuage anxiety.

physical or emotional security Feeling safe from emotional, verbal, and physical assault.

***Pneumocystis carinii* pneumonia (PCP)** Form of pulmonary disease caused by an opportunistic pathogen (fungal protozoan).

polymerase chain reaction (PCR) Laboratory technique using molecular biology to identify the nucleic acid sequence of HIV in the cells of an infected individual. Used in the early detection of perinatally exposed infants and in monitoring persons on clinical trials.

postpartum depression Subgroup of depression occurring 30 days or less in the postpartum period.

preconscious Memories that can be recalled to consciousness with some effort.

precursor Something that precedes. Tyrosine is a precursor to dopamine in the synthesis of dopamine in the body.

premorbid State before onset of the disorder.

prevalence Estimate of the frequency of a disease condition in the population, (e.g., ADHD affects 5% to 11% of school-aged children).

primary appraisal Judgment an individual makes about an event.

primary gain Relief or expression of anxiety through symptoms of disorder.

privacy Allowance of physical and emotional space for self and others.

probable cause Sufficient credible facts that would induce a reasonably intelligent and prudent person to believe that a cause of action exists.

process recording Written record of an encounter with a patient that is as nearly verbatim as possible, including both verbal and nonverbal behaviors of the nurse and the patient.

professional chaplain Also known as a spiritual care professional. One who has extensive postgraduate clinical training to offer spiritual care within a health care organization (see Box 17-4).

projective identification Placement of feelings on another to justify one's own expression of feelings.

proxemics Study of the way in which people perceive and use environmental, social, and personal space in interactions with others.

psychiatric rehabilitation Promotion of the patient's highest level of functioning in the least restrictive environment.

psychoeducation Strategy of teaching patients and families about disorders, treatments, coping techniques, and resources, based on the observation that people can be better participants in their own care if they have knowledge.

psychomotor retardation Markedly slowed speech and body movements.

psychoneuroimmunology Field of research focusing on the interactions of mind, environment, and bodily function, particularly immune system function.

psychopathology Study of underlying processes, both biological and psychosocial, that lead to mental disorders.

psychosis Inability to recognize reality, complicated by severe thought disorder and the inability to relate to others.

psychosocial adversity Environmental conditions such as poverty, unemployment, or overcrowded living conditions that do not support optimal development of a child.

psychotherapeutic management Model for nursing care that balances the three primary intervention modes used by psychiatric nurses: therapeutic nurse-patient relationship, psychopharmacology, and milieu management.

psychotic depression Subtype of depression, in which a person experiences delusions and hallucinations, often misdiagnosed as schizophrenia or schizoaffective disorder.

psychotropic drugs Medications used in the treatment of mental illness.

purge Compensation for calories consumed by self-induced vomiting, laxative abuse, diuretics, or enemas.

pyramidal system Motor system for voluntary movement.

race Breeding population that primarily mates within itself.

raphe nuclei Located along the midline of the brainstem (raphe = seam). Serotonin is synthesized from these cells.

reactive depression Depressed mood related to some life event (e.g., divorce, losing job).

reappraisal Appraisal made after new or additional information has been received.

recreational therapists Assist patients to find leisure interests so they can learn to balance work and play.

relational worldview Grounded in the belief in spirituality and the significance of relationships and interactions among individuals.

religion Defined structures, rituals, beliefs, and values through which communities frequently address to spiritual concerns.

religiosity Preoccupation with religious ideas or content.

resilience Capacity to move forward with development, despite psychosocial adversity or genetic vulnerability.

resiliency Capability to withstand stressors without permanent dysfunction or developmental delay.

respect for the individual Acknowledgment and allowance of the rights of others to be unique.

restraint Physical control of a patient to prevent injury to the patient, staff, and other patients.

reuptake Physiologic process that occurs when a neurotransmitter is taken up into the presynaptic neuron after having been released into the synapse. Some psychotropic drugs are designed to prevent the reuptake of a specific neurotransmitter in order to increase the synaptic presence of that neurotransmitter.

rigidity Assumption of an inappropriate posture.

satisfaction Relaxation of the tension of physiologic needs.

schizophrenia Syndrome, illness, or mental health disorder heterogeneous in cause, pathogenesis, presenting picture, response to treatment, and prognosis. Symptoms generally reflect a progressive deterioration and disorganization of the individual's personality structure, affect, and cognition. The DSM-IV-TR lists the following types: paranoid, catatonic, disorganized, undifferentiated, and residual.

scientific cause of illness Belief that there are specific concrete explanations for every illness and disease. This explanation involves the entrance of pathogens such as viruses, bacteria, and germs into the body.

seasonal affective disorder Subtype of depression occurring in late autumn or winter and lasting until spring.

seclusion Process of placing a patient alone in a specially designed room for protection and close observation.

secondary appraisal Evaluation an individual makes about potential actions to be taken.

secondary gain Attention and support received from others while ill.

selective serotonin reuptake inhibitors (SSRIs) Class of antidepressants. Potent blockers of serotonin reuptake, thus increasing the level of serotonin in the synapse.

serotonin (5HT) Monoamine neurotransmitter from the indolamine family. It is derived from the amino acid tryptophan. Deficiencies of serotonin are linked to depression.

shuffling gait (parkinsonism gait) Style of walking typically demonstrated by individuals whose dopamine stores have been blocked or depleted as a result of Parkinson's disease or antipsychotic medications.

smudging Common sacred rite of purification and cleansing practiced by many North American Indian nations. It includes the burning of cedar and sage for the purpose of fanning smoke with an eagle feather over or near the patient. It is seen as purifying the spirit and preparing the patient for a difficult spiritual journey such as illness or death, as well as being used for other spiritual rituals.

social organization Culture around particular units, such as family, racial, or ethnic groups; religious groups; and community or social groups.

social skills group Help psychiatric patients learn, practice, and develop skills for dealing with people in social situations.

socialization skills Those skills necessary for negotiating everyday interpersonal issues (e.g., acknowledging responsibility for one's behavior, using eye contact appropriately, interacting with others for purposes of sharing and support).

somatic therapy Therapeutic approach that uses physiologic or physical interventions to affect behavioral changes. For example, electroconvulsive therapy is a somatic treatment.

somatization Conversion of mental states or experiences into bodily symptoms; associated with anxiety.

soul Nonphysical, transcendent part of human beings involving their mind and will.

space Distance and intimacy needs of culturally unique individuals in human interaction.

spirituality Awareness of relationships with all creation, an appreciation of presence and purpose that goes beyond the five senses and the physical world, and includes a sense of meaning and belonging. It is often inclusive of religion.

splitting Inability to integrate good and bad aspects of self and others. Views self and others as all good or all bad.

status epilepticus Repetitive seizures; usually refers to repetitive grand mal seizures.

statutory law Statutory law is written law emanating from a legislative body. These laws are written by state and federal legislative authorities and passed in accordance with state and federal law.

steady state Desired state in anticonvulsant and other therapies when the serum concentration of the drug is consistent and is maintained at a therapeutic level.

step system Process by which inpatients gain privileges and responsibilities based on their progress.

stereotyping Assumption that all people in similar cultural, racial, or ethnic groups think and act alike.

stereotypy Continuous repetition of speech or physical activities.

stressor Stimulus perceived by the individual or the organism as challenging, threatening, or damaging.

striatum Basal ganglia that include the caudate and putamen.

substance-induced mood disorder Results from the disturbance or alteration of a person's mood that is due to the ingestion of a prescribed or nonprescribed drug or medication or exposure to a toxic substance.

substantia nigra Literally, black substance. A pigmented area of the midbrain where dopamine is synthesized.

suicidal ideation Individual's thinking about and inclination toward self-injury or self-destruction.

suicidal plan Specific method designed to inflict self-injury or self-destruction as verbalized by an individual.

suicide Self-inflicted death.

sulcus Groove separating gyri. Deep sulci are referred to as fissures.

superego Psychoanalytic structure of the mind equivalent to the conscience (sense of right and wrong). It develops in early childhood and provides the ego with an inner control to help cope with the id.

synapse Microscopic space between two neurons.

tangentiality Inability to have goal-directed associations of thought; never gets to desired goal from desired point.

tardive dyskinesia Extrapyramidal syndrome that usually emerges late in the course of long-term antipsychotic drug therapy. Includes grimacing, buccolingual movements, and dystonia (impaired muscle tonus). May be irreversible.

teamwork Staff working together to achieve agreed upon goals for the unit and for patient care.

terror State of extreme tension.

theist One who believes in God, without necessarily conforming to a particular set of religious beliefs. Based on the Greek word for God, *theos.*

therapeutic In the psychotherapeutic management model, it is the communication of respect, of a desire to help, and of understanding to another person. Understanding includes knowledge of mental mechanisms, coping strategies, and stressors. Active listening is a crucial component of being therapeutic.

therapeutic communication Interactive verbal and nonverbal strategies that focus on the needs of the patient and facilitate a goal-directed, patient-oriented communication process.

therapeutic listening Listening that is focused on the patient and obtains therapeutically useful information about the patient.

therapeutic milieu Treatment environment managed in such a way that the environment itself is therapeutic.

therapy Means, usually with words, to cure or manage the course of another person's mental disorder. Nurses who practice psychotherapy are trained in a specific therapy model (e.g., psychoanalysis, cognitive therapy).

thinking Process of following a goal-directed flow of ideas, symbols, and associations to a logical conclusion in accordance with the person's developmental stage.

thought disorder Thinking characterized by loose associations, neologisms, and illogical constructs and conclusions.

time Either a physical quantity measured by a clock or patterns and orientations that relate to social processes.

time out Disengaging the child from a specific situation (e.g., directing the child to sit in a chair facing away from other patients so that the child might regain self-control).

tolerance Need for increasing amounts of a substance to achieve the same effects.

tonic State of continuous tension.

transference Unconscious emotional reaction to a current situation that is actually based on previous experiences.

tricyclic antidepressants Drug classification of antidepressants that block the reuptake of norepinephrine and serotonin into the presynaptic neuron.

tuberoinfundibular tract Dopaminergic system with neurons in the arcuate nucleus of the hypothalamus that project to the pituitary stalk. This tract controls the secretion of prolactin.

tyramine Substance derived from the amino acid tyrosine and found in many common foods, such as aged cheeses, yogurt, and avocados (see Box 21-4). Tyramine-rich foods can cause a hypertensive crisis in a person being treated with MAOIs.

tyrosine Amino acid that is the precursor to dopamine.

unconscious Memories, conflicts, experiences, and materials that have been repressed and cannot be recalled at will.

undoing Defense mechanism by which a person symbolically acts out to reverse a previously committed act or thought. A common ritual in obsessive-compulsive disorder.

unit norm Expected behavior for a given therapeutic setting.

unnatural cause of illness Belief that outside forces such as a spell or a hex being cast on the sick person is the cause or the source of illness or disease.

validation Process of confirming an individual's intent by questioning the content of his or her message.

vascular dementia Results from the interruption of blood to the brain, which causes anoxia, ischemia, and subsequent infarction.

ventral tegmental area (VTA) Located in the midbrain, this region is dorsomedial to the substantia nigra and ventral to the red nuclei. The nuclei in this area produce dopamine. The efferent pathways from the VTA include the mesocortical and mesolimbic tracts.

ventricle System of connected brain cavities that are filled with cerebrospinal fluid, including the lateral ventricles (in the central portion of the telencephalon), the third ventricle (which runs between the thalami), the fourth ventricle (in the pons and medulla), and the connecting cerebral aqueduct (in the midbrain).

vesicle Storage sac at the synaptic terminal.

voluntary commitment Status in which the patient or his or her conservator or guardian requests treatment and signs an application for that treatment. This person is also free to sign himself or herself out of the hospital.

Wernicke's area Sophisticated auditory association cortex that is located within the planum temporale and interprets spoken language.

Wernicke's encephalopathy Confusion and ophthalmoplegia caused by thiamine deficiency; most common in alcoholics. It results in necrosis and hemorrhage in the mammillary bodies and periventricular structures of the brainstem.

Western medicine Conventional clinicians use this term to describe the medicine practiced by the holders of Doctor of Medicine (MD) or Doctor of Osteopathy (DO) degrees, some of whom may also practice complementary and alternative medicines. Other terms for conventional medicine are allopathic, regular, mainstream medicine, and biomedicine.

white matter Composed of myelinated neuronal axons.

withdrawal (1) Act or process of turning inward to avoid a perceived environmental threat. (2) Physiologic response to cessation of an addictive substance.

word salad Incoherent mixture of words or phrases.

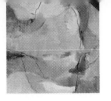

Index

A

Page references followed by "f" indicate figures, "t" indicate tables, and "b" indicate boxes.

Monoamine oxidase inhibitors—cont'd
  classification of, 234b
  contraindications, 250-251
  definition of, 235b, 341b
  description of, 192, 248
  dosage of, 238t-239t
  interactions of, 211
    drug-drug, 248-249, 249t
    food-drug, 249-250, 250b
    nursing considerations for, 250-251
  irreversible, 238t-239t, 251
  mechanism of action, 235
  nursing considerations for, 250-251
  older adults, 250, 616
  overdose, 234b
  patient education regarding, 251
  pharmacokinetics of, 238t-239t, 248
  pharmacologic effects of, 248
  pregnancy uses, 250
  selective, 192
  side effects of, 234b, 239t, 248, 250, 356b
  therapeutic levels, 250
  toxic levels, 250
  tricyclic antidepressants *versus*, 248
Mood
  definition of, 341b, 367b
  description of, 340-341
Mood disorders
  adolescents, 584-585
  biologic causes of, 70-71
  bipolar disorder. *See* Bipolar disorder
  childhood, 584-585
  definition of, 341b, 367b
  depression. *See* Depression
  DSM-IV-TR terminology and criteria, 340-341, 367b
  general medical condition-related, 341b, 367b
  NANDA nursing diagnoses, 367b
  prevalence of, 2t, 306t, 311t, 342t, 367t, 382t, 407t, 432t, 453t
  substance-induced, 341b, 367b
Morphine, 461t
Motor cortex, 56-57
Motor neurons, 67
Moxibustion, 166t, 170
Multidisciplinary team, 111
Multiple sclerosis, 71
Muting, 266
Mutism, 311b
Mydriasis, 220

N

Naloxone, 468, 484
Naltrexone hydrochloride, 463, 484
NANDA nursing diagnoses
  anxiety, 121b, 383b
  bulimia nervosa, 507b
  delirium, 409b

NANDA nursing diagnoses—cont'd
  dementia, 409b
  depression, 342b
  description of, 174
  family nursing, 162b
  generalized anxiety disorder, 383b
  major depression, 342b
  mood disorders, 367b
  schizophrenia, 313, 314b
  spirituality, 179, 179b
  substance-related disorders, 480b
Narcan. *See* Naloxone
Narcissistic personality disorder, 440-441
Narcotics Anonymous, 485-486, 496
Nardil. *See* Phenelzine
National Alliance for the Mentally Ill, 157, 328b
National Center for Complementary and Alternative Medicine, 535, 546
National Institute of Mental Health, 6, 306b
National Mental Health Act, 6
Native Americans
  alternative and complementary therapies used by, 546
  cytochrome P450 system variations in, 171
  mental health descriptors used by, 169
  metabolism variations, 171
  worldview, 168t
Natural cause of illness, 166t, 168
Nature argument, 306b, 307
Naturopathic physician, 534b
Naturopathy, 534b, 541
Navane. *See* Thiothixene
Nefazodone, 235, 238t-239t, 241
Negative consequence, 518
Negativism, 311b
Negligence, 37, 40
Neologism, 311b
Nerve, 54
Neurofibrillary tangles, 413, 415f
Neuroleptic(s)
  adolescents treated using, 588t, 591
  children treated using, 588t, 591
  definition of, 204b, 214b
Neuroleptic malignant syndrome
  antipsychotic drugs and, 222-223, 224b
  definition of, 210b, 221b
  description of, 207
  treatment of, 223
Neuron(s)
  anatomy of, 66
  association, 67
  communication among, 196
  definition of, 54, 66, 196
  dendrites of, 196
  functions of, 66-67
  lower motor, 57
  motor, 67
  postganglionic, 67

Introduction to Psychiatric Nursing

Choose the *most* appropriate answer to the following questions:

1. Approximately what percentage of Americans over the age of 18 is personally affected by mental or addictive disorders each year?
   - _____ 1. 10%
   - _____ 2. 15%
   - _____ 3. 25%
   - _____ 4. 40%

2. The cost of disorders of the brain is very high. Which of the following is closest to the total cost (both direct and indirect) of these disorders (in the millions of dollars)?
   - _____ 1. 100
   - _____ 2. 200
   - _____ 3. 300
   - _____ 4. 400

3. The first state hospitals that Dorothea Dix established were meant to be:
   - _____ 1. Asylums
   - _____ 2. Treatment centers
   - _____ 3. Places of confinement
   - _____ 4. Located near follow-up resources

4. The forces behind deinstitutionalization started gaining momentum during what period?
   - _____ 1. 1940s and 1950s
   - _____ 2. 1960s
   - _____ 3. 1970s
   - _____ 4. 1980s

5. The chief result of the scientific study era was:
   - _____ 1. The asylum
   - _____ 2. Objective study of psychiatric disorders
   - _____ 3. The community mental health movement
   - _____ 4. Homelessness

6. The psychiatrist who has had the most influence on modern psychotherapy is?
   - _____ 1. Bleuler
   - _____ 2. Freud
   - _____ 3. Kraepelin
   - _____ 4. Skinner

7. The number of patients in state hospitals today is approximately:
   - _____ 1. 70,000
   - _____ 2. 200,000
   - _____ 3. 300,000
   - _____ 4. 400,000

Briefly answer the following questions:

8. What are the ABCs of the pre-Enlightenment era?

9. Who were the two men most responsible for the period of Enlightenment?

Match the concept or person with the benchmark in psychiatric history:

_____ 10. Period of scientific study   a. Asylum
_____ 11. Period of psychotropic drugs   b. Freud
_____ 12. Period of Enlightenment   c. Home health
_____ 13. Period of community mental   d. Led to least restrictive alternative or
        health   environment
                                                  e. Deinstitutionalization

Briefly define the following terms:

14. Asylum (first definition):

15. Psychotropic medications:

16. Least restrictive alternative or environment:

17. Deinstitutionalization:

18. "Worried well":

Indicate *T* for true and *F* for false:

_____ 19. Deinstitutionalization is the depopulating of community mental health centers.
_____ 20. Community mental health and home health nursing are directions in which psychiatric nursing is headed.

Chapter 2

Name: _____

Psychotherapeutic Management in the Continuum of Care

Choose the *most* appropriate answer to the following questions:

1. What is the underlying foundation for the components of psychotherapeutic management?
   _____ 1. Knowledge of drugs
   _____ 2. Knowledge of psychopathology
   _____ 3. Knowledge of therapeutic skills
   _____ 4. Knowledge of milieu management

2. Which of the following components of psychotherapeutic management is most important according to the authors?
   _____ 1. A therapeutic nurse-patient relationship is most important.
   _____ 2. Appropriate use of psychotropic drugs is most important.
   _____ 3. A well-managed milieu is most important.
   _____ 4. A therapeutic nurse-patient relationship, psychotropic drugs, and a well-managed milieu are equally important.

3. In making referrals in the continuum of care, which of the following concepts is most important to consider?
   _____ 1. Therapeutic communication
   _____ 2. Least restrictive setting
   _____ 3. Diagnosis
   _____ 4. Family participation

4. The most important dimension of milieu management is:
   _____ 1. Safety
   _____ 2. Structure
   _____ 3. Norms
   _____ 4. Setting limits

5. The milieu management concern of balance has to do with the balancing of:
   _____ 1. Safe versus unsafe behaviors
   _____ 2. Independence versus dependence
   _____ 3. Side effects versus desired effects
   _____ 4. Healthy behaviors versus unhealthy behaviors

6. The psychotherapeutic management intervention, the therapeutic nurse-patient relationship, relies primarily on:
   _____ 1. Administration of appropriate medications
   _____ 2. Use of the nursing process
   _____ 3. Use of words
   _____ 4. Cultural sensitivity

7. Of the many reasons for understanding psychopharmacology, the one that underscores the autonomy of nursing practice is:
   _____ 1. A high percentage of psychotropic drugs are given on a prn basis.
   _____ 2. The issue of drug interactions with over-the-counter drugs is growing.
   _____ 3. Patient teaching always requires a highly individualized approach.
   _____ 4. Nurse practitioners now order more psychotropic drugs than do physicians.

8. Electroconvulsive therapy is:

_____ 1. A component of the psychotherapeutic management model

_____ 2. An important treatment tool but lies mostly outside the psychotherapeutic management model

_____ 3. Best subsumed under the milieu management component

_____ 4. Unrelated to the psychopathology of any given disorder

9. Which of the following is considered a special population in this textbook?

_____ 1. People of ethnic minorities

_____ 2. Older adults

_____ 3. Women

_____ 4. Individuals with mental retardation

Briefly answer the following questions:

10. What are the six environmental elements that nurses must consider in creating a therapeutic milieu?

11. What are the interventions used in psychotherapeutic management?

12. What type of unit might be therapeutic with only the milieu portion of nursing care present? In other words, are there patients who may "misuse" medications and one-to-one interactions?

13. Can you name at least three functions of a nurse in psychopharmacology?

14. What is psychopathology?

Models for Working with Psychiatric Patients

Choose the *most* appropriate answer to the following questions:

1. Mr. Lawrence tells the nurse that he has had three factory jobs in the last 8 months because he was too slow for the assembly line and his co-workers would not help him. He feels alone. He is having difficulty with his ceramics project. With which developmental stage is Mr. Lawrence struggling?
   _____ 1. Autonomy versus shame and doubt
   _____ 2. Initiative versus guilt
   _____ 3. Industry versus inferiority
   _____ 4. Intimacy versus isolation

2. A new patient has had multiple stressors for a long time. You expect this patient to be in the stage of exhaustion (GAS) and show which of the following behaviors?
   _____ 1. Personality disorganization, immobilization, suicide
   _____ 2. Increased alertness, mild anxiety, mobilization of resources
   _____ 3. Problem solving with assistance, somatic complaints
   _____ 4. Task-oriented behaviors, normal weight return

3. Using principles of cognitive behavioral therapy and reality therapy, the nurse working with patients would do which of the following?
   _____ 1. Explain that rational beliefs produce feelings of anxiety or hostility.
   _____ 2. Encourage patients to shift blame to others when possible.
   _____ 3. Support patients' denial so that grief is lessened.
   _____ 4. Teach patients that they are responsible for themselves and their choices.

4. In using the nurse-patient relationship as a means for the patient to improve interpersonal skills, which of the following statements would indicate an appropriate intervention?
   _____ 1. "I would like you to make a list of your irrational beliefs about relationships."
   _____ 2. "What exactly do you want to tell your boss about your new work schedule?"
   _____ 3. "Tell me about the dreams you have had this past week."
   _____ 4. "What do you think will happen if you join your friend in smoking crack cocaine?"

5. On the adult psychiatric unit, you see a patient smoking in her room. Smoking is not allowed on the unit. Which of the following interventions is most appropriate?
   _____ 1. Confront the behavior.
   _____ 2. Tell your supervisor.
   _____ 3. Ignore the behavior unless you see her smoking again.
   _____ 4. Remind all patients about the nonsmoking policy.

6. During a discussion with the nurse, the patient says, "I told you that I do not want to talk about my boss now; maybe tomorrow." The most appropriate nursing response is which of the following?
   _____ 1. "Okay, we can talk about your boss tomorrow."
   _____ 2. "I know it is not easy to talk about your boss, but it is important for your progress."
   _____ 3. "Your boss is a nasty person. I think you can confront him more appropriately."
   _____ 4. "You are suppressing this problem with your boss."

7. In the admission interview, the patient says that she found out that her husband is having an affair but says, "My husband is such a good man. I love him so much." Which of the following statements by the nurse would be appropriate?

  _____ 1. "I wouldn't put up with his affair if I were you."
  _____ 2. "When are you going to admit that a divorce is inevitable?"
  _____ 3. "I know you love him. Tell me how his affair is affecting you emotionally."
  _____ 4. "Are you going to tell him that he has to choose between you and his girlfriend?"

8. A patient tells group members that she feels ashamed about being sexually abused as a child. After the group session, the nurse would make which of the following statements?

  _____ 1. "Tell me more about how you felt when you were being abused."
  _____ 2. "The guy who molested you is the one who should be ashamed."
  _____ 3. "You should have reported the abuse to the police."
  _____ 4. "You need to forget about the abuse and get on with your life."

9. A patient is describing his difficulty in trusting people, especially in social situations. The nurse decides to work with the patient on his anxiety and interpersonal skills. Which of the following statements would indicate the best area on which to focus?

  _____ 1. "Everyone gets uncomfortable in new social situations."
  _____ 2. "So what if everyone does not like you."
  _____ 3. "Just be yourself and everything will be all right."
  _____ 4. "What are you afraid will happen when you meet new people?"

10. While talking with the nurse, the patient reveals that he feels overwhelmed by all the stresses in his life. The nurse decides to encourage the patient to attend groups that will help with his issues. Which of the following groups would be most helpful?

  _____ 1. Arts and crafts
  _____ 2. Exercise group
  _____ 3. Biofeedback training
  _____ 4. Problem-solving group

Case Study: Kim is a 28-year-old legal assistant who is married but has no children. Her husband, Tony, is a 29-year-old lawyer who has told Kim that he is having an affair with Jamie and wants a divorce. Initially, while talking with the nurse, Kim expresses much hostility toward Tony and accuses Jamie of causing it. Then Kim says that there is nothing left to her life and that all she does at home is cry and sleep. Kim describes not wanting to be seen by her friends but, at the same time, wishing that others would tell her that she is still attractive. While showing no emotion, she then says that she just wants the divorce to be over so she can get on with her life. "If Tony can have sex with someone else, so can I." When the nurse suggests to Kim that counseling can help her through the divorce, Kim says that she does not need counseling because her life will be over very soon.

Critical Thinking Questions: On a separate sheet of paper, briefly answer the following questions:

1. Match specific statement or behaviors of Kim with the defense mechanisms that they reflect.
2. Identify Kim's behaviors that suggest developmental issues in Erikson's first three stages.
3. Using principles of the reality therapy model, give examples in which Kim:
   a. Is denying her own responsibility for her situation
   b. Has lost her self-respect
   c. Shows fear of rejection
   d. Is irresponsibly violating her own morals
   e. Is being dishonest about her real needs and feelings
4. Using the principles of the Stress Models, design appropriate immediate and longer-term interventions for Kim.

Chapter **4**

Name: _____

Legal Issues

Choose the *most* appropriate answer to the following questions:

1. Wyatt v Stickney was a court case that considered the issue of:
   - _____ 1. Exemptions from guilt by reason of insanity
   - _____ 2. Right to treatment
   - _____ 3. Right to personal privacy
   - _____ 4. Right to refuse treatment

2. Tarasoff v. The Regents of the University of California was a court case that considered the issue of:
   - _____ 1. The right to refuse treatment
   - _____ 2. The duty to warn of threatened suicide
   - _____ 3. The duty to warn of threatened harm to self or others
   - _____ 4. The right to treatment

3. Individuals can be involuntarily treated for all of the following reasons *except:*
   - _____ 1. Dangerous to self
   - _____ 2. Dangerous to others
   - _____ 3. Gravely disabled
   - _____ 4. Convinced that they are Jesus Christ

4. Margaret Jones is an older woman who was found wandering in the city park. She is disheveled, dirty, and not making much sense when she speaks. She is bothering people trying to enjoy themselves, and, after several complaints, the police pick her up and bring her to the county hospital emergency department. Physical examination reveals a malnourished, dehydrated elderly woman with a suspected delirium superimposed on a form of dementia. She is admitted to the geriatric psychiatric unit. Ms. Jones tells everyone to leave her alone. Which of the following categories best fits Ms. Jones' situation?
   - _____ 1. Voluntary
   - _____ 2. Involuntary
   - _____ 3. Gravely disabled
   - _____ 4. Danger to others

5. Ms. Jones refuses to take any medication. She states that she does not need it. If this response continues, which of the following legal courses can be taken?
   - _____ 1. Force her to take her medication.
   - _____ 2. Hide the medicine in applesauce.
   - _____ 3. Start conservatorship proceedings.
   - _____ 4. Allow her to refuse medication based on her right to refuse treatment.

6. The delirium clears after Ms. Jones has received intravenous fluids and a nutritious diet. A workup results in a diagnosis of Pick's disease, a debilitating dementia. The social worker starts to evaluate posthospital placement. A primary legal concern is:
   - _____ 1. To ensure that Ms. Jones receives treatment
   - _____ 2. To ensure that Ms. Jones' right to confidentiality is not violated
   - _____ 3. To consider her right to the least restrictive alternative or environment
   - _____ 4. To ensure that the appropriate people are warned of her impending discharge

7. Which of the following rights can be suspended with good cause?
_____ 1. The right to treatment in the least restrictive environment
_____ 2. The right to freedom from restraint and seclusion
_____ 3. The right to confidentiality of records
_____ 4. The right to warn others of danger

8. Corporate compliance is best defined as:
_____ 1. A health care provider's responsibility to comply with governmental laws and regulations
_____ 2. A health care provider's policy and procedure manuals
_____ 3. A list of patients' rights
_____ 4. The hospital's mission statement

Fill in the blanks with the best answers from the list of concepts related to patient rights.

9. _____ is an environment that provides the necessary treatment requirements in the least restrictive setting possible.
10. Patient information can be released only with _____ consent of the patient or responsible party.
11. When _____ and _____ interventions are not successful, seclusion alone or seclusion with restraint may be required.
12. In emergency situations, a nurse can approve a seclusion or restraint order when no psychiatrist is available. A psychiatrist must see the patient within _____ hours.
13. A patient in restraint or seclusion must be checked by a registered nurse every ____ minutes.
14. Range-of-motion exercises on joints must be completed on a patient in restraint every _____ hours.
15. When a nonpsychiatrist physician admits a patient, the patient must be seen by the psychiatrist within _____ hours.
16. Providing the patient with information about his or her specific treatments is called _____.

a. Mental Health Systems Act	g. Verbal	n. Probable cause
b. 30	h. Pharmacologic	o. 3
c. 2	i. Written	p. 24
d. Least restrictive alternative or environment	j. Negligence	q. 72
e. Informed consent	k. 1	r. Community Mental Health Centers Act
f. 4	l. 15	
	m. 60	

Match the ruling with its description. You may use some answers more than once.

_____ 17. Tarasoff v Regents of the University of California
_____ 18. Griswold v Connecticut
_____ 19. M'Naghten rule
_____ 20. Wyatt v Stickney
_____ 21. Rogers v Okin

a. Not guilty by reason of insanity
b. Right to personal privacy
c. Right to treatment
d. Right to refuse treatment
e. Right to refuse treatment based on right to privacy
f. Duty to warn of threats to others

Psychobiologic Bases of Behavior

Choose the *most* appropriate answer to the following questions:

1. Schizophrenia may be best thought of as:
   - _____ 1. A neurodegenerative problem
   - _____ 2. A neurodevelopmental problem
   - _____ 3. Overproduction of CSF
   - _____ 4. Decreased serotonin production

2. Cranial nerve XII is part of the:
   - _____ 1. Central nervous system
   - _____ 2. Parasympathetic nervous system
   - _____ 3. Peripheral nervous system
   - _____ 4. Sympathetic nervous system

3. The connecting white matter between the two cerebral hemispheres is the:
   - _____ 1. Corticospinal tract
   - _____ 2. Corpus callosum
   - _____ 3. Extrapyramidal system
   - _____ 4. Internal capsule

4. The white matter of the brain consists of:
   - _____ 1. Myelinated dendrites
   - _____ 2. Myelinated axons
   - _____ 3. Cell bodies
   - _____ 4. Corona radiata

5. The thin outer layer of gray matter is called the:
   - _____ 1. Cerebral cortex
   - _____ 2. Basal ganglia
   - _____ 3. Diencephalon
   - _____ 4. Frontal lobe

6. The area of the brain associated with thought, goal-directed activity, and inhibitions is known as the:
   - _____ 1. Parietal lobe
   - _____ 2. Satiety center
   - _____ 3. Prefrontal area
   - _____ 4. Hypothalamus

7. The system associated with the four Fs, emotions and motivation, and memory is the:
   - _____ 1. Cortex
   - _____ 2. Limbic system
   - _____ 3. Thalamus
   - _____ 4. Hypothalamus

8. When a lesion develops in the Papez circuit, somewhere along its intricate path, which of the following occurs?
   _____ 1. The thirst mechanism is compromised.
   _____ 2. Memory is compromised.
   _____ 3. Fight or flight is compromised.
   _____ 4. Set drive is compromised.

9. Which of the following brain nuclei is involved with pleasure and addiction?
   _____ 1. Red nucleus
   _____ 2. Hypothalamus
   _____ 3. Substantia nigra
   _____ 4. Nucleus accumbens

10. A spinal nerve lesion caused by multiple sclerosis would affect which of the following types of neurons?
    _____ 1. Upper motor neuron
    _____ 2. Lower motor neuron
    _____ 3. Association neuron
    _____ 4. Unmyelinated neuron

11. A specific small lesion of the left precentral gyrus at the level of the homunculus' hand would cause:
    _____ 1. An upper motor lesion
    _____ 2. Loss of coordinated motor movement (paresis) of the left hand
    _____ 3. Loss of the right visual field
    _____ 4. A lower motor lesion

12. What is the neurotransmitter that connects the preganglionic and postganglionic neurons of both the sympathetic and parasympathetic systems?
    _____ 1. Acetylcholine
    _____ 2. Norepinephrine
    _____ 3. Serotonin
    _____ 4. Dopamine

Briefly answer the following question:

13. The Babinski's response is a reflex. Does it occur with an upper motor neuron disorder, such as a stroke, or with a lower motor neuron disorder, such as polio?

Match the following movement disorders with the correct sites of dysfunction.
_____ 14. Awkwardness of gait   a. Basal ganglia disorder
_____ 15. Intention tremor   b. Cerebellar disorder
_____ 16. Parkinsonism
_____ 17. Chorea

Match the following change in neurotransmitter bioavailability with the disorder it is thought to precipitate.
_____ 18. Depression   a. Increased dopamine
_____ 19. Schizophrenia   b. Decreased dopamine
_____ 20. Parkinsonism   c. Decreased norepinephrine
                                d. Decreased serotonin
                                e. Decreased GABA

6-8

Unit II: Continuum of Care

Choose the *most* appropriate answer to the following questions:

1. The patient has been hospitalized for 3 days after a suicide attempt. Suicidal ideation is still present, but the patient no longer has a specific plan. Lack of appetite and disturbance in sleep are present. The patient lives alone, has no support system, and insurance will not cover further hospitalization. Which of the following levels of care would be most appropriate?

   _____ 1. Community outreach program   _____ 3. Subacute care
   _____ 2. Weekly outpatient care   _____ 4. Further inpatient hospitalization

2. In community-based care, which of the following would interfere with the nurse-patient relationship?

   _____ 1. Rapport   _____ 3. Setting
   _____ 2. Time   _____ 4. Medications

3. The recovery model of care emphasizes which of the following concepts?

   _____ 1. The nurse is responsible for the consumer's life goals.
   _____ 2. The psychiatrist controls the consumer's choices.
   _____ 3. The consumer is solely responsible for arranging needed services.
   _____ 4. The consumer controls and is responsible for his or her own life.

4. Which of the following situations is most likely to result in an inpatient stay?

   _____ 1. An older woman who has begun wandering out of the house at night
   _____ 2. An adolescent arrested for drinking at a friend's after-prom party
   _____ 3. A recently divorced man sitting on the railing of a bridge over an interstate highway
   _____ 4. A child who has begun hitting his classmates since his sister was born

5. A 12-year-old boy says he really loves his family, which includes his new stepfather. However, he admits to dreams about his deceased father's words that his son was useless and dumb. Which level of care is most likely indicated?

   _____ 1. Health promotion   _____ 3. Treatment
   _____ 2. Primary prevention   _____ 4. Rehabilitation

6. Which of the following purposes of hospital-based care is most critical?

   _____ 1. Referrals to outpatient services
   _____ 2. Medication and education compliance
   _____ 3. Family education and support
   _____ 4. Safety for the individual and others

7. Which of the following would be a unique and important target issue in programming for older adults?

   _____ 1. Medication education
   _____ 2. Coping strategies
   _____ 3. Death and dying
   _____ 4. Interpersonal relationships

8. An individual is brought to the inpatient unit because she is wandering on the interstate highway in her nightgown. She has a history of prior admissions for psychotic episodes and medication noncompliance. She tells the nurse that she just wants to go home. Which of the following should be the nurse's response?

_____ 1. "You can't go home until the doctor says you can."
_____ 2. "I know you want to go home right now, but we are very concerned about keeping you safe."
_____ 3. "First, we need to get you back on your medicine."
_____ 4. "Since it is the middle of the night, you have to stay until morning."

9. A 46-year-old man, newly divorced, is being assessed by a crisis worker in the emergency room after an overdose and an attempt to hang himself from a backyard tree. He is medically stable but is still distraught about being rescued. Which type of programming is likely to be the most appropriate for the man?

_____ 1. A day therapy program
_____ 2. A psychiatric intensive care unit
_____ 3. An acute-care unit with problem-solving groups
_____ 4. A community living skills program

10. A 14-year-old girl is admitted after 3 months of lack of appetite, decreased sleep, and suicidal ideations. She states to the nurse that she "just wants to be in heaven with her mother." The nurse is likely to seek increased involvement by which of the following team members?

_____ 1. Psychiatrist and neurologist   _____ 3. Activity therapist and pharmacist
_____ 2. Social worker and physical   _____ 4. Dietician and chaplain
           therapist

Case Study: Mary Catherine ("Katie") is an 18-year-old woman who was admitted to an inpatient unit after an overdose of Xanax. During the admission interview, she described many personal and family stressors. She was a freshman in college when she "fell in love" with a student. They had been dating for 6 months when she discovered she was pregnant. When she told her boyfriend he denied that it was his baby and said that he never wanted to see her again. She stopped going to classes and then went home. Katie said that her parents were furious and told her she would have to put the baby up for adoption because "they had enough problems to deal with." This is when she "knew that suicide was the only option." "Unfortunately, my brother found me too soon and here I am." When asked about family stresses, Katie talked about each member.

She described her mother, Mary Elizabeth, as a wonderful person who was overwhelmed, worn out, and depressed again. This circumstance was caused, in part, by having Mary's father in the house for the last 2 years. Katie said her 72-year-old grandfather, Matthew, has been "going down hill" since his wife died 4 years ago. "He probably has Alzheimer's and no longer wants to live. For the last 6 days, he's refused to eat or take any of his medicines." Katie's father, Sam, was described as "an okay father"; but 3 weeks ago, he began drinking again after 11 years of sobriety. "He admits to needing help with all the stress at work and at home. I think he went to the employee assistance counselor last week and an AA meeting." Katie said that her 15-year-old brother, Sam, Jr., was the "wild one." "He parties, has sex, drinks alcohol, smokes marijuana, and doesn't care about school." Mark, her 13-year-old brother, was described as the "good one." "He is good at everything—school, sports, scouts. Even his friends are good kids, but he isn't home a lot."

Katie is now nearing discharge and says she thinks the whole family needs help. When her parents visit that evening, the nurse asks them if they would be interested in having a family conference before Katie comes home. They agree to meet with the multidisciplinary team. In preparation, the nurse outlines the possible needs and potential referrals for each family member.

Critical Thinking Question: If you were the nurse, what referrals along the continuum of care might you suggest for each person? *(Write your referrals for Katie, Matthew, Mary Elizabeth, Sam, Sam Jr., and Mark on a separate sheet of paper.)*

Chapter 9

Name: _____

Communication

Choose the *most* appropriate answer to the following questions:

1. One goal of therapeutic communication is which of the following?
   _____ 1. Assisting patients with learning communication skills
   _____ 2. Allowing the nurse to express feelings
   _____ 3. Becoming the patient's friend
   _____ 4. Developing consistent communication techniques

2. Encouraging a description of perception is reflected in which of the following statements:
   _____ 1. "What do you mean by 'feeling alienated?'"
   _____ 2. "I know what you mean."
   _____ 3. "It sounds as if you have been depressed."
   _____ 4. "What do you think is happening in your marriage?"

3. A major purpose of listening is which of the following?
   _____ 1. Encourages patients to guide the interview
   _____ 2. Allows the nurse to interpret and validate data
   _____ 3. Is easy for most people to do
   _____ 4. Reflects what patients say

4. Which of the following reflects a common interference in nurse-patient communication?
   _____ 1. Discussing fears abut patients with colleagues
   _____ 2. Validating patient information with the family
   _____ 3. Admitting and apologizing to a patient for a mistake
   _____ 4. Avoiding issues that are uncomfortable for patients

5. A patient is describing the reason for his admission. He says, "After I was forced to retire, I didn't know what to do with myself. My wife is still working. I don't feel like much of a man anymore." Which of the following best reflects the content theme conveyed by the patient?
   _____ 1. Dependency
   _____ 2. Sadness
   _____ 3. Worthlessness
   _____ 4. Financial problems

6. You notice a new patient sitting alone in the corner staring at the floor. Using the concept of proxemics, which would be the next most appropriate action by the nurse?
   _____ 1. Walk toward her and ask what she wants.
   _____ 2. Ask her to come to the nurse's station.
   _____ 3. Kneel in front of her and ask her name.
   _____ 4. Sit near her, leaving an empty chair next to her.

7. Which of the following statements by the nurse best reflects therapeutic communication?
   _____ 1. "I think your doctor needs to know that you're not sleeping well."
   _____ 2. "What do you want me to do about your problems?"
   _____ 3. "Sometimes your doctor can be abrupt, even with the staff."
   _____ 4. "No, I don't have to chart what you said tonight."

8. A patient is role-playing using assertive skills with his wife and says, "I'm tired of your nagging all the time." In using the technique of feedback, which would be the most appropriate response?

    _____ 1. "You are still off base."

    _____ 2. "When you said that, I felt like I was being blamed."

    _____ 3. "See? You can do this after all."

    _____ 4. "I can help you do this better."

9. The patient's goal for the day is to decide whether to return to graduate school. Which of the following statements by the nurse would be most appropriate?

    _____ 1. "What would be the advantages of returning to school?"

    _____ 2. "You seem upset about this right now."

    _____ 3. "I think you'll do fine back in school."

    _____ 4. "What does your mother think you should do?"

10. After several days in the hospital, a patient reveals that he has urges to touch his nephew in a sexual way. Which of the following statements would indicate an appropriate nursing intervention?

    _____ 1. "That would be wrong of you to do that."

    _____ 2. "I'll have to report this to your doctor."

    _____ 3. "What would happen if you acted on this urge?"

    _____ 4. "Why would you want to do this to him?"

For each of the following dialogues, indicate whether the nurse's response is therapeutic *(T)* or nontherapeutic *(N)*, and label the technique used. (Therapeutic and nontherapeutic techniques are listed in the chapter.)

Example:

Patient: "I do not know what to say. I can't talk anymore."

  T   "I'll just sit with you a few minutes."

  Offering self_____ *(technique used)*

Patient: "I just can't take it anymore. Losing my wife is impossible to accept."

11. _____ "Everybody has to die sometime."

12. _____ *(technique used)*

Patient: "I hear voices all the time. I can't get them to stop!"

13. _____ "I know the voices are real to you, but I don't hear them."

14. _____ *(technique used)*

Patient: "Things are never going to get better."

15. _____ "It may not seem as if they will, but they will."

16. _____ *(technique used)*

Patient: "I feel as if I am going to clock out."

17. _____ "What do you mean by 'going to clock out?'"

18. _____ *(technique used)*

Nurse-Patient Relationship

Choose the *most* appropriate answer to the following questions:

1. Which of the following best describes the nurse-patient relationship?
   - _____ 1. Based on a single theoretical model that explains the dynamics of the patient's needs
   - _____ 2. Conducted by a nurse psychotherapist who offers specialized techniques for specialized problems
   - _____ 3. Based on a foundation of companionship, mutual support, and interest
   - _____ 4. A series of goal-directed interactions conveying respect and a willingness to help the patient

2. Issues and patient behaviors that interfere with progress in a nurse-patient relationship are handled in which of the following ways?
   - _____ 1. Generally ignored until the patient is more stable
   - _____ 2. Usually not significant enough to address directly
   - _____ 3. Usually assessed and then a specific intervention is designed
   - _____ 4. Generally not charted because of the need for confidentiality

3. Which of the following statements by the nurse reflects therapeutic self-disclosure?
   - _____ 1. "When my mother died, I felt sadness and anger. What have you been feeling since your wife died?"
   - _____ 2. "I'm a nurse on this unit. I will be working with you today with any problems you are having."
   - _____ 3. "I can't be your girlfriend, but I can help you think of ways to find new friends."
   - _____ 4. "I know it's hard for you to change things at home, but I think you are ready to do it."

4. One strategy for helping patients change behaviors is called changing the risk/benefit ratio. Which of the following statements reflects this strategy?
   - _____ 1. Making mistakes provides opportunities for learning new behaviors.
   - _____ 2. Making one's own decisions improves one's self-esteem.
   - _____ 3. Changes are more likely to occur when risks are low.
   - _____ 4. Changes the patient has made are reinforced at discharge.

5. A few patients who do not respond to verbal diffusing of anger may have threatening behaviors. Which of the following is an important precaution for the nurse to take?
   - _____ 1. Avoid arguing with the patient's delusion.
   - _____ 2. Be aware of the patient's beliefs and values.
   - _____ 3. Avoid going into the patient's room alone.
   - _____ 4. Confront the patient's manipulative behaviors directly.

6. When working with a suspicious patient, which of the following is an important intervention?
   - _____ 1. Continue to require that the patient attend groups.
   - _____ 2. Communicate clearly, simply, and congruently.
   - _____ 3. Offer a prn medication regularly.
   - _____ 4. Allow the patient to cry when needed.

7. The desire to change is not always sufficient; one must know how to change. Which of the following interventions reflects this principle?
   _____   1. Offering anger-management classes
   _____   2. Waiting until the patient is ready for change
   _____   3. Recommending an appropriate support group
   _____   4. Facilitating rational decision making

8. Helping patients to be involved in their own care facilitates their progress. One patient says her goal for today is to get out of the hospital. Which of the following statements would reflect the most helpful nursing interventions at this point?
   _____   1. "I realize you want to go home."
   _____   2. "What behaviors do you need to change in order to be discharged?"
   _____   3. "What brought you to the hospital in the first place?"
   _____   4. "I'm sure the doctor will let you go today."

9. A patient finishes a phone call, slams the phone down, and says, "He did it again." To help the patient deal with her feelings appropriately, which of the following actions or statements would be most helpful?
   _____   1. Give the patient time to cool down.
   _____   2. "I can see you are upset. What is happening?"
   _____   3. "Slamming the phone is not going to help."
   _____   4. Tell the patient's nurse what the patient said and did.

10. In a group, a patient states, "I know this divorce is inevitable. I wish someone would just tell me how to get over it." After the group, the nurse decided to use supportive confrontation with this patient. Which of the following statements reflects this approach?
   _____   1. "It seems hard right now, but things will get better in time."
   _____   2. "Do you think it would help you to hear from a member of a divorce recovery group?"
   _____   3. "What do you want me to help you with?"
   _____   4. "I know you'd like easy answers, but you can get support here as you work on your own answers."

Case Study: Arnie is a 22-year-old patient who has been on the unit for 5 days. When he was admitted, the initial patient assessment revealed that he had been arrested by the police for standing in the middle of the street, knocking on car windows, and shouting "messages against the devil." Arnie denied these behaviors and adamantly stated that he did not belong in the hospital. "I need to go back to my corner and tell everyone what God was saying to·me." He admitted to hearing God's voice and to believing that he is "God's special messenger."

On the day after his admission, Arnie became withdrawn in his room and was pacing frequently. He stated, "I am going to go to hell for all this trouble I have been causing."

On the fifth day after admission, Arnie reported feeling better and that God's voice was almost a whisper now. He said, "I guess I'll keep my praying to myself and in church." The psychiatrist agreed to discharge Arnie the next day.

Critical Thinking Question: Using concepts described as part of the phases of the nurse-patient relationship and interactions with selected behaviors, identify issues that apply to Arnie's situation. Then, list statements you might use in talking with Arnie that would address these issues. *(Write your answer on a separate sheet of paper.)*

Chapter 11

Name: _____

Nursing Process

Choose the *most* appropriate answer to the following questions:

1. Which of the following concepts is most accurate about the focus of nursing diagnoses?
   _____ 1. Based on what the patient says are issues that need work
   _____ 2. Specific problems that point to a desired patient outcome
   _____ 3. Specific behavioral goals the patient needs to address
   _____ 4. Based on nursing activities needed to assist the patient

2. In the afternoon after a patient was admitted, the patient is overheard yelling to someone on the phone. The patient had not shown signs of aggression previously. The nurse decides to investigate this patient's behavior. Which of the following factors would be the most important to explore first?
   _____ 1. How the patient might be less aggressive
   _____ 2. What goal the patient wants to accomplish now
   _____ 3. The context or situation that precipitated the aggression
   _____ 4. What the patient will do in the next phone call

3. Which of the following is an appropriate nursing diagnosis?
   _____ 1. Depression related to loss of wife as evidenced by suicidal ideation
   _____ 2. Suicidal ideation related to depression as evidenced by wish to be dead
   _____ 3. Loss of support related to wife's death as evidenced by grieving
   _____ 4. Grieving, dysfunctional, related to loss of wife as evidenced by suicidal ideations

4. A patient who has been making cuts on her wrist when she is angry is admitted to the unit. Which is the most appropriate initial or first outcome or goal?
   _____ 1. Patient will tell the nurse when she is feeling angry.
   _____ 2. Patient will verbalize that she no longer wants to harm herself.
   _____ 3. Patient will sign a contract stating she agrees not to harm herself.
   _____ 4. Patient agrees that she will not threaten the safety of herself or others.

5. During an interview with the nurse, the patient states, "I might as well die. No one cares about me anymore. My suicide would show them." Which of the following describes the themes in this interaction?
   _____ 1. Content—suicidal ideation, revenge; mood—anger; interaction—manipulative
   _____ 2. Content—revenge, suicidal plan; mood—depressed; interaction—withdrawal
   _____ 3. Content—loneliness, hopelessness; mood—depressed; interaction—passive
   _____ 4. Content—suicidal, lonely; mood—guilt; interaction—resistant to help

6. A patient with a broken leg is in the emergency room. He comments to the nurse, "God told me he would protect me from harm, but the devil broke my leg anyway." This statement would be included in a mental status examination in which of the following categories?
   _____ 1. Thought clarity
   _____ 2. Thought content
   _____ 3. Insight
   _____ 4. Judgment

7. Which of the following patient statements would reflect "recent memory?"
   _____ 1. "Are you a doctor or a nurse?"
   _____ 2. "Who knows what I was doing 40 years ago?"
   _____ 3. "I really don't want to share that information."
   _____ 4. "Could it be from the fish I ate yesterday?"

8. A patient has been in the hospital for 2 days. The nurse notices that she has been sitting alone and crying for a few minutes. Which of the following is the most appropriate nurse response?
   _____ 1. Sit down, pause, and then ask her, "What are you crying about?"
   _____ 2. Take her a tissue and say, "I'll be back in a few minutes."
   _____ 3. Let her alone to cry in peace, but be sure to talk to her later.
   _____ 4. Tell her that it is time for group and ask her if she wants to go.

9. After talking with a patient, the nurse wants to chart a quick progress note about the patient's ambivalence about filing for divorce. Which of the following would be an appropriate progress note?
   _____ 1. Patient talked about divorce. Showed anger and confusion. Patient is ambivalent. Patient is told to talk to a lawyer.
   _____ 2. Patient is ambivalent about divorce. Was tearful and sad. Gave patient her prn medication.
   _____ 3. Patient discussed wanting and not wanting a divorce. Was tearful while talking. Patient is ambivalent about possible divorce. Offer support and allow her to express her feelings.
   _____ 4. Patient cannot make decisions. Not ready for discharge. Refer patient to the chaplain.

10. The nurse is ready to discuss the discharge instructions with the patient. Which of the following points should be considered first?
    _____ 1. Assessing how well the patient can read
    _____ 2. Asking if the patient has packed up her belongings
    _____ 3. Making sure the patient has a ride home
    _____ 4. Giving the patient all her new prescriptions

Briefly answer the following questions:

11. A patient has the nursing diagnosis of "high risk for violence, self-directed; related to pending divorce as evidenced by suicidal thoughts." Write a short-term goal for this patient.

12. A patient has the nursing diagnosis of "high risk for violence, self-directed; related to pending divorce as evidenced by suicidal thoughts." Write a long-term goal for this patient.

Case Study: A 20-year-old man in a jogging suit is standing in the corner with his back against the wall. When approached, he says, "I am not going to tell you anything. I didn't tell the police anything either. I don't belong here. It's my wife who should be locked up in this hospital for putting poison in my vodka."

Critical Thinking Question: Given this limited time of observation, how many items of an initial patient's assessment can you list? *(Write your answer on a separate sheet of paper.)*

Anxiety, Coping, and Crisis

Choose the *most* appropriate answer to the following questions:

1. Which of the following criteria influences an individual's definition of an event as a stressor?
   _____ 1. The quantity of anxiety experienced
   _____ 2. The individual's self-concept, skills, and resources
   _____ 3. Whether a stressor is internal or external
   _____ 4. The accuracy of the individual's interpretation of stimuli

2. The characteristics of anxiety have been defined in a variety of ways. Which of the following is not one of the characteristics?
   _____ 1. Part of a process instead of an isolated phenomenon
   _____ 2. A warning sign of perceived danger or threat
   _____ 3. A sense of powerlessness in the face of a less visible threat
   _____ 4. A subjective experience of physical pain

3. Pam is being evaluated in an emergency room for chest pain, elevated blood pressure, and headaches. All the test results are negative. Pam then reports a series of recent stressors. She describes trying to manage her stressors by taking pain pills with alcohol, so she can "just go to sleep and forget it." She admits her strategies are not working. "I wake up, and the problems are still there, and I can't even make it to work on time." The nurse assesses Pam's coping as which of the following?
   _____ 1. Maladaptive
   _____ 2. Palliative
   _____ 3. Dysfunctional
   _____ 4. Adaptive

4. Dan was admitted to the unit a week ago with complaints of fatigue, the inability to get out of bed, and low self-esteem. During a phone call to his wife, Dan begins screaming, "Don't leave me, I need you!" He then throws all of his clothes into his suitcase, starts crying, and says repeatedly, "Home…Jane…she can't…" The assessment and immediate intervention that would be most accurate is which of the following?
   _____ 1. The patient is in crisis. Allow him to cry about what happened. Tell him he cannot leave the unit.
   _____ 2. The patient is angry. Encourage him to discuss his feelings and what he will do during his weekend pass.
   _____ 3. The patient is afraid of divorce. Encourage him to discuss ways to reconcile with his wife while on pass.
   _____ 4. The patient is out of control because of stress. Let him cry for a few minutes, and then teach him assertiveness skills.

5. Anxiety-related responses are crucial for handling dangerous situations. Tolerating fear and pain is made possible by increases in which of the following neurochemical factors?
   _____ 1. Glucocorticoid levels
   _____ 2. Dopaminergic system activity
   _____ 3. Thyroid-stimulating hormone
   _____ 4. Release of endogenous opiates

6. Any coping mechanism can be adaptive or dysfunctional, depending on the situation. The nurse uses which of the following criteria to evaluate the effectiveness of the coping?
   _____ 1. The amount of anxiety remaining
   _____ 2. Increased dopamine release
   _____ 3. The consequences on the patient's relationships
   _____ 4. The patient's resistance to a cold or influenza

7. It is common for the nurse to teach patients new coping techniques. Which of the following would be taught as the most effective technique?
   _____ 1. Relaxation exercises
   _____ 2. Problem-solving strategies
   _____ 3. Protective self-talk
   _____ 4. Appropriate advice-seeking skills

8. A newly admitted patient is very tense and pacing. He is threatening to leave the unit and says, "You can't keep me here. I have special powers to protect the world from aliens." Which of the following interventions would be most helpful?
   _____ 1. Decrease stimuli and pressure. Offer him his prn medication.
   _____ 2. Discuss problem-solving strategies for decreasing anxiety.
   _____ 3. Place the patient in restraints.
   _____ 4. Teach him relaxation strategies.

9. A patient is scheduled for discharge tomorrow. Which of the following statements would indicate that the patient is ready for discharge?
   _____ 1. "I just can't get rid of these thoughts about dying."
   _____ 2. "I have a list of my medicines and have made an appointment with my doctor."
   _____ 3. "I'm glad I'm getting out of here. I shouldn't be here anyway."
   _____ 4. "I know I'm ready to go. I've got everything under control."

10. A patient is admitted in a state of crisis and is at risk for attempting suicide. The most immediate goal for this patient is which of the following?
    _____ 1. Helping her find a better support system
    _____ 2. Teaching her new coping skills
    _____ 3. Insuring her safety and security
    _____ 4. Discussing her short- and long-term goals

Case Study: Jason is a 26-year-old man who was admitted to the hospital after suddenly developing delusions about his wife poisoning his beer every night. He stated that he might need to hurt his wife because she was trying to kill him. He also said that he hears a "voice" telling him that he will fail at everything. His boss told his wife that Jason had become suspicious of a new employee and accused her of being a spy for a competing company.

Critical Thinking Questions: Given this limited data, answer the following questions:

1. What are all the behavioral symptoms that Jason is showing that indicate a +3 anxiety level?

2. Using crisis intervention strategies, what are the most immediate nursing interventions needed for Jason? *(List the interventions.)*

3. What information would you share with Jason's wife about what is happening to him?

Chapter **13**

Name: _____

Working with the Aggressive Patient

Choose the _most_ appropriate answer to the following questions:

1. Which of the following statements about anger is most accurate?
   _____ 1. Open displays of anger should be discouraged.
   _____ 2. Verbalization of anger is detrimental to relationships.
   _____ 3. Anger is a normal response to frustration of desires and needs.
   _____ 4. Suppression of anger helps decrease the potential for violence.

2. Which of the following is the major guide in dealing with overt aggression?
   _____ 1. American Nurses' Association standards for nursing
   _____ 2. Social norms defining assault and battery
   _____ 3. Hospital protocols for seclusion and restraint
   _____ 4. Principle of the least restrictive alternative

3. In a staff in-service program on aggression management, you would emphasize which of the following?
   _____ 1. Verbal aggression is a safe alternative to physical aggression.
   _____ 2. Assertiveness allows for expression of anger while protecting the rights of self and others.
   _____ 3. Passive-aggressive individuals turn their anger inward.
   _____ 4. Passive individuals rarely cause trouble for themselves and others.

4. When a patient has been placed in seclusion and restraints, intensive-nursing care is initiated. This action involves which of the following?
   _____ 1. A nurse continually monitors the patient via a TV monitor.
   _____ 2. A restraint blanket is automatically placed over the patient.
   _____ 3. Range of motions is allowed for one limb at a time every 8 hours.
   _____ 4. The physician must be called within 4 hours for an order for the restraint.

5. When a staff member who was injured by a patient returns to work, supportive interventions are made available. The ultimate goal of these interventions is which of the following?
   _____ 1. Emotional support and debriefing of the event
   _____ 2. Assessment of the staff members needs
   _____ 3. Facilitation of the staff member's return to work
   _____ 4. Emotional resolution and decreased chance of resignation

6. Nursing interventions can prevent an angry patient from becoming violent. When approaching an angry patient, which of the following interventions is most appropriate?
   _____ 1. Assessing the patient's anger-reduction methods before admission
   _____ 2. Determining the patient's reactions to changes in the milieu
   _____ 3. Asking the patient about the cause and target of his or her anger
   _____ 4. Knowing the patient's admitting diagnosis

7. A new patient is brought to the unit in four-way restraints. The nurse would decide that he is ready to have the degree of restraints reduced if the patient states which of the following?
   _____ 1. "Get me out of these. I can't move around enough."
   _____ 2. "Boy, I shouldn't have let myself get out of control."
   _____ 3. "You people can't do this. I know my rights."
   _____ 4. "I'm not going to tell you anything until you release me."

8. A patient's wife and son accompany him to the unit. The son says, "I haven't seen my father act like this with my mom in 20 years. What's happening to him?" Using the developmental view of aggression, which of the following responses would be appropriate?

_____ 1. "Your parents may be getting on each other's nerves lately."
_____ 2. "Society and the media are so full of violence these days."
_____ 3. "As one gets older, there may be a loss of impulse control again."
_____ 4. "Alcohol can have that effect on many people."

9. During the admission interview, the patient admits to making threats toward his ex-wife for the last 2 weeks because she had started dating someone. Which of the following would be the best nursing diagnosis for this patient?

_____ 1. Risk for violence toward ex-wife caused by feelings of abandonment as evidenced by ex-wife starting to date
_____ 2. Aggressiveness related to ex-wife's new boyfriend as evidenced by verbal threats toward ex-wife
_____ 3. Ineffective individual coping related to unresolved anger at ex-wife and her new boyfriend
_____ 4. Risk for other directed violence related to unresolved anger as evidenced by making threats toward ex-wife

10. The physician has just told a patient that she will be discharged this afternoon. While the nurse is discussing her discharge plans, the patient gets restless and tense and says, "I'm not ready. I can't leave now." Which of the following is the most appropriate intervention?

_____ 1. Switch from discharge planning to asking the patient about her concerns.
_____ 2. Tell the patient to go to her room and then talk to her later.
_____ 3. Offer to give the patient her prn injection for anxiety.
_____ 4. Include community resources as part of the patient's discharge instructions.

Case Study: Andrew is a patient admitted to the unit at 3:00 AM after being arrested by the police and treated with an IM antianxiety medication in the emergency department. He is still asleep at 8:00 AM. Given this limited data, answer the following questions:

Critical Thinking Questions:

1. What is the most critical information to try to obtain before Andrew's awakening?

2. After all the information is gathered for question #1, what information would you ask Andrew after he awakens?

3. Later in the day after an upsetting phone call, Andrew is demanding to be released and threatening to "kill everyone who gets in his way." What are the next nursing interventions to be implemented?

4. When it is determined that Andrew is not responding to anger-control strategies and directions given by the nurse, what is the next set of interventions to be used?

Chapter **14**

Name: _____

Working with Groups of Patients

Choose the *most* appropriate answer to the following questions:

1. Which statement is correct regarding the leadership functions of the psychiatric nurse?
   _____ 1. Observed only in formal, planned, and structured group meetings
   _____ 2. Seldom demonstrated in an inpatient unit
   _____ 3. Inherent in the role of a psychotherapeutic manager
   _____ 4. Used only in an outpatient setting

2. Which of the following statements best describes how patients benefit from groups?
   _____ 1. Patients gain support from the group leader only.
   _____ 2. Patients can test out new behaviors when discharged.
   _____ 3. Patient's feelings of powerlessness are not addressed.
   _____ 4. Patients learn how their behaviors affect others.

3. Which of the following groups would be appropriate for patients who are confused and have a short attention span?
   _____ 1. Reality orientation
   _____ 2. Relapse prevention
   _____ 3. Conflict resolution
   _____ 4. Assertiveness training

4. Which of the following groups would most likely be led by a consumer or patient?
   _____ 1. Psychodrama
   _____ 2. Discharge planning
   _____ 3. Alcoholics Anonymous
   _____ 4. Medication

5. Which of the following patients might the nurse include in a group about problem solving?
   _____ 1. An acutely manic patient
   _____ 2. A disoriented patient
   _____ 3. An intoxicated patient
   _____ 4. An anxious patient

6. A patient in a group states, "I don't like people at the group home telling me what to do." Which of the following responses by the nurse would be appropriate?
   _____ 1. "Maybe you don't do what you are supposed to."
   _____ 2. "Next time, tell them to do it themselves."
   _____ 3. "Give us an example of what you mean."
   _____ 4. "I wouldn't like it either."

7. A patient has been monopolizing the group for the last 10 minutes that her physician has treated her unfairly. Which of the following responses by the nurse would be appropriate?
   _____ 1. "You are taking too much of the group's time."
   _____ 2. Say nothing and let the patient continue.
   _____ 3. "I think patients in this group are getting bored with this discussion."
   _____ 4. "You are doing well in contributing to our session today, but I would like to hear what others are thinking."

Briefly answer the following questions:

8. The patient population has a variety of illnesses and problems. Dan has chronic paranoid schizophrenia and is bothered by auditory hallucinations that tell him not to drink milk because it is poisoned. The voices bother him at bedtime, and he has difficulty falling asleep. Barbara is experiencing an episode of recurring major depression and verbalizes derogatory statements about herself. Michael is in a hypomanic state and is thinking about divorcing his wife. Brenda has been abusing alcohol and scratches her arms with paper clips when she is overwhelmed by her emotions. Which groups would the nurse recommend for these patients?

9. The nurse is conducting a psychoeducation group focusing on signs of relapse and relapse prevention. Marla is silent and does not verbally participate in the discussion. Larry periodically walks out of group for a few minutes at a time but always returns and participates appropriately. Joe has a tendency to interrupt others because of his eagerness to participate and desire to be liked. Mona seeks the attention of the group by monopolizing the group session. Hal is verbally aggressive and makes comments that cause others to be silent and uncomfortable. What statements would the nurse make that would be therapeutic for these group members?

Chapter 15

Name: _____

Working with the Family

1. A healthy family has which of the following characteristics?
   _____ 1. The members have the same values and beliefs.
   _____ 2. The members avoid expressing negative feelings.
   _____ 3. The members accept differences among themselves.
   _____ 4. The members keep all information about the family within the family.

2. A young couple with a 2½-year-old child and one on the way are in Duvall's stage of the "Family with Young Children." Which of the following is the primary task of this stage?
   _____ 1. Development of career and marriage is most important at this time.
   _____ 2. Introduction or adjustment of children to systems outside the family takes precedent at this time.
   _____ 3. Giving of selves to the community is important to the family at this time.
   _____ 4. Assumption and development of parental roles is the primary task to be completed at this stage of family development.
   _____ 4. The nurse should indicate to the patient that she must follow family rules.

3. The Burt family had been adjusting to having their college-age daughter, Margo, diagnosed with obsessive-compulsive disorder (OCD). The family acknowledges that Margo was always a "neat freak" but only recently recognized the degree of anxiety and stress she has been experiencing in daily life. The nurse plans to educate the family about OCD. Which of the following plans would be most effective?
   _____ 1. The nurse teaches Margo about her illness and her medications and suggests that she teach her family what she has learned.
   _____ 2. The nurse teaches the family about Margo's illness and medications and suggests that they educate Margo about her disease and the medications used to treat it.
   _____ 3. The nurse directs Margo and her family to other resources to help them learn about the illness and medications to treat it.
   _____ 4. The nurse educates the entire family at the same time about the disease and medications to treat it.

4. An 18-year-old woman, the youngest in her family, is leaving for a college that is a long distance from her home. She will not be able to come home until Christmas. She has been a good student, plans to become a lawyer, and wants to participate in theater while in college. The family is excited but somewhat apprehensive about this transition. Which nursing diagnosis is most appropriate for this family?
   _____ 1. Parental role conflict
   _____ 2. Impaired parenting
   _____ 3. Family coping: readiness for enhanced
   _____ 4. Family processes: interrupted

5. During the assessment phase of a family interaction, the nurse might ask which of the following questions?
   _____ 1. "How do the members of your family express anger?"
   _____ 2. "What would you like to see changed in the family?"
   _____ 3. "How did you feel when you said no to your son?"
   _____ 4. "Can you identify one short-term goal for your family?"

6. What would be an effective nursing intervention when an anxious psychiatric patient is requiring constant attention from family members?

_____ 1. Suggest that the family take care of all of the patient's needs.

_____ 2. Tell the family to refrain from helping the patient.

_____ 3. Medicate the patient whenever he starts getting upset.

_____ 4. Talk with the family about promoting self-care of the patient, but suggest that they help him when he is overwhelmed by anxiety.

7. A nurse is teaching a class about parenting that focuses on productive interaction between parents and their children. Which statement by a group member who is a single parent demonstrates progress in the area of limit setting?

_____ 1. "I told my son he was grounded for 2 weeks because he was on the phone too long last night."

_____ 2. "I discussed my son's phone habits with him last night and told him that he was restricted from the phone this coming weekend because he violated the rules we had established for his phone use on school nights."

_____ 3. "Last night, my son spent all evening on the phone. I yelled at him, but he paid no attention to me. It makes me so mad!"

_____ 4. "I never get to use the phone on week nights because my son is always talking on it. At least he is home and I don't have to worry about where he is."

Case Study: Marla Smith, a 50-year-old divorced factory worker, was brought to the local mental health clinic by her oldest daughter, Trena, who had been visiting her mother for the past week. The interview with Mrs. Smith and Trena revealed that for the past month, Mrs. Smith has been eating only one meal a day and sleeping only 1 to 3 hours per night. When not at work, Marla sits at home crying. She has begun questioning whether she can continue to work. Six weeks ago, her youngest child, Sid, was married and moved out of the house. Marla told the nurse "I thought I was ready for this, that I could handle having him leave, but I'm so sad." Trena comments that she and her mother usually cook and shop when she comes to visit, but this time, her mother has not been able to do any fun activities and just sits around the house. The nurse asks Marla, "How are you feeling?" "Lonely," replies Marla. The psychiatrist prescribes an antidepressant to treat Marla's depression. The nurse works with Marla on psychosocial treatment of Marla's illness.

Critical Thinking Questions:

1. What developmental stresses are facing Marla at this time?

2. Are there any aspects of Marla's situation that lead to her problem?

3. What nursing diagnoses apply to Marla?

4. What are realistic short-term goals (within a week) that Marla can achieve regarding this problem or illness?

5. What are long-term goals (within a month) that Marla can achieve regarding this problem or illness?

6. What interventions would be effective to help Marla achieve the short-term goal?

Chapter **16** Name: _____

Cultural Competence in Psychiatric Nursing

Choose the *most* appropriate answer to the following questions:

1. Culture is best defined as:
   _____ 1. An ethnic group
   _____ 2. A patterned behavioral response that develops over time
   _____ 3. Values, beliefs, and norms
   _____ 4. Biologic variations and psychologic characteristics

2. A nurse providing care to a minority or ethnic population should:
   _____ 1. Explore the beliefs and values of individuals within the population
   _____ 2. Correct the inferior practices of the population
   _____ 3. Implement scientifically proven interventions
   _____ 4. Be trained in self-defense techniques

3. The analytic worldview:
   _____ 1. Values community needs and concerns above individual ones
   _____ 2. Values detail to time, individuality, and possessions
   _____ 3. Values the significance of relationships
   _____ 4. Values the interconnectedness between an individual and the environment

4. When a nurse provides health education to a young African-American patient with a large support network, the nurse should be sure to include the patient's:
   _____ 1. Mother   _____ 3. Grandparents
   _____ 2. Father   _____ 4. Social worker

5. Many Hispanic people seek health care from:
   _____ 1. Church-related agencies   _____ 3. Government agencies
   _____ 2. Emergency facilities   _____ 4. Shamans

6. When providing health care for a Native-American reservation, it would be important for the nurse to be aware of the high incidence of:
   _____ 1. Drug use   _____ 3. Lack of values
   _____ 2. Malnutrition   _____ 4. Alcoholism

7. When teaching patients who use English as a second language, it is most important to:
   _____ 1. Use a loud tone of voice.
   _____ 2. Talk as you would to any patient.
   _____ 3. Speak slowly and use simple words.
   _____ 4. Ask the patient to repeat the instructions.

8. The best option in providing care for ethnic populations in which time and routine is less structured is to:
   _____ 1. Be flexible.
   _____ 2. Be informed of practices and plan accordingly.
   _____ 3. Establish an open-door policy and eliminate appointments.
   _____ 4. Make the population conform to meet the standards of the agency.

9. Socioeconomic factors such as poverty, poor nutrition, and inadequate housing:
   _____ 1. Do not significantly affect mental disorder
   _____ 2. Affect only stress-related disorders
   _____ 3. Are outcomes of mental illness, not contributing factors
   _____ 4. Contribute significantly to an individual's mental health

10. The most common barrier to delivery of culturally competent care involves:
    _____ 1. Provider bias   _____ 3. Miscommunication
    _____ 2. Differences in the patient's and _____ 4. Failure to assess the patient's
             the nurse's worldviews   cultural perspective

11. A person who believes that an illness is caused by a supernatural being is said to have which of the following views of illness causation?
    _____ 1. Natural causation   _____ 3. Scientific causation
    _____ 2. Unnatural causation   _____ 4. Spiritual causation

12. Which of the following ethnic or racial culture might speak of depression as "having heart pain?"
    _____ 1. European American   _____ 3. Hispanic
    _____ 2. Native American   _____ 4. African American

13. A significant number of Asians and Native Americans have a relative deficiency of:
    _____ 1. Alcohol dehydrogenase   _____ 3. Aldehyde dehydrogenase
    _____ 2. Acetaldehyde   _____ 4. Aldehyde

Case Study: Mary is a 36-year-old African-American woman diagnosed with paranoid-type schizophrenia. Mary is a native of New Orleans but has lived in Chicago for the last 6 months. She is married and has two children, ages 10 and 12. Mary has a master's degree in education and is presently employed as a kindergarten teacher in the public school system. Mary has been admitted to the psychiatric unit with the following symptoms:

1. *Delusions:* Mary believes a hex has been put on her, causing her to be unable to organize her thoughts. Mary states she has been unable to locate a voodoo priestess to lift the hex.
2. *Hallucinations:* Mary states that she sees demons and snakes around her.
3. *Other symptoms:* Continuous lip-smacking, grinding of teeth, facial grimaces, and tongue thrusting. Mary believes these symptoms are part of the hex.

Mary has a distinct Southern dialect. When the staff members are unable to interpret what she is saying, she becomes agitated. She has two brothers, four sisters, four aunts, seven uncles, and numerous cousins, all of whom live in the Chicago area and visit her. On occasion, as many as 10 visitors arrive attempting to see her. Mary states that her family has been invaluable to her in her fight to get rid of the hex. Many of her family members have prepared potions, offered prayers, and consulted people who are knowledgeable about the removal of spells. Despite all of these efforts, Mary says that she has not had a moment of relief from the hex in the last 8 to 9 months.

Mary weighs 112 pounds and is 5 feet 2 inches tall. For 6 years, she has been treated with haloperidol (Haldol) 4 md tid.★

Critical Thinking Questions: *(Write your answer on a separate sheet of paper, if necessary.)*

1. As the nurse taking care of Mary, how should you manage the number of visitors wanting to see her?

2. How would you assess Mary's belief in voodoo and hexes?

3. How would you deal with Mary and her family member's beliefs about the necessary treatment of her symptoms?

★From Pool VL, Davidhizar RE, Ginger JN: Cultural aspects of psychiatric nursing. In Keltner NL, Bostrom CE, *Psychiatric nursing,* ed 2, St Louis, 1995, Mosby.

Spirituality

Choose the *most* appropriate answer to the following questions:

1. What is the largest religious group in the United States, with which about four out of every five people identify themselves?
   - _____ 1. Baha'i
   - _____ 2. Christianity
   - _____ 3. Neo-pagan
   - _____ 4. Zoroastrianism

2. What of the following is one of the two general understandings of the term spirituality used in this chapter?
   - _____ 1. Bombastic
   - _____ 2. Futuristic
   - _____ 3. Humanistic
   - _____ 4. Nihilistic

3. A theistic understanding of the term spirituality must include some concept of:
   - _____ 1. Democracy
   - _____ 2. Determinism
   - _____ 3. Hallucinations
   - _____ 4. Higher Power

4. Xavier contrasts "healthy spirituality" with:
   - _____ 1. Being heart healthy
   - _____ 2. Freedom to choose
   - _____ 3. Healthy ego boundaries
   - _____ 4. Sick religiosity

5. Frankl's notion of making meaning through freedom to choose implies that human beings find meaning when they:
   - _____ 1. Commit themselves to something outside themselves
   - _____ 2. Search for their identity
   - _____ 3. Seek revenge
   - _____ 4. Turn on, tune in, and drop out

6. In Loder's notion of a "presence" that orders the world, presence can also be translated as:
   - _____ 1. Absence
   - _____ 2. Face
   - _____ 3. Freedom
   - _____ 4. Tyranny

7. In Groessoehme's study, what percentage of adolescent psychiatric inpatients reported that they had never been asked about their religious or spiritual beliefs by any mental health professional (other than the chaplain)?
   - _____ 1. 5%
   - _____ 2. 25%
   - _____ 3. 60%
   - _____ 4. 95%

8. VandeCreek says that most nurses have little or no time to conduct meaningful spiritual assessments or provide spiritual care because they are:
   _____ 1. Not spiritually minded
   _____ 2. Prohibited from doing so because of separation of church and state
   _____ 3. Too busy because of other nursing responsibilities
   _____ 4. Unaware of a holistic approach to patient care

9. Because religious language is symbolic by nature, psychotic patients need to receive spiritual care in which the language is:
   _____ 1. Ascetic
   _____ 2. Concrete
   _____ 3. Existential
   _____ 4. Symbolic

10. The most spiritually sensitive thing to say to someone who has experienced a loss of any kind is:
   _____ 1. A heart-felt "I'm so sorry."
   _____ 2. "Don't feel that way."
   _____ 3. "God won't put on you any more than you can bear."
   _____ 4. "I know how you feel."

Case Study: Wanda is a 68-year-old African-American woman whose angina led to cardiac bypass surgery. Her parents both died of heart attacks and her husband died of a stroke 21 years ago. Wanda has a history of hypertension and depression, both of which have been medically managed well over the last 20 years. She was compliant with attending an outpatient cardiac rehabilitation program daily. Her family told the rehabilitation team that they thought her depression had grown worse and feared she wanted to commit suicide. Members of the team cite as evidence that she has started giving away items of sentimental value to friends and family members, has written down who should get what things when she dies, and has consulted an attorney about a will. Her family also wonders if she is "crazy" because she talks a lot about "going home," even though she goes back home every afternoon. The next day, Wanda asked her rehab nurse about how to make a living will. The nurse took a few moments to ask about this desire, assessing for symptoms of depression. The nurse detected no other signs of depression or delusional thinking. Wanda said with a smile, "Life is so short. And I'm ready to go home. Are you?"

Critical Thinking Questions:

1. Do you see Wanda exhibiting any signs of depression or delusional thinking?

2. Is it unreasonable that Wanda would want to prepare for death?

3. What do you make of Wanda's talk of "going home?"

4. Why would Wanda's case make for a good presentation at team meeting?

Chapter 18

Name: _____

Introduction to Psychotropic Drugs

Choose the *most* appropriate answer to the following questions:

1. Psychotropic drugs were partially responsible for the development of which of the following concepts?
   _____ 1. Least restrictive alternative or environment
   _____ 2. Psychotherapeutic management
   _____ 3. Psychotherapy
   _____ 4. Behavior therapy

2. Which of the following has been proclaimed as the first legitimately new antipsychotic drug since Thorazine?
   _____ 1. Prozac
   _____ 2. Clozapine
   _____ 3. Zoloft
   _____ 4. Mellaril

3. A substance that changes the resting potential of a postsynaptic membrane is a(n):
   _____ 1. Psychoactive agent
   _____ 2. Cerebrospinal antagonist
   _____ 3. Amino acid
   _____ 4. Neurotransmitter

4. Neurotransmitters:
   _____ 1. Are synthesized from natural precursors
   _____ 2. Are stored primarily in the cell body
   _____ 3. Combine with many different receptors
   _____ 4. Cannot be mimicked by drugs

5. The brain is protected from fluctuations in the body by the:
   _____ 1. Spinal chord
   _____ 2. CNS
   _____ 3. Blood-brain barrier
   _____ 4. Meninges

6. The most important chemical property influencing a drug's ability to pass easily through the blood-brain barrier is:
   _____ 1. Water solubility
   _____ 2. Lipid solubility
   _____ 3. Protein-binding capability
   _____ 4. Bioavailability

7. Which of the following drugs can most easily pass the blood-brain barrier?
   _____ 1. Penicillin
   _____ 2. Potassium
   _____ 3. Dopamine
   _____ 4. Levodopa

8. A protein–bound drug is found:
   _____ 1. In the blood stream
   _____ 2. In tissue fluid (ECF)
   _____ 3. In the brain
   _____ 4. In the urine

Match the term with its definition:

_____ 9. Synapse   a. Part of the neuron that transmits impulses toward the cell body
_____ 10. Axon   b. Storage sac at the synaptic terminal
_____ 11. Vesicle   c. Part of the neuron that transmits impulses away from the cell
_____ 12. Dendrite   body
_____ 13. Precursor   d. Microscopic space between two neurons
                         e. Something that precedes

Briefly answer the following questions:

14. What is the most prescribed class of antidepressants?

15. Name the first traditional and the first atypical antipsychotic drug.

16. State the mechanism of action of MAOI antidepressants.

17. What are the three dimensions of the blood-brain barrier?

18. Wayne, a 32-year-old chain smoker, states, "I can't quit. Smoking is so addictive." Explain why smoking is so addictive.

Antiparkinson Drugs

Choose the *most* appropriate answer to the following questions:

1. Parkinsonian symptoms can be caused by:
    _____ 1. An imbalance between dopamine and serotonin
    _____ 2. Age-related degeneration of the extrapyramidal system
    _____ 3. Dopamine-enhancing drugs such as antipsychotics
    _____ 4. Disruption of the thalamic-hypothalamic pathway

2. A decreased availability of dopamine in the brain is responsible for:
    _____ 1. Parkinsonism
    _____ 2. Schizophrenia
    _____ 3. Tardive dyskinesia
    _____ 4. Anxiety

3. The pharmacologic goal in treating parkinsonism is to:
    _____ 1. Increase acetylcholine to balance GABA
    _____ 2. Increase dopamine to balance acetylcholine
    _____ 3. Decrease acetylcholine to balance GABA
    _____ 4. Decrease dopamine to balance acetylcholine

4. EPSEs are related to Parkinson's disease because:
    _____ 1. Both are related to decreased availability of dopamine.
    _____ 2. Both are related to increased availability of dopamine.
    _____ 3. They are not related.
    _____ 4. Both are caused by degenerative processes.

5. A patient in oculogyric crisis (a severe dystonic reaction) needs immediate intervention. Which of the following drugs is appropriate?
    _____ 1. Artane   _____ 3. Kemadrin
    _____ 2. Cogentin   _____ 4. Parsidol

6. A patient taking benztropine (Cogentin) complains of blurred vision. Which cranial nerve is being affected by benztropine?
    _____ 1. CN II   _____ 3. CN VII
    _____ 2. CN IV   _____ 4. CN III

7. A patient is receiving Haldol 5 mg bid. Knowing that Haldol is a high-potency antipsychotic drug, the nurse is most likely to observe significant:
    _____ 1. Anticholinergic effects   _____ 3. EPSEs
    _____ 2. Sedative effects   _____ 4. Orthostatic hypotension

8. A patient is taking an anticholinergic to decrease EPSEs associated with Haldol. The nurse should instruct the patient to:
    _____ 1. Avoid hot baths and showers.
    _____ 2. Limit fluid intake to approximately 1000 ml/day.
    _____ 3. Have monthly WBCs drawn.
    _____ 4. Stop taking the anticholinergic if the pulse rate falls below 60 bpm.

9. Tardive dyskinesia is probably related to:
   _____ 1. Dopamine receptor blockade in the basal ganglia
   _____ 2. Serotonin receptor blockade in the basal ganglia
   _____ 3. Hypersensitivity of dopamine receptors in the basal ganglia
   _____ 4. Increased levels of acetylcholine

10. A patient with schizophrenia is given one of the antipsychotic drugs. The nurse is aware that, of all the EPSEs, the one that can be most life threatening would be:
    _____ 1. Akathisia
    _____ 2. Tardive dyskinesia
    _____ 3. Acute dystonic reactions
    _____ 4. Drug-induced parkinsonism

Case Study: A 25-year-old woman who is taking an antipsychotic drug (haloperidol) starts to experience psychomotor slowing as she walks down the hospital hallway. Before she reaches the end of the hall, she requires assistance. Within 2 minutes of sitting down, her neck becomes rigidly hyperextended, and the eyes roll upward in a fixed stare. Her breathing becomes labored because of her neck, and she is frightened. Because she is also delusional, it is difficult to imagine what this frightening medication side effect means to her. Benztropine (Cogentin), 2 mg, is given intramuscularly and repeated in 15 minutes because she did not respond as quickly as was hoped. Within another 5 minutes, she was back to her "normal" self.

Critical Thinking Questions:
1. What type of EPSE is she experiencing?

2. Why would it be inappropriate to use trihexyphenidyl?

3. What effect might levodopa produce in a person with schizophrenia?

Critical Thinking Questions: Parkinson's disease is caused by dopamine deficiency. However, because dopamine does not pass the blood-brain barrier easily, its immediate precursor, L-dopa, is given. L-dopa does not cross the blood-brain barrier well either because it is broken down quite readily by an enzyme, dopa decarboxylase.
1. What is a pharmacologic solution to this problem?

2. How are the associated or secondary symptoms linked to the primary symptoms?

Antipsychotic Drugs

Choose the *most* appropriate answer to the following questions:

1. The first antipsychotic introduced in the United States was:

_____ 1. Chlorpromazine _____ 3. Haloperidol
_____ 2. Lithium _____ 4. Clozapine

2. Antipsychotic drugs were first "discovered" in about:

_____ 1. 1945 _____ 3. 1959
_____ 2. 1950 _____ 4. 1963

3. High-potency drugs are more likely to have severe _____ side effects than are low-potency antipsychotics.

_____ 1. Sedative _____ 3. Anticholinergic
_____ 2. Extrapyramidal _____ 4. Orthostatic hypotension

4. Which of the following side effects should the nurse anticipate being particularly bothersome to a 65-year-old man with benign prostatic hypertrophy?

_____ 1. Sedative _____ 3. Anticholinergic
_____ 2. EPSEs _____ 4. Orthostatic hypotension

5. A patient has been taking antipsychotic drugs for years. You notice that he begins to grind his teeth and moves and smacks his lips frequently. Your assessment would include:

_____ 1. Oculogyric crisis _____ 3. Tardive dyskinesia
_____ 2. Gustatory hallucinations _____ 4. Neuroleptic malignant syndrome

6. Which of the following side effects of antipsychotic drugs is most lethal?

_____ 1. Oculogyric crisis _____ 3. Tardive dyskinesia
_____ 2. Gustatory hallucinations _____ 4. Neuroleptic malignant syndrome

7. When drugs are provided without the benefit of a well-managed milieu or a strong nurse-patient relationship, patients will:

_____ 1. Decompensate _____ 3. Be free to grow in their own ways
_____ 2. Be receiving custodial care _____ 4. Be allowed to be creative

8. Which of the following does olanzapine induce more than does risperidone?

_____ 1. Weight gain _____ 3. Akathisia
_____ 2. Prolactin elevation _____ 4. EPSEs

9. Which of the following atypical agents needs several days of titrated doses to reach the therapeutic dose?

_____ 1. Olanzapine _____ 3. Clozapine
_____ 2. Quetiapine _____ 4. Risperidone

Briefly answer the following questions:

10. What is the role of serotonin antagonists in treating negative schizophrenia?

11. Which dopamine receptor subtype is primarily affected by traditional antipsychotics?

Case Study 1: Bill is a 41-year-old man with a long history of schizophrenia. Bill has been divorced for 15 years, has not seen his children for 6 years, and lives in a cheap downtown hotel. He was admitted to your unit 3 days ago after he caused a problem in a 24-hour food mart. He entered the store about 5:00 AM and began shouting, waving his fists in the air, and talking loudly to himself. The police were called, and Bill was admitted to the psychiatric evaluation unit. Several of the questions below are based on this clinical example.

Critical Thinking Questions:

1. Your first nursing intervention should be to:
   _____ 1. Ignore the patient; to attend to this behavior will only reinforce it.
   _____ 2. Call the physician. This case may be a life-threatening side effect of haloperidol.
   _____ 3. Give a prn anticholinergic drug to counteract the effects of haloperidol.
   _____ 4. Give a prn antipsychotic drug to treat this bizarre behavior.

2. Bill was discharged about a month ago. Unfortunately, there were no realistic options for him but to return to his downtown hotel. He does have appointments to see a community mental health nurse on a weekly basis. He complains of hearing voices and admits during one of his appointments that he is not taking his medication. Which of the following medication strategies would best suit a patient in Bill's situation?
   _____ 1. Chlorpromazine once per day at the clinic
   _____ 2. Haloperidol decanoate once every 2 weeks
   _____ 3. Fluphenazine 5 mg tid given to the hotel manager to administer
   _____ 4. Electroconvulsive therapy

Case Study 2: Tyrus, age 29, was first admitted to a state hospital in 1995 and released within 2 months. The admitting psychiatrist diagnosed schizophrenia, alcohol dependence, and dependent-avoidant personality disorder. He reported hearing threatening voices. Within the last year, Tyrus moved to a group home and became depressed to the point that he would not get out of bed. Six months earlier, Tyrus tried to kill himself by drinking a caustic home-cleaning product. A few days later, he poured bleach in his eyes and was readmitted to the state hospital. He is now in a day treatment program for individuals with chronic mental illness. He has several obsessive social fears that, at this point, prevent him from working or even participating in public or social life.

Critical Thinking Questions:

1. What medications would be appropriate for an individual who suffers from the symptoms expressed by Tyrus?

2. How would you link neurotransmitter theories of schizophrenia to the symptoms present in this man?

Name: _____

Antidepressant Drugs

Choose the *most* appropriate answer to the following questions:

1. During the first day of treatment with a TCA, you expect:
   - _____ 1. An improvement in appetite
   - _____ 2. An improvement in mood
   - _____ 3. Anticholinergic side effects
   - _____ 4. Signs of toxicity

Situation: John, a 69-year-old retired truck driver, has been very despondent for some time. After careful assessment, it is determined that John is depressed. The next two questions are based on this situation.

2. Which of the following TCA side effects would be a special concern for John?
   - _____ 1. Mania
   - _____ 2. Sialorrhea
   - _____ 3. Dry mouth
   - _____ 4. Urinary retention

3. Other side effects that might concern John's nurse are:
   - _____ 1. Polyuria
   - _____ 2. A history of herpes
   - _____ 3. Constipation
   - _____ 4. Cataracts

4. Which one of the following statements is true of TCAs?
   - _____ 1. They can be typically given intramuscularly.
   - _____ 2. They have a wide therapeutic index.
   - _____ 3. Beneficial, therapeutic effects occur within hours.
   - _____ 4. Many side effects disappear after 6 weeks.

5. Which TCA is the most sedating (see Table 21-2)?★
   - _____ 1. Amitriptyline
   - _____ 2. Protriptyline
   - _____ 3. Nortriptyline
   - _____ 4. Bupropion

6. Which antidepressant class has the most anticholinergic side effects?★
   - _____ 1. TCAs
   - _____ 2. MAOIs
   - _____ 3. SSRIs
   - _____ 4. Novel antidepressants

7. Which antidepressant enhances the effects of norepinephrine most effectively?★
   - _____ 1. Amitriptyline
   - _____ 2. Desipramine
   - _____ 3. Fluoxetine
   - _____ 4. Paroxetine

8. A depressed patient treated with TCAs should experience a clinical improvement within:
   - _____ 1. 24 hours
   - _____ 2. 1 week
   - _____ 3. 2 to 4 weeks
   - _____ 4. 6 to 8 weeks

9. Bill is placed on an MAOI after TCAs proved to be ineffective. Which of the following should be all right for Bill to take?
   - _____ 1. Aged cheese, figs, certain wines
   - _____ 2. Indirect-acting stimulants
   - _____ 3. Mixed-acting stimulants
   - _____ 4. Direct-acting stimulants

Student: These questions are meant to help you use the text.

10. According to the chapter discussion, TCAs achieve their effect by:
    _____ 1. Blocking the reuptake of serotonin and norepinephrine at presynaptic neurons
    _____ 2. Blocking neurotransmitter metabolism
    _____ 3. Inhibiting monoamine oxidase
    _____ 4. Decreasing acetylcholine levels

11. According to the text, MAOIs achieve their effect by:
    _____ 1. Blocking the reuptake of serotonin and norepinephrine at the presynaptic neuron
    _____ 2. Blocking neurotransmitter metabolism
    _____ 3. Increasing dopamine bioavailability
    _____ 4. Decreasing acetylcholine level

12. The original catecholamine hypothesis of depression considered:
    _____ 1. Dopamine only
    _____ 2. Norepinephrine only
    _____ 3. Serotonin only
    _____ 4. Norepinephrine and serotonin

13. Which of the following antidepressants specifically increases levels of norepinephrine?
    _____ 1. Fluoxetine
    _____ 2. Mirtazapine
    _____ 3. Reboxetine
    _____ 4. Sertraline

14. According to the monoamine hypothesis of depression, depressive symptoms may be expected to be alleviated by:
    _____ 1. Depletion of central norepinephrine
    _____ 2. Depletion of central serotonin
    _____ 3. Inhibition of norepinephrine reuptake
    _____ 4. Inhibition of acetylcholine reuptake

Case Study: Joe, 30 years of age, states he had a normal childhood, had friends, and enjoyed school. However, at an early age, Joe reports being raped by his 20-year-old male cousin and friend. After the rape, Joe did not tell anyone out of both shame and fear. He tried to go on as if "nothing had happened." His life started spiraling downhill shortly thereafter. He started failing school in which he once excelled. By the time he reached junior high, Joe became reclusive, avoided contact with his friends, and was generally fearful and anxious. By his early twenties, he began using an excessive amount of alcohol to fight his fears and social anxieties. Over the years, Joe has received treatment for depression. Recently, he has experienced auditory hallucinations, and he has attempted suicide on three different occasions. Joe is now hospitalized for a recent suicide attempt, which he refers to as an attention-getting gesture. Joe admits to feeling both hopeless and angry with his position in life.

Critical Thinking Questions:
1. If you were prescribing, what psychotropic medication would you give Joe?

2. Do you think a one-time event such as a traumatic rape may cause life long problems as is suggested in this case study? Explain your rationale.

Antimanic Drugs

Choose the *most* appropriate answer to the following questions:

1. Which of the following statements about lithium is *true*?
   _____ 1. Lithium is a naturally occurring element.
   _____ 2. Lithium has always been used as a mood stabilizer.
   _____ 3. Lithium levels are typically drawn once per week.
   _____ 4. A gross hand tremor is an early side effect.

2. The serum parameters for a therapeutic response to lithium are:
   _____ 1. 0.2 to 0.6 mEq/L
   _____ 2. 0.6 to 1.2 mEq/L
   _____ 3. 1.0 to 1.6 mEq/L
   _____ 4. 2 to 3 mEq/L

3. An adverse effect of lithium therapy that is caused by inhibition of antidiuretic hormone is:
   _____ 1. Ataxic toxicity
   _____ 2. Uremic syndrome
   _____ 3. Diabetes insipidus
   _____ 4. Interstitial nephritis

4. A patient is receiving lithium for the treatment of bipolar disorder. When planning for patient teaching about this medication, the nurse knows it is important to include the following information:
   _____ 1. It will be necessary to adhere to a low-sodium diet while taking lithium.
   _____ 2. It will be necessary to take a diuretic with lithium.
   _____ 3. Lithium will need to be taken for the rest of the patient's life.
   _____ 4. Lithium blood levels must be checked periodically even after the patient is stabilized on the drug.

5. The nurse should continually assess the patient for early signs of lithium toxicity, which would include:
   _____ 1. Tinnitus
   _____ 2. Severe tremor
   _____ 3. Akathisia
   _____ 4. Torticollis

6. Losing one's hair can be traumatic. Which antimanic drug is known to cause transient hair loss?
   _____ 1. Carbamazepine
   _____ 2. Lithium
   _____ 3. Olanzapine
   _____ 4. Valproate

Case Study: Billie is a 45-year-old woman living in a residential facility. She attends day treatment 5 days a week. She has a lengthy history of hospitalizations, discharges to outpatient programs, and rehospitalizations. She was in an automobile accident in 1995 that left her with some cognitive impairment and seizure disorder. Her diagnosis is bipolar disorder exhibited by agitation, insomnia, irritability, and grandiosity. She has been placed on a regimen that includes lithium and divalproex sodium (Depakote).

Student: "Billie, is it all right if I talk to you?"
Billie: "Yeah, I know I can trust you. They are coming to get me tonight."
Student: "Who is coming to get you?"
Billie: "The reverend and his son. Why don't you ask me some Godly questions?"

Critical Thinking Questions:
1. How would you assess this patient's mental status to this point?

2. The conversation is picked up a minute or two later:
   Student: "How do you like it where you live?"
   Billie: "I'm isolated, everybody is isolated. They hate me because I am going to heaven."
   What does this response do to your first opinion?

3. A week earlier Billie experienced diarrhea, vomiting, weakness, and a lack of coordination and had a gross tremor. As a nurse, what should be one of your first concerns?

4. Billie is now stabilized but wants to lose weight. What are major considerations for her?

Antianxiety Drugs

Choose the *most* appropriate answer to the following questions:

1. Benzodiazepines are abused because:
   - _____ 1. They increase inhibitions.
   - _____ 2. They blur reality.
   - _____ 3. They can be mixed safely with other drugs, such as alcohol.
   - _____ 4. They improve cognitive processes (i.e., they "enhance clear thinking").

2. Benzodiazepines are thought to work by:
   - _____ 1. Exciting the CNS
   - _____ 2. Stimulating the reticular activating system
   - _____ 3. Increasing inhibitory feelings
   - _____ 4. Enhancing the effects of GABA

3. Benzodiazepines given alone can usually cause all but one of the following:
   - _____ 1. Dependence
   - _____ 2. Withdrawal
   - _____ 3. Death from overdose
   - _____ 4. Abuse problems

4. Valium interacts with alcohol to cause:
   - _____ 1. CNS depression
   - _____ 2. CNS excitement
   - _____ 3. An increase in tolerance to alcohol
   - _____ 4. A depletion of neuronal stores

5. Which of the following benzodiazepines is most often prescribed for older patients?
   - _____ 1. Diazepam (Valium)
   - _____ 2. Lorazepam (Ativan)
   - _____ 3. Chlordiazepoxide (Librium)
   - _____ 4. Alprazolam (Xanax)

6. Which of the following antianxiety drugs shows no cross-tolerance with CNS depressants and no withdrawal symptoms?
   - _____ 1. Diazepam
   - _____ 2. Buspirone
   - _____ 3. Oxazepam
   - _____ 4. Alprazolam

7. The major concern when administering flumazenil (Romazicon) is:
   - _____ 1. It speeds the metabolism of benzodiazepines.
   - _____ 2. It has a short duration of action.
   - _____ 3. Patients may not leave the benzodiazepine-induced state.
   - _____ 4. It causes dependence as well.

8. The drug of choice for obsessive-compulsive disorder is:
_____ 1. Imipramine
_____ 2. Clomipramine
_____ 3. Diazepam
_____ 4. Propranolol

Indicate *T* for true and *F* for false:

_____ 9. Benzodiazepines have been shown to cause fetal abnormalities in pregnant women who take these drugs.

Case Study: John is a 32-year-old man with a history of panic disorder with agoraphobia. He reports being a happy-go-lucky boy until the age of 12 when he experienced very traumatic physical abuse by a stepfather. His stepfather beat him and ridiculed John for not fighting back. John reports becoming more and more reclusive and anxious, and a successful school year deteriorated into failing grades. John states that he got to the point that he hated going to school, but once at school he dreaded going home. He felt confined at school, particularly when he could not select his own seat at the rear of the class. Over and over, he experienced what he can now describe as panic attacks at school. Class tests would push him to a point of a near "nervous breakdown." Nonetheless, he persevered for a while. John was anxious at school and fearful at home. He had a miserable life and he spiraled downward until he gave up on school in the tenth grade. Although John believes that he had the talent to be a "white collar" professional, his work life has been a series of day laborer jobs. John has been prescribed alprazolam (Xanax) 1 mg bid and sertraline (Zoloft) 200 mg per day.

Critical Thinking Questions:

1. What should be a major concern when caring for John?

2. John still complains of anxiety. He says, "These drugs helped at first, but I started getting the shakes again." What would be an obvious place to start when assessing the situation?

3. John receives an increase in his benzodiazepine, but within a few days, he develops dizziness, lethargy, and has a hangover the next morning. He also does not seem as mentally sharp as he has in the recent past. What is going on?

4. Do people like John get appreciably better?

24 Name: _____

Introduction to Milieu Management

Choose the *most* appropriate answer to the following questions:

1. For psychiatric patients, 24-hour care is traditionally provided by:
    _____ 1. Nurses
    _____ 2. Psychiatrists
    _____ 3. Psychologists
    _____ 4. Social workers

2. When only psychotropic drugs are used to treat patients, this approach is considered to be:
    _____ 1. Custodial care
    _____ 2. Milieu management
    _____ 3. Psychotherapeutic management
    _____ 4. Routine nursing care

3. The first professional to conceptualize the need for all aspects of the patient's environment to be therapeutic was:
    _____ 1. Sigmund Freud
    _____ 2. Maxwell Jones
    _____ 3. Emil Kraepelin
    _____ 4. Hildegard Peplau

4. The primary purpose of limit setting is to communicate to patients that:
    _____ 1. Behavior must conform to established norms.
    _____ 2. Inappropriate behavior will be punished.
    _____ 3. Their behavior is wrong.
    _____ 4. The nurse is in charge.

5. Therapeutic community refers to:
    _____ 1. A patient-led government that enforces community rules
    _____ 2. The area surrounding the mental health center
    _____ 3. The meetings of all members of the psychiatric care team
    _____ 4. The physical structure of the unit

6. The most important element of the milieu that overrides all others is:
    _____ 1. Norms
    _____ 2. Balance
    _____ 3. Safety
    _____ 4. Environmental modification

Indicate *T* for true and *F* for false:

_____   7. Milieu management is the purposeful use of all interpersonal and environmental forces to enhance mental health.

_____   8. Consistency is very important in a therapeutic milieu.

_____   9. Psychiatric environments are characterized by their recognition of the need for flexibility.

_____   10. Home health agencies cannot employ milieu principles.

_____   11. Florence Nightingale was the first to recognize nursing's responsibility for creating and controlling the milieu.

Briefly answer the following questions:

12. What are the three essential features of the therapeutic environment?

13. A common criticism of mental health care is that patients who are hospitalized on an inpatient unit in a therapeutic milieu are discharged to the "real world," which does not have the same consistency and structure. Identify at least three ways to help decrease patient problems at discharge.

25

Name: _____

Variables Affecting the Therapeutic Environment

Choose the *most* appropriate answer to the following questions:

1. What effect does burnout have on the therapeutic environment?
    _____ 1. Interferes with development of a therapeutic relationship with the patient
    _____ 2. Causes more rigidity in rules
    _____ 3. Results in premature discharge of patients
    _____ 4. Increases withdrawn behavior among patients

2. In Sayre's study on nurses' use of humor, which of the following is considered detrimental to staff morale and patient care?
    _____ 1. Whimsical humor
    _____ 2. Conflict
    _____ 3. Sarcastic humor
    _____ 4. Rules

3. Which of the following is *true* regarding the influence of management on the nursing staff?
    _____ 1. Rules and efficiency should not be required of professional nurses.
    _____ 2. Management practices can support or hinder nursing practice.
    _____ 3. Nurses must have positive reinforcement from management to provide good care.
    _____ 4. Burnout is caused solely by bad management.

4. JCAHO requires which of the following in the patient's social environment?
    _____ 1. Locked doors
    _____ 2. Telephones in each room
    _____ 3. Closet and drawer space for personal property
    _____ 4. Smoking room

5. Which of the following has been associated with a higher occurrence of assaults on staff?
    _____ 1. Self-reflective style
    _____ 2. Authoritarian attitudes
    _____ 3. Smaller physical size
    _____ 4. Being around patients in the day room

6. Patients with schizophrenia do better in environments with:
    _____ 1. Rigid structure
    _____ 2. Low stimulation
    _____ 3. Support and organization
    _____ 4. High interaction and social contact

7. Clinical supervision facilitates the maintenance of a therapeutic environment by:
    _____ 1. Providing a forum for nurses to examine attitudes, reactions, and conflicts
    _____ 2. Forcing nurses to be open
    _____ 3. Providing time away from patient care
    _____ 4. Allowing nurses to talk about personal problems

Indicate *T* for true and *F* for false:

_____ 8. Management practices have an effect on the therapeutic environment.

Match the term with its description:

_____ 9. JCAHO
_____ 10. Maxwell Jones
_____ 11. Norms
_____ 12. Structure
_____ 13. Balance

a. Evaluating whether to follow a suicidal patient into the bathroom or wait outside the door
b. "Father" of milieu therapy
c. Developed specific criteria for therapeutic environment
d. Needed so as to use all the resources in the environment
e. Clearly articulating acceptable and unacceptable behavior

Define or give function for the following. Give an example.

14. Feedback:

15. Social skills groups:

16. Individual responsibility:

17. Street skills group:

18. Psychoeducational programs:

19. Limit setting:

20. Safety:

Case Study: Julie is a staff registered nurse (RN) on the addiction recovery unit of a large university hospital in which most of the staff members are licensed professional counselors or social workers. Julie's supervisor is an RN; however, a social worker is in the position of unit manager and is functionally also Julie's supervisor. Julie is responsible for monitoring and assessing patients on drug "detox" protocols, obtaining laboratory specimens when ordered, assessing and monitoring any physical complaints patients may experience, and administering prescribed medications. Most of the time, Julie finds herself performing secretarial duties such as answering the phone, taking physician orders, and filing reports completed by the counselors. Julie's input is welcomed at treatment team meetings, but she rarely has time to attend because no one else is available at the nursing station. Julie has spoken to her unit manager about her dissatisfaction with being unable to do other nursing activities with patients and with the treatment team. Julie submitted a proposal for patient education classes pertinent to understanding addiction and issues that occur during the first few years of recovery. Julie also explained that she would like to have more time to talk with patients during which they can talk about their personal issues in treatment. The unit manager explained to Julie that her primary purpose for being there was to satisfy JCAHO legal requirements for an RN on the premises and that she was not really needed for other treatment interventions because these were fully covered by the counselors. Julie has also spoken to her RN supervisor about the problem but was told that she needed to do whatever the unit manager needed her to do because Julie was really not working directly with the nursing staff.

Critical Thinking Questions: *(Write your answers on a separate sheet of paper, if necessary.)*

1. How does the unit manager and RN supervisor's position with Julie affect Julie's work morale and effectiveness with patients on the unit?

2. What actions might the RN supervisor take to support Julie's commitment to providing nursing care to patient's on the unit?

3. What actions might Julie take to reverse the situation?

26

Name: _____

Therapeutic Environment in Different Treatment Settings

Choose the *most* appropriate answer to the following questions:

1. Patients are discussed individually and decisions regarding treatment are developed in:
   _____ 1. A community meeting   _____ 3. A group meeting
   _____ 2. A team meeting   _____ 4. A staff meeting

2. Arts and crafts are most likely used by OTs for which of the following treatment objectives?
   _____ 1. To learn new work skills
   _____ 2. To improve use of leisure time
   _____ 3. To improve attention and concentration
   _____ 4. To develop a method of distraction from anxieties

3. A benefit of psychoeducational groups is:
   _____ 1. It prevents further progression of the illness.
   _____ 2. It prevents recurrence of symptoms.
   _____ 3. It improves self-esteem of participants and family members.
   _____ 4. It improves quality of life, reduces relapse rates, and alters negative family reactions.

4. One function of community meetings is to:
   _____ 1. Handle staff conflicts
   _____ 2. Discuss patient diagnoses
   _____ 3. Discuss individual treatment needs and concerns
   _____ 4. Handle conflicts between patients or between patients and staff

5. An adult patient with depression and a suicidal plan would most likely be admitted to the:
   _____ 1. Open adult psychiatric unit
   _____ 2. Partial hospitalization program
   _____ 3. Integrated medical-psychiatric unit
   _____ 4. Intensive and acute care psychiatric unit

6. One important role of the adolescent psychiatric nurse is:
   _____ 1. Monitoring interactions with peers
   _____ 2. Applying punishment for inappropriate behavior
   _____ 3. Keeping parent and child separated during treatment to decrease conflict
   _____ 4. Avoiding consistent assignments to prevent dependency

7. Which of the following patients might be suitable for an integrated medical-psychiatric unit?
   _____ 1. One with bipolar disorder and hypertension
   _____ 2. One with depression and chronic headaches
   _____ 3. One with psychosis and a urinary tract infection
   _____ 4. One with depression and congestive heart failure

8. The primary difference between state psychiatric hospitals and other psychiatric facilities is:
   _____ 1. Location of the facility
   _____ 2. Types of patients served
   _____ 3. Unique treatments offered
   _____ 4. Length of stay and degree of restrictiveness

9. Community treatment settings are typically less restrictive than are inpatient settings, thus requiring very careful assessment of:

_____ 1. Safety   _____ 3. Living conditions
_____ 2. Social skills   _____ 4. Medication compliance

10. The majority of psychiatric care takes place in:

_____ 1. Hospitals   _____ 3. Institutions
_____ 2. Community settings   _____ 4. Halfway houses

Indicate *T* for true and *F* for false:

_____ 11. Exercise has a beneficial effect on well being and mood.
_____ 12. Psychiatric registered nurses can conduct groups.
_____ 13. Geropsychiatric units require special physical design to address the unique needs of this population.
_____ 14. Forensic psychiatric hospitals mostly treat patients from prisons.

Match the psychiatric team professional with the primary clinical responsibility:

_____ 15. Psychiatrist   a. Applies principles of exercise physiology to clinical
_____ 16. Psychiatric social worker   care of patients
_____ 17. Occupation therapist   b. Assists with self-care activities and the development
_____ 18. Recreational therapist   of leisure interests
_____ 19. Psychiatric nurse   c. Makes diagnoses and prescribes treatment
_____ 20. Exercise therapist   d. Emphasizes occupational and daily functioning
                                          e. Manages the therapeutic milieu
                                          f. Mobilizes community and social resources

Briefly answer the following question:

21. Why is competence in medical-surgical skills essential for the psychiatric nurse?

Case Study: The psychiatric institute is opening as a 26-bed closed psychiatric unit in a large hospital. The unit will serve men and women, and the primary patient diagnoses are expected to be schizophrenia, severe depression, and bipolar disorder. Most patients will be involuntarily admitted or require close nursing staff supervision because of the acuity of their illness. A planning meeting with the architects and senior administration is scheduled to work on the physical design of the unit. Several nursing staff members have been invited to participate in the planning process.

Critical Thinking Questions: In the following questions, if you are able to come up with three to four items, you will demonstrate understanding of the chapter content. With experience, more areas of importance will become apparent to you. *(Write your answers on a separate sheet of paper, if necessary.)*

1. What recommendations would you make for the physical layout of the unit?

2. What impact will the physical layout have on the milieu?

3. What kinds of activities would be appropriate for the mix of patients on the unit?

Chapter 27

Name: _____

Introduction to Psychopathology

Choose the *most* appropriate answer to the following questions:

1. The most common mental disorders are:
    _____ 1. Anxiety disorders
    _____ 2. Chemical dependency disorders
    _____ 3. Schizophrenia
    _____ 4. Mood disorders

2. Approximately what percentage of the population suffers from schizophrenia in any 12-month period?
    _____ 1. 10%
    _____ 2. 5%
    _____ 3. 1%
    _____ 4. 0.5%

3. There are several diagnostic systems available for nurses. The system that is most commonly used in the United States is:
    _____ 1. Feighner criteria
    _____ 2. Research Diagnostic Criteria
    _____ 3. DSM-IV-TR
    _____ 4. ICD-10

4. Signs and symptoms of mental disorders are criteria used by clinicians to establish a diagnosis. When a patient reports hearing voices, the nurse understands this to be a(n):
    _____ 1. Objective sign
    _____ 2. Subjective symptom
    _____ 3. Diagnostic proof of schizophrenia
    _____ 4. Delusional symptom

5. When clinicians state schizophrenia is caused by life experiences, they are supporting which of the following arguments:
    _____ 1. Nature
    _____ 2. Organic
    _____ 3. Biologic
    _____ 4. Nurture

6. When psychopathologic terms are operationally defined, it facilitates:
    _____ 1. Research
    _____ 2. Patient adherence to medications
    _____ 3. Nursing autonomy
    _____ 4. Nurse-patient communication

Briefly answer the following questions:

7. Approximately how many people in the United States are affected by mental health disorders? What percentage of the total population does this represent? Do you believe the researchers are correct?

8. List the five most common mental health disorders in the United States.

9. The cause of mental disorders can be attributed to "nature" or "nurture." Explain each of these terms.

Case Study: Jane is a 22-year-old senior nursing student. You have become well acquainted with Jane because you have shared three clinical rotations with her and have sat near her in several classes. You have noticed that Jane has a very low tolerance to stress. For example, both Jane and Sally failed the last drug quiz; but, although Sally seemed to take it in stride and announced, "I'll be ready next time," Jane fell apart. She was crying and wondering aloud whether she should "just give up."

Critical Thinking Question: Does this situation have anything to do with mental health?

Chapter **28**

Name: _____

Schizophrenia and Other Psychoses

Choose the *most* appropriate answer to the following questions:

1. Schizophrenia may be associated with elevated levels of:
   - _____ 1. Norepinephrine
   - _____ 2. Dopamine
   - _____ 3. Serotonin
   - _____ 4. Acetylcholine

2. The term schizophrenia was coined by:
   - _____ 1. Morel
   - _____ 2. Kraepelin
   - _____ 3. Bleuler
   - _____ 4. Freud

3. The term schizophrenia means:
   - _____ 1. Splitting of mind and affect
   - _____ 2. Split personality
   - _____ 3. Multiple personalities
   - _____ 4. Disturbance (i.e., "schizo") in thinking (i.e., "phrenic")

4. A person brought into the county emergency room is laughing inappropriately, being silly, and not making sense. The patient is dirty, and her clothes are torn. Which DSM-IV-TR diagnostic criteria category would most nearly fit this behavior?
   - _____ 1. Disorganized type
   - _____ 2. Catatonic type
   - _____ 3. Paranoid type
   - _____ 4. Undifferentiated type

5. Which of the following descriptors fits type I schizophrenia?
   - _____ 1. Cortical
   - _____ 2. Hyperdopaminergic
   - _____ 3. Structurally related
   - _____ 4. Does not respond readily to drugs

6. A patient states that he hears voices telling him that he is Jesus. This misperception is a(n):
   - _____ 1. Delusion
   - _____ 2. Hallucination
   - _____ 3. Illusion
   - _____ 4. False belief

7. The patient in question 6 believes that he is Jesus. This symptom is called a(n):
   - _____ 1. Delusion
   - _____ 2. Hallucination
   - _____ 3. Illusion
   - _____ 4. False belief

8. The patient being reviewed during the morning report is described as having bizarre delusions and hallucinations. Based on this limited information, you are:
   - _____ 1. Optimistic because antipsychotic drugs should help these type I symptoms
   - _____ 2. Optimistic because type II symptoms respond well to milieu management
   - _____ 3. Pessimistic because type I symptoms are slow to respond to antipsychotic drugs
   - _____ 4. Pessimistic because the bizarre nature of the symptoms indicates a very sick person

9. Mr. Thomas, an unmarried 40-year-old truck driver, is admitted to the psychiatric unit for the first time. He was at a truck stop when he became very agitated, was talking to himself, and frightening people around him. He arrives on the unit in leather restraints with a police escort. He screams, "Get them away from me! Don't let them kill me!" This symptom is best described as:
   - _____ 1. Regression
   - _____ 2. Flight of ideas
   - _____ 3. Hallucination
   - _____ 4. Delusion

10. Mr. Thomas, during admission processing, tells you that the other truck drivers are against him. He tells you that he has proof that they have bugged his truck. Mr. Thomas's symptoms would probably carry the diagnosis of:
    - _____ 1. Anxiety reaction related to schizophrenia
    - _____ 2. Schizophrenia, paranoid type
    - _____ 3. Schizophrenia, disorganized type
    - _____ 4. Schizoeffective disorder

761

Study Guide

11. Schizophrenia will affect approximately what percentage of the population over a lifetime?
    _____ 1. 1%   _____ 3. 10%
    _____ 2. 4%   _____ 4. 15%
12. Which of the following early scientist had the most pessimistic view of schizophrenia?
    _____ 1. Bleuler   _____ 3. Kraepelin
    _____ 2. Freud   _____ 4. Sullivan
13. Imaging techniques have revealed which of the following anatomic changes in some people with schizophrenia?
    _____ 1. Increased ventricular brain ratios   _____ 3. Decreased ventricular brain ratios
    _____ 2. Increased cerebral blood flow   _____ 4. Synaptic pruning
14. Rigidity and high fever in a schizophrenic patient should cause the nurse to first consider:
    _____ 1. Parkinsonism   _____ 3. Neuroleptic malignant syndrome
    _____ 2. Catatonia related by hyperthermia   _____ 4. Drug interactions or a coma
15. In attempting to distinguish between environmental and genetic etiologic factors for schizophrenia, the best population to study is:
    _____ 1. Fraternal twins   _____ 3. Unrelated individuals
    _____ 2. Monozygotic twins   _____ 4. Siblings
16. The major concern associated with water imbalance among patients with schizophrenia is:
    _____ 1. Hypokalemia   _____ 3. Convulsions
    _____ 2. Hyponatremia   _____ 4. Hypomagnesemia
17. Abnormal involuntary oral-facial movements in schizophrenic patients are usually related to:
    _____ 1. Exposure to neuroleptic medication
    _____ 2. Exposure to anticholinergics
    _____ 3. Younger patients
    _____ 4. Ethnicity of patients

Indicate *T* for true and *F* for false:

_____ 18. The majority of professionals no longer subscribe to theories suggesting that schizophrenia is caused by a dominating mother.

Briefly answer the following question:

19. What are the classic symptoms of the group of disorders known as schizophrenia?

Case Study: T.Z., a 45-year-old woman, has experienced symptoms of schizophrenia since late adolescence. She required several short hospitalizations and also needed commitment to a state hospital 20 years ago as a result of bizarre behaviors and psychotic symptoms, where she remained for 18 years. Her medication regimen includes haloperidol 20 mg, olanzapine 25 mg, and clonazepam 1 mg at bedtime; haloperidol decanoate 350 mg intramuscularly every 4 weeks; bupropion 100 mg in the morning; and propranolol 10 mg tid. Attempts to decrease either formulation of haloperidol has resulted in an increase in psychotic symptoms, sleep difficulties, and increased agitation. She has not required hospitalization for the last 2 years but continues to exhibit psychotic symptoms. She is monitored by the local mental health agency and is seen on a weekly basis.

Critical Thinking Questions: *(Write your answers on a separate sheet of paper.)*
1. Why would a person who still exhibits psychotic symptoms not be in a hospital setting?

2. Is this quantity of medication excessive?

3. What effect on a person would you expect after 18 years in a state hospital?

Chapter 29

Name: _____

Depression

Choose the *most* appropriate answer to the following questions:

1. Which of the following conceptualizations of depressive disorders best explains the effectiveness and appropriate use of antidepressants?
   _____ 1. Depression is related to a change in neurotransmitters.
   _____ 2. Depression is related to alterations in subcortical nuclei.
   _____ 3. Depression is related to intrapsychic conflicts amenable to antidepressants.
   _____ 4. Depression is related to psychosocial stressors, which immobilize the individual.

2. Subjective symptoms of major depression include:
   _____ 1. Alterations in activity
   _____ 2. Alterations in social interactions
   _____ 3. Alterations in affect
   _____ 4. Alterations in eating habits

3. Pessimism, self-blame, self-deprecating thoughts are examples of:
   _____ 1. Alterations in affect
   _____ 2. Alterations in cognition
   _____ 3. Alterations in activity
   _____ 4. Alterations in perceptions

4. Chest pain, constipation, dizziness, and fatigue are examples of:
   _____ 1. Alterations in affect
   _____ 2. Alterations of a physical nature
   _____ 3. Alterations of perceptions
   _____ 4. Alterations of cognition

5. Delusions and hallucinations are examples of:
   _____ 1. Alterations in affect
   _____ 2. Alterations of a physical nature
   _____ 3. Alterations in perceptions
   _____ 4. Alterations in cognition

6. The most important parameters for suicidal patients are:
   _____ 1. Whether they mean to hurt themselves
   _____ 2. Whether they have a plan, have chosen a lethal method, and have attempted to block rescue efforts
   _____ 3. Whether they have a history of suicidal thinking
   _____ 4. Whether the suicidal attempt is a cry for help or represents a manipulation

7. Marilyn is a 73-year-old Caucasian woman who recently lost her husband of 40 years and was just admitted to the unit. Her daughter reports that she will not eat, does not sleep, and seems a little confused at times. The important concern is about:
   _____ 1. Starting her on the correct antidepressant
   _____ 2. Differentiating between depression and dementia
   _____ 3. Addressing her basic needs (e.g., sleep, food, proper elimination)
   _____ 4. Helping her cope with the loss of her husband

8. John, who is 70 years of age, is admitted to the unit for depression. He has been a successful businessman for many years. He complains of weight loss, early morning awakening, fatigue, slowed gait, pain, and feeling sad for months. He cannot think of anything that has happened recently that would make him so depressed. John should be told that:
   _____ 1. Depression can occur "out of the blue" without precipitating life events.
   _____ 2. Depression is a symptom of old age.
   _____ 3. Many people feel sad.
   _____ 4. The depression will probably stop within 2 months.

9. The major biochemical changes caused by early life trauma involve which system?
   _____ 1. The hypothalamic-pituitary-adrenal axis and the corticotropin-releasing factor system
   _____ 2. The hippocampus-thalamic feedback system
   _____ 3. The serotonergic (raphe nuclei) cortical system
   _____ 4. The monoamine uptake system

10. You are wondering if John is suicidal. As a nurse, the first thing you should do is:
   _____ 1. Assess for indicators of suicidal ideations.
   _____ 2. Ask John if he is having suicidal thoughts.
   _____ 3. Talk to the family about John's recent behaviors.
   _____ 4. Place John on level 1 suicide precaution.

11. After antidepressant medications have "stabilized" the patient, the best therapy approach (according to this book) is:
   _____ 1. Psychoanalysis   _____ 3. Interpersonal therapy
   _____ 2. Cognitive therapy   _____ 4. Behavioral therapy

Indicate *T* for true and *F* for false:
   _____ 12. Research has found a role for early life trauma in depression.

Briefly answer the following question:
13. What are the two etiologic categories of mood disorders emphasized in this chapter?

Case Study: Billie first began experiencing symptoms of major depression at the age of 45. She was married at the time. She was hospitalized 6 months after her first episode resulting from the development of delusional thinking, as well as decreased energy, hopelessness, sleep disturbances, appetite disturbance, and an inability to return to her job as a schoolteacher. Her delusion of germs caused her to bathe and scrub herself several times a day. She was prescribed an antidepressant and an antipsychotic while hospitalized. During hospitalization, her husband abandoned their already shaky marriage. Once discharged, she did not follow up with appointments and eventually stopped taking the prescribed medications. After years of being in and out of hospitals, she was referred to a local mental health center. She was diagnosed with major depression with psychotic features and was prescribed different antidepressant and antipsychotic medications. Approximately 4 months after beginning treatment at the mental health center, Billie developed suicidal ideations and was prescribed an SSRI. At age 60, after numerous adjustments and drug changes, Billie is living independently and able to do volunteer work and participate in church activities. She continues to be seen at the local mental health center on a regular basis. Billie has experienced a recovery of sorts but states, "I have little left to live for."

   Critical Thinking Questions: *(Write your answers on a separate sheet of paper.)*
   1. Losing her husband may have been a devastating blow to Billie as she was attempting to recover. If you were the husband, what might be the reasons for the divorce?

   2. In real life, the divorce was not devastating to Billie. What might be some reasons for that unlikely scenario?

   3. Why would the clinician prescribe both an antidepressant and an antipsychotic?

   4. Is it common to switch medications as often as the clinicians did with Billie?

   5. The final statement by Billie is troubling. What do you make of it?

Bipolar Disorders

Choose the *most* appropriate answer to the following questions:

1. Ms. Long is taking lithium and has a lithium serum level of 1.5 mEq/L. Which of the following is expected, based on an understanding of appropriate lithium serum levels?
   _____ 1. Some manic behavior   _____ 3. Mild symptoms of toxicity
   _____ 2. Appropriate symptom control   _____ 4. Significant toxicity

2. Flight of ideas, insomnia, delusions of grandeur, and intense irritability are symptoms that may be attributed to:
   _____ 1. Bipolar I   _____ 3. Cyclothymia
   _____ 2. Bipolar II   _____ 4. Hypomania

3. Which of the following statements best captures a therapeutic approach to a bipolar patient who is reluctant to abide by unit television protocols and wants the period extended 1 hour?
   _____ 1. "The television is turned off at 10:30 every weekday night."
   _____ 2. "Is there something particularly meaningful you want to watch tonight?"
   _____ 3. "I know you are aware of unit policy, so I would like to hear more about your request to have television hours extended."
   _____ 4. "I appreciate you asking, and I think your request is reasonable. Television will remain on until 11:30 tonight."

4. Bipolar I disorders can be distinguished from depressive disorders by recognizing that:
   _____ 1. Bipolar I disorder indicates only manic or hypomanic behavior.
   _____ 2. Bipolar I indicates the presence of one or more manic episodes.
   _____ 3. Bipolar I disorder is a 3-month period of alternating highs and lows.
   _____ 4. Bipolar denotes that the patient has two disorders concurrently.

5. Billy, a patient on the unit, starts saying, "Birds, birds, where is Lady Bird? You ain't no lady." You recognize this as:
   _____ 1. Grandiosity   _____ 3. Delusional thinking
   _____ 2. Distractibility   _____ 4. Flight of ideas

6. Geri has been up and down emotionally for the last 2 years or so. She has never been delusional or suicidal, but her mood swings are starting to take their toll on her personal relationships. The most likely diagnosis, given this limited amount of information, is?
   _____ 1. Bipolar I   _____ 3. Cyclothymia
   _____ 2. Bipolar II   _____ 4. Dysthymia

7. Linking mania to a massive denial of depression is best thought of as:
   _____ 1. A psychodynamic view   _____ 3. A genetic view
   _____ 2. A biologic view   _____ 4. A behavioral view

8. William is pacing back and forth, is talking loudly, appears very agitated, and seems to be angrily talking and making references to another male patient. Which of the following nursing actions would you consider the highest priority?
   _____ 1. Speak very clearly, and ask William to join you on the porch.
   _____ 2. Attempt to reduce the environmental stimuli that are provoking William.
   _____ 3. Be very consistent with William in your enforcement of unit policies.
   _____ 4. Discuss his escalation behavior with him.

9. William appears to be less agitated but is talking continually, jumping from subject to subject. Which of the following is the best intervention?
   _____ 1. Do not interrupt unless it is life threatening.
   _____ 2. Get him involved in the card game in the day room.
   _____ 3. Give a prn dose of lithium.
   _____ 4. Interrupt his flow of words with brief statements.

10. Which of the following meals would be most appropriate for bipolar patient in a manic state?
   _____ 1. Spaghetti and a salad
   _____ 2. A roast beef sandwich and mashed potatoes
   _____ 3. French fries and a hot dog
   _____ 4. Chili and tortillas

Case Study: Toby is a 33-year-old man with a history of disabling bipolar disorder. Toby was adopted at the age of 4 by a dysfunctional family. The adoptive father routinely meted out harsh punishment for what Toby recalls as minor infractions. He also witnessed his adoptive mother sustain severe beatings from this man. Toby has been in and out of hospitals for about 15 years. He has been married four times and is now divorced again. He has one child from these marriages, and the mother of the child will not permit him to see her (the child is in another state). He does relatively well when taking his medications (valproic acid) but has been historically noncompliant to treatment—when he starts feeling "abnormal," he stops taking his medicine. He really enjoys "the way up," but then things "get out of hand." Currently, Toby is angry, volatile, continually pacing, and very verbal. He has not been eating much because he "cannot" sit still long enough to eat.

Critical Thinking Questions:
1. An important nursing diagnosis for Toby would be sleep pattern disturbances related to hyperactivity. Appropriate nursing actions include all except which of the following:
   _____ 1. Increase activities in the afternoon so that Toby will be ready for bedtime.
   _____ 2. Provide a warm cup of cocoa about 8:00 PM.
   _____ 3. Let Toby sleep when he can; his body knows when it needs rest.
   _____ 4. Provide a quiet place to sleep.
2. When patients such as Toby do not take time to eat, an appropriate nursing intervention is to:
   _____ 1. Stay with the patient until everything is eaten.
   _____ 2. Provide high-protein finger foods that the patient can eat on the run.
   _____ 3. Offer foods that the patient likes.
   _____ 4. Use behavior modification to encourage patient to eat.
3. Toby tells the nurse that his third wife had spies following him because she still wants him. He starts sharing with the nurse all of his exploits with women and how he can "get a woman anytime I feel like it." Such statements are best assessed as:
   _____ 1. Paranoid delusions
   _____ 2. Delusions of grandeur
   _____ 3. Nihilistic delusions
   _____ 4. Probably true
4. Toby and other individuals suffering from bipolar disorder often display which of the following communication problems?
   _____ 1. Poverty of speech
   _____ 2. Verbosity
   _____ 3. Alogia
   _____ 4. Terseness
5. What is the most important dimension of patient care for Toby now?

6. What is the best strategy for communicating with Toby when he is experiencing a manic episode?

Chapter 31

Name: _____

Anxiety-Related Somatoform and Dissociative Disorders

Choose the *most* appropriate answer to the following questions:

1. Which of the following refers to secondary gain?
   _____ 1. The benefits received from others while sick
   _____ 2. Decreasing and relieving anxiety
   _____ 3. Increased ability to cope with anxiety in the future
   _____ 4. The benefit received from medication

2. Before patients with anxiety-related disorders can solve problems and develop adaptive coping responses, which of the following actions would the nurse do first?
   _____ 1. Confront patients with their maladaptive behaviors.
   _____ 2. Assist patients with managing and reducing anxiety.
   _____ 3. Administer prn lorazepam (Ativan) to eliminate subjective symptoms of discomfort.
   _____ 4. Help patients develop insight into their illness.

3. The characteristic symptom of ASD and PTSD that distinguishes them from other anxiety-related disorders are:
   _____ 1. Severe depression
   _____ 2. Suspiciousness of others
   _____ 3. Lack of interest in family and activities
   _____ 4. Reexperiencing the trauma in nightmares and flashbacks

4. Which intervention would be most appropriate in planning care for the patient with somatoform disorder?
   _____ 1. Push insight so that the patient connects the conflict with the need for physical symptoms.
   _____ 2. Tell the patient to stop talking about his feelings.
   _____ 3. Allow the patient to focus on physical symptoms.
   _____ 4. Involve the patient in milieu activities.

5. The patient with obsessive-compulsive disorder needs to rearrange his clothing in his closet 17 times each night before he can sleep. The nurse finds the patient arranging his clothing in his room at 11:00 PM. Which nursing action is appropriate?
   _____ 1. Tell the patient to finish arranging his clothing in the morning.
   _____ 2. Give the patient medication to help him sleep.
   _____ 3. Allow the patient to complete his activity.
   _____ 4. Remind the patient that bedtime was at 10:00 PM.

6. One goal of critical incident stress management (CISM) for victims of disasters is to prevent development of ASD and PTSD. Another goal is which of the following?
   _____ 1. A return to a previous or enhanced level of adaptation
   _____ 2. Recovery from injuries or surgery
   _____ 3. Establishment of emergency shelters and food supplies
   _____ 4. Management of information and press releases

7. Nurses working with trauma survivors often need to debrief about their own experiences. This course of action is one way to deal with which of the following concepts?
   _____ 1. Integration of memories
   _____ 2. Vicarious victimization
   _____ 3. Survivor guilt
   _____ 4. Grief and mourning

8. Treatment of ASD and PTSD includes processing of emotions, as well as memories. Which of the following is typically an important aspect of emotion management?
   _____ 1. Teaching about the dynamics of trauma responses
   _____ 2. Reviewing of initial thoughts at the scene of trauma
   _____ 3. Safe verbalization of feelings, especially anger
   _____ 4. Referrals to appropriate support groups

Briefly answer the following question:

9. What two areas would the nurse teach the patient about panic disorder?

Case Study: As you near the nurse's station to begin the evening shift, you hear screams and gunshots. The ex-husband of one of the day-shift nurses has killed his ex-wife, wounded two other staff members, and then killed himself. Hours later, after the police and coroner's investigations are completed, you find one of the day-shift nurses sitting in the lounge, staring at the wall. As you talk with her, you realize that she is having trouble remembering the shootings, is showing no emotions, and is in a daze. With this information, answer the following questions:

Critical Thinking Questions:

1. Using principles of crisis intervention and CISM, list your immediate interventions.

2. As the staff member begins to process the event cognitively and emotionally, plan your next intervention.

32 Name: _____

Cognitive Disorders

Choose the *most* appropriate answer to the following questions:

1. The major symptoms of delirium include:
   - _____ 1. Primarily cognitive disturbances developing gradually with age
   - _____ 2. A widespread cerebral dysfunction affecting thinking, attention, perception, memory, consciousness, and activity level
   - _____ 3. Transient pathologic, neurologic symptoms, such as ataxia and diplopia
   - _____ 4. Changes in motor functioning, rigidity, and tremor

2. The major symptoms of dementia include:
   - _____ 1. Depression, aphasia, restlessness, and wandering
   - _____ 2. Vision and hearing disturbances and ataxia
   - _____ 3. Impaired intellectual function and judgment and changes in personality and perceptions
   - _____ 4. Disturbances in reflexes, memory, and impulse control

3. The percentage of U.S. population over age 17 that has a cognitive disorder is:
   - _____ 1. 1%
   - _____ 2. 3%
   - _____ 3. 5%
   - _____ 4. 10%

4. The incidence of Alzheimer's disease in the U.S. population over the age of 65 is:
   - _____ 1. <1%
   - _____ 2. >5%
   - _____ 3. >10%
   - _____ 4. >30%

5. Donepezil is classified pharmacologically as a:
   - _____ 1. Cholinomimetic
   - _____ 2. Cholinesterase inhibitor
   - _____ 3. MAO–B inhibitor
   - _____ 4. Antipsychotic

6. Over the age of 85 about what percentage of the U.S. population develops Alzheimer's disease?
   - _____ 1. 5% to 10%
   - _____ 2. 10% to 15%
   - _____ 3. 20% to 25%
   - _____ 4. 25% to 50%

7. A serum enzyme that can elevate when using tacrine is:
   - _____ 1. ChE
   - _____ 2. CPK
   - _____ 3. ALT
   - _____ 4. MAO

Match each of the following cognitive disorders with its primary characteristics:

_____ 8. Alzheimer's disease
_____ 9. Parkinson's disease
_____ 10. Huntington's disease.

a. Neurologic disorder causing tremor, rigidity, and weakness in voluntary movement
b. Deterioration of neurologic, motor, and intellectual functions
c. Progressive nonreversible CNS disorder affecting cognitive function

Briefly answer the following questions:

11. What are subjective and objective symptoms of Alzheimer's disease?

12. Name three other disorders or conditions that may present similar symptoms and that should be ruled out before a diagnosis of Alzheimer's disease is made.

13. List and define the four As of Alzheimer's disease.

Indicate *T* for true and *F* for false:

_____ 14. Antipsychotic medications are effective in treating some symptoms of delirium and dementia.
_____ 15. The primary goal of nursing care for a patient with dementia is an individualized approach that maintains an optimal level of functioning.
_____ 16. Huntington's disease occurs most often among young to middle-aged adults.
_____ 17. Seizures are characteristic of Huntington's disease.
_____ 18. Symptoms of Pick's disease are similar to symptoms of Alzheimer's disease.
_____ 19. Antipsychotic or neuroleptic drugs can be effective in treating cognitive symptoms of Alzheimer's disease.
_____ 20. Stress can decrease the functional ability of people who have Alzheimer's disease.
_____ 21. Individuals with cognitive disorders rarely notice changes in their environment, routine, or caregiver.
_____ 22. Wandering is a significant problem among people who have cognitive disorders.
_____ 23. Parkinson's disease is characterized by extrapyramidal symptoms.

Match the characteristic with the term. You may use some answers more than once.

_____ 24. Memory impairment and inability to dress self
_____ 25. Progressive decline of self-care abilities over the last year
_____ 26. Abrupt inability to remember and carry on conversation
_____ 27. Reduced ability to focus and pick up on nonverbal clues
_____ 28. Confused and disoriented

a. Delirium
b. Dementia
c. Both delirium and dementia

Chapter 33

Name: _____

Personality Disorders

Choose the *most* appropriate answer to the following questions:

1. Which of the following statements is accurate regarding individuals with personality disorders?
   - _____ 1. They experience discomfort because of other's reactions toward them.
   - _____ 2. They receive psychotropic medication to eliminate their personality disorder.
   - _____ 3. They are flexible in how they relate with others.
   - _____ 4. They are usually hospitalized for their personality disorder.

2. Which nursing approach is most appropriate for a patient with a paranoid personality disorder?
   - _____ 1. Involve the patient in groups as much as possible.
   - _____ 2. Use a light-hearted manner in interacting with the patient.
   - _____ 3. Confront the patient's use of projection and need to control.
   - _____ 4. Use clear, simple explanations when making requests.

3. A patient with borderline personality disorder uses self-mutilation for which of the following reasons?
   - _____ 1. As a means to get attention
   - _____ 2. To express intense feelings of anger or frustration
   - _____ 3. To express feelings of autonomy
   - _____ 4. As a means to manipulate staff

4. Mrs. Cannon withdraws from everyone on the unit. She refuses to go to activities because no one will like her, and she feels she is unable to initiate conversation with others. Which action would be therapeutic for Mrs. Cannon?
   - _____ 1. Escort Mrs. Cannon to her activity and leave her there.
   - _____ 2. Tell Mrs. Cannon that she should rest in her room until she feels more comfortable with others.
   - _____ 3. Include Mrs. Cannon when the nurse initiates a conversation with the patient's roommate.
   - _____ 4. Suggest to Mrs. Cannon that she discuss these difficulties with her physician.

5. Mr. Brand constantly bends rules to meet his needs and then gets angry when other patients and staff confront him on his behavior. He threatens patients and manipulates the staff to get what he wants. Which is the best nursing approach to use with him?
   - _____ 1. Administer prn medication every time Mr. Brand does not follow the rules.
   - _____ 2. Ignore his behavior and privately tell the other patients to let Mr. Brand have his way.
   - _____ 3. Encourage the other staff members to take turns watching Mr. Brand.
   - _____ 4. Set firm limits for Mr. Brand, and be consistent in confronting behaviors and enforcing unit rules.

6. The patient with borderline personality disorder states to the nurse, "I think I'll go to nursing school." The patient did not graduate from high school. Which statement by the nurse is appropriate?

_____ 1. "Why would you want to do that?"
_____ 2. "What do you need to accomplish before you can do that?"
_____ 3. "Have you told your family?"
_____ 4. "Which school do you want to go to?"

7. The nurse is interacting with the patient diagnosed with major depression and dependent personality disorder. The patient states, "Can you go to my room and get my glasses for me?" The nurse judges this statement to reflect which of the following?

_____ 1. The patient is maintaining her need to rely on others.
_____ 2. The patient is voicing an assertive statement.
_____ 3. The patient is demonstrating signs of autonomy.
_____ 4. The patient is behaving on a level equal to that of the nurse.

Briefly answer the following questions:

8. The nurse admits Ann, a patient with borderline personality disorder, to the inpatient unit. Ann is brought from the emergency room after having both wrists sutured for cuts made with a steak knife. The patient is tearful and angrily states to the nurse, "I wanted to die. My boyfriend hasn't called me for 3 days. No one cares." Which approaches would the nurse immediately initiate to help Ann?

9. A staff member on the unit states to the nurse, "Ann just wants attention. She could have killed herself if she had really wanted to die." How would the nurse respond to the staff member?

10. Ann continues to voice feelings of hopelessness and emptiness. Should Ann receive medication at this time? Why or why not?

Chapter 34

Name: _____

Sexual Disorders

Choose the *most* appropriate answer to the following questions:

1. During the admissions interview, a patient states to the nurse that she has no interest in sexual intercourse with her husband. Which nursing action is best?
   _____ 1. Advise the patient to talk to her physician about this.
   _____ 2. Tell the patient not to worry about it now.
   _____ 3. Direct the patient to discuss another subject.
   _____ 4. Further question the patient about this concern.

2. A patient states to the nurse, "I feel so guilty because I fondled my daughter's 7-year-old friend." Which of the following responses is most appropriate?
   _____ 1. "We can't do anything about that now."
   _____ 2. "Tell me more about what happened."
   _____ 3. "Your guilt will lessen after your medication starts to work."
   _____ 4. "Does your wife know about this?"

3. A patient is an incest perpetrator. In a discussion with the patient's wife, the nurse would do which of the following?
   _____ 1. Tell the wife to divorce her husband.
   _____ 2. Explain that the husband alone needs treatment.
   _____ 3. Recommend a support group for the wife.
   _____ 4. Advise the wife to call the police about her husband's activity.

4. A patient with major depression is also a known pedophile. The nurse includes which of the following strategies in the plan of care?
   _____ 1. Isolate the patient in his room as much as possible.
   _____ 2. Help the patient discuss his feelings about himself and his problems.
   _____ 3. Tell the patient that he ought to be ashamed of himself.
   _____ 4. Advise the patient to discuss his problems openly with other patients on the unit.

Case Study: Jim is a 34-year-old patient who has been visiting the community mental health center for 3 months. His axis 1 diagnosis for major depression was made, and he was prescribed sertraline (Zoloft) 50 mg orally every morning. During a conversation with the nurse, he discloses that he has molested his neighbor's 8-year-old daughter.

Critical Thinking Questions:
1. What is the nurse's legal responsibility in this case?

2. What would the nurse include in the plan of care for this patient?

3. What impact might Jim's axis I diagnosis of major depression and medication have on his sexuality?

Chapter **35**

Name: _____

Substance-Related Disorders

Choose the *most* appropriate answer to the following questions:

1. The primary drug problem in North America is with:
   _____ 1. Alcohol   _____ 3. Heroin
   _____ 2. Cocaine   _____ 4. Marijuana
2. Constricted pupils indicate the use of:
   _____ 1. Mescaline   _____ 3. Alcohol
   _____ 2. Psilocybin   _____ 4. Opioids
3. Alcohol is metabolized at about what rate?
   _____ 1. 15 ml every 60 minutes
   _____ 2. 10 g per 10 kg of body weight per hour
   _____ 3. 5 g per 10 kg of body weight per hour
   _____ 4. 10 ml every hour in a healthy adult
4. Symptoms of alcohol withdrawal include:
   _____ 1. Euphoria, hyperactivity, and insomnia
   _____ 2. Depression, nystagmus, hypotension, and revulsion to alcohol
   _____ 3. Significant disorientation, hyperactivity, and somnolence
   _____ 4. Nausea and vomiting, diaphoresis, and tremors
5. Alcohol is classified as a(n):
   _____ 1. CNS stimulant   _____ 3. Opioid
   _____ 2. CNS depressant   _____ 4. Hallucinogen
6. Which of the following is the best example of denial?
   _____ 1. The patient states that he does not drink.
   _____ 2. The patient claims to drink on the weekend only.
   _____ 3. The patient states that "he can take it or leave it alone" when it comes to alcohol.
   _____ 4. The patient states that he has a drinking problem.
7. A common effect of CNS stimulants is:
   _____ 1. Hypotension   _____ 3. Sedation
   _____ 2. Anorexia   _____ 4. Hypophrasia
8. In which of the following ways does crack cocaine differ from "regular" cocaine?
   _____ 1. Slower but better high   _____ 3. More expensive to purchase
   _____ 2. Stronger effect   _____ 4. More complicated to produce
9. Which of the following is an opioid?
   _____ 1. Cocaine   _____ 3. Quaalude
   _____ 2. Heroin   _____ 4. Ecstasy
10. Opioids are best classified as:
   _____ 1. CNS depressants   _____ 3. Agonists
   _____ 2. CNS stimulants   _____ 4. Antagonists
11. Death from opioids usually occurs from:
   _____ 1. Hypertension   _____ 3. Respiratory depression
   _____ 2. CNS stimulation   _____ 4. Cardiac arrhythmia
12. Withdrawal from barbiturates is:
   _____ 1. About as severe as withdrawal from stimulants
   _____ 2. About as severe as withdrawal from opioids
   _____ 3. More severe than withdrawal from heroin
   _____ 4. Is unpleasant but not life threatening

Study Guide

13. If opioid overdose is suspected, the patient can be given:
_____ 1. Antabuse _____ 3. Elavil
_____ 2. Narcan _____ 4. Librium

14. Which of the following short-term effects have often been found in users of hallucinogens?
_____ 1. Dystonia _____ 3. Sexual preoccupation
_____ 2. Time distortion _____ 4. An increase in goal-directed activity

15. Deaths related to PCP are usually the result of:
_____ 1. Overdose _____ 3. The pain-producing quality of the drug
_____ 2. Perceptual distortions _____ 4. Suicide

16. The safe amount of alcohol for a pregnant woman to drink is:
_____ 1. No drinks _____ 3. Two drinks
_____ 2. One drink _____ 4. Three drinks

17. Addicts prefer inhaling crack cocaine because:
_____ 1. It is cheaper. _____ 3. The high lasts longer.
_____ 2. The high is almost instantaneous. _____ 4. Inhalation does not produce the "yo-yo" effect.

18. Individuals who use amphetamines on a regular basis can have symptoms indistinguishable from which of the following psychiatric disorders?
_____ 1. Social phobias _____ 3. Obsessive compulsive disorder
_____ 2. Paranoid schizophrenia _____ 4. Depression

19. Which of the following statements best defines drug abuse?
_____ 1. Using any drug on a regular basis is drug abuse.
_____ 2. Drinking alcohol on a regular basis at parties is drug abuse.
_____ 3. Drug abuse occurs only if the substance is illegal.
_____ 4. Regularly using a drug for recreation purposes.

Indicate *T* for true and *F* for false:

_____ 20. Overdose of heroin is more lethal than withdrawal from heroin.

Case Study: Terry is a 39-year-old opioid-dependent registered nurse whose presentation in treatment is precipitated by the state nursing board. Nursing was Terry's life, and her identity centered on being a nurse. Reporting that it was not uncommon to "share medication" with patients, Terry told of how easy it was at first to document giving the maximum prn pain medications in a patient's chart, but not always giving them to the actual patient. "I never let one of my patient's be in pain, though," Terry reported.

Terry's supervisor did not suspect a problem until medication became unaccounted for. Terry thought that all areas had been covered but was eventually caught, not because of stupidity, but from the kind of impaired judgment that results from drug use.

Terry's nursing license was put on probationary status. Most facilities were not willing to hire a nurse on probation; the board's limitations placed on Terry were strict. Terry cannot work the night shift and cannot hold the keys to medication storage. Terry must also submit to random drug testing. Without a job, Terry cannot begin to fulfill the conditions of probation.

Terry was hired as a nurse at a health care facility and has 6 months remaining until another hearing date can be set.

Critical Thinking Questions:

1. What are your thoughts about Terry's statement, "I never let one of my patients be in pain, though."

2. Would you be willing to work with Terry?

Dual Diagnosis

Choose the *most* appropriate answer to the following questions:

1. The nurse, in planning care for a patient with dual diagnoses, uses which of the following concepts?
   _____ 1. Patients have the same needs and require the same interventions.
   _____ 2. Patients require interventions relevant to individual needs and their specific mental illness and substance problems.
   _____ 3. Patients should be treated for the mental illness only.
   _____ 4. Patients should be referred to a substance-dependency unit for their alcohol problems.

2. A patient with dual diagnoses is being admitted to the unit. Which of the following diagnoses would the nurse expect the patient to have?
   _____ 1. Chronic paranoid schizophrenia and dependent personality disorder
   _____ 2. Major depression with suicide attempt
   _____ 3. Undifferentiated schizophrenia and alcohol dependence
   _____ 4. Major depression and borderline personality disorder

3. The nurse is leading a group with patients who have dual diagnoses. The nurse would use which of the following approaches?
   _____ 1. Supportive and gentle confrontation
   _____ 2. Intense confrontation with all patients
   _____ 3. Expecting all patients to participate in every meeting
   _____ 4. Requiring all patients to attend every meeting

4. Regarding medication compliance, which of the following patient statements indicates the need for further teaching?
   _____ 1. "I should take all medications as prescribed by the psychiatrist."
   _____ 2. "I need to tell the nurse or doctor about any uncomfortable side effects."
   _____ 3. "I should not stop the medication even though I might be feeling better."
   _____ 4. "I will not take the medication if I want to drink alcohol or use street drugs."

5. A patient with chronic schizophrenia and marijuana abuse will be discharged from the hospital in 5 days. Which of the following actions would the nurse use?
   _____ 1. Tell the patient that follow-up treatment will not be necessary.
   _____ 2. Arrange for outpatient treatment with the help of the social worker.
   _____ 3. Tell the patient to ask his physician about discontinuing haloperidol (Haldol).
   _____ 4. Inform the patient that smoking a little marijuana now and then is safe.

6. The patient with major depression and alcohol abuse states, "When I stop drinking, I feel depressed." Which response by the nurse is the best?
   _____ 1. "Maybe you need a change in medication."
   _____ 2. "It is not unusual to feel that way."
   _____ 3. "Alcohol is a depressant and increases feelings of depression in someone who is already depressed."
   _____ 4. "Don't be discouraged; depression takes a long time to feel better."

Briefly answer the following questions:

7. Mark is depressed and anxious and is prescribed 40 mg of Prozac in the morning. He uses marijuana to forget his problems and to "mellow out." What are the important issues for the nurse to discuss with Mark?

8. Mark tells the nurse that he sometimes feels worse the next day after using marijuana. How would the nurse respond?

Eating Disorders

Choose the *most* appropriate answer to the following questions:

1. The most appropriate, immediate short-term goal for a newly admitted anorectic adolescent with the nursing diagnosis "alteration in nutrition related to refusal to eat as evidenced by loss of 15% of expected body weight" is which of the following?
   - _____ 1. Patient will gain 1 to 2 pounds per week.
   - _____ 2. Patient will discuss her relationship with her parents.
   - _____ 3. Patient will agree never to purge again.
   - _____ 4. Patient will promise not to manipulate staff.

2. Based on the short-term goal selected in question #1, which of the following would be the most effective nursing intervention for the anorectic adolescent newly admitted to an inpatient unit?
   - _____ 1. Contract with patient for a safe minimum weight for the patient to attain and maintain.
   - _____ 2. Communicate empathy and encourage the patient to express feelings.
   - _____ 3. Lock bedroom and bathroom doors to prevent the patient from purging.
   - _____ 4. Discuss the patient's manipulation with her, and assess consequences if she manipulates again.

3. Which of the following questions or statements reflects use of cognitive theory in treating an anorectic patient?
   - _____ 1. "How do you feel about the way your parents treat you?"
   - _____ 2. "Why do you constantly cook food, but never eat it?"
   - _____ 3. "How do you feel about yourself when you have to eat?"
   - _____ 4. "You've said when you get thinner, your problems will be solved; but you are getting thinner but are still not happy. At what point will you be thin enough to be happy?"

4. Which of the following is the primary reason the anorectic refuses to eat, but is preoccupied with thoughts of food and involvement in food preparation?
   - _____ 1. She is slowly attempting to kill herself.
   - _____ 2. She feels pain and discomfort whenever she ingests food.
   - _____ 3. She identifies strongly with thin people.
   - _____ 4. She is afraid of losing control over this one aspect of her life.

5. The parents of an anorectic girl are most likely to describe their daughter with which of the following adjectives?
   - _____ 1. Rebellious and rowdy   _____ 3. Timid and shy
   - _____ 2. Dependable and obedient   _____ 4. Irritable and introspective

6. Erickson would describe an eating-disordered adolescent as being most deficient in which of the following characteristics?
   - _____ 1. Initiative   _____ 3. Autonomy
   - _____ 2. Industry   _____ 4. Intimacy

7. Which of the following medications would be effective in short-term treatment of a bulimic patient?
   - _____ 1. Risperdal or other antipsychotics
   - _____ 2. Xanax or other anxiolytics
   - _____ 3. Cogentin or other antiparkinson medications
   - _____ 4. Prozac or other SSRI antidepressants

8. A nursing diagnosis appropriate for a bulimic patient my be "powerlessness related to inability to control eating as evidenced by bingeing and purging." Which of the following is an appropriate nursing intervention to address the aforementioned problem?

_____ 1. Remind the person to weigh herself daily.
_____ 2. Warn the patient about the health dangers of excessive vomiting.
_____ 3. Encourage the patient to consult with her parents frequently.
_____ 4. Arrange a meeting in which the patient and dietitian can formulate a structured meal and snack plan.

9. Some health care professionals who work with eating-disordered patients believe there is an obsessive-addictive element to the behavior of these patients. In view of this belief, which of the following self-help groups would be most helpful to a bulimic patient?

_____ 1. Overeaters Anonymous   _____ 3. Jenny Craig
_____ 2. Weight Watchers   _____ 4. T.O.P.S. (Take Pounds Off Sensibly)

10. What approach would be most effective in helping an eating-disordered patient hospitalized for extremely low weight who has been sneaking diet pills?

_____ 1. Education about the health risks and dangers of diet pills
_____ 2. Discussion concerning the patient's fears of losing control if she complies with the weight gain recommended in her care plan
_____ 3. Discussion about the fears or worries generated in her physician, her family, and the nursing staff concerning her current health status
_____ 4. Discussion of the patient's lack of need for diet pills because of patient's extreme thinness

Case Study: Nonie is a college freshman who is experiencing difficulties adjusting to college life. She attends school 600 miles away and cannot go home except at semester's end. Her roommate has noticed that she rarely goes to the cafeteria, but when she does, she eats large amounts and later can be heard in the bathroom vomiting. In the evening, she often disappears for hours, saying she's going for a walk. One night, a classmate saw her in the local grocery with a shopping cart full of junk food. Nonie is a ballet dancer who worries constantly about her weight. She says, "If I gain another ounce, my partner won't be able to lift me. They'll throw me out of the company, and then what will I do? I'm no good at anything else!" Nonie faints during one of her school tests and is taken to the college health nurse. The results of a physical examination and tests show abnormalities. Nonie's parents are called and asked to come pick her up. Nonie reveals that she was anorectic from 10 to 14 years of age, receiving inpatient and outpatient treatment. During high school, her weight stabilized. She remained slightly underweight until she began menstruating at age 16 as a result of hormonal therapy. Her weight then gradually increased to normal for her height and remained there until she was accepted into the dance company shortly after being admitted to college.

Critical Thinking Questions: (*Write your answers on a separate sheet of paper.*)

1. List significant assessment data from this case study.

2. List two to three nursing diagnoses that would apply to Nonie.

3. What are one to three realistic short-term goals (within 1 week) Nonie can achieve regarding her problem or illness?

4. List interventions likely to be effective in helping Nonie achieve the short-term goal.

5. How would you evaluate the achievement of the short-term goal?

Study Guide

Chapter 38

Name: _____

Behavior Therapies

Choose the *most* appropriate answer to the following questions:

1. A patient is disrupting a group session. Other patients are encouraging this behavior. You ask the patient to take a "time out" in his room because:
   - _____ 1. Neutral stimulation elicits cooperative response.
   - _____ 2. Social reinforcement is not available in his room.
   - _____ 3. Reinforcers control whether a behavior will be repeated.
   - _____ 4. Deprivation decreases the chance of a behavior occurring.

2. A mother brings her young son to a counselor because of acting-out behaviors. Using operant-conditioning principles, you decided to analyze which of the following?
   - _____ 1. Human reflexes
   - _____ 2. Stimulus generalization
   - _____ 3. Primary and secondary reinforcers
   - _____ 4. Internal factors influencing behaviors

3. You talk with this mother about decreasing her son's behavior by:
   - _____ 1. Developing a self-control program
   - _____ 2. Teaching her son relaxation techniques
   - _____ 3. Reinforcing successive approximations and negative reinforcement
   - _____ 4. Reinforcing opposite behaviors and removing secondary reinforcers

4. You are conducting assertiveness training for a group of patients. Techniques that would be most helpful are:
   - _____ 1. Modeling and shaping
   - _____ 2. Imitation and deprivation
   - _____ 3. Reinforcement and extinction
   - _____ 4. Modeling and negative reinforcement

5. Behavioral modification is an effective treatment strategy in helping patients deal with anxiety and change in their behaviors. However, this technique is typically combined with which of these other treatment approaches?
   - _____ 1. Psychoanalysis and medications
   - _____ 2. Developmental and stress-management approaches
   - _____ 3. Cognitive therapy and medications
   - _____ 4. Interpersonal and reality therapies

6. Positive and negative reinforcements accomplish which of the following goals?
   - _____ 1. Increase the probability that a behavior will recur
   - _____ 2. Reinforce behaviors with food, water, and sleep
   - _____ 3. Decrease behaviors with an incompatible target behavior
   - _____ 4. Suppress a behavior with a consequence such as time out

7. Skills training sessions involve which of the following behavioral strategies?
   - _____ 1. Time-out for undesirable behaviors
   - _____ 2. Modeling of and practicing behaviors in role-plays
   - _____ 3. Relaxation techniques to decrease anxiety
   - _____ 4. Intermittent reinforcement of the target behaviors

8. An example of positive reinforcement on the psychiatric unit is:
   _____ 1. Visiting hours
   _____ 2. Group therapy
   _____ 3. Token economy programs
   _____ 4. Nurse-patient contracts

9. Susan is a 9-year-old girl in the third grade. Her teacher puts a star on a chart in the class-room for each completed spelling exercise. When a student gets 10 stars, he or she can choose a prize from a special box. Five students in the class have already claimed their prizes. Susan has eight stars and is excited about her anticipated reward. The star chart is an example of:
   _____ 1. Intermittent reinforcement
   _____ 2. Shaping
   _____ 3. The Premark principle
   _____ 4. Continuous reinforcement

10. Ellen has become disabled by a phobia during the previous year. She experiences palpitations, dizziness, and fear whenever she hears music. She has been unable to go to the market or almost any other public place. Which behavior therapy might best help her cope with her symptoms so that she can go to public places again?
    _____ 1. Token economy
    _____ 2. Systematic desensitization
    _____ 3. Time-out
    _____ 4. Contingency contracting

Briefly answer the following questions:

11. John is a 52-year-old man who likes to monopolize conversation in group therapy, interrupts other speakers, and makes lists of things to do each day. Can you identify three techniques to decrease his behaviors that interfere with the therapeutic milieu for other patients?

12. What are the components of the behavioral nursing process?

Critical Thinking Question: You are responsible for treatment of 10 patients with chronic mental disorders who will be hospitalized for 1 month. What behavioral strategies would you use and why?

Chapter 39

Name: _____

Somatic Therapies

Choose the *most* appropriate answer to the following questions:

1. Succinylcholine (Anectine) given immediately preceding ECT produces which of the following?
   _____ 1. Muscle relaxation (paralysis)
   _____ 2. Anesthesia
   _____ 3. Decreased amounts of secretions (decreased possibility of aspiration)
   _____ 4. Convulsive activity

2. During effective, modern ECT, the nurse might expect the patient to:
   _____ 1. Have a full grand mal seizure
   _____ 2. Have only a brain seizure
   _____ 3. Become apprehensive immediately before the electrical stimulus
   _____ 4. Have a brief seizure (10 seconds or less)

3. ECT is most often prescribed for which of the following?
   _____ 1. Severe depression
   _____ 2. Catatonia
   _____ 3. Manic-depressive illness
   _____ 4. Movement disorder

4. The most controversial somatic therapy is:
   _____ 1. ECT
   _____ 2. Psychosurgery
   _____ 3. Phototherapy
   _____ 4. Transcranial magnetic stimulation

5. The effect from atropine that is most useful in ECT is:
   _____ 1. Mydriasis
   _____ 2. Dry mouth
   _____ 3. Urinary hesitancy
   _____ 4. Decreased lacrimation

6. ECT is ineffective in treating which of the following?
   _____ 1. Major depression
   _____ 2. Movement disorder
   _____ 3. Catatonia
   _____ 4. Anxiety

7. Typically, how many ECT treatments are given to a patient suffering from major depression?
   _____ 1. Once per week for 3 months
   _____ 2. Six to twelve treatments given on a three-times-per-week basis
   _____ 3. One to four treatments as needed
   _____ 4. One treatment every day for 2 weeks

8. The most common side effect of ECT is:
   _____ 1. Cardiovascular symptoms
   _____ 2. Temporary amnesia
   _____ 3. Permanent memory loss
   _____ 4. Hairline fractures of bones

9. Somatic therapies used to treat depression include all of the following except:
   _____ 1. Psychosurgery
   _____ 2. ECT
   _____ 3. Transcranial magnetic stimulation
   _____ 4. Phototherapy

10. Ruth is extremely suicidal and has not responded to antidepressants. She agreed to ECT this morning but refuses to sign the consent form. What is the best nursing intervention?
    _____ 1. Go ahead with the treatment because she has given verbal consent.
    _____ 2. Inform her husband he must go through the court system before treatment if she will not sign.
    _____ 3. Having her husband sign the consent form as next of kin.
    _____ 4. Tell Ruth she must sign before she can have any more cigarettes.

11. Mrs. Tyler is scheduled for ECT this morning. It is now 2:00 AM, and she cannot sleep. What would be the most appropriate nursing action?
    _____ 1. Sit quietly with her and discuss any concerns she may have.
    _____ 2. Offer her Seconal, which she refused at bedtime.
    _____ 3. Tell her there is nothing to worry about. Many treatments are given everyday.
    _____ 4. Offer warm milk and a backrub.

12. Susan just had her sixth ECT. Which of the following would be your highest priority in her posttreatment care?
    _____ 1. Observe for confusion.
    _____ 2. Reorient to time, place, and person.
    _____ 3. Monitor respiratory status.
    _____ 4. Carefully document type and length of seizure activity.

Fill in the blank to complete the following statement:

13. Somatic therapies use _____ interventions to produce behavior change in people with severe psychiatric disorders.

   Case Study: Penny (see clinical example in text) returned to the hospital emergency department with her daughter 9 months after her successful ECT treatments. She presented with depressed mood, thoughts of suicide, a 10-pound weight loss in the previous month, lack of interest in life, and vocalized guilt related to her husband's death. The attending emergency department physician admitted her to the psychiatric floor.
   Critical Thinking Questions:
   1. Should you be surprised to see Penny back in the hospital again after her successful treatment 9 months previously?

   2. What options might postpone or eliminate future hospitalizations?

Chapter 40

Name: _____

Alternative and Complementary Therapies

1. A popular herbal remedy for anxiety is:
   - _____ 1. Kava kava
   - _____ 2. Gingko biloba
   - _____ 3. St. John's wort
   - _____ 4. Melatonin

2. Gingko biloba should not be taken with:
   - _____ 1. Beta blockers
   - _____ 2. Antidepressants
   - _____ 3. Antacid
   - _____ 4. Anticoagulants

3. Which of the following agencies oversees efficacy studies of complementary and alternative therapies?
   - _____ 1. National Center for Complementary and Alternative Medicine
   - _____ 2. American Medical Association
   - _____ 3. U.S. Food and Drug Administration
   - _____ 4. Holistic Nursing Society

4. Acupuncture has been approved as a complementary therapy for:
   - _____ 1. Substance abuse
   - _____ 2. Schizophrenia
   - _____ 3. Dementia
   - _____ 4. Mania

5. All of the following have contributed to the increasing use of alternative therapies in the United States except:
   - _____ 1. Increase in chronic illnesses
   - _____ 2. Dissatisfaction with traditional health care system
   - _____ 3. Rising cost of health care
   - _____ 4. Proof of safety and efficacy of alternative therapies

6. St. John's wort has been found to be effective for:
   - _____ 1. Dementia
   - _____ 2. Mild-to-moderate depression
   - _____ 3. Depression with psychotic features
   - _____ 4. Depression with suicidal ideation

7. Which of the following interview questions would increase the chances of finding out about a patient's use of alternative or complementary therapies?
   - _____ 1. "Do you use any remedies such as herbs, vitamins, massage therapy, or other therapies besides those prescribed by your doctor?"
   - _____ 2. "Do you ever do anything else to help with your problem that your doctor hasn't approved?"
   - _____ 3. "Have you ever tried any of those Eastern therapies?"
   - _____ 4. "Do you use anything from another kind of health practitioner that we need to know about?"

8. The clinical reason it would be useful to have tighter regulation of herbals is:
   _____ 1. Standardization of doses and purity of contents
   _____ 2. Limiting the amount of money spent on products that are not legitimate
   _____ 3. Controlling access to herbal products that are not proven scientifically effective
   _____ 4. Preventing the sale of herbals in health food stores

9. Relaxation and meditation have been shown in some studies to:
   _____ 1. Reduce circulating catecholamine levels
   _____ 2. Raise dopamine levels in the periphery
   _____ 3. Increase omega-3 fatty acids
   _____ 4. Decrease white blood cells

10. Homeopathic remedies involve:
    _____ 1. Using healing methods within the home
    _____ 2. Manipulating muscles and tendons for relaxation
    _____ 3. Combining pharmaceutical agents with herbal preparations
    _____ 4. Using very dilute quantities of the substance that produces the symptoms as a treatment

11. Which of the following statements is *true* regarding regulation of alternative health care practitioners?
    _____ 1. There are standards of practice for all alternative health care practitioners.
    _____ 2. There is a great variability in the credentialing and licensure of alternative health care practitioners.
    _____ 3. Only licensed physicians may prescribe herbals and other alternative therapies.
    _____ 4. The National Credentialing Board of Alternative Health Practitioners must certify all health care practitioners using alternative health care methods.

12. The American Holistic Nurses Association Certification connotes:
    _____ 1. Nomination by consumers of the nurse's holistic approach to care
    _____ 2. Prescriptive authority for herbals, homeopathic remedies, and acupuncture
    _____ 3. Specialized education in the use of all modalities of alternative health care
    _____ 4. Having met competency standards for integrating the body-mind-spirit connection in their nursing care

Indicate *T* for true and *F* for false:
_____ 13. Because herbals are natural, they are safe for an unborn fetus.
_____ 14. Herbals are beneficial during the first trimester of pregnancy.
_____ 15. In general, it is best to avoid herbal therapies during pregnancy.
_____ 16. Most herbals can be safely used after the first trimester of pregnancy.
_____ 17. Very few people use alternative or complimentary therapies in the United States.
_____ 18. Natural herbs can cause severe reactions, including cardiac arrhythmias, liver failure, and several other potentially fatal reactions.

Chapter 41

Name: _____

Survivors of Violence and Trauma

Choose the *most* appropriate answer to the following questions:

1. Victims of crime experience emotional violation even when there is no physical injury. This violation involves which of the following?
   _____ 1. Loss of trust and sense of autonomy
   _____ 2. Destruction of personal property
   _____ 3. "Blaming the victim"
   _____ 4. Depression

2. Which of the following needs and rights of rape survivors must be addressed immediately during emergency department procedures?
   _____ 1. A medical release to work
   _____ 2. The presence of a representative of the prosecutor's office
   _____ 3. A referral for long-term counseling
   _____ 4. Privacy, confidentiality, and resource information

3. At a workshop on incest that is geared toward schoolteachers, which of the following statements would you present as most accurate?
   _____ 1. Incest involves physical assault and rape by an older relative.
   _____ 2. Most victims report the abuse when they reach adolescence.
   _____ 3. Coercion is the means used to get victims to conceal the abuse.
   _____ 4. It is best for survivors to confront the perpetrators.

4. A close friend describes nightmares that she is having about her father, anxiety when her boyfriend touches her, and a wish to be dead. Your most appropriate question is which of the following?
   _____ 1. "What is wrong with your boyfriend?"
   _____ 2. "Are you afraid of your father?"
   _____ 3. "Was your father sexual with you when you were a child?"
   _____ 4. "Why do you want to be dead?"

5. For most crime survivors, the type of resource needed depends on the stage of recovery with which they are struggling. The most appropriate resource in the recoil stage is which of the following?
   _____ 1. Crisis intervention
   _____ 2. Support groups
   _____ 3. Long-term counseling
   _____ 4. Medical attention

6. A woman calls a crisis phone service. She is crying and saying that her husband is getting drunk and will probably beat her up as usual. Which of the following interventions is the most appropriate?
   _____ 1. Giving her the number for the prosecutor's office
   _____ 2. Sending her information about the dynamics of partner abuse
   _____ 3. Telling her to get rid of all alcohol in the house as soon as she can
   _____ 4. Assisting her to get to a safe place if she is willing

7. A co-worker confides to the nurse that her former husband has been following her everywhere she goes before and after work. Which of the following suggestions would be most appropriate?

    _____ 1. Tell her to tell her former husband to leave her alone, or she will have him arrested for sexual harassment.

    _____ 2. Have her make arrangements to get a ride to and from work every day.

    _____ 3. Encourage her to talk to the employee counselor about options for dealing with the situation.

    _____ 4. Point out to her that her former husband's actions are annoying but not dangerous.

8. The nurse is designing an in-service for the emergency department staff as victims of partner abuse. It would be particularly important to include which of the following factors?

    _____ 1. Leaving an abusive partner is a process over time. Returning to the abuser is typical.

    _____ 2. The victim will need to stay with a relative until it is safe to return home.

    _____ 3. Staff members should include the abuser in the assessment and referral processes.

    _____ 4. Once the abuse is reported to the police, the abuser will no longer risk being abusive.

9. For families, friends, and survivors affected by the terrorist attacks at the World Trade Center and the Pentagon, critical incident stress management was a crucial intervention in the months after the events. Since then, the priority goals for recovery have focused on which of the following?

    _____ 1. Relocation to a community less at risk for terrorism

    _____ 2. Regaining a sense of trust, safety, and security

    _____ 3. Input into the design of a permanent memorial at each site

    _____ 4. Improved and better coordinated disaster plans

    Case Study: On September 18, 2001, Craig was seen in the emergency department with a serious overdose of psychotropic medications (Risperdal, Desyrel, Tegretol, and Catapres). He has been hospitalized in the past for posttraumatic stress, depression, dissociative episodes, self-mutilation, and suicide attempts. He was treated for 2 days in the medical ICU and is being transferred to the inpatient psychiatric unit. The ICU nurse verbally reports on the current status of Craig's medical problems, as well as the following: "He talked incessantly about things like the terrorist conspiracy, the evil in the world, world destruction, not trusting anybody, lack of control over his life, sex, rituals, sacrifices, being in a coffin, and how he just had to die if he didn't kill someone soon."

    Critical Thinking Questions: Given only this information from which to develop a care plan, answer the following questions: *(Write your answers on a separate sheet of paper, if necessary.)*

1. What kind of crimes or traumas and symptoms would you need to investigate with Craig?

2. What nurse-patient relationship strategies would be best to use to enhance your nursing assessment?

3. What short-term goals would you suggest in your treatment plan?

4. What referrals would be appropriate for Craig?

Chapter **42**

Name: _____

Child and Adolescent Psychiatric Nursing

Choose the *most* appropriate answer to the following questions:

1. Which of the following is considered a risk factor for childhood psychiatric disorders?
   _____ 1. Intact family
   _____ 2. Genetic vulnerability
   _____ 3. Social support
   _____ 4. Age

2. The child with ADHD would most likely exhibit which of the following symptoms?
   _____ 1. Anxiety
   _____ 2. Positive peer relationships
   _____ 3. Hostility
   _____ 4. Restlessness

3. Which of the following psychostimulants is falling out of use because of reports of hepatic failure?
   _____ 1. Methylphenidate (Ritalin)
   _____ 2. Amphetamine
   _____ 3. Pemoline (Cylert)
   _____ 4. Methylphenidate (Concerta)

4. According to Rosenbaum, which of the following SSRIs need not be tapered slowly to avoid withdrawal effects?
   _____ 1. Fluvoxamine
   _____ 2. Fluoxetine
   _____ 3. Paroxetine
   _____ 4. Sertraline

5. Many childhood and adolescent psychiatric disorders are more prevalent in boys. Which of the following is more common in girls?
   _____ 1. ADHD
   _____ 2. Depression in adolescents
   _____ 3. Tic disorders
   _____ 4. Conduct disorders

6. Ken's psychiatric diagnosis is ADHD. With the aid of medication, a short-term goal for Ken would be:
   _____ 1. To sit and play with his toys for 90 minutes
   _____ 2. To get along better with other children
   _____ 3. To express his anger in an acceptable manner
   _____ 4. To stop before throwing a toy across the room

7. Carol is exhibiting behavioral changes suggesting obsessive-compulsive disorder. Which of the following would be the primary nursing intervention?
   _____ 1. Assist Carol in identifying events or situations that trigger the urge to carry out repetitive behavior.
   _____ 2. Provide tension-relieving activities.
   _____ 3. Develop a relationship with Carol that promotes trust.
   _____ 4. Help Carol identify angry feelings.

8. What is the most important capacity that a nurse working with adolescents should have?

_____ 1. Denial of personal limitations

_____ 2. Flexibility with predictability

_____ 3. Serious attitude

_____ 4. Ability to challenge

9. Schizophrenia is more common in:

_____ 1. Young children (6 to 12 years)

_____ 2. Adolescence (12 to 16 years)

_____ 3. Young adulthood (17 to 25 years)

_____ 4. Middle adulthood (25 to 40 years)

10. The most commonly prescribed drug for ADHD is:

_____ 1. Methylphenidate (Ritalin)

_____ 2. Amphetamine

_____ 3. Pemoline (Cylert)

_____ 4. Clonidine (Catoptric)

11. Carol is exhibiting behavioral changes that suggest that she is depressed and possibly suicidal. What would be the primary nursing intervention?

_____ 1. Assist Carol in identifying her strengths.

_____ 2. Provide tension-relieving activities.

_____ 3. Develop a relationship with Carol that promotes trust.

_____ 4. Help Carol identify angry feelings.

Case Study: Randy is a 9-year-old boy with ADHD. He is currently in the third grade at the neighborhood public school. According to his teacher, he is defiant and disruptive in the classroom and would do better in school if "he tried harder…." The teacher also notes that the late morning is the worst part of the day—before his noon time medication. At home, his mother notes that he requires close supervision lest he get into trouble with neighbor kids or his younger brother. In her words, "It's always someone else's fault, but if I'm not watching him, look out, trouble is coming." He is quick to perceive hostile intent from others and often acts on that belief, resulting in arguments or fights. He likes sports, but often can't wait his turn.

In addition to hyperactivity and impulsive behavior, his mother also complains that Randy doesn't listen, defies rules, and argues with his mother and father. His father drives a delivery truck and works long hours; therefore Randy's mother is the primary disciplinarian in the family. Over the previous several months, Randy's mother finds herself having to exact increasingly stronger punishments. "I yell and scream, I send him to his room, I take away his toys, I've even spanked him a few times—nothing works." The worst period at home is the late afternoon and early evening.

Randy is healthy with no history of serious illnesses or injuries. He had multiple ear infections as a young child, which was largely resolved following the installation of pressure equalizing tubes. He is average height and slender build, weighing about 65 pounds. The first sign of difficulty emerged in kindergarten when he was unable to remain seated. The first grade went a bit better because there was an aide in the classroom. He was diagnosed with ADHD by the pediatrician and started on methylphenidate in the second grade. He is currently taking 10 mg of methylphenidate twice per day (7:30 AM and 12:00 noon).

Critical Thinking Questions: *(Write your answers on a separate sheet of paper, if necessary.)*

1. Based on data from the MTA study, what medication change would make sense in Randy's case? Why?

2. In addition to medication, parent management training would be an appropriate intervention for Randy and his family. Why would this be an appropriate intervention, and how would the nurse present this intervention to the family?

43

Name: _____

Mental Disorders in Older Adults

Choose the *most* appropriate answer to the following questions:

1. While hospitalized for depression, Mr. Lassern, a 78-year-old Caucasian widower with long-standing diabetes, complains of severe burning pains in his feet. Which of the following nursing actions would be the best?

   _____ 1. Recognizing that older adults often have somatic complaints when they are depressed, engage Mr. Lassern in a discussion of his feelings.

   _____ 2. Recognizing that Mr. Lassern's pain is probably related to his diabetic neuropathy, allow him to remain in bed rather than take part in unit activities.

   _____ 3. Perform a pain assessment.

   _____ 4. Express sympathy for Mr. Lassern's discomfort, but require that he participate in unit activities.

2. The physician places Mr. Lassern on an antidepressant to target his depressive symptoms that include lethargy, hopelessness, and withdrawn behavior. Which of the following antidepressants would you most likely expect to be selected?

   _____ 1. Trazodone (Desyrel)

   _____ 2. Fluoxetine (Prozac)

   _____ 3. Amitriptyline (Elavil)

   _____ 4. Phenelzine (Nardil)

3. Modifying the psychologic assessment to fit the special needs of older adults is useful in which of the following ways?

   _____ 1. List skills and behaviors expected of a person the patient's age.

   _____ 2. Schedule an interview in the late afternoon or evening.

   _____ 3. Discourage reminiscing by using direct questions.

   _____ 4. Compensate for vision or hearing impairments, and allow extra time for patients to respond.

4. On admission, Mr. Lassern's family expressed concern that he might be "drinking too much." Which of the following would be helpful in determining whether alcohol is a problem?

   _____ 1. Using the CAGE or G-MAST in the assessment

   _____ 2. Mr. Lassern's statements about how much he drank

   _____ 3. Mr. Lassern's statement that he didn't drink any more alcohol now than he did when he was 30 years of age

   _____ 4. Mr. Lassern's reassurance that he only drank when he had difficulty sleeping since his wife's death

5. In the first decades after the year 2000, the estimated proportion of the population over 65 will:

   _____ 1. Remain stable

   _____ 2. Decline

   _____ 3. Experience modest growth

   _____ 4. Increase substantially

6. Psychiatric disorders among older adults are:
_____ 1. Generally independent of other health-related problems
_____ 2. Usually associated with other significant health problems
_____ 3. Infrequent and self-limiting
_____ 4. Rampant and inevitable

7. Which of the following is not a barrier to mental health care for older adults?
_____ 1. Family members preferring more personalized services
_____ 2. Discrimination by some health care providers
_____ 3. Attitudes of older adults about mental illness
_____ 4. Failure to detect mental illness

Briefly answer the following questions:

8. The physician places Mr. Lassern on suicide precautions. List at least four factors that place him at risk.

9. In the year 2050, what approximate percentage of the population will be over the age of 65?

10. List the reasons that the treatment needs for mental health services have been underestimated for the older adult population.

11. Depression is the most common mental illness in older adults, yet it is often overlooked, misdiagnosed, or inadequately treated. List at least four consequences of these limitations in contemporary health care.

Case Study: Woody, a 78-year-old widower, is a patient of the geropsychiatric unit. He is withdrawn and angry with his family for "tricking" him into the psychiatric hospital. He thought he was being admitted for assessment of his painful diabetic neuropathy. On the evening shift, the nurse notices that Woody's door is closed. When the nurse knocks and enters, she finds Woody weeping silently and saying, "Dear Jesus, take me. Oh Jesus, Jesus, please don't punish me any more. Oh Lord, Oh Lord." The nurse finds him inconsolable.

Critical Thinking Questions: *(Write your answers on a separate sheet of paper.)*

1. How would you describe what is happening to this patient?

2. You have probably heard about spiritual care in your nursing program, but most care providers are reluctant to have "religious discussions" with patients. Would you be comfortable dealing with Woody's religious expressions? How would you say something meaningful without imposing your own religious views?

3. Legislation and funding for older adults are receiving a lot of attention. Pressure to ensure continuance of social security and increase benefits for Medicare is high. Within the last few years, however, some people have been questioning these efforts; they point out that the most at-risk group in this country include children, who represent our future. Money is critically needed for schools, health care, and safety. These individuals believe that a greater good would be realized by shifting societal support to the young instead of to older adults who already enjoy significant advantages. Which side of the argument do you take? Why? Are there dangers in pitting one group against the other?

Working with Patients with HIV Infection

Choose the *most* appropriate answer to the following questions:

1. What proportion of AIDS cases in the United States is attributable to the risk of behavior of homosexual sex?
   - _____ 1. 15%
   - _____ 2. 25%
   - _____ 3. 45%
   - _____ 4. 75%

2. What is the most common psychiatric disorder among people with HIV disease?
   - _____ 1. Bipolar disorder
   - _____ 2. Major depressive disorder
   - _____ 3. Borderline personality disorder
   - _____ 4. Adjustment disorder with anxious, depressed, or mixed mood

3. The symptoms of HIV-associated dementia most closely mimic the symptoms of which psychiatric disorder?
   - _____ 1. Bipolar disorder
   - _____ 2. Major depressive disorder
   - _____ 3. Borderline personality disorder
   - _____ 4. Adjustment disorder

4. Which of the following is most likely to be affected by discrimination related to HIV status?
   - _____ 1. Overall life satisfaction
   - _____ 2. Medication adherence
   - _____ 3. Sexual risk behavior
   - _____ 4. Severity of disease

5. The most common cause of sexual dysfunction in HIV-positive individuals is:
   - _____ 1. Shame and guilt
   - _____ 2. Anxiety and depression
   - _____ 3. Anemia
   - _____ 4. Hypogonadism

6. Current estimates suggest that up to what percentage of patients receiving HAART is non-adherent to their HIV-medication regimen?
   - _____ 1. 10%
   - _____ 2. 25%
   - _____ 3. 50%
   - _____ 4. 80%

7. Under certain conditions, individuals receiving social security disability income payments who wish to attempt a return to work may work for up to how many months without losing their benefits?
   - _____ 1. 3
   - _____ 2. 4
   - _____ 3. 6
   - _____ 4. 9

8. Which of the following methods for HIV transmission has been virtually eliminated?
   _____ 1. Exchange of blood or body fluids through sexual contact with a homosexual HIV-infected person
   _____ 2. Exchange of blood or body fluids through sexual contact with a heterosexual HIV-infected person
   _____ 3. Parenteral injection of blood or blood products infected with HIV
   _____ 4. Vertical transmission of HIV from mother to baby

Case Study: Laura, a 37-year-old widowed African-American woman, was diagnosed with HIV 1 year ago after the onset of PCP pneumonia and candida esophagitis. She temporarily stayed with her mother while recuperating, but she planned to move back to her home as soon as her condition would allow. Five years earlier, her husband died of AIDS. She has a 10-year-old son who is not infected with HIV. Although she worked occasionally, her primary income was from the death benefits of her late husband. After a slow recovery from PCP pneumonia, HAART was initiated. She regained her energy and moved back into her apartment where she lived with her son. Her weight increased from 96 pounds to 122 pounds. However, Laura did not tolerate the initial therapy, because of an episode of mania possibly caused by the lamivudine, anemia related to zidovudine, and diarrhea related to nelfinavir. She developed peripheral neuropathy when switched to a regimen containing stavudine. Six months after diagnosis, Laura developed major depression. She frequently found that she was unable to stop crying. Owing to difficulties of transportation, she resisted psychotherapy or counseling. Laura did not have a car. Her brother brought her to the clinic, but he had to miss work to do so. A number of psychopharmacologic agents were initiated but discontinued for reasons related to toxicity. Eventually, mirtazapine was instituted and her symptoms of depression abated. Unfortunately, her response to HAART was minimal at best. She remained severely immunosuppressed with a high viral titer. Her nurse practitioner suspected nonadherence, but Laura insisted that she fell asleep or forgot and that she took her medicine most of the time. She estimated that she missed the evening dose of medicine every other day.

On her most recent visit to the clinic, Laura reported that she had tried to work as a part-time cashier to make a little extra money so she could afford some of the things her son wanted before entering school. However, the pain in her feet and the fatigue would not allow her to stand the required 8 hours. She began to sob and stated that she knew "she was getting worse," "was losing weight," and was afraid she "would die soon." She said she thought she needed to move back to her mother's house because she lacked the energy to take care of herself and her son.

Critical Thinking Questions:

1. What educational topics might be appropriate to discuss with an HIV-related patient facing transition to disability?

2. What issues might you expect to be most important when working with HIV-infected mother confronting death when you know she has a 10-year-old son?

3. Identify five NANDA-approved nursing diagnoses that would be appropriate to Laura's current situation, and describe your plans for intervention.

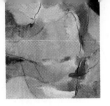

Answer Key to Student Worksheets

Unit I: Introduction to Psychiatric Nursing

Chapter 1: Introduction to Psychiatric Nursing

1. 3
2. 4
3. 1
4. 1
5. 2
6. 2
7. 1
8. Assistance; banishment; confinement
9. Pinel, Tuke
10. b
11. d
12. a
13. e
14. A place of refuge; sanctuary
15. Medications used in the treatment of mental disorders
16. Term used to describe the concept of treating patients where their lives would be less restricted
17. The depopulation of state hospitals
18. Typically healthy individuals experience difficulty coping with their current situation
19. F
20. T

Chapter 2: Psychotherapeutic Management in the Continuum of Care

1. 2
2. 4
3. 2
4. 1
5. 2
6. 3
7. 1
8. 2
9. 2
10. Safety, structure, norms, limit setting, balance, and environmental modification
11. Self, medication, and environment
12. Drug and alcohol treatment programs
13. Examples:
    Dispense medications
    Evaluate need for prn medications
    Assess patient's response to medications
    Plan for a response to medications
    Assess for side effects, treat, and evaluate treatment
    Educate patients on medications and answer questions
14. The study of underlying processes, both biological and psychosocial, that lead to mental disorders.

Chapter 3: Models for Working with Psychiatric Patients

1. 3
2. 1
3. 4
4. 2
5. 1
6. 2
7. 3
8. 1
9. 4
10. 4

Case Study and Critical Thinking Questions

1. *Projection of blame:* Accuses Jamie of causing the divorce
   Denial: Denies her role in the divorce and of the need for counseling
   Intellectualization: Describes situation without showing emotion
   Rationalization: "If Tony can have sex...so can I"
   Regression: All she does at home is cry
2. *Stage I—Hostility:* Toward Tony
   Projection of blame: Accuses Tony
   Dissatisfaction: Nothing left to her life
   Withdrawal: At home, from friends
   Stage II—Dependence on other for approval: From friends
   Self-conscious: Not wanting to be seen by friends
   Self-doubt: No longer thinks that she is attractive
   Stage III—Reluctance to show emotions: "While showing no emotion..."
3. a. Blames Jamie instead
   b. Nothing is left to her life
   c. Not wanting to be seen by friends
   d. "If Tony can have sex...so can I"
   e. "Does not need counseling"
4. *Focus on decreasing anxiety:* Decrease stimuli and distractions, encourage adaptive coping, problem solving, and relaxation.

Chapter 4: Legal Issues

1. 2
2. 3
3. 4
4. 3
5. 3
6. 3
7. 2
8. 1
9. d
10. i

11. g, h
12. f
13. m
14. c
15. p
16. e
17. f
18. b
19. a
20. c
21. d

Chapter 5: Psychobiologic Bases of Behavior

1. 2
2. 3
3. 2
4. 2
5. 1
6. 3
7. 2
8. 2
9. 4
10. 2
11. 1
12. 1
13. Upper motor neuron
14. b
15. b
16. a
17. a
18. c, d
19. a
20. b

Unit II: Continuum of Care

Chapters 6 through 8

1. 3
2. 2
3. 4
4. 3
5. 2
6. 4
7. 3
8. 2
9. 3
10. 4

Case and Critical Thinking Question

Katie: Crises resources if she becomes suicidal again; outpatient counseling (but no medications because of her pregnancy); prenatal care and classes, if she decides to continue the pregnancy, or an abortion clinic, if she does not; parenting classes if she chooses to keep the baby, or adoption resources if she does not; self-esteem and stress management classes.

Matthew: A home visit to evaluate his mental and physical status; possible admission to an Older Adult Unit for a complete assessment and treatment of his medical and psychiatric needs, as well as an evaluation of the family's ability to care for him at home.

Mary Elizabeth: Outpatient evaluations of her possible depression and need for medication and counseling; a home visit to assess her ability to meet Matthew's home safety and care requirement needs, if he is able to stay with the family; a support group for families of those with Alzheimer's disease; respite care resources, if needed.

Sam: Continue seeing the Employee Assistance counselor at work; a 2-week outpatient relapse program in the evenings, if he is willing; frequent AA meetings.

Sam Jr: Outpatient evaluation for possible substance abuse and treatment, if needed; sex education and counseling, if his is willing; self-esteem and stress-management classes.

Mark: School-based counselor for periodic assessment of his needs and counseling, if appropriate; continued involvement with his support system and activities.

Unit III: Therapeutic Nurse-Patient Relationship

Chapter 9: Communication

1. 1
2. 4
3. 2
4. 4
5. 3
6. 4
7. 1
8. 2
9. 1
10. 3
11. Nontherapeutic
12. Giving information
13. Therapeutic
14. Presenting reality
15. Nontherapeutic
16. False reassurance
17. Therapeutic
18. Clarification

Chapter 10: Nurse-Patient Relationship

1. 4
2. 3
3. 1
4. 3
5. 3
6. 2
7. 1
8. 2
9. 2
10. 4

Case Study and Critical Thinking Question

Building trust and beginning assessment: "I'm the nurse who will work with you today, and I would like to help you with any concerns you have. Tell me a little about what you are experiencing right now."

Conveying empathy: "I realize that it is difficult for you to be here without knowing why."

Conveying empathy and managing emotions: "I hear how upset and angry you are. Tell me more about what you are feeling right now."

Providing support and beginning assessment: "You want to go back to your corner and that is important to you. Let's talk about the circumstances that led to your admission."

Providing structure: "You have been pacing in your room for quite a while. I can give you a medicine that will help you relax and feel less worried. Then maybe we can talk together."

Reality testing related to hallucinations: "I know that listening to God's voice is important to you, but I don't hear his voice."

Supportive confrontation: "Telling God's messages on your corner means a lot to you. Where would be a safer place for you to do this?"

Teaching new skills: "I can show you some relaxation techniques to use when you are feeling upset or restless."

Evaluation of progress: "I am glad you have decided to keep praying to yourself and in church. I think this will help keep you out of trouble with the police. What else do you want to work on with your outpatient counselor?"

Referrals: "I have your discharge instructions for you to read and take home with you. It lists your medicines and the time of your appointment with your counselor this Friday."

Dealing with hallucinations and delusions: "Tell me more about hearing God's voice and being his special messenger."

Dealing with denial: "You said you don't belong in the hospital. What were you doing when the police arrived?"

Dealing with suspiciousness: "Since you will be here for a few days, let me tell you about the staff and the activities on the unit.

Chapter 11: Nursing Process

1. 2
2. 3
3. 4
4. 3
5. 1
6. 2
7. 4
8. 1
9. 3
10. 1
11. Patient will sign a no-harm contract within 2 hours
12. By day of discharge, patient will list three names and

telephone numbers of who to call when feeling suicidal again

Case Study and Critical Thinking Question

Demographic data: 20-year-old married male

Admission data: Unknown; brought by police

Reason for admission: Unknown; patient denies need to be here

Drug and alcohol abuse: Unknown; patient drinks vodka

Support systems: Quality of relationship with wife is unknown

General appearance: Wearing a jogging suit; standing back against the wall

Behaviors in interview: Refuses to give information; is withdrawn

Orientation: Aware that he is in the hospital

Memory: Remembers the police

Mood: Angry

Thought clarity: Coherent

Thought content: Denial of problems, suspicious, accuses wife of poisoning his vodka

Insight: Denies he has a problem

Judgment: Unknown; brought by police

Motivation: No motivation for treatment at this time

Chapter 12: Anxiety, Coping, and Crisis

1. 2
2. 4
3. 3
4. 1
5. 4
6. 3
7. 2
8. 1
9. 2
10. 3

Case Study and Critical Thinking Questions

1. Defensiveness, hypersensitivity, thoughts of hurting his wife, delusions, hallucinations, distorted perceptions

2. Decrease his anxiety, contract for safety (No harm contract) of self and others, build trust and offer support, help him manage emotions safely, bolster his sense of security

3. Behaviors that reflect high (+3) anxiety, interventions already done and the next most important interventions planned, Jason's verbal threat to hurt her and how this affects her visiting him

Chapter 13: Working with the Aggressive Patient

1. 3
2. 4
3. 2
4. 1
5. 4
6. 3
7. 2

8. 3
9. 4
10. 1

Case Study and Critical Thinking Questions

1. History of brain dysfunction, intellectual impairments, family violence or gross disorganization, previous incidents of violence and destructiveness, potential triggers of aggression.

2. Current source of anger and target, likelihood of escalation, how well he can talk about anger without losing control, willingness to agree to a no-harm contract.

3. Offer to help him gain control of his angry behaviors. Talk calmly and avoid sudden movements. Ask him to take prn medication and go to his room. Alert staff about what is happening.

4. Ask staff to be on stand-by at a distance. Inform him that staff will take control if he cannot follow directions and control himself. Try to escort him to his room without any bodily contact. Ask him to give staff any dangerous articles in his possession or in his room. Ask him to stay in his room without the door being locked.

Chapter 14: Working with Groups of Patients

1. 3
2. 4
3. 1
4. 3
5. 4
6. 3
7. 4
8. Possible groups that could be beneficial for these patients are a recreation group, such as exercise; creative expression groups (e.g., arts and crafts, music); psychoeducation groups such as illness management, mood management, signs of relapse, and dealing with crisis; medication groups including purpose, therapeutic effects, and side effect management; problem-solving groups such as relationship issues and discharge planning; stress management groups such as anger management, relaxation, and stress-reduction; and social skills groups such as assertiveness training and daily living skills.

9. The following statements would be useful for these patients in this group:

   For the silent or anxious member: "Some of us find it hard to talk in a group but everyone here has something to say that can help someone else."

   For the member who interrupts: "Joe, Larry was talking now. It will be your turn to talk when he is finished."

   For the dominant member: "Mona, you are contributing to our discussion today but I would like to hear what others are thinking."

   For the hostile member: "Hal, you sound angry today. What happened?"

Chapter 15: Working with the Family

1. 3
2. 4
3. 4
4. 3
5. 1
6. 4
7. 2

Case Study and Critical Thinking Questions

1. Developmental stresses facing Marla include:
   a. Empty nest syndrome
   b. Diminishing parental role
   c. Lack of generativity and sharing of life that is expected at the middle adult period of life

2. The fact that Marla is divorced and has no spouse to turn to for companionship and the fact that her last child just left home may make the loss seem greater to her.

3. Appropriate nursing diagnoses would be:
   a. Diversional activity deficit related to lowered mood as seen in sitting around home when not at work
   b. Knowledge deficit (antidepressant medication) related to a new diagnosis of illness, as seen in questions concerning the effects of her medication
   c. Social isolation related to changes in parental role as seen in sadness and crying

4. Short-term goals (STG)
   a. Marla will state the purpose, action and side effects of the antidepressant medication prescribed for her.
   b. Marla will verbally acknowledge the difficulties of adjusting to having all her children gone from home.
   c. Marla will talk with the nurse at least twice about her feelings related to living alone.

5. Long term goals (LTG)
   a. Marla will remain compliant with her medication regimen and report that her appetite, sleep, and mood have returned to normal.
   b. Marla will initiate at least one group activity outside work in which she participates at least once a week.

6. Interventions for STG
   a. Assess Marla's suicidal ideation, and plan to ensure patient safety.
   b. Explore Marla's feelings regarding her son to discover, and assess her feelings regarding the significance of this loss.
   c. Explore interests, past hobbies, and community activities to assess possible areas for the development of leisure activities.
   d. To build self-esteem, offer positive reinforcement for patient's ability to manage day-to-day activities.
   e. Teach desired effects, side effects, and mechanisms of action of the antidepressant that the patient is taking to improve compliance with medication regimen.

Chapter 16: Cultural Competence in Psychiatric Nursing

1. 2
2. 1
3. 2
4. 1
5. 1
6. 4
7. 4
8. 2
9. 4
10. 3
11. 2
12. 2
13. 3

Case Study and Critical Thinking Questions

1. If family visits are desired by the patient and if they do not interfere with the patient's treatment, the family could be allowed to visit with the patient off the unit to avoid disturbing and encroaching on other patients and families. Alternatively, two or three family members could be allowed to visit at one time on the unit on a rotating basis. The important point is to understand that the number of visitors is not uncommon among African Americans; hence, they should be accommodated unless it is harmful to the patient or other patients.

2. The important point here is to assess the patient's "baseline" beliefs about voodoo and other unnatural causation of illness. In other words, is this a manifestation of her illness or a deeply held cultural belief?

3. Although this does not fit with the biomedical understanding of mental illness, dismissing these views would alienate the family. The patient's family's beliefs should be incorporated by allowing the family to pursue cures in alignment with their own belief system, thus resulting in a greater likelihood of compliance. On the other hand, if the patient is not cooperating with the treatment and some negotiation with the family does not occur, perhaps the patient should be discharged. Related is the obvious case of tardive dyskinesia (TD). TD is typically irreversible; more than likely, Mary's symptoms cannot be resolved. Nonetheless, the fact that this was not "caught" earlier is not only evidence of poor psychiatric care, but it potentially undermines her confidence in "traditional" medicine.

Chapter 17: Spirituality

1. 2
2. 3
3. 4
4. 4
5. 1
6. 2
7. 3

8. 3
9. 2
10. 1

Case Study and Critical Thinking Questions

1. Although Wanda has a history of depression, it has been managed well for 20 years. She has began treatment for both depression and hypertension after the death of her husband. At her most recent hospitalization, she sought treatment for angina and was compliant with both the recommendation for surgery and the cardiac rehabilitation. Making preparation for her own death, however, could be one warning sign of suicidal ideation. As for the delusional thinking, it is important for the team to ask her what she means by "going home." This situation clearly calls for further clinical assessment, although her nurse did this only after the patient initiated a discussion about a living will.

2. Not at all. Given her family history, demographics, the reality of her own heart disease, and the fact that her husband died of a stroke, she realizes that she will die one day.

3. To Wanda, "going home" is symbolic language for dying and the after-life. She is not delusional. She is using the language of her faith to express that which gives her meaning and hope. She is also expressing that she is not afraid of death. Furthermore, Wanda does not want to kill herself. If she did, she would probably be noncompliant with treatment recommendations.

4. It is right to do an initial assessment for symptoms of depression or psychosis. Assuming that there is a spiritual care professional on the rehabilitation team (or available to it), this is a perfect opportunity for a referral to this professional. The spiritual care professional can help Wanda explore the issues of death, hope, and meaning. Through the team's intervention, the family can also come to understand that Wanda has reached some resolution about the high probability of her death as a result of heart disease. It is also a teachable moment for the health care team. Instead of assuming depression or psychosis, they can understand that Wanda speaks a spiritual language, and that no cause for further psychiatric assessment exists.

Unit IV: Psychopharmacology

Chapter 18: Introduction to Psychotropic Drugs

1. 1
2. 2
3. 4
4. 1
5. 3
6. 2
7. 4
8. 1

9. d
10. c
11. b
12. a
13. e
14. SSRIs
15. Thorazine, Clozaril
16. Block monoamine oxidase enzymes
17. Anatomic, physiologic, metabolic
18. Nicotine receptors are found at the myoneural junction and on the postganglionic neuron. Also, nicotine receptors modulate dopamine tracts in the pleasure pathway.

Chapter 19: Antiparkinson Drugs

1. 2
2. 1
3. 2
4. 1
5. 2
6. 4
7. 3
8. 1
9. 3
10. 3

Case Study and Critical Thinking Questions

1. Dystonic reaction (i.e., oculogyric crisis and torticollis)
2. Trihexyphenidyl is not available in a parenteral form.
3. Levodopa elevates dopamine levels and could cause exacerbation of psychotic symptoms.

Critical Thinking Questions

1. Sinemet. It contains both L-dopa and carbidopa. Carbidopa inhibits dopa decarboxylase from metabolizing levodopa.
2. Secondary symptoms are derived from primary symptoms. For example, rigidity causes difficulty in swallowing; difficulty in swallowing causes accumulation of saliva, which leads to drooling.

Chapter 20: Antipsychotic Drugs

1. 1
2. 2
3. 2
4. 3
5. 3
6. 4
7. 2
8. 1
9. 2
10. Theoretically, enhance dopamine in cortex and basal ganglia.
11. D_2

Case Studies and Critical Thinking Questions
Case Study I

1. 3
2. 2

Case Study II

1. This person receives both an antipsychotic and an antidepressant. It is not uncommon for both classes of drugs to be prescribed.
2. Positive schizophrenia is linked to excessive dopamine in limbic areas and can result in auditory hallucination (e.g., threatening voices). The withdrawal behavior seems to be more of a negative symptom and theoretically may be caused by decreased dopamine levels in the cortex. Although depression is not typically associated with dopamine fluctuations (actually, it is, but norepinephrine and serotonin get most of the attention), it seems reasonable that some problems with non-dopamine neurotransmitters would occur. Further, as will become clear in the chapter on schizophrenia, depression is relatively common among individuals with schizophrenia.

Chapter 21: Antidepressant Drugs

1. 3
2. 4
3. 3
4. 4
5. 1
6. 1
7. 2
8. 3
9. 4
10. 1
11. 2
12. 2
13. 3
14. 3

Case Study and Critical Thinking Questions

1. Joe would benefit from an anxiety drug such as lorazepam (Ativan) and an antidepressant. An SSRI or one of the novel antidepressants would be a good choice. In this particular case, the patient was prescribed sertraline 200 mg qd. It would also be important to assess whether auditory hallucinations are still occurring. If so, an atypical antipsychotic would be appropriate.
2. This is not clear-cut. Some clinicians believe that a traumatic rape can cause life-long problems. Others may believe that something was "going on with this person already" or the trauma would not have been this debilitating. I believe that some things in life are so hurtful they can follow an individual the rest of his or her life. There is evidence that indicates an individual's biochemistry and "hard-wiring" can change in response to trauma.

Chapter 22: Antimanic Drugs

1. 1
2. 2
3. 3
4. 4
5. 2
6. 4

Case Study and Critical Thinking Questions

1. Of course there is only limited information, but the fact that she would begin the conversation with "Yeah, I know I can trust you. They are coming to get me tonight." should at least trigger the idea that this woman is suspicious and may be delusional. Of course you would not label her as delusional until you had more assessment data, but warning signals should go off.

2. It would probably start confirming your initial thinking. Billie's response sounds paranoid and conspiratorial, which would indicate a full bipolar disorder as opposed to someone who is "only euphoric."

3. I think the best and definitely the safest approach would be to suspect lithium toxicity. The lithium should be held and the patient carefully monitored. When mild toxicity is suspected, giving her a glass of tomato juice with salt will help eliminate the lithium. It would also be important to order tests to determine serum lithium levels.

4. To keep lithium levels consistent, Billie will need to avoid strenuous activity, which causes excessive loss of sodium through sweating, and she will need to stay away from diets that restrict sodium. Sodium loss other than through urination can lead to an increase in lithium levels and a consequent lithium toxicity.

Chapter 23: Antianxiety Drugs

1. 2
2. 4
3. 3
4. 1
5. 2
6. 2
7. 2
8. 2
9. F

Case Study and Critical Thinking Questions

1. There are many concerns, but I think suicide is a possibility because John feels helpless and hopeless. Like many abused kids, John was handed a lousy deal, and as an adult he is still "paying" for it. John realizes he could have been "somebody." I would be concerned that he might finally give up on life.

2. My first thought would be that John is developing tolerance to the dose of alprazolam. Remember, tolerance to the antianxiety effects occur slowly, perhaps over a few months, but they do occur. He may need to have the alprazolam boosted to 1 mg tid. Of course, the sertraline might need to be adjusted as well.

3. My knee jerk reaction would be that the increase to 1 mg tid pushed him into the typical side effect profile and that might be exactly right. But I would be a little surprised given that John had developed tolerance to a dose just a little lower. My suspicious nature might

make me wonder if John was taking a nonprescribed depressant or perhaps even drinking a little alcohol. Either assessment could be correct.

4. Some individuals like John learn to deal with the stressors that trigger some of the worst reactions (e.g., they use avoidance), and they can live a relatively comfortable life. However, drugs alone are seldom the answer. Often, individual therapy or behavior therapy are useful. Unfortunately, some individuals never improve a great deal. They learn to live very confined and, at times, miserable lives.

Unit V: Milieu Management
Chapter 24: Introduction to Milieu Management

1. 1
2. 1
3. 2
4. 1
5. 1
6. 3
7. T
8. T
9. T
10. F
11. T
12. Distribution of responsibility and decision making, high level of interaction with patients and staff, and clarity of role and leadership of the program.
13. Discharge planning is crucial for making the "continuum of care" work. The following issues should be assessed and considered:
    - Home health care
    - Residential facility placement
    - Day treatment
    - Return to work
    - Family support of patient
    - System support of family
    - Outpatient support

Chapter 25: Variables Affecting the Therapeutic Environment

1. 1
2. 3
3. 2
4. 3
5. 2
6. 3
7. 1
8. T
9. c
10. b
11. e
12. d
13. a

14. Articulation of one's perception of what another person has said or meant
15. Learn, practice, and develop certain social skills that are deficient in the patient
16. Holding the individual accountable for behavior
17. Learn, practice, and develop skills required for survival on the street
18. A strategy for teaching patients and families about disorders, treatments, coping techniques, and resources, based on the observation that people can better participate in their own care if knowledge deficits are removed
19. Holding people to established norms with the intent of helping them function more constructively and effectively
20. Making sure that the treatment environment is safe; safety overlaps all other concerns and always should be the highest priority

Case Study and Critical Thinking Questions

1. Julie is in a position with two supervisors, neither of whom are adequately attending to her needs and strengths as a nurse. Julie is working with non-RN staff and has no support from her unit manager or RN supervisor. The nature of Julie's work activities and the staffing arrangement excludes Julie from active participation in the treatment process and in collaboration with other staff. This lack of support from management, separation from other treatment staff, and minimization of her role as RN will likely lead to low morale for Julie and will also diminish her value to other staff. Patients become aware of strained work relationships in such a setting, and this will eventually have a negative affect on the milieu for patients and staff.

2. As the direct RN supervisor for Julie, action must be taken to support and develop the role of an RN in the addiction and recovery unit. It is the responsibility of the RN supervisor to negotiate with the unit manager and possibly other persons in management for the appropriate use of the experience and skills of an RN in the treatment setting. Although this is clearly an issue that should have been addressed before the opening of this unit, it is still possible for the RN supervisor to meet with the appropriate people in management to advocate for Julie's role as an RN. It may be that education regarding the role of an RN is necessary, a matter that can be easily corrected. If the issue is a lack of value for an RN, a different strategy is indicated. In this incidence, meetings among treatment staff may be necessary for the purpose of talking through issues of interprofessional conflict. The important point here is that without the support of her RN supervisor, Julie is paralyzed in her effectiveness as a member of the treatment team.

3. Julie, although somewhat restrained by her supervisors, still has a professional and personal responsibility to fulfill her role on the treatment team. When it is time for treatment team meetings, Julie might negotiate with neighboring units to provide coverage of the nursing station while she attends the meeting. Julie might also request a meeting with someone above the level of her RN supervisor or with someone in human resources. Ultimately, Julie may have to resign this position and seek something more in alignment with her professional abilities. Sometimes, a resignation is the best way to send a message to management that a work situation is not acceptable. If subsequent RNs also refuse to accept the "status quo," management will eventually have to respond because an RN is required on the unit.

Chapter 26: Therapeutic Environment in Different Treatment Settings

1. 2
2. 3
3. 4
4. 4
5. 4
6. 1
7. 4
8. 4
9. 1
10. 2
11. T
12. T
13. T
14. F
15. c
16. f
17. d
18. b
19. e
20. a
21. To treat the patient holistically, the nurse should be able to assess, attend to, and refer for treatment symptoms indicating physical problems. Just as the medical-surgical nurse is expected to meet some psychiatric and mental health needs of patients, the psychiatric nurse is expected to meet some medical-surgical needs of patients. Finally, patients are increasingly more acutely ill and more likely to have or develop concurrent medical or physical disorders.

Case Study and Critical Thinking Questions

1. The doors to the unit should be locked with an access code or keyed entry for staff. Cameras will need to be visible in the halls and corridors to view activity on the unit. The nursing station needs to be centrally located with a view of the entire unit. The nursing station

should have an open appearance with easy access by the patients. Several different treatment rooms and dining areas need to be available for patients. Private visiting areas need to be available. The unit should be attractive but not overstimulating. Soothing colors should be used.

2. An open nursing station creates a more open environment for patients and minimizes the feeling of separateness. This arrangement encourages more interaction between patients and staff. Separate areas for less acutely ill patients will be helpful as a refuge. Patients dealing with depression and anxiety may find the patients with psychosis disturbing or frightening. Research has shown that loud or bright colors are more stimulating, whereas soothing colors have a calming effect on patients. Although opportunities for all patients to interact together need to be available, there needs to be spaces, other than the patient rooms, to serve as a "refuge" from other patients. The same is true for the staff; some space needs to be available where staff members can retreat and regroup as necessary.

3. Some activities can be shared on the unit, such as a therapeutic community meeting or some recreational activities; however, ideally, activities appropriate to the patient's treatment needs should be provided. Patients with depression and anxiety will need more focused classroom educational-type activities, whereas patients with disturbances in thinking will need areas suitable for activities that focus on improving concentration and attention, such as tasks guided to completion (e.g., drawing, categorizing objects, completing lists).

Unit VI: Psychopathology

Chapter 27: Introduction to Psychopathology

1. 1
2. 3
3. 3
4. 2
5. 4
6. 1
7. Over 50 million, about 25%
8. Anxiety disorder, phobias, mood disorders, alcohol disorder, major depression
9. *Nature:* Biology, genetics, neurochemistry, pathophysiology
Nurture: Environment, early life experiences, stressors

Case Study and Critical Thinking Question

First, although we plunked this "case study" down in front of you, we caution you not to succumb to the temptation of "analyzing" your classmates.

Now to address the question: People are different, people handle stress differently, and, quite frankly, some people can just handle more stress. Nonetheless, of the

two students, Sally seems "more together" than does Jane. Although the information provided is limited, it would be only fair to say that Jane is struggling. Obviously, Jane may have situational problems in her life that have her on edge (e.g., financial, relational), or her reaction may be more "organic"; research does show that exposure to certain kinds of stressors in childhood can cause a person to have a decreased threshold for stress later in life. Whether this finding is true for Jane, we cannot tell.

Chapter 28: Schizophrenia and Other Psychoses

1. 2
2. 3
3. 1
4. 1
5. 2
6. 2
7. 1
8. 1
9. 3
10. 2
11. 1
12. 3
13. 1
14. 3
15. 2
16. 2
17. 1
18. T
19. Hallucinations, delusions, disordered thinking

Case Study and Critical Thinking Questions

1. This is a good question, and to answer it, one needs an appreciation of some of the content in Chapter 1 and the "phases" of schizophrenia discussed in this chapter. T.Z. is stable. She is not stable at a high level but stable enough not to need treatment offered in a state hospital. On the other hand, someone requiring this much medication to stabilize should be observed closely. Living in a psychiatric group home and seeing a nurse on a weekly basis is adequate for now.

2. This amount of medication is extraordinary; but some individuals require this dose level to stabilize. This case study represents a real person with some of the information altered for confidentiality purposes. The author has given more haloperidol decanoate than T.Z. is receiving but only a few times in a long career.

3. In a word, institutionalization! Although this phenomenon is not nearly as common as it was years ago, 18 years is a long time. Institutionalized individuals often can no longer adequately perform the things that are required in modern American life (e.g., cooking, cleaning, shopping).

Chapter 29: Depression
1. 1
2. 3
3. 2
4. 2
5. 3
6. 2
7. 2
8. 1
9. 1
10. 2
11. 2
12. T
13. Biologic; psychologic and/or psychodynamic

Case Study and Critical Thinking Questions
1. Living with a depressed person can be very difficult. Reread the situation in the Family Issues box in which Joan and her husband were having difficulties. Whereas we are led to believe that depression is a result of divorce, many of us often believe it is the cause of the divorce.
2. Their marriage had been deteriorating for a long time. Of course, you do not know this fact from a brief vignette, but such a scenario is not uncommon anyway. In this marriage, there had been loud, mean-spirited arguing for some time. In other words, the marital stress exacerbated Billie's symptoms. After the initial shock of the divorce, many individuals thought Billie actually started doing better.
3. Billie was a difficult person to treat, but the principle of working with the patient until an effective treatment regimen is found would be true for any patient with depression.
4. In my opinion, needing to change medications this many times is unusual, but it is not rare.
5. It is troubling and ironic. Billie has basically recovered from depression only to have a life pretty much empty of any meaningful relationship. Although older women are not at particularly high risk for suicide, a person who has fought to regain "sanity" only to be alone is a person to assess for suicidal ideation. This situation is sad but not uncommon for many individuals recovering from mental illness.

Chapter 30: Bipolar Disorders
1. 3
2. 1
3. 1
4. 2
5. 4
6. 3
7. 1
8. 1
9. 4
10. 3

Case Study and Critical Thinking Questions
1. 4
2. 2
3. 2
4. 2
5. The nurse should be concerned with safety issues and compliance issues. Toby is in a vulnerable situation. He is agitated, angry, and hyperactive. These symptoms have the potential to cause problems in several ways. Toby might become injured (e.g., confrontation with others, physical injury in countless other ways) or injure someone else. Toby is also at risk for problems related to sleep disturbance and alterations in nutrition. Developing strategies to help Toby comply with the medication regimen is critical if he is to start recovering.
6. Patients experiencing a manic episode are talkative and struggle to listen to others. As the text recommends, it is important to communicate in clear, concise statements. In addition, the nurse must convey a calm but firm presence. If Toby continues to talk without allowing the nurse to interject, the nurse may need to carefully break into the conversation. This is not the time for a lengthy discussion because the patient simply cannot tolerate it.

Chapter 31: Anxiety-Related Somatoform and Dissociative Disorders
1. 1
2. 2
3. 4
4. 4
5. 3
6. 1
7. 2
8. 3
9. The nurse would advise the patient about symptoms that may be experienced and that the symptoms will subside. The nurse would support the patient by telling him that he is not "crazy" or going to die. The nurse would teach the patient about the purpose and use of medication in blocking symptoms of panic.

Case Study and Critical Thinking Questions
1. Promote emotional security to prevent more decompensation by offering empathy, support, and strategies to decrease anxiety.
2. Help her decide which action would be most helpful to her.
   a. Call her family and tell them what has happened and that she is safe.
   b. See a crisis counselor this evening before going home to her family.
   c. Have the family be with her when she sees the crisis counselor.

d. Arrange for her family to take her home, stay with her, and then bring her to the crisis counselor in the morning.

e. Assess for physical injury. Focus on the fact that she is now safe from harm.

Chapter 32: Cognitive Disorders

1. 2
2. 3
3. 2
4. 2
5. 2
6. 4
7. 3
8. c
9. a
10. b
11. Alterations in memory, abstract thinking, judgment, and perception
12. Delirium, depression, encephalitis, TIAs, anticholinergic reactions, (all of these are potentially reversible)
13. *Amnesia:* Inability to learn new information or to recall previously learned information

   Agnosia: Failure to recognize or identify objects, despite intact sensory function

   Aphasia: Language disturbance that can be exhibited in both understanding and expressing the spoken word

   Apraxia: Inability to carry out motor activities despite intact motor function (e.g., ability to grab a doorknob but not knowing what to do with it)
14. T
15. T
16. T
17. F
18. T
19. F
20. T
21. F
22. T
23. T
24. b
25. b
26. a
27. c
28. a

Chapter 33: Personality Disorders

1. 1
2. 4
3. 2
4. 3
5. 4
6. 2
7. 1

8. The nurse should be emphatic, acknowledge the reality of the patient's emotional pain, and offer support. Because the patient has made a suicide attempt and is voicing suicidal ideation, the nurse provides a safe environment to decrease self-harm and impulsive behavior. Use of a "no-harm" contract would be appropriate. The nurse should also contract with the patient to seek staff members when the patient experiences thoughts or urges to do self-harm.

9. The nurse would respond by saying, "All suicide attempts are serious. Patients with borderline personality disorder who self-mutilate misperceive the lethality of their suicide attempts and are at high risk for accidentally killing themselves. Their suicide attempt is as serious as are those who do not self-mutilate.

10. An SSRI would be appropriate medication for Ann to decrease her suicidality, impulsiveness, hopelessness, and emptiness.

Chapter 34: Sexual Disorders

1. 4
2. 2
3. 3
4. 2

Case Study and Critical Thinking Questions

1. The nurse is legally required to report the incident to legal authorities in the area for further investigation.

2. The nurse would assess Jim for suicide because of his depression and guilt and institute interventions to ensure safety for Jim. The nurse would explore opportunities for Jim to establish age-appropriate relationships through his church or community, including groups and activities at the mental health center. Plans would also include measures to increase his self-esteem, manage his feelings of guilt, and confront other issues related to his depression. Enforcing medication compliance for his depression is necessary. Self-help groups might also help him cope with his illness and daily life.

3. A typical symptom of major depression is loss of libido or interest in sex. A side effect of sertraline (Zoloft) is sexual dysfunction. The nurse would carefully assess and evaluate these medications as possibly affecting Jim's sexual performance. The nurse would also ask Jim if he is taking other medications and determine if sexual side effects are possible.

Chapter 35: Substance-Related Disorders

1. 1
2. 4
3. 1
4. 4
5. 2
6. 3

7. 2
8. 2
9. 2
10. 1
11. 3
12. 3
13. 2
14. 2
15. 2
16. 1
17. 2
18. 2
19. 4
20. T

Case Study and Critical Thinking Questions

1. The correct response labels this statement for what it is: a rationalization and a weak one at that. On the other hand, if it is true, I would not view Terry as harshly as I would a nurse who allowed a patient to suffer (and this has happened many times). What Terry did was unethical, and the punishment was appropriate.

2. Many nurses would not want to work with Terry because they view this behavior as immoral and weak. Furthermore, in some hospitals, the "impaired" nurse can leave the unit for counseling if they feel a need to do so. This absence can sometimes leave the good employees to pick up the slack. On the other hand, many impaired nurses do a good job and have earned the full respect of their peers.

Chapter 36: Dual Diagnosis

1. 2
2. 3
3. 1
4. 4
5. 2
6. 3

7. The nurse would discuss how effective his medication is for the depression and whether he is experiencing side effects or uncomfortable symptoms from Prozac. It is also important for the nurse to discuss what situations prompt him to use marijuana, how he feels afterwards, and what he experiences after he stops using. Teaching Mark about alternative ways of handling his feelings and stressful situations would be helpful.

8. The nurse would discuss the importance of decreasing usage and assess Mark's motivation to change his behavior. The nurse would recommend open-ended dual diagnosis treatment if available. If dual diagnosis treatment is unavailable, the nurse would help Mark with anxiety-reduction strategies and social skills. The nurse would also teach Mark about the effects of marijuana on the body and how it interferes with treatment for his depression and anxiety.

Chapter 37: Eating Disorders

1. 1
2. 1
3. 4
4. 4
5. 2
6. 3
7. 4
8. 4
9. 1
10. 2

Case Study and Critical Thinking Questions

1. Assessment data:
   - Previous anorexia, underweight
   - Obsession with weight gain
   - Delayed menstruation
   - Ballet fuels weight concern
   - Bingeing and purging
   - Menstrual cycles normal in the past
   - Abnormal physical findings
   - Period of weight being stable
   - Separation from home and family
   - Adjustment to college life

2. Appropriate nursing diagnoses would be:
   a. Disturbance in body image, as related to need to maintain a certain weight for ballet as evidenced by bingeing and purging
   b. Disturbance in self-esteem, as related to fear of failure, adjustment difficulties as evidenced by negative comments about own weight and personal abilities

3. Short-term goals (STG):
   a. At the end of 1 week, Nonie will establish an eating contract with the nurse.
   b. At the end of 1 week, Nonie will discuss her adjustment problems with the nurse.
   c. At the end of 1 week, Nonie will state one positive aspect of herself.

4. Interventions for STG:
   a. Nurse will explain the parameters of the nurse-patient relationship to Nonie to promote patient trust and engagement in the relationship.
   b. Nurse will involve Nonie in developing an eating plan that meets both the requirements of weight gain and Nonie's concerns about food to increase chances of success of contract by having Nonie buy into the plan.
   c. Nurse will encourage Nonie's parents to involve her in therapeutic groups addressing self-esteem issues to help her recognize her abilities and positive qualities through the feedback of her peers.
   d. Nurse will have Nonie complete a self-assessment identifying her positive and negative qualities to obtain a baseline of her feelings about self.

e. Nurse will help Nonie identify past successes and current capabilities to help Nonie recognize that she has other abilities.
5. Evaluation of the STG:
a. Review eating contracts with Nonie, and mutually evaluate success in compliance.
b. Discuss progress of nurse-patient relationship; plan for future development of relationship.
c. Discuss referral to therapeutic groups and sessions that have been attended.
d. Discuss current progress and future plans regarding self-esteem issues.

Unit VII: Special Therapies in Psychiatric Nursing

Chapter 38: Behavior Therapies
1. 2
2. 3
3. 4
4. 1
5. 3
6. 1
7. 2
8. 3
9. 2
10. 2
11. Time-out for interrupting others, token reward when he listens to others, and contracting to take turns talking in the group
12. See Box 38-1.

Critical Thinking Question

Operant conditioning: To shape and reinforce positive behaviors, extinguish negative behaviors by withdrawing privileges; skills training for positive behaviors not shown by the patients, a token economy program to reward activities for daily living and expected tasks

Respondent conditioning: To strengthen alternative responses to pain, fear, and anxiety using relaxation techniques (deep breathing, deep muscle relaxation), yoga, meditation, positive imagery, positive self talk, and systematic desensitization for phobic behaviors

Chapter 39: Somatic Therapies
1. 1
2. 2
3. 1
4. 2
5. 2
6. 4
7. 2
8. 2
9. 1
10. 2
11. 1
12. 3

13. Physical or physiologic

Case Study and Critical Thinking Questions
1. Disappointed probably, but surprised no. The temporary nature of ECT effectiveness presents a major disadvantage to its use. Penny responded favorably to the first series of treatments and may respond equally well for another series.
2. Continuance or maintenance ECT, particularly when coupled with antidepressant therapy, should reduce future depressive moods.

Chapter 40: Alternative and Complementary Therapies
1. 1
2. 4
3. 1
4. 1
5. 4
6. 2
7. 1
8. 1
9. 1
10. 4
11. 2
12. 4
13. F
14. F
15. T
16. F
17. F
18. T

Unit VIII: Special Populations in Psychiatric Nursing

Chapter 41: Survivors of Violence and Trauma
1. 1
2. 4
3. 3
4. 3
5. 2
6. 4
7. 3
8. 1
9. 2

Case Study and Critical Thinking Questions
1. Suicidal and homicidal ideation, self-mutilation, post-traumatic symptoms, depression, dissociative experiences, childhood sexual abuse, cult or satanic abuse, and military-political associations and programming (MK-ULTRA)
2. Safety and security, trust building and "prompting" strategies, a nonjudgmental attitude, empathy, and support without confrontation

3. "No-harm" contract (suicide, homicide, self-mutilation), anger or rage management, alternative coping for urges to harm self or others, management of dissociative episodes, identification of support systems and resources, medication management, and protection from outside triggers

4. Community of self-help groups and on-line support for the issues of cult or military-political abuse, childhood sexual abuse, PTSD, and depression, as well as special programs for survivors of torture, SRA, and MC and a psychiatrist for medication management

Chapter 42: Child and Adolescent Psychiatric Nursing

1. 2
2. 4
3. 3
4. 2
5. 2
6. 4
7. 1
8. 2
9. 3
10. 1
11. 3

Case Study and Critical Thinking Questions

1. Add a third dose of methylphenidate in the afternoon, because it is likely that the noon dose is worn off by 4:00 PM. An increase in the morning and noon dose might also be worth considering, given the teacher's observation that the late morning is a time of deteriorating behavior.

2. Parent management training would be appropriate because of the escalating punishment that is taking place in the family. Parent management training approaches behavior modification through establishment of rules, clear limits, positive attention, and predictable consequences. A potential pitfall in communicating the value of parent management training is inadvertently sending the message that the parent is to blame for the child's behavior problems. Therefore the nurse can point out that children with medical conditions or serious psychiatric conditions have special needs. Thus, although the parents are not to blame for the child's behavior problems, they may have to learn specific parenting techniques to promote optimal development.

Chapter 43: Mental Disorders in Older Adults

1. 3
2. 2
3. 4
4. 1
5. 4
6. 2
7. 1
8. White, male, age 78, recent loss of spouse, chronic painful condition

9. 20%
10. Ageism, older adult attitudes about health care, finances, and dementia are overestimated, while depression is underestimated; incidence of alcohol abuse has been minimized; and physician- and patient-induced drug abuse has been only recently recognized.
11. Suicide, somatization, needless suffering, institutionalization

Case Study and Critical Thinking Questions

1. Woody is miserable. He is experiencing tremendous mental distress and perhaps physical pain as well. His plea to God is for a release from the pain and should be heard by the nurse, whose immediate actions should be aimed at providing relief. The nurse should also assess for suicidal ideation.

2. Spiritual assessments are important because they provide information about the meaning of religion in the patient's life, including personal beliefs and practices not revealed by naming a faith or denomination. Woody's religious expressions provide an opportunity for the nurse to explore the role of religion in Woody's life and his current thought processes. Comforting religious platitudes are not helpful in most cases and may be offensive. Instead, a religious conversation exploring the patient's beliefs and experiences might lead to more positive results by helping the patient clarify the current feelings related to punishment or abandonment.

3. Our nation has a diverse population, and each segment has special interests and needs. Children and older adults are both "at-risk" groups that would benefit from increased funding. Children are the future of our country, but with the life expectancy increasing, older adults also have productive years ahead of them. Resources that increase the health, well being, and functional capacity of older citizens promote the positive contributions of our older citizens. For example, many agencies (including schools and youth-focused agencies) rely on volunteers; and older adults increasingly find activities such as these a rewarding way to fill their needs for interaction and productivity. Society is best served by balancing the needs of all rather than focusing resources only on a narrow segment of the population.

Chapter 44: Working with Patients with HIV Infection

1. 3
2. 4
3. 2
4. 1
5. 4
6. 3
7. 4
8. 3

Case Study and Critical Thinking Questions

1. It is important that someone (and in this case, the nurse) discuss realistic goals with the patient, in other words, what is a realistic expectation given the degree of disability? Other important issues include discussion of advance care directives and teaching regarding disability entitlements.

2. It will be important to discuss issues pertaining to her son. Who would she want to take care of him if she is no longer able? Other issues include her prognosis, the likely course of the disease, and palliative measures.

3. Consider diagnoses related to physical, emotional, and spiritual status of someone facing the end-stage of a life-threatening disease.